The
ENCYCLOPEDIA
of
COMMON
DISEASES

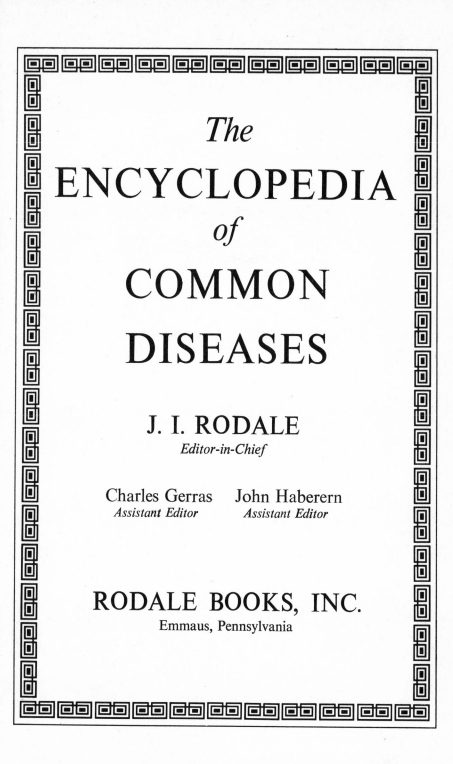

The
ENCYCLOPEDIA
of
COMMON
DISEASES

J. I. RODALE
Editor-in-Chief

Charles Gerras
Assistant Editor

John Haberern
Assistant Editor

RODALE BOOKS, INC.
Emmaus, Pennsylvania

CONTENTS

BOOK ONE

DISEASES AFFECTING SPECIFIC PARTS OF THE BODY

SECTION 1

The Back

CHAPTER		PAGE
1	Backache	3
2	Don't Let Poor Posture Give You a Backache	6
3	Can Exercise Prevent Backache?	9

SECTION 2

The Bones

4	Preventing Osteoporosis	13
5	Osteoporosis and Vitamin C	17

SECTION 3

The Ears

6	How Well Do You Hear?	19
7	Vitamin A and Your Hearing	21
8	Protect Your Hearing!	24
9	A New Approach to Deafness	27
10	Understanding the Misery of Tinnitus	30

SECTION 4

The Eyes

11	Some Questions and Answers about Cataract	34
12	Cataract and Good Nutrition	37
13	Tension Causes Eyestrain	41
14	What Can Be Done for Crossed Eyes?	42
15	Blindness and Glaucoma	45
16	Myopia	56
17	Virus Disease of the Eye	60
18	What Drugs Can Do to the Eyes	62
19	Eyesight and Vitamin Deficiency	65

SECTION 5

The Feet

20	When Your Feet Hurt, You Hurt All Over	70
21	Your Feet Require Special Care	75
22	The Prevention of Foot Disability	78

SECTION 6

The Gall Bladder

CHAPTER   PAGE

23   That Pesky Gall Bladder 84

SECTION 7

The Gums

24   The Health of Your Gums 89
25   Wisdom in Treating Gum Disorders 91
26   Nutrition Should Be Complete for Gum Health 95
27   How to Prevent Pyorrhea 97
28   Bioflavonoids for Gum Disease 104

SECTION 8

The Hair

29   Are You Good to Your Hair? 105
30   Baldness—Some Remedies Worth Trying 109

SECTION 9

Headaches

31   Investigating Headaches 114
32   An Unusual Cause of Headaches 121
33   Headaches from Milk 123

SECTION 10

The Heart

34   Heart Disease 125
35   A Glossary of Heart Disease Terms 166
36   New Findings on Heart and Artery Disease 170
37   Heart Trouble and Your Diet 174
38   Can Fresh Fruit Help Prevent Heart Trouble? 178
39   Vitamin E for Heart Disease 180
40   Vitamin E Used Internationally for Heart Disease 183
41   Is Heart Disease Related to Anxiety? 186
42   How Important Is Stress in Heart Disease? 190
43   Is Too Much Sun Related to Heart Attacks? 193
44   Soft Water and Heart Trouble 195
45   Hardening of the Arteries 201
46   A New Twosome—Goiter and Arteriosclerosis 204
47   Arteriosclerosis and a Fatty Diet 206
48   Metals and Hardening of the Arteries 210
49   Coronary Thrombosis: A Study in Causes 213
50   A Theory of Coronary Thrombosis 218

CHAPTER   PAGE
51   What About Low Blood Pressure? 223
52   High Blood Pressure 226
53   Facts on Salt Eating and High Blood Pressure 231
54   Stroke! 236
55   A Cardiac's Choice of Medications 241

SECTION 11

The Kidneys

56   Kidney Stones 244

SECTION 12

The Liver

57   Liver Ailments 248
58   Liver Health 252
59   Cirrhosis of the Liver 254
60   How Close Are You to Hepatitis? 259

SECTION 13

The Prostate Gland

61   Enlarged Prostate 264
62   A New Theory on Prostate Gland Disorders 269
63   The Prostate Gland and Zinc 272

SECTION 14

The Skin

64   Skin Problems on Contact 275
65   Detergent Dermatitis 279
66   Skin Health and Soaps 281
67   Skin Trouble from the Linings of Shoes 283
68   The Mystery of Psoriasis 285
69   Vitiligo 289

SECTION 15

The Teeth

70   Tooth Decay and Diet 292
71   Sugar, Candy and Caries 295
72   Vitamin B$_6$ Fights Tooth Decay 299
73   A Review of the Theories of Tooth Decay 302
74   Official Statement on the Causes of Tooth Decay 305
75   Can Malocclusion of the Teeth Be Prevented? 309
76   Causes and Remedies for Malocclusion 315

BOOK TWO

GENERAL DISORDERS OF THE BODY

SECTION 16

Alcoholism

CHAPTER		PAGE
77	The Disease of Alcoholism	319
78	Is Alcoholism a Disease of Starvation?	323

SECTION 17

Appendicitis

| 79 | Appendicitis Is Still a Problem | 329 |

SECTION 18

Arthritis

80	Arthritis and Arthritic and Rheumatic Diseases	333
81	Stress	340
82	Rheumatism and Eggs	343
83	Drugs for Arthritis?	345
84	Cherries for Gout and Arthritis	348
85	Sugar and Arthritis	349
86	A Proposed New Diet for Arthritics?	351
87	More on a New Diet for Arthritics	354
88	Vitamin P and Vitamin C for Arthritis	357
89	Arthritis and Vitamin C	359
90	Vitamin D for Arthritis Patients	363
91	Arthritis and Foot Disability	365
92	Preventing Stiff Shoulder	375
93	Sleep and Rheumatism	379
94	Good Posture Prevents Rheumatism	386
95	Mineral Baths for Arthritics	390
96	Physical Therapy Is Effective	393
97	Notes on Arthritis	395

SECTION 19

Asthma

98	Your Enemy, Asthma	398
99	Asthma, Is Climate the Answer?	403
100	Bronchial Asthma	407
101	Asthmatics Might Try Exercise	410
102	A Doctor's Case of Asthma	413
103	The Asthmatic Ordeal of Marcel Proust	415

SECTION 20

Bad Breath

CHAPTER   PAGE

104   A Discussion of Bad Breath 417

SECTION 21

Bed Wetting

105   Enuresis at Teenage 422

SECTION 22

Buerger's Disease

106   Buerger's Disease 425

SECTION 23

Cancer

107   What Is Raising the Cancer Rate? 429
108   Do We Know What Causes Cancer? 432
109   Information on Environmental Cancer Hazards 436
110   Cancer-Causing Chemicals in Food 440
111   Statistics Reveal Some Probable Cancer Causes 443
112   Lung Cancer and Tobacco 446
113   A New Theory on the Cause of Cancer 450
114   Our Poisoned World and Cancer 453
115   A New Approach to the Cancer Problem 457
116   Is Cancer a Virus Disease? 460
117   Your Emotional Make-Up 464
118   Hair Growth and Cancer 468
119   Cancer: Possible Side Effect of Polio Vaccine? 470
120   Experiments Show Heated Fats Can Cause Cancer 474
121   Cancer and Antibiotics 478
122   Rimless Eyeglasses and Skin Cancer 480
123   Is Cancer Related to Nutrition? 481
124   Cancer and Poor Nutrition 486
125   Nature-Conforming Nutrition and Cancer Prevention 489
126   Does Gardening Prevent Cancer? 493
127   Some Facts on Cervical Cancer 505
128   Experiments with Garlic and Cancer 507
129   Vitamin B Deficiency and Cancer 508
130   Is Vitamin C Deficiency Related to Cancer? 513
131   Does Breast Feeding Prevent Cancer of the Breast? 516
132   Krebiozen—The History of a Tragedy 519
133   Cancer and Drosnes-Lazenby Treatment 524
134   Can Cancer Be Prevented? 527
135   Cancer Cures 535
136   The High Risk of Finding a Cancer Cure 538

[ix]

SECTION 24

Celiac Disease

CHAPTER   PAGE

137   Celiac Disease and Whole Wheat 542

SECTION 25

The Circulation

138   Intermittent Claudication 546
139   Vascular Disorders 549
140   Treatment of Vascular Disorders 553

SECTION 26

Cleft Palate

141   Cleft Palate—Heredity or Nutrition? 558

SECTION 27

Colds

142   Colds Are Everywhere 560
143   The History of My Colds 563
144   Colds and Vitamin A 573
145   Ample B Vitamins Protect Against Colds 579
146   Vitamin C Is a Natural Cold Preventive 581
147   Vitamin C and Bioflavonoids 585
148   Stop That Cold With Garlic! 587
149   No Salt for Chronic Cold Sufferers 589
150   Dry Heat and Chilling Are Conducive to Colds 592
151   Breathing 597
152   Should You Take an Aspirin for Colds? 599
153   Shun the Antihistamines 602
154   How About a Shot of Penicillin? 604
155   How Harmless Is Menthol? 605
156   Smokers Have a Higher Percentage of Colds 608
157   Low-Carbohydrate Diets for Respiratory Disorders 612

SECTION 28

Constipation

158   What Is Constipation and What Causes It? 616
159   Constipation Is Related to Other Diseases 619
160   Exercise to Fight Constipation 621
161   Try Natural Foods to Treat Constipation 624
162   Is Water Drinking Important for Preventing Constipation? 627
163   The Relationship between Vitamins and Constipation 629

SECTION 29

Cystic Fibrosis

CHAPTER   PAGE

164   A Chance to Fight Cystic Fibrosis 632

165   The Nutritional Aspects of Cystic Fibrosis 635

SECTION 30

Diabetes

166   Diabetes in Modern Times 638

167   Good News for Diabetics 641

168   A New Diet 644

169   Diabetes and the Weather 646

SECTION 31

Diarrhea

170   Carob Flour for Diarrhea 649

171   Buttermilk or Bananas for Diarrhea and Dysentery 651

SECTION 32

Digestion

172   Some Digestive Tract Symptoms of Vitamin Deficiency 655

173   Garlic 657

174   Garlic Therapy in Diseases of the Digestive Tract 661

175   A Natural Treatment for Intestinal Disorders 665

176   A Low-Carbohydrate Diet 670

177   Diet Care to Prevent Colitis 673

178   Ulcerative Colitis 676

179   Ulcerative Colitis, Bread and Milk 679

SECTION 33

Dizziness

180   Dizziness—A Mysterious Symptom 683

SECTION 34

Epilepsy

181   Epilepsy 688

182   Epilepsy and Other Mental Disorders 696

SECTION 35

Flu

183   The Asiatic Flu 701

SECTION 36

Gangrene

CHAPTER   PAGE

184 Using Vitamin E on Gangrene 703

SECTION 37

Goiter

185 The Riddle of Goiter 705
186 Some Environmental Causes of Goiter 712

SECTION 38

Hemorrhoids

187 Hemorrhoids 716

SECTION 39

Hernia

188 Hernia Is Easily Avoided 719

SECTION 40

Indigestion

189 Avoiding Indigestion 723
190 Garlic Triumphs Over Indigestion 727
191 Dyspepsia from Starch Eating 729

SECTION 41

Insomnia

192 Insomnia Is a Frustrating Problem 732

SECTION 42

Leukemia

193 Leukemia in Infants and Young Children 736

SECTION 43

Lupus Erythematosus

194 The Appearance of Lupus Erythematosus and
    Aplastic Anemia 740

SECTION 44

Mental Illness

195 Mental Illness 744
196 The Nutritional Approach to Nervous Disorders 747

[xii]

CHAPTER   PAGE
197   Retarded Mentality Means Nutritional Need 750
198   Mental Illness and Vitamin B$_{12}$ Deficiency 753
199   The Thyroid 756
200   Blood Sugar and Mental Health 761
201   Low Blood Sugar, Crime and Mental Illness 764

SECTION 45

Miscarriage

202   Preventing Miscarriage 769

SECTION 46

Mongolism

203   Hope Seen for Mongoloid Children 771
204   Mongolism and Fluoridated Drinking Water 774
205   A Treatment for Favorable Change in Mongolism 778

SECTION 47

Mononucleosis

206   Fighting Mononucleosis 782

SECTION 48

Multiple Sclerosis

207   Multiple Sclerosis, the Crippler 784
208   Significant Facts about Multiple Sclerosis 789

SECTION 49

Muscular Dystrophy

209   Muscular Dystrophy—A Multiple Deficiency? 792
210   A Cure for Muscular Dystrophy? 796

SECTION 50

Overweight

211   Overweight Is a Mistake You Can Correct 797
212   Overweight and High Blood Pressure 802

SECTION 51

Parkinson's Disease

213   Parkinson's Disease 805

[xiii]

SECTION 52

Pernicious Anemia

CHAPTER   PAGE

214   Pernicious Anemia   809

SECTION 53

Polio

215   Treatment of Polio Victims   811
216   Polio in Primitive Countries   815
217   Vitamin A vs. Polio   817
218   Infantile Paralysis and Vitamin B Deficiency   820
219   Vitamin E for Post-Polio Disorders   825
220   The Sandler Diet for Preventing Polio   826
221   Garlic Tablets and Polio   830
222   Iodine Against Polio   832
223   The Slow Death of the Salk Vaccine   834
224   Scientific Experts Reveal the Salk Vaccine Hoax   841
225   Confusion Reigns over the Salk Vaccine   848

SECTION 54

Pruritus Ani

226   Pruritus Ani   852

SECTION 55

Rabies

227   Rabies—Fact or Fancy?   854

SECTION 56

Scurvy

228   Scurvy Yesterday and Today   858
229   Don't Wait for a Scurvy Diagnosis   863
230   Modern Infants' Diets Can Lead to Scurvy   866

SECTION 57

Sinusitis

231   The Sinus   869
232   How's Your Sinusitis?   870

SECTION 58

Staph Infections

233   Staph Infections Create New Problems   874

[xiv]

SECTION 59

Tobacco Amblyopia

CHAPTER   PAGE
234   Tobacco Amblyopia   880

SECTION 60

Trichinosis

235   Trichinosis Is a Threat to You   882

SECTION 61

Tuberculosis

236   Tuberculosis and Malnutrition   885
237   Failure of B.C.G., the Anti-Tuberculosis Vaccine   888

SECTION 62

Ulcers

238   Could You Get an Ulcer?   891
239   Views Are Changing on Ulcer Cause and Its Treatment   895
240   Low Blood Sugar as a Cause of Ulcers   898
241   Gastric Ulcers Can Be Prevented   899
242   Potatoes for Ulcer Patients   902
243   Vitamin C Injections for Ulcers   903
244   Bioflavonoids for Ulcers   905

SECTION 63

Underweight

245   The Problem of Underweight   907
246   Too Fat—or Too Thin?   913

SECTION 64

Undulant Fever

247   A New Treatment for Brucellosis   916

SECTION 65

Varicose Veins

248   Varicose Veins   918
249   A New Theory on Varicose Veins   922

[xv]

BOOK THREE

GENERAL DISCUSSIONS OF DISEASES

SECTION 66

CHAPTER		PAGE
250	Bananas and Disease	929
251	Lung Cancer Isn't All A Smoker Has to Worry About	932
252	Vitamin Deficiency Plus Smoking Equals Trouble	940
253	Researcher Cites Smoking as a Cause of Disease	942
254	Do Any Diseases Just Happen?	945
255	Conquering the Infectious Diseases	947
256	Many Disorders Associated with Salt Intake	950
257	Diseases and the Medical Profession	954
258	Drugs Are Doing Us Little Good	959
259	Some Speculations on a Brand New Disease	962
	Subject Index	965

BOOK ONE

DISEASES AFFECTING
SPECIFIC PARTS
OF THE BODY

1. Backache

Today we speak of backache as "low back pain," for generally the severe backaches occur at the bottom end of the spine. A wide variety of possible causes is listed in any medical article on backache. Backache may be the result of arthritis. It may arise from some unusual muscle strain, plus emotional strain. It may result from some recent or long-forgotten bump, jar or wrench occurring especially during periods of fatigue. It may indicate a slipped vertebral disc. An infection of the genital or urinary tract, an acute illness, general ill health, a local infection somewhere in the body or overweight may bring about backache. We are surprised at how often we find physicians indicating that backache may be psychosomatic—a physical symptom of some profound emotional strain or frustration. Finally—and this is the kind of backache that is most common and most easily prevented—it may be simply the result of poor posture, improper furniture or surroundings or the wrong kind of movements in daily life.

Says W. B. Parsons, M.D., writing in the *Canadian Medical Association Journal* for July, 1951, "every joint has an optimum position of function, . . . moderate departures from that position will increase the likelihood of strain and extreme departures will almost inevitably result in pain." The lower part of the back bears almost half the weight of the body, centered chiefly in the lumbo-sacral joint. This joint connects a moveable piece of anatomy—the spine—with a part that is, generally speaking, not so mobile —the pelvic structure. Anatomists seem to feel that the construction of the lower part of the back displays abundant evidence that man is not especially well equipped to walk in an upright position. The animals who walk on all fours do not, we suspect, ever have backaches.

How the Backache Comes About

Dr. Parsons continues: "In people with poor posture, the joints are at or near the limit of normal motion, but are prevented from going beyond this point by muscle power and there is no strain—the fault is compensated. As with the heart, if something breaks that compensation, the joints will be moved beyond the limits of normal, and strain or decompensation results. Clinically this is backache."

Think of it this way, he says: the normal position of the wrist is straight out in a line with the arm. When you bend the wrist as far down as you can, at right angles, there is no pain. You can even push it down with your other hand, and so long as the muscles in the arm can withstand the push,

[3]

there is no pain. But if the weight becomes too great, or if the arm muscles are caught off-guard by a sudden unaccustomed movement and the wrist is bent a little further, there is strain on the supporting muscles, and pain for you. Putting this in terms of the back, you can exert pressure on the low back joint by putting up with poor posture, for perhaps many years. But a sudden unexpected twist, lifting a too-heavy object, an unaccustomed amount of work crowded into one busy day, and there will be strain on the supporting muscles of the back—and backache.

If you drag about day after day with a pretty constant backache, we suggest that you have an examination to find out whether you may be suffering from one or another of the things outlined above. If not, your backache is what doctors call "idiopathic"—a disorder for which they can find no cause. In that case, the cause is probably poor posture, the wrong kind of furniture or the wrong kind of movements.

Your Backache and Your Bed

If you wake up with a backache, chances are very good that your back has not been getting proper rest during the night, due to a bed that is too soft. Look at someone lying in a hammock and you will get an exaggerated idea of what a soft bed does to one's body. If you lie on your back, your chest is constricted and your back curved unnaturally. On your side, the lower half of you is extended too far and the upper half constricted. If you lie on your stomach, the spine and hips are extended into a completely unnatural curve.

Dr. Parsons tells us of a woman who went on a camping trip where she had to sleep flat on the hard ground night after night. She experienced a remarkable recovery from a backache "that had plagued her for years." Your bed should be firm and flat. In most cases, modern springs and mattresses tend to "give" too much which is why many people find it far better to sleep with a fairly thick board between the mattress and springs, so that the bed does not curve beneath your weight, no matter how you sleep. This kind of bed board can be bought or you can make one yourself from a piece of plywood.

We all must know by now that modern living room chairs in which we are expected to "lounge" have an absolutely devastating effect on one's body and one's posture. You were not meant to sit curled in a forward curve, with your knees close to your chin, your chest constricted, your abdomen cramped, your lungs crushed into a tiny space that barely permits them to breathe. Your chairs should be reasonably straight, with a length from the seat to the floor that is comfortable for you, so that your knees don't jut up into the air if you are tall, so that your feet don't hang dangling if you are short. The back of the chair should conform pretty much to the curve of your own back.

If you sit at work all day, the chair you sit in is even more important. Progressive employers today know that workers will work faster and better and there will be less absenteeism if the chairs are fitted to the workers' height and the kind of work they are doing. If you must bend over your work, it will help to raise one foot to a stool or a platform from time to time.

Poor Posture the Most Common Cause of Backache

Tall, thin people are inclined to be more susceptible to backache from poor posture than are short stocky ones. Obviously the muscles that support the back have a bigger job to do—more actual back structure to support and a longer distance over which the support must be given. By and large we moderns have extremely bad posture, which makes us highly susceptible to the backache for which there seems to be no other cause. In the pregnant woman, or the woman who has had children the muscles that support the abdomen are weakened, the abdomen sags, pulling on the back to deepen the curve there and produce a full-fledged case of "sway-back." This can easily be corrected if you catch it soon enough. If not, backache is a likely result.

We have often wondered how many men have "pot-bellies" because they don't wear suspenders. Hence they unconsciously stick out their abdomens to hold up their belted trousers. Teenagers who grow too fast tend to slouch so that their height will not be noticed, rounded shoulders are the result.

All of us should know by now the excessive harm to posture that can be done by wearing high heels. There is no excuse for anyone to wear high heels in these days when low-heeled shoes are so attractive and popular. If you feel you simply cannot get along without high heels, wear them only when you go out in the evenings, for a very few hours at a time, and when you are not going to be on your feet a great deal.

Good posture every day, all day long can do away with backache—the ordinary kind of backache. Good posture is a matter of exercise, very simple exercise. But it is much more a matter of remembering all day to keep your posture good. The exercise will strengthen your muscles. But if you let them sag back to their original sloppy state during the day, you will have all the work to do over again next time you take your exercises. •

Correcting Your Posture

Stand in front of a full-length mirror after your next bath and look at your posture. You know what good posture is—all of us do. You should be able to hang a straight plumb-line from your ear to the ball of your feet, and half of you, perfectly balanced, should be on each side of the line. You can improve the tone of your stomach muscles by lying flat on a bed or the floor and raising up to a sitting position without using your hands or arms. Or you can lie flat and lift one leg after the other into the air, slowly. It's as simple as that.

Or, if you want something even more simple, try exercising your abdominal muscles while you go about your business. Pull up and in on them, tucking your buttocks beneath you. Hold your head high, your chin in, your shoulders up. When you lift something heavy, bend your knees, get close to the object, and when you lift, let your legs do the work rather than your back. When you bend, don't bend over at the waist, with your knees straight. (And incidentally, this kind of bending, trying to touch your toes, with legs straight, is the very worst exercise you can do, if you suffer from backache.) Bend your legs, keep your trunk straight.

Dr. Parsons says "For those who say they get enough exercise all day long in their work, the only answer I know is that practice makes perfect, but not if you practice the wrong way."

2. Don't Let Poor Posture Give You a Backache

If the people of this country who suffer from back complaints of one kind or another ever form a club, they are sure to outnumber the D.A.R., Rotary International and the American Legion combined. That is why an article appearing in the *Canadian Medical Association Journal* of August, 1957, caught our attention. Written by Norman C. Delarue, B.A., M.D., M.S. (Tor.) F.R.C.S. [C], Toronto, the discussion not only suggests several possible reasons for the back pains that plague so many people, but it outlines several preventive exercises which can be done by the layman.

Dr. Delarue offers some very convincing evidence to show that backache is usually traceable to bad posture habits. Once these habits are formed, the body adjusts itself as best it can, but the spinal column cannot function well when it is tilted to an unnatural degree. Edges that were meant to be cushioned from one another by cartilage, meet and scrape, and, in time, pain makes standing erect almost unbearable.

Poor Posture Habits Start in Youth

Most of our poor posture habits are formed in our youth. In school and while working at homework in the evening, the child sits at a flat-topped desk, hunched over and leaning close to his work, deep in concentrated study. No wonder this position becomes second nature to him. In the interests of better posture, Dr. Delarue suggests desks with a tilted writing area and a flat margin above for reference books, pencils, etc. The seats should have contour backs and foot pedestals. These innovations would create in the student a tendency toward good posture as he works because it would be more difficult to slump while using such facilities.

By the time one reaches his late teens his posture habits have been pretty well molded. The male who is by nature less conscious of his appearance than the female, tends to slump at work or when standing, without being aware that he is doing so. The female, on the other hand, is painfully conscious of her developing figure in adolescence. She squares her shoulders with almost military determination to avoid the look of flat-chestedness. At the same time she insists on kowtowing to fashion by wearing high heels. That she doesn't fall flat on her face, thus extended, defies every principle of engineering known to man. Now if she holds her shoulders back, and chest forward, it means that milady must have her torso (and her spinal column) bent like a bow when the high heels are worn, with the rump extended quite beyond reason to act as ballast.

A few years of walking and working in this position would soon have a lady off the high heels and down to earth out of sheer discomfort. However, the tired tummies and protruding posteriors found means of support and disguise in the girdle and corset. So the American lady marches with all determination toward backache.

The male doesn't fare much better. His slumping round-shoulderedness leaves him with prominent thyroid cartilage, a particularly unattractive "Adam's apple," and sagging jowls from the necessity of burying the head lower in the shoulders to allow one to look straight ahead and below, instead of looking to the sky as the forced position of the head would dictate.

But of even more consequence is the fact that the sternum (chest bone) is depressed in the round-shouldered individual, and this interferes with the normal expansion of the thoracic cage. The respiratory bellows are affected, resulting in shortness of breath and inability to sustain any kind of muscular activity.

Exactly How Were We Meant to Stand?

The entire basis for proper posture is the fact that the spinal column is designed to stand in a straight line, with segmented curvatures to provide flexibility and absorb stress from the base of the skull to the pelvis. To maintain this healthful position, the body has several main sets of tools: the abdominal muscles, the gluteal muscles of the buttock and the hamstring muscles of the back of the thigh. All of these serve to keep the pelvis at its proper level, allowing no permanent tilt either forward or backward, and thus offering a steady and level support for the spinal column.

Dr. Delarue gives several rules and exercises for correcting dangerous posture habits before too much damage has been done. These are most effective when used by young people whose muscles and bones are still developing.

For general back hygiene one should observe proper methods of standing, sitting and lifting. When standing or sitting for any length of time, it is wise to flex the thighs comfortably to straighten the pelvic tilt by pulling the rear rim of the pelvis downward. When sitting for a long period, both legs should be supported on something. For standing for long periods without changing position, a leg rest, like the old brass rail in the swinging door bars of the '90's or a step of some kind should be handy.

[7]

The rule for lifting heavy objects from a level lower than the hips should be carefully followed: one goes down on his haunches in a squat, the back is kept straight and the knees are flexed in the lifting. This simple precaution can save one from many other physiological complications not even related to posture and backache.

To maintain the efficiency of the thoracic bellows, avoid a hollow chest and keep the sternum elevated, the following exercise is suggested by Dr. Delarue:

Stand as tall as possible, with the head erect, chin in, chest out, tummy in and buttocks flat. Now square the shoulders, elevating and lowering them while breathing deeply. You can feel those lazy chest muscles working.

Do you have a sag in your sacroiliac? You shouldn't. But here's how you can check for yourself. Stand with your back against a wall with thighs, calves, buttocks, shoulders flat against it. Now see if you can fit your hand between the wall and the small of your back, just above the buttocks. If you can, your posture needs work. Bend slightly forward until the space between your back and the wall is eliminated, then try to straighten up without allowing the space to form. This will take plenty of muscle power in your abdominal region as well as the backs of your thighs and buttocks. If you don't seem to be getting anywhere at first, don't be discouraged. You can work on those muscles till they're strong enough to maintain such a position without your consciously trying.

Exercises to Do

For the abdominals try this: lie flat on your back and hold your legs straight, lifting them slowly to about 60° (or about the number 2 on a watch dial if the subject is lying at number 6), then lower them slowly. Repeat this with one leg, then the other. You should do it as many times as possible until you get tired—not exhausted, just tired. Keep count of the number you do, and try to increase the number at regular intervals, say one or two more per week. In no time you will feel new strength in your abdominal region, and find that standing and walking erectly comes much more naturally.

The exercises to strengthen the back muscles of the thighs (hamstrings) and the buttocks (gluteal) are much the same, except that the leg raising is done while lying face down. Remember to keep the legs straight, as in the preceding exercise. Flexing the knees against resistance, such as your bedroom wall, will also act to strengthen these muscles.

Both of these exercises will give you the muscle power you need to keep the pelvis from tilting too far forward or backward. With the pelvis on an even keel, the rest of the torso will stay that way, too.

We think that there is no better exercise for posture, and for just plain all-around increase in health and well-being than walking in the open air. Editor Rodale arranges his busy schedule to fit in a daily two-hour constitutional, and considers the physical and mental benefits derived from this practice well worth the sacrifice of his valuable time. Do as much walking as you can, and try to practice the tips on good posture offered by Dr. Delarue while you walk. Skip the high heels and the girdles. Give your body a chance to work without such hindrances.

Make sure, too, that your bad posture isn't the result of bad diet. Get plenty of bone-building calcium from supplements such as bone meal, so that your spinal column is made up of firm, hard bones. For the muscles, vitamin E and wheat germ for strength, and vitamin C from rose hips and fresh vegetables and fruits for healthy muscular tissue. Plenty of protein in the diet is important, too, for this is the very stuff of which muscles are made.

Good posture is not possible without good nourishment, and lack of good posture is almost sure to lead to backache at some later time in life.

3. Can Exercise Prevent Backache?

By RICHARD A. HAMILTON, D.C.

Chronic pain will develop sooner or later in posture-poor spines. Gravity and age are ever present, tending to worsen the condition. After the distortion is forced beyond its margin of safety, pain and stiffness show themselves. At this stage, most people seek temporary relief with belts, aspirin or heat therapy.

This type of backache resembles pain from organic disease, so it would be wise to have a complete examination in order to eliminate this possibility. Naturally, the cause of postural backache must be removed before results are achieved. Posture improvement must be worked at with systematic perseverance by the patient. Nobody else can help you but yourself, so learn what you must do and stick to it.

The only way to improve poor posture is with the proper exercise and constant spinal discipline. The plan of attack is to find out where there is a lack of support and which set of muscles are weak. After these facts are known, we must equalize the foundation with professional help, for this may necessitate surgery, manipulation, a shoe lift or a brace. Now we go to work to improve the posture by strengthening the weak muscles. Acute postural troubles are usually due to muscle tension, not weakness, and shouldn't be subject to exercise.

In corrective exercise we consider the back muscles as opposing the abdominal muscles and the right spinal muscles as opposing the left spinal muscles. The distortions pictured in Figure 1 are the 3 typical posture defects that result either alone or in combination.

[9]

EXERCISE CHART AS DESCRIBED IN TEXT

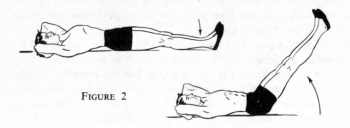

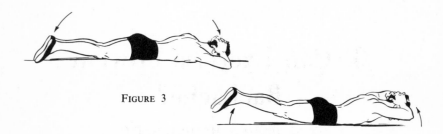

Figure 2

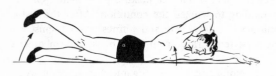

Figure 3

Figure 4-A

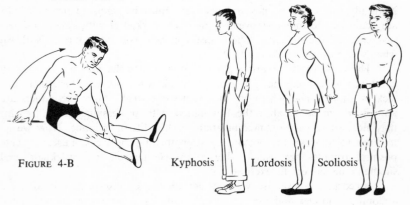

Figure 4-B

Kyphosis Lordosis Scoliosis

Figure 1-A Figure 1-B Figure 1-C

Weak Abdominal Muscles Must Be Strengthened

Weak abdominal muscles are seen in a person with lordosis. (See figure 1B.) The person has a flabby abdomen which protrudes and sags. His abdominal organs being unsupported in time "fall," giving rise to disease and disorder. The sway-back can cause kidney neurosis besides increased muscle tension, with the weight carried on the heels and transmitting shock waves up the spine. This in turn thins the spinal discs, causing many places along the spine to be tender trouble spots. High heels should never be worn by anyone with this tendency as they tend to increase the arch of the back.

The correct exercise is lying on the back and doing leg-ups. (See figure 2.) This should not be overdone at first, but gradually increase the time you spend on it, so that you stop each time just before fatigue sets in. You must use good judgment along with perseverance in muscle building. It will take time, so apportion a regular routine for yourself each morning and night. This exercise may begin with a couple of minutes and work up to 15 minutes each day and will pay off in from two to three months, if a certain amount of effort is made to keep the stomach sucked in when you stand and walk. Doing the exercise on the floor will give a firm base on which to flatten out the sway-back condition when the legs are raised.

Weak Back Muscles Can Be Corrected

The slouch posture is seen more today than ever before because of our sedentary lives and monotonous occupations. (See figure 1A.) Fatigued muscles are caused by inactivity and nervous strain and need proper exercise to overcome their state of toxic laziness. We grow fat and lethargic like pumpkins, ride to work, bend over a desk or bench all day and sit in an easy chair to watch TV in the evening. No wonder our backs are weak and unstable from much misuse and little use.

The typical slouch can have quite a variable posture, but in general his head will droop forward and his chest sink in. This phlegmatic fellow usually has a list of complaints and really never feels good. And no wonder! His chest is resting on crowded abdominal organs, and his neck is under constant strain trying to hold his head up. His back is beset with weakness and tenderness with the many accompanying disorders. Yes, this is the lazy man's posture and is definitely a basic cause of many diseases.

Yet it could be prevented by thinking, sitting and standing tall, plus regular moderate exercise. Actually it is much easier to hold the head up in a balanced position rather than in a strained "hang-dog" way. It is also much easier to sit with your back well supported in a sensible chair than slumped over in some overstuffed monstrosity. It is easier to stand erect with chest held high, but for some reason we give in to gravity, developing all sorts of distortions. A little strenuous work or exercise will many times be the straw that breaks the camel's back and leads to further back trouble, so avoid overdoing in all irregular activities.

The exercise in this case is merely one of lying face down on the floor with the hands behind the head and doing backbends (see figure 3). This should be done for only short periods at first, increased as strength returns. Never overdo, but always stop before fatigued.

One-Sided Spinal Weaknesses

One-sidedness seems to go hand-in-hand with restricted occupational habits and routines. Lack of exercise and favored motions are the culprits in this case. Occasionally malformations or bone disease exist. For these we should seek professional aid.

Scoliosis is the curving of the spine to either the right or left side of the body (see figure 1C). This type of posture defect eventually brings pain and pressure at the apex of each curvature. The distortion worsens with age and is definitely one of the main causes of organic pain and neurosis. The weak side can be detected by comparing the size of the spinal muscles and the weight carried by each foot.

Having ascertained the side of weakness, we should then endeavor to build it up with the proper exercise. As equal tone returns, the tipping and rotation of the vertebrae will slowly normalize. Manipulation will hasten the procedure and is sometimes absolutely essential for correction of longstanding curvatures.

The cervical spine or neck is the most critical area in the entire back and trouble here can refer pain and disorder to almost any part of the body. In view of this, particular care should be taken to specifically correct any distortion existing in the upper spine, especially of the first two vertebrae. Correct all faults wherever they exist and don't overlook them. This should be heeded by both patient and doctor.

Concerning the one-sided spine that comes as a result of an acute temporary condition, we should attempt to relieve the pain, whether from pressure or tension, by rest, heat, massage and manipulation. Only after the muscle spasm and acute pain have ceased should exercise be attempted.

In a scoliotic or one-sided spine the chronic weakness of the muscles on one side allows for the resulting curvatures. The symptoms that develop will cease as the distortion diminishes and the one-sided posture improves. To build up the weak side, lie face down and lift the outstretched leg in a single leg-up and at the same time, with the weak-side hand on the back of the head, lift the elbow and shoulder up from the floor. This exercise is a one-sided back bend (see figure 4A) and should never be overdone, but you can gradually increase the length of time you practice it.

The second exercise for improving scoliosis is to do sit-ups with the weak-side hand touching the opposite foot. (See figure 4B.) This also should be pursued with an intelligent long range program for best results.

4. Preventing Osteoporosis

An article by B. E. C. Nordin, M.D., which appeared in the *Medical Press* for February 10, 1960, speaks of the causes of osteoporosis. He says that the condition affects far more women than men, possibly because of the greater proportion of older women in the population. Although this ailment may occur at any age, it is especially common in older age groups. Supposedly there is a relationship between the occurrence of osteoporosis and the menopause. However, we do not know very clearly just what this may be. One reason for its much greater incidence in women appears to be the demands made by childbirth. In one survey which was done, it was found that in a certain group of patients 40 per cent of those women who had not borne children had osteoporosis against 72 per cent of those who had borne many.

The disease may make itself known when a bone breaks, perhaps the hip bone, an accident which causes such discomfort and complications among older folks. More commonly, says Dr. Nordin, the complaint is backache which may occur in one spot or generally all over the back. The backache may be related to exercise; it may be aggravated by rest in bed; it may radiate down both thighs.

Bones Have Porous, Sponge-Like Appearance

The disease actually consists of an enlargement of the spaces in bone so that its appearance becomes porous. What looked before like a rock now appears like a sponge, with holes growing larger all the time. Since bones are important chiefly for support, you can easily see what difficulties would result. A backbone that cannot support the weight of its owner will produce pain, undoubtedly. Bones which are full of air holes are more likely to break in a fall than solid, staunch bones. Hence the many incidents of broken hips, arms and legs among older people whose steps may be unsteady or whose sight may be dim.

Protein is involved in the formation of bone, says Dr. Nordin, and it has been fashionable in past years to think of osteoporosis as a disorder involving protein rather than calcium. We know that one needs protein to form bones. On the other hand, breakdown of the structure of bones must result from lack of calcium. That is, calcium that should appear in bones has disappeared, leaving the holes which bring on the osteoporosis.

[13]

Getting and Keeping Calcium Is Important

The relationship of osteoporosis and calcium, or lack of it, in the diet is clearly shown by the results of many surveys. The *Lancet* for May 7, 1955, reports that in a group of 33 patients over the age of 68, those with a calcium intake under 500 milligrams of calcium daily had a 74 per cent incidence of osteoporosis whereas those who took over 500 milligrams of calcium daily had an incidence of only 14 per cent.

About 99 per cent of the body's calcium is stored in bone. An article by J. M. Finlay in the *Canadian Medical Association Journal* for May 15, 1956, tells us that bone is not a hard, impermeable substance. Instead, all the substances in it are constantly being exchanged, replaced and absorbed into other tissues. The bones of the average person weigh most at about 25 to 30 years of age. Thereafter they decline in weight indicating that minerals are being lost from them.

Calcium Sufficiency Depends On Three Big Factors

Whether or not one has enough calcium depends upon 3 things, according to Dr. Nordin: How much calcium is in one's food, how much one absorbs and how much one excretes. He goes on to say that the average intake of calcium in England, where he is writing, is 1,000 milligrams of calcium a day. However, he admits that such a figure contains much variation. It is true, he says, that some people do not get this much calcium and still they remain healthy. These folks can apparently adapt to a smaller amount of calcium and not excrete so much in their urine. However, it seems that one's body does not preserve calcium as it does some other minerals. The excretion of sodium can be reduced to almost nothing if one is eating a low-sodium diet. The amount of potassium excreted depends to some extent on how much is taken in. But it appears that the body is quite wasteful of calcium. You go right on excreting a considerable amount of calcium even when you are getting not nearly enough in your food.

"It is possible," says Dr. Nordin, "that the conservation of calcium, of which there are large stores in the skeleton, has been less vital to the organism in evolution than that of sodium, potassium, phosphate and nitrogen." It seems to us that this reluctance of the body to store and save calcium more carefully is an excellent reason to make certain you are getting plenty of it every day.

What about people who don't absorb the calcium they do get? About 15 per cent of these cases suffer from a disorder called steatorrhea, which involves quite distressing diarrhea. In diarrhea, of course, minerals are lost, rather than being absorbed, because they do not stay in the digestive tract long enough to be absorbed.

"The majority of patients with osteoporosis (those with steatorrhea excepted) go into strongly positive calcium balance when given calcium supplements," says Dr. Nordin. In other words, as soon as they begin to

[14]

get more than enough calcium, all their calcium needs are taken care of, even though they continue to excrete the same amount of calcium.

However, he goes on, it seems that no matter how much calcium is given, new bone matter is not formed in older people. Taking calcium supplements appears to relieve pain and to stop the progress of the disease, but cannot make any change in the way the bone looks under an X-ray. This may be the reason there is so much osteoporosis these days.

Your Calcium Intake Must Be Constant

People who, generally speaking, get enough calcium in their food, probably vary their intake from week to week, says Dr. Nordin. When their intake falls below their requirement, their bones suffer, for calcium apparently is withdrawn from the bones. At other times, when they get more calcium, isn't it possible for this part of the bone to be rebuilt? It seems not, says Dr. Nordin, when the people involved are elderly. It is not at all certain, he says, that people beyond middle age have the power to reconstitute this lost bone. So it becomes vitally important for such people to keep their calcium intake high at all times, for harm done by even a short period of having too little can apparently result in damage that can't be repaired.

We think it is startling to find in the pages of a medical magazine a suggestion that even a short period of living on a diet too low in calcium can result in irreparable harm. Surely here is a challenge for real preventive medicine!

Two other aspects of osteoporosis are stressed by Dr. Nordin. First the importance of vitamin D for the proper absorption of calcium. Vitamin D occurs most plentifully in fish liver oils, which is why we recommend that they be a part of everyone's daily food supplements. But, in the case of people who cannot absorb vitamin D (diarrhea or other conditions resulting in malabsorption) sunlight is the best source of vitamin D. We do not advise long hours of baking in the sun. The resulting tan means that your body can absorb no more vitamin D. We recommend rather outdoor exercise in the shade, for plenty of vitamin D is around outdoors in the summer. In winter, getting enough vitamin D is a real problem for northerners. Go south if you can. If not, spend as much time as possible outdoors on sunny days. In any case, take fish liver oil, summer and winter, to get the maximum amount of vitamin D.

One other suggestion. Steatorrhea, mentioned by Dr. Nordin as a possible contributing cause of osteoporosis, is frequently involved with difficulties in eating wheat and rye gluten. In other words, it may be the wheat or rye products in one's diet that cause the diarrhea which results in loss of calcium and other precious minerals. If you have any tendencies this way, we advise eliminating cereal products from your diet—all breads and breakfast cereals included. Most of us eat far too much cereal anyway, in comparison to the amount of fresh fruits and vegetables, eggs and meat that we eat. If you are suffering from steatorrhea, your doctor has undoubtedly already given you a diet containing no wheat or rye. If not, why not try doing without cereal products for a time just to see if you don't feel better?

Every article that we read on osteoporosis stressed strongly the necessity of physical activity in the prevention and treatment of osteoporosis. Says Benjamin B. Wells in the *American Practitioner and Digest of Treatment* for April, 1956, "diminished physical activity and loss of muscle strength are undoubtedly contributing factors in senile osteoporosis. Partial or total immobilization of any kind must be combatted with every means at our disposal." He also says that studies have indicated that older people need more calcium than younger people to maintain their "calcium balance."

Vitamins Are Important, Too

Dr. Wells stresses vitamin C. "There is no doubt," he says, "that vitamin C is necessary for the normal mineralization of bone and teeth." Out-and-out scurvy, resulting from complete lack of vitamin C, is rare in old people, but deficiency in vitamin C which we know is very common, must be closely associated with the incidence of osteoporosis, according to Dr. Wells. He also makes one very provocative statement about the possible relation of lessened blood supply to osteoporosis. He says, "One wonders about the possibility of diminished blood supply secondary to arteriosclerosis (hardening of the arteries) as a factor limiting the production of bone in aging persons. No positive evidence is available." We'd add—taking vitamin E supplements will lessen the possibility of poor circulation. We would say that vitamin C is extremely important for the prevention of osteoporosis and vitamin C is known to be lacking in most American diets, especially those of older folks—the very ones who need it most. Your richest supply is in fresh raw fruits and vegetables, and rose hips—the concentrated natural supplement made from the fruit of rose bushes.

The *Journal of the American Medical Association* for December 26, 1959, carries an article by James A. Nicholas and Philip D. Wilson of New York, who report on 105 patients who had spontaneous fracture of vertebrae —that is, a bone in their spines just crumbled without any accident or fall being the cause of it. They found that 18 patients had an average of less than 500 milligrams of calcium per day; 22 had between 500 and 800 milligrams and 15 had over 800 milligrams. Thirty-one had gall bladder and other digestive disorders which might result in being unable to absorb what calcium was in their diets.

The authors go into great detail about the various treatment given these patients in the way of casts, exercise, hormone treatment, etc. If they gave them any calcium at all, or took any special care to see that they got plenty of calcium in their diets, no mention is made of it in the article. Doesn't this seem strange?

And, finally, nowhere in any of these articles is there any suggestion that one can get too much calcium. Quite the contrary seems to be true: the problem is always how to get enough. If your mechanism for excreting calcium is working properly, you will always excrete any excess. If it is not working properly, you will get accumulation of calcium, whether you get much or little calcium in your diet.

Bone meal is your best source of calcium. It is made of powdered bones of young cattle. It contains not only calcium but all the other minerals in bone—phosphorus, potassium, iodine, magnesium and so forth. Take bone meal every day. You can take it in tablet form or, much less expensively, as a powder which you can use in food, in omelets, in fruit drinks, on salad and other foods.

5. Osteoporosis and Vitamin C

Osteoporosis, as the name suggests, is porous bone, bone in which the spaces between deposits of mineral have become so large that the bone looks honeycombed. Such bone is, of course, soft and easily liable to fracture. The disease is especially common among older people.

An article in the *American Journal of Clinical Nutrition* for November-December, 1957, indicates that chronic lack of vitamin C may be related to this disease. Say the authors, Dr. H. Grusin and E. Samuel, "There is a wealth of experimental evidence to support the view that vitamin C is essential for the formation of osteoid (bone) tissue." This is rather surprising for we generally think of bone only in terms of minerals and vitamin D. And we generally think of bone as being something formed in childhood which does not change from then on. This is not the case, of course, for bone reacts to body conditions just as any other part of the body does. In osteoporosis the bones are decalcified—that is, calcium has been lost from them. This is part of the reason why they are so weak and yield so easily to breakage.

The Link between Scurvy and Osteoporosis

The 16 patients described in this article were all African Bantus. Perhaps the most revealing aspect of the study is that 9 of these patients were suffering from acute scurvy when they entered the hospital. Scurvy is the disease of vitamin C deficiency. Two other patients had either some symptoms of scurvy or a past history of scurvy. So 69 per cent of the patients were or had been scorbutic.

The surprising thing about this fact is that both scurvy and osteoporosis are uncommon diseases at this hospital, yet they were frequently found together in the same patient. The main symptom of all patients was backache. X-rays of spines showed that much calcium had been lost and fractured vertebrae in all cases.

Treatment with vitamin C did not bring the spines back to normal, with one exception. This patient was kept in the hospital for a year and was given a full hospital diet along with rest and massive doses of vitamin C. The other patients continued to eat their usual diet and returned home to hard physical labor (especially carrying heavy loads on their backs) much sooner than that.

The authors conclude that in such an African community there are many factors which might be responsible for osteoporosis. The diet contains little calcium and not too much in the way of animal protein. However, everyone in the community eats this same deficient diet and osteoporosis, as well as scurvy, are found very infrequently. When they do occur, they often occur in the same patient. Say Dr. Grusin and Samuel, "It is suggested that these osteoporotic patients may have suffered from chronic scurvy or minor attacks of scurvy without being incapacitated and that their chronic vitamin-C deficient state eventually led to osteoporosis."

It was those words "chronic or minor attacks of scurvy . . . without being incapacitated" that caught our attention. We have found evidence that many people in America, especially older people, are suffering from these same conditions—minor attacks, or chronic scurvy, evidenced by loose teeth, bruise marks, swollen or inflamed or bleeding gums. In addition, lack of calcium is tragically obvious among our senior population. Could the osteoporosis not be related to these two important deficiencies?

As the doctors in Africa found out, it was not possible to cure the osteoporosis with even large doses (500 milligrams) of vitamin C. But a patient given a good all-round diet and rest, along with the vitamin C, showed improvement. We have in this article only a theory without the painstaking work that is necessary to establish a new principle in nutrition.

But it is enough, we think, to serve as a warning to those of us who are not getting enough vitamin C. Osteoporosis is a painful and often crippling disease. If you can prevent it by eating lots of fruit and vegetables, raw rather than cooked, and by taking additional vitamin C and calcium in natural food supplements (bone meal is the best source of natural calcium and other minerals), don't you think it's worth the effort?

6. How Well Do You Hear?

According to the American Hearing Society, there were in 1952, 1.3 million children in this country up to 14 years of age with sufficiently impaired hearing to warrant further study. Furthermore, there were 250,000 to 500,000 Americans under the age of 21 with hearing loss serious enough to be called a handicap.

It is difficult to collect statistics on hearing loss, for many people apparently endure gradual loss of hearing over a period of years without becoming concerned enough about it to see a doctor. So we do not really know how much more extensive deafness and defects in hearing may be.

We, of course, are interested in what can be done to prevent defects in hearing. Since our hearing apparatus is part of our nervous system, part of our epithelial system, part of our skin system and our bony system, it seems likely, doesn't it, that many of the same rules for health for other parts of the body would apply in the case of the ear.

For instance, we know that vitamin B is perhaps the single most important element in food so far as the health of the nerves is concerned. We know that, lacking the B vitamins, dispositions get frayed, mentality becomes cloudy, memory fails, eyesight is affected and sometimes numbness and paralysis attack arms and legs. All these are simply the result of nerves lacking the nourishment they must have and can get only from the B vitamins.

Nerve Deafness

Hearing, of course, depends on the efficient working of a nerve—the one called the eighth cranial nerve which carries sounds from the inner ear to the brain. Not all forms of deafness are caused by damage to the nerve of hearing. The various other parts of the ear apparatus may be involved, too. But, for what is called "nerve deafness," there seems to be no doubt that lack of vitamin B may be a very important cause.

What evidence do we have that this is so? In the book, *Nutritional Disorders of the Nervous System,* by John D. Spillane, M.D. (published by Williams and Wilkins Company), we read of cases of beriberi and pellagra in which deafness is one of the symptoms. These are both diseases of vitamin B deficiency. By that we mean that they afflict only people who do not get in their food enough of the B vitamins. Pellagra and beriberi have killed hundreds of thousands of people in the Far East and in our own southland where a combination of poverty, ignorance and a food pattern in which refined corn products loom large, made pellagra an epidemic disease for many years.

Says Dr. Spillane, tinnitus (ringing in the ears) develops before dermatitis sometimes. A certain kind of dermatitis or skin disorder is one of the sure symptoms of pellagra. Owing to the listless or positively demented condition of many patients with advanced pellagra it is difficult to tell whether or not they are deaf. However, he does give reports of some cases where the following percentages were definitely noticed: 5 cases of deafness out of 46 patients; 8 cases out of 60 patients; 7 out of 9 cases.

Of beriberi (caused by deficiency in thiamin, another of the B vitamins) Dr. Spillane says that deafness is probably uncommon in well-advanced cases and may be unnoticed in the acutely ill patient. However, he says that the auditory nerve is mainly involved *in the mild latent form of the disease.* In other words, individuals suffering from a mild deficiency (just as many of us undoubtedly are) might notice the "nerve deafness" without the other symptoms of beriberi.

Dr. Spillane goes on to tell of prisoners of war who had beriberi because of the inadequate diet in the prison camp. Of these there was temporary deafness in many. A few became quite deaf. Of 38 Chinese women being treated for polyneuritis (another symptom of vitamin B deficiency) two were deaf and seven had persistent tinnitus or ringing in the ears. There seems to be no doubt that lack of vitamin B may be related to many cases of noises in the ears.

In a number of cases of neuritis found in Jamaica, the symptoms were numbness in feet and legs, difficulty in walking, incoordination of muscles, deterioration of vision and deafness. The deafness was of the "nerve type" and it was found when these patients were autopsied that the auditory nerve, which carries sound impressions from the ear to the brain, had deteriorated greatly, due undoubtedly to lack of vitamin B. In prisoners of war we are told that tinnitus was a common complaint, frequently followed by deafness which came on gradually. The deafness usually afflicted both ears and began with a feeling of "fullness" in the ears. It is interesting to note that many of these same prisoners who were deaf also had "spots before the eyes"—*scotomata* as the doctors call them.

Lack of Vitamin B and Nerve Deafness

Catharyn Elwood in her excellent book, *Feel Like A Million,* tells us more about nerve deafness and vitamin B. She reminds us that no refined sugar can give us one ounce of energy unless thiamin is present to break it down from pyruvic acid to energy and carbon dioxide and water. The accumulation of pyruvic acid (for lack of vitamin B) is responsible for many ailments—"among them chronic fatigue and a certain type of deafness due to nerve disturbance."

Furthermore she says that deposits of cholesterol collecting in the walls of the tiny blood vessels may have a lot to do with deafness, especially in

[20]

persons over middle age. Several of the B vitamins (inositol and choline) are powerful against the formation of cholesterol deposits. Lecithin and the unsaturated fatty acids (found in vegetable oils, not in animal fats) also emulsify cholesterol and keep it from depositing where it is not wanted.

Miss Elwood tells us of one experiment where two sets of laboratory rats were fed the same diet. One set was given brewer's yeast in addition. The second was not. At autopsy, the rats which got no yeast showed very few hearing cells—a perfect picture of so-called "nerve deafness." The rats which had the brewer's yeast showed no abnormality of the ears. Remember that yeast is rich in protein and minerals, as well as the B vitamins.

If you fear deafness or if you notice that you are just beginning to have difficulty hearing what people say to you, don't you think it would be wise to add brewer's yeast in quite a large quantity to your food supplements? Brewer's yeast is food, you know, so there is no need to worry about getting too much of it. However, don't make the mistake of taking synthetic B vitamins which can easily result in an imbalance of these important vitamins —that is, you may suffer from a deficiency in those which are not included in the synthetic preparation you take.

7. Vitamin A and Your Hearing

"The results of treatment and prevention of chronic progressive deafness have been very disappointing. This is evidenced by the fact that there are approximately 18,000,000 deaf people in this country," say Drs. Hyman W. Bau and Louis Savitt in an article in the *Eye, Ear, Nose and Throat Monthly* for February, 1951. They go on to say that much of this deafness in adults has been progressive from childhood. Preventing hearing impairment, either in children or in adults, is, of course, the solution to the problem, for after the hearing apparatus has been damaged, it is apparently quite difficult to bring it back to anything like good working order.

Drs. Bau and Savitt gave massive doses of vitamin A to their patients with chronic progressive deafness and tinnitus. They injected the vitamin because they knew that often vitamin A and other fat-soluble vitamins are not absorbed in the digestive tract. Then, too, if vitamin A is given in its vegetable form (that is, carotene such as appears in carrots and so forth), the liver must transform it into vitamin A. And this may overtax the liver. The researchers used 50,000 units of vitamin A in each injection.

They excluded certain kinds of deafness and concentrated on others. After giving extensive tests to a group of 24 patients, they made injections every two weeks for a period of 6 weeks. Of the 24 patients, 8 showed no improvement at all. Seven patients showed an improvement of from 5 to 10 decibels; 7 others from 10 to 20 decibels; and the remainder showed an improvement of more than 20 decibels. (Decibels are units for measuring the loudness of sounds.)

So far as tinnitus (ringing in the ears) was concerned, 9 patients complained severely of this symptom, and 6 of these experienced a decided improvement from the therapy. The researchers conclude their article by saying that they consider the tests successful, and they recommend the use of massive doses of vitamin A as a "valuable therapeutic agent" in the treatment of chronic progressive deafness.

Several months later, in May, 1951, the *Archives of Otolaryngology* published an article by M. Joseph Lobel, M.D., of New York who has done considerable work with nutrition and deafness. Dr. Lobel reviews some of the theories and experiments with vitamin A that have gone before. He quotes one investigator, Barlow, as saying that a deficiency in vitamin A which causes changes in the mucous membrane of the throat might produce changes in the middle ear which could become permanent. Another researcher, Cody, tells of impaired hearing in laboratory rats made deficient in vitamin A. In 1933 Rosenfeld gave cod liver oil (rich in vitamins A and D) and calcium to patients with otosclerosis and improved the hearing of many of them. The noises in the ears of which they had complained were either greatly improved or disappeared entirely.

Experiments with Vitamin A

Sir Edward Mellanby, one of the greatest nutritionists of our time, reported in 1934 that he could produce deafness in laboratory animals by depriving them of vitamin A. Lack of the vitamin, he explained, caused an overgrowth in the small bones of the ear which prevented the transmission of sounds. Dr. I. H. Jones in 1940 reminded his medical colleagues which vitamins are concerned with the different parts of the body. Vitamin A affects the ectoderm and the endoderm—those are the parts of the body from which are developed the central nervous system and the mucous membrane. So we can assume with complete assurance that vitamin A is of vital importance to the tissues of the inner ear as well as the throat and chest.

Dr. Lobel tells us of another researcher, Hollender, who gave 100,000 units of vitamin A daily by mouth, along with pituitary extract once a week. He got good results. Another physician recommended 25,000 units of carotene a day along with brewer's yeast 3 times a day plus pituitary extract. Of his patients, 85.5 per cent showed a hearing gain; 13.4 per cent showed a hearing loss and about one per cent remained the same. In another experiment, volunteers were deprived of vitamin A. They showed considerable loss of hearing. When they were further deprived of the vitamin, their hearing became worse. It improved considerably when vitamin A was added to their diet.

Dr. Lobel himself reports on many patients he treated with injections of vitamin A so that there would be no chance of poor absorption in the digestive tract. Results in 300 patients indicated an average gain of hearing in the left ear of 18.9 per cent and in the right ear of 17.3 per cent. Fifty-one patients failed to benefit from the treatment. Two hundred and forty-nine showed very definite gains in hearing conversational tones. Ringing in the ears was benefited, or ceased entirely in the same proportions. Dr. Lobel believes that his study shows that vitamin deficiency and hearing loss are "in some manner related," and he urges that someone make further trials of vitamin therapy.

Finally we come to the work of a San Francisco physician who wrote much earlier on vitamins and hearing disorders. Dr. Grant Selfridge, writing in the *Annals of Otology, Rhinology and Laryngology* for September, 1940, tells us that many diseases formerly thought of as due to infections may now be found to be related to nutritional deficiencies. He quotes Mary Schwartz Rose in *The Foundations of Nutrition* who says that lack of vitamin A is most important for the health of epithelial tissues, like those of the ear. She says, "After damage due to an inadequate supply has been done, dosing with the vitamin will not guarantee a cure, although it may help to hasten such recovery as the tissues are still capable of."

A professor of the School of Medicine at the University of Rochester found that among 317 cases of infants, severe infections were twice as frequent in those whose previous diet lacked vitamin A. We know that infections of the middle ear are thought to be one of the chief causes for loss of hearing. Of 92 laboratory animals on a vitamin A deficient diet studied by another researcher, 20 per cent had infections of the middle ear. And it seems, from Sir Edward Mellanby's studies, that enough vitamin A must be present for the eighth nerve (the nerve of hearing) to be healthy.

Using Vitamin A with Deaf Patients

J. R. Anderson, using Dr. Lobel's method of giving injections of vitamin A and experimenting for 6 weeks only, reports on 30 patients with varying degrees of hearing impairment. In the *Eye, Ear, Nose and Throat Monthly* for February, 1950, he tells us that 50 per cent of the patients showed definite improvement in hearing, both objective and subjective, that is, they themselves thought they had improved and, tests showed that they had. In addition, 17 out of 23 patients with tinnitus or ringing in the ears showed definite improvement and in some cases, complete cure.

We found other information on vitamin A and deafness in our files. But, in general, it is along these same lines. We also found some reports of failure in vitamin A therapy. But we think that the very encouraging results some of these researchers had should encourage us to try vitamin A for the prevention of hearing defects.

Not much mention is made of age in relation to hearing in any of these reports. But we know that, generally, a decline in hearing ability is accepted as part of growing old. We know, too, that as we grow older, we need more vitamin A and our diets tend to have less of the vitamin in them.

[23]

The raw fruits and the green leafy vegetables may be replaced by stewed fruits and cooked vegetables; the two or more eggs a day may be replaced by refined cereal or toast. Changes like these deprive us of vitamin A and present us with a quite serious problem of vitamin A deficiency unless we take a food supplement, high in the vitamin, as part of our daily health routine.

Should our readers take injections of vitamin A in the hope of curing deafness? This is out of our field, which is prevention, not cure. If your doctor believes that you may have difficulty absorbing vitamin A (and if you have liver trouble, you certainly would), he may wish to give you injections of vitamin A. We would suggest that, if you are going to experiment with injections of massive doses, you should certainly take, in addition, generous amounts of the other vitamins—brewer's yeast or wheat germ for vitamin B, rose hip preparations for vitamin C, vitamin E and bone meal for minerals.

If you are interested in preventing hearing defects, and we believe that you should be, no matter what your age, then make certain you are getting enough vitamin A in your diet, and by all means take a vitamin A food supplement. Fish liver oil is rich in both vitamin A and vitamin D. Add it to your supplements. Even though the daily minimum requirement has been set at 5000 International Units, we believe from the research we have done that far more than this is necessary for good health, and especially for the health of the mucous membranes. It is possible to get too much vitamin A, yes. Amounts over 100,000 International Units can be dangerous.

One final caution. Mineral oil destroys vitamin A and all other fat soluble vitamins in the digestive tract. Could the widespread use of mineral oil in this country be largely responsible for our terrible statistics on deafness and hearing defects? Mineral oil is a vitamin enemy—never forget that.

8. Protect Your Hearing!

Throughout our research on the study of deafness, we were constantly impressed by the number of times we ran across statements like this (from an article by Grant Selfridge, M.D., in the *Archives of Otolaryngology* for July, 1941). "More evidence is accumulating that the time to begin the prevention of deafness is really 6 months before conception. Each parent should be taught that an optimum diet, containing the essential food factors (vitamins) is necessary in order to beget a healthy normal child and that such a diet should be carried out by the pregnant mother. The same careful supervision should be given to the diet of the child through infancy, babyhood, childhood and adolescence."

Most writers on hearing and nutrition stress the fact that no one or two vitamins can be held responsible for the health of this bodily mechanism—all of them are important, because all of them have something to do with the health of tissues, bones, nerves, cells or intercellular material—all of which are involved in hearing.

For instance, Dr. Selfridge reminds us in the article mentioned above that vitamin C is an important ingredient of the cementing substance that occurs between all the cells of the body, also that its lack causes bones to decalcify and "has to do with the formation of adhesions." Lack of vitamin C will also, he says, produce a swelling throughout "Corti's organ" which is in the very innermost part of the ear canal. He reminds us, too, that vitamin C has something to do with the health of the nerves and, of course, this means the nerve of hearing as well as all the others. "It is hardly conceivable," says Dr. Selfridge in another article on the subject, "that all the cranial nerves participate in the degenerative processes in certain dietary deficiencies and that the eighth nerve (the nerve of hearing) should be exempt."

Speaking of vitamin C, Dr. Selfridge quotes an article in the *Journal of Laryngology and Otology,* Vol. 54, p. 256, 1939. This author, Adam, speaks of a very low vitamin C level in the urine of several patients he was treating for Meniere's disease—a disorder of the middle ear. In 4 such cases he found that the patient had not been getting nearly enough vitamin C. Three of these were cured "largely by attention to vitamins." The fourth case was that of a woman who had such severe attacks of the disease that they sometimes rendered her unconscious. She had purposely not been eating fresh fruits, believing that they contributed to heartburn. On this doctor's suggestion, she persevered in taking vitamins and conquered the dizziness that is a symptom of Meniere's disease, though the deafness and tinnitus in one ear remained.

Another researcher, Chimani, mentions in the *Journal of Laryngology* for May, 1939, 18 cases of chronic middle ear infection who were given large doses of vitamin C in addition to local treatment; most of these cases showed considerable deficiency in the vitamin. In 10 instances the infection cleared entirely. In the others there was a lessening of the discharge. Study of the middle ear mechanism of a laboratory animal showed that *the tissues of the middle ear store vitamin C.*

Vitamin C is Stored in Vital Organs

This last fact seems to us of utmost importance. Vitamin C is stored in the lens of the eye, in the adrenal glands, the pituitary gland, the liver and other important organs of the body. We are gradually discovering more and more about the meaning of this storage. It appears to indicate that these parts of the body need more vitamin C than other parts. If this is so, then one fearing deafness should be especially certain he gets a diet rich in vitamin C so that the vitamin can be stored in the proper tissues of the ear.

Reviewing an article by 3 other researchers, Dr. Selfridge tells of their study of 53 children, all suffering from chronic middle ear infections. It was found that half of the children showed very little resistance to infections and they were, in general, in poor nutritional condition. More than a third had diseased tonsils and adenoids as well. More than half had a decided deficiency in vitamin C.

In another series of cases it was found that 45 per cent of all those studied who were suffering from "conduction deafness" were below normal in their vitamin C and *mineral* level. In some of these cases vitamin C in large doses brought about normal hearing.

An interesting angle to the whole problem of getting enough vitamin C is that this vitamin is used by the body to fight poisons. Dr. Selfridge in an article in the *Annals of Otology, Rhinology and Laryngology* for September, 1939, tells of a study made at the Southern Pacific General hospital where a number of minerals not known to be useful and possibly even toxic were found in the blood of the patients studied—strontium, arsenic, titanium, chromium, tin, antimony, zinc and lead were some of these. "It is important to know their source," says Dr. Selfridge, "how they gain access to the blood stream and whether they are damaging to nerve tissue." The implication is, of course, that our daily exposure to such substances constitutes a hazard which is undoubtedly minimized by a healthful intake of vitamin C—that fighter against poisons.

One final note—this time not on vitamins. G. R. Gordon, M.D., writing in the *Journal of the Medical Association of Alabama* for April, 1948, tells of giving amino acid preparations along with vitamins. He tells us that during a course of treatment with vitamin B and amino acids for things like anemia, nervous exhaustion and digestive disorders, it was found that patients who had not previously noticed any decline in hearing gradually began to notice an increase in their hearing acuity.

Amino Acids Important for Good Hearing

So a series of studies was started at the Hard of Hearing Clinic at the Medical College of Alabama. Amino acids, as you know, are forms of protein and one of these seems to be particularly important for nerves—glutamic acid. This was given along with other amino acids, brewer's yeast and liver extract "to supply all the vitamin B factors" says Dr. Gordon. In addition, vitamin C was given, too. Since this was a test with a definite time limit where the most had to be made of different kinds of medication, there were injections as well as pills to be taken by mouth.

Says Dr. Gordon, "Those patients whose history revealed deficiency diets or imperfect digestive function and absorption showed the greatest response. An interesting observation was the gratifying increase in the general well-being, mental and physical, as seen in the majority of patients under therapy. This was evidenced by increased appetite, improvement in sleeping habits, greater energy and a marked decrease in fatigability."

Fifty six per cent showed considerable improvement, 20 per cent showed some improvement and 24 per cent showed no improvement. The best gains were in the hearing of high tones which Dr. Gordon says is particularly advantageous since these are the ones used in saying consonants. Many patients, he says, would complain, "I can hear you but I can't understand what you are saying," the reason being that they could not hear the high tones in which consonants are spoken.

Says Dr. Gordon further, "Frequently hearing disorders are associated with personality changes. Anything tending to benefit the whole personality as evidenced in increased sense of well-being and an impression of strength will have an effect on the patients." The diet, high in amino acids and vitamins, apparently had this effect on the patients. Dr. Gordon says that the great majority of the patients maintained their initial gains. Those who regressed never went back to their original low level of hearing.

Back in 1941 when Dr. Selfridge wrote we did not have the large amount of research on vitamin E that we have today. But even then he tells us, it had been discovered that a deficiency in vitamin E produces a marked degeneration of the nervous system in animals. Dr. Selfridge gave his patients vitamin E in addition to the other vitamins he was giving them.

Does it appear, then, that we can prevent deafness, tinnitus (ringing in the ears) and diseases of the middle ear with good nutrition? Yes, it seems that we can, and it seems that the many millions today who suffer from deafness or are hard of hearing may be able to incriminate as the cause of their condition, a diet lacking in important things. Amino acids (at present sold in concentrated forms) are proteins. Is your diet high in proteins— meat, eggs, fish, unprocessed seeds? Are you getting more than enough of vitamins A, B, C and E? You can't, you know, unless you take natural food supplements, for the food you buy in the store these days simply does not contain enough vitamins to keep you from deficiency. Do you eat refined and processed foods—prepared cereals, white bread, white sugar? Every mouthful of food such as these robs you of essential vitamins. Cross them off your list.

9. A New Approach to Deafness

Have you heard of Dr. Curtis H. Muncie? Most people have not, and it is strange that this is so, for he should be famous. Almost 50 years ago Dr. Muncie discovered a means of curing many types of deafness considered, then and now, to be absolutely incurable.

During the 1920's Dr. Muncie did his best to let the world know of his discovery. He toured the United States and several European countries, holding free clinics and giving demonstrations of his new-found technique for increasing the ability to hear in deaf people, whose auditory nerves had not degenerated completely. There was publicity aplenty, and many foremost specialists conceded that Dr. Muncie had indeed found something new and effective. Yet the therapy was never incorporated into the course of study in our medical schools, due perhaps to the nature of the treatment, and its dependence upon a long term of practice for acquiring the "feel" necessary in shaping the involved organs properly. At last Dr. Munice gave up his public clinics and retired into private practice at his Park Avenue office in New York City, New York, where he still restores hearing to a large roster of patients who have been given up by doctors who rely on conventional methods.

Eustachian Tubes Hold the Key

Quite accidentally Dr. Muncie stumbled onto the fact that the Eustachian tubes are basically involved in most cases of deafness. The Eustachian tubes (see figure 5) are canals which connect the throat with the middle ear, and it is their function to equalize air pressure in the middle ear. When one swallows, the tubes open and allow air to enter, and it is for this reason that one experiences relief by swallowing during quick changes of altitude. The changes in air pressure outside the body are matched inside when the swallow opens the Eustachian tubes and allows air into the middle ear.

If this system is working properly, the adjustment is almost automatic. One notices a feeling in the ears much akin to the one felt when water

FIGURE 5: DIAGRAM OF EAR

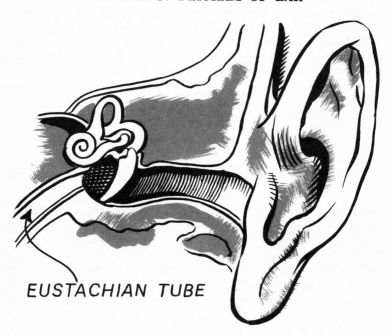

EUSTACHIAN TUBE

has somehow stopped them up. Sounds become dull and distant, until, with a swallow, "your ears pop" and you hear normally once more. If one's Eustachian tubes do not work properly, the "pop" doesn't come. The dull distance in your hearing persists. You are deaf to a greater or lesser degree.

Dr. Muncie found that many cases of deafness were due to Eustachian tubes that were somehow malformed. This interfered not only with air pressure in the middle ear, but also with blood and lymph circulation to different sections of the inner ear. The development of disease in the organ of hearing which resulted in deafness, tinnitus and vertigo, was encouraged by this condition.

An Accidental Discovery

A simple operation to remove the adenoids of a boy previously deafened as a result of scarlet fever was the scene for Dr. Muncie's discovery. The doctor had discovered by exploring with his fingers that several lateral adenoids remained after the others had been removed. He proceeded to break these down with his fingers until one finger slipped into a depression, and with slight pressure, the finger could be pushed further for the distance of about ¾ of an inch. When the boy awoke after the operation, his parents were amazed to find that his hearing was considerably improved.

Dr. Muncie was puzzled, for he was sure that the opening he had entered with his finger was the Eustachian tube, yet all medical textbooks showed these tubes to be about the width of a sipping straw, much too narrow for such an insertion. But this information was based on the observation of dead bodies. Could the Eustachian tubes in living persons be wider? It was so! In live subjects the tubes were found to be formed of malleable cartilage and the first inch was large enough to allow the entrance of one finger.

Hundreds of Comparisons Made

Dr. Muncie then began to examine the Eustachian tubes of hundreds of patients with normal hearing for comparison with hundreds of deaf patients. His fingers soon developed a sensitivity which could quickly distinguish different tubal deformities. He found Eustachian tubes in deaf persons to be markedly different from normal ones in size, contour and tone. It was also true that the type of tubal deformity was usually characteristic of the type of deafness. There were 8 basic types of deformity and Dr. Muncie developed specific techniques for the correction of each.

Series of 50 Cases

As a means of demonstrating the effectiveness of the technique he perfected, Dr. Muncie once took a series of 50 cases which had been diagnosed as Meniere's disease by two or more specialists. None of the 50 had been permanently relieved by traditional methods of treatment, and 29 had even been advised to have brain surgery. On first examination of this group, Dr. Muncie found their average hearing capacity to be about 47 per cent. On completion of treatment, the average ability to hear had been increased to 91 per cent of perfect hearing.

From the evidence we've seen, such results are typical of those achieved by Dr. Muncie's methods.

Dr. Muncie has taught his son Douglas, who practices in Miami, Florida, what he knows, and these are the only two men in this country, perhaps in the world, who practice and can pass on this ability to manipulate the Eustachian tubes to their proper shape.

Now you know why we think Dr. Muncie's name should be better known. Let an athletic record be broken, and the hero's name is a household word; let a women be chosen Mother of the Year, or a man fly a plane higher or faster than any other, and their names fill the papers and radio. But, after all, these feats are not really important to anyone in the world but those immediately involved. Yet here is an accomplishment which can be important to thousands of suffering people and these two men are the only ones able to implement it, still their names are news to most of us. Without magazines such as the *American Mercury*, PREVENTION and a few others, the story of Dr. Muncie's discovery would be buried in his files and in the grateful letters of the patients who have found a new life through his treatment. Strange and sad to think such a situation exists, isn't it?

10. Understanding the Misery of Tinnitus

Describing the misery of tinnitus (ringing in the ears) is not easy, so we doubt that persons who suffer from this malady ever get the sympathy to which they are entitled. Because they do not have great pain, or a wound that is visible, the victims are expected to overcome the discomfort they experience by sheer willpower. The truth of the matter is that they seldom can. There is actually a physical basis for most tinnitus, and one can no more will it away than talk oneself out of a broken leg.

Various Sounds Heard

The sound is constantly there—all day, all night. There is no time, in the patient's conscious moments, that he does not hear what has been described variously as: ringing, buzzing, a noise like a waterfall, a jet of steam, a saw or an engine, a splash, ringing of bells or the telephone, chirping, grasshopper or cricket sounds, whistling, etc. That means that to go to sleep you must overcome the noise. When in conversation you hear it; if you're listening to music or watching television, reading or working this distracting, distressing, maddening noise is ever present. Is it surprising

that the patient is tormented with depression to such a degree that it sometimes leads to suicide?

The condition, as discussed in great detail by Jean-Pierre Taillens in
Review Medicale de la Suisse Romande (80/2:65-78) indicates an abnormality in the auditory canal at some point of its course. The where and
why create a serious problem for the doctor. Sometimes the reason is in-
solvable, the causes can be many and/or unrecognizable.

The Pulse Is Noisy And Is Heard by Ear

In nature absolute silence does not exist. Normally the ear detects the
sounds of the internal life when external sound is absent. As an illustration
of this we are told by Dr. Taillens that the noise one hears when holding
a conch shell to the ear is actually the echo of the sound of the blood
stream running through the capillaries of the cochlea (a spirally wound-
tube which is a part of the inner ear). One researcher (Békésy) claims
that the minute sound of the constant spontaneous movement of the cells
of the body is enough to stimulate a resonant vibration in the ear. The cells
move in a range of one ten millionth of a millimeter. This might give some
idea of the extreme delicacy of the auditory make-up we have, and at the
same time help us realize the possible loudness of the ringing sound we've
been discussing here.

The types of tinnitus fall into 3 general categories. The first is "exotic
or periotic." This comes from disorders of organs near the auditory apparatus. These sounds actually have an observable physical basis. The doctor, using a stethoscope, can hear them as well as the patient. One cause of
these noises is due to the contraction of one of the ear muscles, or to alternating contractions of the soft palate, of the tongue or the uvula. Another is chronic catarrh, which can cause hollow noises, like snapping
when swallowing, due to the separation of the tubular wall when congested.
Noises also occur sometimes at the movement of the jaw bone.

Vascular noises are truly the most common of all, and result from
some physical incapacity. For example, sufferers of pernicious anemia or
chlorosis are likely to hear a whirring sound of the jugular vein, like a
turning wheel or a loud noise. Persons suffering from impairment of the
heart, or carotid, or from arterial trouble near the ear get a noise connected with the throbbing of the pulse. It occurs at regular intervals along
with the pulse beat. Combinations of arterial and venous disorders can also
occur, having manifestations in the persistent sounds of the inner ear.

Any Disorder Can Cause Tinnitus

A different type of tinnitus is called "entotic tinnitus." Here the sounds
are heard only by the patient; they are completely subjective. The sounds
are accompanied by deafness which is an important factor in diagnosis. In
the external ear, accumulation of wax, foreign objects, bony growths, etc.
often cause dizziness and tinnitus. When any of these is removed, the symptoms disappear.

[31]

Where the middle ear is concerned, just about any disorder can cause tinnitus—that includes all types of infections and inflammation. The same is true of the inner ear; however, the possible sources of the trouble involve many parts of the body and make tracing it very difficult. Tumors of the acoustic nerve cause tinnitus; in Meniere's disease even cutting the cochlear nerve won't stop tinnitus and no one seems to know what will. Certain glandular disorders can cause tinnitus and so can high blood pressure. The list of possible causes has never been fully defined.

Drugs Can Cause Tinnitus and Deafness

There are, however, some commonly accepted causes of tinnitus. The internal ear is an organ which is most sensitive to poisons of all kinds. Tinnitus is often one of the first symptoms indicative of and preceding deafness due to poisoning. One of the poisons which can cause such injury is quinine, often used as a medication for malaria. Another is salicylate, a part of most aspirin compounds. It can produce both a congestion of the middle ear and the labyrinth, where a bloody discharge can be noted. If the drug is stopped early enough, says Taillens, tinnitus will disappear; if not, the noises can persist indefinitely. There is room here for speculation on chronic arthritis and headache victims who saturate themselves with aspirin. How many have experienced tinnitus and not been aware of the reason?

There is a long list of drugs which can bring on acute tinnitus when given in large doses: barbiturates, aureomycin, streptomycin, therapeutic arsenic, cocaine, opium and their derivatives. Dehydrostreptomycin (found in combiotic) injures the internal ear even in small dosages. Some persons are especially susceptible. Stopping the drug and protecting the cochlea by means of the administration of vitamin A, prove to be the only effective remedies against this condition.

Deafness and tinnitus can result from exposure to certain chemicals connected with one's occupation. These can be aniline, arsenic, benzene, mercury, lead, carbon monoxide, illuminating gas, phosphorus and sulphur. Gas station attendants are exposed to lead and carbon monoxide frequently; dry cleaners are constantly breathing the toxic benzene fumes, etc. Each of these workers should be using large amounts of vitamin A and vitamin C to offset these exposures.

Tinnitus and deafness often act as a clue to other serious systemic defects. Diabetes, chronic nephritis, a faulty fat metabolism are 3 such conditions, and one should have one's blood examined for sugar, urea and cholesterol count if tinnitus occurs. Virus infections are also likely to result in this type of ear trouble.

Tinnitus From a Tight Collar

One aspect of tinnitus has especially intriguing overtones—reflex tinnitus. It's a sort of sympathetic reaction to the strangest types of stress. One reported case had tinnitus relieved upon the patient's having his glasses adjusted; another had a denture refitted with a resultant tinnitus cure; still another responded to the enlarging of a tight collar. The list is quite long and leads to the conclusion that reflex tinnitus can be caused by anything from an aching tooth to an arthritic joint.

The final type of tinnitus, "central tinnitus," is the most frightening, actually the most serious of all. The victim hears sounds of all kinds which seem to be coming from the central auditory canal. They are intolerable and violent. They spread over everything and echo throughout the head. The noises are heard in both ears which hampers any classification of the cause. Furthermore, the noises resist everything and persist over a similar sound produced by the audiometer, even with greater intensity than ordinary subjective tinnitus. Such a condition is often the sign of the development of a serious disorder, and calls for a complete neurologic examination.

It should be said that there is such a thing as auditory hallucination. While this condition persists the patient hears articulate sounds, bits of phrases or melodies. At this point the problem is considered to be psychiatric, and should be treated accordingly.

The problem of tinnitus is certainly better defined than the cure. Throughout Dr. Taillens' paper we saw only one definite therapeutic suggestion—vitamins. The doctor suggested vitamins A, B and C as a means of both forestalling the development of tinnitus and the means of curing it once it has occurred. We believe that these supplements should be included in everyone's diet, even those who feel they are in perfect health. They are vital in the prevention of many diseases, and if tinnitus can also be avoided as a result of their use, then one is certainly wise to take advantage of the nutrients for that reason, if for no other.

[33]

11. Some Questions and Answers about Cataract

What is Cataract?

Cataract is a disorder of the lens of the eye, generally spoken of as a "degenerative disorder"—that is, it results from things wearing out and breaking down, rather than "catching something" or being injured.

In the eye with cataract, the lens becomes opaque, like a misty or fogged windowglass. The lens is that part of the eye which gathers the rays of light and focuses them on the nerve endings behind it (see figure 6). Apparently what happens in cataract is that cells die or become damaged, turning white in the process. Clusters of these white cells are what you see in the eye with the fully advanced cataract. Cataract is not a "growth" —that is, it is not in the same class with tumors. It does not represent cells growing abnormally. It appears to represent rather cells dying off and becoming useless.

FIGURE 6: CROSS-SECTION OF THE EYE, SHOWING LENS

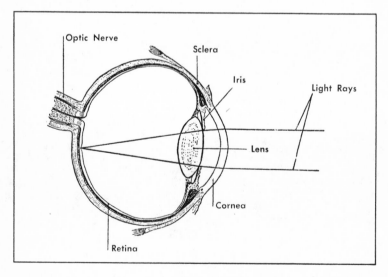

[34]

Is There More Than One Kind of Cataract?

Yes, there are several. Senile cataract is the commonest—the one most people mean when they speak of cataract. The word "senile" is used here because this kind of cataract usually afflicts people who are advanced in age, although, just like gray hair and wrinkles, it can occur in quite young persons as well.

Congenital cataract occurs in babies at birth. Diabetic cataract sometimes afflicts diabetics of any age. It is believed to go along with degenerative changes in blood vessels that also occur in diabetics.

Does Cataract Cause Blindness?

It does. It is the first and most important cause of blindness in this country today. It is estimated that 49,000 Americans are sightless because of cataract. This does not mean, of course, that everyone who gets cataract will become blind; quite the contrary is true. Modern surgery can remove the lens of the eye on which the cataract is spread, replacing it with a powerful lens in spectacles. The patient then can see so long as he has his glasses on. When the cataract is fully developed, light cannot pass through the opacity, so there is no way for an individual with a fully developed cataract to see, so long as the cataract remains on his lens.

Is the Operation for Cataract Painful and Risky?

No. It seems that the biggest hazard is the patient's frame of mind. He may have worked himself into such a state of dread and anxiety that it takes him a long time to recover his peace of mind after the operation. But the time in the hospital is, it seems, far pleasanter than for most operations. Generally a local anesthesia is given so that the discomforts of general anesthesia are avoided. The percentage of failures is apparently very low. If there are no other complications, there is every chance that the patient will be able to see quite well after the operation is over and the new lenses have been made.

We are not of course, enthusiastic about surgery. We believe that cataracts can be prevented by proper diet and care of the eyes. But, if one has *not* prevented the cataract and is in imminent danger of losing his sight, it does seem sensible to think calmly about an operation.

What Causes Cataract?

We do not know. Oh, of course, we do know of some circumstances that appear to be related to the formation of cataracts. Men who work in extremely high temperatures, exposed to the blasting heat of great furnaces, are especially susceptible to cataracts and it is assumed that these cataracts are occupational diseases. Dinitrophenol is a drug taken as a reducing aid. It increases the basal metabolism rate so that the patient can lose weight. Cataracts are quite common, we are told, among women past 40 who have taken this drug to reduce. And cataracts can be produced in animals by giving them this drug. (Isn't it amazing that women would take such a dangerous drug and risk blindness rather than reducing sensibly?)

We know, too, that smoke may have a lot to do with causing cataracts—cigarette smoke and smoke from fires. The Hunzas, for instance, a perfectly healthy nation otherwise, suffer from eye disorders because of the arrangement of their houses where there is not much room for the smoke from their fires to escape. When one considers the thick pall of tobacco smoke in which many of us pass our days (whether we smoke ourselves or just spend our time with those who do), it is not surprising that cataracts are so common, for the tobacco smoke is highly irritating to the eyes.

It has been suggested that long-exposure to bright sunlight may have something to do with producing cataracts, for people living in India are especially susceptible to them. And rural folks who work outside a lot seem to have more than those who work indoors. However, we must not forget that other things may be responsible as well. One researcher tells us that the average cataract patient in India is suffering from a number of different deficiency diseases. Perhaps the cataract is just one of these.

The tendency in old age is to harden, according to one authority. Cataract is another manifestation of this tendency, he says. The blood vessels harden, the muscles become stiff, the skin becomes horny, and the lens of the eye becomes opaque, says he. It's just another indication of old age and nothing can be done about it. This does not, of course, explain the many young people with cataracts, nor yet the babies who are born with cataracts.

We believe that the cause of cataracts is faulty nutrition. We were astonished to find that many, many scientists and physicians admit that cataract is a result of poor nutrition, but very few of them suggest correcting or preventing it by diet!

Before birth, blood is brought to the human lens by a blood vessel which withers away before the baby is born. So the lens, which is bathed in the fluid of the eye, has no way of getting nourishment except from that fluid. Hence it cannot rebuild itself as well as tissues in other parts of the body can, well nourished as they are with food brought by the blood. It gradually becomes brittle and inelastic. The center of the lens gets less nourishment than the edges, so generally the cataract starts in the center and spreads out gradually.

How Can I Tell Whether or not I have a Cataract?

You can't actually. Many cataracts are undetected by the individuals who have them until they begin to interfere with vision. If you notice any peculiarity of vision, it would be best to have your eye doctor check your eyes. Sometimes cataracts produce foggy vision which gradually becomes dimmer. Sometimes bright light is painful. There may seem to be bright-colored rings around lights at night. If you want to be reasonably sure you don't develop any of these symptoms, regardless of your age, we'd suggest

[36]

that you start now to improve your nutrition, which will automatically improve the nutrition of the lens of your eye which must certainly remove you farther and farther from the danger of cataract.

Why Are Cataracts Called This Peculiar Name?

Cataracts have been known for thousands of years. The ancient Greeks "had a word for it." They thought that a cataract was a flow of cloudy fluid in front of the lens. So they named it just that—a waterfall. We have kept the name, even though we know there is no actual flow of water involved.

12. Cataract and Good Nutrition

It is impossible to say categorically that this or that vitamin, mineral or food is "good for the eyes." The eyes like other parts of the body, must be nourished by all the various parts of food that make it nutritious. Vitamin A is extremely important for good eyesight. Deficiency in vitamin A can cause night blindness which means that you have difficulty in adjusting to light after darkness, or darkness after light. The B vitamins (especially riboflavin) are extremely important for healthy eyes. A kind of twilight blindness and a very definite fear of bright light result from not getting enough riboflavin. Vitamin C is important for good eyesight, as it is important for every other function of the body. Calcium is needed in the fluids of the eye. Protein is needed to replace eye tissues that have been broken down. And so it goes.

Are any of these important for the prevention of cataract? All of them are, for they are all necessary to good eye health. You cannot imagine a wonderfully healthy eye, strong, efficient, never giving any trouble, with a cataract beginning to cover the lens! Of course not! What is good for the rest of the eye is also good for the lens. And vice versa.

But we know that certain vitamins may have a somewhat greater importance than others in preventing cataract. For instance, vitamin C is concentrated in the lens of the healthy eyes. Why? We do not know. It is also concentrated in certain tissues in other parts of the body—the adrenal glands, for instance. We cannot help but believe that this concentration of the vitamin must mean that it is needed in that spot especially for some good purpose. Now when we find out that the lens that has a cataract contains very little or no vitamin C, this seems to indicate something very important. Is the lack of vitamin C responsible for the cataract or is the cataract responsible for the lack of vitamin C? If cataract were a contagious disease spread by germs, we would certainly think that the vitamin C had been used up fighting the germs. That's what vitamin C does, you know. But there is no germ involved.

[37]

How then can we explain this peculiar lack of vitamin C in the lens with cataract? One function of vitamin C is to keep repairing the cement between the cells. Could it be that lack of vitamin C has caused these cells to degenerate and form the cataract? It seems likely. And sure enough, we find that in laboratories, researchers have produced cataracts in laboratory animals and then slowed down their growth by giving vitamin C at the same time.

Rats fed large amounts of *dinitrophenol* (the reducing drug that produces cataract, you will remember) responded very rapidly when they were given vitamin C. Other rats developed cataract when they were fed enormous doses of galactose, a form of sugar. If the vitamin C was given along with the sugar, the appearance of the cataracts was delayed. We have this information from a book called *The Newer Knowledge of Nutrition* by McCollum, Orent-Keiles and Day. (Published by Macmillan Company, New York, New York.)

We also know that when scurvy (the disease of vitamin C deficiency) is produced in guinea pigs, there is a marked decrease in the vitamin C of the lens. And it is sometimes possible to produce cataracts in guinea pigs on what is called a scorbutic diet—that is, a diet containing little or no vitamin C. We rather suspect, however, that the reason this is difficult is because cataracts may result from deficiency in several different vitamins—not just vitamin C. And so the guinea pigs whose diet contains plenty of the other vitamins may not get cataract.

McCollum and his associates also tell us that they have a report from a Dr. Josephson indicating that he gave from 15 to 300 milligrams of vitamin C daily to patients with cataract with marked improvement. Within a week mature cataracts became transparent enough to allow some vision.

Riboflavin Important For Eye Health

Vitamin B_2—riboflavin—is extremely important for eye health. The eye is one of the most sensitive organs in the body to a deficiency in riboflavin. In fact, if you are suffering from any peculiar eye symptom, we'd suggest taking many times the minimum amount of riboflavin each day, no matter what medical treatment you are getting for your eyes. The riboflavin is bound to help. And it's very scarce in most of our diets, so there's a good chance that we may be short.

In one experiment rats kept on a diet containing no riboflavin got cataracts—almost 100 per cent of them! It occurred only in rats who were deprived of the vitamin at an early age, not those who got the deficient diet after they were mature. Could it be that the very widespread incidence of cataracts today is the direct result of lack of riboflavin in the diet of folks who were growng up 50, 60 or 70 years ago? In other experiments these clear-cut results have not been secured. It is believed that possibly these laboratory diets were not as deficient in riboflavin as the investigators thought. However, nutrition books in general relate deficiency in riboflavin with cataract.

Could it be possible that cataracts in newborn babies are caused by lack of riboflavin and vitamin C in the mother's diet? There seems to be no reason why not. The mineral calcium is also related to the formation of cataract. Cantarow in his book, *Calcium Metabolism and Calcium Therapy* (Lea and Febiger, 1931), says that a lack of calcium in the diet allows the cataract to form. He also says that calcium seems to be necessary for the body to use vitamin C correctly. Remember what we said about not just one but many, many elements being important for any body function?

Finally we have abundant evidence that a diet low in protein is likely to make one susceptible to cataract. Researchers have been able to produce cataracts in animals by feeding them diets in which one or another of the important amino acids (forms of protein) is lacking. The essential amino acids work together—one cannot function without all of them. Adding the missing amino acids to the diet delayed the appearance of the cataracts.

Treating Incipient Cataract with Diet

Now listen to what one practicing M.D. has to say about preventing and treating cataracts, for this gentleman has been doing wonderful work among cataract patients. Dr. Donald T. Atkinson of San Antonio, Texas, wrote in the February, 1952, issue of the *Eye, Ear, Nose and Throat Monthly* an article entitled "Malnutrition as an Etiological (causative) Factor in Senile Cataract."

He tells us first that there has been a lot of discussion about the possibility of cataract resulting from dehydration of the lens—that is, perhaps the water has been extracted from it. Cholera patients, it seems, go blind in the last stages of their illness because the lenses of their eyes dry out. A frog placed in salt water soon develops cataract because the salt extracts the water from the lens of the eye. Put the frog back into fresh water and the cataract disappears. Dr. Atkinson does not mention the danger of too much salt in the diet of human beings, but his story about the frog makes us wonder whether the vast amount of over-salting we do has anything to do with cataract.

Dr. Atkinson became intensely interested in the relationship of diet to cataract when he was treating the wife of a young physician for cataract. At about the same time, he says, there were numerous other cases of cataract among young people in that part of the country. He remarked to himself that all these young people seemed to be remarkably badly nourished, including the physician's wife.

All of them lived mainly on corn products and salt pork. Their principal beverage was coffee; they drank little water. Fresh foods were almost non-existent in their diets. As for bread, they ate refined wheat and corn bread raised with bicarbonate of soda—not yeast. The soda rapidly destroyed whatever vitamins might have remained in their bread. And the lack of yeast removed the one last source of B vitamins that might have remained to them.

So Dr. Atkinson began to suggest to his patients who were just beginning to get cataracts that they adopt diets rich in some of the vitamins, especially vitamin C—cabbage, oranges, carrots, tomatoes, rutabagas, turnips and so forth. Result? Several patients who really followed the diet found that their cataracts were getting no bigger; in some cases they improved.

The other food factor that Dr. Atkinson used in treating his cataract patients was chlorophyll. He reminds us that green plants are more nutritious than dried ones; that animals do better on green pasture than dried hay, as evidenced by their half-starved looks in early spring, and the rapidity with which they recover once they begin to eat green grass again. The chemical properties of chlorophyll, the green coloring matter of plants, are almost the same as the properties of hemoglobin, the red coloring matter in the blood. The chemical formula differs only in the fact that in the hemoglobin molecule, an atom of iron corresponds to the atom of magnesium in the chlorophyll.

"It is a very engrossing fact," says he, "as it now appears, in the retardation of cataract that the formula of chlorophyll and hemoglobin are so nearly alike. Willstatter found carotin, a type of chlorophyll in the body of fresh carrots, and he suspected that its administration had a wholesome effect on vision. So far as I know I was the first to prescribe a diet of green tops of garden vegetables to cataract patients and I still find that this diet has its advantages in incipient cataract cases."

Will Not Such a Diet Prevent Cataract?

This is the kind of diet Dr. Atkinson uses in cases of cataracts: a greatly increased intake of water—from 8 to 10 glasses a day in addition to the tea, coffee and whatever other beverages the patient is drinking. From a list of the green tops of 6 selected garden vegetables he has them add one as "greens" to the diet daily. We suppose they can choose which ever they like best. Then in addition he gives them chlorophyll tablets, large doses of vitamin C—we mean as much as 1000 milligrams a day. Then he gives them 200,000 units of vitamin A every day. Each patient is required to have a pint of milk and two eggs daily. (Look over this diet if you are worried about cataract and see whether *your* daily diet is this good.)

At the time he wrote this article, 1952, Dr. Atkinson had 450 patients with elementary cataract. Over a period of 11 years in a number of these the cataract had shown no progress. Formerly his patients went through the regular routine with cataract—letting it mature, then having an operation. Now, he tells us, only a limited number have had to have operations.

We think we know another reason for the success of Dr. Atkinson's diet, quite apart from the amount of chlorophyll in it. It contains plenty of vitamins A and C. The green things from the garden are rich in vitamins A and C as well as riboflavin—the B vitamin we found in our research to be important for the prevention of cataract. There is calcium, too, in those green leafy vegetables—lots of it. Then, too, when one is eating plenty of fresh vegetables and fruits, he just can't water his diet down with a lot of white bread and rich desserts. He just hasn't the room. And this is bound to be helpful, too.

We would add to Dr. Atkinson's diet for preventing cataract brewer's yeast, which is the richest possible source of riboflavin and all the other B vitamins. We would certainly add bone meal for additional calcium and other naturally occurring minerals. And we would add vitamin E, to preserve the health of blood vessels, thus assuring better nutrition for all the tissues of the body.

13. Tension Causes Eyestrain

By DR. J. M. WEBER (Optometrist)

Nervous tension may affect your eyes in many strange ways because anxiety and nervousness stimulate excessive eye muscle activity. This in turn gives rise to symptoms of eyestrain.

Take the case of Mrs. G., a storekeeper. She suffered with many signs of eye trouble. Blurred vision, headaches, and burning and itching sensations in her eyes and eyelids. However, a thorough eye examination showed conclusively that she did not need eyeglasses.

"I have this eye trouble mostly at the end of the day," she said. "Usually after figuring my daily business and going over the bills."

Further investigation revealed that she found bookkeeping a complicated and distasteful chore. She also was having difficulty in meeting her bills, which further agitated an already tense situation. After assigning her book work to someone else, and making more convenient arrangements with her suppliers, these symptoms disappeared. Eyestrain commonly is experienced by those who live in a state of nervous tension. This is because slight defects of the eyes, normally tolerated by calmer persons, become aggravated in nervous people.

If you are nervously inclined, and suffer the symptoms of eyestrain because of tension, you may be able to overcome these symptoms by simply relaxing. The first step is to plan a daily relaxation period. Seek quiet, comfortable surroundings, preferably at the same place and the same hour every day. Close your eyes lightly and allow your mind to relax completely. If your eyes sting or itch you can help them relax by applying hot compresses. A daily relaxation period will not only aid your eyes, but the rest of your body as well, because anxiety and tension adversely affect all body organs.

14. What Can Be Done for Crossed Eyes?

We call the condition crossed eyes, the medical books call it strabismus. Whatever the name it is given, the problem is a serious one to those afflicted, and to their families. Science has come up with 4 general courses of treatment which are of greater or lesser efficiency. They include glasses, a patch over the good eye, exercises for the eyes and surgery. There are other approaches to the problem but these are the most favored.

The physical cause of crossed eyes lies in the muscles surrounding the eye. These muscles are equally long and are balanced in equal strength when vision is normal, so that the eye is held in a more or less central position. When one wishes to look to the right or left, or up or down, the muscles contract on one side and expand on the other to complete the action. Of course, one who has normal vision is not aware of any effort put forth to accomplish this movement. The adjustment is made almost subconsciously.

How the Eye Muscles Pull

In cross-eyed individuals, the muscles are not of equal length or strength. For example, when the eye tends to "look" inward, toward the nose, it means that the muscle on the nose side of the eye is shorter and stronger than the muscle on the outer side of the eye. The inner muscle is exerting a force on the eye which the outer muscle cannot match, hence the eye is always looking toward the nose. It is as though the two muscles were engaged in a perpetual tug of war, with the outer muscle always losing.

According to a book by Dr. G. B. J. Keiner, which was reviewed in the *British Medical Journal* (September 6, 1952), all children are potential cases of strabismus at birth. This is due, says Keiner, to the fact that the myelination, or protective covering for the visual paths (optic nerves and muscles) is not yet complete at birth. Usually, by the age of 6 months, the process is completed. If it is still far from complete, the child is blind; if it is slightly delayed, strabismus and squinting are likely to follow. If the nerves are exposed due to a lack of myelin, the body loses its complete control over them, and, in turn, control over the muscles which regulate the eyes' position.

It is obvious that, in Dr. Keiner's view, the prenatal diet of the expectant mother is important in the proper development of what he calls the "ocular paths." It is at this time that the foundation for good eyes is formed. As Keiner says, "The development of the complex reflexes on which orientation of the eyes and binocular vision depend is possible only if the structural framework for adequate functioning is available to the central nervous system." In other words, without the raw materials provided by good nutri-

tion in the prenatal period, a properly finished product, good eyes, can hardly
be expected.

What the Patient Sees

When the eyes are crossed, the victim usually sees two objects rather
than one, because the eyes view the same objects from two widely different
angles. He squints and tilts his head, unconsciously trying to combine the
two images, or to ignore one of them. Of course, neither attempt fully
succeeds. Eventually he may give up the effort of trying to see with both
eyes. He begins, again subconsciously, to look at things with only one eye.
He is rewarded in this by seeing only one image. He becomes so accustomed to using only one eye that the other eye soon becomes incapable of
seeing anything. It is functionally blind.

It is with this danger in mind that eye specialists warn parents not to
ignore young children's crossed eyes in the mistaken hope that the child
will outgrow the disability. Chances are very slim that this will occur.
On the contrary it is much more likely that the condition will worsen to a
point at which it cannot be corrected. The earlier correction of crossed
eyes is attempted, the more chance for success. One expert says that if a
child is old enough to squint—an indication that he is attempting to
reconcile the double image he sees—he is old enough for corrective
measures to be begun.

The therapy used by a doctor who is consulted in a case of crossed
eyes is aimed at one thing; that is, to equalize the pull of the eye muscles
so that the eye in repose is directed straight ahead. The method employed
to accomplish this depends upon the severity of the condition. In some
cases glasses will be enough to force the crossed eye into better focus merely
by using lenses ground in such a way that only a small effort will move the
eye enough to improve the visual picture. Then, as the eye muscles grow
stronger, they begin to take on more of the work and the lenses can be
made weaker and weaker until they are no longer necessary. Complete
success with this method is not too frequent, and one would assume that
crossed eyes treated early, while the condition is new and muscles are
pliable, would be most likely to respond to glasses alone.

Eye Patch and Surgery

Another device used in correcting crossed eyes is an eye patch. One
eye is covered forcing the weaker one to do all of the sight work. The
confusion of the double image is resolved, and it is expected that with
increased work the vision of the weaker eye will be improved.

When an operation is indicated, the surgeon attempts to lengthen or
shorten the eye muscles, and thereby equalize the tension on both sides of
the eye, bringing it into straight focus. Sometimes several operations might
be required to achieve the proper alignment of the eyes.

An auxiliary to the above treatments is eye exercises. To strengthen
the eye muscles, prescribed sets of exercises are used, much as one would

[43]

do setting up exercises to tone up other parts of the body. And, as is the case with setting up exercises, the repeated use of the muscles, and the gradual strengthening and stretching of them, makes the performance of feats which were once considered impossible, quite easy. These exercises for the eye consist of such things as bringing small objects close to the eye, then far away, with the weak eye trying to follow the movement; or one closes the eyes, then opens them, trying to view a far away object at once and thereby forcing the eye into a difficult focussing process. The exercise is, of course, geared to the disability. There is an entire system of such exercises, called the Bates System, in which a series of basic exercises for eye strengthening is prescribed and then more specific ones are worked out for individual types of eye disability. This type of therapy has been successful in itself and as an auxiliary to the other treatments for crossed eyes. Its effectiveness depends to a great extent upon the ability of the patient to practice with regularity over a long period of time.

21 Per Cent Psychologically Originated

One of the most arresting theories of what can cause crossed eyes, was advanced by Dr. Ernest Rappaport in the *Eye, Ear, Nose and Throat Monthly* (June, 1959). He believes that there is a psychological cause behind many cases of crossed eyes. He reminds us that several of our expressions of anger, frustration and irritation tied in with the crossed eyes. When one is angry one is "cross," gets so angry that one is cross-eyed, etc. Dr. Rappaport believes then that the mind and emotions could be responsible for a case of crossed eyes in a susceptible individual. He tells a case history of a young lady who underwent surgery for crossed eyes. The operation appeared to be successful, but the condition worsened once more and another operation was indicated. Two days before the scheduled operation, the patient visited the doctor and told him that she no longer needed the operation. An examination proved this to be the fact. Somehow the eyes that had been disastrously crossed a week before, were better than they had been before. The woman told the doctor that her superior at work, with whom she frequently had violent disagreements, had been transferred to another department just two days before. She remembered that her sight had improved almost the moment she knew about the exchange.

Another example of this is described by Dr. Rappaport. It concerns a teenage boy whose family history was so emotionally and psychologically unhealthy, that the result of this environmental turmoil was, for him, crossed eyes. The complications are quite Freudian and confusing to the layman, but Dr. Rappaport shows quite conclusively that nothing else could have caused this case of crossed eyes. Dr. Rappaport quotes another expert, Pugh, as saying that an analysis of 500 crossed-eye-squint patients showed that 21 per cent were due to psychological causes.

As with most physical disabilities, the prevention of crossed eyes is always easier and more reliable than the cure. Prevention in this case must

[44]

mean prenatal care. The normally developed baby is born with eye muscles of the proper strength, and once he learns to focus them they do their job completely and competently. If he is not born with this equipment, whose fault is it? The mother's, of course. Has she been eating sufficient protein, vitamin-rich foods to insure strong muscle tissue and nerves for control?

Once crossed eyes have occurred in an individual, protein, for building the muscles needed to pull the eyes into proper alignment, seems to be the only specific nutritional prescription possible. As always, all nutrients are necessary for good vision, and eyes that have a good protein supply, but no vitamin A, are not likely to do the good job nature intended them to do. So insure your baby against eye trouble, if you are an expectant mother, by eating carefully of a diet high in protein especially, as well as other nutrients. If you wish to help your child to respond to treatment for crossed eyes, be sure his diet is rich in protein so that he is equipped with healthy muscles that can be made strong enough to hold the eyes in their proper position.

15. Blindness and Glaucoma

Glaucoma is the single greatest cause of blindness in the United States. About 13 per cent of all blind persons lost their sight as a result of this disease. And it has been estimated that in the age group from 35 to 44 the incidence of glaucoma is 1.5 per cent among Americans generally, while in the age group over 65 the incidence is about 3.7 per cent. Many of these cases are unsuspected and undiagnosed.

Possibly the most frightening thing about glaucoma is the fact that it can cause complete blindness within a matter of days after the first noticeable symptoms appear. However, if the disease is discovered and treated in time, even acute cases which require immediate attention can be saved from blindness, so the situation is not as frightening as it might at first seem. Of course, our concern is in preventing glaucoma.

What Is Glaucoma and What Causes It?

We quote from a two-page leaflet published by the Eye Foundation of Santa Barbara, California. "Glaucoma means increased pressure inside the eye and may lead to serious loss of vision without the individual ever suspecting anything is wrong. The eye has its own built-in mechanism which secretes a watery fluid called 'aqueous'; this 'aqueous' is important to the nourishment of the eyes. Just as there is a secretion mechanism within the eye, so also is there a drainage channel to allow a steady flow of the 'aqueous' out of the eye. If this drainage channel is inadequate or gets plugged up for some reason, the fluid collecting within the eye can't get out readily enough, and the pressure inside the eye gets higher and higher. It is as if a rubber balloon is being filled with more and more air and the walls of the balloon are subjected to greater and greater pressure. So with the eye when the fluid pressure inside the eye becomes greater (see figure 7). There is more strain on the wall of the eyeball. Especially vulnerable is the optic nerve which is located on the back wall of the eyeball. Increased pressure on the optic nerve causes damage to the

FIGURE 7: THIS IS WHAT IS HAPPENING TO YOUR EYES

EYE   AUTOMOBILE TIRE

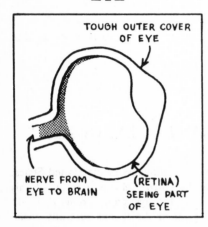
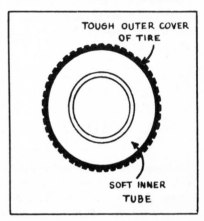
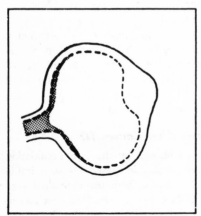
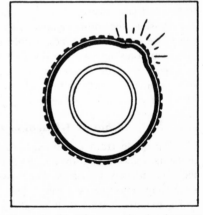

The eyes have become harder than they should. They are harder because there is too much pressure inside them, just as an automobile tire can get too hard from too much pressure. Too much inside pressure harms the eyes by squeezing the seeing parts which can be damaged.

FIGURE 8:

THIS MAY HAPPEN TO YOUR SIGHT—IF NEGLECTED

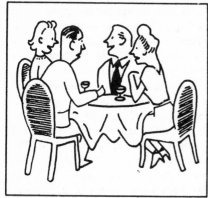 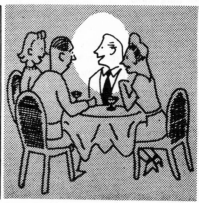

Even in early Glaucoma you can look straight ahead and still see objects out to each side. While looking at the person's face across the table this man can see all the dishes on the table and also the people sitting around it.

Neglected Glaucoma has squeezed this man's sight so that when he looks at the man's face, he cannot see the other people at the table, nor foods passed him until they are placed or passed directly in front of him.

optic nerve fibres; as a result of this damage, the person's vision slowly decreases. The loss of vision may be so gradual that the person himself isn't conscious of it until a great deal of damage has occurred."

Symptoms of Glaucoma

Sometimes there are warning symptoms of early glaucoma. These include:

1. Pains in the eyes, often especially in the early morning.

2. Attacks of blurred vision which may or may not be accompanied by redness of the eyes, pains, rainbow halos around lights at night, headaches, vertigo or nausea.

3. Inability to adjust to darkened rooms, such as theaters, TV showings and so forth.

4. Loss of peripheral vision—that is, vision at the sides—the range of vision has become so narrowed that one can see only the object at which he is directly looking (see figure 8).

5. Difficulty with vision which makes one try frequent changes of glasses, none of which is satisfactory.

Can Be Controlled If Treated Promptly

An editorial in the *New York State Journal of Medicine* for January 15, 1956, tells us that "Chronic simple glaucoma in its early stages can usually be controlled without serious loss of vision. It is a progressive disease, and the later the discovery, the less likelihood for maintaining useful vision. The bitter thing about the disease is the usual absence of warning signs until the condition has progressed to the point where vision is affected. Usually the only early sign is increase in intraocular pressure or tension (that is, pressure within the eyeball). This sign, in turn, is often intermittent in character. When intermittent, it is more likely to be present at periods of stress or emotional anxiety. The patient would be unlikely to call upon an ophthalmologist during the early stages of the disease."

Here, then, is one disorder where early detection is the most important thing. An ophthalmologist can easily test the pressure of the eyeball with a mechanism called the tonometer. In some parts of the country, detection clinics have been established to aid individuals in discovering what the actual state of their eye health is, where glaucoma is concerned. We quoted above from a pamphlet put out at the Glaucoma Detection Clinic of Santa Barbara, California, which is sponsored by the ophthalmologists of that city, to warn of the dangers of unsuspected glaucoma and to discover any unsuspected cases which need treatment.

In California "Glaucoma days" have been organized of which advance notices are read from pulpits, and announced over radio and TV. In 11 such drives, 12 per cent of those tested by general practitioners were referred to ophthalmologists for further tests and, of these, 3.7 per cent were found to have glaucoma.

Is Glaucoma Related to Stress?

An article in the *British Journal of Ophthalmology,* Vol. 1, p. 42, 1958, also relates the incidence of glaucoma to stress. E. Gordon Mackie writes that doctors in glaucoma clinics have reported that there is a high ratio of "stress" among their patients. The apparently quiet, efficient person with glaucoma is often an over-conscientious, over-working perfectionist. He should be encouraged to abandon his over-zealous tendencies, says Dr. Mackie, shed responsibility but continue to exploit the acquired skills which give him pleasure. Interestingly enough, he mentions that tight collars should be avoided when tests for glaucoma are being given. (Is it possible that tight collars, or tight girdles or even such a thing as tight garters or shoes might have something to do with causing the eyeball pressure in glaucoma?)

He also mentions that movies and TV, especially if subjects highly charged with emotion are shown, can precipitate attacks. Beer, tobacco and caffeine should be avoided, he says. In cases of senility a high vitamin intake should be prescribed, he goes on, with special emphasis on vitamin A.

There is also the possible connection between coffee-drinking and glaucoma. Dr. Rolf Ulrich in a book, *Coffee and Caffeine,* reports that a book entitled *The Nature and Treatment of Glaucoma* by Schieck states:

[48]

"There is no narcotic stimulant so injurious to a glaucomatous eye as caffeine-containing coffee, as caffeine combines paralysis of the vaso-constrictors with a rise in blood pressure, so that the blood flow to the eye is increased." In glaucoma it is the inner pressure on the optic nerve that causes the problem. It is only logical, then, that increased blood pressure, generated by caffeine, should aggravate the condition.

If the eye doctor finds that you have glaucoma in either the acute or chronic state, he cannot "cure" it in the sense that after a few treatments your eyes will be normal again. You must have treatments for the rest of your life, just as diabetics must. Eye drops, which are drugs, of course, can reduce the pressure inside the eyeball. But one must resort to this treatment always.

It is possible in some cases to have an operation in which the back of the iris of the eye is "nicked" to make an escape valve for the collected fluid. Sometimes such an operation relieves the pressure for good and in other cases, further operations are necessary.

We do not counsel our readers to have operations or to take drugs except in matters of life or death. However, faced with a choice of total blindness or using eyedrops which will prevent the blindness, even the most health-conscious person will not choose to go blind. He will, we hope, while he is controlling his eye pressure with eyedrops, make every effort to improve his health to such an extent that whatever caused the glaucoma in the first place will be corrected. Incidentally, no one has ever discovered the cause of glaucoma. However, there seems to be no doubt that the individual whose body is perfectly coordinated and attuned does not get such a disease.

Stress Causing Glaucoma Possibly Related to Diet?

We quoted above a statement from the *New York State Journal of Medicine,* showing that stress and emotional anxiety seem to have some-thing to do with bringing on attacks of glaucoma. We want to go into this in a little more detail. In an article by J. E. Martin, "Fear and Glaucoma," in the *Practitioner* for April, 1958, Dr. Martin tells us that "following the German occupation of the Channel Islands I was impressed by the dis-proportionately large number of cases of simple glaucoma which I was asked to see, some of them in a much younger age group than usual. In addition, many of them had progressed to a late stage of the disease before being first seen. After one or two attendances, and having gained their con-fidence, these patients volunteered a history of protracted distressing anxie-ties which seemed to be much more vivid and terrifying than those of pa-tients with other eye conditions which were being seen at the same time."

There were many things to be afraid of in that locality at that time. Dr. Martin says he did not have opportunity to make careful studies which would prove his case, but he says he feels that his observations show certain-ly some relationship between long-continued fear and the onset of glaucoma. He quotes Duke-Elder's book, *Parsons' Diseases of the Eye,* as saying that glaucoma is seen particularly in those who are "highly strung, anxious in disposition and sympathicotonic in type." That word "sympathicotonic" refers to a person's physical reaction to stressful situations— with things like goose flesh, increased blood pressure and so forth. Excessive fear, stress and anxiety may result from errors in diet. We know, for instance, that just not getting enough of several of the B vitamins for a few weeks will make cringing cowards out of brave men, and that the fatigue and nervousness that accompany shortages of the B vitamins can bring on feelings of inadequacy, anxiety and strain.

Glaucoma And Diet

The suggestion that emotional strain may play some part in glaucoma stimulated us to searching for information relating the disorder to diet and we found something which we feel is most significant.

The *Sight Saving Review* for spring, 1955, published a careful study of the diet of 62 glaucoma patients. This suggests, in itself, that deficiencies in diet have been seriously considered by researchers. Ethel Maslansky, nutritionist, of the New York City Department of Health, was responsible for the survey.

She tells us that the age and occupational categories of the patients studied indicate that their need for high calorie foods was not great. They were mostly older people who were not working, hence were sedentary. Ninety-four per cent of the men and almost 96 per cent of the women were 40 or over, about half of all the people interviewed were 60 or over.

The people interviewed were asked to list all the foods they had eaten the day before they visited the glaucoma clinic at the Presbyterian Hospital. From each patient two to 20 sample menus were collected from which the final estimates of daily diet were made.

The food elements for which recommended daily allowances have been established, were then figured. Here is the comparison of the amount of these elements in the diets of glaucoma patients compared to the recommended daily allowances:

TABLE 1: DIETARY CHART OF GLAUCOMA PATIENTS

	Women Patients		Recommended Allowances		Men Patients		Recommended Allowances	
Protein	65.9	grams	55	grams	64.1	grams	65	grams
Calcium	.51	grams	.80	grams	.59	grams	.80	grams
Iron	9.9	mg.	12	mg.	9.3	mg.	12	mg.
Vitamin A	6528	I.U.	5000	I.U.	5102	I.U.	5000	I.U.
Thiamin	.78	mg.	1.40	mg.	.86	mg.	1	mg.
Riboflavin	1.26	mg.	1	mg.	1.39	mg.	1.60	mg.
Niacin	12.5	mg.	10	mg.	11.2	mg.	10	mg.
Vitamin C	83	mg.	70	mg.	66	mg.	75	mg.

The nutritionist who wrote this article says as follows about this chart: Protein, vitamin A, niacin are provided in ample amounts to satisfy the daily recommended allowance. Calcium, iron, thiamin and riboflavin are lower than they should be. The men patients were not getting enough vitamin C.

The trend in food consumption on the part of glaucoma patients suggests better than average practices as known to the nutrition clinics in several ways, says Miss Maslansky. "Green leafy vegetables and yellow vegetables were eaten several times a week and at least one source of vitamin C was used every day—usually citrus or citrus juice. The frequency with which carrots appear in these dietaries, particularly in the female group, would suggest a magical association of carrots with good eyesight in the minds of some of the glaucoma patients."

Of course, there's nothing wrong with believing in magic where food is concerned, provided that the magic has a sound basis in scientific fact. In this case carrots may be providing ample vitamin A and they may not. It is well known that carotene, the substance found in carrots and other yellow and green foods, is transferred into vitamin A inside the body— in the liver, to be exact. Those patients who had disordered or inefficient livers (and such conditions are extremely common beyond middle age) may have benefited not a whit from all the carrots they were eating—so far as vitamin A is concerned.

A reliable source of vitamin A itself—not just carotene—would certanly be a better assurance of ample vitamin A in the diet. Fish liver oil is just such a source. And vitamin A is vitally important for the health of eye tissues.

Interestingly enough, the "recommended daily allowances" with which the glaucoma patients' diets were compared have been established by the National Research Council who say, "the allowance levels are considered to cover individual variations *among normal persons as they live in the United States subjected to ordinary environmental stress common thereto.*"

Meaning of Ordinary Stress

What is "ordinary environmental stress"? We would certainly consider such a disease as glaucoma more than "ordinary stress"—wouldn't you? Wouldn't it be obvious, too, that something in the environment—some kind of stress in the general sense—must have brought about this eye disorder? Wouldn't you say, too, that just getting old is a form of stress? Experts on the subject tell us that it is. So in many ways the glaucoma patients studied are not typical Americans living under "ordinary stresses."

We know—and certainly nutritionists should know—that any and every stress laid upon an individual demands more in the way of nutrition if that individual is to survive. Even such mild stresses as heat and cold, fatigue and anger, anxiety and pain make greater demands on the person who is experiencing them—nutrition-wise. This has been shown many times

[51]

in laboratory experiments. So it seems to us that the suggested daily recommendations are completely inadequate when one is dealing with sick people or old people.

But even if these were young, perfectly healthy people whose diets were being studied, look at the important points at which the diets are inadequate—calcium, iron, thiamin, riboflavin and vitamin C. Calcium is important for every cell of the body every moment of the day. Iron is absolutely essential if the blood is going to do its job of supplying nutriments to tissues. Thiamin and riboflavin are two B vitamins of utmost importance to nerve tissues. Deficiency in these leads one to conclude that other important members of the vitamin B complex—not studied in the survey—are also present in insufficient quantity. This would include choline and inositol, both essential if the body is going to use fat properly, para-amino-benzoic acid, pyridoxine, vitamin B_{12} and all the rest of the B vitamins which are apparently deficient in these patients' menus, since they occur, generally speaking, in the same foods in which the listed B vitamins occur.

Nutritionists agree that vitamin C protects one against many different stresses and poisons in his environment. It is used or oxidized in the process. Therefore, sick people need more of it than well people. Yet the women in this survey were getting only 13 milligrams more than the recommended amount and the men 9 milligrams less than the recommended amount. The author uses official estimates of the amount of vitamin C in the vitamin C-rich foods the patients say they ate. We do not know, however, whether the orange juice which supposedly contained the daily ration of vitamin C had been standing in the refrigerator for several days, in which case it would have lost most of its vitamin content. We do not know whether other fruits counted on for vitamin C content may also have been exposed to the air so long that their vitamin C content was practically nil. With such a narrow margin to get by on, doesn't it seem possible that the actual level of vitamin C in the blood of all these patients may have been far below normal?

Be Sure Diet Is Nutritionally Balanced

The author of the *Sight Saving Review* article says, in conclusion, "On an individual basis it is safe to say that only a few dietaries reflected adequate intake in all the nutritional components . . . Other groups of approximately the same age, and socio-economic status seem to share similar dietary deficiencies, the most prevalent being calcium. In this limited study no gross deficiency could, therefore, be correlated with glaucoma." And later . . . "The economic factor plays a large part in this age group, the stress and strain of the process of aging may indicate greater needs for some of the nutrients."

We say "amen" to that. Furthermore, we say to readers, especially those over middle age—are you sure that you are getting enough of all the important vitamins and minerals—but especially those which this survey proved to be in short supply—calcium, iron, the B vitamins and vitamin C? Foods rich in these elements are fresh raw fruits and vegetables, unrefined seed products like sunflower and pumpkin seeds, nuts, liver, eggs, wheat germ and of course food supplements like bone meal (for calcium and other minerals), brewer's yeast and/or desiccated liver for B vitamins and iron and rose hip preparations or some other source of natural vitamin C with the bioflavonoids that go along with it.

Other Theories on Glaucoma

We found several other interesting theories on glaucoma in medical literature. There was an article from a French journal, *Bulletin des Sociétiés d'Ophthalmologie,* for October, 1954, by M. J. P. Levy, on the subject of sleep therapy for glaucoma patients. Dr. Levy believes that glaucoma is at least partly a psychosomatic disease. He says that we have known for many years that emotion plays a big part in causing this ailment. We have pointed out that people who get glaucoma seem to be, in general, people who are anxious, over-conscientious, "high-strung," etc. One may, of course, conclude, as Dr. Levy does, that patients of this emotional make-up tend to bring the disease on themselves. Of course, one could also assume, as we do, that the same unhealthful practices that produce this kind of personality also produce the glaucoma.

However, Dr. Levy treats patients with long, long hours of sleep, carefully induced by sedatives, over a period of two weeks. Actually, the patient sleeps from 16 to 20 hours daily, waking only a few hours a day for meals and personal hygiene. The sleeping pills are tapered off at the end of the treatment.

Reporting his observations on 5 patients, Dr. Levy tells us that, in general, results were good. He says that sight was improved, the size of the visual field was increased and some of the other symptoms were improved. None of the patients, incidentally, was a long-time sufferer. Dr. Levy points out that this kind of treatment can be used only for patients who have early symptoms of the disease.

Certainly, no one could treat himself with this kind of therapy. And we do not approve of taking sleeping pills for any reason. We have never heard of this method being used at all by American doctors. It is much more the kind of thing European doctors like to try. However, the experiment does suggest one important item. Rest and relaxation are essential for the prevention of glaucoma. Certainly if 15 days of practically nothing but sleep will bring about improvement in glaucoma cases, then regular relaxation should play some part in preventing this condition. This means not just plenty of sleep, but interesting hobbies, satisfying vacations and, perhaps most of all, a calmer, more casual attitude toward one's everyday work and responsibilities.

[53]

Is Climate Important for the Glaucoma Patient?

Another French writer discusses climate in relation to glaucoma treatment. Dr. M. M. Collier and his associates state in *Bulletin des Sociétés d'Ophthalmologie* (January, 1956) that acute glaucoma attacks are more frequent in winter and during the passage of a weather "front"—that is, when the weather is changing and we have wind, storms and so forth. Citing only the case of one patient whose malady improved when she went to a resort, they don't make much of an argument for their theory. However, they do point out that, for the glaucoma patient who has the means to travel and can select where he wants to live, it would seem wise to live in some section of the country where violent changes of the weather are not the usual thing—and this, of course, suggests the south rather than the north.

Is Glaucoma a Deficiency Disease?

Finally, an American ophthalmologist, M. J. Schoenberg, believes that glaucoma may be a deficiency disease—in the same sense that scurvy is a disease of deficiency in vitamin C, beriberi results from a vitamin B deficiency and so forth.

In an article in the *American Journal of Ophthalmology* for December, 1943, Dr. Schoenberg describes the various kinds of glaucoma patients. He says there is, first, the pre-middle-age group in which the disease is frequently a familial one; the middle-age group, between 44 and 55 years, when the aging processes throughout the entire organism play a leading role. Then there is the group between 50 and 70 in which nutritional disturbances and the consequences of long-standing infections may add what he calls "an additional burden" to the glaucoma problem. Finally, old age, which, he says, may begin as early as 45 or as late as 80 years, brings degenerative changes of the lenses, the circulatory system and the optic nerves. He also tells us that the placid, calm, inert individual in whose life fear and worry play a minor role is much less of a problem than the alert, emotional, over-anxious one. (Everyone seems to agree that emotions and personality play a big part in glaucoma!)

Dr. Schoenberg then proceeds to describe how an impulse is transmitted from nerve terminals to muscle cells, to activate the muscle cell and cause something to happen. It seems that a chemical substance is secreted which converts the nerve impulse into motion.

There are evidences, he says, that lead us to believe that in glaucoma there exists a disturbance of this whole process. To compare this situation with the situation in scurvy—the teeth become loose and the gums bleed in scurvy because the cement that holds cells together is inadequate for its job. The reason is that vitamin C must be present for this cement to be manufactured. In some such way, the substance necessary to complete the chemical mechanism of nerve impulses to muscle is not present in glaucoma, Dr. Schoenberg believes.

He goes on to say that the drugs given to glaucoma patients for dropping into their eyes approximate this chemical substance, in that they seem to bring about a temporary restitution of the function of that part of the eye. They must be dropped into the eye at regular intervals, the dosage must be exactly right and one must expect the hypertension of the eye to return shortly after medication is stopped.

So it seems, Dr. Schoenberg believes, that there is a similarity here to conditions like goiter, diabetes, night blindness, pellagra, scurvy. For goiter can be controlled with thyroid extract, which is not present in sufficient quantity in certain kinds of goiter. In diabetes, there is not enough insulin, which is a body secretion. If insulin is supplied regularly at the proper time, diabetes can be controlled. Night blindness results from vitamin A deficiency. It can be completely cured by taking vitamin A and it will return if one becomes deficient in the vitamin again. Pellagra and scurvy are diseases of vitamin B and vitamin C lack, respectively.

Dr. Schoenberg states that the situation in glaucoma is much the same. He does not hazard a guess as to what the missing substance may be in glaucoma. Is it a vitamin that one can get in food or is it a hormone like insulin, produced by the body?

In any case, deficiency diseases are best prevented by diet rich in all good food elements, for the very term "deficiency" implies that something is missing in diet. Dr. Schoenberg's conclusions are that in glaucoma patients the doctor should think first of eliminating all disturbances due to ill health, then he should advise patients repeatedly about ways of maintaining good health. He should pay utmost attention to *minutest details* and he should always *consider the possibility that glaucoma is a deficiency disease.*

Summary of Our Findings

To summarize all the information we have presented, then, it is important to:

1. Check often for symptoms of glaucoma, especially after one has reached middle age. Get speedy help from an ophthalmologist if he finds you have glaucoma.

2. Eat the best possible diet and take diet supplements. Once again, this is especially important after middle age, as Dr. Schoenberg points out. Vitamins A, B and C are especially important for eye health. The B vitamins will contribute to the well-being of nerves so that a "high-strung" person, inordinately susceptible to glaucoma, need no longer be "high-strung." Vacations, rest, relaxation, enjoyment of leisure time and a confident attitude toward one's responsibilities are essential here.

3. Seek, if possible, a temperate climate, with weather that is warm and uniformly serene.

4. Heed the lesson of the survey which indicated that diets of glaucoma patients may be low in calcium, iron, thiamin, riboflavin and vitamin

[55]

C. Food supplements like fish liver oil, bone meal, brewer's yeast and/or desiccated liver and natural vitamin C from rose hips or green peppers will provide these vitamins and minerals every day. And a good diet, high in protein and fresh foods and vegetables is essential.

All sketches used by courtesy of The National Society for the Prevention of Blindness.

16. Myopia

Myopia is nearsightedness, a condition in which the individual can see clearly things right beneath his nose, but cannot see things farther away— across the street, for instance. The myopic eye is like a camera permanently focused for a close-up.

Myopia generally becomes apparent when one is a child or perhaps in the teens. It is caused by an abnormal enlargement of the eye in the diameter from front to rear. This greater length of the diameter of the eye causes the image of what is being seen to be focused in front of the retina rather than on it. As the child grows older, this enlargement process gradually ceases.

Many things are blamed for myopia—posture, light used for reading, heredity, diseases and diet deficiencies. According to an article in *Coronet* for September, 1959, more and more children are found to be nearsighted. In 1925 only about 20 per cent of high school and college students wearing glasses were nearsighted. Today more than 30 per cent have been diagnosed as myopic.

The article quotes Sir John H. Parsons, an English ophthalmologist, as believing that in days to come myopic sight will be considered "normal." Our eyes are adapting to modern conditions, he says. Whereas our forefathers had to scan horizons, look out over wide fields, seas and rivers, we must spend our lives in narrow rooms, peering at something on our desks in the way of reading material—lists, charts, books, blueprints, reports or something of the sort. This must be why there is so much more myopia among our young people than there used to be, in the opinion of several experts.

It seems to us that this is a very shallow argument indeed. For it suggests that the body is able to re-adapt the focusing of its eyes within about 50 years, whereas for thousands and thousands of years before this, the eye has been adapted for far-seeing. It does not seem possible to us that such a big change could possibly take place within so short a time. Our bodies are not equipped to make this kind of change in adapting to our environment within a space of time so short. Changes like this take many generations.

Aside from this is the fact that there are still millions of people who must use their eyes largely for seeing at great distances. Have they or their children also begun to experience more myopia? We are not told and we doubt that anyone has done an investigation of this.

Our Food Lacks Valuable Vitamins

It seems to us, rather, that exactly the same things in our environment are responsible for increased myopia as those which are causing our children's jaws to be too small for their teeth, causing degenerative diseases like cancer to take a terrible toll among young people and causing almost 50 per cent of our young men to be rejected for military service for physical and psychological reasons—namely, our processed and devitalized modern diets.

We were delighted to find in a French medical journal, *Presse Médicale*, for April 25, 1959, an article by two Paris physicians who have been giving vitamin E to their myopic young patients with remarkable success. Drs. C. and G. Desusclade tell us that they have been giving vitamin E for the past 10 years and that they can generally stop the process of the disease, or maladjustment so that the young patient does not become any more nearsighted. Checking on their early patients after 8 years, they found that the effects are lasting.

Not satisfied with mere success, they then decided to find out why vitamin E produces these results. For this, it would seem to be necessary to understand how and why myopia occurs. They had long known, they tell us, that vitamin E can be used to treat diseases of the connective tissue— the collagen diseases. Could this be what was involved in their treatment of myopia? They believed, they tell us, that the collagen fibers of the eye may lose part of their physical qualities and become abnormally distended so that they cannot give the support they should. In other words, the ligaments become lax.

In 1956 another researcher, Garzino, using an electron microscope, discovered that the fibers of collagen (that is, the connective tissues) in the eye of a myopic individual have a smaller diameter than those of the normal eye and that they are bathed in a more abundant liquid than is present in the normal eye. The two Paris doctors think this is ample proof of their theory that vitamin E helps in cases of myopia because myopia is a disease of the connective tissue. Their conclusion is that myopia is something which has a definitely mechanical *and nutritional* base.

They tell us that myopia is due to the feebleness of the conjunctive "shell" of the eye. This feebleness may have been acquired in some cases before birth, during growth inside the womb, but usually it is acquired during childhood and adolescence.

"What is the cause? Lack of vitamin E or perhaps an exaggerated need for this vitamin or a lack of ability to assimilate the vitamin properly," they declare. They continue, "Proof of the vitamin E treatment lets us verify not only the complete stoppage of the development of a case of myopia, but also the improvement of those little, more general symptoms that are so often associated with it—little disorders of the joints, slight glandular upsets, retarded development of puberty."

How Much Vitamin E Will Prevent Myopia?

The treatment they give their young patients is as follows: one or two 50 milligram tablets of vitamin E (alpha tocopherol acetate) first thing in the morning every day for 3 months. After this 3-month treatment, a lapse of several weeks is allowed and then another 3-month series is given. According to Drs. Desusclade, this stabilizes the improvement. It is well to repeat the treatment every year, they believe, while the child is growing up.

Our authors warn against the installation of atropine in the eyes, and the use of eye exercises. They say that while some good results are obtained through exercise, they believe that they are dangerous. Exercises done before treatment with vitamin E may pull on the delicate tissues of the eye, since they are unused to this kind of exercise. After the treatment, however, Drs. Desusclade believe that eye exercises are helpful, for they permit the now strengthened muscles to help in shortening the too-long diameter of the eyeball which has been causing the trouble.

In stressing how important it is to discover myopia and begin treatment with vitamin E at once, the authors remind us that certain kinds of myopia may lead, in later life, to detached retina which can be a cause of blindness. Myopia is not, then, just a slight disarrangement which can easily be corrected by glasses, but, in one form at least, is something which may turn out to be quite serious in terms of health.

The researchers tell us that they usually had better results in their vitamin E treatment if they gave other vitamins and also amino acids at the same time. Amino acids are forms of protein.

High Protein Diet Prevents Myopia

This information does not surprise us. A British researcher, Dr. P. A. Gardiner in *Food Field Reporter* for April 27, 1959, reported finding that myopic children who are given increased amounts of animal protein in their diet have decreased rates of deterioration in eyesight compared to children who do not receive the increased protein.

Dr. Gardiner used two groups of children for his research. All were nearsighted. In one, the control group, no effort was made to change the usual diet the children had been eating all their lives. The second group of children were given increased amounts of animal protein—we suppose, meat, eggs, fish and other protein foods.

Results were startling. In the 5-7 age-group, the untreated children's visual deterioration was 4 times greater than that of the children getting the high protein diet. In the 8-9 year group, the deterioration in the untreated group was 3 times greater. In children over 12, actual improvement in nearsightedness occurred in those cases taking the largest quantities of animal protein. We are told that the Nutrition Foundation is planning further investigation into this finding.

What does such a report mean to you, as you are planning your family's meals? It may mean that the child who goes off to school without breakfast may develop myopia and the child who eats a good breakfast may not. The difference between a breakfast of eggs and one of cereal may be important in preventing myopia. The child who eats a pick-up lunch of potato chips and a sundae and the child who eats a well-planned lunch containing plenty of meat, eggs or fish may show clearly the difference, not just in general health, but also in susceptibility to myopia.

In this regard it is well to keep in mind that vitamin E is destroyed in the presence of rancid fats. Potato chips, salted nuts and many fried foods are dripping with rancid fats. If you fry foods in fats that are used over and over again, it is practically certain that these fats are rancid and are a serious threat to your family's health.

Vitamin E Not A Medicine

So far as the findings about vitamin E are concerned, we were disappointed to note that the French researchers thought of vitamin E only as a medicine to be given to combat a condition and, even though they themselves said that myopia is caused by a deficiency in vitamin E, at no time did they suggest simply making vitamin E supplements a regular part of the child's diet! Instead they recommended giving a series of doses of the vitamin, then skipping a few weeks, then giving another series. Doesn't this seem to be very shortsighted?

Our own Food and Drug Administration has shown a similar shortsightedness in making a recent announcement about vitamin E in which they "warned of false claims for the product." Beware! said our Food and Drug Administration. "Any claim in the labeling of drugs or of foods offered for special dietary use by reason of vitamin E that there is need for dietary supplementation with vitamin E will be considered false." There is plenty of vitamin E in our diets, the report went on. Now, just when the Food and Drug Administration checked the individual diet of every individual American, we do not know. But it seems that a great many French children are deficient in vitamin E, according to the article we have quoted above. And it does not seem unlikely that the same is true of many American children, considering the fact that every single survey done indicates that they have serious shortages in other vitamins and minerals, and considering the fact that all of the vitamin E has been removed from our best source— cereals and other seed foods.

Incidentally, the "warning" which the FDA issued appears in a press release in which they announced that vitamin E is now officially recognized as being essential for human nutrition. It is a great victory for those of us who have been saying this for years. So, to confuse people and make it appear that vitamin E is actually not very important, the press notice contained the "warning" which was, of course, played up prominently by most newspapers.

Here are the foods richest in vitamin E. How many of them does your child eat daily? Beans, beef liver, whole grain cereals (not refined or processed in any way), wheat germ, eggs, green peas, sweet potatoes, turnip greens and salad oils such as corn oil, cottonseed oil, peanut oil, and all seed foods such as sunflower seeds, nuts and so forth. Do you think these foods play an appreciable part in the diet of the average American child? Don't you think their lack constitutes probably the most important cause of the great increase in myopia which we mentioned at the beginning of this discussion? The eating of enormous amounts of fried foods containing rancid fat must also be responsible for our national deficiency in vitamin E.

Make certain your children take vitamin E supplements along with the other food supplements they take. Make certain their diet is high in protein and vitamin E.

17. Virus Disease of the Eye

During World War II, at a time when efficient production was all important, an epidemic of a curious eye disease broke out in many industrial plants, costing many man hours and causing much concern among defense officials. The puzzling thing about this disease was that it struck almost exclusively among industrial workers, and didn't seem to be transmitted to any of the family members nor to other close contacts the victims might have. The most spectacular of its early appearances occurred at the Naval Shipyards at Pearl Harbor in Hawaii in the summer of 1941. At that time 10,000 workers were afflicted, and yet the disease was seen hardly anywhere else on the islands. The disease was typified by a swelling of the eyelids, pain, intolerence of light and constant tears. This was followed by superficial pitting of the cornea and finally deeper spots of cloudy tissue in the cornea which might persist for up to two years.

Spreads to the Mainland

While researchers were still puzzling over the cause of this ailment, it began to appear on the mainland of the United States. Once more its prime target was seen to be shipyard workers, although the disease was also observed in other industries. It was for this reason that it came to be known as Shipyard Eye. Several thousand cases were diagnosed and Shipyard Eye soon came to be recognized as a serious threat to the war effort. But, try as they might, scientists could not discover the cause of this phenomenon. Research did offer one bit of information: the origin of the problem was not bacterial, so a search for a virus began.

Intensive work by Dr. Murray Sanders resulted in isolating what he believed to be the virus, and he found injections of it to be fatal to mice, rabbits and some monkeys. Inoculations of the substance into volunteer human beings resulted only in swelling of the eyelids, but no pitting or clouded spots on the cornea, as in classic cases of this disease, which Sanders had named epidemic keratoconjunctivitis, or E.K.C. In the midst of his work, Sanders was taken into the service, and the method for isolating the virus was somehow lost, as were the samples which had already been isolated.

Once more the search began, but this time more consideration was given to the question of how the disease was transmitted within such narrow limits. Why hadn't it gone beyond the gates of the shipyards and factories? Why was it not seen in children, except on several very rare occasions?

Outbreaks in Hospitals

The first break in the pattern showed itself when outbreaks began to occur in hospitals where eye surgery was performed and in patients who visited opthalmologists' offices. While the laboratory under the direction of Ernest Jawetz, M.D., Ph.D., whose account of this search appears in the *British Medical Journal* (April 4, 1959), was working on the problem of E.K.C., one of the technicians who worked there contracted the disease. Her case was classic in its symptoms, and afforded an excellent opportunity for investigation. It was believed that she was infected in the course of repeatedly inoculating large volumes of infective tissue culture, containing the suspected adenovirus type 8 into experimental rabbits. In spite of the fact that she was married and the mother of 4 small (7-12) children, and made no effort to shield her family and close associates from contamination, not one of her contacts contracted the disease.

Tissue cultures were taken from the eyes of the affected technician and analysis showed them to contain only the minutest trace of the infective adenovirus type 8. It soon became clear as to why the disease was not transmitted from one person to another in casual contact. The author, Dr. Jawetz, is of the opinion that because of the tiny concentration of the virus, only an actual insertion of the virus into the eye, by means of fingers, instruments or solutions can cause the disease.

Why Only Industrial Workers?

With this assumption to go on, the question of why shipyard and industrial workers contracted it so freely was examined once more, and Dr. Jawetz's astonishing guess seems to be the only logical explanation. He notes that, in shipyards and similar plants, the workers are constantly exposed to many chemical and mechanical irritants which bring many of them to the dispensary. Once there, the examination of the eye by a physician using instruments is almost automatic, and the use of some ophthalmic solution is also likely. Thus virtually all persons exposed to the manipulations of an intense eye examination are susceptible to infection, and if a doctor should disseminate this virus, it is easy to see that an explosive epidemic could follow. This explained the outbreak of the disease in eye hospitals and ophthalmologists' offices.

It is truly amazing to discover that in Europe and North America the main point of transmission for a disease well known for over 70 years should turn out to be the doctor's office. (Editor's Note: In the Orient this virus is stronger and more prevalent, and can be transferred through respiratory or fecal excretions.) It is obviously important, therefore, that in choosing a physician for an eye examination, the cleanliness of his office and the attention he gives to proper sterilization of his instruments be considered. Don't take these things for granted. Even doctors are sometimes careless, or in too much of a rush to bother with details which might mean the difference between contracting and avoiding a serious illness for you.

18. What Drugs Can Do to the Eyes

The world of drugs, in which medicine has largely taken up residence, has shown that it can be valuable in treating emergency cases when death is close and there is no time to consider the dangerous side effects of the drugs. But such successes have led doctors and some patients into the error of believing that drugs are the only answer to disease, that they should be used first when disease strikes, and that nothing else can be effective.

This attitude has done a great deal of harm. It has led to the use of drugs at times when their use was not indicated, and when other treatments would have been more effective. It has resulted in the use of powerful drugs for minor illnesses. The frequently serious side effects have often done more damage than the original illness. Penicillin is the favorite example: it is often given by doctors in cases on which it could not possibly have an effect; it is powerful, and frequently has dangerous side effects; in persons allergic to it, it has been known to cause death many times.

This talk of the use of drugs, and the unexpected effects they can have, came about as the result of an article which appeared in the *Medical Press* (December 16, 1959), written by Dr. Frank W. Law, Surgeon at Moorfield's Eye Hospital in London. Dr. Law talks of the various effects on the eyes which commonly used drugs can cause. For example, it is interesting to find that swelling of the eyelids and surrounding tissues may be caused by iodides and arsenicals. These are two commonly used ingredients in today's drugs. Is it not possible that swelling and irritation could also be caused by these in delicate tissues throughout the body which are not so readily visible?

Dr. Law tells us that, in the past, in order to eliminate these symptoms, double dosage of the offending chemical was given. Mercifully, this practice is no longer commonly followed.

Thiouracil is a commonly used drug for depression of an overactive thyroid. It has also shown itself as an enemy to the eye. Thiouracil has caused paralysis of the muscles of the eye, paralysis of the muscles of the eyelid, causing it to droop and causing deviation of the focusing power.

Similarly, a disturbance of ocular movement may be caused by curare-like drugs, specifically, d-tubocurarine.

Drugs Change Eye Color

One of the most unusual and disturbing phenomena of drug therapy reactions is the change of color, either in the eye itself or in what the eye sees. For example, prolonged use of acetophenetidin, a common aspirin ingredient, may cause the eyes to take on a mauve coloring. This can also occur in prolonged use of sulphanilamides. In the case of chloroquine and amodiaquine, two drugs used to treat malaria, arthritis and some skin diseases, not only the color of the eye may be changed, but deposits may occur on the cornea, and blurring of vision and light halos can result. Though it is rare, muscular degeneration of the eyes has been reported from the use of chloroquine.

Atropine is one of the drugs frequently used in eye examination, as well as in gastrointestinal disorders and for travel sickness. It changes the size of the pupil and interferes with the eye's accommodation to light and darkness as well as distance. Severe poisoning may follow atropine's external use. The most striking symptom is a peculiar delirium. At first it shows itself in profuse and senseless talkativeness, later there is complete confusion, often with hallucinations, sometimes becoming maniacal. Fortunately, recovery can usually be expected.

Physostigmine is a drug which came to us from the Calabar coast of Africa. It was used there by the natives who considered its ingestion an ordeal. It could kill a guilty man or merely cause an innocent man to vomit. It was later discovered that, if the bean were used fresh, it acted as an emetic, older beans could cause death. Its use in modern medicine is to contract the pupil of the eyes in glaucoma, and to relieve pain in rheumatism, bursitis and arthritis and myasthenia gravis (severe muscular fatigue and exhaustion marked by progressive paralysis of the muscles). It can cause myopia, or near-sightedness and myosis, an excessive contracting of the pupil.

Potassium iodate is known chiefly as an antibacteriant, and is used in tubercular inflammations of the nose and larynx, as well as for inflammatory conditions of the mucous membranes. Doctors who use it should know that potassium iodate can cause degeneration of the retina. Some tranquilizers can effect a similar degenerative result, usually preceded by an upset of the dark adaptation of the eye.

Quinine, famous for its action against the symptoms of malaria, and

[63]

used as a diagnostic agent for suspected myasthenia gravis, as well as a treatment for myotonia congeneta (a disease characterized by spasm and rigidity of certain muscles), has some supremely dangerous side effects. Excessive doses can cause extreme dilation of the pupil, swelling of the retina, sudden and complete loss of vision, ringing in the ears and deafness. The blindness is sometimes permanent, and should sight return, it is incomplete and never really good.

Chloramphenicol is a very powerful drug whose serious side effects are warned against in *The Dispensatory of the United States*. It is used against typhoid, urinary and respiratory infection, venereal diseases, etc. After prolonged administration of the drug, the patient may experience degeneration of the optic nerve. Vision often does not return. It is also presumed to act upon the intestinal flora, interfering with the assimilation and synthesis of the B vitamins .

Digitalis, long used as a treatment for heart disease, in spite of the dangers involved, threatens the user with a unique side effect to the eyes. Vision may become monochrome. Everything is one color—red, yellow or green. Digitalis has also been cited as a cause of visual hallucinations.

The effects we speak about here do not take into account what is happening to other parts of the body. What happens to the brain, the lungs, the heart or liver when a drug strong enough to cause blindness or paralysis of the optic nerve is administered? No one knows, in many cases. Nor are doctors always aware of how much residue of each drug dose remains in the body. It is for such reasons that we are against the use of drugs in all but the most emergent circumstances. They should be a last resort, and should be used with full awareness of the serious danger involved. A person should be told that a drug injected to ease arthritic pain frequently results in mental breakdown, and that tranquilizers sometimes cause degeneration of the retina. Perhaps such a reminder would act as a brake on both patient and doctor in choosing drugs without considering other therapeutic possibilities.

19. Eyesight and Vitamin Deficiency

There are many parts of your body which act as sentinels—that is, they will give danger signals when things are not going well. We all know that a doctor looks at your tongue when he is diagnosing your ailment. He may also examine your fingernails and lips. But if he is a good doctor and, especially if he is very conscious of the importance of good nutrition to health, he will probably also examine your eyes for symptoms that will indicate clear as a bell what may be causing your difficulty.

Deficiency in any of the major vitamins results in eye symptoms. In one way this is good, for those of us who study nutrition can be aware of these symptoms, and if we find them in ourselves or in members of our family, we can hazard a pretty sound guess that vitamin deficiency may be responsible. For instance, burning, itching eyes that are frequently bloodshot may indicate eyestrain. True, this may mean that you are using your eyes too much or that you may need glasses. But if you get the glasses and use your eyes a lot less and the symptoms still continue, we would suggest sitting down and going over a week's menu with a certain vitamin in mind. If you find, as you are likely to, that you have been steadily skipping this important vitamin without even being aware of it, then is the time to become very conscious of it, reorganize your menus to include it and then watch for improvement in the eyes.

An interesting article in the *Medical Press* for June 4, 1952, summarizes the effects of the deficiency of various vitamins on the eyes and indicates how to remedy these conditions. The author of the article is A. J. Cameron, M.D., Ch.B., D.O.M.S., FRCS, a surgeon at the Royal Eye Hospital in London, England. Dr. Cameron tells us that for the last 50 years amblyopia has been reported which seemed to be due to nutritional deficiency. Amblyopia means simply dimness of vision that is not caused by an organic disease of the eye or some defect in the eye mechanism. In England, before the war, says Dr. Cameron, nutritional deficiency was unusual. But after the war it became quite common to find the symptoms of a partial vitamin deficiency which showed itself in delayed healing of wounds, tardy return to health after an illness and extension of the time an infection might be expected to run its course.

In these cases of more or less slight vitamin deficiency it is not unusual to find definite changes in the cornea, lens and retina of the eye. Of course, this does not always indicate simply that the necessary vitamin or vitamins are lacking in the diet. It may mean instead that the person is unable to assimilate them, no matter whether he has plenty of them at hand. Pregnant women and nursing mothers are more liable to this kind of deficiency because of the drain on their own body resources. Usually deficiency of one vitamin alone does not occur. An individual deficient in one is almost certain to be deficient in others as well. This is one reason why we stress a wide variety of diet. It is also one very good reason for never taking synthetic vitamins. It is hardly possible, for instance, to be deficient in just one of the B vitamins. Taking a synthetic B vitamin is quite likely to lead to a deficiency in another of the B vitamins. Dr. Cameron tells us that the vitamins most important from the point of view of eye health are: vitamin A, the B vitamins, vitamins C and D.

Vitamin A Deficiency and Eye Health

Most of us know that lack of vitamin A causes definite eye symptoms. There are night blindness, xerophthalmia and keratomalacia. Xerophthalmia is a dry and thickened condition of the conjunctiva or eye tissues, which sometimes follows conjunctivitis or a disease of the tear glands. Keratomalacia is a softening of the cornea.

It is known that the normal retina and the choroid (an eye membrane) contain enormous amounts of vitamin A. Apparently, vitamin A is necessary for the process that goes on inside the eye when your body moves from darkness to light, or from light to darkness. So a lack of vitamin A would hinder this process.

It has been found that night blindness resulting from vitamin deficiency may be accompanied by scotomata—that is, dark spots in the field of vision. We know that both these conditions are caused directly by too little vitamin A and can be cured by increasing the amount of vitamin A available for the use of the body.

Often night blindness is accompanied by dryness of the cornea and the eye tissues, with triangular spots, silver gray and shiny which are called Bitot's spots, after the physician who first studied them. The area that is affected by this dryness feels gritty, as if there were grains of sand on the eyeball. Then, too, as if there were a film of oil over it, it cannot be "wetted."

Keratomalacia is an advanced and much more serious state of either or both of these two first conditions. Dryness is first noticed, followed by a softening of the cornea which becomes gray, dull and cloudy. Since this condition is an indication of severe vitamin A deficiency, other tissues in the body also suffer and may finally be so starved for vitamin A that the patient dies.

Vitamin B is Important, Too

It seems that most of the B vitamins, as well, are necessary for eye health, and that even partial deficiency in one or more of them results in symptoms that can be recognized by physicians. Serious lack of thiamin (one of the B vitamins) may bring on beriberi or neuritis. In the eyes, this takes the form of retrobulbar neuritis, or pains behind the eyeball. There may also be many dark spots on the field of vision, probably near the center of this field.

In describing cases of repatriated prisoners of war from the Far East, Dr. Cameron tells us that he found 3 different kinds of symptoms: 1. Dark spots in the center of the field of vision; 2. General lack of clear vision in the entire visual field; and 3. Psychogenic symptoms—that is, examination could discover nothing wrong with the eyes, but the patients complained of sight disorders. These soldiers who had been imprisoned, eating completely inadequate diets, found that their symptoms persisted for as long as 8 to 12 months, and when they returned to a good diet they very often found that for a while the symptoms grew worse. Then, of course, the addition of the necessary B vitamins in large enough amounts brought about a cure of all symptoms.

Riboflavin, niacin, pyridoxine, pantothenic acid and folic acid, other B vitamins, are also concerned in eye health. In certain forms of pellagra, for instance, giving just niacin will not cure the disease. These other members of the B family of vitamins are necessary as well. In pellagra there is inflammation of the eyelids and loss of eyelashes, erosion of the eye tissues and clouding of the cornea. When riboflavin is lacking in the diet, the eyelids may smart and itch, the eyes grow tired, vision may be poor and cannot be improved by glasses, it may be difficult for the individual to see in dim light and there may be extreme sensitivity to light. This does not mean that the patient cannot stand any light at all, but rather that he suffers actual physical discomfort in the presence of bright light.

Adelle Davis in her book, *Vitality Through Planned Nutrition*, gives more details about eye conditions that result from lack of riboflavin. Dr. Day at Columbia University produced cataract in rats who were deficient in riboflavin. If they were not given riboflavin, they eventually became completely blind. Dr. Sydenstricker of the University of Georgia studied 47 patients all of whom lacked riboflavin. They suffered from a variety of visual disturbances. They were sensitive to light, suffered from eyestrain that was not relieved by wearing glasses, and had burning sensations in their eyes and visual fatigue. They were sensitive to light and their eyes watered easily. Six of them had cataract. Within 24 hours after the administration of riboflavin, symptoms began to improve. After two days, the burning sensations and the other symptoms began to disappear. Gradually all disorders were cured. When the riboflavin was taken away from them, the symptoms gradually appeared again and once again were cured by riboflavin.

Very often patients with such disorders will get glasses and continue to wear them even though they notice no improvement. Children do not generally suffer from riboflavin deficiency as much as adults, for American children generally drink lots of milk which is rich in riboflavin. But after we are grown, we must become conscious of other sources of riboflavin, if we would avoid these eye disorders.

Vitamin C Is All-Important for Eye Health

Vitamin C, also called ascorbic acid, is one of the most important elements in a diet for good eye health, and one of the most difficult to obtain in abundance. Vitamin C is not stored in the body, so you must eat foods containing vitamin C every day. In scurvy which is the disease indicating severe vitamin C deficiency, there are hemmorrhages of the eyelids and eye tissues. The eyes have a tendency to water, the conjunctival membranes grow dry and there may be softening or ulceration of the cornea. There are large amounts of vitamin C in the lens and other parts of the normal eye. In cases of cataract the amount of vitamin C is diminished. We do not know, says Dr. Cameron, whether it is lack of vitamin C that brings on the cataract or the cataract that results in lack of vitamin C. Adelle Davis tells us that the blood and urine of individuals suffering from cataract contain far less vitamin C than that of people the same age who do not have cataract. She also tells us that large doses of vitamin C have brought about improvement in cataract patients.

Vitamin D is that vitamin which our body manufactures from the ultraviolet rays of the sun. It is necessary for the proper use of calcium and phosphorus by our bodies. Rickets is the disease resulting when there is not enough calcium, phosphorus or vitamin D. In some kinds of rickets, a cataract of a certain kind develops. Ample vitamin D in the form of fish liver oils or sunshine will forestall rickets and also this kind of cataract, if there is also enough calcium and phosphorus. Adelle Davis tells us that myopia or near-sightedness has been developed in puppies by depriving them of vitamin D and calcium. Vitamin D has also been used successfully in preventing and curing near-sightedness in children.

Dr. Cameron mentions that vitamin E as used by Dr. Shute and his co-workers in their treatment for heart disease and high blood pressure results in improvement of the inflammation of the retina that may accompany hypertension. Vitamins K and P are frequently used with vitamin C to prevent or improve hemorrhages in various parts of the eye. In fact, Dr. Cameron tells us that two European surgeons are in the habit of giving vitamin C for two or three days before and 10 days after an operation for cataract.

Dr. Cameron's observations and conclusions on the subject of vitamin deficiency in relation to eye health are that treatment for these various symptoms should be begun within two months of the time they first appear. Although there may be a great improvement in vision, he says, small dark spots in the field of vision may persist indefinitely.

Planning Your Diet For Eye Health

It is not easy, of course, for a lay person to recognize these eye symptoms in himself. And there is no reason to become alarmed and decide one is suffering from severe deficiency if one's eyes get tired and irritated after a day of reading in a library, for instance. On the other hand, eye symptoms may come gradually, so gradually that you are hardly aware of them and by the time you have a fully developed case of night blindness or spots before your eyes, the deficiency may have reached such proportions that it will take a long time of concentrated attention to diet to bring you back to normal. So the wise precaution is to prevent any of these symptoms from ever appearing. A fully adequate diet will do it. This means ample protective foods—meats, eggs, green leafy vegetables, yellow vegetables and fruits (for vitamin A), all kinds of fresh vegetables and fruits for vitamins B and C. And we can't stress too strongly how necessary it is to eat fruits and vegetables raw whenever possible. Heat and exposure to light and air are not friendly to B vitamins and vitamin C. So the more cooking, shredding and storing you put your foods through before eating them, the less of these two vitamins you will have. If you live in the north, it is hardly possible to get enough vitamin D in the winter, unless you supplement your diet with fish liver oils. Never take synthetic vitamin D.

Fish liver oils contain larger amounts of vitamin A than any other food, so they are, we think, an absolute necessity for eye health, especially if you aren't willing to make a conscious effort to eat lots of yellow vegetables such as carrots and sweet potatoes. The B vitamins are those neglected orphans, so scarce in our present-day diets which include so much of white bread, cake, refined cereals and white sugar. You must eat completely whole grain cereals, lots of fresh vegetables and fruits and organ meats, such as liver and kidney, if you want to get even a smattering of the B vitamins you need. In addition, we strongly suggest supplementing your diet with desiccated liver or brewer's yeast for those extra B vitamins. Don't take synthetics, which may contain only one or only a few of the B vitamins. You must have them all, for they work together in your body's chemistry and if you are short of one, you are almost bound to be deficient in others, too. Brewer's yeast and desiccated liver contain them all.

Finally just a few extra cautions on vitamin C. Over and over again it has been brought to our attention that aging goes hand in hand with vitamin C deficiency. Maybe we need more vitamin C as we grow older. Perhaps we just gradually stop eating vitamin C rich foods after middle age. At any rate, cataract, along with so many other diseases of old age, is closely related to vitamin C deficiency. Is there any logical reason why we should look forward to an old age clouded by cataract, when all kinds of vitamin C rich foods are available to us the year 'round? We think not. And this is why we dwell so persistently on the importance of vitamin C in our diets. Don't shove aside that decorative bit of parsley on your plate. Parsley is rich in vitamin C. Eat it by the handful every day. Buy water cress whenever you can find it, or grow your own if you live in the country, and get used to the idea of whopping big tossed salads that are green with water cress, endive, raw spinach and any other greens you can find. Bleached vegetables have few vitamins. Shun them. And finally, because we are sure you are not getting enough vitamin C every day of your life, take rose hips as a food supplement. They contain more vitamin C than any other food and are rich in vitamins A, E, K and B as well. For nibbling between meals, you won't find anything more delicious or better for your eyes than sunflower seeds. . . . Here's health to your eyes!

20. When Your Feet Hurt, You Hurt All Over

Human hands appear to be marvels of fine workmanship and design. What miracles may not be accomplished by a human hand, trained in some delicate skill or made powerful by practice for anything from violin playing to carpentry! But it seems that our hands are mere slabs of insensitive flesh compared to our feet. Dr. Frederick Wood Jones of the University of Manchester says that man's hand is a "ridiculously simple and primitive appendage . . . (but) man's foot is all his own. It is the most distinctive human part of his whole anatomical makeup." He adds that the foot is man's crowning achievement, his finest piece of adaptation.

The 52 bones and 214 ligaments composing our two feet are small, delicate and finely balanced. Yet they carry our weight over the 8 miles or so that most of us walk in a day, they endure, for the most part uncomplainingly, hours of standing on hard floors or walking on hard sidewalks. No human engineer could construct so efficient a machine for weight bearing and motion.

Yet we esteem our feet so little, treat them so badly and neglect them in such a wholesale fashion that something like 75 per cent of us suffer from some foot disorder, of which we may or may not be conscious. For evidence of foot troubles does not necessarily appear first in the feet. Pain in your legs, your back, your neck or your head may be coming from your feet. Poor posture may be the result of faulty foot function and likewise painful feet may result from poor posture. Your weight is important, too, for it goes without saying that every extra pound adds to the work your feet must do.

Consider for a moment how feet were made to be used. Primitive man walked barefoot. His feet were adjusted to soft earth which he could grasp with his toes as he walked. Today even those of us who live in the country spend much of our time walking on hard level floors. City-dwellers pound the hard sidewalks every time they step outdoors. Practically none of us who are adult ever go barefoot, preferring to wear slippers even for that short walk from our evening bath to the bedroom. From the time we are toddlers our feet have been shod in shoes—usually badly fitted shoes. The women of modern times have earned (and we believe they deserve them) countless foot disorders because of their vanity in selecting shoes that look small and flattering regardless of what they do to feet. There is no engineer, physician or chiropodist who could find any excuse for high heels except vanity.

The way we stand and walk has more to do with the health of our feet than any other one factor. The weight of your body should be borne on the outside arch of the foot which is made of bone for the express purpose of bearing weight. The inside arch is made mostly of ligaments and muscles. When we walk incorrectly and stand with an incorrect posture, the weight is thrown instead on the inside arch. Muscles and ligaments endure all they can, and then give way, resulting in fallen arches which is one of the most painful conditions known, and may involve all kinds of dreadful apparatus necessary to bring relief. The purpose of these contraptions is, of course, to take the place of the muscles that have collapsed. Exercise is important, too, in curing fallen arches, as well as specially designed shoes. All of them are very expensive and very painful.

Good Posture Helps Prevent Foot Trouble

What can we do to prevent foot trouble? As you might expect, we should concentrate our preventive efforts in childhood and much of the literature dealing with foot health concerns training and proper shoeing of children. We must be aware of the fact that foot disorders are very often not apparent for years and a child's foot may become deformed so gradually that he experiences no pain and his parents may not suspect that anything is wrong. Posture is of utmost importance. One's feet should at all times be straight—that is, parallel to one another, rather than turned out or turned in. Pigeon-toes suggest immediately that something is wrong and the pigeon-toed child will usually be taken to the doctor. But until quite recently it was considered genteel to turn the toes out in walking and many of us suffer today as a result of this fad. When the toes turn out in walking or standing, the weight of the body is thrown on the inner arch which sooner or later is bound to give way. So the first and most important exercise for healthy feet is learning to walk and stand with feet parallel. When we take a step the weight should be first on the heel, then as we go forward, it is transferred to the outer arch and finally to the great toe.

But it is, you will agree, impossible to walk correctly unless you have comfortable shoes. We will not even discuss trying to walk in high heels, for this comes under the heading of "hobbling" rather than walking. It is impossible to walk correctly in high heels. Regardless of whether you are holding your feet correctly parallel, they must slip forward in your shoes due to the height of the heel. And many of the foot troubles of modern women are concentrated in the forepart of the foot which is, of course, that part which is twisted and deformed by high heels.

High heels aside, there is considerable controversy as to what constitutes correct shoes. They should, of course, be big enough and right here is where so many foot troubles have their start in childhood when little feet are growing rapidly, getting too big for shoes long before the shoes wear out. In a school survey in England, reported in the *Medical Press,* June 18, 1952, we learn that 61 per cent of the boys and 83 per cent of the girls were wearing shoes that were too short for them. Corns and calluses were practically universal on all children over the age of 10. A foot health program examining school children in Massachusetts in 1943-44 discovered that 75 per cent of the children were wearing improperly fitted shoes. The number of incorrectly styled shoes increased with age, as did the foot defects. Eighty per cent of the stockings or socks were too short, resulting in just as much discomfort and deformation as too-short shoes; and children 5 to 10 years of age were 40 to 50 per cent foot defective, while high school children were 80 per cent defective, for they had corns, calluses, ingrown toenails, hammertoes, bunions, etc.

Children Outgrow Shoes Rapidly

An active youngster takes 30,000 steps in one day. If his shoes do not fit properly, is it any wonder that his feet soon suffer from all kinds of ailments? Children's shoes should be replaced as soon as there is any indication they are too small. The fitting should be carefully made, with the child standing, so that the full weight is on the feet. There should be the width of an adult's thumb between the toes and the end of the shoe. And since you never know how fast your child may be growing during any given time, you should make frequent examinations between shopping trips, just to make sure that junior's feet still have enough room inside his shoes. In general, it appears that shoes should be firm enough to give support, yet should not be made of stiff unyielding leather which might be appealing because of its durability. Nor should sneakers be worn a great deal of the time. If your child finds that sneakers are comfortable during the summer, make sure that he wears leather shoes part of the time, for sneakers or tennis shoes do not give enough support for constant wear.

Until the age of 16 or so, children's shoes should be renewed every 3 or 4 months, if you want to be certain their shoes are not too small. Hand-me-downs are an excellent way to save money on clothes, but poor economy in shoes. No one, child or adult, should ever wear shoes that someone else has been wearing. Heels should be straightened whenever they seem to be run over. And, incidentally, heels worn down either on the outside or the inside are an indication that posture is poor and feet are not functioning as they should.

The first evidence of badly fitted shoes appears on the skin—redness or blisters anywhere on the foot indicate friction or pressure, which mean poor fit. Corns and calluses may develop in a person with foot deformity who wears perfectly fitting shoes and also in a person with perfect feet who wears badly fitting shoes. However, in general, preventing corns and calluses is simply a matter of making sure your foot-gear is not causing friction or pressure at any one point and throwing away any pair of shoes that cause trouble. One of the major causes of foot trouble in housewives is wearing old shoes to do housework and saving the comfortable good ones for going out. Any housewife knows that she walks miles during the average work day using her feet constantly. So she should make certain that everyday shoes are the most comfortable ones she has—of course, with low heels. And always remember that properly fitting stockings and socks are just as important as properly fitting shoes.

A New Kind of Shoes

We received some time ago a most interesting book on the subject of shoes which presented so revolutionary a view of what proper shoes should be that we want to share it with you. Written by a professional skater who decided to make his own shoes when he could not find any that were comfortable, *Shoes and Feet to Boot* by Alan E. Murray tells the story of his search for correct footwear. Suffering tortures from painful feet which were also his only means of livelihood, Mr. Murray set out to make his own shoes and, after years of experimenting, designed what he calls the "Space Shoe." It is a shoe that apparently meets all requirements in that it lets you walk as primitive man walked. That is, the shoe fits your foot almost as tightly as your own skin; each toe is outlined. And you walk on a soft platform. Your toes can sink in as they do when you are walking on the sand of a beach.

As you might expect, such revolutionary shoes do not look like ordinary shoes. One commentator tells us they look more like a catcher's mitt. Yet these shoes are being worn today by countless people who have formerly suffered agonies from painful feet. They are worn by dancers and actors, by waiters and nurses, by salesgirls and barbers and other people who must stand or walk the greater part of the day. Arthur Godfrey and Robert Cummings wear Space Shoes. Each shoe is made individually from a plaster cast of your individual foot. After you get used to the strange sensation of "walking on air" which the shoes give you, you find that your foot defects begin to disappear and gradually your feet are remolded into the perfect shape which hard sidewalks and floors have so cruelly deformed. The testimonials in the book tell almost unbelievable stories of pain relieved and many varied ailments cured—ailments that at first glance seem to have nothing to do with feet.

Rules For Foot Health

Here are some rules for foot health as outlined by the United States Public Health Service:

1. Select shoes and hose that fit properly. Tight shoes cause pressure and shoes that are too large cause friction. The heels of shoes should be kept straight.

2. Shoes should be well supported through the arch of the foot, particularly for children, whose feet tend to flatten when they stand up.

3. The growing child should be taught the importance of foot cleanliness and how to protect the feet against ill effects of what may seem to him to be minor injuries.

4. During adult life, foot trouble may be a part of a general bodily condition where attention should be directed toward the improvement of general health.

5. When standing for long periods, place the feet 2 to 4 inches apart, point them straight ahead and support the weight on the outside of the feet. (When walking, keep the feet parallel and pointed straight ahead.)

6. In stepping forward, the weight should fall first on the heel, whereupon the body is carried forward over the foot, weight being applied along the outside of the foot from the heel to the small toe and finally across the forward part to the great toe.

7. The toenails should be cut straight across and not too short.

8. Frequent cleansing, and careful drying of the feet, together with frequent changes to dry hose and shoes may aid in relieving excessive perspiration.

9. Prompt care of all wounds and blisters on the feet may prevent serious consequences.

10. Fallen arches are the result of weakened leg muscles which allow the main or lengthwise arch in the foot to sag. An orthopedic surgeon should be consulted about this condition, as special treatment is indicated.

11. The feet should be bathed at least once a day with soap and warm water and then thoroughly dried. (We say: Omit the soap. Your skin is naturally acid and soap makes it alkaline, resulting in an unhealthy condition where all kinds of germs can take hold.)

12. Exercise the feet. The arches may be strengthened by bending the toes—best accomplished by picking up small objects such as marbles, with the toes.

We would add two last suggestions: Take off your shoes whenever you can and walk around in your bare feet, especially if you can walk in a yard or on a sandy beach. When you are tired, rest with your feet up, or lie for a half hour or so with your feet higher than your head, on a slanting board or with pillows beneath your legs.

21. Your Feet Require Special Care

If there is a comforting thought about foot trouble, it is that no one who has it is suffering alone. Experts estimate that 80 per cent of the women in the United States, and 60 per cent of the men, suffer from disorders of the feet. Most of them are painful enough to keep corn plasters and bunion pads moving off the drug store counters at a very fast pace. Many victims are driven to more drastic attempts at self-help, and risk serious infection by razor-blade surgery. When foot problems reach those proportions, it is safer and more helpful to consult a chiropodist, or podiatrist, a doctor who specializes in diseases of the feet.

Chiropodists have had more good fortune than chiropractors in ingratiating themselves with organized medicine in America, and their efforts are supported and recognized by the American Medical Association. Chiropodists have much the same educational requirements as chiropractors: one or two years of college required before entry into one of six approved schools, and the courses require 4 years for completion. In these 4 years the student attends 4200 to 4400 hours of classes in the usual medical school courses such as bacteriology, pathology, dermatology, plus special courses in foot gear, foot orthopedics, etc. This appears to qualify the chiropodist to work side by side with a medical doctor, in the same way that a dentist does.

Shoes Create Need For Chiropodists

If there is one factor in modern life, one single thing which has made the doctor who specializes in foot disease indispensable, it is shoes. Women are especially at fault here. It would appear that they love to suffer. Not only do they wear high heels which tilt them forward into an awkward and unnatural position, but they defy all logic by actually narrowing the shoe where it should be widest, at the toe, the foot's widest point!

The surest indication that there is something basically wrong in our approach to foot coverings is the large number of children who suffer from foot disorders. It might be understandable that an adult, after 30 or 50 years of poor posture, job peculiarities requiring use of the feet, or constant walking on incompatible surfaces, would develop foot trouble, but why should a child have such a problem? Except, of course, for the small percentage of congenital deformities, the foot disorders of children can be blamed almost entirely on the shoes they wear. Are there so many such cases as to cause concern? Well, judge for yourself. In 1944 the National Association of Chiropodists examined 20,000 children in New York City. Of these, 60 per cent were found to have simple foot disturbances (problems which one or a few treatments could correct), and 20 per cent were found to have advanced disorders (problems which would require extended treatment). This leaves 20 per cent or 4,000 of 20,000 children whose feet were considered healthy and normal. The very same ratio was the result of a survey in Hartford, Connecticut, by that city's Chiropody Society. This time 1,674 school children of all ages were examined and only 20 per cent emerged with a clean bill of health. One-third of the children were found to be wearing improper shoes at the time of the examination. Forty per cent of the children had already developed bone abnormalities of the foot. Foot problems have become so common among children that some states require an annual examination of the feet for all school children.

Improper Styling and Fit of Shoes

The experts tell us that any of a number of factors can mean trouble with the feet. Improper styling, which includes pointed toes, high heels, etc., has received a large share of the blame, and rightly so. Poor fit, even in a properly styled shoe, can cause severe discomfort, as well as future woes. When one is buying shoes the salesman should take a measurement of the feet as the purchaser is standing, for the foot broadens considerably under body weight. In trying on a shoe, one should walk in it, to see how it "rides" on the foot. It should fit snugly, without pinching. If the shoe is too big, it will cause trouble by rubbing against the heel or instep of the foot until soreness develops. Loose shoes are frequently responsible for as many foot problems as shoes which are too tight.

Materials and Workmanship

The materials of which a shoe is made can have a great deal to do with foot health. Many synthetics have been used lately, and they have one basic fault. They don't "breathe" with the foot. In leather there are many minute air holes which permit some circulation for air around the foot. Many synthetics do not allow for this, and the climate is ripe for infection in a foot that is so confined.

The construction of the shoe usually varies with the price. In well-made shoes, inner seams are finished so that the welting is at a minimum. Protrusions, such as nails from the heels, are never felt. The lining is securely anchored and not likely to fray. All of these things conspire to make a shoe comfortable and to spare you trouble with your feet.

Even if the material of the shoe is the finest, individual peculiarities often enter into the problem. Sensitizing and irritating chemicals such as monobenzyl ether of hydroquinine, used to prevent rubber oxidation, frequently have a bad effect on some feet. The dyes and resins can cause sensitive feet to burn intolerably. If such problems beset you, and you can see no visible reason for the trouble, change the brand of shoes you use. Different manufacturers use different chemicals and formulae for dyes, and a change of maker could solve the problem.

Must We Wear Shoes?

Why don't we just go without shoes, as nature obviously intended? The hard floors and sidewalks of civilization have just about eliminated that possibility. Bare feet would be brutally ruined by these hard surfaces. When man was walking on resilient earth and grass, bare feet were able to hold their own without damage. Now, life without some foot protection and support would lead to serious breakdowns of foot comfort and health. It is significant, though, that foot disorders seen among shoe-wearing people are not known among barefooted races.

The American Podiatry Association has made some worthwhile comments on the most common foot problems we run into as shoe-wearing Americans: Corns and calluses are symptoms of ill-fitting shoes, or malformations of the foot bones. They should never be cut with a razor blade or any other non-sterile instrument. Foot infections can easily result and force long periods of inactivity. If such a condition becomes painful enough to cause you to contemplate cutting it out, see a podiatrist who is trained to care for such conditions properly.

Ingrown Toenails, Bunions and Athlete's Foot

Ingrown toenails, says the Association, are caused by ill-fitting shoes and stockings, or by improper trimming. This last cause is the most common one. Something seems to make most persons think that trimming toenails without rounding the corners is not neat, so they clip off the corners. When growth begins again, instead of growing straight out, the tapered nail takes a new path—inward, and begins to cut painfully into the flesh of the toe.

Bunions, a severe swelling and tenderness of the joint of the big toe, are caused by a weakness of the ligaments and muscles of the foot and leg, says the Association. This problem sounds much like bursitis to us, and might yield to vitamin B_{12}, as the common shoulder bursitis has been known to do.

Athletes foot, also called ringworm, is a skin disease caused by a fungus. Fungus thrives best in a warm, moist, dark environment—just the kind the inside of a shoe provides. The raising of the skin's resistance by using food supplements rich in vitamins C and A is one of the means of avoiding this problem. Another is frequent soaking of the feet, and fresh socks or stockings daily so that the feet will stay dry in the shoe. This measure is also most effective in eliminating offensive foot odors.

The feet require special attention if they are to stay trouble free. Their unnatural confinement in shoes makes them doubly suceptible to problems. Give them a break by buying comfortable, sensible shoes, and taking extra sanitary precautions to prevent infection.

[77]

22. The Prevention of Foot Disability

By SIMON J. WIKLER, Doctor of Surgical Chiropody

Infants

Infants' toes and feet should be regarded as carefully as their hands and fingers. Just as mothers would not dare constrict the fingers or hands, so must the feet be left free. Swaddling, binding, placing tight stockings on, and tucking blankets firmly over the feet are all reprehensible practices. Feet should be perfectly free to twist and turn at a baby's will, at least in the first year of life. If a parent is particularly anxious about keeping a baby's feet warm, elevations or cradles should be placed in the crib under the blankets in the vicinity of the feet so that no constrictions are caused. Parents too often imagine that baby's feet suffer cold as readily as their own do. A baby as yet undeformed by shoes needs to have its feet protected from cold no more than its hands.

Prewalking babies under no circumstances need shoes. The bronzed baby shoes, which some parents are proud to exhibit, should be nothing more than a reminder of the first deformity they inflicted on the child. Stockings for warmth may be needed in cold weather, but even this type of clothing is used more frequently than necessary. When the parent does not consider gloves necessary for the baby, stockings are likewise unnecessary.

When the infant first begins to stand and walk, indoors at any rate, shoes are not necessary. In a playpen or in the house where the floors are clean the child is more comfortable when barefoot. In the winter, when floors are cold, woolen stockings are more practical than shoes. Above all, it should be recognized that infants are starting to develop their bones and muscles. Deformity to the feet of babies is most serious. The first purchase of shoes should be avoided as long as possible.

Growing Children

For growing children the most important consideration is the proper selection of shoes. If a shoe fits a growing child when it is purchased, in a very short time it will be too small for him. Shoes should therefore be purchased larger than the fit. In the lives of children there are periods in which they grow very rapidly. At such times the shoes will be rapidly outgrown. Parents should teach themselves what a good fit in shoes is so that they can constantly check on the fit rather than rely on the occasional visit to the shoe store or the judgment of a shoe clerk.

The design of a modern shoe which brings its "toe" to a point makes the first half inch useless. For a growing child there should be at least an adult's thumb width of length extra; some free space should exist on either side of the toes. The feet should be examined frequently, and when this distance is diminished the shoes should be discarded. Regarding width, some free space should exist on either side of the ball with just enough purchase between the eyelets for the shoes to be laced firmly; or, in the case of sandals, the shoe should be wide enough to fall off the foot at each step when they are not fastened.

If some parents are surprised at having such large shoes for children recommended, they may be interested to know of the practices of cobblers before the manufactured shoe. These now extinct artisans would have the child stand on a piece of sole leather, draw an outline around the foot with extra room for a winter's growth, and hand-make the shoe with assurance that no deformation would result until the child could go barefooted again the following summer.

Arch support shoes are never advisable when recommended by a nonprofessional, and in this author's opinion only a small fraction of the arch shoes recommended even by professionals is justified. Often expensive shoes have arch support features only to justify their prices, and for this reason expensive shoes are sometimes more deforming than inexpensive ones.

Stockings are a necessary evil because of the moisture and filth which accumulate during the wearing of a confining shoe. Modern stockings, like shoes, have no relation to the true structure of the foot. Instead of expanding at the toes, stockings become pointed at the toes. For this reason stockings should be worn about an inch and one half longer than the ends of the toes, and the added length of stocking should be pulled to fit in the unused toe portion of the shoe. When a child's stocking becomes less than three-fourths of an inch longer than the longest toe, it should no longer be worn by the child.

In spite of all the precautions that one might take with shoes and stockings, the design of modern shoes makes some deformity inevitable. If, however, for a growing boy or girl the pointed-toe styles are avoided, and, for girls, the change to a high heel is postponed as long as possible, deformity to the feet will be kept to a minimum.

Prevention of Foot Deformity in Women

When it comes to considering the deforming styles in women's shoes, some authorities throw up their hands in despair and say, "Here is a situation that defies all reasonableness or hope of solution." They are mistaken, and the ladies themselves have proved them to be. Within recent years the young girls have taken to wearing shoes that are less deforming.

It must be remembered that the ready-to-wear clothing industry is only eighty years old. For many centuries the only people who could dress in the height of fashion were the rich. When the invention of modern shoemaking machinery made it possible (some eighty years ago) for women of the middle and lower income classes to be shod like the women of wealth, they literally were crazed at the opportunity. Girls who had to stand on their feet all day in shops, housewives doing their scrubbing of floors, all wore the high-heeled pointed shoes approved by the women of leisure. Women were so enamored of their newly won privilege that they would not lay the harmful shoes aside except at bedtime.

The entire female population, wherever manufactured shoes could be obtained had their feet cruelly mutilated. Telling a woman that for her health's sake she should stop wearing fashionable shoes was the same as telling her that she must sacrifice glamor. When modern industry made it possible for every woman to be shod like a Cinderella, such an opportunity could not be laid aside by a mere desire to avoid corns, bunions and fallen arches.

However, the young ladies of today are not aware of the passions which motivated their grandmothers to dress like a duchess. The tiny, useless feet which were considered a mark of distinction by former generations are now considered freaks by our present day girls. Today girls are not ashamed to wear utilitarian clothing, and flat shoes. Consequently, after another few decades have passed, the institution of grossly deformed feet may come to an end.

Housewives should be encouraged to do their daily chores either barefoot or in cloth scuffs. Occasionally to don high-heeled shoes can do no harm, but on a shopping expedition, for example, wearing fashionable shoes is a mistake. Women who are employed in offices often wear fashionable shoes to and from work but change to flat slippers in the office. Women are beginning to find out that the bare healthy foot is an attractive attribute. Trends in shoe fashions have been exposing more and more of the bare foot, and it is hoped that such styles are a prelude to the demand for non-deforming sandals such as the ancients used.

Prevention of Foot Deformity in Men

There has been hardly any change in the deforming characteristics of men's shoes. It is quite difficult to find men's shoes of a good grade that are not stylishly pointed. The few shoes that are available in the broader-toed designs seem to have arch-support features which negate any value a broad-toed shoe might have. Until men recognize how undesirable the present shoes are and demand better ones, the shoe manufacturers will continue using their great investment in lasts, dies and patterns. The writer has successfully developed a functional shoe for adults. To widely distribute such a product requires capital and business ability beyond this author's capabilities.

There are certain customs in foreign lands that our men would do well to emulate. The Japanese, for example, remove their shoes on entering their houses. The Mohammedans consider it sinful to wear shoes in their mosques. Men on reaching home after a day's work should lay aside their shoes and go either barefoot or in stockinged feet. For constant wear around the house the newly invented slipper sock would be an ideal type of footwear. The English custom of changing to slippers on arriving home from a day's work is a good one.

For those who are imbued with love of exercise, the best exercise is going barefoot. The Hawaiians play football and soccer in bare feet. On playing fields free of cinders and glass we would do well to try the same thing ourselves. A walk on a sandy beach barefoot can be stimulating for the feet. Men who look fondly back to their barefoot boyhood would find it healthful to drive their cars to some country dirt road, take off their shoes and socks and stroll about for an hour or two. Once while playing golf in the West Indies I envied the caddies who went barefoot. Playing golf barefoot became a newly found delight for me.

Non-Deforming Shoes

While human beings should go barefoot more often, shoes are of course necessary articles of clothing. The rigors of some weather and terrains, together with the need of protecting the feet from contact with disease-producing agents, make protection with foot covering mandatory. For example, the disease of hookworm is definitely due to the contacting of bare feet with filth. Even the primitive Indians who were very close to nature wore footgear, though theirs was of a non-deforming pattern.

The Indian moccasin was a simple form of footgear that could be easily and quickly made from hides. The sole and upper was one continuous, flexible piece of leather, with a small piece sown across the top to hold the covering on the foot. The modern manufactured shoes that are called moccasins are misnamed, for they are usually made with separate soles and uppers, heels, steel shanks, and Goodyear-welt construction, and they are deforming in the usual manner. Some few manufacturers will make a true moccasin, but then they spoil the flexibility of their product by making it from too rigid a leather or by stitching on an extra sole. Other manufacturers have their false-moccasin-type shoes hand-sewn through the vamp, and they advertise that as an advantageous feature. But if a shoe is of inflexible construction, hand-sewing the vamp has no value. True moccasins would be excellent and practical footgear. If the public should understand what a true moccasin is and should insist on the stores carrying the real product, the shoe manufacturers would make this desirable shoe.

Thong-Type Sandal

The thong-type sandal was extensively worn by the ancient Greeks and Romans, and it is still widely used throughout Central and South America, and in the Far East. The thong sandal, when it is properly made is truly non-deforming footgear. The thong between the great and second toe permits the toes perfect freedom and expansibility. In recent years thong-type sandals have become popular as women's beach wear. Nevertheless, if

[81]

leather is used the usual sole leather is not satisfactory, for, unless leather permits flexibility throughout the foot, the musculature soon suffers. Flexible belt leather should be used for the sole.

Thong-type sandals are easily made. A single layer of belt sole leather should be cut out to an outline of the bare foot increased on all sides by a quarter of an inch. With a chisel two slits, three-sixteenths of an inch apart, are cut in the sole space between the great and second toe. Slits are cut on the edge of the sole on either side of the foot, behind the great and little toe joints respectively. Two other slits are cut on the edge of the sole in front of the ankle bones. Strap leather thongs are then woven through the slits and the foot is firmly bound to the sole. Factory methods are not necessary to make this type of footgear. Families would save a good deal of money and avoidance of foot trouble if the thong-type sandal were made either at home or by the local cobbler.

Non-Deforming Footgear in Other Lands

The Japanese tabiis are a non-toe-compression form of footgear. The tabi is a thong-type wooden clog in which the wood is cut in a number of places to give it a degree of flexibility. Chiropodists are unknown in Japan because the injury of the forefoot does not occur in their native shoes and there is no occasion for development of corns, etc. In the large cities, however, the Japanese are commencing to wear the American-type shoe. If this new custom is adapted very widely, the Japanese will soon suffer the frequency of our degenerative diseases. That the custom of wearing American shoes is not likely to take hold among the masses of the people may be illustrated by the following experience of an American Army officer in Japan. A group of Japanese laborers were working on an American construction project. The supply officer had a surplus of G.I. shoes and, much to the initial delight of the Japanese, he distributed a pair to each of them. Yet their satisfaction was short-lived, for their undeformed wide feet hurt unmercifully when they wore the American shoes. Of course the shoes were discarded, and the laborers resumed their tabiis or went barefoot.

Certain tribes in the Philippines wear a wooden-type sandal that has a single strap across the instep to hold the sandal on the foot. Nevertheless, this strap is not very secure and, in order to keep the sandal on firmly, the wearer must grip with the toes at each step before putting the foot down on the ground. Continuous exercise of the toes in this way makes the foot strong. An orthopedic surgeon who was stationed in the Philippines stated that the people in the tribes who wore this type of shoe were the most handsome he had ever seen, the women retaining their symmetrical postures until an advanced age.

The fabulous beauty of the ladies of the Island of Bali may be said to be largely influenced by their custom of going barefoot. Their well formed breasts are the result of good posture induced by sturdy, un-

[82]

deformed feet. Cancer of the breast in these women is rare. In the rural areas of India people either go barefoot or wear thong-type sandals. In spite of semi-starvation and unhygienic conditions causing many to suffer early deaths from infections and deficiency diseases, these peoples nevertheless have excellent postures and are largely free of degenerative diseases. All this may be said to be due to their custom of not deforming their feet.

A New Shoe

This author developed a non-deforming shoe for children and had it patented. It has no heel elevation and is twice as wide through the toes as in the heel, the dimensions required by a normal foot. The sole fans out from the heel in two straight lines, since it is maintained that the indentation made on the inner and outside of modern shoes unnecessarily constricts the musculature of the foot. Without a heel, the shoe does not need an inflexible shank to bridge the difference in height, which is the function of the shank in a heeled shoe. The toe area of the shoe broadens out so the toes can be spread within the shoe. The shape of the front of the shoe is like the natural conformation of the child's toes, making it possible for the foot to grow unconstricted to the very end of the shoe. There are no stiff counters in the heel, because the counters in ordinary shoes prevent a shoe from fitting firmly around the heel, the one place that a shoe should fit well. There are no arches or any other supportive devices in this shoe, since for a growing child a shoe should act as a spacious covering for the foot and nothing more.

The shoe was placed on one child when he was two years of age. Prior to wearing the shoe he complained about walking and insisted on being carried. The boy seemed perpetually tired, and was subject to a never-ending series of colds and sniffles that the pediatrician had diagnosed as an allergic condition possibly brought on by undue fatigue. The toes of the child were curled and deformed from an obviously too narrow shoe, in spite of the fact that the mother had purchased Triple E shoes in the child's shoe length. The toes were thin and weak and the boy was hardly able to bend them at all. The musculature on the bottom of the feet was sparse and the bones could be felt through the flesh. After wearing the new shoes for one year, the child walked more freely and displayed agility on his feet far superior to his playmates who wore the usual shoes. The perpetual tiredness disappeared and the allergic type of colds no longer affected him. His toes took on a sleek strong appearance. The flesh on the bottom of his feet became dense and bones could no longer be felt through it.

Another child to whom the new shoes were given had previously suffered the same symptoms as the above mentioned child showed, with the additional fact that he was constantly falling and kept his feet pointed outward in a 45 degree angle. The boy's father, who was a physician, had used expensive shoes but, in addition, had prescribed an extra piece of

[83]

sole leather on the inside of the shoes ostensibly to support the arch, though it gave the child no opportunity to use his foot muscles. After 3 months of wearing the new shoe he gained balance, he pointed his feet straight ahead when walking and standing, and his toes and foot musculature, which had formerly been weak and helpless, took on strength.

The one objection mothers have to the described shoe is that it looks different. They are so accustomed to seeing a pointed shoe that a shoe the width of a child's foot appears strange. But pointed shoes have not always been in vogue. As a matter of fact, during the reign of King Henry VIII the style in shoes had become so wide that it became necessary to restrict the width of a shoe to 6 inches, by royal decree.

With the recognition of the value of unhampered and undeformed toes, the style in shoes may change to make it possible for people to wear a non-deforming shoe and still be fashionably dressed. With adults, that state of affairs will probably take some time to come, but with infants and children, where style to the point of sacrifice of health should be no great consideration, non-deforming shoes should be adopted without delay.

SECTION 6: THE GALL BLADDER

23. That Pesky Gall Bladder

One adult in every 5 may eventually have gallstones. At least half of the women living into their sixties will have them. And any woman has 8 times as much chance as a man to hear a surgeon say, "Better take it out." Operations seem to be the prized answer of medical science to problems of the gall bladder.

This tendency is apparent in medical books and journals. Descriptions of gall bladder trouble are lengthy, talk about operations and possible complications of surgery is ever-present. But when you look under "Gall Bladder Disease, Therapy" you find only a few half-hearted suggestions on diet, on which there is considerable disagreement, and nothing much else.

Tucked under the right lobe of the liver, the gall bladder is, we think, quite an important organ, although one of the authorities we consulted referred to it as a "side pocket" for which the body has no use, like an appendix. This hardly seems reasonable to us since all of us come equipped with such a gadget and since it has a definite function to perform which is certainly done much less effectively should the gall bladder be removed. The gall bladder stores bile, a substance manufactured by the liver to help digestion. The liver makes bile all the time, but it is needed only when there is some fat in the intestine to be digested, so the reserve stocks of bile are sent to the gall bladder which concentrates them and keeps them until they are needed.

Bile does not actually digest fat. But it encourages the digestive action of pancreatic juice, stimulates intestinal action and aids in emulsifying fat so that it can be used by the body. How, then, do all the folks whose gall bladders have been removed get along? The bile ducts or tubes that lead from the liver to the gall bladder and then into the intestine enlarge so that more bile can flow through them. And some of this is apparently stored there. But of course this is not as efficient a system as the original one. So naturally it is best to keep your gall bladder if at all possible, and to keep it in the best possible health.

Cholecystitis and Cholelithiasis

Cholecystitis (from chole, the Greek for bladder) is the word meaning inflammation of the gall bladder. Formerly it was thought that this condition resulted from "germs" in the gall bladder. At present this theory is out of date. But inflammation of the gall bladder can be and is dangerous and painful with or without gallstones.

Cholelithiasis is the medical name for gallstones. What causes them? Many possible causes have been mentioned down through the years. There seems to be no doubt, however, that the formation of gallstones is intimately related to diet. Those who have trouble with their gall bladders are usually overweight. This means, of course, that they overeat. Or at any rate, that they eat more than they should of certain foods. Usually, too, they are over 40, although recently more and more cases of gall bladder trouble are occurring in younger people.

The flow of bile may be obstructed in cases of overweight people and pregnant women, where the actual weight of the fleshy tissue stops off the flow of bile in the little ducts. This causes it to back up into the gall bladder, and trouble ensues. Then, too, it seems that gallstones may be caused by what is called "disturbed metabolism" of cholesterol. Cholesterol is a fatty substance that exists in fatty foods of animal origin—eggs, butter, fat meat and so forth. Most gallstones contain cholesterol and it seems obvious that the stones would not have formed in the first pláce had not something gone wrong with the way the body is supposed to use cholesterol. Apparently the amount of cholesterol in the diet has little to do with the formation of stones. Yet the favorite diet given to gall bladder patients for relieving gallstones is a cholesterol-free one.

An article in Today's Health for March, 1956, explains the formation of gallstones like this: "The materials which go to produce gallstones are made when your body burns fat. The way your body burns fat depends on your glands. The amount of fat it has to burn depends on your diet. If anything is wrong with either, gallstones are much more likely."

Risk Appraisal, a book for the insurance companies and their doctors, has this to say, "Coronary disease affects many individuals with gall bladder disease." The author, Harry Dingman, thinks this may be because the individual with heart trouble becomes sedentary and often fat and this makes it more likely that his gall bladder ducts would become sluggish and stones would result.

True. We too, are constantly pointing out the wisdom of daily exercise for everyone and especially for those who fear heart trouble. But isn't it also true that the very same inadequate diet that brings on the heart complications may be responsible, too, for the gall bladder trouble? So mightn't the same diet that prevents heart and blood vessel diseases also prevent gall bladder disorders? We think that it may.

You Must Have Certain Foods to Use Fat Properly

What are the various elements in the diet that are most involved in the way the body uses fat? Almost everything in the way of vitamins, so it becomes perfectly obvious that the vitamins in one's diet are of utmost importance—far more than the amount of fat or cholesterol one eats.

For instance, choline, a B vitamin, is used in the body to transport digested fats from the liver to the various fat deposits in the body. A complete deficiency in choline produces high blood pressure in laboratory animals within a week. Replacing choline in the diet reduces the blood pressure. Removing all choline from the diet of rats (from a cancer-susceptible line of rats) causes the death of the rats within a short time. Putting back just enough choline to keep the rats alive results in 50 times more cancer than would normally have occurred on a diet rich in choline. How can we possible overlook choline as one of the most important single items in the diet so far as fat metabolism is concerned? Yet it was not mentioned once in all the material we read on gall bladder disease.

Inositol, another B vitamin, is intimately involved with the way the body uses cholesterol, this dangerous fatty substance from which gallstones are chiefly made. Here is one experiment showing the relationship. Rats fed a regular diet and large amounts of cholesterol were divided into two groups. One group got, in addition, added inositol. At the end of the experiment, the rats who got just regular diet and the cholesterol had a cholesterol increase of 337 per cent in their blood. The rats which got the inositol (along with just as much cholesterol) had an increase of only 181 per cent. Would you say, therefore, that inositol is important if you are going to be sure that the body uses fats, and especially cholesterol correctly? We have never seen it mentioned in connection with gall bladder trouble.

Biotin, another B vitamin, is directly involved in the assimilation of fat by the body. It must be present in the intestine in ample quantity or fat cannot be digested. Would you say that it is important for the prevention of gall bladder trouble?

Please don't write in and ask where you can get choline, inositol and biotin. You can't get them, so far as we are concerned, except in food, for we believe that taking these 3 B vitamins apart from the other B vitamins is a serious mistake. In food you can get them most abundantly in eggs, liver, wheat germ, beef heart and brewer's yeast. They have been carefully removed from all processed foods, such as white flour and white sugar.

The Importance of The Fat Soluble Vitamins

The fat soluble vitamins, (A, D, E and K) must be considered when you are planning a diet to prevent gall bladder trouble. First of all, they are present in fatty foods, and if you should decide to go on a low-fat diet to prevent gall bladder trouble, you are likely to run into serious difficulty because you will simply not get enough of the fat soluble vitamins. And vitamin K is directly affected by anything that goes wrong with the gall bladder. Bile must be present in the intestine or vitamin K cannot be absorbed by the body. Vitamin K is responsible for the proper coagulation of the blood. Could a lack of vitamin K caused by gall bladder disorder be partly responsible for today's tragic incidence of cerebral hemorrhages or "strokes"? We think it might be.

We are also told that a lack of vitamin A may affect the lining of the gall bladder. This seems likely since vitamin A is important to the health of all the membranes of the body, but especially the linings of organs and passageways.

Vitamin C and Gallstones

Now we come to the theory of W. J. McCormick, M.D., of Canada whose work with vitamin therapy is well known. Dr. McCormick, in the *Medical Record* for July, 1946, presented the theory that lack of vitamin C may be responsible for the formation of "stones" of various kinds in the body. He tells us that more than a hundred years ago "stones," especially kidney stones, were much more prevalent than they are today. He reminds us that more than a hundred years ago, vitamin C was in very short supply in the diet, especially in the wintertime. Scurvy, which is the disease that comes when vitamin C is completely lacking, was a common disease then. People died of it. Today it is almost unknown. Why? Because these days we have fresh raw fruits and vegetables throughout the winter months and we know, at least most of us know, that we must eat a certain amount of such foods to be healthy. Still we have gallstones and kidney stones and tartar on the teeth, which, according to Dr. McCormick, is another evidence of lack of enough vitamin C.

Dr. McCormick, giving massive doses of vitamin C along with a liberal amount of vitamin B, found that, among his own patients, he could clear up evidence of deposits in the urine and at the same time his patients remarked on their freedom from tartar.

There are two ways, he says, in which lack of vitamin C may bring

[87]

about the formation of stones. Vitamin C is absolutely necessary for the health of tissues. It must be present to form the cement that holds cells together. When there is not enough of it, cell material flakes off and forms a kind of garbage which has no place to go. In the genitourinary tract these provide the nucleus for kidney stones which bring a certain amount of infection and begin to collect layers of other materials around them.

In support of his theory, Dr. McCormick describes one country after another where "stones" are almost universal—and vitamin C is almost completely lacking in the diet. Among Tibetans and Szechwanese, he says, almost everyone has gallstones and inflammation of the gall bladder. The diet of these people consists of butter, tea, barley flour and rice, with little or no fresh fruits or vegetables. The high fat content of the diet, with practically no vitamin C to counteract it, may well be responsible for the fact that gallstones rather than kidney stones are the common ailment.

Dr. McCormick's theory is only a theory. We have yet to hear of a doctor putting his patients on a diet high in vitamin C to prevent or cure gallstones. We long for the day when we will read of such a doctor. But meanwhile, and especially since vitamin C is just about the most important single item in anybody's diet, regardless of his health, why not give the theory a try? There is nothing to prevent you, and a world of good health to gain.

Rely On Diet and Diet Supplements

And what of the other vitamins we have mentioned? They are all necessary and highly important. Where do you get them? First, in a well-planned diet, high in protein (meat, fish, eggs, nuts) and fresh fruits and vegetables—a diet that has no room at all for foods made from white flour and white sugar, a diet that is not watered down to little more than calories by the inclusion of candy, soft drinks, doughnuts and all the other treacherous sweets that spell disaster. Isn't it significant that the chief common characteristic of gall bladder sufferers is obesity? The very same foods that made them fat give them the gall bladder trouble.

In addition to a good diet (*every day—no exceptions for weekends or holidays!*), you need food supplements for vitamins and minerals—fish liver oil for vitamins A and D, brewer's yeast, and/or dessicated liver for vitamin B, rose hip preparations for vitamin C, natural vitamin E and wheat germ oil, bone meal and kelp for minerals. If you fear gall bladder trouble, or if you want to reduce safely and surely, this is the diet and these are the diet supplements for you!

24. The Health of Your Gums

Why do we get what dentists call "periodontal disease"—or disease of the gums? How does it happen that more teeth are lost from gum disease than from all other reasons combined? In recent years the science of periodontistry has achieved ever greater importance, for many Americans, especially those who are past middle age, are faced with the prospect of losing all their teeth, not because of diseases of the teeth but because of unhealthful gums!

Dr. Sidney Sorrin, D.D.S., Associate Professor of Periodontia at the New York University College of Dentistry, has done excellent work in discovering and presenting to the dental profession many highly significant facts about the how and why of gum disease.

Causes of Gum Disease

In an article in the *Journal of Dental Medicine* for January, 1955, Dr. Sorrin and his associate Dr. Marvin Simring list the possible causes of gum disorders. They may come under the heading of functional—that is, how one's teeth perform their functions of biting and chewing. Teeth that are too big or too small for their supporting gum structure, teeth that do not meet properly in a "bite" so that much of the force of the bite is lost, teeth that are clenched or ground because of nervous habits are likely to be responsible for lots of gum trouble.

In addition, irritants on the inside of the mouth may help to bring on gum disorders. Impaction of food, tartar on the teeth, mechanical irritants such as dentures that don't fit and hence rub against the gums, chemical irritants, atmospheric irritants (mouth breathing), improper tooth brushing—all these may help to bring on trouble with gums. Then, too, there are the possible systemic reasons—having to do solely with bodily health—faulty nutrition which may mean that the body is too acid or too alkaline; that there is vitamin or mineral deficiency or both; chronic diseases; gland disorders; anemias; allergies or sensitivity to drugs; pregnancy; psychological causes.

Vitamin C is the single most important food factor for gum health, vitamin A and vitamin B being almost as important, as well as calcium and the other minerals that are so necessary for bone health. (Much of our trouble with gums arises from the fact that jawbones disintegrate and wear away so that the whole mouth and tooth structure are thrown out of alignment. American diets are notoriously short on calcium, so necessary for healthy bone structure.)

[89]

Here is one of Dr. Sorrin's case histories—a woman patient, aged 39, who came to him with an extremely bad case of gum disease. Her gums had receded and eroded, they bled at the slightest touch and they were filled with pus. He tells us that this patient had always used an upward, downward and circular method of tooth-brushing. She had the following abnormal habits: pencil-biting, bobby-pin biting, bone chewing, hangnail biting, biting on nuts. Her diet was unbalanced, with large quantities of cake, pies, pastries and candies being eaten. She also told Dr. Sorrin that she had pains in her elbows and knees, slight heart trouble and used laxatives constantly. Furthermore, she had high blood sugar, low blood pressure and anemia. So it seems that her gum disorder sprang from completely inadequate diet, poor mouth hygiene, especially so far as tooth-brushing was concerned and bad habits of which she was probably unaware but which apparently had a lot to do with the poor condition of her gums.

As for the habits that can be so harmful to teeth, here is a list of the commonest ones. Check over it carefully. And better check with your family, too! Perhaps you actually do some of these things without being aware of it.

Habits That May Do Serious Damage

First of all, Dr. Sorrin cautions against the use of dental floss, saying that you may do far more harm than good by using it. You may defeat your own purpose by injuring the gums further. Dental floss should be used only by dentists, says Dr. Sorrin. Now check your score on these:

1. *Neurotic habits:* lip-biting, cheek-biting, toothpick-biting, tongue pressure against teeth (that is, pressing or thrusting your tongue against your teeth), fingernail-biting, pencil-or pen-biting, biting on ear parts of eyeglasses, playing with bridges or dentures (slipping them nervously in and out of place), clenching teeth for control of emotions, biting on straws, matches, etc.

2. *Occupational habits:* Thread-biting, keeping pins or needles in the mouth, holding nails between teeth, cigar-biting (cigar workers may do this), using a reed in playing a musical instrument, any occupation in which the patient grinds his teeth in rhythm with the work at hand, package-wrappers who constantly keep cord between their teeth while packing parcels, stone-cutters, bricklayers, plasterers (dusts erode their teeth), bending wire with teeth while making artificial flowers, etc., etc., etc. Probably every manual occupation carries some risk, if at any time you hold anything in your teeth while you are working.

3. *Miscellaneous habits* (and these are the ones most of us are guilty of): pipe-smoking, biting on various objects such as safety pins and hair pins, biting or chewing a cigarette holder, opening tops of bottles with the teeth (yes, apparently there are some people who do!), cracking nuts or bones with teeth, chewing of cigars and/or tobacco, abnormal sleeping or reading habits (with the fingers pressed against the teeth), mouth breath-

ing which dries out the mucous membrane in the front part of the mouth, pressure on the teeth from the hand when the head rests on the hand (how often do all of us do this, when we are sitting at a table!), thumb-sucking, chewing on one side of the mouth only (a very common habit), wedging of toothpicks between teeth, opening bobby pins with the teeth, biting the end of a tobacco pouch string (where the individual closes the pouch by holding one end of the string in his mouth while he is rolling a cigarette or filling his pipe).

It seems surprising, doesn't it, that a learned dental researcher should have to take the time to point out in the pages of a learned dental magazine that such habits are harmful and very destructive to teeth and gums alike! Yet how often are any of us conscious of doing any of these things? How many of us had any idea of the harm they might do?

Dr. Sorrin says, to the dentists to whom he is addressing his remarks: "The eradication of an established habit is easier if the patient becomes conscious of the involuntary habit, realizes its harm and cooperates in its elimination by the exercise of will power or by the adoption of a harmless substitute. After the habit is discovered, the means of correction must then be determined. In some instances, for example, the teeth can be ground so that it will be impossible for the patient to resume the abnormal position of the teeth."

A word to the wise is sufficient. We are sure that readers will make every effort to correct habits such as these and will watch their children and other members of the family to make sure that such habits do not develop.

25. Wisdom in Treating Gum Disorders

The use of natural methods in treating and preventing disease has many champions among doctors and dentists whose learning and skill are respected throughout the world. The value of their influence on the thinking of laymen, as well as that of other medical men, cannot be overestimated. We think it is important, then, to give our readers a glimpse of the writings of practicing doctors who use vitamin therapy and good diet to achieve their results, and who publish reports of their work in journals not ordinarily accessible to lay people. It is from these men that we get the reassurance we need to continue in our pursuit of good nutrition for our families, as well as the effort we put forth to convince our friends of the importance of carefully selecting the foods they eat.

It is for this reason that we applaud the work of Dr. Harry Roth, B.S., D.D.S. Dr. Roth is Assistant Professor of Periodontia at the New

York University College of Dentistry, and has had papers printed in just about every recognized dental journal in the United States. As you can see, his opinions are respected by his colleagues. But more important to us, his opinions are largely our opinions. Dr. Roth is strongly in favor of good nutrition as a means of acquiring and maintaining healthy teeth, tongue, lips and gums. We have read and analyzed a fairly representative group of articles written by Dr. Roth, alone or in collaboration with colleagues. In each case, you will note that his treatment was based on an analysis of causes, and that the remedy was one not merely intended to relieve, but to cure—usually by adding missing nutrients and eliminating harmful foods. There is much to be said for this type of treatment, and we know that the advantages will become increasingly clear as the deadly effects of modern drugs continue to show themselves.

Dentistry Has an Obligation to the People

Doctor Roth's general attitude toward dentistry and its obligation to the people is best expressed in an article by him which appeared in the *Journal of the American Dental Association* (January, 1945). "Dentistry," he said, "has up to the present failed to fulfill its full obligation as a health service. . . . The discovery of nutritional deficiencies by means of routine oral examination and the institution of vitamin therapy and improvement of dietary intakes are important responsibilities of the dentist."

It is Dr. Roth's belief that the dentist has marvelous opportunities for diagnosis and treatment of disease in its early stages. He reminds us that most dental patients appear to be well and are not under the care of a physician. The dentist has the opportunity in the course of his examination to spot the signs of nutritional deficiencies, many of which make their appearance in and around the mouth, and to begin treatment by which he might be able to forestall future complications of a more serious nature.

Why Some Dentists Fail with Nutritional Therapy

Dr. Roth has had gratifying results in treating disease conditions of the mouth with therapy based on nutrition. He freely admits that many of his colleagues have not been so successful, but he feels that the failure of their patients to respond is due, not to the need of some other treatment, but to inexperience through which the dentist fails to consider certain factors. First of all, sufficient dosage of vitamins must be maintained over a long enough period. For example, Dr. Roth sometimes prescribes 500 milligrams of vitamin C per day for a full year. Another mistake often made is the attempt to treat long-standing vitamin deficiencies by ordinary dietary means. If essential vitamins are lacking, heroic dosages are often necessary to repair damage before any normal maintenance of good health can be hoped for. The dentist must also consider conditions present in the body which might interfere with the proper absorption of the prescribed vitamins by the tissues. If such a condition is present, the vitamins administered, no matter how badly they are needed, simply don't get a chance to work, and, therefore, don't seem to relieve the patient's condition.

Eight Out of Nine Improved

Dr. Roth has demonstrated the effectiveness of his theories many times. In the magazine, *Oral Surgery, Oral Medicine and Oral Pathology* (June, 1957), he reported on the results of treating bleeding gums in 3 sets of experimental patients. The first set consisted of 9 patients who were given 6 tablets of an ascorbic acid (vitamin C) bioflavonoid formula per day. The second group of 8 people received 6 tablets per day which contained no active ingredient at all, and the third set of 8 people received no tablets at all.

The 3 groups were examined bi-weekly for 3 months. At the end of that time, there was improvement noted in 8 of the 9 persons getting the vitamin supplement, while only 3 of the 8 who received the inactive tablets were improved and only 3 of those receiving nothing had improved. It was concluded, however, that vitamins were not the only factor in this experiment's results. Stress and mental state seemed to have an effect, too. Still it is obvious that chances for recovery were greatly enhanced by the vitamin therapy used.

Even Biting a Sandwich Caused Bleeding Gums

To get down to a more particular case history, consider the report by Dr. Roth, carried in the *New York State Dental Journal* (May, 1950). It discusses the case of a young man of 19 whose gums were so tender and bled so readily that blood would be found on his pillow in the morning. Even biting into a sandwich would cause them to bleed, as would tooth-brushing. A blood specialist was consulted, and blood transfusions were administered to control the blood losses the patient had sustained. A weekly dose of mineral oil (1½ ounces) was prescribed to relieve the patient's constipation complaint, and he also began to take some vitamin C.

When his condition persisted, he consulted Dr. Roth. Dr. Roth believes the history of the patient's illnesses, habits, diet, type of work, etc., to be of great value in determining the cause of his condition. In the course of giving this history, the patient disclosed that he ate 12 to 15 breakfast buns with coffee each day of the 5-day working week. He explained that they were given to him in exchange for errand-running for a local restaurant-owner.

Diet Radically Changed

One of the first things Dr. Roth prescribed was the discontinuance of all refined carbohydrates (cakes, pies, candies, sodas, white bread and alcohol), and the substitution of whole wheat bread, cereals, fruit-juices, milk, eggs and raw salads. Also, 600 milligrams of vitamin C per day were added to the patient's diet. After only two days on the diet, the bleeding onto the pillow stopped and the bowel action showed improvement. In two weeks, the bleeding that occurred when the patient would chew his food stopped. Even biting into an apple caused no bleeding. The patient's employer testified that the boy's work was improved, too.

After 4 weeks, the doctor prescribed 3 multiple vitamin capsules per day and 18 desiccated liver capsules (for B vitamins) per day, as well as the maintenance of the new diet the patient had been eating. There was no other treatment, yet in 4 months from the start of treatment, the patient's mouth and gums were completely healed.

A similar case is recorded in the *Journal of the American Dental Association* (April, 1951). This time Dr. Roth made the report in collaboration with Dr. Stone. This patient was an attorney of 39 who complained of bleeding, painful gums and bad breath. Upon the simple administration of 1000 milligrams of vitamin C per day, the following results were evident: bleeding stopped, there was improvement in gum tone, a discoloration of the tongue disappeared, the pain in the gums was gone and there was a reduction in unpleasant taste and mouth odor.

The lawyer discovered that all of the symptoms returned as soon as the vitamin C therapy was discontinued.

Mental Stress Can Cause Mouth Problems

Dr. Roth found that mental attitude or stress can cause peculiar symptoms, quite aside from a need for dietary supplementation. In the *New York Journal of Dentistry* (January, 1957), he discusses several mechanical manifestations of stress, such as gnashing and grinding of teeth, or clamping them tightly shut in sleep or when awake. He tells us that these are expressions of nervous tension, conscious or unconscious aggressive tendencies. They can have quite harmful effects on the teeth and gums.

Dryness of the mouth in which the mucous membranes of the lips and cheeks cling to the teeth, causing both pain and annoyance, can have a psychic origin, too. An illustrative case is offered of a woman of 43, unmarried, who complained of just such a dryness. The only treatment given her, after examination disclosed no deficiencies that could be responsible, was a vitamin pill and an inactive pill containing no medication to be taken on regular schedule. The symptoms were soon relieved, and it was the physician's opinion that the useless daily pill and the advice and reassurance gained from consultation were largely responsible for the lady's recovery.

Careful History-Taking Reveals Bad Biting Habits

Another possible cause of aggravation of diseases of the teeth and gums is abnormal biting habits. Here again the patient's history is important, for if the dentist fails to investigate a patient's personal habits, he may fail to unearth one of these important causative factors. For example, a male patient of 19 complained of recurrent abscesses in the maxillary molar regions of his mouth. The teeth there were loose, and the area was very painful. Questioning the patient revealed that the patient had a habit of chewing prune pits and other fruit pits as well as match sticks. He chewed a pencil or a pen during his college lectures and study periods. It was concluded that such chewing was the cause. The patient desisted from the habit and the condition cleared up.

You will notice that in each of the above cases, a natural solution was found. The core of the problem was explored and treated, not only the symptoms. Pain killers and drugs seem to have little place in Dr. Roth's practice. He substitutes diet and food supplements.

The procedure Dr. Roth follows is easy enough for anyone to adopt. If you are having any gum problems, you haven't got much choice. Get the refined carbohydrates out of your diet and fill it in with unprocessed, wholesome foods; then add vitamin supplements such as desiccated liver or brewer's yeast and vitamin C. Unless yours is a structural difficulty of the jaws, you'll see the difference, and soon.

26. Nutrition Should Be Complete for Gum Health

Dental caries is, of course, one of our foremost health problems, but there seems to be an increasing incidence of other troubles about the mouth and especially the gums. Bleeding gums seem to show an almost immediate response to vitamin C and the bioflavonoids, according to many dentists whose writings on the subject have appeared in noted professional journals. Several other doctors have written that their success in treating mouth disorders, aside from tooth decay, is due to a conditioning of the patient with vitamin C and a multiple vitamin preparation, before any other work is done. Whatever the approach, many doctors and dentists agree that the problem is nutritional.

In the July, 1958, issue of *Parodontopathies,* Joseph C. Muhler wrote that he does not believe that a single nutrient lies at the bottom of every problem involving the gums and mouth. He offers a good bit of evidence to show that nutritional needs are multiple in these cases. Complete nutrition, he says, is especially important in maintaining good resistance to disease in the tissues. Most workers today, says Muhler, are of the opinion that protein deficiency results in increased incidence of periodontal (gum) disease due to reduced resistance to infection and impaired healing. When one considers that protein actually supplies the raw materials for building tissue in the same way that bricks provide the raw material for building a wall, its importance in maintaining healthy gums becomes clear.

Fats and Calcium

A factor that receives very little mention in discussions of this topic is the part dietary fats play. Recent studies have shown a relationship between capillary resistance (of major importance where bleeding and bruising are concerned) and the fats one eats. Fats are also related to the body's proper use of certain essential minerals. Interestingly enough, the use of minerals such as calcium and phosphorus is not exclusively concerned with the teeth and bones, for a study has shown that the lower the calcium intake of the subjects, the greater the degree of periodontal or gum disease. Not only, then, is it necessary to maintain a good intake of minerals but a proper balance of dietary fats must be present to make use of them.

Blood studies were done on a group of periodontitis patients to determine deficiencies of specific nutrients in the blood. A greater percentage of nutritional shortages was seen in these subjects than in a control group. An examination of the food intake of both groups indicated that a large percentage of the individuals fell below recommended standards for calories, calcium, protein, phosphorus, iron and the B complex. Vitamin C was especially low in the blood serum of a large number of the periodontitis patients, though they were considered to have taken an adequate amount of this vitamin. Dr. Muhler suggests that this vitamin was, for some reason, not being properly utilized.

Emotions May Play a Part

The interaction of the various parts of the body, one on the other, is illustrated by Dr. Muhler's contention that the emotions and mentality are involved with some cases of periodontitis. He says that almost every case of sudden serious tissue destruction of the gums is connected with emotional disturbance and/or certain personality variables. As proof he offers the record compiled at Camp Kilmer, New Jersey, during an 8 week period of study. All patients referred to the periodontics section of the dental clinic were included in the study. Sixty-six patients who showed either serious tissue destruction of the gums, or mere inflammation of the gums, were tested and interviewed. Patients with the more severe gum problem tended to have the most disturbed personality adjustment. Prior to the occurrence of their current problem these men had had some emotional stress which could have brought on the condition. Of those with the serious acute tissue destruction, 41 per cent had either severe or moderate stress prior to their illness, while only 15 per cent of those with the painful, but less serious, inflammation of the gums had had any recent emotional difficulty.

Dr. Muhler's final observation is concerned with enzymes. He has seen evidence of the efficiency of enzymatic medications in promoting the healing of open wounds by the speedy elimination of pus, which makes far better and faster granulation of tissue. It follows from this that proper enzyme supply in the body will prevent, or at least promote the healing of, disorders of the gums.

The whole of Dr. Muhler's paper is a statement of our belief: complete nutrition is necessary for complete health. Each of our organs is somehow dependent upon the function of the other, and, while specific nutrients are known to have "specialities" in aiding the workings of certain parts of the body, they always rely on the presence of other nutrients for their best effects. This is one reason for the slow acceptance of nutrition as a treatment for disease among many patients and physicians. While oftentimes it is possible to achieve startling results with a single vitamin or mineral, sometimes a general reworking of the entire dietary system is required before results begin to show. But when they do show, the results are lasting, as compared with the temporary relief sometimes following a quick injection of the common antibiotics or hormones.

Whether the problem is sore and bleeding gums, skin problems or colitis, the cure lies in a program of complete nutrition, not just one vitamin for a few weeks, but all of the vitamins all of the time—either in the foods we eat or natural supplements.

27. How to Prevent Pyorrhea

Would you be very much surprised to learn that more teeth are lost because of pyorrhea than because of tooth decay? One authority (Don Mosher, D.D.S. in the *Military Surgeon* for April, 1942) tells us that more teeth are lost from the ravages of this disease than from all other sources combined. Pyorrhea has been known by physicians since the days of Hippocrates—the fifth century B.C. The Egyptians, the Greeks, the Romans and the early Chinese suffered from pyorrhea, judging from descriptions of the disease in their medical literature.

Dr. Mosher goes on to tell us that the beginning of pyorrhea can be detected 5 years before it becomes serious—by the use of X-ray. The disease resembles tuberculosis in that it progresses very slowly, giving no warning by pain or discomfort. Normal gum and mouth tissues are light pink, firm and in firm contact with teeth, all spaces between teeth being neatly filled in with gum tissue. Pyorrhea might be defined as chronic gingivitis or gum disease. In pyorrhea the gums are swollen and red, they bleed easily and are tender to the touch. As the disease progresses, the gum tissues detach themselves gradually from the teeth, the gums become thick, hard and leathery and eventually the bony foundation of the tooth roots is destroyed, the teeth become loose and must be extracted. Tooth decay is a disease of youth, claiming the majority of its victims among teenagers. Pyorrhea is a disease of middle age and old age, which leads us to believe, of course, that it is a degenerative disease and hence that it *can* be prevented.

Some Reasons For Pyorrhea

Very often pyorrhea is not accompanied by tooth decay. It can occur in mouths which have been carefully tended from the point of view of hygiene. Apparently there are mechanical reasons for some cases of pyorrhea. Chewing always on one side of the mouth can bring it on. Malocclusion (and most of us suffer from some degree of malocclusion) can produce pyorrhea, because the stresses and strains of chewing can work havoc with teeth and gums alike when teeth are not arranged in the proper pattern to share these stresses. Excessive tartar can cause pyorrhea by accumulating along the gums and irritating them until pus pockets are formed. Yet we are acquainted with people who take meticulous care of their mouths, brushing their teeth carefully after each meal and these folks still have excessive tartar on their teeth. Hence they are likely candidates for pyorrhea. Periodontists have developed many treatments for dealing with gum disorders caused by malocclusion, such as filing off any teeth which may be out of line just enough to throw the rest of the teeth "out of occlusion."

There are other gum diseases, among them Vincent's disease or Trench Mouth (so-called because during World War I it was common among soldiers). Trench mouth begins with a germ that may be passed from person to person on cutlery or dishes. It results in ulcers of the gums, mouth and throat, which are extremely painful and pus-laden. The business of curing it may take weeks or even months for, if the victim is to go on eating, it is impossible to keep the inside of his mouth sterile.

In spite of all the wonders of modern medicine, tooth decay, which affects almost everyone in civilized countries is still a mystery. We do not know what causes it. Some scientists claim that it is caused by the acid formed when carbohydrates are eaten, some say it is the result of refining foods so that we do not have as much chewing to do as our ancestors had, some say it results from lack of calcium and other minerals, some persist in affirming that brushing teeth faithfully will arrest tooth decay. Pyorrhea presents us, we believe, with a much easier problem to solve and we are convinced we know how pyorrhea can be prevented. If you have pyorrhea already, your dentist is probably giving you treatments. You should by all means continue with these treatments. But this does not prevent you from undertaking a health program of your own which may make the dentist's treatments unnecessary! Look at the evidence we have assembled on preventing pyorrhea and judge for yourself.

Vitamin A Is Important

J. A. Sinclair, D.D.S., in an article in the *Journal of the American Dental Association* for October, 1939, tells us, "Experiments conducted by May Mellanby showed that pyorrhea develops readily in dogs on diets deficient in vitamin A, while on similar diets with this vitamin added the gums remain normal. 'The fact that nerves are affected by a vitamin A deficient diet' she writes, 'suggests that possibly diseases of the gums develop in the first place as the result of loss of neurotrophic control (that is, the control of the relationship between nerves and nutrition) and later lead to pyorrhea'." Dr. Sinclair reminds us that just getting enough vitamin A in the diet is not enough. We must be sure, too, that the vitamin is being absorbed and properly used. In cases of digestive and liver trouble, vitamin A may not be assimilated. In youngsters who are growing fast, more vitamin A is needed. In patients with severe infections, vitamin A is used up so rapidly by body tissues that there is never enough left for ordinary functions.

Paul E. Boyle, D.M.D., Otto Bessey, Ph.D., and Burt Wolbach, M.D., writing in the November, 1937, issue of the *Journal of the American Dental Association,* tell us that "experimental rickets and vitamin A deficiency in laboratory animals have been shown to affect the paradental (gum) structures," although they believe that these disorders are not similar to human gum disease. J. D. King, Ph.D., D.P.D., L.D.S., in the *Medical Journal of Malaya,* December, 1946, has this to say about vitamin A and pyorrhea: "As regards the use of vitamin A in the prevention and treatment of human paradental (gum) disease, little reliable information is available. On the basis of the animal investigations, however, we should be well advised to insist on a liberal supply of this food factor in the dietary of the expectant and lactating mother and of her offspring at least up to puberty, in order to insure that the gum epithelium and alveolar bone are properly formed."

Vitamin B and Pyorrhea

The relation of vitamin B to healthy gums is discussed at length by Dr. Sinclair who reminds us that Vincent's disease occurs often among people afflicted with pellagra—a vitamin B deficiency disease. He describes cases in which the redness and soreness disappeared almost miraculously within a day after the pellagra patient was given niacin—the B vitamin most concerned in pellagra. He also tells us that a gangrenous condition of the gums was produced in monkeys on a diet deficient in vitamin B. And once again, he mentions that it is not enough just to get ample vitamin B in the diet—there are times when a great deal more is needed. "Certain patients who preoperatively showed few or no signs of vitamin deficiency developed frank deficiency following operation. Fever increases the vitamin B requirement and in an individual whose vitamin intake has for any reason been impaired prior to operation, fever occurring postoperatively may result in a very rapid development of deficiency, particularly if the intake of food is inadequate during this time. We have noted that patients with achlorhydria (lack of hydrochloric acid in the stomach) show evidence of deficiency even when the dietary intake is adequate."

Dr. Sinclair tells us, too, that sensitivity of teeth and gums to thermal changes and to instruments seems to depend entirely on their supply of vitamin B. Time and again, he says, patients who could not drink hot or cold liquids and suffered anguish at the touch of a dental instrument were relieved of all these symptoms by a large dose of vitamin B. He has found that in every case of Vincent's disease and pyorrhea, his patients who were treated with vitamins A, B and C responded well.

Dr. King has personally treated 500 patients with Vincent's disease, using niacin (one of the B vitamins) which, he says, seems to restore some link in the chain of tissue respiration. He once gave himself Vincent's disease so that he might observe it first-hand. And he came to the conclusion, he says, that "the condition is likely to occur only in persons whose general resistance is depressed by defective nutrition or other illness." . . . We were glad to find, too, that Dr. King agrees with us as to *how* one should take vitamin B. . . . "One important point of agreement appears to be that in many animals the sum of the known vitamin B_2 components in their synthetic state is by no means as effective as the whole complex in the form of less artificial products, such as yeast and liver preparations." If you are not getting enough vitamins in your daily meals, take natural food supplements in which these vitamins are concentrated—but don't take synthetic vitamins!

Relation of Vitamin C to Pyorrhea

It seems to us that any researcher seeking to prevent or cure pyorrhea would think first of vitamin C, because of the serious gum disease that accompanies scurvy. And so we find that a great deal of constructive work has been done along these lines. We know for instance that pyorrhea is almost universal in Newfoundland and is accompanied with heavy deposits of tooth tartar. The diet of Newfoundland is remarkably lacking in fresh fruits and vegetables which, of course, contain vitamin C. In the British West Indies, on the other hand, where vitamin C-rich fruits are eaten in great quantity the year 'round, there is little or no pyorrhea.

Dr. Sinclair reminds us that vitamin C deficiency destroys the body's ability to rebuild tissues and fibers such as the tissues of the gums. He tells us that he completely cured two patients of pyorrhea by giving them 150 milligrams of vitamin C daily for 30 days. Dr. Boyle tells us that among 66 patients examined at the Harvard Dental School, more than half had far less vitamin C than normal in their blood. And all of these patients had marked disease of the gums. "Ten of these patients in the low level range were given pure vitamin C by mouth and showed clinical improvement in the periodontal structures coincidental with increase in the blood ascorbic acid (vitamin C)."

In another *Dental Association Journal* article (October 1, 1944) J. S. Restarski, M.D.S., D.D.S., and M. Pijoan describe an experiment in which they induced scurvy in 6 volunteers. The diet was complete in every way, except that it lacked vitamin C. Within 5 or 6 months, these subjects showed the classical signs of scurvy—hemorrhage, fatigue, etc.—but did not seem to have any gum disorders. From this Dr. Restarski and M. Pijoan conclude that, while gum diseases might have developed if they had been left on the diet longer, a lack of vitamin C cannot be taken as one of the causes of pyorrhea. Of course, we differ in this conclusion. Let us relate one more experiment and then we'll tell you why we disagree.

C. D. Marshall Day, Ph.D., D.M.D. and K. L. Shourie, M.B., B.S., describe in the *Indian Journal of Medical Research* an experiment at an orphanage in India. All the children were on the regular orphanage diet —high in cereals and low in fruits and vegetables. Many of the children suffered from gingivitis and tooth tartar. Fifty of them were given 100 milligrams of vitamin C per day for 100 days in addition to the regular diet, while 50 others who acted as controls, ate the regular diet with no added vitamin C. The results were disappointing, say Drs. Day and Shourie. There was some slight improvement in the children taking the vitamin C, but not enough to make much difference.

What is your conclusion? Do these two experiments prove that vitamin C is not important in preventing pyorrhea? To us they prove exactly the opposite—vitamin C is vitally concerned in the prevention of pyorrhea, *but*—pyorrhea is a disease of several deficiencies, not just vitamin C! The volunteers who gave themselves scurvy did not get pyorrhea because their diet contained ample vitamins B and A and other important factors. The Indian children were already eating a diet so low in vitamins A, B and C that the mere addition of one of these—vitamin C—could not stop the disease. On the other hand, Dr. Sinclair brought about astounding cures by giving his patients large doses of all 3 vitamins! And mark that fact well—Dr. Sinclair did not just tell his patients to eat a well-rounded diet and let it go at that. He took for granted that they were simply not getting enough of these 3 important vitamins in their diet and he gave them *large doses* of all 3 vitamins.

Minerals Are Involved, Too

Other researchers have turned up valuable material concerning mineral deficiency and pyorrhea. First Lieutenant William A. Musgrave, D.D.S., writing in the *Military Surgeon* for February, 1941, tells us that the calcium-phosphorus balance is an important consideration in pyorrhea patients. Testing his patients for the amount of calcium and phosphorus in their blood, he found that by far the largest number of those with pyorrhea had a high phosphorus-low calcium ratio. That is, their diets contained far too much phosphorus in relation to the amount of calcium they obtained. Meat and cereals are high in phosphorus. Milk and green leafy vegetables contain calcium, so it is not surprising to find many American soldiers with their calcium-phosphorus balance upside down.

Dr. Musgrave found congested, bleeding gums, soft tissue pocket formation and excessive tartar deposits above and below the gums. "The high phosphorus pulls the calcium out of the body with loss of bone density" says he, "if the calcium leaves the body by way of the saliva, heavy salivary and serumal (serum) deposits are found on the teeth. If the calcium is lost by way of the urine, the saliva may be so low in calcium that erosion or gingival caries may result with very little tartar found." He advises diets with meat and eggs 6 times per week, whole grain cereals, very little candy or sweets, one raw salad per day, one or two non-starchy cooked vegetables per day, raw fruits for dessert, plenty of cheese and butter, and one or two glasses of raw fruit or vegetable juices per day. (We believe one should avoid all sweets as well as all dairy products.)

Allison G. James, D.D.S., of Beverly Hills, writing in the *Annals of Western Medicine and Surgery,* September, 1947, states, "With the understanding that nutrition is the process by which growth is promoted and health maintained, and that disease represents disturbed nutrition of the cells, part or organism affected, dental pathologic lesions receive a more logical consideration than is possible from the mechanistic point of view." Dr. James believes that the inclusion of refined foods and sugars in our diet is responsible not only for pyorrhea but also for tooth decay. Here are the conclusions he comes to: "1. Inclusion of a proportion of refined grain and sugar products in the diet beyond the tolerance of the patient appears as the chief causative factor in dental caries and paradentosis (gum disorders). 2. Proportionately as the phosphorus intake increases beyond the one and one-half ratio to calcium, the vertical atrophy (disease) of paradentosis increases. 3. For prevention and control of dental disease, diets of 2000 calories may not safely be diluted by refined grains and sugar products."

Our Conclusions

In conclusion we want to quote from a most encouraging and sensible article by Anna P. Boudin, D.D.S., which appeared in the *Medical Woman's Journal* for April, 1943. It is especially gratifying to know that this article was written 18 years ago when vitamin research had not progressed nearly to the point where it is today. Yet Dr. Boudin courageously lays the entire blame for tooth and gum disease right where it belongs—in faulty nutrition. She describes an experimental study in which 4 groups of monkeys were maintained on different diets. The first group ate a regulation laboratory diet, supplemented with *all the vitamins.* They showed no gum disease, even though the germs of gum disease were found in their mouths. Their good nutrition enabled them to withstand these germs. The second group had a diet deficient in vitamin C, with added supplements of vitamins A and D. They all developed diseases of the mouth and lost their teeth. The third group was given a diet deficient in vitamin C plus supplements of vitamins A and D and several of the B vitamins. They developed "slight to moderate" diseases and all showed a definite increase in the number of germs present. The fourth group was given a diet deficient in one of the B vitamins, but with plenty of vitamins A, C and D and other members of the B group. Fifty-four per cent of them developed gingivitis in addition to anemia, loss of appetite, weakness and diarrhea. Germs from the mouths of diseased animals were transferred to the mouths of the first group on the full diet with all the vitamin supplements. These well-nourished animals did not become diseased and the injected areas healed promptly.

Dr Boudin says, "It has been found that a diet completely lacking in vitamin C produces extensive gingivitis (in guinea pigs, monkeys and man). However, vitamin C therapy alone failed to produce a cure. Generally, when the vitamin C intake is low, multiple deficiency may be present. Therefore, each patient suspected of vitamin C deficiency should be studied from all aspects."

It seems to us that any reasonable person, studying the evidence we have presented, can come to only one conclusion—pyorrhea is indeed a deficiency disease—not a disease involving deficiency of one food element but many. So, if you wish to prevent pyorrhea as you grow older—and remember, it destroys more teeth than all other causes put together—do not decide to do it by taking one food supplement alone. That won't work. Vitamins A and D are contained in fish liver oil. All the B vitamins are in brewer's yeast and desiccated liver. Vitamin C is most abundant in rose hips and other natural vitamin C supplements. The proper ratio of calcium and phosphorus is found in bone meal, along with other important minerals. You can't get along without *all* of them. And by taking just one or just two of these supplements, you may be leaving out the very vitamin or mineral in which you are most deficient.

If you possibly can, get all your vitamins and minerals in your daily food. But because most of us must eat some food that has been refined and denatured and hence, is lacking in vitamins and minerals, we believe sincerely that most of us should take natural food supplements which will guarantee rich amounts of all the important food elements. Certainly, if you suspect that your gums are not as healthy as they might be—and remember pyorrhea progresses silently and without warning—be sure to supplement your meals with the food supplements we have mentioned above.

28. Bioflavonoids for Gum Disease

In an article in *Dental Digest* for August, 1956, on the subject of bioflavonoids for periodontal disease, Joseph D. Lieberman, D.D.S., of New York tells us that diseases of the gums (such as pyorrhea) cause the loss of far more teeth than all other dental diseases combined. Soft, swollen, tender, reddened gums that ooze blood or bleed profusely at the slightest touch of a toothbrush—these are symptoms of periodontal disease.

Says Dr. Lieberman, "Among the nutritional disturbances prominent in relation to nutrition and gingival (gum) health are those associated with ascorbic acid (vitamin C) deficiency. This may be demonstrated by the frequent occurrences of a low-grade infectious gingivitis among school children which McCall points out may be the result of, or at least associated with, subclinical vitamin C deficiency."

For his investigation, Dr. Lieberman gave a bioflavonoid-vitamin C-vitamin K preparation to 101 patients, ranging in age from 22 to 84 years, for whom the "usual conventional methods of treatment" had been unsuccessful. The patients were given 8 tablets daily for the first 10 days (two tablets 4 times a day). For the next 3 weeks the dose was reduced to 4 tablets daily (one tablet 4 times a day). No other treatment was given.

Analyzing 11 typical cases, Dr. Lieberman finds that the treatment resulted in controlling the bleeding and restoring the gums to an "essentially normal healthy condition," in about 90 per cent of the cases within 10 to 30 days! The tablets which Dr. Lieberman used in this experiment contained 50 milligrams of (synthetic) vitamin C, 2 milligrams of (synthetic) vitamin K and a total of 72 milligrams of the various parts of the bioflavonoid complex of substances. As you can see, such a preparation would give only 400 milligrams of vitamin C per day and a similarly small amount of the bioflavonoids. But even these doses were effective against an ailment that affects almost everyone in our land over middle age!

Note, too, that the tablets contained synthetic vitamins. We are convinced that far more impressive results can be obtained using natural vitamin preparations. Why? The story of the bioflavonoids is the best answer to this question. For many years we have known that vitamin C is necessary for good health and powerful against many human disorders. But our scientists did not even know of such a substance as bioflavonoids until recently.

But health-conscious people who were taking natural vitamin preparations all along got the bioflavonoids along with their vitamin C, so actually they had the benefit of this scientific discovery long before it was made, for the simple reason that they believed that nature knows best and that taking food in natural forms is best. What other food elements are there that naturally go along with vitamin C and the flavonoids? Scientists do not know as yet, but you will be getting them all in natural food supplements such as rose hips and, of course, in your daily meals, chiefly in fresh raw fruits.

~~~~~~

SECTION 8: THE HAIR

~~~~~~

29. Are You Good to Your Hair?

Probably the loudest hue and cry about "good looks" comes from the womenfolk—and understandably. But noise or no noise, the men also have their share of concern when it comes to hair, particularly the loss of it.

Baldness

Though there are cases of women losing their hair, they are rare, and the problem of baldness usually confines itself pretty much to men. Specialists, over a long period of time, have tried to find the cause of the general pattern of loss of hair in middle age, and have come up with an amusingly large and varied number of answers. Some say it is purely hereditary; others attribute it to disease of the scalp or some vitamin deficiency, or dandruff. But to most of these reasons, the question can usually be asked: "Why does it not happen to women?" Women may have poor circulation, they wear hats more frequently than men, often, and their scalps are not always models of health or free from dandruff.

We, unfortunately, cannot supply the answer, but probably, as Dr. James B. Hamilton of the Long Island College of Medicine, states, the basic reasons are due to 3 principal factors: genetic inheritance, age and the presence of a plentiful supply of male hormones. Perhaps, as Dr. Marion Sulzberger (who is bald), of the New York University Postgraduate Medical School, humorously reasons: "Perhaps hair, like tails, is something left over from man's early ancestry. Perhaps we baldheaded men are a step higher on the evolution ladder than our wives." In any case, it seems right to assume that it is a natural phenomenon, which, unless a method is found to prevent it, is bound to occur in many a male.

However, in this matter of prevention, we should not scoff too heartily at all the theories and reasons for its existence as they can give us clues as to possible cures, and eventually prevention itself. In an article in

[105]

Science News Letter, for November 10, 1951, an account is given of the findings of Dr. Peter Flesch and associates at the University of Pennsylvania in Philadelphia, which state: "Men get bald because the male sex hormone stimulates oil-producing glands in the skin to change the amount or quality of the oil they produce. . . . The skin oil is technically termed sebum. When painted on the skin of rabbits and mice, all the rabbits and many of the mice lost their hair in 10 days." In his experiments, Dr. Flesch also found that excessive amounts of vitamin A taken over a long period of time may lead to loss of hair, particularly in children. As with his experiments with sebum, Dr. Flesch and his staff painted vitamin A on the skins of their laboratory animals, with the result that the animals lost their hair. Next, the doctors hope to be able to find a way to check baldness in humans.

Since there is evidence that few Americans get enough vitamin A, there seems little chance that too much vitamin A would be causing the widespread baldness among American men, especially since baldness is unknown among many peoples whose vitamin A intake is far greater than ours.

In the matter of circulation nothing has actually been proved, but it is generally believed that regrowth can occur through massage, frequent brushing and methods of bringing the blood into the hair region. Charles V. Ferrante, in his book, *Baldness—Its Cause—Its Prevention,* published by the author, after examining many theories for baldness, arrives at the simple conclusion that lack of exercise of the scalp is the sole cause of men's loss of hair on the crown of the head. He states that women do not lose their hair because they have always had to "exercise" it from earliest childhood, while men's hair needs no such tending, for appearance's sake. The reason men do not lose their hair on the sides and in the back is that these regions receive friction from the pillow at night, while the crown does not. He discredits the male hormone theory, citing the lack of baldness in male Indians.

We have two more suggestions—just suggestions—as to why men may become bald while women do not. Could one reason be the tight collars men wear, which women do not? Or could it be the fact that women, in general, have wider arteries than men? We have heard that this is so and it occurs to us that this may result in better circulation in general among women.

Graying

Graying is another hair problem which men share with women, and causes them the same concern. Is gray hair a necessary part of growing old? Can it be prevented, and what about the cases of gray, or even snow white hair which occur at a much earlier age? Though the experiments have dealt mainly with animals, diet has been found to be the key to the problem. Animals have been fed diets in which one or another of the vitamins is lacking. Then they have been observed to see whether there is a loss of hair color. If so, the vitamin is then replaced in the diet to see whether the color will return.

Dr. James Hundley, of the National Institute of Health at Bethesda, Maryland, found significant results when he experimented with rats a few years ago. Reporting to the International Physiological Congress in Copenhagen, Denmark (*Newsweek,* August 28, 1950), he stated that in his studies of some 200 black rats he had found copper to be a necessary element in the diet for normal hair growth and color in rats. When Dr. Hundley increased the amount of copper in the diets of rats whose hair had turned gray from inadequate diets, the hair suddenly started darkening in 5 days, and a complete change back to black hair occurred in 3 months.

In experiments by Dr. Douglas V. Frost and F. Pierce Dann, reported in the *Journal of Nutrition,* for May, 1944, laboratory animals were fed good diets which contained also synthetic B vitamins—thiamin, riboflavin, niacin, pantothenic acid and pyridoxine. Within two to eleven months the animals' hair began to gray. Weight decreases, anemia and other indications of ill health accompanied the grayness. None of the female animals came in heat or could be bred successfully during this time. No change took place even when 3 other B vitamins were added—inositol, para-amino-benzoic acid and choline. Then the experimenters took whole liver and, by chemical means, separated out those vitamins mentioned above, and fed the animals the remaining part of the liver, the "filtrate factor." Others they fed whole brewer's yeast. Almost immediately rejuvenation of the hair began, as well as improvement in hair growth, weight, appetite and muscle tone. So it was found that something in liver and yeast, aside from the known vitamins, brought about the change.

There are many other theories about the cause of loss of color in the hair, for example the effect of sulfa drugs. It is believed they rob the body of its store of pantothenic acid, another B vitamin. This is discussed by Harold D. West and Raven Rivera Elliott in *Archives of Biochemistry* for January, 1948. Dr. E. Geiringer, of Edinburgh, suggests in the *Revue Medical de Liège,* October 15, 1950, that vitamin C may play an important role in the preservation of hair pigment.

When all the evidence is in, the major guilt seems to lie in diet. We cannot say, after hearing all the testimony, that we can be sure of any one vitamin or food factor as being the single cause of grayness. But we do believe it is obvious that when grayness occurs some one or a variety of the valuable food elements is missing. *We* recommend the following food supplements if there is a suspicion of deficiency in your diet: Fish liver oil perles for vitamins A and D; desiccated liver and/or brewer's yeast for all the B vitamins; vitamin C from natural food supplements and minerals from bone meal.

Care of the Hair

The question has often been asked as to the damage done by hair dyes and permanent wave lotions and chemicals. We believe that nothing should be put on the scalp—creams, lotions, soaps, even water—as they tend to alkalize a normally acid scalp and destroy the natural oils. But medical verdicts have proclaimed that no serious harm is *normally* done when these substances are cautiously used. Though beauty-parlor treatments and home permanent-wave sets have been thoroughly tested for the *average* effect, they do not claim to avoid causing a harmful reaction in certain cases of sensitivity.

Some enlightening remarks are given by John Goodwin Downing, AMA of Boston University School of Medicine and Tufts College Medical School, Boston, Massachusetts. Writing in the *Archives of Dermatology and and Syphilology*, Vol. 63, p. 561, May, 1951, he says that there are both mechanical and chemical dangers to scalp health. Metals used in connection with the hair may cause trouble. In the case of the chemicals, most of the dangerous and irritating ones have been removed by the industry, but they cannot, of course, remove all the substances to which individual persons may be sensitive.

He states further that there are many chemicals used that may cause trouble—the oils in bay rum, the synthetic perfumes in brilliantine, the various oils and resins in creams and wave preparations. The scalp lotions and tonics contain irritants and other substances that may sensitize individuals. Shampoos contain perfume and various sulfur mixtures, coconut oil shampoos are perfumed with several synthetic oils, any one of which may be harmful to individual users. "Hair dyes and rinses are the oldest but still the most dangerous hazard of the hairdressers' trade," he says.

Reporting on the ultra-fashionable fashion in 1950, *Time* magazine had an article on the latest hair style—the "chignon," or false buns, braids or curls. Speaking of the hair used for such glamorous creations, Joseph Fleischer & Company, in Manhattan, made this interesting comment: "Only hair bought from European women has the quality necessary for good chignons . . . the hair of American women is damaged by too much pampering, tinting and shampooing (all the things the beauty shops do to it). The hair of European women is like a well-manured garden. The quality is good, but sometimes it doesn't smell too well."

We believe that the hair will keep its health and natural lustre, and hence its beauty, if it is allowed to grow unmolested by any solution or process, letting the natural oils do the work, along with frequent brushing and exercising of the scalp. Editor Rodale does not wash his hair, but cleans it with vigorous brushing. His barber has remarked that he has a very clean and healthy scalp.

Combined with this, as a "beauty prescription" we heartily advise a well-balanced diet, rich in the essential vitamins and minerals. The hair, like the rest of our bodies, must be fed, and, similarly, it responds best to those elements of food which are vital to its life and health.

30. Baldness—Some Remedies Worth Trying

Baldness is usually good for a laugh with everyone except the man who has lost his hair. He is usually busy investigating every theory on how baldness occurs and how regrowth of hair can be accomplished. We have long held that careless diet is the underlying cause of baldness, that somehow or another the man or woman who is a victim of baldness is short of some food element which is a vital part of the body's hair-growing formula. Sometimes putting such an element back into the diet can result in restoration of hair, but inclusion of foods in the diet which might affect hair growth is much more effective in keeping hair than in getting it back.

New theories on what makes hair grow crop up continually. Some are the result of elaborate tests and scientific observation, while others are merely guesses from old-timers who have a full head of hair and are convinced that they owe their good fortune to never having ridden on an escalator. None of these suggested preventives or cures seems to be universally applicable, but we have tried to print all that sound sensible in the hope that someone might benefit.

Flex Your Scalp Muscles

An arresting theory on baldness which might offer a simple clue for avoiding same was contained in the *New York Times* (May 5, 1957). The article described studies by Dr. M. Wharton Young of Howard University, Washington, D.C. which indicated that chances of avoiding baldness are pretty good if one has muscles under the scalp.

To prove his theory, Dr. Young applied electrodes (a means of transmitting electrical current) to hairy and hairless parts of the scalps of bald humans. These electrodes were connected to an electromygraph (a machine which records the electrical response of contracting muscles). The balding subjects were then instructed to try to move their scalp and to try to move their ears. Electrical responses, typical of the activity of muscles, were registered in areas that had hair, while bald spots showed no muscle activity at all. These results confirmed previous studies which showed that muscles under the scalp have a rich supply of blood vessels which bring additional blood for hair follicles in a healthy head of hair.

This theory of blood vessels under the scalp for healthy hair is one basis for the massage therapy often recommended for a good head of hair, or as an antidote for falling hair. However, if the theory of muscles under the scalp is correct, massage ignores one elementary need, and that is actual exertion of these muscles to strengthen them. It would be a wise form of self-help and preventive medicine to exercise the scalp muscles every day. Simply try to move your scalp consciously by wrinkling your forehead and attempting to move your ears for a few minutes in the morning and at night. It won't cost you a thing, and scientific evidence says it should help you to retain your hair.

A person once suggested to us the novel idea that men suffer from baldness far oftener than women because they cut their hair short while women wear theirs considerably longer. During sleep, while the head is moving around on the pillow, the strands of women's hair pull at the scalp, exercising it in a healthful way, according to this theorizer. Men, with their much shorter hair, do not get the benefit of this unconscious exercise and massage.

A B-Vitamin Helped Many

In her book *Let's Eat Right to Keep Fit,* Adelle Davis recommends the use of the B vitamin inositol, in combination with other sources of B vitamins, in treating baldness. She writes that in almost every case in which inositol therapy was begun, the patient reported that his hair stopped falling out. In some cases new hair growth was obvious within a month. Miss Davis tells of one man of 48 who had been bald for years and grew hair so thick that it looked like rabbit fur. But, she admits, some men grew not a single wisp of hair in spite of their intake of inositol.

We know that the B vitamins are vital to bodily health, especially for nerves and internal organs. New areas of their usefulness are being discovered every day, and their function as a deterrent to baldness is not at all unlikely. Extra intake of B vitamins in the form of brewer's yeast, wheat germ, kidney and liver can only bring added good health whether your baldness is affected or not, so what can you lose? Try inositol as a weapon against baldness that has already begun, and make sure your diet is rich in B vitamins, even if you are not plagued with falling hair, as a preventive measure.

Baldness and Mental Agitation

It has been suggested, and borne out by experiment in many cases, that one's mental state can be responsible for baldness. The *American Practitioner and Digest of Treatment* (April, 1956) carries a report on a study made to determine the frequency and severity of mental illness in patients who come to skin specialists to consult on baldness problems. Out of 44 patients in the study, 32 were psychoneurotic, 9 had some degree of psychotic involvement and only 3 were entirely free from mental illness. It was admitted that the mental stress experienced by these people was made worse by the problem of baldness, but in no case did a previously healthy person become neurotic because of hair loss.

This theory of some baldness being due to mental stress is backed up by an article in *Modern Medicine* (April, 1951), as well as a newspaper column by Gladys P. Thomas, carried in the (Allentown, Pennsylvania) *Evening Chronicle* (August 28, 1958). Miss Thomas, in quoting Dr. Howard Berman, dermatologist, on increased baldness in women of today, blames this fact on women's battling for a place in a man's world. In Dr. Berman's opinion, the cultivation of aggressive masculine traits in women seems to influence their glandular make-up. Such women, he says, are more susceptible to ulcers, high blood pressure, heart disease and male patterned baldness.

Male Hormones Blamed

Many researchers point to the undeniable fact that men are far in the lead when it comes to baldness problems. They connect this fact with an over-production of male hormones, and blame the occasional baldness in women on too many male hormones also. In the previous chapter we have already discussed *Science News Letter's* (November 10, 1951) article on this viewpoint based on work by Dr. Peter Flesch of the University of Pennsylvania in Philadelphia.

Good Health magazine (July, 1950) carried a similar opinion. It said that baldness in the male is due to genetic inheritance, age or a too plentiful supply of male hormones. The article discouragingly states that boys begin to lose hair at their temples from the age of puberty, and that the process continues from there, lifelong and irreversible.

The *Archives of Dermatology and Syphilology* (60: 1116-1119, 1949) prints the finding that tight braids, metal curlers and excessive brushing of hair may lead to traumatic (i.e. due to injury) baldness. Such baldness is usually temporary, unless the injurious practice is continued indefinitely.

The pony-tail hair-do may cause a receding hairline, according to Science Service in the *New York Times* for August 8, 1958. An Austrian physician says that a symmetrical loss of hair at the borderline can be seen in some of the girls and women who wear the pony-tail. A Scandinavian study showed that Eskimo women who combed their hair backward and tied it in pigtails had spots of reduced hair growth in certain areas of the head. Sometimes examination of the hair roots reveals that the hair follicles are regressed, degenerated or inflamed.

Tonics and Lotions Are A Waste of Money

It is the opinion of most experts that there is nothing you can rub on your head, paint on your head or spray on your head that will bring back lost hair. If you insist on treating your baldness from the outside, you might as well settle for a toupee, or hairpiece, as they are now known, because it's the only way you'll ever cover your scalp with hair. If you are willing to try nutrition, you might be successful in growing new hair or halting the mass desertion that might be going on by reducing your salt intake. Perhaps the increase in inositol recommended by Miss Davis, which has worked for some, might work for you. If it doesn't save your hair, you can rest assured that the money was not wasted, for the inositol will be working toward the health of some other part of the body. And exercising the scalp muscles isn't a bad idea either. Exercise of any tissue is healthful and therefore worthwhile; doubly worthwhile since the possibility of its effectiveness in preventing baldness is backed up by scientific research. These are the things to try if baldness threatens, not worthless, sometimes harmful tonics, lotions and cosmetic preparations. Nature meant you to have hair, cooperate with her and you'll keep it—maybe even get it back if it's gone!

Salt and Falling Hair

The dietary culprit that we know as salt has a gift for popping up in the least likely places. Scientists study physiological problems for years, testing the most exotic components of our diets without results, when all of a sudden someone thinks to try testing salt, and finds his answer in that common chemical. This has been the case in heart disease, all types of edema and now salt has shown itself as a contributory cause of baldness.

The concern expressed by people who find they are going bald is often a source of amusement for others. To the true scientist baldness is nothing to laugh at. He is not concerned with the looks of the balding person at all. He is anxious to know if aging, of itself, has anything to do with loss of hair. It is not unreasonable to hope that observations on the nature of baldness might throw some light on other aspects of aging.

Salt in the Scalp Tissues

Eugene Foldes, whose report appeared in *Acta-Dermato-Venereologica* 35: 334, 1955, worked under this hope. He knew that under certain conditions an excess of electrolytes—mainly, sodium chloride (salt)—may accumulate in some tissues and may interfere with the proper function of these tissues. Could it be possible, Foldes wanted to know, that baldness develops when an excess of salt is present in the scalp tissues and actually disturbs or thwarts the function they have of growing hair? Could this function be improved by reducing the amount of sodium chloride in these tissues? He would attempt to do so by administering diuretics which would help the body expel extra fluids and, with them, salt.

Finding a way to scientifically measure this information was truly a challenge. Dr. Foldes decided to consider the number of hairs shed during the experiment as an indication of baldness. Should there be a reduction in the number of hairs falling during the experiment, it would be considered an indication that the therapy was effective. The hairs that fell from the experimental patients were carefully counted, but it was found that the daily hair loss fluctuated regardless of outside influences. This divergence in the numbers of falling hair seemed to even out into a weekly figure that varied less than 10 per cent, and a daily average was then arrived at from the weekly figure.

Shampoo Increases Loss

It was also found that shampooing is accompanied by a larger than average hair loss. This is a factor which balding persons might bear in mind in the interests of preserving what hair they have.

In one case, the patient was a woman of 62 years of age who complained of loss of hair. She was given the diuretic in the form of rectal suppositories, and abstained from shampoo during the period of observation. In her first 3 weeks of therapy the woman reduced her average daily hair loss approximately 46 per cent.

A young male patient had similar results. He had noticed an excessive loss of hair during the last two or three years. In approximately two months his hair loss was reduced from an average daily count of 188 to 74, a decrease of about 60 per cent.

Drugs Only for Experiment

It was found that a tolerance to the drugs being used was likely to occur, and that the drug would then prove to be ineffective in preventing future hair loss.

Though we carry the report of Dr. Foldes' work, it should be understood that we would be strongly opposed to the common use of drugs to prevent baldness. The drugs employed by Dr. Foldes were used only as a means of controlling the salt supply in the tissues of the scalp for experimental purposes. We are certain that he would be against the use of these drugs as a standard treatment for baldness just as we are. What is interesting is that the reduction of salt in the tissues did affect the loss of hair. And it follows that a lower intake of salt would reduce the amount of this chemical in the tissues of the scalp without any drugs at all. Dr. Foldes' theory should then be just as effective concerning a scalp which is kept free of salt in its tissues, as it is where the salt already there has been driven out by the use of drugs.

The balding person who gives up the use of salt in his diet will be doing himself a few other physiological favors aside from holding on to his hair. In past years salt has shown itself to be involved in diseases of the kidney, as well as liver, dropsy, difficulty in childbirth, deafness, headaches and others.

[113]

31. Investigating Headaches

A common ailment, common in fact to about 65 per cent of Americans, an ailment for which individuals seldom seek medical help, but an ailment that afflicts perhaps one per cent of us every single day of our lives—this is headache. Our figures come from a carefully conceived and supervised survey done by Henry D. Ogden, M.D., of New Orleans and presented at the annual meeting of the American Academy of Allergy in New York, February 5, 1951. In his survey Dr. Ogden studied 4,634 individuals whose answers to his questionnaire appear in an article in the *Journal of Allergy* for January, 1952.

These were not patients of the doctor. They were farmers, housewives, students, laborers, salespeople, clerical workers and so forth, selected at random and given a questionnaire to fill in or interviewed by a professional interviewer. The questionnaire included almost every conceivable question that might be asked about headaches, including the subject's own opinion as to what might be causing his headaches.

This is quite a large group of people to be interviewed on one subject and we feel that the answers give a representative picture of what the situation nationally is in regard to headaches. Results showed 64.8 per cent of the 4,634 subjects suffer from headaches. People with headaches have a higher incidence of various respiratory symptoms than people who don't have headaches. There is also quite extensive history of family complaints of allergy of one kind or another among people who have the most headaches. Only 18 per cent of headache sufferers go to a doctor for their headaches. Pain in the front of the head is the commonest kind of headache. There is more headache among women, younger adults, single people, educated individuals, executives, students and professional people. Dr. Ogden also concludes from his survey that along with emotional and occupational problems allergy should be investigated by physicians dealing with headache patients.

We found several other significant things in the results of the survey. Over one per cent of the people interviewed said that they have daily headaches! The percentage of headaches present when the individual wakes from sleep in the morning was 13.3 and 10.2 per cent reported that their headaches appear in the afternoon. Headaches are not so frequent among older people. Of the women answering the questionnaire, 71 per cent had headaches, whereas only 50.7 per cent of the men did. Manual laborers have a very low incidence of headaches. Fatigue and eyestrain are the two most common causes of headache in the opinion of the individuals themselves.

Using figures in a much smaller survey, we find that one doctor questioned 400 adults as to when their migraine headaches began and found that 34 per cent of them reported that they had migraine headaches before the age of 15.

Drugs Are Not the Answer

We have an enormous file of medical articles and articles that have appeared in general magazines on the subject of headache. Most of them consist of discussions of the different kinds of headaches, and there are many, the possible causes, and there are at least 30 of these, and cures ranging all the way from neck stretching to drugs to high protein diet.

We will not discuss the subject of drugs at all. We believe that drugs do not cure and do not prevent headaches. They may of course relieve pain, but they surely do not remove the cause, and in killing the pain, they may well bring about aftereffects or side effects that are as bad as or worse than the headaches. It is pretty generally agreed among members of the medical profession that the worst way to treat a headache is to dose yourself with the advertised headache remedies, without going to a doctor or trying to discover what is causing the headaches. There are many reasons for this. The patent medicine remedy may relieve the pain of your headache and you may postpone indefinitely finding out what causes it . . . a serious mistake. The headache remedy, as in the case of salicylic acid, which is in aspirin and other remedies, may do you serious harm. And, by the constant use of headache remedies, you may develop a genuine drug addiction that will be harder to cure than the headaches.

There May Be An Emotional Basis For Headaches

Most writers on headaches pay some attention to the possible emotional causes. In this, of course, we are not speaking of headaches that have a definite organic cause. Migraine headaches in 15 children studied by 3 physicians of the Headache Clinic of the New York Montefiore Hospital and reported in the *New York State Journal of Medicine* for October 1, 1950, showed that 9 of these children demonstrated definite neurotic tendencies which were apparent just on questioning by the doctors, without the aid of any psychological tests. Only 3 of the remaining 6 children appeared to be well adjusted to their environments. A sample case history is given of a 13-year-old girl whose headaches started at the age of 18 months. In this case the obvious difficulty was the child's relationship with her mother which was tempestuous and violent. They battled constantly, and yet the child was so dependent on her mother that she had few friends, stayed home with her mother whenever she was not at school and went out of the house only in her mother's company. It is easy to see how such a situation could result in chronic headaches with nausea, vomiting and severe prostration, which occurred every 10 weeks with such regularity that future headaches were marked on the calendar for months in advance.

Other observations made during the study indicated that various conflicts in the children resulted also in temper tantrums, unreasonable fears, frequent nightmares, bed-wetting, nail-biting, thumb-sucking and other personality difficulties that go with maladjustment. It seems quite possible to us that when these children grow up they may learn to control the outward manifestations of neurosis such as we have just mentioned, but would not this very suppression of emotion probably bring about even more violent headaches? In other words, the adult cannot fling himself on the floor in a temper tantrum, so, holding in his rage and frustration, may he not develop even worse symptoms?

A physician who writes in the *Medical Journal of Australia* says yes, and he speaks from his own experience in trying to cure his own headaches. J. Bostock, M.D., first experimented on his eyes, purchasing glasses to correct his astigmatism. This had no effect on his headaches. He believed that focal infection might be causing them and had his tonsils removed, with no effect on the headaches. He had read that constipation, resulting in "auto-intoxication" could cause headaches. Keeping his digestive tract completely unobstructed with laxatives made no difference to the headaches. Then it occurred to him that headaches might be caused by "repressed hate" as he calls it. There is a war in the mind between what you want and what you can obtain. In the ensuing frustration, the victim feels that he is in a trap and the headache appears. Dr. Bostock feels that the term "migraine" should be re-defined to include a consideration of this psychological factor.

What About Eyestrain?

It is noteworthy that fatigue and eyestrain are the principal reasons for headaches, according to the people interviewed in our original survey. Some medical opinion agrees with this, other doctors disagree. Francis M. Walsh, M.D., of the University of Minnesota, and Leon D. Harris, M.D., of the Lutheran Deaconess Hospital, Minneapolis, writing in *Modern Medicine* for March 1, 1952, say that actual eye disorders are quite infrequent among children brought to them. Studying 100 young patients from 4 to 17 years of age, they found that 46 had "depressed" vision, but were free from any other symptoms. The remaining 54 had normal vision without glasses, but were brought to the doctor complaining of headaches, eyes that hurt, being slow readers and holding books close to their eyes while reading.

"Children with good vision may complain of headaches or eye pain to gain parental attention," say these physicians, "the first born whose place is usurped by a new baby . . . . may feel neglected and sometimes resorts to this stratagem." In the opinion of these doctors, slow reading and holding books close to the eyes are caused by other things entirely and they seem to feel that getting glasses for the child will not affect cures. "Emotional origin" is a far more common cause for headaches.

On the other hand, Dr. Albert D. Ruedmann, Professor of Ophthalmology at Wayne University School of Medicine declared in the October 14, 1952 issue of the *Journal of the American Medical Association* that 25 per cent of all headaches are caused by eye difficulty. He said that eyes are overworked, overused and used under poor working conditions (bad light, etc.). He gave as examples the child who is inattentive, the businessman who has a headache at noon which is relieved by lunch and then has a recurrence about 3 or 4 o'clock in the afternoon, the convalescent patient who reads in bed and so forth.

They may require, he said, medical exercises, surgical treatment, glasses or all 3. He also believes that pains in the neck which may lead to headache are caused by imbalance in the muscles of the eyes. The neck muscles function chiefly to move the head so that the eyes are in a good position to see. If there is a disorder in the balance of the eye muscles, the neck muscles must be strained to get good sight.

Low Blood Sugar and Headaches

We are interested in that businessman mentioned by Dr. Ruedmann— the man who gets a headache around noon which stops when he has his lunch and begins again around 3 or 4 P.M. We are interested in him mostly because of another clipping in our file in which J. A. Harrill, M.D., writing in the *Laryngoscope* for February, 1951, gives the case histories of 72 patients whose headache and dizziness were caused by low blood sugar and completely relieved by a high protein diet. The headache was described as dull and throbbing, often present at night and often related to meals.

There is a fascinating and provocative book on the subject of blood sugar by E. M. Abrahamson, M.D., and A. W. Pezet, *Body, Mind and Sugar,* published by Henry Holt and Company. In this book we find that the patient with low blood sugar is apt to feel worse in the early morning hours (3 or 4 A.M.) or after he gets up in the morning. This is because he has not had any food for so long that his blood sugar is especially low. If he eats little or no breakfast and especially if he eats carbohydrates for breakfast (cereals, toast, waffles, coffee) his blood sugar drops again before lunch and again in the late afternoon. Now in our original survey on headaches we found that the two commonest times for headaches to appear are upon arising in the morning and again in the afternoon. It seems seldom that anyone gets a headache in the evening, unless it is the direct result of eyestrain or a particularly fatiguing day. In the evening, after a big dinner, with plenty of protein, blood sugar level is high.

We do not say or imply that all unexplained headaches are caused by low blood sugar, but we do earnestly suggest that if you suffer from head-

[117]

aches, and especially if they occur in relation to the time you get up and the time you eat meals, you should certainly get Dr. Abrahamson's book and try the high protein diet which he recommends. It is not a difficult diet to follow and it may produce startling results.

Just two further comments on the subject of high protein diets in relation to headache. Dr. Abrahamson found that so-called "allergic" conditions responded very well to his diet. He regularly cured asthma and hay fever patients with it. We saw in our initial survey that people who suffer most from headaches also have a higher incidence of respiratory disturbances and a family history of allergy. Can these disorders also be caused by the same low blood sugar that is causing their headaches?

Then, too, we constantly encountered mention of neurosis in connection with headaches—especially migraine headaches. We know that a high carbohydrate diet (which is also an inexpensive diet) requires lots of B vitamins for its proper digestion. We know, too, that all of the B vitamins have been removed from our popular processed carbohydrates such as breakfast cereals, white sugar and white flour. In addition, we know that the B vitamins are responsible for morale.

Anyone who does not get enough B vitamins suffers from "nerves," depression and even neurotic symptoms. Can it be that a diet high in refined carbohydrates is responsible for both the migraine headaches and the nervous, tense, hypersensitive personalities that go with them?

Other Possible Causes For Headaches

Other physicians have developed theories on the relation of muscles to headache. In *Münchener Medizinische Wochenschrift,* a German medical publication, we find C. Baeckmann writing of what he calls "myogenic headaches" which occur most frequently in women of middle age, with pain at the base of the skull leading to a stiffening of the neck. Dr. Baeckmann believes that the various household chores that women perform in cramped positions such as sewing, knitting, peeling potatoes and so forth may well result in "an unnoticed and lasting" elevation of the shoulders, caving in of the chest and sway-back, which lead to stiff neck muscles and so to headache. He suggests massage of these neck muscles and relaxing exercises, application of heat, and, of course, postural exercises to correct the various postural defects the years have brought. R. J. Dittrich, writing in the *Lancet* for February, 1951, describes a lower back pain that frequently leads to headaches. The lower back pain resulted from "abnormalities of subfascial (under the muscles) fat in the lower back," and although it is not clear just how the headache could result from low back pain, Dr. Dittrich says that apparently it did.

The *New York State Journal of Medicine* for March, 1953, claims that neck-stretching is the cure for "most headaches." Two surgeons who have treated more than 500 chronic headache cases report that they cured 60 per cent, achieved real improvement in 30 per cent and failed in only

10 per cent by using "traction" on the patients' necks. They continue their treatment for several months, even if the headache has disappeared meanwhile. It is not a remedy you could try at home, for it involves stretching the patient's neck with a series of weights varying from 5 to 60 pounds.

Aniseikonia, An Unusual Eye Disorder

We cannot leave the subject of headaches without telling one story from our own experience. A friend of ours had headaches for 20 years—blinding, searing, nauseating headaches that put her to bed at least 3 or 4 days out of every month. She had taken 30 or 40 different treatments all to no avail. Her glasses (for astigmatism) were changed regularly and each time her glasses were changed her headaches grew worse. Her friends began to believe the headaches must be a sign of neurosis. She herself was at the point of complete desperation and had made arrangements to have an examination for brain tumor.

A neighbor who was an optometrist asked if she would stop in at his office before she went out of town for her examination. Figuring that she had nothing to lose, she did. With a series of curious and very complicated machinery, Dr. Benton Freeman of Allentown, tested her eyes and told her she had aniseikonia, a maladjustment of eyesight. Over a period of 6 months he adjusted and re-adjusted a set of curved lenses. When they were perfectly adjusted, for the degree of aniseikonia that she had, he made permanent lenses for her. This all took place 5 years ago. From the time the first aniseikonic lens was placed in the frame of her glasses, she has not had a headache. What is perhaps even more surprising, she continually bit her fingernails down to the quick during the years when she had headaches. A month after the headaches stopped, she found to her amazement that she had stopped biting her nails.

Aniseikonia is an eye disorder in which each eye sees objects at a different distance and different position in space. The effort made by her brain in trying constantly to adjust these two images was the cause of our friend's headaches. The aniseikonic lenses cannot cure this maladjustment of her eyes, but so long as she wears them she is free from all symptoms. In her case, each time her lenses were adjusted for astigmatism, her aniseikonia became worse, because then she saw each of the two images even more clearly.

Aniseikonia was discovered at Dartmouth a number of years ago and research and experimentation were done on a grant from John D. Rockefeller whose headaches were cured by aniseikonic lenses. It is estimated that more than one per cent of our population may have aniseikonia. There are only about 25 doctors in the country who have the equipment to test for it. They can tell you in a half hour whether you have aniseikonia or not and if you have, they can, without fail, prescribe lenses to correct it. It is a lengthy procedure, but certainly well worth the time and money.

[119]

Dr. Freeman has patients from all over eastern United States, some of whom must be brought to his office in an ambulance, if they happen to break their lenses, for their symptoms are so violent without their glasses. Many ophthalmologists refuse to believe in the existence of such a disorder, even after they have interviewed these same patients, some of whom cannot stand on their feet or sit in a chair without falling, once they take off their glasses. If you believe aniseikonia may be causing your headaches, we'd suggest that you write to Mr. Rodale and ask for the name of the doctor nearest to you who can test you for it. Address J. I. Rodale, Rodale Press, Incorporated, Emmaus, Pennsylvania.

Other Aspects of Headaches

There are several other aspects of headache that we should mention, although they seem to be quite obvious. If you suffer from sinus trouble, this can be a cause of headache. Impacted teeth may press against a nerve and cause agonizing headaches which have no apparent cause, if the impacted tooth is undiscovered. Eyestrain is something we should all avoid. And this means simply: don't read or do close work over too long a period or in a light which is not adequate.

Allergy can cause headaches. One of the articles in our file relates the story of a man who always got a headache when he went to New York. His trips to New York were the only times he ever ate lobster. He was allergic to it. Bright's disease, uremic poisoning, tuberculosis, malaria, fevers and infections may cause headaches. There is a headache called the "hypertension" headache suffered by patients with high blood pressure. "Nervous" headache may be just the result of a busy, busy day when you are trying to accomplish more than is humanly possible and this in the midst of strain, noise and hurry. The obvious preventive is relaxation and a reorganization or change of work to eliminate the strain.

Our Suggestions

If you still have headaches and have eliminated any of the above as possible causes, we'd suggest:

1. Check on your emotional state. See if you can discover whether some actual frustration or repressed "hate" or intolerable personal dilemma is responsible. If so, either resign yourself to chronic headaches, or change the mental attitude or situation, no matter how impossible it may seem at first glance. You may need the help of a psychiatric counsellor.

2. Correct your posture. There are many good books on this subject available at your local library. Check on your posture often while you are working, and guard against working in a position that cramps or tires you.

3. Take better care of your eyes. During an evening of television, rest your eyes frequently and be sure you are sitting far enough away from the screen. Don't read or work in inadequate light. Get plenty of vitamin

A and vitamin C in your diet—two food elements that are mighty important for eye health.

4. If you have violent headaches that resist all diagnosis, write to Mr. Rodale for information about aniseikonia.

5. Read up on blood sugar. You will find information on the subject covered in later chapters in this book. Or ask your library to get a copy of Dr. Abrahamson's book on the subject.

32. An Unusual Cause of Headaches

Does anyone in your family grind his teeth? This activity has a scientific name, "Bruxism," which means, literally, to gnash, grind or clench the teeth. Surprisingly enough, it is a fairly common practice, especially among people who are under emotional tension. Some of them have gotten into the habit of clenching or grinding their teeth in sleep, so that the only way they know this is happening is that the edges of their teeth show evidence of wearing down because of the constant pressure on them.

Fifty Per Cent Suffered More Than Five Years

Considering that any activity of the teeth involves many muscles in the face, head and temples, it is not surprising to find that chronic headaches frequently result from bruxism. The *Lancet* for August 6, 1960, carried an article by Ragnar Berlin and Leopold Dessner, medical doctors at a Swedish hospital, relating their findings with 62 patients who came in complaining of chronic headache. Most of them were between 15 and 30 years of age. Eighty per cent had had the headaches for more than a year and 50 per cent for more than 5 years. Most of them had already consulted several doctors without gaining more than temporary relief at the very best.

Drs. Berlin and Dessner outline the process by which grinding or clenching of the teeth for long periods of time can result in headache. The chewing muscles are involved, the muscles of the temple and, often, the muscles that control movements of the head, especially the one which is used in drawing the head back. The tension of these muscles over long periods of time produces eventual lack of oxygen in the surrounding area, and pain soon results due to the collection of unoxidized materials, which stimulate the ends of nerves, causing pain. In addition, the muscles pull on

[121]

tendons and supporting tissues. All these factors combine to produce a pain which is felt as a headache.

Head Pains Felt As Dull Pressure

According to our authors, the pain is usually felt as a dull, pressing headache, situated toward the front, behind the eyes, in the temples or on top of the head. It may also appear at the back of the head. Sometimes it appears only on one side.

They believe that the original cause for clenching or grinding the teeth is usually some disturbance in the "bite." We assume this means anything in the teeth or mouth which makes biting uncomfortable or awkward —for instance, a new denture or partial denture, a tooth filling which is too high or otherwise uncomfortable and other things of this kind. The patient usually wakes up with a headache, if he grinds his teeth at night. If his bruxism occurs during the day, the headache seems to grow worse after a period of exacting work or mental stress. He may be able to feel definite tenderness in his teeth and in the chewing muscles and those at the temple.

Patient May Be Unaware Of Clenching

A doctor or even a member of the family may be able to perceive that the patient is grinding or clenching his teeth when he is unaware of it. If the habit results from unconsciously trying to readjust his "bite" which has been thrown out of kilter, it can probably be corrected with a visit to the dentist who can smooth off fillings, adjust ill-fitting dentures and so forth.

The Swedish doctors used a plastic plate which they inserted into the mouths of their patients which kept them from clenching their teeth. The patients wore these for as long as 6 months—that is, at least 4 or 5 months after the disappearance of the headache which should occur within 4 to 6 weeks. Of the 62 patients they treated, 87 per cent were completely cured or considerably improved. The other 13 per cent were either slightly improved or not at all.

Our authors believe that some cases of headache from bruxism can be relieved by general relaxing exercises. These would involve, we suppose, exercises for the body in general, as well as for the head and neck.

Uncomfortable Conditions Cause Tooth Grinding

An article in the *Annals of Otology, Rhinology and Laryngology* for December, 1959, relates the experience of a dentist of Orange, New Jersey, Dr. Woodrow S. Monica, who treated several patients who suffered from bruxism after they were fitted with partial dentures. When it became apparent from the condition of their mouths that these patients were actually grinding their teeth in an effort to make their mouths more comfortable, he inserted a splint, similar to a boxer's mouthpiece, which was worn at night and which apparently cured the headaches.

[122]

Dr. Monica used the same splint on another patient who had headaches without any evidence of bruxism. The splint did not help at all in this case.

It seems to us, readers can make use of this information in two ways. First, if you or some member of your family suffers from unexplained headaches, bruxism may be the cause. It would be well to check. And on the other hand if you notice that you or someone else has the habit of grinding or clenching teeth, it would be wise to get over the habit if possible, by constant reminders and relaxing exercises. It would be interesting, too, to bring up the subject with your dentist. He may have patients suffering from this complaint.

33. Headaches from Milk

Headaches from milk? Surely we must be mistaken. But no. We find quite an extensive literature on the relation of milk to headaches. We think it is important, first because of the number of people who suffer from headaches these days, and secondly because of the fact that an astonishingly large number of adult individuals are living on milk exclusively these days. We refer to ulcer patients, of course.

Our most unusual case history is that of a graduate nurse who had "sick headaches" from the age of 14. While she was a student nurse, she lost about one-third of her time because of headaches. A typical attack began with a sense of pressure and pain, her eyelids dropped and twitched, and the headache went into high gear with severe throbbing around the right temple and ear. She also suffered from dizziness, loss of appetite, nausea, vomiting and inability to endure light. Sometimes she lost consciousness! Sometimes she couldn't keep on her feet. She had difficulty enunciating words during the time the headache was most severe.

The headaches varied from two hours to 10 days and left her completely exhausted. Her rest at night did not improve the exhaustion. An operation was performed to cut an artery which resulted in freedom from the headaches but gave her a new kind of pain near her ear. Another operation gave her complete relief from all pain for 5 weeks after which the headaches returned as bad as ever. She had been in the habit of drinking a quart of milk a day and she ate more beef than any other meat. She was put on a diet eliminating milk, and a number of other foods as well. Then after a time, the attempt was made to return the various foods to her diet. She took her first glass of milk for breakfast. The second glass was followed in 40 minutes by an excruciating headache during which she was only half conscious. The headache persisted for 48 hours. Eating beef produced the same kind of symptom. Milder reactions followed when she attempted to drink tomato juice, chocolate and grape juice. Aside from these, and, of course, milk, she is now able to eat anything and she remains free from headaches. It is interesting to note that many of her friends and medical advisers thought her headaches were psychosomatic.

A Different Kind of "Nerves" Brought on by Milk

In another case, reported by A. Alvin Wolf and Leon Unger in the *Annals of Internal Medicine*, for May 1944, we read of a woman who had "sick headaches" for over 30 years and hives for two or three years. She had the headaches at intervals of every week to every month. And they were so severe that she could not work and indeed had to remain in bed. She was tested for a number of foods to which she suspected she might be allergic. For the milk test, she was put on a milk-free diet for one week, then given 10 ounces of milk. Ninety minutes later she became very ill, developed a severe headache, nausea and vomiting. She vomited for an hour and was not entirely free from headache symptoms for 24 hours. By going on a diet completely free from milk she remained free of headaches. The report was written two years after the tests were made and there had been no headaches at all.

A different kind of upset, characterized as a "nervous storm" is described by Walter C. Alvarez, M.D., of the Mayo Clinic in *Gastroenterology*, August, 1946. This patient, also a woman, had alarming and prostrating attacks which came every two or three weeks. Symptoms were: rapid heart beat, pain in the left arm and left side of the neck and chest, weakness and breathlessness, a sense of trembling in the abdomen, perhaps diarrhea, gas, chilliness in the hands and feet, headache, sometimes a little fever and profuse discharge from the vagina. She had had these spells for 15 years or more. Between spells her health was good and physical examinations did not show anything wrong. "The diagnosis made by most physicians consulted was functional storm of some kind," says Dr. Alvarez.

It occurred to one physician finally that she might be allergic. Skin tests showed that she was allergic to cheese. She eliminated it from her diet and improved but still had the spells. Gradually she became worse and lost 25 pounds. She was then advised to skip milk as well. She did. Months later, she reported that she had had only one attack when she had eaten an ice that probably contained milk. Dr. Alvarez seems to feel that all her troubles were over, so long as she omitted milk and cheese from her meals.

Dr. Alvarez believes that headaches from milk may result from unchanged protein getting into the blood stream. He says in a communication to the editor of the *Journal of the American Medical Association*, for March 14, 1953, "Years ago Hinshaw and I questioned 500 consecutive patients seen at the Mayo Clinic and found 26 per cent who knew that they were sensitive to cow's milk, ice cream or milk products." Then he tells of a fellow physician who had to have many blood transfusions. He was allergic to beef protein and could always tell when the donor of the current transfusion had been eating beef, for he got an immediate reaction.

If you or someone in your family suffers from unexplained headaches, don't hesitate to try a completely milk-free diet for a few weeks at least. And remember this means that no milk can be used in other foods. And, if you want the test to be conclusive, make certain you eat no cheese or butter either.

SECTION 10: THE HEART

34. Heart Disease

By J. I. RODALE

I have had some experience with heart disease, as I've been a "case" since a boy. But I've never had a heart attack! I have had a heart murmur for as long as I can remember, and the stethoscope today sometimes emits sounds that are strange to a practiced medical ear. But I am in wonderful health just the same.

I can run up and down the two flights of stairs leading to my office 10 times a day; I have reduced my blood pressure to a normal of 120 over 70 (when I was 21, it was 145 over 75), I have never had digitalis, nitroglycerine or any other medication and have worked out a system that makes me look forward to a long, pleasant, un-senile life, without a cardiac incident or clinical episode, as the medical practitioners would say.

It was done by a *method,* of course, and I would like to share the *method* with as many persons as possible—not only heart cases, for the adoption of this *method* can prevent heart disease also.

First, we must understand that the heart is *the* most important organ in the body. It maintains the circulation of the blood by its pumping action. Therefore it must be kept in a high state of "condition."

There are two ways by which you can keep the heart in a healthy state. One is by nutrition. The diet is of terrific importance in the efficient operation of the heart. This is only common sense, but there are many factors involved. One of them is the question of protein-carbohydrate ratio of the food eaten. Since all the body's organs are made up mainly of protein, we can see how important it is to consume enough of this dietary substance. Can you visualize the make-up of the heart chemically when the

[125]

body is taking in too much carbohydrate? It has been shown that the physical matter of perhaps over 90 per cent of the body changes and is replaced every year, so you can imagine how easy it would be to improve the physical structure of the heart by good nutrition.

We must not overlook the fact that the arteries are part of the system that contributes to the operation of the heart. Since the health of the arteries will deteriorate due to an overconsumption of fat, it is of vital importance to learn where the danger point is in regard to the consumption of fat.

Heart cases, as well as those who do not wish to develop into one, should observe all the rules of good diet. They should eliminate artificial sugar and salt from the diet. This means cutting out soft drinks, candy, pastries and sugar in coffee or tea. If overweight they should reduce, making less work for the heart. The heart movement continues, but the force required for every beat is greatly reduced. They should not eat the preserved and smoked meats such as ham, bacon, frankfurters, corn beef, salami, sausage, etc. These are loaded with salt and preservative chemicals. They should eat plenty of fresh vegetables and fruit, and *no canned goods.* A good rule is *not to eat food* that has gone into factories. This permits only fish, meat, fruits and vegetables. I would go strong on white potatoes baked in their skins. They are not fattening if eaten in a diet (with no eggs) of a low-fat content. I would also exclude all dairy foods of every kind.

Now let us dwell on the aspect of exercise and physical activity, for this is a matter of life and death to all of us. Our sedentary way of life is killing us long before our time.

The heart is an organ that is in constant motion, expanding and contracting to cause a pumping action. It never rests, except between beats for a split second, and it thrives on motion. It demands the stimulation of body movement for many reasons, one of which is to prevent infiltration of fat into the heart muscle, thus hindering its efficient operation. One must keep in motion as much as possible, exercising, walking, going up and down stairs, etc. Playing golf on weekends is not sufficient. There must be enough physical activity every single day. This is a *must* to a heart case. The heart like a limb of the body must get its share of the effect of exercise, otherwise it will lose its tone. Non-exercise of a hand or a foot will cause stagnation in it.

Vitamin E

In my program for a heart case I would give number one position to the taking of vitamin E, because this vitamin oxygenates the tissues and also has anti-bloodclotting ability. This is important to prevent death through thrombosis, or a blood clot. This anticlotting quality of vitamin E was discovered by Drs. Zierler, Grob and Lilienthal, and their findings were written up in the *American Journal of Physiology,* Vol. 153, p. 127, 1948.

In the case of a thrombosis, the taking of sufficient vitamin E can save lives, by preventing blood from forming clots. A standard practice in certain heart cases is to administer the drug heparin for this purpose, but vitamin E has other purposes also and is a much more valuable and safer tool. The *Annals of Surgery,* Vol. 131, p. 652, reports that vitamin E and calcium appear to be helpful in the treatment of vascular diseases. Dr. A. W. Allen of Boston, commenting on this article tells us that he has used vitamin E on a number of patients and can report that 50 of these who were "vulnerable," that is susceptible to thrombosis, escaped this serious condition. This seems to us particularly important, for in these cases vitamin E was used to prevent rather than to cure, and 50 lucky patients continued in good health. Dr. J. C. Owings of Baltimore comments that he has treated many leg ulcers due to phlebitis with a combination of rutin and vitamin E, all of which remained healed, so long as the patient continued to take the vitamins.

Drs. W. E. Crump and E. F. Heinskell, writing in the *Texas State Journal of Medicine,* Vol. 11, 1952, agree that the use of the regular anti-coagulants for routine prevention of clotting diseases in patients after operations is too dangerous for general use. In most cases where these medicines are used, as many patients die of hemorrhage as might have died of clots and 16 per cent of other cases develop non-fatal bleeding complications. When vitamin E was used as treatment by these physicians, no bleeding occurred and only minor side reactions were noticed.

I would like to quote from a speech delivered by Dr. Evan S. Shute of the Shute Foundation of London, Ontario, Canada, to show how vitamin E acts in the body:

"The power of vitamin E to treat and prevent heart disease of all types, whether coronary or rheumatic, depends upon 4 chief characteristics:

"1. Vitamin E seems to be a natural anti-thrombin in the human blood stream. It has been found by Zierler of Johns Hopkins and the United States Navy Research Department and Kay at Tulane to be a substance normally circulating in the blood of all men which prevents clots occurring inside the vessel. It is the only substance preventing the clotting of blood which is not dangerous. It does not interfere with the normal clotting of blood in a wound and with the normal healing process. Indeed it actually accelerates the healing of burns and wounds.

"2. The second important effect of the use of vitamin E is oxygen conservation. It is a natural antioxidant in the body. It has been shown by Houchin and Mattill, and this has been confirmed by many workers, to decrease the oxygen requirement of muscle by as much as 43 per cent and makes the narrow stream of blood which gets through the narrowed coronary artery in many heart patients adequate to prevent the occurrence of anoxia (lack of oxygen), which is the trigger that sets off anginal or heart pain. Consequently, we have patients in Montreal who were once unable to walk half a block without the occurrence of angina pectoris but are now able to climb Mount Royal. Indeed, there is present in my audience today at least one such patient.

"3. The third major function of vitamin E is the prevention of excessive scar tissue production and even, in some instances, the ability to melt away unwanted scar. It has been proven to function in this way in many areas of the body—from the hand, in Dupuytren's contraction (Rochester, New York)—to urinary tract strictures (Johns Hopkins).

"4. It is a dilator of blood vessels. This was beautifully demonstrated by X-ray in rabbits injected before and after the administration of vitamin E by two workers in Florence, Italy. It opens up new pathways in the damaged circulation, therefore, and bypasses blocks produced by clot and hardened arteries.

"These 4 functions, all of them extensively confirmed in animal experimentation and human clinical work, make it the most valuable ally the cardiologist has yet found in the treatment of heart disease. It has no rivals. No other substance has this array of needful properties. This drug then becomes the first safe drug which can be given to patients suffering from the results of a clot in a coronary artery. There has been and still is no treatment at all for this kind of case except two mildly useful drugs, which can be administered with great peril to the already precarious patient. Vitamin E replaces 'rest and reassurance,' which have no authentic basis, with real help to the damaged, laboring heart itself. It is the key both to the prevention and treatment of all those conditions in which a lack of blood supply due to thickened or blocked blood vessels or a lack of oxygen is a factor or the whole story of the disease. As I have said, it has no rivals. No pharmacologist or internist can suggest another substance with all the properties and power of this vitamin. God made it unique and we ignore it at our peril."

High Blood Pressure

If I was a heart case and had high blood pressure I would do everything in my power to quickly get it down to normal, which is about 120/70, because high blood pressure, or hypertension, in a heart case is only asking for trouble. This fact is generally accepted by the medical profession. For example, Benjamin F. Miller, M.D., in *The Complete Medical Guide* (Simon and Schuster) says (p. 608): "High blood pressure places an increased strain on the heart and blood vessels," and he comments further that 65 per cent of the people with high blood pressure die of heart attacks.

Dr. Louis Tobin in a symposium on arteriosclerosis at the University of Minnesota, September 7, 1955, said that hypertension accelerates hardening of the arteries which is one of the main causes of heart disease deaths.

What is a normal blood pressure? Some say that anything over 150 is abnormal. But I see no reason, barring organic trouble, why it could not be brought down to 120/70. That is what I have done, from a blood pressure of about 170, 8 or 9 years ago.

How does one go about reducing one's blood pressure? There are two ways. First, the method of the average physician, which stresses the low-salt diet plus a dozen or more high-powered drugs, each with its particular harmful side effect. Second, the nutritional method—a low-salt diet, the taking of garlic pills and rutin. The latter is used in hypertension to a great extent today by the medical profession.

First let us discuss the low-salt diet. To some people, eating without salt is the end of the world. As Kipling has said, "Being kissed by a man who didn't wax his moustache was like eating an egg without salt." I learned to eat eggs without salt many years ago and have cultivated a taste for egg, not for salt.

That salt eating is a cause of hypertension was proven by a recent survey. At a meeting of the American Society for Experimental Pathology in Atlantic City, New Jersey, Lewis K. Dahl and Robert A. Love of the Brookhaven National Laboratory told of their findings in cases of 448 patients. Of these, 55 were salt abstainers, 186 ate an average amount of salt and 207 sprinkled salt liberally on their food. There was no one with high blood pressure among the abstainers. There were 12 hypertensives in the intermediate group and 20 among those who used salt liberally. The researchers declare that this is not just pure chance. They claim that a certain level of salt is necessary for the development of high blood pressure.

There is an important item in the January 15, 1955, issue of the *Journal of the American Medical Association* in the Queries Department. In reply to a doctor's question about the value of a low-salt diet, the editor recommends it most highly, then states, "It seems rational that the diet that is effective for treatment should also be effective for prophylaxis." Prophylaxis means prevention. In other words, a low-salt diet is recommended for everyone who is healthy, in order to prevent hypertension. The editor finally concludes, "It has been asserted that congestive failure never develops in any patient with hypertension (even of the seemingly 'refractory' class) if he is kept on a correct low-sodium diet."

I think I have submitted sufficient evidence to prove that whether you have heart disease or high blood pressure, or whether you merely wish to prevent these two diseases, it is highly advisable to be on a very low salt diet. Incidentally, if you are healthy and feel that your body needs some salt, may I assure you that practically every item of food contains salt in its natural make-up—some more than others.

I had a very interesting experience with salt that I must relate. I discontinued it in 1940, but a few years later I began merely to gargle with salt water. Mouth sores developed that went away on discontinuance of the salt, which makes me think that the tissues of salt users are pickled with the effects of the salt.

Now, what about rutin and garlic? Rutin is a product made from the

[129]

leaves of the buckwheat plant. It can help to maintain the walls of the blood vessels so that they do not become fragile.

Since, it would seem to me, the condition of the vessel walls is a factor in blood pressure, because the force of the blood is exerted against those walls, it would be a wise course for everyone, from childhood on, to take some rutin every day so that the structure of the artery walls might be kept in the best of shape.

No one can dispute the fact that garlic is a specific as a means of lowering high blood pressure. Unfortunately, it is not much used in the United States, where physicians would rather depend on the complicated action of high-powered drugs. But in Europe it is quite a common medicament for many purposes and diseases, but especially for reducing blood pressure.

I would like to talk about my own experience with garlic. When my blood pressure was about 170, I began to use garlic perles with good results. These are made so that they do not dissolve until they are in the stomach, and if a person does not belch there will be no odor. Later, however, when I had to take vitamin E in large doses to control my heart condition, I found that I could not take garlic. It seemed to reduce the effectiveness of the vitamin E, bringing back some chest pressure pains on walking uphill. But since my blood pressure was now perfectly normal, that is, 120/70, I no longer needed the garlic, and have discontinued it without experiencing any increase in the blood pressure. In the taking of vitamins one must watch for these antagonisms by a process of trial and error.

Besides garlic, no salt and the taking of rutin, there must also be good general nutrition—no white sugar, or refined foods, a good part of the vegetables should be eaten raw, plus raw fruit, no overeating, plenty of exercise, no smoking, etc. A healthy body, from every point of view, will not tolerate a condition of high blood pressure.

Obesity

One medical writer has described it thus: "A pump built to irrigate 10 acres will wear out more quickly if compelled to provide ample moisture for a larger area. The heart ceaselessly forces blood through miles of microscopic tubes. Every additional pound of flesh adds millions of extra cells that must be provided with air and food conveyed in the blood. Supplying these superfluous cells wears out the heart prematurely."

There are dozens of separate medical studies that have been made, which indicate that obesity is very bad for the heart; I will present a few of them.

In a bulletin of the Metropolitan Life Insurance Company appears the following:

"The death rate is one-third higher among those whose body weight is 20 per cent above the average. The death rate from coronary artery disease is 50 per cent greater among the overweight. Among those with 25 per cent excess body weight the death rate from diabetes is 8 times higher than among persons of normal weight. "For every inch the waist measurement exceeds the chest measurement the person may substract two years from his life expectancy."

The following is from *Medical Times* of December, 1956.

"About one-fifth of the population of the United States is obese. There are many social, economic and medical complications to being obese. Recent actuarial studies by life insurance companies have starkly documented the risks of being obese. One 25 year study covering 25,000 men and 25,000 women revealed a 150 per cent mortality rate above the expected among the obese. Conversely, substandard policy holders who decreased their weight had a significant drop in expected mortality. Obese army officers had 1½ times the expected retirement rate. Obesity adds to the morbidity of the degenerative diseases of middle life. Hardening of the arteries, the top cause of death in the United States, was found to account for 50 per cent of the deaths among the obese, 149 per cent above the expected incidence."

There can be no question that being fat is deadly to a heart case. The life insurance companies know this, and will make fat people pay higher premiums for life insurance.

Although we have already discussed blood pressure earlier, brief reference must be made to it here since overweight, blood pressure and heart disease go together.

In a book entitled *Risk Appraisal,* published by an insurance organization known as the National Underwriter Company, the author Harry Dingman, shows that blood pressure is in general higher when a person's weight is higher. In an analysis which was done of 9,926 unselected life insurance policy holders, it was found that all of them showed an increase in blood pressure with increasing age and weight.

For example, at age 50 the average of underweights was 128, normal weights 133 and overweights 137 systolic blood pressure. At age 60 the average of underweights was 135, normal weights 145 and overweights 152. Mr. Dingman says that in the obese, when there is a reduction in weight there is usually a reduction in blood pressure.

So there you have it in plain, blunt figures. To be a heart case and to be overweight is to be shamefully negligent. If you are even only 10 pounds overweight and are a heart case, you may pay for it.

How To Diet

Here is my method of reducing weight. Of course, it may not work for everyone. There is a certain amount of experimenting that one must indulge in to determine what is the best way for each individual, but one should continue trying and experimenting until the gluttonous appetite is subdued.

First, there is the question of how much and what kind of starchy food should be in the diet. My opinion is, and it is based on long study and observation in myself and others, that all wheat products should be completely eliminated from the diet of a heart case, and I include in this taboo even whole wheat bread, organically grown. This includes also all cereals, but does not apply to rice. Of the latter a moderate amount may be taken, as well as a little corn (maize).

When you cut out bread, you are also eliminating the salt that is in it, which is a factor in weight reducing. Incidentally, I don't believe that it is only the salt in the bread that causes the increase in the weight. There is something more, probably the gluten, which makes the bread suitable for baking. That is why other forms of starch that contain no gluten, such as potatoes and bananas, are not nearly as fattening. Also bear in mind that wheat contains 2½ per cent fat, bananas only ½ of 1 per cent, white potatoes 1/10 of 1 per cent and sweet potatoes 1.1 per cent fat.

As a heart case you owe it to yourself to eliminate all wheat products and see what happens. This means complete elimination—not even a slice of toast a day, and absolutely no sandwiches of any kind. In my own case, I keep my heart condition in wonderful control with a breadless diet and heavy doses of vitamin E. Sometimes, when I break the rule and indulge in bread, there have been some slight heart symptoms within a short time. In the last few years I have rarely broken the rule because I am so convinced of the harmfulness of wheat products to the well-being of a heart case.

The heart case should consume a low-fat diet. It is important to reduce the total amount of fat in the diet of a person with a heart condition, but in making the decision as to which types of fat to retain in the diet, bear in mind that the egg is a whole food, out of which a living thing will emerge. It has the germ of life in it if it is a fertile egg. There just isn't any comparison with milk and dairy products. The egg is by far superior from every point of view, besides containing a large quantity of lecithin which is the antidote to the cholesterol that the egg contains. To cut down on eggs is a terrible dietary blunder even where there is hardening of the arteries.

Of course, one cannot cut out fats altogether. If one does, one may become the subject of feelings of depression. Once I tried this as an experiment and my head began to feel kind of peculiar. Fat is necessary for the proper absorption of carotene which is the first step in the body's manufacture of vitamin A.

Skipping breakfast as a means of losing weight is not desirable. That is the opinion of many medical experts. The consensus is that you will be so hungry that you will eat more the rest of the day. In my case, the heavy breakfast lulls my appetite the rest of the day. I thus found it easy to eat very light lunches—one-half the amount of food I used to eat; and when I eat a light breakfast, for some mysterious reason I have a strong desire to nibble after supper and before bedtime. There is much medical evidence in experiments with rats proving conclusively that reduction in daily calories adds years to the life. But this is especially important to a heart case because the heart is overtaxed in helping to digest heavy meals. Cut down on the amount of food you eat and eliminate entirely fried foods, coffee or tea or maté, soups, bread and flour, dairy products, sugar and salt. And remember, vitamins should be taken with meals because they aid the digestion. I have found it much easier to take off pounds if I am taking vitamins at every meal. By aiding the digestion, the vitamins seem to break down or homogenize the fats so they are not stored as fat. This is of terrific importance in a reducing program.

Fats and Cholesterol

The most common kind of heart condition is caused by atherosclerosis, or hardening of the arteries. It is not really heart disease, but a disease of the arteries. It is a condition caused by fatty deposits containing cholesterol which thicken the artery walls, thus reducing the amount of space in the arteries for the blood to circulate. If this happens in the big arteries that feed blood into the heart, it creates an impediment to its flow, and if it occurs during an emergency or severe activity, when the blood need increases, it will bring about heart symptoms such as the chest pressure pains and angina.

Cholesterol is nothing new. It has been known for several hundred years. It is found only in animal fat. Vegetable fat does not contain it, but the body can make it from sources other than fat. Cholesterol is a compound which is a constituent of gallstones. In reasonable amounts it is needed by the body. It is an important part of the nerve tissue. It also opposes those elements which destroy red blood corpuscles. It is the substance that reduces the wateriness of cells, giving them a semi-solid character. It has other important functions, but when it increases too much and accumulates in places where it has no business to be, it can be a great hindrance to the proper circulation of the blood.

Latest researches seem to indicate that one need not worry about cholesterol as such, but rather should be concerned about the total fat consumption. Dr. Charles F. Wilkinson, Jr. of New York University Postgraduate Medical School said, "There is no evidence from studies in human patients that fat in the diet, is the cause of coronary disease." But he is in the minority. On the other hand, doctors like Norman Jolliffe, M.D., of the New York City Department of Health, hold, "No prudent person who has had, or wishes to avoid, coronary heart disease should eat a high fat diet."

If you examine all the evidence, you will come to but one conclusion. Our prosperity is causing us to live on the fat of the land, the fat is clogging up our arteries and the result is deaths from heart attacks. We have the highest heart disease rate of any nation on earth, and we con-

[133]

sume a higher per capita amount of fat than any other country. Forty years ago 30 per cent of our diet was fat. Today it is 40 per cent.

In the war years, when some of the European countries drastically cut their fat consumption, deaths from atherosclerosis declined considerably. For example, in France the death rate from coronary thrombosis from 1941 to 1945 was 20.6 per 100,000 of population. But after normal fat consumption was resumed, in the years from 1945 to 1949, the mortality rate from this disease went up 25.5. The same condition held in Sweden, Finland, Norway and Italy. But in the United States, where there was no drop in fat consumption, there was a rise in the deaths from coronary diseases during the war years. It is not only from this study but from a large mass of scientific medical data that proof has been found that there is a direct relation between fat consumption and artery health.

In reference to the animal versus vegetable type of fat, permit me to quote from the *Science News Letter* of April 28, 1956, which discussed the Bronte-Stewart-Ancel Keys researches among the Bantus of South Africa. It says: "The fats that put a lot of cholesterol in the blood are animal fats, or hard fats. Beef drippings, butter, eggs and beef lead to a prompt and significant increase in blood cholesterol, Dr. Bronte-Stewart and associates found by diet experiments with humans in South Africa.

"When they fed vegetable oils, such as olive oil, sunflower-seed oil and ground-nut (peanut) oil in equivalent amount, blood cholesterol did not increase."

To sum it up, may I quote from *Borden's Review of Nutrition Research* of January, 1956:

"A considerable literature suggests that a large intake of dietary fat may produce atherosclerosis. Keys and his associates in particular have been proponents of this point of view. The literature until the past few years tended to indicate that fats of all kinds were equally 'bad' in this regard. Recently, Kinsell and his associates have shown that chemically constant diets, containing large amounts of vegetable fat not only produced no increase in plasma cholesterol and other lipids (fats), but were associated predictably with a striking decrease in plasma lipids as compared to the levels on an average mixed diet. Replacement of the vegetable fat by animal fat in experimental diets, resulted in a prompt return of the lipids to levels noted on an average diet. These results have been confirmed by Ahrens et al, and by Beveridge et al."

So, we know now that animal fats should be on the low side in the diet, and that we can be fairly liberal with vegetable fats, especially corn, soybean, sunflower and fish oils, for these are noted for their ability to reduce the cholesterol in the blood.

Vitamin C and Cholesterol

There were several researches performed in the last few years which prove that vitamin C is an important factor in keeping down the cholesterol in the blood. One of the most remarkable of them has recently come out of Russia and was written up in *Terapevtichevski Archiv*. Vol. 28, p. 59, 1956. (The translation was done by Julius Nemetz of Allentown, Pennsylvania.) This article proves that vitamin C is both a preventive and a cure of atherosclerosis. According to it, Dr. I. A. Miasnikov was able to prove that within a few hours after administering vitamin C (ascorbic acid) her patients showed a sharp decline in the cholesterol level of the blood. In 1952 she proved graphically that vitamin C could stop artificially induced atherosclerosis. These observations were confirmed by coworkers L. A. Tiapinoi, G. N. Loubman and E. M. Berkoviskin.

Here is part of Dr. Miasnikov's report regarding the effect of this vitamin. First, the amount of cholesterol in the blood was checked, before administering the vitamin C, and then the amount of cholesterol was determined after the first, second, third and fourth hour, after giving the patients one-half gram of ascorbic acid (vitamin C). Of the 35 patients, 28 had an excess of cholesterol and 7 had between 150 and 180 milligrams of cholesterol. In those 7 patients whose cholesterol was normal, the use of ascorbic acid did not change the level of cholesterol. But in those with high cholesterol, the level was lowered considerably. In 15 patients the percentage of cholesterol came down 15 per cent. In 8 patients it came down 16 to 30 per cent; in 5 patients, 31 to 50 per cent. A definite sharp decline of cholesterol in the blood was noted within a 24 hour period after the use of ascorbic acid, and a normalizing effect by the end of the experimental period.

In summary the article says:

1. The literature and our observations indicate that ascorbic acid normalizes the level of cholesterol in the blood. From the first dose of one-half gram of ascorbic acid, there is a sharp decline of cholesterol in the blood.

2. It is possible that periodic use of ascorbic acid will prevent the development of atherosclerosis in healthy people of advanced ages.

3. Large doses of ascorbic acid under hygienic regimes produce good therapeutic results in people suffering from atherosclerosis.

4. Some patients suffering from atherosclerosis develop high blood pressure. With the use of ascorbic acid and the hygienic regime, a reduction of the blood pressure takes place and the pressure becomes normal.

To me this is a terrific piece of research, and it adds another honor to this wonderful vitamin. I have seen vitamin C cure cases of arthritis and acne, as well as other skin conditions. We know that this vitamin is good for the teeth, gums, bones and eyes, that it protects against infections and colds, that it causes wounds to heal quickly. But that it would be helpful in reducing the blood cholesterol comes indeed as a pleasant surprise.

I said I was pleasantly surprised about discovering that vitamin C was effective in reducing the body's cholesterol, but I had overlooked the fact that in my booklet, *How to Eat for a Healthy Heart* (Rodale Books, $1.00) I had covered the subject with 3 references. Here is one of them:

I refer to a research written up in the *American Journal of Physiology* (December, 1950, p. 708). Dent, Booker, Hayes, Harris and Greene of the Department of Pharmacology and Oral Medicine, Howard University, Washington, D.C., in experiments with dogs found that the presence of cholesterol reduces the amount of vitamin C in the blood and the blood cells, and the more cholesterol given to the dogs, the greater the vitamin C excreted in their urine. This creates a vitamin C deficiency. It has also been found that the reverse is true, namely, increasing the vitamin C reduces the cholesterol.

There is, therefore, plenty of evidence that vitamin C should be a specific in the prevention and cure of atherosclerosis, but you do not see this mentioned in the newspapers, and I wonder how many doctors prescribe it for atherosclerosis. On the contrary, the newspapers and the physicians are ready to shout "food faddist," regarding anyone who would take vitamin C without a doctor's prescription. Yet here is a vitamin that is quite safe to take in highly excessive quantities, for it is water-soluble and any excess is excreted from the body.

Besides reducing cholesterol, vitamin C plays a tremendous role, directly and indirectly, in preventing or curing heart disease generally. This vitamin maintains the blood vessels and connective tissues in good condition, preserving the strength of the capillary walls. This one function of vitamin C is of great importance in considering the underlying causes of heart disease.

Vitamin B and Cholesterol

There are many parts of the vitamin B complex that have been shown by medical research to be of value in the prevention and cure of atherosclerosis. Included in this group are choline, pyridoxine, inositol and thiamin.

Choline is a lipotropic agent, which means that it combines readily with fats or oils, and thus hastens the removal of fat deposits. In the *Proceedings of the Society of Biology and Medicine* (73: 37-38, 1950) there is an article describing a study of the effect of choline on 230 patients, done by Dr. L. M. Morrison, and W. F. Gonzales of the College of Medical Evangelists, Los Angeles, California. It was summarized in in *Modern Medicine* as follows: "Half the patients were given conventional medication but no choline after discharge from the hospital; the other half received choline daily for 1 to 3 years. Among the untreated patients, the 3-year death toll was about 30 per cent, while only 12 per cent of the choline-treated patients died."

It seems that pyridoxine is also involved in the process by which the body uses fat. In an article that appeared in the *Journal of Chronic Diseases* for July, 1955, there is an article called "Is Atherosclerosis a

[136]

Condition of Pyridoxal Deficiency?" written by Henry A. Schroeder, M.D., of the Department of Internal Medicine, Washington University School of Medicine, St. Louis, Missouri. In this article Dr. Schroeder tells us that too little pyridoxine in the diet of monkeys produces, in general, the same condition as human hardening of the arteries. He says also that a deficiency of pyridoxine in rats causes high blood pressure. There is evidence, he says, that the whole process takes place in the blood vessels of these animals very much as it does in those of man.

Dr. Schroeder gives us an excellent estimate of the amount of pyridoxine in the average American diet. About half the pyridoxine in grain is lost when the grain is processed. Canned vegetables contain little, although fresh vegetables and fruits are quite rich in it. The processing of milk and meat, cooking and stewing food result in substantial losses of the vitamin. Any amount of heat or light damages pyridoxine.

According to many independent medical observers, inositol, another fragment of the vitamin B complex, is concerned in some way with the metabolism of fat, as well as cholesterol. There have been numerous researches on animals as well as on people that have proven that the daily taking of the vitamin inositol will result in a lowering of the cholesterol content of the blood.

An article in *Newsweek* for September 11, 1950, describes the experiments of Dr. Louis B. Dotti, Dr. William C. Felch and Miss Stephanie J. Ilka of St. Luke's Hospital, New York, who experimented with feeding two groups of rabbits a capsule of cholesterol daily. One group of rabbits received just cholesterol and a regulation diet. The other group of rabbits got, in addition to the cholesterol, a capsule of inositol. At the end of the feeding period the first group of rabbits showed an increase of 337 per cent in the cholesterol content of their blood. Those who had received inositol, too, showed an increase of only 181 per cent.

Thiamin is stolen from our bodies by the robber foods—white sugar, synthetic sugar, white flour, prepared cereals and many other refined and processed foods. If you eat carbohydrates in natural forms you do not experience any thiamin deficiency because the thiamin to digest the sugar or starch is present in the natural food. When you eat white sugar in coffee, cakes, candies, pies, ice cream and soft drinks, you are presenting your digestive tract with large quantities of sugar to be digested and no thiamin or other B vitamins to aid in the process. In order to handle this sugar at all, the body must steal thiamin from other processes and from its storage places in the liver, kidney and heart. This means that if you eat much white sugar, if you eat some of it every day, you are almost bound to suffer from thiamin deficiency. If you are a heart case, such dietary habit is cold suicide.

In a book called *The Avitaminoses* by Walter H. Eddy, Ph.D., and Gilbert Dalldorf, M.D. (published by the Williams & Wilkins Company), appears the statement, "Thiamin deficiency impairs the function of the heart, increases the tendency to extravascular fluid collections and results in terminal cardiac standstill." The authors show how the famous English research physician, Sir Robert McCarrison, in experiments with pigeons, produced cardiac (heart) changes in them by feeding them a vitamin B deficient diet. Eddy and Dalldorf describe another experiment in which congestive heart failure was produced in pigeons and then cured by thiamin.

We can see, therefore, that if we assure ourselves sufficient vitamin B, preferably in the form of supplements to the regular diet, such as brewer's yeast, desiccated liver, wheat germ and blackstrap molasses, we will be moving in the right direction towards preventing undue accumulation of fatty deposits in the artery walls.

Saturated and Unsaturated Fatty Acids

What do we mean by unsaturated fatty acids? How are they different from the saturated ones?

Fatty substances are made up of various atoms of carbon, hydrogen and oxygen, linked together like chains. Some are long, meaning they have many atoms linked together; others are short. Some kinds of fats have open links, you might say, where other atoms can be attached to them. These are called the "unsaturated fatty acids." By "unsaturated" we mean that these open links in the chain are there, ready to be filled or "saturated" with an atom of some other substance.

Linolenic, linoleic and arachidonic acids are just such "unsaturated" fatty acids. That is why they are so extremely valuable to good health. What do we mean by that? Well, you see, since they have open links in their chain of atoms, they are ready, willing and able to combine with other substances in the big chemical laboratory that is the body. So they take part in all kinds of different things that go on. They can combine with other parts of food; they can help to carry these other parts of food through the miles of blood vessels and they are used in building cell structure. They can do all this because—and only because—the open links in their chains of atoms invite other substances to join with them in various chemical combinations.

Well and good, you may say, so all we have to do is eat plenty of fat and we'll get enough unsaturated fatty acids to be healthful. Of course, it's not that simple. First of all, certain things can happen to these *unsaturated* fatty acids that change them to *saturated* fatty acids before we eat them. In this case, the open chains have already been filled with some other substance and there is no chance that this kind of fat can take the active part it should take in the body's laboratory.

When oxygen is combined with the unsaturated fatty acids, an atom of oxygen moves into the empty link, joins itself chemically with the other atoms and what happens? The fat becomes rancid. When hydrogen is added, it moves into the empty link, joins itself to the other atoms and we

[138]

have what is known as "hydrogenated fat"—a thick, almost solid, substance like lard. In both cases, of course, since the empty links have been filled, the fat can no longer fulfill its duties inside the body, because it is now "saturated"—there is no place for body substances to join with it and help in the work of the body.

Naturally nobody ever purposely makes fats rancid, for the taste is unpleasant and, as we have discovered, rancid fat in the diet is responsible for the destruction of fat-soluble vitamins. So rancid fats should be carefully avoided. Natural fats in their natural state, such as those in sunflower seeds, for instance, carry along with them substances called antioxidants which prevent oxygen from turning the fat rancid. But in many of the processes to which our table and cooking oils are subjected today, the antioxidants are destroyed.

People who depend on processed foods for their unsaturated fatty acids are just not going to get them. And people who are told by their doctors to eat a fat-free diet are not going to get them. People who eat diets high in animal fats are not going to get them, for they are most abundant in vegetable and cereal fats, and not at all plentiful in animal fats, such as butter, eggs, milk and meat fats.

Lecithin for Heart Patients

The treatment for high cholesterol content of the blood has been, among some physicians, to tell their patients to cut out all foods that are high in cholesterol. This would include: brains, egg yolk, fish roe, kidney, liver, sweetbreads—foods especially high in cholesterol.

A far better point of view, it seems to us, is to study everything about the patient's diet and see if perhaps he is getting too little of something else which is the very thing he needs so that his body can use cholesterol properly and it will not accumulate in his blood vessels or gall bladder. Is there such a substance? A great many medical researchers believe there is and they have years of hard work to prove their theories.

The substance that apparently protects against accumulations of cholesterol is lecithin. It is pronounced *less-i-thin* with the accent on the first syllable. The word comes from the Greek *Lekithos,* meaning *the yolk of an egg,* for lecithin is most abundant in egg yolk.

How does it happen that the lecithin occurs in egg yolk where cholesterol also is plentiful? Doesn't it sound like another of Mother Nature's provisions for good health? Cholesterol without lecithin can be harmful. So they are both included in this one especially healthful food. Why then should we have any trouble with cholesterol—aren't we all getting enough lecithin in our food?

Apparently not, and the reason is that the processing which our various fats and oils go through before they appear on grocery shelves destroys the lecithin content, but leaves the cholesterol. Hydrogenated fats, for instance—the shortenings used in pastry and for frying—do not contain lecithin, for it has been destroyed in the hydrogenation process. What happens as a result? The lecithin was put there by nature to act as an emulsifying agent for the cholesterol.

This means simply that when the cholesterol tends to coalesce or lump together, the lecithin breaks it up, mixes with it and keeps it finely divided so that it can be circulated throughout the body as a perfectly stable "emulsion" that will not solidify or congeal. Once the lecithin is removed, there is nothing to keep the cholesterol moving along through the blood stream—it cakes; it gathers in lumps.

H. D. Keston and R. Silbowitz reported in the *Proceedings of the Society of Experimental Biology and Medicine,* Vol. 49, 1942, that feeding lecithin to rabbits who were receiving large amounts of cholesterol kept the cholesterol from collecting in the blood and in the blood vessels and prevented hardening of the arteries in the rabbits. G. L. Duff and T. P. B. Payne wrote in the *Journal of Experimental Medicine,* Vol. 92, 1950, that they had shown in laboratory animals that the amount of cholesterol taken is *not* the important thing in hardening of the arteries—*the important thing is the instability of the cholesterol.* That is, when the cholesterol is not emulsified, it deposits on artery walls. Lecithin, of course, emulsifies it.

Lecithin is made in the liver, provided certain ingredients are present there. Why, then, should we have to get it in food—why not manufacture our own? One of the B vitamins, choline, and the unsaturated fatty acids (sometimes called vitamin F) must be present for the liver to make lecithin. We have done our best to remove both these substances from our national diet, so our supply of lecithin suffers. Get lecithin in your diet from such natural sources as seeds (melon seeds, sunflower seeds, cereal seeds and so forth), cold-pressed oils and food supplements.

Human Specific Gravity

A subject never discussed in connection with heart disease is the specific gravity of the human body. But it is of paramount importance with regard to the working of the human heart. In consideration of obesity, attention is given usually to a reduction in the food intake, rarely to the effect of exercise on the specific gravity of the body. Both of these are equally important in a reconstruction of the human body in order to prevent a heart attack.

But first let us see what we mean by specific gravity. According to the dictionary, specific gravity is the weight of a given volume of any kind of matter as compared with the weight of an equal amount of water. Specific gravity is a measure of the density of a substance, and for convenience it is contrasted with the density of water as a standard of comparison.

If the specific gravity of something is said to be 1.50, it means that a certain volume of it weighs 50 per cent more than a similar volume of water. If the specific gravity of fresh water is 1, then the specific gravity of sea water is about 1.026. Expressed another way this means that sea water is about 2½ per cent heavier than fresh water. This is due to the fact that sea water contains more minerals than fresh water.

If a substance floats on water, it means that its specific gravity is less than that of water. If it sinks, then its specific gravity is higher than that of water. A fat person, for example, would have a lower specific gravity than a muscular person. This means that a cubic inch of fat tissue weighs less than a cubic inch of muscular tissue. The muscular tissue is more compact. The fat tissue less compact. Low specific gravity, that is where the tissue weighs less, per cubic inch, is very disadvantageous from a health standpoint.

In considering the subject of specific gravity as it affects the human heart, John Davy said that organic disease of the heart cannot take place unless the specific gravity of the heart goes down. The higher the specific gravity of the heart, the less chance of it going bad. A high specific gravity for the heart means that it is all muscle. If the body becomes fat, some of it overflows into the heart muscle and impedes its efficiency. The heart can perform its work easier if it is all muscle, the way nature intended. But you cannot selectively remove the fat from the heart unless you remove it from the entire body.

In this connection I would like to relate a personal experience. I have a heart condition, and when I am overweight, I experience the typical angina chest pressure pains on undue exertion, such as walking up a hill. I found, however, due to a long program of walking an hour a day, that my specific gravity increased. I could tell it by measuring my chest-abdominal difference. This higher specific gravity caused my pressure pains on exertion to be much less severe. But they were still there to a certain limited extent.

However, when I got my weight down below 164, I found that I could walk uphill without any symptoms at all. One-hundred sixty-four seems to be some kind of threshold in my body.

When my weight goes above 164, excess fat probably spills over into the arteries and into the heart muscle, causing trouble. It has happened 3 or 4 times in getting my weight above and below 164. Each time I get below 164 I find I can do vigorous exercise without experiencing any heart symptoms. I imagine that every person has some kind of threshold weight figure below which his heart functions more efficiently. An attempt, therefore, should be made in heart cases to find out what this figure is. I am certain that in my case the improved effect was not only a reduction in my weight effected by dieting, but an increase in my specific gravity due to walking an hour a day.

You may never have thought of your body as a work of engineering. but it is, and you are the engineer. You may make that body healthier by bringing its specific gravity up to the ideal figure for its best operation. You can break that body by letting its specific gravity run down. Basically there are two ways to bring up a low specific gravity. One is by your diet, the other is by exercise. But it should be exercise that must be taken every single day. I like walking for that purpose, and it should be for a minimum of an hour a day. Walking is the great elixir of human life! You cannot imagine how important it is.

Alcohol and the Heart

There is a generally held belief that a little alcohol taken every day will open up the coronary arteries, and that, therefore, it is advisable for heart cases to take a little nip of liquor every day. According to revised medical opinion, this is not so, and it is quite dangerous to indulge in this practice. In the first place, alcohol destroys vitamin B in the body. Secondly, it damages the nervous system and the brain. It affects the liver, many of the glands, destroys red blood corpuscles and is generally harmful to the metabolic processes of the body. In addition, alcohol is a poison. In fact, the word intoxicated means being "poisoned." Alcohol by medical agreement is a definite, dangerous poison, and is the greatest single cause of insanity. And yet the public as well as most physicians are in full accord with the fact that a little alcohol every day is desirable for older people and for heart cases. However, I have seen several of my relatively young friends die of heart attacks, who were following their doctors' instructions to drink a little liquor every day to open up their arteries.

I was sailing along agreeing with the popular stream of thought about this "little bit of daily liquor," when in reading the July 14, 1956, issue of the *Medical Journal of Australia,* I came across an abstract of an article that had appeared in the January, 1956, issue of *Diseases of the Chest.* It was as follows:

"A. M. Master and H. L. Jaffe . . . believe that a low-calorie diet should be given in coronary thrombosis because such a diet diminishes the work of the heart and prevents gastrocardiac reflexes. Whiskey should not be given, because it may increase the pulse rate. Smoking should be prohibited."

This gave me a little jolt! This was the first negative word I had ever heard against whiskey in a heart condition. I, therefore, decided to investigate further, searching in indexes and medical books. My search was finally rewarded when I found a piece of medical research that was so convincing that never again will I remain quiet when I hear a person say that a small amount of alcoholic liquor is advisable for a heart patient or for an older person.

The work of this research was done by 3 United States Public Health Service doctors who wrote it up in the May 27, 1950, issue of the *Journal of the American Medical Association.* Their names are Russek, Naegele and Regan. The article about it in the *Science News Letter* of June 3, 1950, carries the following title: "Alcohol No Heart Remedy," and the subheading: "The past practice of giving alcohol in cases of the heart disease known as angina should be changed. Alcohol does not dilate the heart arteries as once thought."

[142]

The 3 researchers screened out a large number of heart cases and from them chose 5 who, from a technical point of view, would be preferable for the electrocardiographic readings. On certain occasions each one of them was given some glycerol trinitrate, a type of drug usually given when angina or chest pressure symptoms occur. On other occasions the same persons were given 1 or 2 ounces of whiskey. In each case an electrocardiographic reading was taken a little afterwards, the person being made to do some exercise first. Only one test was given in any one day. Say the authors: "The results of this study clearly indicate that a misconception exists regarding the value of whiskey in the treatment of coronary disease." It was found, however, that although the electrocardiographic reading showed that alcohol did not do anything for the arteries, it did prevent somewhat the pressure pains of angina, but it did this by sedative action, not by opening up the arteries. The article states that since its pharmacologic action on the coronary circulation is so different from that of glycerol trinitrate, alcohol can no longer be advised for the purpose of opening up the coronary arteries.

The authors wind up by saying that alcohol is not a coronary vasodilator and that if it is employed regularly it will create a false sense of physical fitness and security that could lead to fatal consequences.

My suggestion: If you're a heart case, become a teetotaler and observe the law of not even one. If you won't take the first drink, there will be no second. At the same time give up coffee, tea and tobacco.

Heart Disease and Smoking

A person who has heart disease is committing slow suicide if he is a smoker—whether it be of cigarettes, cigars or a pipe. Something in tobacco prevents the heart from functioning properly. There is so much clinical evidence of this that it should convince even the most skeptical.

I will submit a few items from a bulging file of medical researches and investigations. In 1954 the American Cancer Society reported on a survey of almost 200,000 people, consisting of smokers and non-smokers. In this group of smokers (a pack of cigarettes or more a day) there were 344 deaths from heart disease. Only 171 would have died of this cause if their mortality rates had been the same as the men in this group who never smoked.

An editorial in the *Journal of the American Medical Association* (November 8, 1952) tells us that cigarette smoking causes a definite constriction of the blood vessels, that it raises the blood pressure and the pulse rate. These effects are extremely detrimental to heart cases, or to persons who are susceptible to cardiac trouble.

In the *Connecticut Medical Journal* for January, 1957, there is a report on 20 young men (from 20 to 40 years old) who had heart attacks due to hardening of the coronary artery. Of these, 14 were heavy smokers (using between 40 to 100 cigarettes a day); 4 were moderate smokers (using 10 to 20 cigarettes daily); and only two did not smoke. The authors state that this is a higher number of heavy smokers than would be found among a group of young men chosen at random, that is, men without hardening of the arteries.

Dr. McCormick speaks about the effect of tobacco on the vitamin reserves in the body. He refers to two medical investigators, Onastel and Wheatley, who have shown that tobacco causes a vitamin B_1 deficiency in the body. Dr. McCormick has also proven in his own clinical researches that smoking causes serious deficiencies in vitamin C.

Says Dr. McCormick, "Recently Patterson has called attention to the low vitamin C status of coronary thrombosis cases. He found that 81 per cent of such cases in hospital practice had a subnormal blood-plasma level as compared to 55.8 per cent in a corresponding group of general public-ward patients. He . . . suggests that patients with this disease be assured of an adequate intake of vitamin C."

Most Americans are aware these days of the controversy that rages over the fact that an overabundance of cholesterol in the blood stream appears to be intimately related to hardening of the arteries and thus to heart disease. Earlier we showed how vitamin C is able to reduce the cholesterol in the blood stream. Now, if smoking reduces the supply of the body's vitamin C, one can see its danger to a heart case—smoking would tend to cause an increase in the cholesterol content of the blood.

An article in the *New York Times* for September 6, 1955, tells of definite research relating smoking to fatty particles in the blood.

"Men who smoke cigarettes regularly run a 40 per cent greater risk of dying of coronary heart disease than do non-smokers," says the article.

". . . the link has been established between smoking, the presence in the blood stream of giant particles of fatty materials, and the development of coronary heart disease. This affliction is one of the leading causes of death in the nation today. Heart diseases are now the leading cause of death in the United States; coronary heart disease alone accounts for nearly half of all deaths due to heart and blood vessel diseases in general."

Doctors have warned heart patients for years against the effects of smoking. In March of 1955, the *Journal of the American Medical Association* ran an editorial which erased all doubt as to the official position of doctors on smoking and heart disease. "There seems now to be definite evidence that smoking, even though it may not directly affect the coronary arteries, can have a damaging effect on the myocardium (muscular wall of the heart). . . . No patient with coronary disease should incur the added risk to his heart imposed by smoking . . ."

The data I have presented isn't one-tenth of what we have in our files regarding the dangers of smoking to a heart case or to one who fears to contract this condition. But it should act as a warning to smokers and should discourage non-smokers from ever considering the adoption of this dangerous habit. In the great controversy now raging over whether smoking causes cancer of the lungs, this other aspect—that smoking causes heart attacks—seems to be completely ignored.

The Heart and Coffee Drinking

It is important that a heart case give up coffee drinking, so as to insure that no other pathological conditions will arise to impose an additional burden on the heart. But coffee drinking is bad for the heart itself, as you shall see.

Of all the harm that coffee drinking does, its ability to prevent iron from being utilized in the body is one of the more serious disadvantages. A doctor writing to the *Lancet* (December 7, 1957) says, "It is indeed rather difficult to understand how people who take tea or coffee with every meal can ever absorb iron from their food at all." This could lead to anemia which is a rather unpleasant complication for a heart case.

Then there is the question of a possible vitamin deficiency caused by coffee drinking. Walter H. Eddy, Ph.D., in his book, *Vitaminology* (Williams and Wilkins), says it may be that large amounts of caffeine in coffee may create an inositol deficiency. Inositol is one of the B complex vitamins. The coffee bean contains from 1 to 2 per cent caffeine. It has been reported, says Dr. Eddy, that when commercial coffee was added to the basal diet of dogs, a paralysis resulted that was curable by inositol. An eye condition also occurred that could be corrected by giving biotin, another of the B vitamins. The suggestion is that the inclusion of caffeine in the diet can creat a biotin and inositol deficiency.

Drugs and certain soluble chemicals have been known to use up some of the body's vitamin resources. Chlorine uses up vitamin E, alcohol vitamin B, tobacco vitamin C. Now we see that caffeine has a similar power, and for that reason it is absolutely contra-indicated to a heart case, for such deficiencies can cause serious disorders in the body that may make it more difficult for the heart to function efficiently.

Caffeine as a drug is used by the medical profession in certain cases of heart trouble. It dilates the coronary arteries, and furnishes a better blood supply to the heart. Many heart cases will experience a sense of comfort with coffee, but this is the short-term effect. What is its effect on the long-pull?

In this respect I would like to relate my own experience. For a long time I came to lean rather heavily on coffee, drinking 8 cups a day, and it worked wonderfully as far as my heart condition was concerned. When I gave it up on several occasions, I would begin to experience chest angina pains on exertion. But when I went back to coffee, this condition would miraculously clear up. Of course, basically it was the vitamin E that I was taking that prevented these symptoms, but coffee was doing its share, too. One seemed to be no good without the other. So I went about singing the praises of coffee, and feeling that perhaps it was saving my life.

But something was happening to me that made me question the use of coffee. In the first place, I was becoming very nervous. Secondly, I seemed to be experiencing difficulty in remembering things. I would meet a person on the street whom I knew rather intimately and for the life of me, I wouldn't be able to think of his name. Caffeine, I knew, destroys nerve cells and I could see that it was beginning to do a rather good job on mine, especially the ones in my brain.

Now I began to realize that drinking coffee could be a powerful contributor to the senility of old age, the doddering of the mind and the body in general. Dr. Frederick C. Swartz, of Lansing, Michigan, in a discussion of physical health at the University of Michigan recently said that if a person wished to avoid shaky hands and a tottering gait in later life he should give up drinking coffee.

As far as my heart was concerned, coffee drinking didn't seem to hurt it. On the contrary it seemed to help. It didn't raise my pulse even one beat a minute. But I feared some hidden damage that it could be doing which would make my heart suffer later in the period near the last lap when my heart would want every organ of my body to play ball properly.

I decided to cut out drinking coffee for the third time. I watched for the return of my heart symptoms as had occurred twice before, but this time I did not experience them. Evidently my program of healthy living, daily exercise, walking an hour a day, taking my vitamins and following a generally healthy nutritional program had strengthened my heart, so that this time it didn't require coffee as a prop. And slowly my nervousness began to disappear and my ability to remember improve. As the months go by, I feel better and better, but it will take many years to do away completely with the damage that coffee did to my body.

H. M. Marvin, M.D., in his book, *You and Your Heart* (Random House, 1950), states that the effect of coffee varies among different individuals. Some find that their heart beats faster, but others do not. Some people seem to develop a tolerance for coffee, but there are hidden effects that may not appear on the surface. One can "get away with" coffee drinking up to a certain age perhaps, but what is the cumulative effect of the caffeine at later ages, and exactly what is the danger point as far as age is concerned?

A heart case should be very careful how he cuts out coffee drinking, if he has come to depend on it. If he experiences any symptoms, then he must go on a rigorous program of developing his body the way I did. Temporarily, he might have to reduce the number of cups a day, or drink half cups. But gradually, through careful body conditioning, he is bound to conquer the habit without distressing his heart.

The Pulse

In the consideration of heart disease one of the most important factors is the pulse (a high pulse being very dangerous in such a condition). Very little, however, is heard about this subject when heart disease is being discussed. In my treatment of the subject of heart disease, therefore, I intend to go into the subject of the pulse in some detail.

According to the *Encyclopedia Britannica,* "The normal average pulse rate is 72 per minute, in women about 80; but individual variations from 40 to 100 have been observed consistent with health."

When we use the word *pulse* we are talking about what is called the heart rate, or the rate at which the heart pumps the blood. While the body is at rest, the heart will pump at an average rate of 90 gallons of blood an hour. During violent exercise it will pump at the rate of 450 to 600 gallons an hour, which means that the pulse goes up. But the rate at which the heart will pump differs in different people. For example, taking arbitrary figures, in one person it might take 100 beats to pump a gallon of blood while in another it might have to be done with 200 beats. The pulse beat represents the rate at which the heart pushes the blood through a network of vessels in the body that average 168 million miles in length. There are many factors involved in this work, but I will state as a general rule that the lower the pulse, within reason of course, the better it is for the health of your heart.

Drs. Raymond Pearl and W. Eden Moffet in a report to the National Academy of Science in 1940, reported that in studying the lives of 386 men, they found that those lived longer who had a lower pulse by about 4 beats a minute than the shorter-lived ones. The long-lived group lived on an average 26 years longer than the short-lived group. Incidentally, the long-lived group had a weight of 6 pounds each less than the short-lived group. The interesting fact in this study is that if only a 4 beat difference had such a significant effect, what would be the effect of a greater difference? For example, by certain methods, I reduced my own pulse from 85 to about 68. The method will be explained later.

Now suppose you suddenly discover that your pulse is high. Is there anything you can do about it? The answer is a definite yes. How does one go about reducing one's pulse? There are several things you can do.

First, you must reduce the quantity of food you eat per day. This should apply mainly to overweight persons so that if you are underweight, you would have to get special advice in this category.

A second means of lowering the pulse is to avoid emotional storms. Dr. William Dock, Professor of Medicine at State University of New York College of Medicine, at a meeting of the New York Academy of Medicine in 1951 said, "Cardiac acceleration is a common sequel of anger, apprehension and related moods, so that heart failure may be precipitated by emotional storms, just as it is by fever and other conditions . . . which accelerate the pulse."

A third means of lowering the pulse, if one is a smoker, is to eliminate that habit. Nicotine causes a shrinking of the arteries and will raise the pulse from 5 to 20 beats a minute. Fourth: Avoid the use of drugs. Physicians have observed very high pulses in persons taking antihistamines. Many persons take this type of drug for hay fever. Many sulfur-containing drugs will heighten the pulse. Digitalis, given to prevent a heart attack, has been known to accelerate the pulse. Desiccated thyroid substance will increase the heart rate, as will certain preparations used to cure the tobacco habit. A person can easily check the pulse effect of any drug he is taking. Most of them are bad for the pulse, which means bad for the heart.

High temperature may raise the pulse. If a person has a heart condition, he should not work in front of a steel furnace, or in a bakery where the heat is high. It will raise the pulse by 10 or more beats a minute.

There are two other means of reducing the pulse which are extremely important. One is exercise, and the other is a study of one's diet to eliminate particular foods that have a propensity to raise the pulse. It is a form of allergy. The science of ascertaining these pulse-irritating foods was developed by Arthur F. Coca, M.D., and will be discussed in the following pages along with a description of how I reduced my pulse by means of exercise.

The Coca Method

Several years ago I was extremely fortunate in discovering Dr. Arthur F. Coca's work in curing allergies through the observation and control of the human pulse. Up to this time the procedure, in checking for a person's allergies, was to scratch the skin with a needle, but Dr. Coca obtained the same results, even more correctly, by observing the effect of each food on a person's pulse. If, when a person ate only of one particular food, it was observed that it abnormally raised the pulse, then there was an allergy to that food. Dr. Coca found that the average sick person's pulse was high because in his diet there were usually included 5 or 6 foods which were difficult for his digestive system to handle, the theory being that in such cases the heart had to work harder to bring extra pressure to bear to complete the digestion of those foods.

In following Dr. Coca's system you choose a time about an hour and a half after you have eaten and eat a small portion of a food that you wish to test, taking your pulse immediately before the test. You then take your pulse a half hour later, and again a half hour after that, recording the figures in a ruled blank book, with the date, time, etc., leaving room for a list of the food eaten, and other comments. It will become a valuable record for later study.

I found that the average food raised the pulse from 3 to 5 points per minute, although there were some that did not raise it at all, but that when a food caused the pulse to run up 8 or 9 points, it was usually one of the allergy-causing ones. In my own case I discovered that figs, honeydew melon, hot chicken soup, onions, whole wheat and fried foods of any kind were the basic trouble-makers. It was absolutely fascinating the fun there was in checking them down. For example, at first the indication showed that chicken raised my pulse unduly. But after I had accumulated sufficient records, showing in each case whether the chicken had been fried or broiled, I found that my pulse went up only when I ate fried chicken. I could eat broiled chicken without any trouble at all.

The whole thing is terrific in its implications! When one considers what a reduction of the pulse means to one's well-being and longevity, it is to wonder that so little work has been done in connection with researches on the human pulse. In my own case, merely by cutting certain items of food out of my diet, my pulse was reduced by 15 beats per minute.

If you decide to make a pulse study, my suggestion is first, for about a week, to keep a record of your pulse before and after whole meals. Take the pulse a half hour and an hour after your regular meals, without attempting to cut anything out of your diet. Later, after you have learned what foods are irritating your pulse, and have eliminated them, do the same, and observe the difference in the pulse increase, before and after meals.

For a heart case it is of the utmost importance to make use of the Coca system for reducing the pulse, for the heart will have far less work to do if the pulse is significantly lowered.

I would like to describe another bit of personal research that was an outcome of my pulse experiments. I noticed that after one particular meal my pulse shot up much more than it should have, and for no accountable reason. After a bit of reflection, however, I recalled that I had overlooked taking my vitamins at that meal. In other words, I figured, in some way, vitamins added to food at meals cause it to be more thoroughly digested.

What is the reasoning behind this statement? Digestion requires the aid of the pump—the heart. If there is some difficulty at a particular meal, the heart has to pump more, which is reflected in more beats of the pump per minute. Could it be possible that vitamins act as catalysts with food, causing it to be more thoroughly digested and absorbed by the blood stream, thus putting less of a load on the heart? If this is so, think what a help the taking of vitamins at meals could be to the average heart case! The important point at issue is, that if the results I have obtained are generally applicable, then it is extremely important that we divide our daily vitamin ration into 3 portions, taking some at breakfast, some at lunch and some at dinner.

The Reduction of Pulse by Exercises

Before I became aware of the power of exercise to bring the pulse down, I was the most typical example of the sedentary businessman you could find. But after writing my series called *This Pace Is Not Killing Us,* I began to realize that unless I went in for exercise, my physically inactive life would surely kill *me* before my time.

But here I was with a high pulse which had to come down by means of exercise, or else my life would be shortened, and, on the other hand, a heart condition which might not respond too well to exercise. I had always heard that a heart case must rest as much as possible. So I decided to approach the matter warily. The first day I walked for only 10 minutes. Nothing happened! I was still alive. For the next few days I

[149]

walked 10 minutes each day. Then I upped it to 15 and in about a week I was doing a full hour every morning, covering a brisk 3 miles, and enjoying it immensely.

One day during this hourly walk it seemed that my heart began to pound a little, so I stopped and took my pulse. To my surprise I found it to be 112. As my pulse at rest was between 76 and 80, I came to the conclusion that it was the exercise of walking that was making my heart work harder. A few hours later at rest my pulse was back to about 78. In other words, the demands that my walking made on my heart had raised it about 35 beats a minute. An interesting bit of knowledge, I thought.

Thinking that danger might be concealed somewhere in this fact, I decided from this point on to keep a record of my pulse during these walks.

A word about the method of taking my pulse. When I stop, I wait about 20 seconds, and then count the beats of my heart as I note the ticking off of 30 seconds by the watch. I then take the count of the next 30 seconds and that is the one I record. This, of course, is then multiplied by two. I stop for a rest of about a half minute to a minute, halfway between each pulse stop, thus making about 20 stops in all. However, if I experience any pressure symptoms, I will stop for a moment wherever necessary. Remember, I am still a heart case.

As my walks progressed, from day to day, there occurred a reduction in the pulse, and a development gradually of a sense of well-being towards the end of each walk. This indicated possibly that the flabbiness of the heart was turning into muscle. But there was still something wrong either with the heart, or the arteries leading in and out of it, that gave me the pains during the first 15 minutes of walking each day. Then these practically disappeared, and at the same time there is a sizeable increase in the pulse. Does this indicate a second step in the rebuilding process? Have the heart muscles become so strong that they can do some function that they could not do before? Have they been able to close some kind of gap? Have they engaged in some additional physical building of something in the heart, an action which required the help of the whole heart to pump more blood for its accomplishment? Such a project would definitely raise the pulse.

Then the thing is done. The heart goes back to its previous pace. It goes down as precipitately as it went up. Is this fantastic reasoning? Perhaps. But it will have to do until someone works out a better reason. Perhaps it was not the heart alone. Is it possible that my lungs were strengthening themselves, being able to perform more efficiently so as to give more oxygen to the heart with less physical action of taking breaths?

During my daily walk, I perspire profusely. Perspiration is one means the body employs to rid itself of toxins, or poisons. Is it possible that such poisons, remaining in the body, because of a sedentary daily regimen, make the heart work harder to rid the body of them through other means and channels?

Is it also possible that these toxins by remaining in the body and distorting the blood chemistry on a permanent, continuing basis, further interfere with various internal processes, which throw additional strain onto the heart, thus forcing it to pump more rapidly in an attempt to reduce the condition?

Not every heart case will be permitted to do what I have done. The physician must be the judge in each case. There may be serious cases where extreme caution will be in order. There are damaged hearts, and those that have experienced thrombosis, occlusions and surgery. These persons must depend on their physicians for guidance.

The Width of Arteries

Wide, roomy arteries are a tremendous advantage in going through life, and people that are so endowed can go at a faster pace than people who have narrow arteries.

The disadvantage of narrow arteries is that if a narrow-arteried person gets cholesterol deposits on the walls of his blood vessels, the space in them is cut down to such an extent that a serious blood blockage could result. On the other hand, if a person has wide arteries and cholesterol deposits pile up, there is still enough room for the blood to course through them freely.

Dr. Edgar Rentoul of Houston, Renfrewshire, England, in a special communication to the *Lancet* of December 12, 1953, was skirting around this field of speculation. He said,

"1. A few people are so genetically constituted that their coronary arteries are resistant to all adverse factors.

"2. In the remainder the principal factors are of a simple mechanical nature: (a) the bigger the coronary arteries, the more room there is to have atheromatous plaques without disastrous results; (b) the faster the blood goes through the coronary arteries, the less likely it is that they will develop obstructions in their walls.

"3. Assuming these statements to be correct, then the part played by exercise is clear. The more you exercise, the bigger your coronary arteries: the more you exercise, the faster the blood flows through them, the more difficult it is for an obstruction to develop on the walls.

"4. I think that the exercise, to be really effective as a protector of the coronary arteries, must be fairly vigorous. The round of golf once a week is not much use."

I would like to compliment Dr. Rentoul on his observations. Under number (1) above he says that some people are born with such a physical heritage that they can go along under adverse conditions and not have a heart attack. These people have wide arteries. He confirms this thinking under number (2a) when he says that where the arteries are wide, even though they are coated with cholesterol, there is still plenty of room for the blood to circulate. Under (2b) he says that the faster the blood goes

through the coronary arteries, the less likelihood there is that a fatal blockage will result. Then under (3) he states that exercise not only widens the
arteries, but makes the blood flow faster in them.

I know this from my personal experience. When I go on my daily
one-hour walk, sometimes under adverse conditions, I may experience slight
chest heart symptoms, but this will occur only at the beginning of the
walk. What is the reason for this? Evidently a failure of the arteries to
feed the blood fast enough to the heart, due to narrow arteries. But as I
keep moving, my coronary arteries open up, and the blood flows faster. The
result is that I never experience these symptoms after the first 10 or 15
minutes of the walk. So it seems that continuous exercise over the years
could be a powerful factor in gradually widening the arteries.

The Villains—Starch and Sugar

The book, *How to Prevent Heart Attacks,* by Benjamin P. Sandler,
M.D. (Lee Foundation for Nutritional Research, 2023 West Wisconsin
Avenue, Milwaukee, Wisconsin), is based on the theory that low sugar in
the blood is the cause of heart disease. Dr. Sandler is connected with the
Veterans' Hospital at Oteen, North Carolina.

Dr. Sandler does not believe that the fat content of the diet is responsible for the recent increase in heart disease. This sounds incredible, based
on the huge amount of research that has been done on cholesterol and
fat, but perhaps eventually it may be found that Dr. Sandler's low carbohydrate diet will be more effective in curing heart disease than the low fat
diet. Probably a combination of both will be found to be the answer.

The proof of the pudding is in the eating, says Dr. Sandler, because
the low carbohydrate diet he devised has been successful in many cases in
giving relief from attacks of heart pain, and to prevent their occurrence.
One of the clues that convinced Dr. Sandler of the dangers of carbohydrates and sugar to heart cases was the fact that in diabetics heart disease
is more serious, occurs at an earlier age and is more common.

Dr. Sandler draws attention to the fact that 100 per cent of the
carbohydrate food (sugar and starch) one eats, turns to sugar. Such food
items as bread, macaroni, rice, spaghetti and cereals are typical starchy
foods. So, in order to keep the sugar consumption low, we must be extremely cautious with respect to the carbohydrate content of our diets. A
high consumption of sugar and starch will lead to a low level of sugar in
the blood, and that is what leads to heart symptoms.

How does a high sugar diet lead to a low level of sugar in the blood?
When one ingests sugar, or starch that turns to sugar, insulin is secreted in
the pancreatic gland in order to prevent it from raising the level of sugar
in the blood. The function of the insulin is to keep the sugar down. But
if too much insulin is secreted as occurs where large amounts of sugar are
ingested, then the sugar in the blood declines considerably. The liver,
certain glands and part of the nervous system also enter into the process,
but it is the insulin directly that lowers the blood sugar.

In order to understand how this theory works we must know the effect of sugar on the heart's action. "The heart muscle is made up of innumerable muscle cells," says Dr. Sandler. "Like all muscle tissue, it needs certain nutrients to perform its work of contraction and relaxation. The chief nutrients are sugar and oxygen, both of which are brought to the muscle by the blood. . . . In the muscle cells, the sugar and oxygen react chemically to yield the necessary energy needed for the work of contraction. . . . Among the many varied and complicated chemical reactions that occur during (heart) muscle contraction, is the production of lactic acid. . . . Under certain conditions, lactic acid may accumulate in abnormal quantities in a muscle, including the heart, and it is believed that this accumulation of lactic acid along with a few other acid metabolites produced during muscle contraction is responsible for the heart pain. One of the conditions that may cause this abnormal accumulation of metabolites is the . . . abnormally low sugar utilization by the heart muscle. . . . Any significant interference with the supply of sugar or oxygen will embarrass heart action, and the degree of interference will determine the degree of embarrassment—from a mild fleeting chest pain to the severe crushing pain of the fatal heart attack."

But it isn't merely the low blood sugar that does the harm. Dr. Sandler has found from experience that it is the violent fluctuations in the blood sugar that create trouble. Eating a meal rich in carbohydrates will do that because first it raises the blood sugar, then it lowers it. "The rapid rate of change in the downward direction results in a severe environmental change for the heart muscle to which it fails to accommodate readily and so the muscle is embarrassed and the symptoms of pain are felt by the patient."

In addition to sugar, as has already been said, oxygen is important to the healthful operation of the heart muscle. Quoting Dr. Sandler, "It has been shown that a cell utilizes oxygen in proportion as it utilizes sugar. But oxygen is useful to the cell only if there is some fuel to burn (oxidize) for the production of energy. The blood may be normally saturated with oxygen but if the blood sugar level is half of what it should be, the body will consume less than normal oxygen. . . . It has been accepted by many that the immediate cause of heart pain is an acute oxygen lack on the part of the heart muscle."

Stresses and Strains

The fact that stresses that arise in our daily lives can be a factor inimical to good heart health came forcefully home to me one day at the Hialeah race track at Miami, Florida. Some friends had dragged me there and under conditions of propinquity I put $25 on a horse. He was a 10 to 1 shot, and as I saw him edging ahead, and realized that I might win $250, I began to experience some terrific angina pains. It wasn't the money, it was the excitement of winning. My horse *did* win by a good margin, but it was a rather close call for me. Had it not been that I am a regular taker of heavy doses of vitamin E, along with eating what I consider the proper

[153]

diet for a heart case, and walking an hour a day, I believe my number would have been up that day. So, today, when I read that stresses and strains are a factor in heart disease, I pay attention.

Let us see what some physicians think on this subject. Dr. Herman T. Blumenthal, Laboratory Director of St. Louis Jewish Hospital, as reported in *Newsweek* for April 16, 1956, believes that emotional stress is the main cause of arteriosclerosis, or hardening of the arteries. For what reason? He claims that stress raises the blood pressure. It is not normal high blood pressure that damages the artery walls, but the characteristic fluctuations in it, caused by stress and strain—the ups and downs. Fluctuations of blood pressure against artery walls cause injuries and hardening. To be healthy, artery walls should be elastic. A significant remark made by Dr. Blumenthal: "Except for a small number of persons who have inherited abnormal amounts of fat in their blood stream, cholesterol is the result, not the cause of the disease."

Dr. Hans Selye in his famous book, *Stress* (Acta, Incorporated), states that emotional excitement leads to the increase of the pulse rate and blood pressure and causes a shrinking of the arteries. Fear will markedly reduce the flow of blood in the body. In experiments, says Dr. Selye, repeated emotional stimuli caused an inflammation of the external sheath of arteries which is the reason why various stresses cause angina pains. "Many other experimental and clinical observations suggest that nervous strain can cause arteriosclerotic lesions."

Situations provocative of frustration and anger raise the blood pressure, says Dr. Selye, and reduce the blood flow to and from the kidneys. Studying 695 men of an armored brigade which took part in desert warfare for one year, it was found that 27 per cent had high blood pressure at rest for months after this period.

In the *Journal of the American Medical Association* of June 12, 1954, Smith and Chapman write of a simulated heart disease caused by anxiety. In other words, some persons are talking themselves into having symptoms of heart disease. According to one authority, 90 per cent of the soldiers in British army cardiac (heart) hospitals during World War I had no organic heart disease. The patient's fears and anxieties cause him to think he has heart disease—any minor discomfort is interpreted as a sign of disease. Such persons actually develop palpitations, chest pain and difficulty in breathing.

According to these authors, the best treatment for such cases is in some way to relieve their anxiety, to decrease their tensions. In my opinion, if vitamin E were prescribed, it would be far better, especially if it were accompanied by a thorough description of what it could do for the patient. That would be an effective way to subdue his fears and decrease his tensions. Perhaps the fact that these people worry easily may be due to the fact that they have many vitamin and mineral deficiencies, and the prescribing and use of a whole set of vitamins and minerals will give them a sense of physical well-being that would preclude the harboring of such imaginary anxieties.

Vitamins B and C especially are very important to counteract the effects of stress on the body. This subject is covered in the *Merck Reporter*, October, 1952, in an article by Drs. Goodhart and Jolliffe. According to this article, vitamin C is found in large amounts in the adrenal glands and is needed in additional amounts in adaptation to stresses. It states that the requirement for the B vitamins rises during stress.

If one has a heart condition or the symptoms just described, one must go into training so as to be able to cope with the occasional stresses that may arise. I follow and do all the things suggested in this book and feel certain that they will protect me under conditions of heavy mental and emotional strain.

Exercise

There was a time when I used to pooh-pooh the value of exercise and used to tell the story of Chauncey Depew, the famous financier of the last century, who lived to be way over 90, and who always deprecated the importance of taking exercise. "The only exercise I get," he used to say, "is to act as pallbearer for friends who used to take exercise."

Perhaps he didn't take exercise as such, but I'll wager he was a big walker, for those were the days before the auto was known. He was a stockholder in many corporations and was known to attend many board meetings, going from one to another, sometimes merely to show his face and to collect the director's fee. But there is a reason why some persons live to 90 without exercise, and why others die at 50. It is a matter of the vitality endowment at birth, the condition of the glands, chest expansion, width of arteries, etc. If a man has chosen the right ancestors and received a good share of their physical perfection through the accident of birth, then he can break many health rules and still live to a ripe old age.

One need not spend hours in daily calisthenics. Walking furnishes a very interesting form of exercise, although at least 10 minutes of daily setting-up exercises can be very valuable. I strongly recommend a walk of at least an hour a day. Some people seem to forget that they have feet. They forget that there is such a thing as walking. The other day in visiting a hospital I walked down two flights of stairs, and a nurse remarked, in amazement, "Are you *walking* down?"

A doctor in a medical journal says, "The popular picture of the coronary heart disease victim is that of a burly business or professional man, fat and soft from overeating and lack of exercise." Another expresses it this way, "Motion is the essence of life. Like all things pertaining to life, we know little concerning it. It is an inherent characteristic of all animate things to move through space with ease and power, not only for protection but for the pleasure of doing so." I have learned to love my daily hour's walk, and wouldn't miss it for anything except rain or snow.

Dr. Paul D. White, a world renowned heart specialist, told a House

Appropriations Subcommittee, "Coronary thrombosis is an epidemic. . . . Wise exercise is one remedy."

As far as I'm concerned, I'm conscious of the fact that I have to move about as much as possible, in order to keep the fat out of my heart muscle. I have my telephone at another desk. Every time it rings I have to walk 15 feet to it and 15 feet back. My office is on the third floor and every day I walk up and down to and from it at least 4 or 5 times—sometimes more, because I purposely do not have a buzzer system. When I want to talk to one of my people, I go to them. I do not make them come to me.

John Homans, M.D., in the *New England Journal of Medicine*, January 28, 1954, said, "The prolonged sitting position occasions a degree of dependency stasis that may result in the rapid development of a quiet type of thrombosis in the deep veins of the calf. From this, a propagation of clot and pulmonary embolism may immediately follow . . . Such matters are important enough to suggest the advisability of making movements of the toes, feet and lower legs when one is sitting for long periods and of getting up and exercising when opportunity offers. The right leg seems more susceptible than the left. There is evidence that persons over 50 years of age should have this particularly in mind and that physicians should be alert to recognize the significance of lameness after airplane flights, automobile trips and other occasions of a prolonged seated position."

Dr. Edward P. Luongo of Los Angeles in a report to an American Medical Association convention described a study of 100 heart cases in the 40-to-50-year-old age group, and stated that 70 of them showed no regular exercise patterns either at work or away from their jobs. Dr. Charles H. Bradford, at an Eastern regional meeting of the International College of Surgeons in 1957 said that "Nature did not intend the intricate cardiac mechanism to serve a sedentary body. Certainly, the stimulus of natural exercise plays a wholesome part in regulating metabolic disorders."

Many physicians advise their patients against climbing stairs. Except in rare cases, according to the best opinion today, this is a great blunder.

I am a heart case and as I have said a few moments ago, I climb two flights of stairs 4 or 5 times every day, and have hardened myself because of it. I can now accomplish it without becoming winded. So many of my visitors come up to my office puffing terribly. It is a sign that they don't exercise every day.

Dr. Richard T. Smith, Director of the Department of Rheumatology, of the Pennsylvania Hospital, said that human life may well be shortened below its potential by lack of both physical and mental activity. He said, "The heart is a muscle and must have maintenance of tone. It is not the athletic heart that kills us, but lack of it."

Is this enough? I can give you much more on the dangers of a sedentary life, but there are more aspects of the general subject of exercise which will have to be covered. So, whether you have heart disease or not, get out and move. Walk, do setting-up exercise, go window-shopping—any kind of movement will suffice. You will never regret it.

Exercise—*What It Does*

The most important thing that exercise does is to oxygenate the body which is most desirable to a heart case, for it is lack of oxygen which is an important element in inducing a heart attack. Oxygenation of the body may be compared to the draft of a boiler which burns up the refuse and slag in the body.

Dr. William B. Kountz, Professor of Clinical Medicine at Washington University, at a public meeting said that the medical profession has long been aware that a decline in the body's oxygen consumption causes such ailments as hardening of the arteries, heart disease, body-wasting and other typical manifestations of old age. This is important, he said, in the maintaining of the burning or oxidative process of the body. The *Journal of the American Medical Association* of September 15, 1956, states that when the oxygen supply to the tissues goes down, the number and size of the cells also decreases. This causes tissue atrophy, or aging. Thus, by taking exercise, and insuring the oxygenation of the body, one ages gracefully.

Angina pectoris, a disease marked by a sudden or periodic chest pain, sometimes with a feeling of suffocation and impending death, is due most often to lack of oxygen in the muscular substance of the heart; that is, the heart muscle.

Another effect of exercise is to maintain the general muscular tone throughout the body. This includes the heart muscle, the importance of whose tone can well be realized. An important muscle is the diaphragm which, if its muscular tone improves, will enable a person to breathe more efficiently. This means healthier lungs. The diaphragm is like the piston of a pump in its action, and if it has good tone, it can more efficiently cause the suction of blood into the heart via the great veins. Exercise breaks up congestion in the lungs. Breathing becomes easier.

The effect of exercise is to quicken the circulation. *Science News Letter* of November 3, 1951, says in this respect:

"In a man at rest about a gallon of blood is circulated every minute . . . approximately the entire blood supply visits the tissues once every minute. With vigorous exercise these visits may be 8 or 9 times as frequent. The blood, instead, of traveling at a rate of 55 feet a minute in the large arteries may move 450 feet a minute. This makes possible a more rapid and complete removal of waste from all parts of the body, and increases the amount of oxygen in parts of the body depending on it. Exercise taken simply and regularly tends to keep the arteries soft, warding off arteriosclerosis or other old age conditions."

Dr. Paul D. White, mentioned earlier in this chapter, in a medical article (*Journal of the American Medical Association*, September 7, 1957) stated that exercise improves bowel function and digestion. It also helps to induce sleep, more "than any medicine, highball or television show." It controls obesity, and, most important takes the fat out of the walls of the coronary and other important arteries. This is one of the most important rewards of exercise. It reduces the cholesterol level of the blood.

Besides lowering the cholesterol level of the blood, exercise increases the specific gravity of the body, making the tissues more compact. This is highly desirable in connection with the body's general economy, but especially in regard to the functioning of the heart.

Dr. William Brady, in the *Chicago Daily News* of January 2, 1958, says that daily exercise—a brisk walk of several miles—causes the body to store up calcium. In other words, walking or other exercise promotes calcium metabolism. The reverse, says Dr. Brady, is also true. Prolonged confinement to bed or too much resting depletes the calcium reserve. That is why in so many cases a hip is broken after a bed-fast patient begins to move about. Many very old persons fall down and it is thought that as a result they break their hip. Now it is believed that the hip is broken first, which then causes the fall.

Exercise causes added vitamins to be absorbed by the body, especially vitamin A (*Journal of Nutrition*, April 10, 1958). This is probably due to better oxygenation and through improved digestion.

According to the *Journal of the American Medical Association* (October 5, 1957), "The greatest value (of exercise) lies in its stimulating effect on endocrine (glands) activity, perhaps the thyroid in particular, and in overcoming the tendency to sleep and snooze, too much a counterpart of obesity." When the endocrine glands are reduced in efficiency, a common occurrence with old people, it contributes to the fatigue of old age, which shows the importance of regular exercise for older persons.

There isn't a part of the body that doesn't seem to be aided by exercise and muscular activity.

Is Exercise Harmful To a Heart Case?

Is it dangerous for a heart case to exercise? To answer this question we must first analyze what is included in exercise. I think common sense would dictate that we should eliminate its more strenuous forms, such as tennis, basketball, etc. In our discussion we will include for our purposes such exercises as walking, golf, horseback riding, setting-up exercises, etc. To answer the question in the first sentence on this basis, I would say that 99 per cent of heart cases can safely exercise.

It used to be thought that the average heart attack came in the throes of severe activity, but recent studies indicate that this is not so. *Time*, of October 19, 1953, throws some light on the subject:

"Coronary patients who think they can stave off further attacks by unnatural idleness are mistaken," said Manhattan's Dr. Arthur M. Master. "Of 2,200 heart attacks, he found 23 per cent occurred during sleep, 29 per cent while at work, 24 per cent during mild activity, 13 per cent during walking at an ordinary pace, 9 per cent during moderate activity and only two per cent during unusual exertion."

Dr. Master found that "the percentage of attacks that occurred during sleep, rest, mild, moderate or severe activity coincided with the proportion of the day usually spent in these states. The occurrence of coronary occlusion thus seems to be coincidental with what the sufferer is doing when the attack occurs," Dr. Master said.

On page 1264 (April 2, 1955) of the *Journal of the American Medical Association* appears the statement: "Stout thus summarizes the matter: 'The mass of evidence indicates that work and exercise do not precipitate coronary thrombosis, coronary occulsion, or myocardial infarction.'" All 3 are forms of heart attacks.

Thus, we have shown that it is not exercise that is the cause of a heart attack. Now I would like to show, on the other hand, that exercise is a form of insurance to prevent a heart attack. In this respect I would like to consider a series of studies that were made in London, the results of which appeared in the *Lancet* for November 21 and 28, 1953, under the title "Coronary Heart Disease and Physical Activity of Work." The occurrence of coronary heart disease was studied in drivers and conductors of buses, trams and trolley buses, in motormen and guards on subways, a group comprising 31,000 men between the ages of 35 and 64.

Peculiarly it showed that "coronary heart disease behaves differently in the drivers and in the conductors . . . the immediate deaths accounted for 31 per cent in the drivers as against 19 per cent in the conductors.

"Is this a chance phenomenon? . . . the greater physical activity of 'conducting' (on these double-decker vehicles) is a cause of the lower incidence and mortality in the conductors . . . the underground railwaymen had a pattern of disease similar to that of the road vehicle drivers . . . the physical effort in the conductors' work may be a protective factor, safeguarding them in middle age from some of the worst manifestations of coronary heart disease suffered by less active workers."

An article in the *British Journal of Industrial Medicine* (10: 245, 1953) by doctors Morris and Heady also discusses a study which revealed that deaths from coronary heart disease "in middle age may be less common among men engaged in physically active work than among those in sedentary jobs. . . . It was found that the mortality from coronary heart disease at 45 to 64 years of age among the heavy workers was rather less than half that of the light workers."

The question may naturally arise whether there are certain kinds of heart conditions where caution should be the rule on the question of exercise. There are a few. Where there has been some kind of incident in connection with the heart, conservatism would call for prudence in connection with exercise. In such cases the physician will usually advise the proper course. Dr. U. L. Brown, in the *Medical Journal of Australia,* February 13, 1954, gives some good advice in this respect. He says: "Every case must be individually assessed, and you must steadily avoid the far too common and equally ignorant assertion that the manifestation of coronary disease marks the end of a man's useful working life. . . . A man may do in safety anything he can do in comfort, and he is well advised to remain active within his limits of comfortable exertion, rather than sink into himself and lead a life of invalidism. If he remains active, I believe that the development of the collateral circulation is assisted by the increased blood flow which accompanies effort, whereas it is probably hindered by the stagnating blood flow of ill-advised rest."

Diseases Caused by Lack of Exercise

Exercise is of most tremendous importance to the heart, but it is also effective in maintaining the health of the organs of the body. If you get sufficient exercise, every gland and organ of the body will benefit and be strengthened. A chain is as strong as its weakest link. If any organ is sick, it makes that much more work for the heart.

In the *American Practitioner and Digest of Treatment*, (July, 1956, p. 1114) appears the following: "Towbin has shown that the incidence of pulmonary embolism (the blocking of an artery in the lungs) is probably much higher than generally supposed. Many aged persons who supposedly die from cardiac (heart) disease probably die as the result of pulmonary embolism. Thrombophlebitis (a condition in which inflammation of the vein wall has preceded the formation of the clot in the vein) of the legs with its resultant pulmonary embolism is caused to some extent by lack of exercise. The evils of bed rest include the development of negative nitrogen balance and calcium loss through the kidneys with its possibility of development of kidney stone."

The article goes on to say: "Exercise may be important as an adjunct for mental health. Nervous tension can be released at times by exercise either in the form of specific muscular exercise or through some form of athletics."

Speaking about phlebitis mentioned above, I once had a friend, Dr. Otto Meyer, of New York, who died a few years ago, and who specialized in this disease. He effected miraculous cures by injections and bandaging of the feet of the patient and then advising him to walk a great deal every day. Dr. Meyer's patients were usually people who stood a great deal but did not move around much, such as dentists, floorwalkers, priests, etc. He claimed that it was lack of movement that was at the bottom of phlebitis.

In arthritis or rheumatism and gout we have the same thing. While there is a dietary incriminating factor, and possibly one of climate, there can be no question that the average arthritis and gout sufferer is a person who takes very little exercise.

In connection with arthritis let us consider the fact that after a few minutes of walking or other exercise the body begins to make cortisone. In people who have arthritis the body does not make sufficient cortisone for its needs, so the doctor prescribes it. But the doctor's cortisone and the body's cortisone are not the same. In the case of the former, there are terrible side effects. Such cortisone sometimes affects the mind, and softens the spine. Far better to do an hour of walking a day as an insurance against arthritis and other diseases.

Hypokinetic diseases are caused by general inactivity. *Hypokinetic* is a word meaning decreased motor functional activity, which means that hypokinetic diseases are those in which body movement is restricted. Dr. Hans Kraus, in *Modern Medicine*, April 15, 1956, says, "Physical inactivity is a large factor in a number of disease entities (hypokinetic disease). Muscle tests may thus become a means of predicting the incidence of this disease group in a population. Expectancy of hypokinetic disease in the United States is probably about 5 times as great as in other countries. Study, treatment, and prevention of physical inactivity as an important factor in disease are imperative for our national welfare."

Prostate disease, which occurs in 60 per cent of men over 50 years of age, is in part due to lack of exercise. Dr. John Nesfield, in the *British Medical Journal*, January 19, 1957, said, "I suggest that the prostate has a definite function, and that it is our civilized mode of life that leads to its giving trouble in old age. Veterinary surgeons tell me that prostatic troubles are common in pampered house dogs but unknown in foxhounds, working farm dogs, sheep-dogs, etc."

The evidence is unmistakable. Exercise is of terrific importance to the health of the body, especially the heart. If you want to prevent disease, eat right, take the necessary vitamins and mineral supplements, keep a happy frame of mind and move around a lot.

Walking for the Heart

The historian, George Macaulay Trevelyan, once said, "I have two doctors, my left leg and my right"—a very witty statement, but powerfully true. In the case of a heart condition, these two doctors can save the life of the patient. Movement, that's what a heart case needs. Keep the heart pumping and teach it to like it.

People have said to me, "I'm so busy, when will I have the time to walk?" Squeeze the time out somehow. Everything else will get done, you will see. Here is an interesting plan for the beginning walker. Start off by walking 15 minutes before going to work. Then do 15 minutes during the lunch period, and 15 minutes before or after the evening meal. Slowly these periods can be lengthened until one finds that he is doing two hours a day without any trouble at all.

If there is something about your kind of heart condition that you think contra-indicates walking, you will know it after your first 15 minutes. But it would be best to clear it with your doctor first—and then follow some kind of plan.

At the beginning it would be best to search out a flat terrain, otherwise heart cases will experience angina symptoms. Expect also that you will have more difficulty at the beginning of a walk than in the second half. If pressure pains occur, rest a moment or two. At the beginning of muscular exertion, time is required for the adjustment of the circulation to the increased oxygen demand. But this initial period of oxygen deficiency soon passes. The taking of vitamin E, which increases the oxygenation of the body, is very helpful to walkers.

There's a great advantage to heart cases in walking regularly, rather than merely at week ends. Give the heart a daily treatment. It is just like taking vitamins—you must do it every day. The cumulative effect on the heart's action will soon be noticeable. After a while you will develop a kinesthetic sense, that is, a sense of surefootedness, a sense of perception of muscular movement. It will create grace in the motions of the body.

Here are a few cautions about walking. If you walk in the sun, do not wear rimless glasses. Have glasses with dark rims. Cancer of the skin has been caused by the sun penetrating through the unrimmed glass and shining on the skin in the manner of a magnifying glass, which, by means of the sun's rays, can set fire to a piece of paper.

How about walking in city streets which are polluted with gasoline and chimney vapors? If the country or large parks are not available, I walk in the city, but take large doses of rose hip vitamin C and desiccated liver. These are known to aid the body in getting rid of toxic substances. If you have a highly nutritious diet, if you avoid the dangerous things like sugar, factory chemicalized foods, etc., if you indulge in plenty of walking and do everything possible to harden your body and make it healthy, the polluted air will not hurt you . . . much.

When I walk in Allentown, I have worked out routes that take me for the most part through narrow alleys, where there is very little auto traffic or gasoline odors.

In walking keep your head up, don't drag your feet on the ground and do not keep your feet too far apart.

I am also a believer in moderation where the sun is concerned. Get a reasonable amount of sunlight, but at times choose the shady side of the road, or wear a protective covering for your head. In some cases too much sun has attacked the nose, creating tiny pimples which could be symptoms of something more serious—probably cancer.

If you walk a lot, you will become a happier as well as a healthier person. It is a remarkable tonic for the nervous system. Unhappy people who go to psychiatrists should try walking. It is far better medicine for the sick of mind and for those with sick hearts. Walking is as important as food.

Colds and Their Effect on the Heart

It is a well-known fact that disease in other organs of the body can affect the heart, but I did not think that such a minor form of sickness as the common cold could influence it. But as one physician has expressed it in a medical journal, "In general, *any* infection in patients with heart disease is hazardous, and demands prompt treatment, or better still, prevention."

I was very much surprised to come across a medical commentary regarding the effect of colds on heart disease. It was in a publication called *Arteriosclerosis* (September 7, 1955) and was a review of an article in *Diuretic Review*. The commentary follows:

"The question, 'How important are respiratory infections as a cause of heart failure?' is examined in a recent issue of *Diuretic Review*.

"Recently published papers in the professional literature point to general agreement, *Diuretic Review* reports, that respiratory infections, particularly colds, are the most common irritating and aggravating factors in congestive heart failure.

"In a study of more than 300 cases of heart failure, a British medical investigator found more than half with some type of respiratory infection.

"Furthermore, it was established that the infection was the precipitating cause of decompensation in 156 of the 300 cases. In a similar study conducted by 3 investigators and reported in the *American Journal of Medical Science,* a direct relation was found between the frequent occurrence of heart failure among cardiac patients and onset of 'even minor colds.'

"The British investigator, Dr. F. J. Flint, believes respiratory infection in the person with a weak heart may initiate cardiac failure by causing damage to the heart muscle or by favoring congestion of the lungs.

"Under any circumstances, *Diuretic Review* points out, these studies emphasize the importance of looking for and treating respiratory infection in cardiac patients."

To prevent colds, practically no bread or other rye or wheat products should be eaten. In my own experience the fact has been corroborated that the elimination of wheat and rye products goes a long way towards the complete annihilation of the common cold.

Another preventive measure is the taking of vitamins A and D in the form of halibut liver oil perles. This has the effect of strengthening the mucous membranes all over the body. When this happens in the nasal regions, it makes it that much more difficult for disease germs to breed there.

But of all the vitamins, C is the most important in the prevention of colds. Our HEALTH BUILDER contains quite a bit of medical data, the work of many physicians all over the world, which shows that vitamin C can not only prevent colds, but if given in tremendous amounts after a cold has started, can abort it within an hour or two. In the *British Medical Journal,* April 21, 1951, appeared a letter from Drs. John and Isabel Fletcher, who stated that in their practice they have found vitamin C an excellent preventive of colds. They tell of experiments in Holland, Germany and Australia, in which colds were prevented by the administration of vitamin C. In the German experiment there was a marked fall in the extent of colds over a period of 8 months among factory workers given 100 to 300 milligrams of vitamin C a day, a benefit not found when they were given 20 to 50 milligrams.

The amazing part of all is the fact that so many of the things that will prevent colds are also good to keep the action of the heart healthy, namely:

No bread and sugar
Calcium
Vitamin B
Vitamin C

Miscellany

Here is a potpourri of factors in heart disease, each one of which does not contain enough data to make up a whole section.

Aluminum Utensils

Dr. Arthur F. Coca, in his book, *Familial Nonreaginic Food Allergy* (Charles C. Thomas), has shown that eating food cooked in aluminum utensils will raise the pulse of many people. In other words, these people are allergic to the aluminum, some of which gets into the food.

In my own case, many years ago when I was drinking coffee, I proved that when it was made in an aluminum pot, it raised my pulse, but when it was made in stainless steel, it did not.

Tallness

Tall persons are more prone to have high blood pressure, they more often have trouble with their backs and they tend to die of heart involvement at a lower age than the rest of the population. It stands to reason that it takes more work for the heart to pump the blood to the head and feet of a tall person.

Posture

Dr. Ian Stewart writes a letter to the editor of the *British Medical Journal* (July 27, 1957) in which he says that heart disease "seems to be most prevalent in countries where bodily comfort is most readily achieved, and I would like to suggest that the slouching position achieved in the ordinary easy chairs may have something to do with the appearance of atheromatous lesions (hardening of the artery) in a site usually about 1½ centimeters from the origin of the left coronary vessel."

Constipation

There are many references in medical literature to the effect that constipation can produce on a heart case. I will refer to one. In the *Cincinnati Journal of Medicine* for August, 1958, there is an article entitled "Constipation and Sudden Death," which is startling to say the least. It states: "At the fourth annual meeting of the American College of Angiology it was revealed that excessive straining during bowel functioning may cause a series of circulatory changes that might end with the dislodging of a thrombus.

"Hundreds of patient observations indicate that straining can initiate an automatic cycle of extreme fluctuations in blood pressure and circulation. . . . It will occur if the air pressure in the chest cavity is raised forcibly 40 millimeters of mercury or more and maintained for 8 to 10 seconds.

"A dramatic rise in venous pressure may result—up to 40 or 50 millimeters over resting levels—that is followed by an abrupt drop on sudden release of strain. The result may be a suction action that may detach a bland thrombus. Should the clot lodge in lungs or heart, death would follow.

"Another pertinent disclosure was that 50 to 60 per cent of all adults of middle age or older harbor asymptomatic, detachable clots in the veins of their feet or calves."

Reversal of Body Processes

Here is some very encouraging news for people with a heart condition. At a meeting of the American Medical Association in Miami, Florida, in 1954, 4 doctors from New York Medical College state that, starting at age 60 and going to 75, there is a reverse biochemical and physical process which can then enable a person to survive to 100. They obtained their information from a study of 1,000 old persons between the ages of 80 and 100. They found that after the age of 75 cholesterol and other fatty substances in the blood went down instead of up. Between the ages of 60 to 75 they discovered that "the percentage of increase of aortic calcification over the preceding decade also reversed itself."

In assessing these findings, one of the doctors, Eiber said: "In other words, during the age period 60 to 75, which we refer to as the 'threshold age,' certain biochemical and physical processes reverse, and instead of continuing their upward trend, actually reverse and go down. What the mechanism of this threshold period is, has not been fully worked out, as yet. It is some invisible, not clearly understood barrier.

"Most of us die before reaching that barrier, or while going through it. But, once we get through, our chances of living to be 100 years are good."

In closing, I would like to quote from a remarkable editorial that appeared in the *Medical Journal of Australia,* of April 6, 1957. It contains so many of the recommendations offered in this discussion that it will make a fitting ending for it. Here are quotations from it:

"The study suggests strongly that the total caloric intake is a factor in the prevention or postponement of coronary disease." In other words, do not overeat.

"There was a close relation between overweight, excessive total caloric intake and lack of exercise in the coronary disease group.

"A history of the taking of tobacco and alcohol did not suggest that these substances played any part in the causation of coronary disease, although when the disease is developed the use of tobacco may be harmful.

"A point of some importance in the early diagnosis of coronary disease and in the detection of probable candidates for the disease in the future is the observation that there is a sustained rise of pulse rate (15 to 30 beats per minute) and of diastolic pressure (10 to 30 millimeters of mercury) on the average of 2 to 5 years prior to attack.

"From the data collected it would seem that sedentary living and poor health habits are the real culprits in coronary disease, and not hard work, overexercise or occupational stress.

"On the nutritional side, apart from consumption of excess calories, present indications point strongly to the consumption of excess fat as a causal factor in coronary disease.

"There is now overwhelming evidence that the dietary intake of polyethenoid fatty acids seriously interferes with the metabolism of at least 15 species of animals. This may be due to destruction of vitamin E by the highly oxidizable polyethenoid fatty acids, at any rate the metabolic injuries can be corrected by giving vitamin E."

I would like to end on that note . . . namely, that vitamin E can correct metabolic injuries of the body. The medical profession generally has been averse to recommending vitamin E. We think that it is the one thing, above all others, that is of the most extreme importance to a heart case.

35. A Glossary of
Heart Disease Terms

What does your doctor mean when he says you have a cardiac infarction? Or angina pectoris? Or endocarditis?

Here are the explanations of some of the terms used in referring to heart and circulatory disorders.

Arrhythmia. This is an increase in the rate of heart beat when you breathe in, a decrease when you breathe out, caused by interference with breathing out. Usually this condition has no adverse significance but it may be aggravated by rheumatic heart.

Auricular fibrillation. This is the rapid and irregular quivering of the auricles (or upper chambers) of the heart. The pulse becomes completely irregular with a beat as high as 150 to 160 per minute. Causes may be rheumatism, hyperthyroidism, acute infections like flu or pneumonia, poisons like tobacco, emotional strain. If one does not have heart disease, there is probably no danger. The condition may go on for many years without harm.

Auricular flutter. Much the same except that the contractions are regular. This condition is rare.

Bradycardia. Slow heart beat. Any pulse rate under 60 per minute is classed as bradycardia. If one's heart normally beats slowly this is an extremely healthful condition. But slow heart beat resulting from interference with the nerves to the heart is quite serious. Present in a fairly young person and causing fainting spells and epileptic-like convulsions, this is called Stokes-Adams syndrome.

Coronary disease. This covers a number of different disorders. *Coronary sclerosis* is the hardening of the arteries that lead to the heart. This may cause *coronary occlusion* which is the obstruction of the coronary artery by a blood clot or embolism. Occlusion occurs suddenly and is accompanied with severe pain and shock. *Coronary insufficiency* is a partial blockage of the coronary artery so that some blood gets through but not enough to nourish the pericardium (the sac in which the heart is enclosed). This then becomes diseased—and the name of this condition is *coronary infarction. Angina pectoris* is mild coronary insufficiency, that is, a lack of blood getting through causes trouble.

Dextrocardia. The heart is on the right rather than the left side of the chest. Apparently this causes no impairment to health.

Dropsy or edema. This is the abnormal accumulation in the tissues of fluid that has escaped from blood vessels. It usually indicates heart disease or circulatory obstruction of some kind. When it occurs in the abdomen it is called *ascites.* In the brain—*hydrocephalus.* In the chest—*hydrothorax.*

Effort syndrome. This means simply weakness of the circulatory system. Breathlessness, heart palpitations and rapid heart beat are symptoms. Individuals with this condition become exhausted where ordinary persons would be merely tired.

Endocarditis, acute. This is acute inflammation of the lining of any membrane of the heart. Usually it is present in cases of rheumatic fever.

Endocarditis, bacterial. This is inflammation caused by some bacteria. It may be streptococcus. The acute form involves chills and fever. The chronic form may show simply fatigue, loss of weight, breathlessness.

Endocarditis, chronic. The commonest cause of this is rheumatic fever. Sometimes it is called chronic valvular heart disease. The valves in the heart become warped or shrunken and let the blood flow backward.

Heart enlargement. Such a condition might occur when one is doing extremely hard physical work (an athlete for instance) for which the heart increases in size to accommodate the extra work. Usually it is from other causes, however—to compensate for such conditions as valvular

[167]

disease, kidney disease and so forth, where the load on the heart is greatly increased. *Fatty* heart is an enlargement of the heart, usually of those who are sedentary and obese.

Heart murmur. "Probably no single objective finding ocurs that leads to more false diagnoses of cardiac disease than a murmur." The diagnosis depends on the ear of the doctor listening to the heart. Organic heart murmur indicates that at some time some infection has inflamed the lining of the heart.

Myocarditis. Inflammation of the myocardium or heart envelope. It is usually due to rheumatic fever. *Chronic myocarditis* and *myocardosis* are in much the same category as heart disease with great enlargement.

Neurosis, cardiac. Symptoms may be dizziness, nervousness, weakness, sleeplessness, palpitation—all these without any apparent cause. The assumption is that such symptoms may be imaginary or neurotic. We suggest getting plenty of B vitamins, vitamin E and calcium if you have difficulties of this kind.

Palpitation. This is a consciousness of your heart beat, whether it is slow or fast, regular or irregular. It may sometimes pound or thump. It may come from fatigue or overexertion, coffee, alcohol or tea. It usually is not serious.

Pericarditis. This is the inflammation of the pericardium or heart envelope.

Pulse, alternating. Strong and then weak beats. The heart is trying to rest with every other beat. *Assymetrical*—strong one side of the body, weak on the other side. *Bigeminal*—two regular beats, a pause, two regular beats, a pause, etc. *Dicrotic*—this means a double beat. *Intermittent.* Sometimes called *extrasystoles.* This means dropped or skipped beats, or pauses instead of beats. Often this is not associated with heart disease, but may result from fatigue, emotion, worry, coffee or tobacco. If heart action is speeded up with exercise, extrasystoles may disappear. If they do not, myocardial heart trouble may be present. *Irregular*—loss of rhythm of pulse. If this is chronic it may denote something quite serious.

Tachycardia. Rapid heart action. Fast pulse. A beat of 90 or higher per minute. The heart must work faster to do the work done by other hearts with 70 beats a minute. It may be a symptom of infections, or may be emotional or neurotic.

*   *   *

So much for the heart. Now for definitions of some blood vessel terms.

Acrocyanosis. A bluish discoloration of the skin (fingertips usually) which indicates lack of blood. It may be the beginning of Buerger's disease.

Acroparesthesia. A feeling of pins and needles in the finger tips.

Acrosclerosis. Raynaud's disease—see the later definition of this.

Aneurysm. This is a blood-containing tumor in the wall of a blood vessel. The wall is weakened but does not burst.

Anigoma. A tumor formed of a blood vessel. These are seldom dangerous unless they are exposed to injury.

Apoplexy—stroke. A hemorrhage in the brain. The term may be used also for hemorrhages in other parts of the body.

Arteriosclerosis. Hardening of the arteries. A degenerative disease with a thickening of the walls of the arteries because there is an increase of tissue there.

Atherosclerosis. Hardening of the arteries with fatty deposits on the lining. Cholesterol usually forms the fatty deposits.

Buerger's disease. Also called *thromboangiitis obliterans.* This is the inflammation of the inner lining of small blood vessels with constriction and clogging due to blood clots. Because of impaired circulation, the feet or hands become cold and tender. More than any other reason, tobacco appears to play a large part in causing this disease.

Claudication, intermittent. A spasm in the artery, causing muscle cramping in the legs, with pain and limping. There is a diminished blood supply to the legs. We have published information indicating that vitamin E helps.

Embolism and thrombosis. Embolism is obstruction of a blood vessel by a clot or foreign substance. Thrombosis is formation of a clot. If the thrombus or blood clot tears loose from the blood vessel wall and arrives eventually at a blood vessel too small for it to pass through, there will be an embolism at this point.

Periarteritis nodosa. Inflammatory condition of medium-sized arteries. This results in the formation of a series of nodules in the middle and outer coats of arteries.

Phlebitis. Inflammation of a vein. *Thrombophlebitis* is phlebitis with blood clots. Frequent causes are injury, infection, childbirth and varicose veins. Once again, vitamin E has been used with great effectiveness.

Raynaud's disease. Constriction of the blood vessels causing impaired circulation in the hands, feet, ears and nose. The hands are affected most often. They may become pallid, numb and purplish. Vitamin E has been mentioned here, too.

Varicose Veins. Dilated and swollen veins. May come from an infection. Fat persons are more susceptible than thin ones. Standing for long hours is undoubtedly one of the causes. Vitamins E and C are effective preventives. But mistreating your legs by standing for long hours is inviting trouble.

36. New Findings on Heart and Artery Disease

One of the clearest and most sensible interpretations of the controversy over fats in the diet and their relation to heart and artery disease appeared in the *Royal Society of Health Journal* (England) for May-June, 1960. It was written by H. M. Sinclair of Oxford University, one of today's giants in nutrition research.

Dr. Sinclair begins by defining coronary heart disease. It is caused by the thickening of the walls of the blood vessel leading to the heart—the coronary artery. This is what doctors call atherosclerosis and we generally speak of as hardening of the arteries. It is not exactly "hardening." It involves the deposit of a "mush" of certain substances—fats, protein and minerals—on the inner wall of the artery. Such a thickening causes the narrowing in the passageway so that not enough blood reaches the heart. Medical terms used for various aspects of this disease are ischemic heart disease, myocardial infarction, coronary heart disease, coronary thrombosis or heart attack.

The increase in the disease has been astonishingly rapid during the twentieth century. Dr. Sinclair quotes a noted physician of the past century who stated that he did not see a single case of this disease during 10 years of practice at a Montreal hospital. At present it is the commonest single cause of death in Western countries. The apparent increase in deaths from heart disease in men in England and Wales, for instance, is nearly threefold since 1940. In 1921 the death rate from angina pectoris was 41, whereas in 1957 the rate was 2,209.

Studying the incidence of the disease in various countries, Dr. Sinclair tells us that many interesting facts come to light, none seeming to point to any one factor which is responsible. Why should the Japanese in Japan have a lower death rate from heart disease than Japanese in Hawaii? Why should Japanese living in California have a higher rate than those living in either Hawaii or Japan? Why should Mexico have the lowest death rate from heart disease, while France stands lower in scale than the United States, England or Finland?

Looking for a nutritional cause of heart disease has preoccupied Dr. Sinclair for many years and he insists that the cause is dietary. The past few years have made almost everyone of us aware of the word "cholesterol" used in conjunction with heart and artery disease. Cholesterol is a fatty substance which is an important part of human cells. It is made in the body by various tissues; we do not have to get it in our food. But fatty foods of animal origin contain cholesterol.

We have known for a long time that in certain diseases the amount of cholesterol in the blood is increased: diabetes, deficiency in the thyroid gland and a kidney disease known as nephrosis. In these conditions hardening of the arteries and heart disease are unusually common. Carefully accumulated statistics show that men aged 40 to 60 who had a cholesterol level in their blood below 210 suffered only about half as many heart attacks as men whose levels were higher than 210. There seems to be good evidence, says Dr. Sinclair, that a high cholesterol level in the blood may indicate a susceptibility to heart attacks.

Another angle of the controversy over fats in the blood involves a different kind of fat—the unsaturated fatty acids. These are a kind of fat found most plentifully in vegetable and cereal foods. One of them, linoleic acid, is called an "essential" fatty acid, because it cannot be manufactured by the body, but must be supplied in the food we eat. Research seems to show that considerable animal fat in the diet (butter, cream and fat meat, for instance) increases one's need for linoleic acid. Also—and we think this point is very important—eating a great deal of carbohydrate (starchy or sweet) food from which the body can make the wrong kind of fats *increases the need in the diet for the essential ones.*

Relationship Between Amounts of Each Fat

It sounds confusing, but actually all we are saying is that the more you eat of animal fats, the more you need of the other kind of fats—the ones found mostly in cereals and vegetables. So both aspects of diet are important—how much animal fat (and hence cholesterol) you get, and how much you get in *relation to how much you get of vegetable fats.* If you are a person who normally eats a diet very low in animal fats (no dairy products, no meat but very lean meat) and very low in starches (no desserts, no bread or other starches like macaroni and noodles) then you may need very little of the unsaturated fats to balance the amount of animal fats you get. But if you eat, as most Americans do, large amounts of animal fats, and/or large amounts of starchy foods, then it seems that you will need larger amounts of the unsaturated fats to balance the intake of those fats which are called "saturated."

Dr. Sinclair feels certain that this is the answer to hardening of the arteries and heart trouble—this important relationship between the two different kinds of fat in your diet. If there is not, in your blood, enough of the unsaturated fats, or if there is too much of the saturated ones, then the proper substances cannot be formed so that cholesterol can be absorbed properly into your tissues and it will accumulate. The accumulation of these cholesterol deposits occurs mostly in parts of the blood vessels which have been weakened by high blood pressure or undue strain—and sure enough, these are the areas especially subject to hardening of the arteries.

You will remember that we quoted earlier figures on heart disease among men. They are much higher among men than among women in younger age groups. In the light of such figures, it is interesting to find that the requirement for unsaturated fats (linoleic acid) is much greater among

[171]

male laboratory animals than among females, during the earlier years of life. Does it not seem that this might be a very significant aspect of the problem?

Is Chlorinated Water Part of the Cause?

Another angle—and we think this one is extremely important—Dr. Sinclair tells us that he has been doing some "preliminary work" experimenting with chlorine and mice. He has found that free chlorine can combine with the unsaturated fats, thus increasing the body's need for these essential ingredients of food. Does chlorinated water have the same effect? He feels that research is urgently needed. "It is possible, for instance," he says, "that one of the greatest public health measures ever introduced—the chlorination of public water supplies—could assist the disease." We know that chlorine destroys vitamin E as well. Is it not possible that drinking chlorinated water may make the city dweller more susceptible to heart disease than the country dweller? We know that the disease is far commoner in urban communities. We agree with Dr. Sinclair that research is urgently needed on this subject. No one has ever done any research on the possible effects of drinking chlorinated water over one's lifetime. This fact comes to us from the *Journal of the American Medical Association,* July 28, 1951. Isn't it about time we find out how much of our terrible heart disease mortality may be at least partly caused by chlorinated water?

Overweight and lack of exercise are two other certain causes of heart trouble, according to Dr. Sinclair. "Much evidence is available," he says, "that men who are overweight tend to have higher mortality from coronary thrombosis than men who are underweight." The danger may lie in the process of *becoming* fat, Dr. Sinclair believes. One researcher has found that, if exercise is sufficient to prevent weight gain, diets high in calories and fat can be fed without increasing the blood cholesterol levels. So exercise and overweight and cholesterol levels are closely related. If you eat too much, especially of fat and starches, and get too little exercise, you are more likely to have too much cholesterol in the blood. If you eat and exercise moderately there is less chance. And even if you eat more than you should, but don't put on weight because you "work" it off with exercise, your cholesterol level will probably remain low. Perhaps this may be another reason why country folks have less heart disease than urban folks. Even with today's mechanized farming, country people surely get more physical exercise than city people.

McDonald and Fullerton, writing in the *Lancet,* Vol. 2, p. 600, tell us that high-fat meals cause the blood to coagulate more rapidly. This might explain a number of heart attacks and "strokes" caused by blood clots. However, these two researchers found that moderate physical exercise abolished this threat. The blood did not coagulate too rapidly in those who exercised.

Another angle to the heart disease problem is smoking. Dr. Sinclair tells us that there is no doubt there are more deaths from heart disease in men of 45 to 62 among those who smoke than among those who do not smoke. The levels of cholesterol in the blood are also higher in smokers. Interestingly enough, one investigator has found that smokers consume more fat in their diets than non-smokers! This may play some part in the picture.

What about "stress"? Do we have more heart attacks because we are living at a faster pace than we used to? Investigators have found that, during periods of stress, the blood cholesterol level rises. Students tested just before examinations, soldiers tested during periods of stress, have been found to have high cholesterol levels during such times. So, during periods of personal stress, one should take special pains to eat healthfully and exercise faithfully. So far as today's "pace" is concerned, Editor Rodale has shown in his book, THIS PACE IS NOT KILLING US (Rodale Books, Incorporated, Emmaus, Pennsylvania. Price $1.00) that we actually live much more easily today than at any time in the past.

Diet Is the Most Important Cause of the Disease

To return to Dr. Sinclair's basic theory, he believes that the most important factor of all to be considered in heart disease is diet and the most significant item in the diet is its fat. There is still plenty of controversy among nutrition experts as to which kind of fat does the damage. A famous American researcher, Ancel Keys, believes that the total amount of fat in the diet is the important thing. All fats in the diet raise the level of cholesterol in the blood, says he. But, says Dr. Sinclair, other researchers have shown that vegetable fats (salad oils, nuts, seeds, avocados) tend to lower blood cholesterol, while animal fats raise it. In addition, they have found that some vegetable fats raise cholesterol and others lower it, while some fats from fish (fish liver oils and food fish that are fatty) lower the cholesterol level. So it seems that the secret of which kind of fat has a beneficial effect on the cholesterol level involves the unsaturated fatty acids. Those foods which contain it (most vegetable and cereal seeds and oils and the fats from fish) lower cholesterol. Fats from animal sources (low in the unsaturated fatty acids) and a few rare fats among vegetable foods raise the cholesterol level.

Finally, the research done up to now seems to show that the important thing for heart and blood vessel health is not how much or how little of either kind of fat you get—but how much of the vegetable fat you get *in relation to how much of the animal fat you get.* The more animal fat you eat, the more vegetable fat you need. The less animal fat you eat the less vegetable fat you need.

An additional finding is that starches and sugars in your diet can be changed into the wrong kind of fat and hence, if you eat lots of these foods, you need more vegetable fats to balance the other fats. It is well to keep in mind, too, that the hydrogenation of fats destroys the valuable fatty acids. Hydrogenating fats makes them solid at room temperatures.

[173]

Margarine contains hydrogenated fats. Most commercially sold peanut butter contains some hydrogenated fat; modern lard has been hydrogenated.

So far as processed foods are concerned, all of these probably contain the harmful fats—prepared mixes, prepared foods like frozen fried food, pies, pastries, salted nuts, crackers, pretzels—most of the foods most of us eat every day have been made using the wrong kind of fats.

Some Recommendations

What are the only answers to which Dr. Sinclair's stimulating article directs us? Regardless of what future research may show about fats in the diet and other aspects of modern life which may be involved in heart and blood vessel trouble, we can at least begin to practice prevention by taking careful note of the following:

1. The kind of fat you eat is important. We would advise eating as little animal fat as possible—no dairy products or fatty meats. Lean meats and eggs we feel are basic essentials.

2. Get as much as possible of the vegetable fats and the one animal fat rich in unsaturated fatty acid—salad oils, wheat germ oil, wheat germ flakes, avocados, fish liver oils. And raw, unprocessed seeds and nuts—especially sunflower seeds.

3. We recommend shunning all processed foods that may be loaded with the wrong kind of fat. This means no prepared foods like bakery products, crackers, salted nuts, margarine, candy, ice cream, packaged mixes, commercial peanut butter and so forth.

4. Exercise is important to health and is especially important for those who cannot regulate their diets properly. If you are not getting enough exercise to keep your weight where it should be, you're courting trouble. Walking is the best exercise there is. Walk every day.

5. Avoid drinking or cooking with chlorinated water. If you live in the city, buy bottled spring water or get spring water from a friend who lives in the country. If you cannot do either, at least draw your water and let it stand 12 hours or so before you are going to use it. Some of the chlorine will evaporate.

6. Don't smoke.

37. Heart Trouble and Your Diet

Now that we have all become familiar with the word "cholesterol"—at least to the point of being able to pronounce it correctly—the experts have come up with a new (to them) explanation of what causes fatty deposits in the inside of blood vessels. A researcher at the Rockefeller Institute, Dr. Edward H. Ahrens, has found that a diet rich in carbohydrates and low in fats tends to raise the level of fats in the blood.

As reported in the *New York Times* for May 4, 1961, Dr. Ahrens has spent 9 years testing various diets on 15 volunteers. He announced that 13 of those tested developed the highest levels of blood fat *on the diet that contained no fat at all,* and the lowest levels on a diet which contained 70 per cent fat. In addition, he added, it did not seem to make much difference whether the fats in the diet were saturated (as in animal products and hydrogenated fats) or unsaturated, as unprocessed vegetable, seed, cereal and nut fats are.

Volunteers Reacted Differently to High Fat Diet

Two of the volunteers reacted to the high fat diet differently. In these two, the fat level in the blood rose on this diet. It was found that these folks lacked a certain enzyme, a substance which is necessary to break down fats in the blood. Thus, they did not react to the two diets as did the other 13.

Dr. Ahrens believes that there are, therefore, two different kinds of conditions resulting in high fat in the blood. The one shown by the two human guinea pigs, caused by the lack of an enzyme, is probably inherited and very rare. (He does not explain how, if it is rare, he happened to have two such people in a small group of 15.)

The 13 other persons eating the experimental diets seemed to be demonstrating only a simple principle that has long been known—that starches are turned to fats by the body, for storing in the blood. The accumulation of the fats in harmful deposits inside the arteries indicates, he says, "an exaggerated form" of this perfectly natural process.

In other words, we were meant to eat carbohydrates and they were meant to turn into fats in our blood. The fact that today they are turning into harmful fats that cannot be handled properly by the body seems to us to indicate that there is something very wrong with the kind and amount of carbohydrates we are eating these days.

The diets used in the experiments were the exaggerated kinds used in many experiments where the researcher wants to emphasize greatly one aspect of what he is investigating, so that there can be no possible doubt as to what his results mean. One of the diets eaten consisted of 85 per cent carbohydrate, 15 per cent protein and no fat at all. Another consisted of only 15 per cent carbohydrate, 15 per cent protein and 70 per cent fat. It is most unlikely that any of us would be eating such diets since they are so far removed from the kind of food one gets in everyday meals, but they certainly show that when Dr. Ahrens says a certain thing about a diet high in carbohydrates, he indeed has tested just such a diet.

We think it is extremely interesting that Dr. Ahrens found one thing to be true for 13 people and something quite different for the remaining 2. This shows once again that we are all different. No one rule can be laid down for everyone. "Biochemical individuality," as Dr. Roger Williams of the University of Texas calls it, proves conclusively that, even though one person is not harmed by a given thing, someone else may be. It shows as well that what may be an ample amount of a given food element for one person may be completely inadequate for another. And so on. We are glad to know that more and more researchers are coming around to the conclusion that present-day carbohydrates may be as responsible as the fats in our diet, or more so, for hardening of the arteries and other vascular disorders.

Other Scientists Show Dangers of Carbohydrates

In 1958 John W. Gofman, Alex V. Nichols and E. Virginia Dobbin, of the University of California, wrote a fine book, *Dietary Prevention and Treatment of Heart Disease* (G. P. Putnam's Sons) in which they talked extensively about the possible role of carbohydrates, along with fats, in forming unwanted fatty deposits on artery walls.

In answering the question "How is it that dietary intake of carbohydrates, a foodstuff class which is wholly different from fat, has the ability to raise the amount of certain of the fat-like materials in the blood?" these authors say, "The final answer to this question is not available. We know that the effect does occur . . . One . . . possibility is that when the person is taking in a great deal of carbohydrate, and thus making sugar available in fair quantities, the metabolism of the body may use the sugar preferentially as a fuel for energy. Thus the rate at which certain fat-like materials are used for energy purposes may be slowed down, allowing a build-up in the amount of these fat-like materials in the blood stream. This, of course, is a deleterious result from the point of view of arterial thickening since it is the amount of the fat-like substances *of the blood* which is important!"

The book written by these investigators contains valuable charts giving the carbohydrate content of foods, showing those containing 0-9 per cent carbohydrate, those containing 10-19 per cent carbohydrate and those containing 20 per cent and more carbohydrate, also charts showing the saturated and unsaturated fats in various foods.

In general, the charts show that the 20 per cent and more carbohydrate foods are cereals, bakery products, desserts and prepared, sugared or dried fruits, almost exclusively. Those below 20 per cent carbohydrate are the other fresh fruits and vegetables which we always recommend. Saturated fats occur in greatest quantity in processed foods, desserts and those in which lard, butter, milk or hydrogenated shortenings have been used. Unsaturated fats occur in fruits and vegetables, whole grains and seeds and vegetable and cereal oils.

Blood Sugar Influenced By Carbohydrate Intake

Another worker in this field is Benjamin Sandler, M.D., of Veterans Hospital, Oteen, North Carolina. Dr. Sandler's book, *How to Prevent Heart Attacks* (published by Lee Foundation, Milwaukee, Wisconsin), discussed in great detail the relation of blood sugar levels to heart pain and

[176]

attacks. The author states, "The patient with heart pain experiences all of the ill effects of reduced oxygen inhalation whenever the blood sugar level is abnormally reduced. Hypoglycemia (low blood sugar), absolute or relative, means reduced oxygen consumption by all cells that require sugar for energy purposes. The heart muscle suffers an oxygen lack of varying degree every time the blood sugar falls at an abnormally rapid rate."

What causes the blood sugar to fall? Habitual consumption of too much carbohydrate-rich food in relation to the amount of protein and fat consumed. So Dr. Sandler is saying, in another way, just what Dr. Gofman and his associates and Dr. Ahrens are saying—if you would be free from heart and artery trouble, shun the carbohydrate-rich foods—those are the real trouble makers.

The basis of Dr. Sandler's recommended diet for preventing heart trouble is protein. All foods of animal origin may be eaten in unlimited quantities, including eggs. Any food containing sugar is forbidden—that is, all desserts, soft drinks, jams, pastries, ice cream and so forth. The starchy foods are to be eaten in reduced quantities: all foods of the spaghetti-noodle variety, beans and potatoes. Fruits with high-sugar content should be eaten in limited quantity. All other fruits and vegetables may be eaten in unlimited quantity. Dr. Sandler does not forbid or limit fats. Nor does he make a distinction among different kinds of carbohydrates. We believe that the carbohydrates in fresh fruits, bananas, for instance, have a quite different effect from those in cereals, especially the refined cereals. Nor do we object to the starches in vegetables like potatoes.

We feel that one should cut down on animal fats and should avoid entirely the processed and synthetic ones, like margarine and hydrogenated shortenings.

In France, an article in *Archives des Malaises du Coeur* for March, 1960, by E. Hoareau and G. Delanoe, tells of their studies of 738 heart patients in Morocco. Of these, 111 had hardening of the arteries. Comparing their observations with those of other French researchers, they found that heart diseases due to hardening of the arteries were 4 times less frequent in Morocco than in Paris. Figures on heart diseases due to hardening of the arteries did not run parallel to those for cholesterol, seeming to indicate that these heart patients in Morocco had normal levels of cholesterol.

The French researchers believe that a deficiency in protein food plays a major part in the occurrence of heart conditions due to hardening of the arteries. Moroccans do not have enough protein in their diets, especially protein of animal origin like meat and eggs. The French scientists believe also that an excess of calories from white sugar and white flour products might have the effect of causing deposits on the artery walls, resulting in artery "hardening," as we call it.

One might decide that such could not be the case in America where there is plenty of animal protein available. But there are infallible statistics

[177]

showing that about one-half of the calories of the American diet derive from white sugar and white flour products.

Many surveys have been done showing that individual diets may be seriously lacking in animal protein and very high in refined carbohydrates. Every survey we have seen which dealt with the diet of teenagers testifies eloquently to the serious deficiencies of most teenage diets. Cake, cokes, white bread, candy, all easily available and inexpensive, form far too large a part of the diet of young folks. Among older people, starchy and sweet foods are popular because they are easy to prepare, tasty and soft.

Substitute Proteins for Starches and Sweets

We think there is a valuable lesson to be learned from all the information we have presented above, indicating that starches and sweets are certainly one of the evils, if not the main evil, in hardening of the arteries and heart disease. The lesson is that, if one wants to prevent heart disease, he will automatically eliminate the refined sugars and starches from his meals, he will substitute for them lots of protein foods of animal origin—meat, fish, poultry, eggs. He will eat plenty of fresh fruits, vegetables and nuts. Just to be on the safe side, he will also go easy on animal fats like butter, and will shun entirely the processed fats like margarine and the solid white shortenings.

38. Can Fresh Fruit Help Prevent Heart Trouble?

It's only a crumb of nutritional knowledge, but it comes from one of the world's experts whose pronouncements on things having to do with nutrition and health are listened to respectfully by specialists from great universities. Dr. Ancel Keys, Director of the Laboratory of Physiological Hygiene at the University of Minnesota, stated on November 10, 1960, at a meeting of the American Heart Association that pectin in the diet seems to have a small but definite effect in lowering blood cholesterol.

So, above the din and clamor about dietary fats and cholesterol in their relation to heart and artery disease, we have this word from a man who has been in the thick of the fight. Dr. Keys' statement is so important that we want to print it here exactly as he sent it to us:

"The risk of coronary heart disease is increased in men who have a high concentration of cholesterol in the blood. Follow-up studies in Massachusetts, New York and California, show the frequency of heart attacks is two to four times greater among middle-aged men who have high cholesterol levels than among men of the same age who have lower levels. Accordingly, there is great interest in discovering ways of lowering the blood cholesterol level.

"A reduction in the saturated fats in the diet lowers the blood cholesterol and comparisons among populations show that those who eat diets low in saturated fats have lower blood cholesterol values and a lower incidence of heart attacks than populations who eat diets, such as the usual American diet, which are high in saturated fats. But controlled dietary experiments on man show that the fats in the diet do not fully account for the difference in blood cholesterol among populations.

"Various experiments indicated that besides fats, something in the carbohydrate fraction of the diet has an effect. Further controlled experiments on man have shown that pectin in the diet has a small but definite effect in lowering the blood cholesterol level. In these experiments, carried out on 4 groups of middle-aged men in a State Hospital, the addition to the daily diet of 15 grams (about ½ ounce) of pure pectin caused the blood cholesterol to fall by an average of about 5 per cent. When the pectin was removed from this diet, the blood cholesterol promptly rose to the pre-pectin level.

Pectin Helps Reduce Blood Cholesterol Level

"Pectin is a complex carbohydrate which is naturally contained in many fruits and berries, notably apples. The amount of pectin used in the Minnesota experiments (15 grams daily) would be provided by about two pounds of apples.

"Whether a smaller amount of pectin, or the daily consumption of a couple of apples, would have a similar favorable effect on the blood cholesterol level is not known.

"It appears probable, however, that the high consumption of fruits, including apples, by some populations, helps to explain the low blood cholesterol values in those populations. However, fats remain as the major dietary factor controlling the blood cholesterol concentration."

Our Recommendations

Housewives who make jelly know that pectin is the substance which makes jelly gell. Before it was available commercially, cooks used to combine apples with whatever fruit they were using for jelly and jams, because there was enough pectin in the apples to cause the fruit and sugar mixture to gell.

Is Dr. Keys' statement an excuse for readers to begin to eat jelly and jam? Certainly not, because the sugar or honey these contain represent too much concentrated sweets. And the amount of pectin one would get in the average serving of jelly or jam is inconsequential. Should one, then, take commercial pectin which is used today for jelly-making? Under no circumstances! The preparation contains, aside from "highly refined" fruit pectin, lactic and citric acid (added synthetically), plus potassium citrate and sodium metabisulfite added as preservatives.

[179]

How, then, can you put this discovery of the value of pectin to good use, from the health standpoint?

Eat Lots of Apples, Raw and Unprocessed

Eat apples. Eat lots of apples. Eat them raw and unprocessed. By this we do not mean that you should eat apple pie, or apple jelly, or apple pudding, or apple juice, or apple sauce, or apple dumplings or apples fixed in any other way but raw. We think you should peel them because, unless they are organically grown, they have been heavily sprayed.

Peel them as you eat them. If you let them stand after peeling, the browning that takes place indicates that vitamins and enzymes have been destroyed. If, because of some condition of health, you are unable to chew raw apples, liquefy them in a blender just before eating them. If you have no blender, scrape the cored, peeled apple with a dull knife and eat the scrapings. You will find that raw apples are wonderfully satisfying to eat—so satisfying that you won't want to eat the pastries and other desserts that contain the overload of fat which everybody, including Dr. Keys, believes is so destructive to health.

Other fresh, raw fruits and berries contain pectin, but apples are by far the richest source.

39. Vitamin E for Heart Disease

"A dose of alpha tocopherol calculated by Skelton on the basis of his dog experiments and much higher than had ever been used in clinical medicine before, viz., 200 milligrams per day, was given to the patient, whose myocardial failure quickly vanished. . . . Encouraged by this I next treated my barber, who was dying from a recurrent coronary thrombosis and was in the terminal stages of heart failure with status antinosus. In 3 weeks' time he was playing the tympana in the local theatre. Next my mother's severe angina pectoris disappeared on alpha tocopherol therapy. Then Dr. Wilfrid Shute and I recalled our first successful angina patient of 1936 and the 4 other patients treated at that time. Accordingly, we began with the assistance of Dr. Vogelsang, to collect the series of observations on cardiovascular patients that we may presume to say have changed the face of cardiology." So begins the saga of alpha tocopherol, vitamin E, as related by Dr. Evan Shute in the book on the subject, *Alpha Tocopherol in Cardiovascular Disease,* published by the Shute Foundation for Medical Research, London, Ontario, Canada.

It is an amazing story—the story told in this book—exciting, inspiring, at times heroic, but also completely scientific and objective. The Shute brothers take the reader on a tour of their file of case histories—

well over 10,000 patients treated for heart and vascular disorders with vitamin E. Of particular interest is a chapter by Dr. Wilfrid Shute on classical cardiac therapy—that is, the treatment other than vitamin E that has been used up to now for heart trouble. He discusses digitalis, quinidine, mercurial diuretics and other drugs.

He quotes a member of the Texas Heart Association who said in the *Texas State Journal of Medicine* in 1951, "More than 637,000 deaths annually in the United States from cardiovascular disease account for about 44 per cent of all deaths. . . . When a physician makes a diagnosis of organic heart disease, he realizes that in the care of the patient he has begun a losing fight. In the earliest stages he offers general advice: 'Avoid strenuous activities; live sensibly; watch your weight; don't worry; the heart is a wonderful organ.' Before too long symptoms develop and the doctor braces the patient with digitalis or other drugs, restriction of usual activities, more rest and more encouragement. Again, before long, more urgent symptoms force a retreat. Bed rest, low sodium diet, diuretics and other well known measures are brought to the front and the line is stabilized. But not for long. All too soon increasing pressure bends the line and retreat begins again. Now there are left no more reserves—no more in the heart and no more in the hands of the one trying to help the heart. Then only surrender remains. Not infrequently the enemy strikes suddenly with overwhelming power, and surrender occurs before the doctor can mobilize his forces." How indeed could one better describe the usual case of heart disease treated by the usual methods?

This is, this *has to be,* the point of view of doctors using the time-honored prescriptions against this mysterious and deadly disease. How heart-warming and encouraging, then, to turn the page and find cheering, confident and convincing evidence of the marvelous effectiveness of vitamin E in heart and vascular cases! There are chapters in this book on the use of vitamin E in coronary sclerosis, coronary occlusion, rheumatic heart disease and hypertension. In the chapter "Tailoring the Dose" full instructions are given for using vitamin E in heart therapy, with descriptions of the various categories of patients and the characteristic problems they present in treatment.

Vitamin E to Prevent Heart Disorders

Furthermore, there are chapters on the cardiovascular aspects of diabetes, indolent ulcer, arteriosclerosis, thromboangitis, peripheral thrombosis, geriatrics (the study of old age) and finally a chapter on the use of vitamin E in veterinary medicine.

In the last chapter called "Hopeful Margins," Dr. Evan Shute lets his hopes and his dreams envisage the thought of the other benefits that may in time come to be proven from the use of vitamin E in ophthalmology, diabetes, peptic ulcer, varicose veins, intracranial birth damage, dermatology, hypertension. He also discusses the use of vitamin E as a prophylactic measure for preventing cardiovascular disease long before it rears its lethal head. He says, "We have long urged the prophylactic use of alpha tocopherol (vitamin E) rather than its administration only to people already showing cardiovascular disease. Habitually, food factors such as the vitamins prevent what they relieve. With that in mind the Profession has long urged the prevention of beriberi, peripheral neuritis, pellagra, scurvy, rickets and hemorrhagic disease of the newborn by the timely use of the appropriate vitamin—long before any frank evidence of scurvy or rickets or the rest could possibly appear. . . .

"Now one of the outstanding characteristics of the cardiovascular diseases . . . is that they are long-term degenerations or that chronic degenerations lay the groundwork for their appearance. . . . The average person in this country is exposed to a slow though much less pronounced deprivation of alpha tocopherol than is developed in the laboratory. . . . Whatever harmful results are thus produced may not reveal their existence for years—perhaps for decades. But just as these degenerations come on so slowly and insidiously as to escape recognition until well advanced, so appropriate preventative measures have years in which to get under way, and need never be radical or extensive if undertaken in time. It should demand but little in the way of substitution to remedy a food deficiency which is only partial.

". . . Why need alpha tocopherol be added to diets from which it first has been carefully extracted by modern milling processes? Why should the latter not be revised until foods are no longer alpha-tocopherol-deficient? This would seem to be the logical approach to the question and one in which the aid of such governmental agencies as the Food and Drug Administration of the United States should be enlisted.

"It is commonly said that the average diet in this country contains adequate amounts of tocopherols. This is misleading. Such observations are based upon total tocopherol content, much of this consisting of the relatively inert gamma form (a second part of vitamin E as opposed to *alpha* tocopherol). But if one investigates alpha tocopherol values in the average diet, as two groups of workers have, the results are much different. It then appears that the average diet in Europe or America contains only 10 to 90 per cent of the normal requirement. This, too, is vitiated by intakes of rancid and unsaturated fats. It is obvious that slow alpha tocopherol starvation is the rule, not the exception, and is found among the wealthy quite as often as among the poor."

40. Vitamin E Used Internationally for Heart Disease

The Bulletin from the Vitamin E Society of Canada brings us news of cures worked by the powerful alpha tocopherol (vitamin E) in other countries. It is an impressive story, well worth carrying with you to show to dubious friends, who may doubt the potency of vitamin E because it sounds too easy. "What," they may say, "a mere vitamin given in its natural form, can cure phlebitis, Buerger's disease, heart disease, thrombosis? Impossible. You are being taken in."

Well, folks, here is the record. And at the risk of cluttering up our pages with a series of long, academic-looking words and foreign words, we are giving you the full names of authors, periodicals, volume numbers, dates and countries from which this information comes. If your own physician should tell you he doubts that vitamin E can really be of any benefit in heart and vascular conditions, perhaps he is sincerely unaware that so much research has been done. Perhaps he does not really know what wonders have been worked in recent years with vitamin E. Physicians are busy men with little time to study. But they are receptive to new ideas if they come from dependable sources. If he is doubtful, show your physician these references. Ask him to write to the Shute brothers in Canada (pioneers in vitamin E therapy) and obtain even more information.

In the *American Journal of Physiology,* Vol. 153, p. 127, 1948, K. L. Zierler, D. Grob and J. L. Lilienthal describe laboratory experiments in which they discovered that vitamin E has a profound effect on the blood, especially the clotting of the blood. It has a strong anti-clotting effect both in laboratory experiments and in the veins and arteries of human beings. Now there is a special natural substance in the blood called heparin which is made in the liver, whose job it is to prevent the coagulation of blood. In their tests these scientists found that the action of vitamin E on the blood takes place regardless of how much or how little heparin is present in the blood stream of the patients. So there can be no doubt but that the anti-coagulating action is the result of the vitamin E and nothing else.

In an Italian journal, *Bollettino Societa Chirurgia* Vol. 18, p. 155 (1948) R. Castagna and G. Impallomeni report on 7 patients with phlebitis (inflammation of a vein) and one 71 year old woman who had had an ulcer measuring 5 by 3 inches on her lower leg. The phlebitis responded dramatically to the use of vitamin E alone. The woman patient's ulcer healed in 26 days. The authors have also used vitamin E in treatment of vascular disease (any disease of the blood vessels) and for "strokes." They tell us that in thrombophlebitis (inflammation of the vein in which a blood clot is involved) the improvement by using vitamin E is extremely rapid. In addition, they say, treatment with vitamin E does not require a rigid blood control as do other medications.

Reports from Foreign Countries

The conservative British medical publication, *Lancet* Vol. 2, p. 132, 1949, carries an article by A. M. Boyd, A. H. James, G. W. H. and R. P. Jepson saying that clinical results with vitamin E are far better than any obtained with any other treatment in cases of obliterative diseases of the blood vessels. It can be used most successfully for the relief of cramps in the calves of the legs. "May we repeat," say these authors, "that it is our considered opinion that the clinical observations so far made warrant the continued use of vitamin E therapy."

A Norwegian physician, H. Sturup, writing in *Nordisk Medicin,* Vol. 43, p. 721, 1950, tells us he has seen a number of cases of thrombosis helped by vitamin E therapy. He discusses in detail the case of a 33-year old patient who had chronic phlebitis of the left leg, 5 years after an operation. This patient was not even confined to bed, but took vitamin E daily and within 6 days the pain and swelling disappeared.

The *Annals of Surgery,* Vol. 131, p. 652, 1950, reports that vitamin E and calcium appear to be helpful in the treatment of vascular diseases. Dr. A. W. Allen of Boston, commenting on this article tells us that he has used vitamin E on a number of patients and can report that 50 of these who were "vulnerable"—that is susceptible—to thrombosis escaped this serious condition. This seems to us particularly important, for in these cases vitamin E was used to prevent rather than to cure, and 50 lucky patients continued in good health. Dr. J. C. Owings of Baltimore comments that he has treated many leg ulcers due to phlebitis with a combination of rutin and vitamin E, all of which stayed healed, so long as the patient continued to take the medication.

Postgraduate Medicine, Vol. 10, p. 794, 1951, carries a report by A. Ochsner who believes that vitamin E is the best preventive of a blood clot, because it is a natural substance, so there is no hazard involved in its use. The use of other anticoagulants is dangerous and tying off veins should not be practiced because it will not protect against the detachment of clots. He states that he does not know whether vitamin E combined with calcium is the final answer, but adds that it seems to be best, because it is perfectly safe and does not bring any danger of producing bleeding.

Medical Thesis, published in Paris, Number 471, 1951, quotes a physician as saying he has found vitamin E and calcium useful for preventing blood clots after surgery. M. Reifferscheid and P. Matis writing in *Medizinische Welt,* Germany, Vol. 20, p. 1168, 1951, announce they have found vitamin E to be definitely protective against vascular clotting. They found that large daily doses were necessary. They describe 5 cases of diabetic gangrene, 9 cases of Raynaud's disease (a gangrenous condition) 7 cases of Dupuytren's contracture (contraction of tissues under the skin of the palm) and 14 cases of hemorrhagic (bleeding) diseases all yielded to treatment with vitamin E.

Dr. W. E. Crump and E. F. Heiskell, writing in the *Texas State Journal of Medicine*, Vol. 11, 1952, agree that the use of the regular anti-coagulants for routine prevention of clotting diseases in patients after operations is too dangerous for general use. In most cases where these medicines are used, as many patients die of hemorrhage as might have died of clots and 16 per cent of other cases develop non-fatal bleeding complications. When vitamin E was used as treatment by these physicians, no bleeding occurred and only minor side reactions were noticed. When cases of phlebitis occurred during treatment, they were mild and had no complications. There were no lung clots, fatal or non-fatal, in patients being treated with vitamin E. Dr. Terrel Speed, commenting on these statements, says, "considerable evidence is accumulating to substantiate the value of this therapy. However I have gradually expanded its use and now it is used routinely in essentially the same group of cases mentioned by the authors. If the promising preliminary results are borne out, relative protection against one of the most feared complications of surgery will have been obtained."

Fair Consideration Asked for Vitamin E

In spite of this kind of evidence that has accumulated in increasing quantity over the years, some medical journals are still taking pot shots at vitamin E therapy and spreading doubt as to its effectiveness. Such an article appeared in the *British Medical Journal* for December, 1952. It was answered promptly by Dr. Evan S. and Dr. Wilfrid E. Shute, the two Canadian doctors who have specialized in the use of vitamin E in the treatment of vascular cases. Say these two doctors: "The leading article on 'The Therapeutic Uses of Vitamin E' (December 20, 1952) certainly calls for comment by us, the proponents of the use of alpha-tocopherol in cardiovascular disease.

"Such an article might conceivably have been written in 1948 or 1949. However, the picture has changed so rapidly since that time that your leading article now simply does not reflect the findings of investigators in this field. This is best illustrated perhaps by the current issue of our medical journal, *Summary*, which contains the abstracts of 122 reports which have appeared in the medical literature supporting our original contentions. It seems that alpha-tocopherol shares with Christianity both its beneficence and the observation that those who say it has failed have rarely tried it. Since the American Aristotles first condemned it, too many doctors have dropped a pebble from their own towers to make that condemnation stick.

"Briefly, our current *Summary* records that 17 reports have supported us in the use of alpha-tocopherol for the menopause; 5 in its use for nephritis; 6 for kraurosis vulvae; 4 for capillary permeability; 4 for purpura; 5 for vascular dilatation; 11 for Buerger's disease; 10 for vascular sclerosis; 15 for thrombosis; 3 for muscular power; 20 for indolent ulcers; 14 for diabetes; 4 for Roentgen tissue damage; 4 for incipient gangrene; 2 for wound healing. Finally 46 reports have supported us in the use of alpha-tocopherol for heart disease.

"It is difficult to believe that all these investigators have duplicated an error. Certainly it is cavalier to dismiss such work in one paragraph. Fortunately, our forthcoming book should help to keep the record straight and we will recommend it to your perusal. Also, as Auden, one of your poets, has said,

'One notices, if one will trust one's eyes,
The shadow cast by language upon truth.'

Wilfrid E. Shute
Evan *V. Shute"

41. Is Heart Disease Related to Anxiety?

"There is no evidence that stresses cause heart disease." So says Kurt Aaron, M.D., of East Brisbane, writing in the November 14, 1959, issue of the *Medical Journal of Australia*. He goes on to show, however, in this most interesting article that stress of certain kinds can cause certain heart symptoms in patients whose hearts are perfectly normal.

He quotes A. M. Master who wrote in the *Journal of the American Medical Association* that in collected cases of heart disease, the number of functional heart disturbances not due to any organic disease varies between 20 per cent and 50 per cent. Of 1,000 consecutive patients in his heart practice, he found 38 per cent *without any organic heart disorder.*

Glandular System Triggered By Crises or Emergencies

From time immemorial, Dr. Aaron tells us, we have associated the heart with our emotions. Language is full of phrases like "heartfelt," "lion-hearted," "broken-hearted," etc. We know, too, that the heart is actually associated very closely with the emotion of fear and its natural accompanying physical preparedness. Physical response to danger requires increased blood supply to the muscles, dilation of the small arteries that lead to the muscles, the release of the gland secretion, adrenalin, and an increase in the "output" of the heart—that is, the heart must beat harder, faster or both.

In earlier days, of course, danger meant the same thing it means to animals—one had to fight or run. So these body preparations took place to give strength for fighting or swiftness for escape. It is true, that the clotting time of the blood is shortened when one feels fear, anger or hostility. This means the blood tends to become thicker—apparently as an adaptation to protect one if he is wounded, so that he will not bleed to death. Today most of us are far removed from danger of actual physical wounds, yet fear and anger still produce today this same reaction—a thickening of the blood. One can easily see, therefore, that chronic fear or anger may lead to dangerous blood clots.

Memories and Emotions Can Affect Action of Heart

It is true, too, says Dr. Aaron, that recalling an event that made one fearful or angry will produce the same body reactions as if the event were taking place in the present. One's heart beats faster, or harder, one feels the rush of blood into muscles and the stimulation given by adrenalin which moves swiftly to all parts of the body to ready it for an emergency. Undoubtedly, people with very vivid imaginations must go through almost the same sensations of fright when they are telling or re-living some fearful event.

However, the perfectly normal patients who came to doctors with complaints of heart symptoms are suffering from something else, says Dr. Aaron. They have a neurosis, which does not mean that their difficulty is imaginary. It's real enough, all right, but it is the result of something in their personalities—nothing in their heart physiology.

Symptoms of the Neurotic Patient

What are some of the symptoms of the patient he means? Heart palpitations, difficulty in breathing, pain in the chest and fatigue. Any one of these singly or in conjunction with some other symptom like frequent urination, indigestion or headache constitute the major complaints of patients who have nothing wrong with their hearts.

Dr. Aaron then describes these symptoms. We think his description of heart palpitations is particularly good. He says, heart palpitation is "the consciousness of the heart beating." It is usually painless and may be felt in the chest or over the heart. The heart may seem to be pounding very hard, it may seem to be beating in places removed from it or the tissues directly around it. Beats may occur that are out of step with the preceding beat or following beats. Or the heart may beat very rapidly.

Palpitations may not be felt in times of real stress or crisis, he tells us. But usually patients feel the palpitations while lying in bed recalling difficult situations.

Breathlessness or labored breathing is another symptom. Dr. Aaron describes this as follows: "the patient calls it shortness of breath and means two varieties. The first is an increase in respiratory rate and the second is the feeling of inability to take a deep breath, as if he could not get enough air into the lungs. Yet this particular type of breathing is associated with deep sighing respiration. It is a feeling of oppression as if something was stopping the thoracic (chest) cage from expanding. I find it a particularly useful symptom in favour of the diagnosis of neurosis, of which it is characteristic. It occurs at any time, has no relation to effort, and is particularly prone to happen in association with recall of fearful and unpleasant situations. It often occurs at night, waking the patient in a panic."

Chest pain, another symptom, can cause a lot of diagnosis trouble for both patient and doctor, for how can you tell it from the pain of angina pectoris? The kind of pain Dr. Aaron is talking about does not occur as a result of effort on the patient's part. It may go on for days. It may yield to rest, but it may be necessary to rest for several hours. One patient told Dr. Aaron that he would have to go to bed for the rest of the day to get relief from his pain caused by visiting the doctor in the morning. It is hard to describe pain. Patients may have read accounts of the pain experienced by angina patients and may confuse their own pain with this.

Why We Get These Symptoms

What causes such heart symptoms, if there is nothing organically wrong with one's heart? Although he is not a psychiatrist, Dr. Aaron believes that emotional happenings in one's past life are responsible. Recalling situations that frightened or angered one stimulates the same physical reaction throughout one's body as if one were frightened or angered.

Says Dr. Aaron, "I have no doubt that most, if not all, patients suffering from anxiety states have gone through prolonged periods of fear without relief in action. An insecure childhood is the most common factor, particularly mother-deprivation, a violent alcoholic father or over-strictness of well-meaning parents. These features are almost always found in the history of these unfortunate persons . . . My conception of the etiology (cause) of these disabilities is, then, conditioning of prolonged anxiety and insecurity as a rule in childhood up to the age of 18 years, resulting in unduly violent emotional reactions to later stresses. These may be every-day stresses of life, recall of difficult life situations, dreams or new severe emotional upsets. The reaction remains the same—stimulation of the auto-matic nervous system. If the fear of heart disease is superimposed on this, the threat to life is added and a vicious circle is established."

Dr. Aaron tells us that it is also possible for people with organic heart disease to have also heart symptoms that arise from anxiety neuroses. In such cases, he says, the doctor must first treat the organic heart trouble, then, if the symptoms persist after the actual working of the heart has been corrected, the patient must work to correct the emotional background that is causing them.

Do emotional stresses cause heart disease? Not according to Dr. Aaron. He takes up the commonly held, widely held, notion that executives have more heart attacks because they "worry more." And asks, "What about the executives in Japan and other countries where heart attacks are comparatively low? Do their executives worry less?"

An investigation by Lee and Schneider in 1958 showed that among a large group of white collar workers in New York there were just as many cases of heart attacks among the employees as among the executives, even though the executives are supposed to be under so much more stress.

Are mental symptoms the result of heart disease? So far as neurosis is concerned, Dr. Aaron believes that people who have heart disease and know that it may get worse and eventually cause a heart attack usually become adjusted to this idea and do not worry greatly about themselves. He says, "The patient with advanced heart disease has reason to worry about his state of health and the eventual outcome; yet it is surprising how well adjusted most of these patients are, and how infrequently they show neurotic traits."

However, he admits that mental symptoms are frequent in association with advanced heart disease, especially in the elderly. Difficulties in sleeping, nightmares, disturbing dreams—all these may contribute to the distress felt by these patients.

Doctors Play a Part in This Kind of Heart Trouble

Finally, Dr. Aaron talks about the patient who has been made fearful about his heart by a doctor. "It is stated," he says, "that some doctors, through ignorance, carelessness or failure to recognize the mental state of the patient, diagnose organic heart disease where no such disease exists, and cause severe disability in these patients who consequently believe themselves to be suffering from serious heart disease. There is no doubt that this occurs. Of 631 persons referred to a work classification unit for assessment because of the presence of heart disease, 175 had no heart disease at all."

Later he says, "I recall a number of patients requesting examination of their hearts who, when told that I could not find any evidence of heart disease, informed me that they had been told that they had heart disease but did not believe it." He is sure, he tells us, too, that there are many people who are made ill by a doctor through misinterpretation of what he tells them about symptoms.

Dr. Aaron's conclusions are that neurosis is a common cause of certain symptoms which appear to be symptoms of heart disease. Adjusting to life situations rather than taking medicine is the cure for such symptoms. He does not suggest how to adjust oneself. This is in the field of mental rather than physical health. He does believe, however, that there is no evidence that stress can cause genuine heart disease. Severe shocks can bring about heart attacks in a person whose heart is already abnormal. Heart disease symptoms, brought on by a doctor's wrong diagnosis, can occur, although Dr. Aaron believes, they generally occur only in individuals who are emotionally unstable. The well adjusted person presumably does not get upset when his doctor tells him mistakenly that he has a bad heart.

We want to add one note to Dr. Aaron's observations. Mental health is closely related to diet. The B vitamins and calcium especially are essential for the maintenance of good mental health. In times when these elements are almost completely absent from the average diet, people are bound to become neurotic. Malnourished people cannot adjust to difficult emotional situations as successfully as well nourished people. Heart palpitations, breathlessness, fatigue are symptoms of lack of B vitamins and calcium, as surely as they are symptoms of a neurotic preoccupation with heart disease.

42. How Important Is Stress in Heart Disease?

It is typical of our society that we insist on simple answers to complicated questions. This is especially so in questions of health. When people ask what causes cancer, they don't want to be told that it is due to a combination of things, such as ingested poisons, food that is denatured, missing nutrients, etc. They want a pat answer—one thing: smoking, liquor, polluted air or fried foods. They want to be assured that if they avoid any one of these, cancer will pass them by. The attitude is similar for all of our major diseases.

In the field of heart disease research, the answers seem to be more confusing than in any other, because the emotions are involved as well as diet, exercise and other factors. An article in the *Journal of the American Medical Association* (October 3, 1959) describes one of the scientific studies which showed emotional strain to be a force involved in the onset of heart disease. It is not the only cause, and may not be a cause at all in some individuals, but observations indicated to Dr. Henry I. Russek, M.D., that one who suffers from emotional strain is more likely to suffer from coronary disease than one who does not. As a matter of fact, Dr. Russek's findings put emotional stress above diet, smoking, heredity, obesity and lack of exercise as a cause of heart trouble.

Responsibility and Personality Patterns

How Dr. Russek arrived at this conclusion is interesting. In association with a colleague, he carefully assessed the background of 100 heart patients under 40 years of age. In 91 per cent of them prolonged emotional strain associated with job responsibility preceded the attack. In a group of 100 patients suffering from diseases other than heart disability, and used as controls for comparison, only 20 per cent were found to be under similar strain preceding the serious attack of their particular illness. Further study of Dr. Russek's findings leads one to believe that a heart disease victim follows a definite pattern of personality. For example 46 per cent of the 100 heart patients worked 60 or more hours per week; aside from this group, another 25 per cent were holding two jobs at the time of the attack. In another 20 per cent there was unusual fear, insecurity, discontent, frustration, restlessness or a feeling of inadequacy in relation to employment.

Further comparison between the heart patients and controls revealed that the heart cases more frequently held positions of responsibility or jobs involving pressure due to deadlines than did the controls. However, in some cases cause of stress was laid not to the type of work, but to too many hours of work a week, or to secondary stresses in so-called leisure time.

The theory of work-approach-heart-disease relationship was studied from a different angle by Friedman and Roseman. They compared groups of men selected solely according to behavior pattern routinely shown at work. Group I showed intense striving, an inclination to compete, desire for recognition, unusual mental and physical alertness and involvement in deadlines. Group II had a behavior pattern opposite to Group I. Group III was similar to Group II, but complicated by a chronic state of anxiety or insecurity.

Visible Mannerisms and Characteristics

Friedman and Roseman found coronary disease 7 times more frequent in Group I (the anxious ones) than in Groups II and III. It is noteworthy that 80 per cent of this group showed obvious characteristics that were easily connected with mental attitudes, such as rapid body movement, tense facial musculature, explosive conversational intonations, hand or teeth clenching, excessive unconscious gesturing and a general air of impatience.

Dr. Russek's findings were contrary in the latter respect. While some of the 100 patients showed some or all of these characteristics, most had a striking degree of self-control, dignified reserve and complacency.

Essentially, over-conscientiousness and taking their work too seriously were the marks of Dr. Russek's 100 heart patients. Either a desire for recognition or a deep sense of obligation to employer or family could be found in most of them. They were generally too concerned about time, overmeticulous, concerned about trivia, impatient with subordinates, worrisome, unwilling to delegate authority. Responsibilities on domestic, occupational and social levels were assumed by these people beyond the dictates of good judgment, and they were prone to neglect the prudent rules of good health.

Low Fat Diet Helps

Is diet not involved at all? Dr. Russek says it is a factor. He advocates a low fat diet, especially for one involved in a stressful situation, either occupationally, domestically or socially. By way of illustration he points to Norway and the Netherlands during World War II. It was a most stressful time for the people of these countries, yet there was no increase in the death rate due to cardiac disease. Dr. Russek regards the fact that fat foods were not generally available to the people at that time, as a partial explanation. In America today the cardiac death rate goes up steadily and and it could be due to stress complicated by the fact that many Americans indulge in the readily available high fat diet.

That factors other than stress can influence the onset of heart disease is not disputed. Of the 100 heart patients observed by Dr. Russek, every one had a high fat diet, heredity factor, or emotional strain in his background. Of the controls, 24 per cent were entirely free of any of these. The heart patients were found to have two of these major factors in the background of 95 per cent of the 100 cases. Of the controls, only 12 per cent had two such factors.

How About Smoking?

Dr. Russek checked on smoking and found that not only was smoking more prevalent in the coronary group, but twice as many of the coronary patients, as compared with the controls, were heavily addicted to the use of tobacco. It was undecided by the author whether the smoking brought on the heart disease, or whether it was a manifestation of the inner tensions usually present in a coronary-prone subject. Nervous smoking, as well as eating and drinking, may be the result of stressful situations. Social activities can often breed the feeling that only a cigarette, a drink or food will fill the anxious or boring moment. If one is continually thrown into such situations, the habit is easily formed which eventually affects one's health and perhaps one's heart.

If Dr. Russek's deductions on the basis of observing 100 cardiac patients are not scientifically absolute, they certainly are indicative of stress as a factor in heart disease. He even quotes authorities to show that the cholesterol level of the blood rises strikingly during stressful situations. Emotional episodes call forth rapid mobilization of fatty acids from body tissues into the blood stream. Stress is related in this, and other known and unknown ways, to changes in the body's workings. It is not difficult then to attribute heart disease to a steady disruption of normal body functions by constant and unrelieved stress.

Can You Control Emotional Stress?

We have often emphasized the connection between the emotions and diet. The B vitamins have been shown time and again to have an almost miraculous control over healthy mental attitudes. If tenseness and emotionalism seem to be creeping into your make-up, if you find yourself slipping into the personality pattern described above, check into your diet. Do you include brewer's yeast, desiccated liver, wheat germ and the organ meats, all rich in B vitamins? Do you find yourself eating more and more

[192]

refined foods, starches, bread and sweets which are devoid of these precious nutrients or rob the few you've managed to acquire? Are you hurrying through breakfasts of coffee and sweet rolls, and lunches of sodas, sandwiches with jelly or processed cold cuts, and a candy bar? Is dinner a starchy frozen meat pie or spaghetti topped off with pie and ice cream? This kind of eating does not prepare one to deal calmly with the stresses of family and job. This kind of eating can lead to heart disease.

43. Is Too Much Sun Related to Heart Attacks?

Warnings about over-exposure to the sun are usually confined to care about sun poisoning, sunstroke and possible skin cancer. These are certainly serious enough conditions, and would be enough to make most prudent persons think twice before baking themselves in pursuit of a tan. However, an even more serious illness, myocardial infarction (a clot at the heart wall) is believed by John C. Ham, M.D., and Alton M. Paull, M.D., to be directly due in some cases, to over-exposure to the sun's hot rays. Writing in the *Rhode Island Medical Journal* (October, 1958) these two gentlemen presented some very impressive evidence to give weight to their theory. After reading it, we wonder if you will still feel that it's perfectly safe to lie in the sun, scorching your body until you become bronze tan like the models in the lotion ads.

Two cases of myocardial infarction occurring in rapid succession, and associated with intense exposure to the sun, led the authors to investigate the possibility of naming such exposure as a definite cause of heart attack. Research soon brought out the fact that exposure of the body to heat produces changes in the physical and chemical characteristics of blood in animals and man which might tend to slow the coronary circulation and to favor blood clotting.

Rabbits and Dogs Affected

Experiments with rabbits, overheated for short periods of less than two hours, showed that the rhythm of their heartbeat was altered, the valves of the heart were disturbed and coronary circulation and myocardial function were abnormal. In overheated dogs, it was found that the blood chemistry was very definitely altered—the blood sugar level was changed and the salt content increased.

Ham and Paull cite a study of 44 human cases of heat stroke. In all of them the blood chemistry had spontaneously changed, and in some cases, signs of heart failure or circulatory failure, appeared. Another report tells of 3 cases of heat stroke observed at various periods of time following a long march in hot weather. The subjects, all male, were 22, 23 and 30 years of age, respectively. Their symptoms included a pressure and oppressive feeling in the chest in one and a sudden loss of consciousness in another. The third patient showed strong symptoms of myocardial infarction.

Dallas Records Indicative

Supporting the supposition of Ham and Paull even further, are the findings of H. E. Heyer, et al, (*American Health Journal*, 15:741-747, 1953). Heyer's study was of the relationship between the incidence of myocardial infarction to different months of the year in Dallas, Texas. It was found that the incidence was considerably higher in the months of July and August than in the cooler months. The daily temperature readings in Dallas during these months usually exceed 95 degrees, and often 100 degrees Fahrenheit. Heyer suggested that the profound physiologic adjustment one must make to maintain constant body temperature under such conditions may be a causative factor in the incidence of myocardial infarction. In none of the patients included in this study was there frank heat stroke, but a mild degree of heat exhaustion is common in Dallas. Adjustment to such a climate does cause an increase in cardiac work, often with increased output of blood volume, and transmission of a larger portion of blood through to the skin to promote heat loss. Such activity, according to Heyer, is quite likely to lead to myocardial infarction.

The authors offer a case history. The patient was a sun worshipper who had advanced, inactive heart disease. One day, after baking in a hot summer sun for a prolonged period with a great part of his body exposed, he suffered an oppressive feeling in his left chest that persisted all evening and prevented his sleeping. It lasted about 24 hours, then he was not bothered for 10 days. On the eleventh day, the patient once more sun bathed with his chest bare. This time the suffering was worsened. He had such pain in the upper torso that morphine was required on two occasions. He was advised to avoid such continuous periods of sun bathing.

The subject had no more episodes of chest pain, but he died a few years later of congestive heart failure. Among other difficulties with his heart and circulatory system, an autopsy revealed an acute myocardial infarct.

Also interesting is the case of a 50 year old man who had no predisposition whatever to heart disease. He was admitted to the hospital on July 30, 1956, with strong symptoms of heart disease—chest pains, weakness, coughing, chills and a choking sensation. Examination showed no physiological indications of heart trouble. Rhythm was regular, no murmurs, no enlargement of the heart, no friction-rub or gallop, no pulse change and the blood pressure was normal. Outwardly the man was a well-developed, well-nourished, *deeply tanned* male.

After a few weeks' rest in the hospital the patient went home and

[194]

resumed mild activity. He felt fine until, after eating a light meal, he developed a squeezing sensation in the chest, with an oppressive feeling and radiation of pain to the shoulder and neck. After a few days in the hospital, the patient developed symptoms not unlike pneumonia. After this phase, X-ray revealed slight enlargement of one of the valves of the heart.

Investigation later revealed that immediately prior to both attacks the patient had sun bathed in a pair of trunks for from 1½ to 2 hours in the hot sun, perspired profusely and then felt chilled. For several years he had been accustomed to a great deal of sun bathing.

The authors are careful to say that there is no proof that a heart condition will result in every case of sun bathing. They do, however, warn that the indications as to a relationship between over-exposure and heart disease should result in a cautious attitude toward sun bathing.

We believe that the sun is a powerful, not completely harmless, influence on good health. Prolonged exposure to its hot rays is dangerous and foolhardy. Don't be careless about it—especially at midday in the summer months.

44. Soft Water and Heart Trouble

The dialogue about the value of hard or soft water has been going strong now for at least 10 years. We know it is obvious that hard water, (water with a high calcium and magnesium content), is more inconvenient to work with than soft water. The water softener companies advertise that they can correct this with ease. Health-conscious people know, however, that most commonly-employed means of water softening involve a transfer of two parts of sodium to the softened water for every one part of calcium or magnesium removed. The danger represented by the added sodium in the water far outweighs any convenience factors that might be present.

There was considerable speculation, too, that hard water might even be of nutritional value due to the minerals it could supply to the body. This theory was given some support by an article which appeared in the *New York Times* (May 7, 1961). The headline said, "Water is Linked to Heart Deaths—Mortality Found Higher in Soft Water Regions."

In some detail the story told of a British research team whose findings indeed confirmed the headline. Drs. J. N. Norris, M. D. Crawford and J. A. Heady of London Hospital Medical College studied the relation between death rates and hardness of water in the country boroughs of England and Wales. Their finding: "The softer the water supply in the country boroughs of England, the higher the death rate from cardiovascular disease tends to be. . . . What this means is not at present clear, and further investigation is indicated."

The team agreed that the main problem was to decide whether there was a cause-and-effect relationship between heart disease and soft water. They were not sure if the minerals in the hard water actually had some preservative effect. Or it is also possible that soft water, either natural or treated, carries harmful trace elements which have an adverse effect on the heart. Whatever the reason, it is obvious that to trade hard water for soft is to invite increased likelihood of heart disease. Either something in hard water protects against heart ailments, or something in soft water water causes them, according to these scientists.

Similar Findings in the United States

Their work, it turned out, was a British version of work done in the United States by Dr. Henry Schroeder, reported in the *Journal of the American Medical Association* (April 23, 1960). Dr. Schroeder found that, in general, the watershed areas of the Mississippi, Missouri and Ohio Rivers had hard water and lower death rates and that the Atlantic and Pacific Coast states had softer water and higher death rates. Dr. Schroeder found the connection between cardiovascular disease and soft water to be significant, though not proved. "It seems to me to be fairly well established —not that soft water is the cause of cardiovascular disease, but that it has some influence on death rates."

What about the question of water softening apparatus? There exists the logical danger of exposing individuals to added sodium intake, when these individuals might be suffering from some disease in which even a very little sodium could cause serious harm. This, of course, does not deal directly with the findings of the British scientists or Dr. Schroeder. In their research only naturally-occurring waters were considered. Their contention is that any soft water is less safe than hard water. But if that is true, then artificially softened water, because of the added sodium, is even more of a hazard.

Why We're Afraid of Sodium

The case against sodium is very forcibly presented in these pages in Editor Rodale's "Heart Disease and Its Control" (See chapter 34). Salt (sodium chloride) is, of course, a major source of sodium intake for most people. Salt-free diets are very often recommended by doctors treating patients who have heart disease, dropsy, etc. Salt increases the volume of the blood, and therefore raises the blood pressure, which is the force produced by the work of the heart muscle and transmitted to the blood vessels.

In the January 15, 1955, issue of the *Journal of the American Medical Association,* Editor Rodale found this comment in answer to a question about the value of a low-sodium diet: "It has been asserted that congestive failure never develops in any patient with hypertension (even in the seemingly refractory class) if he is kept on a correct low-sodium diet."

Dr. Frederick Allen, who introduced to this country the low salt diet for high blood pressure, was quoted in the *Journal of the American Medical Association* (June 4, 1949) as saying, "My conclusion based on unique experience in several thousand cases during 28 years, is that saltless diets, especially when begun reasonably early, can specifically arrest progressiveness, prevent complications and thus provide the first real control of deaths from hypertension."

Dr. Leo A. Saperstein of the University of Southern California, wrote in the *Proceedings of the Society of Experimental and Biological Medicine* (73: 82-85) of his experiments which showed that feeding salt to rats induced high blood pressure, and enlarged their hearts and kidneys.

These are just a few of the many recorded experiments which have shown sodium to be a serious threat to circulatory health, as well as to other functions of the body. It is obvious that any unnecessary sources of sodium should be avoided. The sodium in artificially softened water is certainly a hazard that no one need be exposed to.

Manufacturers of water-softening equipment are quick to minimize any danger involved with the use of their product. But we continually come across authoritative evidence that proves there is something to be concerned about if you are considering the installation of a water softener.

In the *Canadian Medical Association Journal* (February 25, 1961) there appeared a letter from David J. Bryant, M.D., of the Province of Saskatchewan. In it Dr. Bryant told of his hospital's experience with softened water. "During the fall of 1960 a water softener, using zeolite as an absorbant, was installed in the local Dinsmore Union Hospital, all the water being used in the hospital being routed through the softener. It was noticed that saberetics, such as hydrochlorothiazide, used in the treatment of hypertension and edema of congestive heart failure, etc., were suddenly found to have little or no expected effect . . . it was recognized that the water softener was converting the water used in the hospital for every purpose into a mild saline solution, and as a result had all of our hospital patients on a fairly high sodium diet!"

Dr. Bryant's hospital was lucky to discover the cause of the problem before any serious damage to the patients (at least Dr. Bryant didn't mention any). We wonder though about the aftereffects on patients who were hospitalized at the time. How many were potential heart cases for whom the extra sodium acted as a trigger to heart complications to be seen in a month or a year? Think of the number of patients in a hospital who are on a salt-free diet for one reason or another. At Dinsmore Union they were leaving sodium out of the food, and putting it into the water!

Think of the hospitals in the United States and Canada which might be using softened water and still be unaware of the sodium in it being added to the patients' diets. If hospitals, whose main concern must be for patients' health, are taken in by the safety claims of water softener salesmen, what chance has the average layman? If hospitals, with staffs and equipment for scientific evaluation, can make a mistake about the value of a water softener—or even neglect to investigate it at all—how can the average home owner be expected to know what he is getting into when he signs up for its installation?

Every Installation Different

It is not possible to set up a definite schedule for the exact amount of sodium one will get with a water softener, and the salesman who says it is, is at best, mistaken. Dr. Henry Schroeder, the expert on water softness mentioned before, was consulted on a question printed in Questions and Answers in the *Journal of the American Medical Association* (May 20, 1961). A Jacksonville, Florida, doctor wanted to know if a water softener is likely to put sufficient sodium in the water for it to be harmful to a patient on a low-sodium diet. Dr. Schroeder said first that the amount of sodium put into the water would vary with the hardness of the water "and the present efficiency of the softener." (The efficiency varies with the amount of time the softener is in use.) He also noted that the amount of sodium which is naturally present in the local water supply is different in different places. Then, too, some municipalities soften hard water at the water treatment plants, with zeolite soda lime, "which can add a large amount of sodium."

Dr. Schroeder gives, as an indication of the high sodium content possible in the water we take from the tap, the reading for the water supply at Sarasota, Florida (530 milligrams of sodium per liter after softening), which he characterizes as "extreme." Dr. Schroeder points out that anyone who drinks that water would disrupt a diet aimed at restricting sodium intake to 200 milligrams or even 500 milligrams of sodium per day. Some waters, of course, add only a few milligrams of sodium a day.

Analysis May Be Needed

"If one suspects that tapwater contains enough sodium to affect the total intake," says Dr. Schroeder, "analysis and decision on using bottled water for drinking and cooking should be made. Values for sodium in municipal water can be obtained from treatment plants." Now this presupposes two rather unlikely possibilities: 1. that the average householder would get to wondering about the sodium value of his tap water, when he is probably unaware that it is being softened at all, by the city, hence unaware that extra sodium is coming his way; 2. that he would take the time to call the treatment plant for the information, or have the background needed to relate the information they give him to its importance in *his* life.

You see, most Americans are not likely to suspect danger from softened water. Rather they would be inclined to give the water bureau a rousing vote of thanks if it were to soften the municipal water supply. This is the miracle that was accomplished by advertising in our country. We have been schooled to the attitude that only those who cannot afford to have water softeners are willing to do without them. Softeners have become a status symbol. So you can imagine the gratitude of citizens who find that their community is willing to shoulder the expense of supplying them with softened water. They aren't likely to protest it; they welcome it!

Your Right to Pure Water

Dr. Schroeder, in discussing Sarasota's water, remarks that "Such saline water should probably not be used for cooking." This means, we presume, that Sarasota citizens must, or should, have at hand a separate water supply for cooking, if they wish to remain healthy. What right has any municipal government to tamper with the public water supply to a point at which its use for human consumption is unhealthful? It is the fluoridation story once more. In water softening we have the proven medical fact that sodium intake is closely related to heart disease, and commercially softened water means added sodium. The softened water is obviously dangerous to all who drink it, but especially to persons with circulatory disorders.

Convenience is not a worthy reason, indeed there is none, for adding sodium to the community water supply. That water is intended to be as pure as possible. It is to be treated only in the interests of purity and freedom from disease-carrying bacteria. It is not intended to act as a vehicle for medication or convenience factors. If one wants softer water, one is at liberty to alter one's own water supply at one's home; why should the whole town have to drink water that has been treated for softness? Softening of municipal water supplies, especially when the result is the staggering sodium count in Sarasota water, is certainly an infringement upon one's rights to a safe water supply.

It is interesting to note that we have in our file 3 letters, which were published in the *Journal of the American Medical Association*, on the hazards of water softeners. In each case, the expert called upon to comment on the problem made mention of some danger involved. Still we see no official stand on water softeners by the medical fraternity. In the January 31, 1951, issue the *Journal's* answer referred to a rather well-known water-softening system, which employed the action exchange principle, in which the calcium and magnesium responsible for hardness are replaced by sodium. In other words, the harder the water you use, the more sodium there will be in it when it is softened. The water-softener salesmen never mention this.

More Sodium, Less Nutrition

In the *Journal* (August 8, 1953) the question of Arthur W. Anderson, M.D., concerned danger, benefit and effect on nutritive value of foods when cooked in softened water. The answer largely minimized any danger from softeners, but included these comments: "It is true that well-softened waters employed in cooking extract a higher percentage of the minerals of vegetables and possibly of the vitamins, but this is not characteristic of ordinary chemically softened waters."

If the minerals, calcium and magnesium, are already filtered out of the water, and cooking removes still more of these minerals from the main remaining source, vegetables, where is one to get the necessary minerals? If cooking them in softened water can also remove more vitamins from vegetables than hard water would, where is one to get one's vitamins? And if this is "not characteristic of ordinary softened waters," who is to know if yours would be "ordinary" or not? Will the water softener salesman tell you that *your* water when softened will rob vegetables of their vitamins and minerals when they are cooked in it? Not likely. Will you be able to check up for your own satisfaction? Not unless you are a chemist with the necessary equipment, or can hire one.

Following the publication of that letter, the *Journal* received a related communication which was printed in the October 17, 1953, issue. Alan W. Shewman, M.D., wrote: ". . . The process of water softening is replacing magnesium and calcium with sodium. Hence the water has a high sodium content. That is why patients suffering from vertigo or dropsy often improve after combining distilled water with their medication."

Dr. Shewman means that the added sodium caused trouble for people suffering with these two physical problems. He used distilled water to avoid the sodium; we say bottled spring water is safest and probably better, healthwise, than distilled water, since, in its preparation, all the healthful minerals are removed from distilled water.

Would Your Doctor Warn You?

How many people drinking softened water have a doctor who will consider the type of water they are drinking in relation to their worsening illness? How many people have become ill due to increased sodium in their tissues, and have no inkling that the softened water they drink to help them take their pills is the very reason for their problem?

Manufacturers of water softeners argue that, aside from the inconvenience of washing with water that won't make suds and leaves rings in the bathtub, hard water can lower efficiency of water heaters and plug up piping and other plumbing. Says *Consumer Bulletin* (February, 1960): "Another disadvantage (aside from the health question) of completely softened water, and this includes naturally soft water too, may be a tendency to increase corrosion of piping and water tanks, particularly in hot water systems. Removing the scale-forming compounds, which afford a degree of protection to the metal from the corrosion due to water, may hasten the rusting of steel pipes and tanks (even so-called glass-lined tanks) and in some cases produce active corrosion even of copper piping. . . ."

We believe that the information we have presented here is enough to convince anyone who is conscious of the value of good health, and how hard it is to retain good health in today's world, that water softeners are still another threat to it. Researchers conclude that naturally soft water is, somehow, able to affect, adversely, your chances of long life. Of course, people who have jobs and families in soft water locales cannot simply move

[200]

out, but they can use bottled spring water for drinking and cooking, to minimize the risk.

With this evidence before us, the very idea of paying to soften the water artificially is truly appalling. Not only do we invite the newly-exposed danger of natural soft water, but we add to it the danger of added sodium in the system.

If you insist on using a water softener to make life easier, make certain that it affects only the hot water line, that which you use for dishes and laundry. Leave the cold water line, which is normally used for cooking and drinking, alone. Experts seem to agree that cooking with and drinking hard water will help you live longer.

45. Hardening of the Arteries

Every once in a while we happen on an article in a medical journal that seems to us so sensible, so practical and so worthwhile that it almost makes up for the volumes of unintelligent and unintelligible gibberish that passes for scientific lore in many instances.

Such an article appears in the *Journal of Chronic Diseases* for July, 1955. It is called "Is Atherosclerosis a Conditioned Pyridoxal Deficiency?" and it was written by Henry A. Schroeder, M.D. The title sounds forbidding until you translate it into simpler words. Atherosclerosis is another word for hardening of the arteries. Pyridoxine is one of the B vitamins. Dr. Schroeder is asking simply, is it possible that hardening of the arteries may result from lack of some of the B vitamins in the diet.

He starts out by telling us that too little pyridoxine (vitamin B_6) in the diet of monkeys produces, in general, the same condition as human hardening of the arteries. A deficiency of pyridoxine in rats causes high blood pressure. There is evidence, he says, that the whole process takes place in the blood vessels of these animals very much as it does in those of men. Pyridoxine is involved in the process by which the body uses fat. We all know that magazines and newspaper articles have recently been declaiming far and wide the fact that fat in the diet has a lot to do with blood vessel and heart disorders. Could it be that deficiency or abundance of pyridoxine in the diet is one of the determining factors, too—perhaps one of the important ones?

Dr. Schroeder gives us an excellent estimate of the amount of pyridoxine in the average American diet. About half the pyridoxine in grain is lost when the grain is processed. Canned vegetables contain little, although fresh vegetables and fruits are quite rich in it. The processing of milk and meat, cooking and stewing food result in substantial losses of the vitamin. Any amount of heat, or light, damages pyridoxine.

[201]

Our Diets Lack Pyridoxine

It is estimated that an adult may need from two to three milligrams of pyridoxine daily. Losses after processing and cooking may make it impossible for us to get enough of the vitamin, especially during winter.

"Therefore from the incomplete data in the literature, it is entirely possible that the American adult is maintained on a marginal intake of this important coenzyme (pyridoxine) during periods of the year in which fresh vegetables and fruits are not available and processed foods and meats are widely used." Of course, too, one must take into account the quite considerable group of people who simply do not eat fresh raw fruits and vegetables even when they are available. Such folks would be bound to be lacking in pyridoxine the year round.

Now for the part pyridoxine plays in fat metabolism. Part of its job is to assist the body in using the unsaturated fatty acids—those important kinds of fat which occur in unhydrogenated vegetable oils and not in animal fats to any great extent. If there were a shortage of these unsaturated fats in the diet, one might need even more of the B vitamin pyridoxine than otherwise; if there were plenty of these fats in the diet, then one might need less pyridoxine. The American diet is notoriously lacking in liquid vegetable and cereal oils, especially as compared to other countries where little animal fat is eaten and liquid oils are used exclusively for cooking and for baking. We know that cholesterol, the fatty substance that collects on artery walls in hardening of the arteries, is dissolved by the unsaturated fatty acids. Dr. Schroeder also tells us that the cholesterol levels in the blood of monkeys deficient in pyridoxine is higher than that of monkeys which are getting plenty of the vitamin, which seems to indicate that pyridoxine plays a part, too, in the whole complicated business of how the body uses fats—for good or for harm.

Incidentally, we found one note in Dr. Schroeder's article which we have not found in any other material dealing with unsaturated fatty acids. Fish need them *in order to remain pliable.* "Even warm-blooded animals fed . . . saturated acids (rather than unsaturated ones) may become stiff," says Dr. Schroeder. Is it possible that the unsaturated fatty acids are essential for preventing arthritis and other forms of stiff joints? Is it possible that it is the unsaturated fatty acids in fish liver oil and wheat germ oil that render them powerful agents against arthritis stiffness in many cases?

Are We Getting Abnormal Amounts of Trace Metals?

To get back to pyridoxine, Dr. Schroeder tells us that it is necessary for certain minerals to be present, too, for the vitamin to function at top efficiency. Going a little deeper into this subject he found that there are many "abnormal" metals or minerals present in the tissues of modern Americans.

What does he mean by "abnormal?" Well, we know that iron, copper, zinc, cobalt and manganese are trace minerals that play a very important part in the activities of the human body. But others apparently do not. And the traces of them that are found in the human body are apparently deposited there when people are exposed to them daily during everyday activities. For instance, an examination of human tissues revealed little or no cobalt (which is absolutely essential for health) but relatively large amounts of nickel and chromium. Where could the nickel come from? One very possible source is hydrogenation. When vegetable oils are hydrogenated (that is, solidified), their precious unsaturated fatty acids are destroyed. That is why we advise our readers against using any form of hydrogenated fats. But now we have an additional reason for alarm. Says Dr. Schroeder, "It is interesting that nickel catalysts are used in the hydrogenation of edible vegetable fats." Could this be the main reason why, in a table Dr. Schroeder gives, showing the minerals present in human tissues, there should be, in general, such large concentrations of nickel, especially compared with the amounts of the essential minerals like manganese and cobalt?

Why should there be such large amounts of aluminum unless because of the widespread use of aluminum cooking utensils? Why should concentrations of tin be so high, except for our constant exposure to this metal in the processing and preparation of foods? Is it not possible that concentrations of these metals that are not essential to human beings may displace the mineral that is supposed to act along with pyridoxine in metabolizing fat in the human body, asks Dr. Schroeder.

"Civilization" Is Responsible

It sounds, actually, a lot more complex than it is. What Dr. Schroeder is getting at is expressed very directly in his summary. The trend of the incidence of hardening of the arteries and high blood pressure is consistent with the accumulation of some substance in the body over a period of many years. In countries where there is little "civilization" as we know it, these disorders are almost unknown. "Civilization" is responsible for removing the pyridoxine from our food and, in the process of solidifying vegetable fat, is also responsible for destroying our chief source of the valuable unsaturated fatty acids. In addition, says Dr. Schroeder, the inhabitants of different countries "differ in their exposure to trace metals in canned and processed foods, in the products of petroleum combustion and water piped through metal pipes."

There are 3 stresses, according to Dr. Schroeder, which "civilization" imposes on the human organism which may account for the high rate of hardening of the arteries:

1. Exposure to abnormal amounts of trace metals.

2. Excessive eating of hydrogenated fats which do not contain the unsaturated fatty acids.

3. Too little pyridoxine. He admits that there are many unknown links in the chain of theory which he has presented in this article. But, says

he, there is little or no experimental evidence against it. "Most of what is known appears to fit."

Getting Enough Pyridoxine Is Important

We think it is one of the most sensible theories we have listened to yet, especially since it takes up the importance of the harmful metals. What can readers do to safeguard themselves against the 3 "stresses" which Dr. Schroeder says may be responsible for hardening of the arteries?

1. Avoid hydrogenated fats like the poison they are. This means any and all of the solid shortenings or margarine. Don't eat factoryized food. Much of it contains hydrogenated fats. Crackers, pastry, "mixes," commercial peanut butter, anything fried in deep fat. Avoid all these.

2. Get plenty of pyridoxine. It comes along with the other B vitamins in fresh raw fruits and vegetables (not cooked, mind you), in liver, heart, wheat germ, whole wheat, peanuts. As you might expect, brewer's yeast—that rich, rich source of B vitamins—contains far more pyridoxine than any other food.

3. Avoid the contaminating of food with metals—tin, aluminum, nickel and so forth. Use glass, enamel or stainless steel utensils rather than aluminum. Don't eat factoryized food or food that comes in a can.

46. A New Twosome—Goiter and Arteriosclerosis

A definite connection seems to exist between disease of the thyroid gland and hardening of the arteries. Of all of the glands of the body, the thyroid seems to be the most complex and far-reaching in its effects. It rules the rate at which we grow, our metabolism (the rate at which we burn our food for energy), as well as our emotions and personalities, so it is not too surprising to find that it influences the way the body handles cholesterol.

As you are probably well aware, iodine is an important raw material for the thyroid gland. From its supply of iodine and a protein, tyrosine, the thyroid manufactures its hormone, thyroxine. When the supply of iodine is short or somehow interrupted, the thyroid strains itself to make thyroxine, often enlarging until a goiter is formed. The goiter, which is simply a swelling of the thyroid gland, is usually a positive sign of a shortage of iodine in the diet.

A Finnish doctor, who reports his findings in the *Lancet* (July, 1958), noticed that persons who die from coronary sclerosis, or hardening of the arteries that lead directly to the heart, often have goiter. More study disclosed to him that goiters were significantly more frequent in such cases than in those dying from other causes. It was this researcher's opinion that the relationship between arteriosclerosis and goiter might be due to underproduction or overproduction of thyroxine stimulated somehow by the pituitary gland.

Body's Thyroxine Output Decreased With Age

Dr. Murray Israel, in a speech to the Andiron Club of New York City, April 18, 1958, told of similar findings. He relates this experience in treating a 60-year-old woman who was dying of generalized hardening of the arteries. She also seemed to have a severe thyroid deficiency. Though the treatment, in such a case, was unheard of at the time, Dr. Israel administered a dose of thyroxine mixed with brewer's yeast to the dying patient. He continued the medication through the day, then the week, and the response was so gratifying that the lady continued to use the thyroxine-brewer's yeast formula for the rest of her life—another 20 years! In trials with many other patients who used and responded to this treatment for hardening of the arteries, Dr. Israel concluded that the secretions of the thyroid gland decrease with age, sometimes diminishing to the extent that the body's needs are not met.

In recent years, the famous Doctor Wilhelm C. Heuper developed a similar opinion concerning the connection between the thyroid and hardening of the arteries. It was his theory that hardening of the arteries occurs when a metabolism failure allows cholesterol to collect in the arteries, instead of using or expelling it from the body. Since the thyroid gland is largely concerned with metabolism, the connection is readily apparent. Chances are that a lack of hormone from the thyroid gland is responsible for the inefficient operations of fat metabolism which, in turn, lead to heart problems in many instances.

Prevention of Iodine Shortage Is Our Concern

While the drastic measure of injecting thyroxine directly into the blood stream was effective for curing disease when used with B vitamins by the experimenting doctors, we are more concerned with measures for preventing the lack of thyroxine in the first place. This is best accomplished by making certain that the thyroid gland has enough iodine to manufacture thyroxine naturally. It has been shown time and again that certain localities simply do not get enough iodine from the food the people eat there or the water they drink. The resultant outbreak of goiter in these areas is so predictable that the term "goiter belt" has been applied to them.

The remedy for this situation is, of course, a deliberate intake of iodine. Years ago when the connection between iodine and goiter was first established, the "powers that be" decided to put iodine in salt so that anyone who bought and used this fortified product would not run any risk of an iodine shortage. Much of the salt used in this country today is iodized.

[205]

As always, it is our belief that the body's nutritional needs should be met by natural food sources, not doctored-up drugs such as iodized salt. In our opinion, the perfect source of iodine is kelp, or seaweed.

The plants and creatures of the sea are all quite rich in minerals, because they get their nourishment from the sea, which abounds with them. Kelp is rich in all of these elements, but its supply of iodine is staggeringly higher. Used as a condiment, in the same way as salt, dried kelp gives about 10 times as much iodine as the same amount of iodized salt. There is salt in kelp, among other minerals, but because it occurs naturally and in combination with so many other nutritional factors, we do not believe it to be harmful. Therefore, kelp is a boon to the person who cannot do without table salt regardless of how it affects his health. Dried kelp sprinkled on his food not only offers the flavor he craves, but will give him many valuable minerals in good quantity, some of which are extremely scarce in the average diet.

Other Iodine Foods

Iodine is also contained in other foods, though often in lesser amounts. Among those richest in iodine are: asparagus, dried beans, spinach, Swiss chard and most sea foods, especially oysters, lobster, haddock and flounder. Those who find these foods on their menu with some regularity are likely to be well supplied with iodine. If you intend to add fish to your diet, be sure to use salt water fish, for they are sure to be uncontaminated by the chemicals that find their way, or are poured, into our lakes and rivers. If your diet can't be changed, and iodine-rich foods are lacking, or even if you do eat a considerable amount of fish, look to kelp for a strong assist in avoiding goiter or the possible complication of hardened arteries from a malfunctioning thyroid gland.

47. Arteriosclerosis and a Fatty Diet

One of the most exciting and hopeful suggestions on the subject of diet and hardening of the arteries is made in the pages of an important British medical magazine by an M.D. who, after announcing the theme of his article, says, "Your readers with stereotyped minds should stop reading at this point." So we are given ample warning that his theory is daring and provocative. It is also one of the most sensible ideas we've run across in a long time.

As it appears in the *Lancet* for April 7, 1956, the idea of Dr. H. M.

Sinclair goes like this: cholesterol deposits on the walls of the arteries may be caused by two circumstances relating to diet in modern civilized countries:

First, our diets are deficient in the *unsaturated* fatty acids which are necessary to keep cholesterol on the move.

Second, our diets are rich in *saturated* fatty acids, whose sources are the large amounts of animal fat we eat and the processed fats—the hydrogenated vegetable oils and the fat heated to a high temperature as in deep-fat frying.

A third angle to his theory is that one of the B vitamins, pyridoxine, is closely related to the chemical activities of all these fatty substances. It is vitally important for us to have plenty of pyridoxine in our meals. But modern refining removes most of it.

Sounds complicated, doesn't it? But actually it is not. Basically all that Dr. Sinclair is saying is that modern food processing may be almost entirely responsible for the disease that is today's number one killer in "civilized" countries.

An experiment with laboratory rats led Dr. Sinclair and his associate, Dr. V. Basnayake, to their theory. They fed the rats a diet that contained no fats at all, but which was a good diet in other respects. What did they find? Large cholesterol deposits in the arteries of the animals. The longer the diet went on the more cholesterol accumulated. Now we are told that cholesterol deposits come from too much fat in the diet. How then could these rats, who were getting no fat at all, develop cholesterol deposits? Dr. Sinclair tells us that their bodies were manufacturing it—and we know that cholesterol is indeed manufactured in our bodies as well as coming from our food. And the reason that it accumulated had to be simply that a fat-free diet prevented the rats from getting any of the unsaturated fatty acids, which must be present in order to keep the cholesterol from depositing where it is not wanted.

It is impossible for us to imagine a daily diet for human beings entirely free from fat, so there is little danger that we may have the same experience the rats had. But, as Dr. Sinclair goes on to say, the more cholesterol and the more *saturated* fat you have in your diet the more *unsaturated* fat you need, if you want to avoid cholesterol deposits. Then, too, if you have enough pyridoxine in your diet, you are likely to avoid trouble, for this vitamin can help out when the important fatty acids are not there.

What Kind of Diets Produce Cholesterol?

So, says Dr. Sinclair, we might expect cholesterol deposits (which we speak of generally as atherosclerosis or arteriosclerosis, or hardening of the arteries) when the diet is high in cholesterol or unnatural fats, low in the unsaturated fatty acids, and/or deficient in B vitamins. "Are such diets encountered?" he asks.

We believe that such diets are the usual ones in this country, rather

[207]

than the exception. Dr. Sinclair says "For many years, and particularly in recent years, animal fats and more especially vegetable fats have become increasingly oxidized and deprived of E. F. A. (Essential Unsaturated Fatty Acids) before being eaten. Vegetable oils, in many cases rich in E. F. A., are hardened by hydrogenation; margarine and shortenings are produced by hydrogenation of cottonseed and soybean oil, some peanut-oil and certain other oils; during this hydrogenation much of the E. F. A. are destroyed and unnatural *trans* fatty acids are formed. Unnatural fatty acids are formed not only during hydrogenation but also during the practice of deep-frying."

How else do we lose these important food elements? Well, they occur in the germ of cereals which our food processors carefully remove and discard when they make white flour and packaged cereals. In addition, the flour "improvers," the bleaches, and many other chemicals that go into baked goods these days undoubtedly have some destructive action on the fatty acids. We have no idea how extensive this may be. In addition, when foods are refined, pyridoxine, the B vitamin, that might get in a few good licks to help the situation, is also removed and discarded.

The next time somebody tries to tell you that "enriched" cereals are just as good as completely whole grain ones, remember what we have said above. Remember how complex the whole thing is and how little of it we understand as yet. The only thing we know for certain is that the essential unsaturated fatty acids and the B vitamins are intimately and certainly involved in what happens to cholesterol in your body. Once you have deprived your body of these two precious food elements, you can expect the worst.

Dr. Sinclair tells us that he worked with Dr. Ancel Keys (one of the world's greatest authorities on the subject of fat in nutrition) and Dr. Keys came to the conclusion that the total amount of fat in the diet was responsible for hardening of the arteries and also coronary thrombosis, or heart attack. Dr. Keys said, in essence, "it doesn't matter what kind of fat it is—we must stop eating so much fat. If we cut down on the fat in our diets, we will cut down on the cholesterol deposits in our arteries."

The Kind of Fat Is the Important Thing

Dr. Sinclair tells us that he now believes this theory is wrong. "What matters," he says, "is, I believe, the amount and structure of the dietary fatty acids." That is, the important thing is *not how much* fat you get but *what kind*. In the final paragraphs of his article Dr. Sinclair pleads for more research. Heart and vascular diseases are wiping out hundreds of thousands who might still continue to live healthy lives if research showed the truth of Sinclair's theory. At any rate, he pleads, let us not make matters possibly worse by taking even more of the B vitamins and fatty acids from our flour and our processed fats.

Dr. Sinclair, handicapped as he says he is, by lack of time and a laboratory to continue his researches, can only urge British medical men to listen to his theory and, if possible, do more research along these lines. And he has already met with opposition. Dr. Ancel Keys, with whose theory he disagreed, replied to him in the April 28, 1956, issue of the *Lancet*. Dr. Keys says that a number of other researchers have had Dr. Sinclair's theory, but he still does not agree with it and he devotes a page and a half of very small type to disagreeing. He does admit that the more sophisticated, richer nations consume more fats of all kinds and he says, "The problem has been complicated by the enterprise and ingenuity of food producers and technologists who provide a superabundance of all kinds of fats and then persuade us to eat them." But what are we going to do, he asks. Are we going to persuade them to add unsaturated fatty acids to their processed products? Or are we going to try to persuade people to eat lots of vegetable, cereal and fish oil, "fresh and in the virgin liquid state"?

We don't know what Dr. Keys or Dr. Sinclair plan to do. We do know what we plan to do about a theory like Dr. Sinclair's. We think that the theory makes very good sense. It adds still another weapon in the war we are conducting against processed foods. It provides still another possible explanation why civilized diet produces diseases unknown among more primitive people.

And this is what we are going to do about it. We are going to urge readers, especially those who are worried about hardening of the arteries and heart disease, to adjust the fatty part of their diets, to *eliminate all processed fats* and to make sure they are getting enough of the unsaturated fatty acids and the B vitamins.

How can you best do this? First of all, cross off your grocery list permanently anything that has been "hydrogenated." The label will tell you. Solid shortenings are hydrogenated. Commercial peanut butter is. Margarine is. Furthermore, factory-made foods contain hydrogenated fats. Don't eat them. This means crackers, prepared "mixes," noodles, roasted and salted nuts, popcorn and so forth. It means any foods fried in deep fat—potato chips, French fries, doughnuts and so forth. Before you buy anything in a grocery, stop and consider whether or not it may contain hydrogenated or highly-heated fats. And don't buy it if it does.

What can you do if you eat in restaurants? Don't order anything fried. Don't eat anything which might contain the wrong kind of fat. What do we mean by that? The crackers that come with your tomato juice or soup, for instance. Muffins, roasted nuts, piecrust, cake—these are not for you.

On The Positive Side

On the positive side—how can you be certain you are getting enough of the essential unsaturated fatty acids? Regardless of how much or how little fat you eat, get unhydrogenated vegetable fat somehow in your diet —eat sunflower seeds or other raw seeds, like wheat seeds. Take wheat germ oil and fish liver oil—both rich sources of unsaturated fatty acids, or take a food supplement made up chiefly of unsaturated fatty acids. Lecithin contains the unsaturated fatty acids. Take a food supplement containing lecithin.

What about salad oils—rich sources of the unsaturated fatty acids? Cold pressed oils—available so far as we know, only from health food stores —are best. If you can't get these, buy and eat the regular salad oils your grocery carries—corn oil, peanut oil and so forth. We are assured by the people who make these that they contain the essential unsaturated fatty acids.

One last thing—the B vitamins. Even though you pay the strictest attention to your diet from a health standpoint, we don't believe it's possible for you to get enough of the B vitamins unless you take a natural supplement that contains them—brewer's yeast, wheat germ or desiccated liver. Although there is no official standard, it has been estimated that we need from ½ to 5 milligrams of pyridoxine alone, every day. A natural food supplement is your best source.

48. Metals and Hardening of the Arteries

Almost everyone seems to think that hardening of the arteries is a condition of old age or middle age in which calcium deposits on the inner lining of the arteries, narrowing them to such an extent that the normal volume of blood can no longer pass through and hence there are gradual difficulties with blood pressure and with disorders resulting from poor circulation.

We have had many letters from people indicating that they are worried about getting too much calcium in their diets. Their doctors have told them that the more calcium you get in your diet, the more calcium is likely to deposit on artery walls, resulting in arteriosclerosis or hardening of the arteries. It is our belief, well buttressed by much research material, that one cannot get too much calcium; that, instead, most of us need far more than we get.

We believe, too, that the way the body uses calcium decides whether one will have unwanted calcium deposits. If all regulatory glands are functioning healthfully, if the diet contains plenty of the necessary vitamin D, vitamin C, phosphorus and calcium, harmful calcium deposits will not form, either in artery walls or elsewhere in the body.

Poisonous Metals In Our Environment

Earlier we discussed the ideas of Dr. Henry A. Schroeder who believes, among other things, that one cause of hardening of the arteries may be "abnormal" metals or minerals present in the tissues of modern Americans. Now we encounter a question to the editor of the *Journal of the American Medical Association* for December 10, 1960, inquiring as follows: "In a current study of the metal content of aging aortic tissue (the aorta is the important large blood vessel leading to the heart) it was noted . . . that the metal that contributes to aging change is probably not calcium but rather aluminum, manganese or copper. What is the biochemistry and enzymatic chemistry involved in this aging process? From what sources would the aluminum probably come?"

The authority assigned by the *Journal* to answer the question does not answer it, to our satisfaction at least. He states that it is difficult to determine just how much any given tissue contains of trace minerals. But he believes that trace minerals which are not easily assimilated would tend to accumulate in the body. He says that little is known about the function of aluminum in the body. "It is undoubtedly poorly absorbed," he goes on, "but estimates of 100 micrograms have been made for the average amount absorbed per day. . . . Certain plants accumulate aluminum salts and these salts are present in small concentrations in drinking water, usually much less than one part per million."

We sent for a copy of the article referred to by the *Journal* questioner above—"The Metal Content Correlation in Aging Aorta," by H. H. Zinsser and two associates at the University of Southern California Medical School. The article appeared in the *Journal of the American Geriatrics Society,* January, 1957. The authors state that there seems to be abundant evidence that the aorta, the important big artery leading to the heart, becomes increasingly less elastic with age. Using an electron microscope these researchers found, they say, that the accumulation of minerals did not appear to be calcium. They found that, for all metals except manganese, there was a definite increase with age. For calcium, copper, iron and lead there were fairly large increases with age. Deposits of aluminum were significantly increased in all the samples.

Discussing the quite large amounts of aluminum that they found, the investigators go on to remark that aluminum is used commercially in certain combinations of chemicals *specifically for the purpose of giving rigidity.* Thus it seems that it may be responsible for just such a result in the human blood vessel.

Our authors remind us that they have subjected only a few blood vessels to the exhaustive, exacting trial tests they outline here. They state that more researchers should take up the question of the accumulation of metals in the arteries. But they also state: "There are good reasons for minimizing the key role that calcium has been given in the development of the elastic changes in the aging aorta . . . Aluminum would account most satisfactorily for the multiple bonding and increases in rigidity. . . . Manganese and copper remain possible agents."

Aluminum Is Dangerous

As many readers know, we believe that aluminum is too soft a metal and too active a metal to be used for the many things we use it for today, in relation to food. Aluminum cooking utensils are particularly suspect, we believe, because when foods, especially acid foods, are heated in such utensils, they take up aluminum from the pans. There seems to be no doubt that this is so, but we have always been told by "the authorities" and the Better Business Bureau that such contamination of food by aluminum could not possibly be harmful in spite of the evidence Editor Rodale presented in his booklet, *Poison in Your Pots and Pans* (available from Rodale Books, Incorporated, Emmaus, Pennsylvania, Price $1.00). The canning industry has gone ahead with manufacture of food cans of aluminum rather than tin. Aluminum foil is used to wrap many of the things we buy, in addition to being very inexpensively available for home use.

Now we have what we believe is another excellent reason for shunning aluminum products in the kitchen. If indeed aluminum is not easily absorbed by the body, if it accumulates in arteries, as the studies above seem to indicate, then by escaping as much aluminum exposure as we can, we may be able to postpone longer that gradual process of hardening which creates such difficulty for our heart and circulatory system. Perhaps aluminum is only a small part of one aspect of this problem. Perhaps the widespread home use of copper water pipes with its slight contamination of drinking water with copper contributes its part, as well. And undoubtedly other metals which are ingested in water and food contribute to the whole picture.

But if we can avoid even a small part of this dismal accumulation of trash in the linings of arteries, we will be doing ourselves a favor. If, in addition to avoiding contamination by metals we also follow the best possible diet—getting plenty of the B vitamins and the right kind of fats and shunning refined carbohydrates and processed fats—perhaps we can avoid the almost inevitable hardening of the arteries altogether.

In making decisions as to whether to buy things made of metal, we think the criterion to apply to aluminum and other metals is: do they actually contaminate things that I eat or drink? Obviously an aluminum chair or roof or a copper bottom on the outside of a kettle do not contaminate food or drink. So we say, use these metals in any way you wish, *except in a way which might contaminate food or drink.* We are especially pleased with the new ceramic wares that can be taken from the freezer right to the oven because they are so hard and so resistant to heat and cold.

49. Coronary Thrombosis: A Study in Causes

By J. W. McCORMICK, M.D., Toronto, Canada

Since the beginning of the present century diseases of the heart and blood vessels have been steadily assuming a more prominent place in our vital statistics, and in this group we find coronary thrombosis in the lead. (Coronary thrombosis is the formation of a blood clot in the coronary artery leading to the heart. We sometimes call it a "stroke.") So rapidly has the mortality from this disease risen in recent years that it is now the principal cause of death for all past 50 years of age.

For some time the increasing toll taken by heart disease has been attributed to the increasing tempo and stress of modern life. Recently, however, a more attractive explanation has attained general acceptance— the theory that our aging population, due to the average increase in life span, results in more people reaching the age in which diseases due to senility take their toll. Both these theories are conducive to medical complacency. A striking example of this tendency was manifested in a public lecture in Toronto recently by a leading health authority in the statement that "there are few more creditable things for a city to have than a high cardiac death rate." In further explanation the speaker said, "The city with the best public health always has the highest cardiac death rate, because the one-hoss-shay has to give out sometime and it is the most natural way to pass out between 60 and 70," the implication being that in such a city a larger number of people must have lived to the age of 60 or more.

Unfortunately, however, this specious theory does not harmonize with the facts for the following reason: 1. Coronary thrombosis, the form of heart disease chiefly responsible for the rising mortality, is not a senile disease, since it takes most of its victims between the ages of 45 and 55 and not a few below the age of 40. In the case of the "one-hoss-shay" it "went to pieces all at once and nothing first." 2. This theory does not explain the unprecedented increase in heart disease relative to pneumonia and cancer, both of which it has superseded as causes of death in recent years. 3. While it is true that the average span of life has doubled in the last half century, this has been accomplished mainly by reduction in infant and child mortality. The toll of degenerative diseases of middle life, however, has not been reduced or postponed. Accordingly, post-65 life expectancy has only slightly increased. 4. The rate of increase in heart disease, particularly coronary thrombosis, has been disproportionately greater than the rate of aging of our population. Vital statistics of deaths of American physicians from 1933 to 1940 inclusive, indicate a rise in cardiac deaths from 33 per cent to 41 per cent of total deaths. Obviously the aging of the medical profession in this short time could not possibly account for such an increase, particularly the relatively higher increase in coronary deaths from 3 per cent to 19 per cent in this same period. Neither is it reasonable to believe that improved methods in diagnosis could have brought about such a change in so short a time, since the electrocardiographic method of diagnosis has now been in use for fully 40 years and physicians as a rule have consultations with leading specialists in their own illnesses.

Study of Coronary Thrombosis Group

In an effort to discover the nature of this insidious causal factor I have made a survey by means of a questionnaire mailed to the widows or next of kin of middle-aged males who have recently died suddenly in the Toronto district, assuming that many of these would be coronary thrombosis cases. It was thought that the widows of these men would be best qualified to supply detailed information regarding their personal living habits—diet, exercise, use of narcotics, age, height, weight, etc. After ruling out deaths due to accidents and infectious diseases there were 269 replies suitable for tabulation. Of this number 151 were found to be cases in which a definite diagnosis of coronary thrombosis had been made by the attending physician or coroner. The remaining 118 cases included non-coronary heart disease, cerebral hemorrhage, cancer, anemia, nephritis, diabetes, etc.

In the coronary thrombosis group (151 cases) the average age at death was found to be 52 years, the average weight was 168 pounds. Sixteen were 200 pounds and over, one being 295. Ninety-four per cent were reported as tobacco smokers and 6 per cent as non-smokers at the time of death. A further check on the latter elicited the fact that a number of them had discontinued smoking a month or so before death, either on their own volition or on medical advice. Fifty-eight per cent of the smokers were rated as "heavy smokers" and 42 per cent as moderate or light smokers. Fifty-five per cent were addicted to alcohol as well. The average age of the heavy smokers at death was 47 years, that of the moderate and light smokers was 58½ years, that of those addicted to tobacco and alcohol was 47½ years (apparently the addition of alcohol, as advised by some writers to counteract the vasoconstrictor effect of nicotine, did not prolong life in these cases.) The two youngest in this group, who died at 27 and 29 years, were heavy users of both tobacco and alcohol.

In the non-coronary group as a whole (118 cases) the average age at death was 60½ years. Sixty-six per cent of this group were addicted to tobacco and 29 per cent to alcohol as well.

Nutritional Habits of These Thrombosis Cases

Regarding the nutritional habits of the coronary-thrombosis group, it was found that as a whole there was a marked tendency to deficient intake of the B and C vitamins, in that nearly all were predominantly white-bread users and low in their use of fresh fruits and salads. The ingestion of milk was also suboptimal, the principal liquids being tea, coffee, alcoholic and soft drinks.

The most striking feature in the above findings and that providing the most obvious etiological clue (that is, clue as to its cause) is the higher incidence of tobacco smoking and the use of alcohol in the coronary-thrombosis group, 94 per cent and 55 per cent respectively, as compared to the combined non-coronary group, 66 per cent and 29 per cent respectively. The breakdown of the age figures in the coronary-thrombosis group also provides evidence of the precipitating effect of narcotic addiction in this disease, the average ages at death being as follows: Forty-seven and one-half years for those addicted to both tobacco and alcohol, 52 years for those addicted to tobacco only and 59½ years for those not addicted to either. The definite correlation of the life span and the degree of narcotic addiction is also most significant, the heavier addiction being associated with a corresponding drop in average age at death.

The Role of Tobacco in Thrombotic Diseases

A correlated study of other thrombotic disease processes may help to clarify the possible . . . role of tobacco. Another form of arterial thrombosis, known as . . . Buerger's disease, has long been recognized as being . . . related to tobacco smoking. Silbert says, "The importance of tobacco as the exciting cause of this disease must be stressed. The evidence in support of this contention is overwhelming. In over a thousand cases of this disease studied by the writer a typical case in a non-smoker has never been seen. Cessation of smoking regularly arrests the disease, while continued use of tobacco is coincident with progression."

(Dr. McCormick then explains exactly what happens in the human being who had just raised a cigarette to his lips. When the nicotine encounters the sympathetic nervous system, the adrenal glands release a substance into the body, which in turn produces a release of blood sugar from the liver, resulting in temporary hyperglycemia—or too much sugar in the blood. What happens then? The sudden increase in blood sugar is a warning to other organs that a poison is present and must be dealt with. Digestion, and stomach and intestinal movement are slowed down, blood shifts from abdominal organs to heart and lungs, causing increased heart action and respiration. The spleen discharges extra red blood corpuscles and platelets which increase the oxygen-carrying ability and the coagulability of the blood—as an emergency protection in case of hemorrhage. This increase in the blood-coagulation rate may have a great deal to do with the development of thromboses, especially considering how often this reaction is repeated in an individual who smokes steadily, day after day and year after year. Dr. McCormick tells us that a similar reaction occurs in post-operative conditions, as a result of the shock, loss of blood and effect of the anesthetic. This reaction would explain the frequency of thrombosis after operations.)

Effect of Tobacco on Nutrition

There is still another approach to this problem—the indirect effect of tobacco and narcotics in general upon the nutritional status, particularly the vitamin reserve and the possible influence of such effect upon the development of thrombosis. Quastel and Wheatley have shown that narcotics (which would include tobacco and alcohol) greatly increase the bodily requirement of vitamin B_1, thus increasing the tendency to deficiency of same. The tissue concentration of vitamin C is also known to be rapidly depleted in toxic conditions (whether their source is within or without the body). When thus utilized, less of the vitamin remains for physiological needs, thus accentuating the (unhealthy) effect. To illustrate, I have found in clinical research that the smoking of one cigarette increases the bodily requirement of vitamin C by 25 milligrams, or the vitamin C content of one orange, thus precluding the likelihood of any heavy smoker ever attaining an optimal tissue level of this vitamin. Recently Patterson has called attention to the low vitamin C status of coronary thrombosis cases. He found that 81 per cent of such cases in hospital practice had a subnormal blood-plasma level as compared to 55.8 per cent in a corresponding group of general public-ward patients. He . . . suggests that patients with this disease be assured of an adequate intake of this vitamin.

Cholesterol and Hardening of the Arteries

(Dr. McCormick reminds us that a discussion of hardening of the arteries and heart disease would not be complete without some mention of cholesterol, since recent research has shown a definite relationship between this substance and the disease. It is quite true that a high level of cholesterol in the blood is generally associated with heart disease, but it seems quite possible, says Dr. McCormick, that this condition may be caused by an inability to assimilate this substance in the body rather than too much of it in one's food.

A deficiency of the B and C vitamins may result in liver damage so that the cholesterol cannot be assimilated by the body. Patients afflicted with high cholesterol blood content are usually advised not to eat liver, eggs and other cholesterol-rich foods. On the other hand, when patients are given a diet that contains ample vitamins B and C, and then are given desiccated or cooked whole liver, there is usually a dramatic decrease in the blood cholesterol, in spite of this much larger intake.)

Sex Distribution of Coronary Thrombosis

Relative to the predominant male-sex incidence of coronary thrombosis Levine says: "The sex distribution of this disease is most striking—a ratio of three and one-half males to one female. It is difficult to explain the great frequency of coronary disease in the male. One may ascribe it to the greater amount of work that men do, although some might question this and maintain that the humble housewife does just as much work in her home. . . . Another factor that may be mentioned is the possible role of tobacco. . . . Certainly the consumption of tobacco has been in the past almost entirely confined to men, and has been one of the few acquired differences in habit between the sexes. It is therefore logical to suspect this habit of playing some possible role in producing such a male preponderance of susceptibility to this disease. A more definite answer may be apparent before long if the coming generation of women continue the smoking habit that seems to have become so general." This forecast was made in 1929 and already the anticipated answer seems to be in evidence. Prior to 1929 the sex ratio of incidence of coronary thrombosis has been estimated as high as five males to one female. However, recent figures supplied by the Toronto Health Department indicate that the present ratio in this disease is two males to one female. Apparently the rising tide of tobacco addiction in women is exercising a leveling action on the sex ratio of incidence of this form of heart disease.

Tobacco Consumption and Coronary Thrombosis

It should further be noted that the rising incidence of coronary and other forms of thrombotic disease has been closely concurrent with the increase in tobacco consumption. Cigarette consumption in Canada has risen from approximately 5 billion in 1935 to 18 billion in 1951, an increase of over 350 per cent, while in the same time the population has increased about 50 per cent. During this same period the incidence of coronary thrombosis, Buerger's disease and post-operative thrombosis has shown a closely proportionate increase. A closely parallel situation prevails in United States where the tobacco per capita consumption is about double that of Canada. One thing is certain, there has been no such increase in the consumption of cholesterol-rich foods by the populace at large during the same period, as would be expected if the cholesterol-ingestion cause of this disease is sustained. On the contrary, statistics indicate a noticeable drop in the per capita consumption of such foods (milk, butter, eggs and meat) during the period in question.

In recent years much stress has been given to the deleterious effects of involuntary inhalation of toxic elements in industrial smoke and fumes ("smog"), tetra-ethyl lead in gasoline, DDT, etc. These are all undoubtedly pathogenic, but with the redeeming feature that they are usually taken in a high degree of atmospheric dilution. On the contrary, little or no attention is given to the voluntary inhalation of toxic fumes in concentrated form in the smoking of over 400 billion cigarettes annually by the people of America. We "strain at a gnat and swallow a 'camel'."

[217]

50. A Theory of Coronary Thrombosis

By ERNEST KLEIN, M.D.

It is early in the morning and I have just had one of those tragic cases of coronary thrombosis. The man was 46 years old and his wife called me up because her husband, who had always been in perfect health, did not feel well. It was about 5 A.M. When I arrived, the patient was dead. He had had a periodic check-up once a year in his place of employment. I tried to find out what had happened. The periodic check-up did not reveal any heart disease.

It happened that the man, a clerk in the Stock Exchange, bought a new home a few weeks before. Since his new house was just around the corner from the old one, he carried most of their belongings himself to the new house. Last night, after dinner, still in perfect health, he went bowling.

What Happens During a Heart Attack

To start at the beginning, let us describe just what happened inside this patient's body before he died. A blood clot closed up the heart artery— that is, the artery that supplies the heart with blood. Fifty per cent of the victims of a "heart attack" (the common name for coronary thrombosis or infarction) survive the attack. Those who survive have a damaged heart muscle. Many people blame the heart itself in cases of "heart attack." This is a wrong conception. The heart is usually in good condition. Generally the blood is at fault. The blood normally flows easily and steadily through all the arteries and veins, carrying nourishment to all parts of the body. If this flow of nourishment stops for some reason, the tissues starve. If the flow stops entirely, they die. In most parts of the body, if the flow of blood stops, another blood vessel tries to replace the disordered one, so that the blood can continue to flow to the starving part.

There is no replacement for the artery that flows into the heart. If this is closed by a blood clot, the heart tissue starves. There are, however, many branches of the coronary (or heart) artery. If a blood clot slips into the coronary artery the result depends on whether it blocks the main artery or one of the many branches. If it blocks the main artery partially, the attack is not fatal. If it blocks it completely, it is. If it blocks a small branch artery, then the part of the heart that receives nourishment from this branch dies. The name for this is "occlusion of the coronary artery" or "coronary occlusion." Another name for it is "infarction."

One of the unsolved mysteries of the whole process is why the blood clots or coagulates inside the veins. And one of the common treatments for a patient surviving a heart attack is to give him anti-coagulants—that is, drugs that will prevent his blood from clotting too readily.

Now going back in my own personal history, let me tell you of my first observations concerning the blood, which resulted in my conclusions as to how to prevent thromboses or blood clots.

Observations on Many Coronary Cases

As an admitting physician during the last war, I had the chance to observe many coronary occlusion cases. It was routine to take a sample of the patient's blood and examine it. When I took samples of the blood from coronary thrombosis patients, I found that it coagulated so rapidly that I could not get it out of the little glass instrument I was using—a pipette. It stuck to the walls of the pipette so closely that I could not remove it even with peroxide. The pipettes were ruined and I had to discard them all. I made this observation on about 60 or 70 patients. When I eventually found a way to push the blood out of the pipette so that I could examine it, I was surprised to find that the hemoglobin was in all cases up to 150 Sahli. And the coagulation time was only a few seconds, whereas normally it is about two minutes.

To explain the above, Sahli is the name of a physician who discovered a way of measuring the hemoglobin. Hemoglobin is the red coloring matter in the blood—a very complex substance containing iron. Because it readily holds oxygen, the greater part of the oxygen in the blood is combined with the hemoglobin. This oxygen is distributed to the various organs of the body and is re-supplied to the blood as it passes through the lungs.

The simple apparatus needed to make the Sahli test can be handled by any physician or lab technician. In normal individuals the Sahli test is about 85. But in these coronary thrombosis cases it was up to 150! And, in addition, the time it took the blood of these patients to clot was only a few seconds, compared to the normal two minutes. My conclusion was that the high hemoglobin number together with the short clotting time may be important factors in coronary thrombosis. I believe that my observation could be used to prevent coronary thrombosis, if you can discover the abnormal thickness of the blood before the clotting starts.

Among patients having coronary thrombosis, there are, of course, exceptions. Those suffering from severe changes of the inside walls of the blood vessels may not have a high hemoglobin number and may suffer from a clot anyway caused by the condition of the blood vessel walls. Then, too, patients who have been given anti-coagulant drugs for a former heart attack will not have the high Sahli hemoglobin number and the short coagulation time, for the drugs will have prevented this.

Experimenting with Diet

In order to work further on my theory, I went to the blood donation center of the famous Post-Graduate (now University) Hospital in New York where I was put in charge of testing the hemoglobin, the condition of the heart and so forth, of all donors. For 3 years I had the opportunity of examining the blood of perhaps several hundred people a day. And I had the chance to get their cooperation in testing out various diets to find which diet would reduce a high Sahli number and lengthen a short coagulation time. At the end of a few days or weeks I could once again test their blood and determine whether or not the diet had accomplished what I wanted.

I came to the conclusion that 1/3 natural fruit juice, 2/3 water, some sugar (according to the taste of the individual) and a small amount of salt (to retain the fluid in the body) are the most suitable liquid foods to drop the hemoglobin number as quickly as possible to the normal level. (*Editor's Note:* It goes without saying that we do not believe in adding sugar to anything, least of all fruit juice, or salt, which we believe is harmful in the amounts in which we usually eat it.)

At the same time, everything that is dry, like bread, potatoes, cake and so forth should be restricted, because this kind of food seems to use up body fluid. The proportion of fruit juice and water can be changed to ¼ juice and ¾ water or ½ juice and ½ water, according to the taste of the patient. Pure fruit juice or plain water seem not to be of any help. Water is not retained by the body for a longer period and concentrated fruit juice seems not to agree with most of the test persons if it is taken in the amount necessary to "thin-down" the blood.

All the foods that build up the blood in anemic patients should be restricted or eliminated if we want to get the opposite effect—that of reducing hemoglobin. Then, too, meals with too much steak, liver and eggs push the hemoglobin number still higher.

Publication Led to Loss of Job

In January of 1949 I decided to present my observations to the staff of the Post-Graduate Hospital, but I found out that there was no way for me to do this. I might either publish my findings without any support or approval, or forget about everything I had done in the past years to fight coronary occlusion and to find a way to prevent the most dreadful disease of our times. I decided to write a short article and take the risk of being fired from the hospital. I believed that it was more important to attract the attention of progressive physicians who could help me finish the work I considered so important than to keep my discovery a secret and keep my job at the hospital.

After four months the committee of physicians of the Medical Society of New York accepted a very short version of my article and published it in *New York Medicine* for May 20, 1949. This is a reputable medical journal of the highest standing. On May 21, 1949, I was fired from my position at the hospital. My daughter, who also worked there, was fired, too. This is the story of my contribution, or let me say attempted contribution, to the fight against the most successful killer—heart disease.

The Danger Signal

How to recognize the danger and prevent the clotting of the blood by thinning it down to the normal concentration (85 Sahli) is the important thing for the prevention of coronary thrombosis. Diagnostic laboratories should be located all over the country and periodic tests of the "thickness" of the blood will reveal the danger of clotting before it is too late. The hemoglobin number (Sahli) is one of the most important parts of this laboratory test, the prothrombin (coagulation) time is the other. Either test can give us a warning signal that clotting of the blood may occur. Loss of body fluid may occur in many different ways. Two of these are perspiration (many heart attacks in the hot weather) and too little intake of fluids to replace the loss. If the blood concentration is high, the chance of being a victim of coronary thrombosis is greater.

To return to the patient whose story opened this article—in all probability his blood concentration was high. The heavy activity of moving his furniture from one house to the other caused him to perspire freely, depriving his body of fluid. Later when he went bowling, he lost more fluid and the hemoglobin of his blood probably shot up to 135 or 145 Sahli—the danger point at which one may develop thrombosis. It need not be in the heart artery. A clot in a brain artery causes sudden paralysis of an arm or leg or loss of speech, depending on which part of the brain is supplied with blood by the affected artery.

Had this patient been given laboratory examinations showing the two factors I have mentioned—hemoglobin and clotting time of the blood, he might have "thinned" his blood to such an extent that he would not have had the thrombosis. The proper diet for him then would have been vegetarian without any starch or with very little starch and an additional 8 to 10 glasses of the water-fruit-juice mixture. You may ask why water or tea would not fill the bill in a person whose hemoglobin level is high. Water quenches the thirst but is eliminated into the bladder within 20 to 60 minutes and does not "thin down" the blood for a longer period. The blood holds the fruit-juice-water mixture as a liquid food and keeps it to thin down the blood. The volume of blood increases. This can be shown by determining the blood volume, by taking the hemoglobin number or by observing the weight of the patient. A drop from the dangerous 140-150 to the normal 85 in hemoglobin may take place in some patients within a few days or weeks or it may take years. Even if all or nearly all starches are eliminated from the diet, even if all meats and eggs are strictly avoided, the weight increases 2 to 6 pounds. This weight increase must be due to the increase of blood volume caused by the intake of plenty of fruits, plenty of salads and plenty of water-fruit-juice mixture.

In the individuals at the blood donation center who tried out my vegetarian-fruit diet I found that there was a drop of 30-40 points in the hemoglobin. Another group was asked to eat nothing but steak, liver and eggs. Liquids were mostly eliminated. Small sips of water were permitted.

The hemoglobin number went up quickly and the coagulation time was rapidly shortened. If persons of this group were sent to a Turkish bath, the perspiration robbed the circulatory system of body fluid and the hemoglobin number went sky-high within a short period. Frequent heart attacks while in Turkish baths or while engaged in strenuous exertion could thus be explained.

I also discovered that starchy foods like bread, cake, cereal, cookies, pretzels and so forth take away body fluid and are to be considered harmful unless the intake of this kind of food is compensated for by the intake of plenty of liquids. The more cake, cookies, etc. you eat, the more fruit-juice-water mixture you have to drink to prevent dryness in your circulation. This dryness causes an increased concentration of the blood thereby raising the hemoglobin number and causing a decrease in the blood volume. The decrease in blood volume causes the blood cells to move closer together and this increased concentration of the blood cells causes the high hemoglobin number and the shortened coagulation time of the blood. This favors clotting of the blood.

To summarize, coronary occlusion or thrombosis is preventable. The thickness of the blood may be measured with the hemoglobinometer (the Sahli test) and so be discovered before the heart attack. It may be prevented by using liquid food (natural fruit juices plus water) for the purpose of thinning down the blood.

This mixture must be taken 6 to 10 times a day. Fruits and salads should form the largest part of the solid food. Meat and eggs should be reduced. Starches of any kind take away body fluid when they are digested, thereby causing further concentration of the blood. They should, therefore, be restricted or temporarily eliminated.

Editor's Note: We have presented Dr. Klein's article as an instance of the kind of observations and deductions that many and many a physician has probably made throughout a long and busy practice. We presented it to show the difficulties faced by such physicians when they try to get help for continuing their research, even when the subject under investigation is as important as coronary thrombosis. We do not believe these conclusions are final—and we are sure Dr. Klein would be the first to agree with us on this. Surely a subject as new and startling as this needs a great deal more laboratory work and closely-controlled experimentation before we know the final answer. But the point is that Dr. Klein apparently cannot get this kind of research help. How many other would-be researchers are in the same fix? And what can be done about it?

We have suggested to Dr. Klein that he try vitamin E therapy in conjunction with his diet for patients whose tests indicate that they may have too high a Sahli number and too short a coagulation time, and hence may be heading for coronary occlusion. As we have shown earlier, the effectiveness of vitamin E therapy in heart cases has been demonstrated in many thousands of heart patients.

51. What About Low Blood Pressure?

The individual who worries about his low blood pressure gets scant attention from medical researchers. Leafing through medical lists which contain just about all the medical articles published in the world, we page through whole sections devoted to high blood pressure—every aspect of it. Turning to "Low Blood Pressure" we find no articles at all listed. Apparently, down through the years, no one has considered low blood pressure of sufficient concern to do any investigating at all on the subject.

The viewpoint of the medical profession is that low blood pressure is a blessing, for if you have it you will probably never be afflicted with all the unpleasant symptoms of high blood pressure. Some physicians believe that a blood pressure of 90 is so low that something should be done about it. Others feel that a pressure of 100 to 110 is an indication that something is wrong. The insurance companies believe that a pressure as low as 100 or even 80 is perfectly compatible with good health, if that has always been your blood pressure. But if you average pressure is 120 and suddenly it goes down to 90 or 80, then probably there is something wrong.

Edward P. Jordan, M.D., expresses the feeling of the medical fraternity in his book, *You and Your Health* (G. P. Putnam's Sons, 1954), when he says, ". . . most of those with low blood pressure are well off and can expect a long life. There are few exceptions; there is a condition known as Addison's disease which, among other symptoms, is characterized by low blood pressure, but this is rare and there are only a few other things which have any serious significance . . . In most cases of below-normal blood pressure the cause seems to be exceptionally elastic arteries and this is a good thing. This generally means that hardening of the arteries will be slow to develop and this in turn has much to do with the expectation for a longer life."

Other medical books tell us that low blood pressure may be simply an indication of poor nutrition and it is often accompanied by low blood sugar, low basal metabolism, sub-normal temperature, anemia, or hypothyroidism (that is, a thyroid gland which does not send out enough of the gland secretion). In general, low blood pressure seems to go with people who do less of everything than other people do. That is, they may not eat enough or exercise enough which causes their glands to slow down and decrease their secretions. In cases of outright starvation, of course, the blood pressure is always low.

One kind of low blood pressure has been dignified with a medical name—postural hypotension. Hypotension is, of course, low blood pressure, the opposite of hypertension or high blood pressure. Many of us are inclined to feel dizzy or lightheaded when we stand up or sit up from a lying-down position. But the individual with postural hypotension is quite likely to have these symptoms to a serious degree. Any sudden change in posture necessitates a change in blood pressure all over the body. In some people the mechanism which adjusts this change is disordered. So, when they rise suddenly from a prostrate position, the blood does not reach the brain rapidly enough, and they may faint or blackout.

We must conclude, then, that hypotension is not a disease, but is rather a symptom that something may be wrong. Blood pressure may be low after a serious illness, such as an infectious disease, an acute fever or heart failure. In these cases, it disappears when the disease has been cured.

But suppose you are one of those people who feel weak and tired all the time, and suppose your blood pressure is low. The doctor may tell you that there is nothing to worry about. But do you want to go on feeling "all dragged out"? If there is indeed no disorder that is causing your low blood pressure, it seems quite possible that good nutrition can easily raise it to the point where you will no longer feel tired.

In an experiment made about 19 years ago it was shown that lack of a B vitamin (thiamin) can cause low blood pressure. In this experiment, reported in the *Archives of Internal Medicine,* Vol. 69, 1942, a number of volunteers agreed to live on a diet in which there was no thiamin. They ate a diet which many people live on in America today—white bread, canned fruits and vegetables, meat, potatoes, sugar, coffee and so forth. The doctors who conducted the experiment even gave them brewer's yeast so that they would not be deficient in the other B vitamins. But they destroyed the thiamin in the brewer's yeast. In addition, the volunteers got supplements containing vitamins A and D, iron, calcium and phosphorus.

The results were astounding. Without exception the volunteers suffered from personality changes as well as physical symptoms. They became tired, grouchy, inefficient, forgetful. Physically, they became constipated and sleepless; they developed neuritis. Their hearts beat abnormally and became enlarged. Their digestive tracts developed all kinds of disorders. Most important of all, from the point of view of our discussion, *they all developed low blood pressure.* The experiment had to be stopped in less than 6 months for it would perhaps have been fatal had it been carried on longer. As soon as they took some thiamin, the symptoms began to disappear and before long they all felt fine once again.

High Protein Diet Important

The second wrong diet that can produce low blood pressure is one in which there is not enough first-class protein. The blood vessels are made of protein, remember, as are the other parts of the body and if enough protein is not available in the diet to keep them from being flabby, they will gradually waste away, just as muscles do. By protein, we mean chiefly protein from animal foods—meat, fish and eggs, because these are the proteins that contain all of the essential amino acids or building blocks which our bodies need. Protein from vegetables, fruits and nuts is good, too, but these foods are not so rich in protein as the foods from animal sources and, too, they do not all contain all of these essential amino acids. If you eat a diet which is lacking in protein, you may possibly invite a shortage of thiamin—so there would be two good reasons for low blood pressure. For, on a low protein diet, you are bound to eat more starchy and sweet food, if you are eating anything at all. Starches and sweets must be accompanied by thiamin so that your body can use them. Hence the more starches and sweets you eat, the more thiamin you need. If you eat refined carbohydrates (white flour, white sugar and processed cereals) then you are bound to be short on thiamin, for the thiamin has been removed from all these foods along with other vitamins and minerals.

What We Recommend

If you are worried for fear your blood pressure is too low, we would suggest first of all that you make certain you have no underlying disorder that is responsible. If there seems to be no good reason for your hypotension, then concentrate on your diet and make it a good one. From the Superintendent of Documents in Washington, D. C., you can secure Agriculture Handbook Number 8 (Composition of Foods) which lists all the common foods according to protein content, giving as well their content of starch, fat, vitamins and minerals. With this book at hand you can easily figure out just how much protein you get a day and incidentally how much thiamin.

The official recommendation from the National Research Council is 70 to 100 grams of protein a day. But it is pretty generally agreed that this is a low estimate and that most of us would be a lot healthier if we got more, especially if we have had a deficiency in it. Sit down with your Handbook and a pencil and figure out everything you eat in one day in terms of its protein content. You will probably be surprised to find that you are getting far less than you should.

As you increase the protein in your diet, you will automatically increase the B vitamins, too, for they occur in foods that are high in protein —liver, eggs and fish. And, too, if you eat a lot of protein you will simply not have room for all the sweet and starchy foods that are bad for you. Take to serving nuts and sunflower seeds for dessert. Eat two eggs for breakfast instead of one. These are suggestions for improving the protein content of your meals which is bound to improve your general health and hence your blood pressure.

[225]

52. High Blood Pressure

High blood pressure—hypertension—is for many of us a menacing demon skulking in the background, ready to leap upon us when we pass middle age. Or, for others of us, it is a devastating reality—an ever-present shadow that dogs our days with headaches, heart palpitations, nervousness, fatigue and the constant threat of a stroke or a heart attack.

Garlic in the Treatment of Hypertension

One of our earliest discoveries was the wealth of material in medical literature of the past 50 years on the subject of garlic and high blood pressure. So much research has been done on the subject of garlic and hypertension that writers are not concerned these days with whether or not garlic improves high blood pressure. Instead they are now disputing exactly how garlic achieves the improvement. In an article in a European publication *Praxis* for July 1, 1948, F. G. Piotrowski, visiting lecturer and member of the faculty of medicine at the University of Geneva, writes of his experience using garlic on about 100 patients.

Dr. Piotrowski believes that garlic improves the blood pressure picture by dilating the blood vessels. He says, too, that it is difficult to conduct experiments with high blood pressure patients and hard to interpret results, for high blood pressure may be the result of a wide variety of causes.

He eliminated from his experiment any patients whose conditions might further confuse the results—that is, those whose pressure dropped when other medicines were given, those who had kidney trouble and so forth. He tells us that Schlesinger, another investigator, secured a drop in pressure after 15 days of treatment with garlic. Pouillard claimed a drop within an hour after the first dose of garlic. Dr. Piotrowski claims no such sensational results and he tells us that he believes intermittent dosage with garlic just for the purpose of obtaining a drop in pressure is not wise. He prefers to administer garlic oil for 3 weeks. He has obtained a drop of at least 2 mm. in blood pressure in 40 per cent of the cases. These were all patients in which the drop could not possibly be attributed to any other cause. All were going to work regularly, so not even special rest could have been responsible.

He says that good results do not occur simply if the patient is young or if his pressure is not especially high. The expected drop takes place after about a week of treatment, regardless. Dr. Piotrowski gave his patients fairly large doses of garlic at first, then gradually decreased the dose over the period of 3 weeks. Then he gave smaller doses throughout the rest of the treatment.

The "subjective" symptoms of high blood pressure began to disappear within 3 to 5 days after the garlic treatment was begun. This means such things as headaches, dizziness, angina-like pains and pains between the shoulder blades. Most of these symptoms were relieved in many cases. Patients said, too, that they could think much more clearly and concentrate better. Piotrowski's conclusions are that garlic certainly has useful properties in the treatment of high blood pressure. It usually causes a drop in the pressure and even when it does not, its use is justified by the relief it brings for the uncomfortable symptoms the hypertensive patient has had.

Vitamins B and C Are Useful, Too

It seems that vitamin C, too, may have a great deal to do with lowering blood pressure that is too high. We know that the body needs more vitamin C under conditions of stress. In *Metabolism*, a medical journal, Vol. 1, p. 197, 1952, Dr. C. L. Pirani discusses the relationship between vitamin C and stress. He says that under conditions of acute or chronic stress the vitamin should be taken in the relatively high dosage of one to two grams daily during the acute stage and as much as 300 milligrams per day thereafter.

In the *Canadian Journal of the Medical Sciences* for August, 1951, Doctors Heroux, Dugal and Paul describe investigations which show that vitamin C given in large doses reduces high blood pressure. They also give an account of their own experiments showing the same thing. In *Clinical Medicine*, Vol. 50, 1943, p. 152, Doctors Davis and Poser describe the results they got in reducing hypertension by giving their patients vitamin C.

In this same magazine for July, 1952, W. J. McCormick, M.D., shows that a diet containing plenty of vitamin C and the B vitamins brings about a dramatic decrease in the blood cholesterol. This substance has been blamed for clogging up arteries and playing no small part in the tragedy of strokes, heart attacks and other heart and blood vessel "accidents," as they are called. So vitamin C contributes to the health of the blood vessels in two ways—first by its ability to build up the actual blood vessel tissues themselves so that they are strong and flexible and its ability to decrease collections of cholesterol.

At least one of the B vitamins has been shown to be involved in the proper adjustment of blood pressure. The *American Journal of Physiology* for December, 1950, reports the production of high blood pressure in rats following only one week of deficiency in choline, one of the B vitamins. As soon as the choline was restored to the diet, the pressure fell and could be kept at normal *unless large amounts of salt were fed which caused the pressure to rise again.* More of that later. Interestingly enough, another researcher at the Alabama Polytechnic Institute experimented with choline deficiency and cancer. His laboratory rats died in from 6 to 12 days when all the choline was removed from their diets. If he added just enough choline to keep them alive, 50 to 60 out of every 100 developed cancer— about 50 times more cancer than might otherwise have appeared. Brothers and sisters of these same rats eating a normal diet developed no cancer at all. Now, of course, none of our diets is absolutely lacking in choline. All of us get some of it every day. But no one knows how much we need for good health. These are the foods richest in choline. How much of these do you get every day? Snap beans, soybeans, beef brain, egg yolk, kidney, heart, liver, peanuts, peas, wheat germ, brewer's yeast. How often a week do you eat many of these foods?

Vitamin E and High Blood Pressure

Drs. Evan and Wilfrid Shute of Canada, world authorities on the use of vitamin E in heart disease, tell us (in their book, *Alphatocopherol in Cardiovascular Disease*) of some of the benefits their heart patients (who were also high blood pressure patients) derived from taking vitamin E.

Of 158 moderately hypertensive or severely hypertensive patients, some 56, or 35 per cent showed some improvement. Six of these returned to normal pressure. And in a period of a year's time only two patients died. In a group of 39 mildly hypertensive patients, 49 per cent showed some benefit. About 14 of these returned to normal pressure. There were no deaths. Most of these patients had heart difficulties as well. And, say the Drs. Shute, their heart symptoms improved so much more than their blood pressure symptoms that they are inclined to overlook the lesser benefits of vitamin E so far as blood pressure is concerned.

Incidentally, folks with high blood pressure should be wary of taking vitamin E in large doses when they begin to take it. Its effect on muscle tone seems to be so striking that it may increase the force of the heart beat and produce a temporary rise in blood pressure. So the Drs. Shute never start a hypertensive heart patient with more than 100 international units (milligrams). Then they keep close watch on his blood pressure and increase the dosage of vitamin E ever so gradually until he may be able to take 150 to 400 units a day.

They believe that the hypertensive patient should take alpha tocopherol or vitamin E if he fears a stroke or a heart attack. They say, vitamin E, being the world's safest anticoagulant, can prevent this. "Here is the best insurance against cerebral or coronary accidents that he can take himself with minimal medical supervision," they say, "the mortality figure in our series speaks for itself. Alpha tocopherol therapy is indicated for hypertensive patients, largely, perhaps, on account of this protective factor."

Rutin is Effective

There is another factor, more recently investigated, which is also important for the health of the blood vessels—rutin, a food substance which is part of a complex "something" we call vitamin P. Doctor H. K. Hollerstein, M.D., and his colleagues at several hospitals in Illinois and Ohio experimented by producing in laboratory animals blood pressure high enough that it ruptured the small blood vessels which hemorrhaged. To one group of animals they gave rutin 10 days before they induced the high blood pressure. According to the *American Heart Journal* for August, 1951, those animals which received the rutin showed no evidence of hemorrhaging. An eye doctor, Dr. L. B. Somerville-Large, gave rutin to his patients to forestall hemorrhaging of the blood vessels in the eye. He says that high blood pressure actually has no relation to the fact that blood vessels may be fragile. But he says that a considerable percentage of hypertensives who do have delicate blood vessels eventually have hemorrhages in the eye or the brain.

Vitamin P and rutin are present in fresh raw fruits and vegetables, along with vitamin C. It is interesting to note that those of us who take natural food supplements like rose hips get all the parts of vitamin P such as rutin in our supplement right along with the vitamin C. Folks who take synthetic vitamin C are getting just that—synthetic vitamin C and nothing more. Now no one knows when, some day, scientists will discover even more valuable food elements in this complicated vitamin C-vitamin P combination. Once again, those of us who take natural supplements will have been getting this substance all along. While those who take only synthetic vitamin C plus rutin will have what? Only vitamin C and rutin.

When we were talking about choline we mentioned that lowered blood pressure in laboratory rats almost immediately shot up again when they were given large amounts of salt. Throughout all of recent medical literature you will find saltless or salt-poor diets, recommended in the treatment of high blood pressure. Probably the most famous diet of all is the Kempner Rice-Fruit Diet which, incidentally, should be undertaken only under the supervision of a doctor. This diet consists of literally nothing but rice and fruit, with some sugar and vitamin supplements. It is believed that the extremely low sodium content of the diet is responsible for the lowered blood pressure that does result from following the diet. Sodium is, of course, the dangerous part of sodium chloride or table salt. The chloride part of it does you no harm. But it seems that we civilized people, with all the salt available that we might want, have taken to using too much of the stuff. It is not a food, you know. It is the only thing we eat which comes from neither animal nor plant. And the food we eat every day (especially if we eat lots of animal protein) contains plenty of sodium. We need no more for good health.

Food Allergies and Hypertension

Dr. Arthur F. Coca has a different idea as to why the rice-fruit diet is successful in lowering blood pressure. Dr. Coca believes that the foods allowed in the rice-fruit diet are foods to which most people are not allergic. That is why the diet is so successful, he says. In an article in the *Medical Record* for December, 1950, Dr. Coca tells us he believes that hypertension is caused by allergies to food. By taking one's pulse after eating a certain food one can see if the food increases the pulse. If so, this food should be omitted. By carefully testing each and every food and not eating

[229]

those that raise your pulse, you can keep your blood pressure low, says he. He describes 42 hypertensive patients who were "treated" by avoiding the foods that raised their pulses. In almost every case the blood pressure was permanently reduced to a low average not attainable with any other kind of treatment.

If you would like to try out Dr. Coca's method, it goes like this: choose a time about an hour and a half after you have eaten and eat a small portion of one food that you wish to test, taking your pulse immediately before the test. Then take your pulse a half hour later and again a half hour after that. Take your pulse at your wrist, using two fingers from the other hand. You may locate two or even many more foods that cause your pulse to race. Eliminate these from your diet and watch the effect on your blood pressure.

Two other reminders for those who want to avoid high blood pressure. Overweight goes along with it, ever so often. Overweight is unhealthy. We all know that. But its particular effects are shown up mercilessly in the statistics which show that overweight individuals are far more likely to suffer from hypertension, heart trouble and all the other heart and vascular disorders. If you are overweight, you *should* worry about the possibilities of high blood pressure. The first and best preventive is to get back to your normal weight. Without any if's, and's and but's. Skip the desserts and the white flour products. Eat meals high in protein. Take your food supplements.

These same rules hold true for those who fear hypertension whether they are overweight or not. High blood pressure is a modern disease and we can't help but feel that the largest part of the responsibility for this killer must lie in our modern devitalized, refined diets. Shun processed foods—white flour, white sugar, packaged, canned, prepared foods. Eat fresh foods—out of your own garden if it is at all possible. Cook foods simply, with as little heat as possible. Eat everything raw that can be eaten raw. Take your food supplements: fish liver oil for vitamins A and D, brewer's yeast and/or desiccated liver for all the B vitamins, rose hip preparations for natural vitamins C and P, wheat germ oil for natural vitamin E and bone meal for minerals.

53. Facts on Salt Eating and High Blood Pressure

Is it dangerous to cut down on the amount of salt you eat without advice from a doctor? Isn't salt absolutely essential for good health? Don't animals travel miles to find salt licks? How can you possibly eat food that hasn't been salted? Isn't it tasteless and dull? Why should you cut down on salt, anyway—is there any proof that reduction will benefit you in any way?

These are some of the questions people ask. We are glad to report that we have found yet another well-documented, scientific report on salt-eating, its effects on the human body and the results of eliminating it from the diet.

Lewis K. Dahl, M.D., of Upton, New York, writes on *Salt Intake and Salt Need* in the June 5 and June 12, 1959, issues of the *New England Journal of Medicine*. His studies on salt eating and how it affects people were made in a metabolic ward of the Medical Department of the Brookhaven National Laboratory. There was no possible chance to cheat on diets, for they were weighed and prepared in the diet kitchens and the patients who took part in Dr. Dahl's studies had no opportunity to add extra salt at any time. Exhaustive tests on all the patients were done in the laboratory, all of which showed just one thing—that the reduction of salt in the diet brings only benefit and that, in cases of hypertension, or high blood pressure, reduction of salt produces an almost magical reduction of pressure to normal levels.

Dr. Dahl says that many groups of primitive people have remained healthy, generation after generation, without ever eating salt at all; that explorers like Stefansson find it difficult to do without salt for a week or so after they begin such a diet but that they gradually become accustomed to saltless food, prefer it and live in perfect health without salt, that only grass-eating animals ever seek out salt licks—those which eat meat apparently never feel the need for salt—that additional salt in hot weather appears to be not necessary at all, except under conditions such as steelworkers encounter at blast furnaces.

All of these facts have been known to science for many years. It is surprising how often they are ignored by popular medical writers, especially syndicated columns by physicians which appear in our daily papers. These gentlemen frequently take off in long, unscientific and undocumented harangues on salt-eating, insisting that nature demands that we add large quantities of this white mineral substance to our food or we cannot survive, let alone be healthy.

How About Doing Without Salt?

Dr. Dahl tells us that no one really knows very much about the amount of salt modern Americans eat because few studies have been done. By reviewing some of these studies, he shows that the available evidence suggests that, whereas metabolic balance can be maintained on sodium intakes of only a few hundred milligrams, or less, the average intake in contemporary American society is 20 times as much.

He tells us, too, that studies made of many groups of primitive people show that they do not suffer from high blood pressure. The studies showed that the amount of salt eaten by these people was extremely low, at a level of one or two grams a day or less. Negroes living in West India, on the other hand, eat a diet high in salt. They have a much higher incidence of high blood pressure than people living around them who do not eat so much salt.

It has been known for some time, Dr. Dahl tells us, that high blood pressure can be produced in animals by injections of certain substances. But, for the high blood pressure to occur, salt (sodium chloride) must also be present up to at least two to four per cent of the daily diet. In addition, studies of animals show that continual, lifetime ingestion of excessive amounts of salt leads to a condition in rats similar to high blood pressure in human beings.

In 1954, Dr. Dahl tells us, he published evidence indicating that high blood pressure is much more frequent among people who eat lots of salt. Among 1,346 adults who were studied, 135 had a low intake of salt, 630 an average intake and 581 a high intake. Sixty-one persons among the high-intake group had high blood pressure, 43 of those who ate an average amount had high blood pressure and only 1 among those who ate little salt.

Is Low-Salt Intake Harmful?

Dr. Dahl tells us of a woman patient whom he has observed for a total of 4 years, during which time she has been on a diet extremely low in salt. She had been taking as much as 4,000 milligrams of sodium when she came under Dr. Dahl's care. She was seeking relief from high blood pressure. The salt in her diet was reduced to 100 to 150 milligrams a day. "She remains the same active, intelligent and somewhat aggressive woman that she was before sodium restriction, although her blood pressure has been normal for several years. Her numerous daily activities include two walks of one and three miles in length on the laboratory grounds."

We want to note here that perhaps the walks partly helped in reducing the high blood pressure.

Low-Salt Diet and High Blood Pressure

In a later issue of the *Journal* (June 12, 1958), Dr. Dahl gives us details of an extremely complicated and convincing experiment which he carried out to find out all he could about restricting salt in the diet. He was particularly interested in the relation of salt-restriction and reducing. He reminds us that reducing diets may sharply limit the amount of salt eaten, simply because less food in general is eaten—therefore, less salt is eaten.

Hence, it must also be true that the salt-eating overweight person must get lots more salt than the average simply because he eats more of everything. Studying patients in a hospital ward where food was measured and no other source of food was available, Dr. Dahl found that simply reducing the weight of patients by diet did not produce a fall in their high blood pressure. Restricting salt intake, however, caused a lowering of the blood pressure in both obese persons and those of normal weight.

Was Such Drastic Salt Reduction Harmful?

Dr. Dahl has performed every imaginable test on patients of his who were on reduced salt intake. He tells us that, over the years, he has found that from 1/4 to 1/3 of his patients with high blood pressure showed a significant fall in the level while they were eating less salt. In only one case was there a slight decrease in a normal blood pressure. Improvement in heart size was found among patients who had enlarged hearts. No other physical changes could be found in these patients, no matter how long they remained on the low-salt diet.

Elaborate chemical tests which were carried out also revealed nothing but changes for the better among people whose salt intake was restricted. Dr. Dahl had psychological tests made of his patients, since it has been suggested that eating a lot of salt is what keeps us on our toes, capable of meeting successfully all the complex problems of modern society. He found without fail that there were no undesirable changes in the patients' characters and, in fact, there were some improvements. A number of his patients reported that, after they had become accustomed to their low-salt diet, their friends, relatives and, particularly clerks in stores, seemed less irritating than they had before. He did find that, for the first 10 days on the low-salt diet some patients might complain that they felt depressed or nervous. But this disappeared very quickly.

Dr. Dahl's own answer to the question "Is there potential harm from a widespread reduction in salt consumption?" is as follows: "The evidence that has been presented here indicates that it is possible for individuals and races to live for years and generations on intakes of only several grams of salt a day." He then takes up the several serious disease conditions in which salt loss is so great that a low-salt diet is not advisable—Addison's disease, severe burns, diabetic acidosis, severe vomiting or diarrhea— but he adds that "if excess dietary sodium (salt) plays the primary part in the etiology (cause) of hypertension (high blood pressure) the possible harm from salt restriction in persons with relatively uncommon ailments must be weighed against the radical decrease in the incidence of the second most common cardiovascular disease in Western society"—that is, of course, high blood pressure.

How Can You Get Used to a Low-Salt Diet?

Dr. Dahl has devoted years to studying patients on low-salt diets. He tells us that he has found no evidence of salt craving among his patients on drastically reduced amounts of salt. They complained for a week or so that food tasted flat but after that they became used to the taste and there were no more complaints. This suggests, he says, that the salt appetite was acquired in these people. It is the result of social custom—not an inborn appetite or a basic physiologic need. "This does not mean," he says, "that the custom or appetite will be changed any more easily than that of smoking tobacco or drinking alcohol, but it seems very important to indicate that *salt appetite* is not to be equaled with *salt requirement.*"

We want to add one word to Dr. Dahl's thoughts about getting along without salt. After you have drastically reduced the salt in your diet, you soon begin to find that you never really tasted food before. What you tasted was the salt. You will experience a revival of interest in your meals when for the first time you enjoy an egg, a baked potato or a piece of meat, without salt.

How Much Salt Should You Eat?

Should you try to cut out all salt from your diet, as patients who are on the Rice-Fruit Diet do? No, we don't think so. Such heroic measures are not necessary. Surely the salt you get in natural food will not harm you. It's the salt you *add* that does the harm.

Dr. Dahl says that, in the presence of existing high blood pressure there is seldom a reduction in pressure unless the salt intake is reduced below one or two grams. He suggests a maximum salt intake of about 5 grams per day for an adult without a family history of high blood pressure. This could be done by omitting frankly salty foods and using the salt-shaker sparingly if at all. He reminds us that an intake of 5 grams of salt per day is at least 10 times the amount upon which one can live healthfully in good balance.

For people with a family history of high blood pressure, Dr. Dahl recommends the immediate adoption of a diet low in salt—500 to 1,000 milligrams a day at the maximum. This should not be difficult to do, he says, once you have become convinced that it is the best plan. He reminds us, too, that increasing the potassium content of the diet may help, since potassium seems to cancel some of the bad effects of sodium in the body. Foods high in potassium are fruits, vegetables, nuts and seed foods.

Suppose you are worried about high blood pressure or suppose you merely want to cut down on salt so that you won't ever have to worry about high blood pressure—how do you go about it? How do you know how much salt you are getting every day and how can you reduce it? We include at the end of this chapter a chart giving the salt content of common foods in terms of the average serving. You can check through this and easily note which are the foods high in salt.

You will notice that all the foods listed here are natural foods, except for cheese, some of the cereal products, powdered milk and bacon. You will see, too, how easy it is to control salt intake at a low level when you are eating only natural, unprocessed foods. Making up menus from

TABLE 2: SALT CONTENT OF SOME COMMON FOODS

Meats:		*Salt in Grams*	*Vegetables:*		*Salt in Grams*
Bacon	3 slices	1.200	Artichokes	1 medium	.018
Beef	1 serving	.057	Asparagus	10 stalks	.060
Chicken	1 "	.048	Beets	2/3 cup	.100
Duck	1 "	.040	Brussels sprouts	2/3 cup	.070
Goose	1 "	.060	Cabbage	2/3 cup	.020
Ham	1 "	1.6 to 2.0	Carrots	¾ cup	.060
Lamb Chop	1 "	.057	Cauliflower	½ cup	.060
Lamb Roast	1 "	.067	Celery	¾ cup	.060
Turkey	1 "	.040	Corn	¼ cup	.020
Veal Roast	1 "	.057	Cucumber	10 slices	.050
			Egg plant	½ cup	.040
Fish:			Endive	10 stalks	.275
Bass	1 "	.069	Greens, dandelion	½ cup	.168
Cod	1 "	.066	Lentils	¼ cup	.030
Haddock	1 "	.057	Lettuce	10 leaves	.120
Mackerel	1 "	.076	Lima beans	¼ cup	.030
Oysters	1 "	.050	Peas	¾ cup	.006
Salmon			Peppers	2 medium	.020
(canned)	1 "	.059	Potato	1 medium	.160
Trout, shad	1 "	.061	Pumpkin	½ cup	.060
			Spinach	½ cup	.120
Dairy Products:			Squash, summer	½ cup	.010
Cheese (Amer-			String beans	2/3 cup	.040
ican)	1 inch cube	.164	Tomatoes	1 medium	.060
Cheese (cot-	2 tablespoon-		Turnips	½ cup	.070
tage)	fuls	.280	Radishes	5 medium	.024
Cheese (cream)	¼ cake	.250	Water cress	10 pieces	.025
Eggs	1 whole	.088			
Buttermilk	½ cup	.160			
Milk, whole	½ cup	.175			
Milk, powdered	2 tablespoon-		*Cereals:*		
	fuls	.080	Bread, graham	1 slice	.230
			Bread, white	1 slice	.130
Fruits:			Cornbread,		
Apple, baked	1	.008	(without salt)	1 piece	.001
Apricots, fresh	3	.003	Farina, cooked	¾ cup	.038
Banana	1 small	.206	Macaroni	½ cup	.024
Cranberries	2/3 cup	.015	Oatmeal	½ cup	.033
Figs, fresh	1 large	.005	Shredded wheat	1 biscuit	.034
Grapefruit	½ small	.008	Rice	½ cup	.027
Grapes	24	.010			
Grapejuice	½ cup	.003			
Muskmelon	½ cup, cubes	.030			
Oranges	1 medium	.010	*Nuts:*		
Peaches	1 medium	.010	Almonds	14	.009
Pears	1 medium	.020	Peanuts	9	.010
Pineapple	1 slice	.080	Pecans	12	.024
Prunes	6 medium	.019	Walnuts	3	.010
Rhubarb	¾ cup	.059			
Strawberries	¾ cup	.010			
Watermelon	1 serving	.010			

Note that, in general, foods high in salt are those foods which we do not recommend: dairy products (except eggs), cereals, bacon and ham.

these foods you will never get near the limit of 5 grams of salt a day suggested by Dr. Dahl if you avoid the processed foods. They all have added salt. In addition, there are many foods that are little else but carriers of salt—olives, pickles, relishes, luncheon meats, dried beef, cheeses —all those foods whose taste is definitely salty are not for you.

What about salt substitutes? We have never seen any research done on the effects of salt substitutes on health, but we are inclined to counsel against them. In general, the commercially available ones are just a mixture of chemicals and many of them contain quite large amounts of sodium (which is what you are trying to avoid). Besides, using a salt substitute is cheating. What you want to do is to get away from the whole idea of "seasoning" your food. Why not enjoy the taste of the food for a change? If you feel that you must use a salt substitute, we suggest powdered kelp which is a purely natural food. Although it contains salt, it contains, too, all the other minerals that occur in sea water, all of which are valuable for you.

54. Stroke!

What is a "stroke"? Why should the aftereffects of this sudden "striking down" kill about 200,000 Americans a year and incapacitate hundreds of thousands of others? Because a stroke does the worst of its damage within a matter of moments or hours, doesn't it seem that prevention might be the very best protection anyone could devise against strokes?

We believe this is especially true in the case of strokes. The many warning signals which generally precede the actual stroke seem to provide the perfect means for prevention of a serious stroke. So we want to talk mostly about these warning signals and what can be done, when they occur, to lessen the chance that they will develop into more serious complications.

A "stroke" (we used to call it apoplexy) may be the result of several different malfunctions or disorders in the blood vessels. One kind of stroke is caused by blood vessels in the brain breaking or giving way so that there is a hemorrhage throughout the brain's tissues. A stroke may be caused, too, by a thickening or a clot in a brain blood vessel which prevents the blood supply from entering the brain. Or it may come about as a result of a floating blood clot which lodges in a brain capillary or artery shutting off the supply of blood. The brain requires enormous amounts of oxygen for proper functioning—about 20 per cent of all the oxygen required by the body. Shutting off this supply of oxygen for even a few minutes results in damage.

Each part of the brain is involved with a different part of human activity; one section is necessary to control speech, another the movement of the arms or the legs on one side of the body, another controls the muscles of the mouth or the eyes and so forth. So damage from a non-fatal stroke is immediately reflected in some other part of the body. There may be extensive paralysis of a limb or limbs. There may be paralysis of a facial muscle; or lasting sensations of numbness in certain parts of the body. There may be difficulty with speech, sometimes involving frightening complexities—for instance, the afflicted person may not be able to associate words with objects so that he calls a table a tree, or a chair a house; he may not be able to write sentences in proper order or may omit important words; there may be "thickness" of speech.

During the months or perhaps years that may be necessary to rehabilitate a victim of stroke, his family may be convinced that his mind is permanently afflicted; whereas the sufferer thinks as clearly as ever, but simply cannot communicate well. Crippling of an arm or a leg may follow a stroke if the affected part of the body is not immediately given good, intensive physiotherapy to keep muscles from deteriorating. An excellent booklet on caring for a stroke patient is available from the Superintendent of Documents for 40 cents. The title is *Strike Back at Stroke*. Although it is prepared for doctors to give the families of their stroke patients, anyone may get a copy and *use the booklet as his doctor orders*, for the exercises described are specific ones and should not be used without instruction from a doctor. Order from Washington, D.C.

However, we are concerned with prevention of stroke. It seems that many of us have warnings of the possibility of major strokes by the occurrence of "little strokes" which indicate that all is not well inside the blood vessels that feed oxygen to the brain. If we are warned by these little strokes and act wisely and promptly, we can perhaps prevent the "big stroke" which paralyzes or permanently injures.

What Are the Symptoms Of Little Strokes?

Dr. Walter Alvarez, M.D., of Chicago, seems to be an authority on "little strokes." Writing in the *Journal of the American Medical Association* for April 2, 1955, Dr. Alvarez states, "One of the commonest diseases of man is that in which, over the course of 10 or 20 years, a person is gradually pulled down by dozens or scores of thromboses (clots) of little arteries in the brain." Although these little strokes are so common, many physicians never think of diagnosing them as such, partly because patients just don't give their doctors all the symptoms or because the physician is not familiar with all the bizarre, peculiar things that can happen to an individual as the result of a little stroke.

Dr. Alvarez tells of a friend who had been incapacitated by a pain in the abdomen (no ulcer was present) and by a slowing down both mentally and physically. The man's wife remembered that the trouble had begun one morning when, for 20 minutes, her husband had been confused and unable to talk. Since then he, who had always been kind and understanding, had become unreasonable and irascible. He was so changed his wife hardly knew him. Dr. Alvarez believes that the man suffered a little stroke on that morning which was responsible for the symptoms that followed.

He tells us that little strokes are episodes in a long illness. "Often when a suspicious episode is seen, if only the physician would ask the relatives to remember some peculiar spell followed by changes in character and ability, they will tell him that the disease must have started many years before." Physicians rarely see more than one episode in the illness.

Here are some of the many, many symptoms of little stroke that Dr. Alvarez has observed in his years as a doctor. See how many of these resemble things that have happened to people you know. Acute indigestion which does not seem to be related to any overindulgence in food or eating any food that disagrees. Temporary weakness in one leg which occurs suddenly when one awakes in the morning. Sudden unexplained clumsiness of one hand; mental or nervous disability that is all out of proportion to the little stomach or chest pain that may be there. A nervous breakdown or queer group of symptoms that come on suddenly—on one day. A sudden dizzy spell, a blackout or a fall after which the patient shows changes in character or ability to work.

Sudden drops in a formerly high blood pressure may indicate a little stroke. Sudden spells of crying unaccompanied by any feeling of sadness. Sudden changes in handwriting or composing sentences in a letter; difficulty in finding words to express oneself; sometimes difficulty in swallowing so that food will go down "the wrong way" and cause choking; the saliva may be thick and ropy; some may drool out of the corner of the mouth.

After a little stroke there may be a sudden burning pain in the hand, wrist or forearm. There may seem to be sudden arthritic changes in a hip or wrist. A fall which the patient says was caused by blacking out may be the result of a little stroke.

Is It a Stroke or a Heart Attack?

"Today, I think most little strokes, if noticed at all, are called 'heart attacks' by physicians," says Dr. Alvarez. "Not having been trained to think of disease of the brain, we rarely do. Also, seeing that persons feel disgrace in having a stroke and none in a heart attack, many physicians, when in doubt, make the diagnosis that will not offend the family."

A sudden pain shooting down through the chest may be almost certainly a stroke, if there is no evidence of shortness of breath or heart difficulty when walking. However, it is perfectly true that the same disordered vascular system that results in strokes may produce heart emergencies, too. Pain shooting into the abdomen may indicate a little stroke, if it comes on suddenly and if no stomach or digestive symptoms are present. Sudden brief attacks of nausea and vomiting may be little strokes. Most elderly people with supposed "Mèniére's disease" may have no trouble at all with their ears so that the dizziness they experience comes from the brain instead—a little stroke.

Burning of the tongue or mouth, bad taste in the mouth, especially if it occurs only on one side, a burning of the skin or scalp or a feeling of extreme heat or cold on skin or scalp. In rare cases sudden blindness in one or both eyes, or even seeing double for a day or two. An old case of migraine headache may be reactivated by a little stroke. A stroke can bring a psychosis. Tendencies toward depressive feelings or suspicions of others, no longer closely controlled, can completely overtake an individual after a little stroke and change him into someone unfamiliar to his family.

These are some of the symptoms that may indicate that a little stroke has taken place. Undoubtedly there are many more. There seems, however, to be one circumstance common to all—the change comes about suddenly. Symptoms can be traced to the happenings of one day when the stroke took place even though at the same time it was not recognized as such.

However, as Dr. Alvarez says, the little stroke is merely one part of a long-term disease. The unhealthy condition of the arteries and capillaries which prevails when the little stroke occurs almost always involves hardening of the arteries and may involve high blood pressure. It is reasonable to assume that arteries whose inner walls are thickened and coated with deposits of minerals and fats are more likely to become clogged with blood clots. It seems obvious, too, that arteries whose walls are weakened and sick will be more likely to rupture, causing hemorrhages.

A Program of Prevention Is the Answer

So the lesson to be learned from the little stroke is to institute immediately a program for a healthy system of blood vessels and a healthy heart. Here is a brief summary of information along these lines, all of which is carefully documented with references to medical and scientific investigations.

1. The use of salt in large quantity by modern Americans has been shown to be closely related to high blood pressure, as well as many other body disorders. We recommend eliminating salt from kitchens and dining rooms and avoiding food already salted like pickles, salt meats, etc.

2. Hardening of the arteries seems to be closely related to our excessive intake of fat, which encourages the formation of cholesterol plaques in the blood vessels, especially fat of animal origin and hydrogenated fats. Fats from nuts, vegetables and wheat germ seem to encourage the proper use of the troublesome substance, cholesterol.

3. An abundant intake of the B vitamins is important, too, for the health of the arteries. One of these, pyridoxine, is directly involved in the body's use of fats. The B vitamins occur abundantly in liver and other fresh meats, fresh raw fruits and vegetables and whole grains. They are

almost wholly absent from all that part of modern diet which consists of refined starches, cereals and processed foods and desserts.

4. A healthy thyroid gland is important for healthy arteries. Several researchers have found that by giving thyroid gland preparations they can improve the working of this gland, which tends to slacken as we grow older. Ocean fish are a good source of iodine which helps keep the thyroid gland healthy, and kelp is the best food supplement to add to one's store of iodine, as well as many other helpful minerals.

5. Vitamin C and the bioflavonoids seem to be closely related to the health of the blood vessels. Blood pressure has been reduced by adding lots of vitamin C to the diet. It is well known that plenty of vitamin C and the bioflavonoids which accompany the vitamin in foods and in natural food supplements prevent hemorrhages by keeping the walls of blood vessels strong and healthy. Rutin is one of the bioflavonoids. Certainly vitamin C and the bioflavonoids are of the utmost importance. Get them in fresh raw fruits and vegetables and in natural supplements made from rose hips, green peppers, etc.

6. Garlic has been used in the past to bring down high blood pressure. We think you should use it in food. Garlic perles are food supplements, tasteless and easy to take.

7. Overweight is a powerful factor in high blood pressure and heart conditions. Keep your weight at or below the optimum weight for your age and height. A diet which ignores refined starches will help.

8. Vitamin E is probably the most important single item for preventing strokes. Because of its important oxygen-regulating function, vitamin E has immediate and far-reaching effects on the entire heart and circulatory system. Taken in adequate dosage it prevents blood clots, keeps the blood in a normal state so that neither clots nor hemorrhages occur. It strengthens the heart and the blood vessel walls. It has beneficial effects on other conditions, such as phlebitis, Buerger's disease, varicose veins and so forth. By all means, if you have suffered the warning symptom of a "little stroke" don't delay in getting vitamin E and taking plenty of it every day. We think wheat germ products are helpful, too, but we believe that each of us should be taking vitamin E as such.

9. Editor Rodale has written a book, How to Eat for a Healthy Heart, which contains much more information about all the above and includes, of course, much information on arteries and the rest of the circulatory system. This is available from Rodale Books, Incorporated, Emmaus, Pennsylvania. (Price $1.00)

55. A Cardiac's Choice
of Medications

The results of vitamin E therapy in circulatory disorders are gratifying, and are convincing more and more doctors of the worth of this nutrient. The cautions for its use are few and specific, as advanced by the greatest living authority on vitamin E, Dr. Evan V. Shute. The thing to remember is that all of us get and require some amount of vitamin E in our diets, so basically it is not harmful to the body. Most persons should get much more than they do. However, Dr. Shute advises that hyperthyroid patients should not use large doses of vitamin E. Those suffering from chronic rheumatic heart are warned by Dr. Shute that almost no one with this condition can take more than 150 units (or milligrams) of vitamin E per day.

Those who take digitalis for the heart or insulin for diabetes should know that the requirements for either of these may be suddenly reduced by the intake of vitamin E.

Start Using Small Amounts of Vitamin E

In cases in which high blood pressure is already present, it has been found that vitamin E in large doses may cause the blood pressure to rise even higher. This rise does not necessarily occur in every such case; quite the contrary, in most cases, the blood pressure is lowered through the use of vitamin E. It is important, however, that the high blood pressure patient start using vitamin E in small amounts as suggested on the label of the container. This is usually 50 or 100 milligrams per day, the amount believed by nutritionists to have been contained in the average diet before refining of foods became such a general practice. One can safely judge the effect of the vitamin in this way, raising or lowering the dosage upon observing the results.

Doctors who cite the required precautions for using vitamin E as their reason for avoiding it, do not hesitate to prescribe the new and old drugs used for the same purpose, whose side effects are notably severe. The truth of the danger involved in using these drugs is emphasized by an article appearing in the *Illinois State Medical Journal* (June, 1959), by Arnold S. Moe, M.D. Dr. Moe briefly surveys the drugs most commonly used in the treatment of heart disease, and lists the problems that can arise in their use.

Digitalis Must Be Watched Carefully

Digitalis is the old standby used by most physicians in treating heart disease. The main danger involved here is that most doctors think of digitalis as a completely harmless drug, and once they have prescribed its use they relax and let the patient go on using it indefinitely on a maintenance dose. Dr. Moe quotes the *Texas Medical Journal* (October, 1956) as carrying the account of 100 cases of digitalis poisoning. It was found that .2 milligrams of digitalis, taken as a daily maintenance dose, proved to be toxic. Twenty-seven of the 100 patients died (presumably from their heart ailments) and 7 of these deaths were directly attributed to digitalis. The heart patient who is receiving digitalis must be watched carefully. In the *Journal of the American Medical Association* (April 26, 1958) an article touching on the subject, by L. Craig and his colleagues, contained this statement: "Average dose formulas, as well as other dogmatic oversimplifications in prescriptions of digitalis drugs, disregard biologic variability. In other words, it is not likely that the same continued dosage will be beneficial for a man weighing 200 pounds, and for a woman weighing 98 pounds, even though their blood pressure readings might be similar. One is bound to be getting too small a dose, or the other too much. Great discretion and careful observation for effects should characterize all digitalis prescriptions."

How Digitalis Can Backfire

An illustration of how the use of digitalis can get out of hand is offered in Dr. Moe's case history of a 60 year old male patient who came to a physician's office complaining that he had suffered a "heart spell," characterized by rapid beating of the heart. Digitalis was prescribed at first, and later the man was put on a maintenance dose of one and one half tablets of digitalis per day. He was under instructions to increase the maintenance dose by one tablet if the heart should begin beating rapidly again. About a month later he noticed that he had begun to speak nothing but nonsense, sometimes for a day or two at a time, but he could not control what he was saying. His eyes became irritated and were playing color tricks on him. Visits to several eye specialists showed no physiological disturbances of the eyes.

The patient began to suspect that the digitalis was the cause of his new difficulties, but his doctor seriously warned him against lowering or discontinuing his digitalis dosage. The patient had a thorough physical examination, and there was no abnormality of any organ. Even the heart did not show any serious defect. Digitalis was discontinued. In 6 days the patient felt his color vision was improving and in 6 weeks he felt it was back to normal. The pulse rate also returned to a normal range as did the blood pressure. It was concluded by the last physician he saw that the patient's "heart spell" was nothing more than palpitations, a common heart-pounding sensation which is not always an indication of heart disease.

The Odd Effects of Quinidine

Quinidine is another popular drug used in treating circulatory disorders, especially where irregular heart beat is a factor. It is often employed in an attempt to prevent heart failure. Dr. Moe tells us that a single small dose of this drug, improperly administered, might be fatal. More commonly the toxic effects of quinidine are: nausea, vomiting, epigastric distress, headache, diarrhea, apprehension and ringing in the ears. Sometimes visual disturbances, fever and skin rashes result from its use.

In *Circulation* (November, 1956) G. W. Thompson reported on 611 cases collected from literature, and, of these, death in 2.1 per cent was attributed to quinidine. Quinidine is known as a classic drug for treating excessively rapid heartbeat. A case history of a 53 year old male heart patient shows the danger of depending exclusively on such a drug. The man observed episodes of this rapid heartbeat for 5 years. He was admitted to the hospital when one such episode lasted much longer than usual. Quinidine, the classic drug in such cases, was prescribed in increasing doses. It almost killed the patient. His pulse rate went from 146 to 240 per minute. Digitalis was employed as an alternate just in time, and the patient recovered.

Drugs as Dangerous as the Disease

Hexamethonium was widely used, at first, to lower blood pressure. It works, but the toxic effects that accompany its use have cut its popularity considerably. Treatment with it can bring constipation, blurring vision, paralytic ileus (bowel obstruction), prostatic obstruction, salivary gland obstruction and, worst of all, a sudden and extreme drop in blood pressure when a patient with advanced hardening of the arteries rises to a standing position.

Hydralazine is a drug used especially for hypertension cases. The list of side effects includes the usual dizziness, rapid heartbeat and headache. But the most alarming discovery is the fact that hydralazine has been known to *produce* angina pectoris in some patients.

Rauwolfia, the father of the tranquilizers, is being used extensively in one form or another for relief of hypertension. The *Journal of the American Medical Association* (September 8, 1956) reported on 56 cases treated with rauwolfia. Four of these developed severe anxiety, agitation and depression. As for the other side effects, 82 per cent of the 56 patients developed drowsiness, fatigue, weight loss, loss of initiative and nightmares.

Test Shows Rauwolfia Drug Doesn't Work

The clincher to the use of rauwolfia drugs comes in the *American Journal of Medical Science* (August, 1956) in which Bello and Turner showed, by means of a double-blind test, that reserpine (a rauwolfia drug) caused neither consistent nor adequate blood pressure reduction. Two-thirds of the cases used in the test showed the common rauwolfia side effects.

So these are the drugs used by most physicians in treating heart disorders. True, there are times when their effectiveness cannot be denied, but it would be difficult, in the face of the evidence provided by Dr. Moe, to insist on their absolute safety. Further, to refuse to use vitamin E, due to concern over its side effects, and then to use any of the drugs mentioned above instead, is hardly consistent. American doctors will soon be giving vitamin E more chances to prove itself, and we are sure it will emerge as one of the best of all treatments for cardiovascular disorders.

SECTION 11: THE KIDNEYS

56. Kidney Stones

A century or so ago kidney stones were an important cause of illness especially among young people. Today kidney stones are far less prevalent in this country and the emphasis has shifted from youth to age. Today kidney stones are a disorder of older people. But in some parts of the world this condition exists among most of the population. Such a background cannot help but lead one to believe that the development of kidney stones shows a background of poor nutrition.

No one knows exactly how or why the stones are formed, but it is generally, if grudgingly, agreed among the experts that diet plays a part. It is known for instance that stones formed chiefly of calcium oxalate may be related to a high content of oxalic acid in the diet. In Bridges' *Dietetics for the Clinician*, (Lea and Febiger, 1949), the editor Harry J. Johnson, M.D., F.A.C.P., says, "It is a matter of common observation that calcium oxalate sediments will appear in the urine of nearly every patient in a ward after ingesting oxalate-rich food as spinach and rhubarb." Now most of us don't eat enough spinach and rhubarb to cause this kind of trouble. But there are other foods rich in oxalic acid that we do eat in quantity, perhaps every day. Chocolate, for instance, and cocoa both contain lots of oxalic acid. Plenty of children (and adults, too) have a cup of cocoa for breakfast, chocolate milk for lunch and dinner and possibly a couple of chocolate bars or chocolate cupcakes between meals. So it is well to keep in mind this possible cause of stones. Oxalic acid foods are undesirable as well because they cause the body to lose calcium.

Dr. Johnson goes on to say that vitamin deficiencies probably contribute to the formation of stones. The effect of vitamin A on the cells lining various passages in the body such as the urinary passage is well known and an adequate amount of the vitamin must be ingested in order to keep the urinary mucous membrane in good condition. Urinary stone occurs frequently following peptic ulcer therapy and the dietary restrictions involved.

Rose's *Foundations of Nutrition,* a classical nutrition textbook (The Macmillan Company, 1944) says that when animals are kept for some time on diets low but not entirely lacking in vitamin A, kidney and bladder stones are frequently found. They have not been found in animals on other types of deficient diets. According to McCarrison there are certain areas of India which are known as "stone areas" because of the prevalence of kidney stones among the people. It is a poor man's disease occurring among those whose chief dietary staple is cereal of some sort, but is most frequent where vegetation is relatively scanty, where grazing for cattle is poor and where wheat is the chief food crop. McCarrison has produced stones in rats in 90 days from weaning time on diets low in vitamin A and consisting chiefly of wheat.

W. J. McCormick, M.D., of Toronto, who has done matchless work on vitamin therapy, has something further to contribute in the way of dietary prevention of stones—whether they form in kidneys, bladder, gall bladder or elsewhere. Dr. McCormick points out in an article in the *Journal of the Canadian Dental Association* for August, 1946, that vitamin A was the only vitamin known during some of these early investigations. Hence researchers who had removed all the vitamin A from the diet of their laboratory animals might think they had the answer, when as a matter of fact, they had also removed other necessary vitamins at the same time. He says that McCarrison found that if vitamin C were also removed from the diet, kidney stones were more likely to be produced. He reminds us that the diet of the Tibetans, the people of West China, India, Labrador and Newfoundland is almost completely lacking in vitamin C, and among these people kidney stones are common. The Easterners live on rice, barley flour, butter and tea with few or no vegetables and fruits. In Labrador and Newfoundland white flour, fish, game, lard, oatmeal, tea and sugar make up the bulk of the diet and here again fresh fruits and vegetables are all but unknown.

Retarding Calcium Deposits with Vitamin C

Dr. McCormick tells us further that the teeth of people living on these diets are covered with tartar. Even very young children have heavy tartar deposits on the teeth. This might happen, he says, because lack of vitamin C leads to a breakdown of the body tissues, including those of the mouth. The mucous lining scales off and, mixing with remnants of food, creates the unsightly and unhealthy deposit that clings so tenaciously to the teeth, resulting in pyorrhea and inflammation of the mouth tissues which have already been seriously weakened by lack of vitamin C.

Is it not possible, he asks, that the urinary tract goes through the same process when there is not enough vitamin C in the diet—the mucous lining scales off and forms the nucleus of the stones? And if this is true of kidney stones, might it not also hold true for gall bladder stones, and stones in the appendix, pancreas, prostate gland, mammary glands, uterus, ovaries and even the calcium deposit that brings about hardening of the arteries and arthritis?

Observing his own patients, Dr. McCormick found that cloudy urine containing phosphates (which constitute some kinds of kidney stones) and pieces of sloughed off mucus from the walls of the urinary canal went hand-in-hand with vitamin C deficiency. Giving large doses of vitamin C (much larger than one would get even in a daily diet relatively high in vitamin C) he could clear the urine within a matter of hours. During this treatment his patients reported to him that the tartar deposits were clearing from their teeth and dentures. Nurses in hospitals reported that patients whose urine had formerly caused calcium deposits on the urinary utensils now found that the utensils remained free from deposits. He interjects at this point a reminder that these particular patients were also getting a diet and dietary supplements high in the complex of B vitamins but his investigations seemed to show that it was the vitamin C that was responsible for the change in the appearance of the urine.

If Dr. McCormick is correct in his theory that ample vitamin C in the diet prevents the formation of stones and tooth tartar, how should we interpret the fact that Americans as a whole have less trouble of this kind than formerly, and the age accent has shifted from youth to middle age? It's very simple, says Dr. McCormick. American mothers these days have had it drummed into their heads that their children must have vitamin C. Summer and winter, infants and youngsters must drink their orange or tomato juice, and eat other fresh raw fruits. But how many of their fathers and mothers get a sufficient amount of vitamin C? We add that adults today are subjected to hundreds of substances that rob them of vitamin C. Smoking one cigarette, as Dr. McCormick himself has demonstrated in his laboratory, uses up 25 milligrams of vitamin C from the blood stream. Drugs, insecticides, minor infections, sleeping pills and scores of present-day industrial products (such as lead, paint and benzene) are enemies of vitamin C. So, while we protect our children from scurvy by giving them fresh fruits and vegetables, we forget that adults need vitamin C in even larger amounts than children. Might this not explain very satisfactorily why the incidence of kidney stones has shifted from children to adults?

Correcting Vitamin C Deficiency May Be the Answer

McCormick quotes J. W. Joly in his book, *Stones and Calculus Disease of the Urinary Organs* (C. V. Mosby Company, 1929): "I believe the hypothesis that stone is a deficiency disease is the most plausible and probable that has yet been advanced. It explains not only all the principal features of the conditions today, but also the changes in incidence during the past years. I believe that vitamin starvation acts primarily on the renal epithelium (the lining of the kidneys) and through it on the colloidal mechanism of the urine; also that once this mechanism is deranged, stone formation must follow as a direct result of the laws of physical chemistry."

Since the time of the early Roman scientist Pliny, physicians have been searching for the cause of kidney stones, looking generally for some medicine that could be taken orally that would dissolve the stones. Pliny's remedy was the ashes of snail shells. One of the main causes for surgery during the past century, stone formation has been so common a disorder that there are in medical dictionaries some 80 words beginning with "lith" which is the prefix referring to stone formation.

Yet how simple the answer may be! And not just for kidney stones, but, as Dr. McCormick suggests, for every kind of unhealthful calcification process that takes place in the body! At first glance it may not seem easy to get enough vitamin C. The vitamin is extremely perishable. It disappears from food in the presence of heat and water. Fruits and vegetables that lie for a long time on the grocer's shelves lose vitamin C with every passing hour. Exposure to air, when you are chopping or slicing foods, destroys vitamin C. It is wasted when cooking water is thrown away. You must get a supply of it every day—your body cannot store it.

Yet, if you should decide that from now on you are going to get enough vitamin C, it isn't really an impossible task. Fresh raw fruits and vegetables are the answer—and the sooner you can eat them after they are picked, the more vitamin C you will have. Citrus fruits are rich in vitamin C. We do not advise eating too many citrus fruits. Eating whole oranges and grapefruit is much better for you than drinking juice, for the vitamins are concentrated in the tissues of the fruit. But cantaloupe is rich in vitamin C. Broccoli, mustard greens, kale, green peppers, turnip greens, water cress, parsley, strawberries, Brussels sprouts and cabbage are good sources.

Pyorrhea and deposits of tartar on teeth are so common in this country as to be almost universal. No one has ever been able to find that you can get too much natural vitamin C. So why not get rid of that ugly scum on your teeth right away and prevent the possibility of pyorrhea and stones forming later on, by being sure you get many times more than the accepted daily minimum requirement of vitamin C which is about 75 to 100 milligrams. Even if you eat ample amounts of the vitamin C-rich fruits and vegetables, take a natural vitamin C food supplement made from rose hips or green peppers . . . just to be sure. You'll find it's well worth it.

57. Liver Ailments

Mrs. B., aged 51, was admitted to the hospital, her stomach swollen grotesquely, her limbs were also outsize, due to an accumulation of liquid in the tissues. She was in great pain, and surgeons sought to relieve her, somewhat, by puncturing the abdominal wall to release the large deposit of pus-like fluid lodged there. They tried every known treatment, including several more draining operations, but the patient continued to sink, eventually became mentally confused, began involuntary bodily twitchings and lapsed into coma, dying shortly thereafter.

For some time previous, Mrs. B. had suffered from lesser abdominal swellings, and swelling of the extremities, as well as networks of broken capillaries on the face and upper torso, pink palms, a muddy yellowish complexion and easy bruising. All of these were common symptoms of liver trouble. The ordeal in the hospital was the expected course of a severe and serious liver breakdown.

Mrs. B. was one of a growing number of liver disease victims. The Metropolitan Life Insurance Company has listed liver disease fourth, among the top 10 causes of death in the country. When we consider that filtering poisons which come into the body through drugs, industrial fumes, additives, pesticide sprays, etc., is one of the liver's functions, the reason becomes obvious. With the steady increase in exposure to such poisons that is part of modern living, the liver is overworked to the point at which its efficiency in its other duties is likely to be seriously impaired.

Jack of All Trades

These other jobs done by the liver are equally important, and we are struck by the amazing versatility of this organ when we are reminded of them. The liver is the largest gland in the body. It fills the upper right portion of the abdominal cavity. (See Figure 9.) After the food we eat has been acted upon by the stomach acids and broken into its various elements, it is absorbed through the intestinal wall into the blood stream. Many of these digested elements are then brought to the liver for an inspection, as it were, before they are allowed into general circulation. This organ functions as a combination food processing plant and sewage disposal plant, breaking foods down even further for use in the body, or for elimination.

The liver processes waste nitrogen in the body into urea for excretion, it is instrumental in regulating the balance of salt and water in the body by building amino acids into albumin, it balances the sex hormones to

FIGURE 9: INTERNAL ORGANS

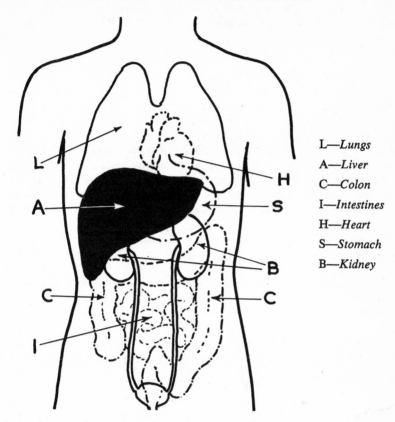

L—*Lungs*
A—*Liver*
C—*Colon*
I—*Intestines*
H—*Heart*
S—*Stomach*
B—*Kidney*

keep the sexual urge from increasing or decreasing abnormally. (In men, cirrhosis of the liver often causes feminizing manifestations; in women, liver difficulties often lead to menstrual pain and irregularity.)

When the skin is broken, the liver is called upon to control the bleeding by clotting, yet it must also help to prevent a dangerous thickening of the blood in the arteries. As food is digested the liver releases energy from it; sugars are extracted, fats are stored, certain vitamins are packed away for release when needed. Even our bones are dependent upon the liver, for the bile it releases contains an enzyme found to be vital for bone formation.

To these abilities can be added others, no doubt, which have not yet been traced by scientists. It is easily understood, then, why a breakdown in the liver's operation can be such a catastrophe. In view of its importance, it is comforting to know that the liver has the unique power of regeneration. In experiments with animals it has been found that large parts of the liver can be removed, and that it will grow back to its original size.

[249]

Presumably, this would also occur in human beings, if the need arose for removal of a part of the organ. We have not, however, seen any literature reporting such surgery. The damaged liver also responds to careful nutritional treatments.

Ways in Which Liver Is Affected

With these powers of recovery, how can the liver fall victim so frequently to fatal disease? There are several ways in which the liver can be seriously affected, the most common are a virus infection and cirrhosis of the liver. The virus causes an inflammation of the liver known as infectious hepatitis. Cirrhosis is characterized by a rapid dying-off of the liver cells, at too swift a pace for regeneration, and the replacement of these dead cells with a hard, fibrous mass of connective tissue. The reason for the occurrence of cirrhosis is believed to lie basically in malnutrition. Alcoholism commonly leads to cirrhosis. It is believed that this is so because alcohol is known to rob the body of B complex vitamins which have proven to be essential to liver health.

Liver damage in heavy drinkers has also been related to a change in the body's metabolism of the trace mineral, zinc. Below normal amounts of zinc are found in the blood streams of alcoholics, and above normal amounts are excreted in the urine. Though it has not yet been proven, studies suggest the possibility that daily doses of zinc might improve liver function in alcoholics. According to the *New York Times* (November 29, 1957), alcohol is known to rob the body of B complex vitamins which have proven to be essential to liver health. Lesser known accompaniments to cirrhosis are various heart disorders (*Medical Science,* May 25, 1959).

Overweight and Liver Damage

Obesity and liver damage also go hand in hand. *Gastroenterology* (34: 586-593, April, 1958) reported on an observation of 18 obese patients, all of whom were 25 per cent to 110 per cent above ideal weight. Liver function tests were given, and all but one of the patients showed some type of liver abnormality. None of these obese patients had any history of a previous disease which might have affected the liver.

The *Lancet* (June 9, 1956) says that severe liver abnormalities can be produced in animals by abnormal diet. The article goes on to say that nutritional liver disease is nearly always due to protein deficiency. The *Canadian Medical Association Journal* (March, 1954) agrees, adding that a lack of the sulfur-containing amino acids is especially dangerous.

Aureomycin Is a Particular Enemy

While most drugs are known to give the liver extra work, and can therefore be instrumental in causing damage and failure, aureomycin seems to cause more trouble than the rest. The *British Medical Journal* (April 4, 1953) tells of the surprise of the early workers with the drug in noting its damaging effect on the liver. Given orally, the antibiotic's action was not so perverse as when given orally in combination with injected dosage. Seven of 14 patients treated with intravenous-oral doses of aureomycin, by Lepper and Associates, showed unfavorable action on the liver. This same pattern of liver damage, resulting from aureomycin treatment, was consistently repeated in experiments with animals. Similar effects were seen in experiments reported in the *New England Medical Journal* (Vol. 247, p. 797, 1952) by Rutenburg and Pinkes. Aureomycin was given, as a post-operative infection-fighter, to 89 patients who had absolutely no history for liver damage or impaired function. Fifty-nine of those patients (roughly, two-thirds) developed some evidence of liver damage. To test further, 20 perfectly well and healthy volunteers were given 500 milligrams of aureomycin twice a day for 3 days. Thirteen of these people developed liver abnormalities.

Protection and Treatment the Same

Knowing the valuable service the liver performs in keeping our bodies functioning, and being apprised of the fact that a complete breakdown of this organ would mean death in less than two hours, our major concern should be how to prevent liver damage, and keep the organ healthy. In this, just about everyone is agreed that nutrition is the best protection, and treatment. In *Medical Science* (May 25, 1959), Charles S. Davidson, M.D., says the diet of patients with liver disease is most important. Agreement follows in an article by Paul de Kruif (*Reader's Digest*, January, 1958) in which the story of the work of Dr. Arthur J. Patek of New York City is related. Dr. Patek, in his fight against liver malnutrition, has restored many cirrhosis patients to health, even though others had given them up, by the use of proper nutrients. His treatment is very simple: rest and a highly nutritional diet, plus plenty of liver extract, brewer's yeast, B complex and other vitamins. Of course, no alcohol is permitted.

The same article quotes the treatment Dr. Fred Steigmann developed in the course of dealing with over 1,000 serious liver cases. He gives his patients a diet high in calories, average-to-high in protein, high carbohydrates, and average fats. Supplementing this are vitamin C and the B complex, especially vitamin B_{12}. Liver extract is given to severely ill patients, not only for the B complex, says Dr. Steigmann, but because of possible vitamin factors not yet defined.

In the *Texas Medical Journal*, Vol. 50, p. 809, R. D. Haines and J. A. Coleman make similar recommendations, and add that adequate unsaturated fatty acids should be included and sodium should be avoided. They end up by saying, ". . . There seems to be an increased need for practically all vitamins in patients with hepatic (liver) insufficiency."

The implication made by these authorities' recommendations is clear: if liver disease is present only nutritional therapy is effective; if one would avoid liver trouble, be sure to maintain good nutrition. It means that a good supply of B vitamins must be present, plus plenty of vitamin C and other vitamins and that one should avail oneself of organ meats for "possible vitamin factors not yet defined." Equally important is the avoidance of those items which might rob the system of the B vitamins already there. (Both alcohol and smoking are known to do this.) And smoking is especially destructive of vitamin C. The B vitamins are richly contained in the organ meats, as well as brewer's yeast, desiccated liver and wheat germ. Vitamin C comes in fresh fruits and vegetables, and in rose hips. Keep your liver healthy by means of good nutrition. The rest of your body will benefit, too.

58. Liver Health

We think of vitamin C in connection with the health of the skin, teeth and gums, blood vessels and other tissues. We know it is related to eye health, it helps fight infections and poisons from the outside. We know, too, that it is rapidly destroyed in the process of fighting poisons. In other words, the more chemicals, sprays, insecticides and other poisons you are subjected to, the more vitamin C you need to stay healthy.

Vitamin C is extremely important to good health for another reason, too—one we would never have suspected. It is necessary for the well-being of the liver—that most important organ of all, the organ without which no one has ever lived longer than a few moments.

The researchers who discovered this fact tested carefully to make certain that some other element in the diet might not have influenced their conclusion—one of the B vitamins, for instance, like choline, which is very important for liver health. Choline prevents livers from becoming "fatty" so it is spoken of as a "lipotropic" substance—that is, something which is attracted to fats and hence is useful in helping the body to manage them properly.

G. C. Willis, writing in the *Canadian Medical Association Journal* for June 15, 1957, tells us that early researchers showed that the liver was affected in scurvy, the disease of vitamin C deficiency. Later on, the subject of vitamin C in relation to the liver was somewhat neglected, mostly because scientists were using for their dietary experiments animals that can make their own vitamin C. (They all can, you know, except guinea pigs, man and the ape family.) Research with the B vitamins showed clearly that fatty degeneration of the liver occurs when choline is lacking in the diet. Several other circumstances have been investigated, too, in regard to fatty liver—the amount of vitamin E in the diet, the degree of unsaturation of the fatty acids in the diet, any antibiotics used by the patient, thyroid and antithyroid drugs being used. None of this uncovered any further information about vitamin C and the liver.

Experiment Proves the Point

So Dr. Willis set up an elaborate experiment in which he fed a total of 115 guinea pigs different diets, to take care of all the different combinations he wished to try—diets that would produce scurvy, but were rich in the B vitamins, scurvy-producing diets to which certain B vitamins had been added, etc. By this means he believed he could finally discover whether vitamin C alone is necessary to prevent fatty degeneration of the liver.

It is. Passing over all the elaborate calculations made and the many examinations of the condition of different livers, we see that there can be no doubt that a lack of vitamin C in a diet which is otherwise healthful can and will produce a fatty liver. It also appears to be true that giving ample quantities of vitamin C causes the harmful deposits of fat to disappear rapidly. Furthermore, Dr. Willis showed that fatty degeneration of the liver can occur in as little as 3 weeks from the onset of a diet *low in fat* but deficient in vitamin C.

Note the kind of diet given—one *low* in fat, so you could not possibly assume that too much fat in the diet brought about the trouble in the liver. Giving the animals choline, the B vitamin which orders fats around like a top sergeant in the body, did not relieve the condition. Giving vitamin C did. So we can conclude, says Dr. Willis, that vitamin C and choline have two entirely separate functions so far as fat is concerned.

"This is not the first time it has been shown that ascorbic acid has lipotropic properties," he goes on. Then he quotes an earlier research showing that the deposits of cholesterol present in human hardening of the arteries can be dissolved by vitamin C.

How Vitamin C Preserves Liver Health

In the case of the liver, lack of vitamin C apparently causes the same condition this deficiency causes in other parts of the body. The intercellular material begins to dissolve and collapse. Giving vitamin C immediately causes the liver to begin to reconstruct these cells once again. Dr. Willis tells us medical literature contains a reference to a 7-month-old child who suffered from scurvy and who had an extreme case of fatty degeneration of the liver. Incidentally, the child had been given milk since birth, but it was obviously milk from which all the vitamin C had been removed by processing or by boiling.

Now you can be even more confident about the benefit you reap, from taking great care about this one aspect of your diet. If you are getting plenty of vitamin C, there is far less chance that you are going to develop hardening of the arteries with all its accompanying effects on the heart and the blood vessels. And there is far less chance that whatever fat you eat is going to collect in your liver to do perhaps deadly damage there.

Vitamin C occurs most abundantly in fresh raw fruits and vegetables. It is highly perishable and disappears rapidly from foods as they wilt or rot.

It is washed away completely when you soak foods in water before cooking or eating them. And it is so sensitive to heat that much of it is lost from cooked fruits or vegetables. So even though you are careful to eat large quantities of raw fruits and vegetables (especially green leafy ones and tomatoes) do take extra vitamin C in the form of a natural food supplement. They are made of rose hips (richest natural source of vitamin C), green peppers or other natural foods.

59. Cirrhosis of the Liver

Cirrhosis of the liver is now among the 10 leading causes of death in the United States, according to the Metropolitan Life Insurance Company. In the age group 45 to 64, it is outranked only by heart disease, cancer and cerebral hemorrhage as a cause of death.

According to *Science News Letter* for August 31, 1957, exactly what causes the disease is still unknown. About one-fourth of the deaths are reported to be associated with alcoholism. If the disease is recognized early and proper treatment begun, recovery can be expected. And what is the treatment? Diet and diet alone. Patients are "urged to eat a diet rich in meat, milk, fish, eggs, fruit and green vegetables," says *Science News Letter*.

A glance at the dining table in the average family reveals why cirrhosis of the liver has leaped so far ahead in the mortality figures. As our food becomes more highly processed every day, our diets contain less and less of the food elements needed by the liver to carry on its work. At the same time the daily dose of poisons becomes more formidable with every passing day. So the detoxifying work of the liver mounts.

Alcoholism, B Vitamins and the Liver

The relation of alcoholism to liver disease is an obvious one. The alcoholic subsists mostly on carbohydrate, for alcoholic beverages are pure carbohydrate. Furthermore, his normal appetite has been so perverted by alcohol that he sometimes goes for long periods of time with no food at all. Then, too, for the body to handle the pure carbohydrate of alcohol, B vitamins must be provided, for they are an essential part of the metabolism of carbohydrates. They are practically nonexistent in the alcoholic's diet, so they are stolen from his body—nerves, muscles, brain tissue and digestive tract. Another good reason for liver trouble dogging the steps of the alcoholic. Several of the B vitamins are of the utmost importance to the health of the liver—especially choline and inositol, two B vitamins most concerned in the handling of fat by the body.

Another very significant aspect of liver health is the matter of taking isolated parts of the B complex of vitamins. It is common practice among medical men to prescribe such B vitamins as thiamin, or riboflavin or pyridoxine each by itself apart from the rest of the B complex. But in the case of the liver, this practice simply won't work out. The *Canadian Medical Journal* for March, 1954, tells us that Gyorgy and Goldblatt noted that in a number of rats maintained on a diet deficient in the entire B complex but supplemented with thiamin, riboflavin and pyridoxine a few died of acute liver damage. Others showed considerable damage.

It seems evident that this occurred because of the lack of other members of the B complex of vitamins. The 3 that were given were not enough. Indeed, it is possible that giving these 3 synthetic vitamins alone may have thrown off the balance completely and made things even worse than they were. Thousands of synthetic vitamin preparations are today being taken by Americans. They couldn't possibly contain all of the B complex of vitamins as it occurs in yeast, wheat germ and liver, because we have not as yet discovered all the parts of the B complex, although we know certain facts about them. Is it possible that taking synthetic vitamins has something to do with the present-day increase in incidence of cirrhosis of the liver?

Protein Essential for Liver Health

According to an article in the *New England Journal of Medicine* written by Dr. Charles S. Davidson and Dr. George J. Gabuzda, cirrhosis of the liver is a widespread disease in parts of the world where there is little animal protein in the diet; that is, the people eat largely carbohydrate diets. And it does not seem to matter how fine a source of carbohydrate they may have or how natural all of their foods are. If animal protein is lacking, cirrhosis of the liver is most likely to occur.

How many folks do you know, especially older folks, who try to get along on little or no animal protein—that is, eggs, meat, poultry or fish? Do you see what a grave danger is stalking these folks? Here, in a land where there is plenty of protein available, cirrhosis of the liver has now climbed to tenth place among diseases that kill. How can this be? Look at the people about you who have a cup of coffee for breakfast, a sticky bun and a cup of coffee for lunch and perhaps only a couple of grams of protein for dinner. According to the official recommendation, children should have from 40 to 100 grams of protein every day. Adults should have from 60 to 70 grams.

Here is a sample of the protein content of some of the foods highest in it. One egg contains about 12 grams of protein. The average serving—about ¼ pound—of meat, poultry or fish, contains about 10 to 25 grams of protein. So one serving of meat a day plus an egg for breakfast will not by any means give you your full quota of animal protein for the day.

It is also true that persons who are badly nourished are much more likely to be affected by liver poisons. We believe that present-day Americans are, generally speaking, very badly nourished. In this connection it is in-

[255]

teresting to note in the *New England Journal* article that people who are on starvation diets or eating very little food seldom show liver damage. *Harm to the liver comes from eating too much of the wrong kind of food.* Experiments with animals have shown us several startling things about liver health. According to an article in the *New York Times* for May 14, 1950, the liver has great power for regenerating itself. Following surgery it builds itself up to approximately 85 per cent of its normal tissue within a period of 14 days. *Regeneration of the liver depends largely on the amount of protein in the diet.* When experimental animals are protein-starved for only two weeks, the shrinkage of their livers amounts to 40 per cent. The protein of meat and eggs seems to be best for rejuvenating the liver. In another clipping sent in by a reader (*Kansas City Times,* September 24, 1957), we are told that by feeding two pounds of sugar to a hog 3 hours before slaughter, the weight of the liver of the hog will increase by 20 per cent. Whether or not this is being done we do not know. But it certainly indicates the very dangerous and almost immediate effect on the liver of that white drug, sugar, against which we have fired so many salvos.

Poisons Damaging the Liver

What are some of the poisons that are peculiarly damaging to the liver? Anesthetics are one. Several of the antibiotics are known to be poisonous to the liver when they are taken by mouth and injected at the same time. Inorganic copper is a liver poison. Does this mean that copper water pipes are a hazard? We think that they are, although the information we got on copper is in relation to alcohol. Say Dr. Charles S. Davidson and Dr. George J. Gabuzda in the *New England Journal of Medicine,* "Copper may play an important role (in liver disease). The copper content of the brain at post-mortem examination has been found to be 5 to 10 times higher in Wilson's disease (one form of liver disease). . . . Liver injury may be produced by alcohol or some substance present in alcoholic beverages—for example, copper."

Other poisons must be treated by the liver to render them harmless before they are excreted. Some of the poisons particularly destructive to the liver are: chloroform, bromide, arsenic and antimony, cinchophen, picric acid, poisonous mushrooms and carbon tetrachloride. It seems impossible, with our present knowledge, that anyone would be exposed to these poisons to such an extent as to harm the liver. But how do we know how much harm may be done to the liver by small doses of these over a long period of time?

Arsenic, for instance, is widely used in insecticides of which a residue is bound to stay on the fruit. How much must accumulate in the body before damage is done to the liver? We don't know. Bromides are used in sleeping pills and sedatives. The number of such medications taken in our country every year is almost astronomical. How much does it have to do with the rising incidence of cirrhosis of the liver?

Other Diseases May Affect Liver

It is well to remember that other diseases may contribute to liver trouble. Impaired digestion, such as ulcerative colitis patients suffer from, brings about such a deficiency in many valuable food factors that the liver cannot continue to function properly. A lack of appetite can bring about the same condition. An overactive thyroid may burn up an abnormal amount of food and thus deprive the liver of badly needed elements. Disorders of other glands may have the same effect.

Dr. A. C. Ivy, former Vice President of the University of Illinois and head of its medical department, writes on liver disease in the August, 1951, issue of *Life and Health*. He tells us that the sedentary lives we lead may have as much as anything else to do with the condition of our livers. Says he, "In some cases of bile obstruction there is evidence that the posture habitually assumed by the patient in his occupation is a contributing factor. Here again, the hygiene of the liver is the hygiene of the body as a whole. Proper diet, posture, rest, habits of living, exercise—these help keep not only the liver healthy but the whole person. Like the entire body, the liver is endowed with wisdom of its own so great as to pass our understanding. The least we can do is to apply what common sense we have in working along with it."

Our file on liver disorders contains much more that is interesting. Since they are covered in another chapter, we have not touched on the so-called infectious liver diseases—hepatitis and homologous serum hepatitis. The incidence of these is rising too at an alarming rate. We have not talked much about "fatty liver," or "liver spells," or billousness related in most people's mind with liver disorder. We have talked mostly about cirrhosis because this is the most serious liver disease one can have, the one most likely to be fatal, the one most likely to lead to cancer, the one that indicates the most serious disruption of orderly body processes.

In general, however, what we say about preventing cirrhosis of the liver applies to other liver disorders as well. If you keep your liver healthy you are not going to take to your bed with any of the diseases we have mentioned above. And it is surprising how much agreement there is among authorities as to the best safeguards for the liver. Medical opinion is practically unanimous. What you eat and do not eat and what poisons you are exposed to—these are the important factors in liver health.

Recommendations for Liver Health

1. *PROTEIN.* A diet containing ample complete protein is essential for liver health. Most foods (except white sugar) contain some protein. But you need complete protein—that is, protein in which all of the essential amino acids or forms of protein are present in the right proportions. Foods of animal origin provide this almost exclusively. It is difficult to arrange a good high protein intake on a vegetarian diet. It is impossible on a diet in which there are refined carbohydrates—white sugar, white flour, pro-

[257]

cessed, devitalized foods. You need 60-70 grams of complete protein a day, every day. If you have not been getting this much, you can probably take up to 150 grams advantageously.

2. *VITAMINS.* Research has shown that all the vitamins are necessary for liver health. The fat soluble ones, like A, K and D are stored in the liver. Vitamin E apparently is extremely important for the liver. But the B vitamins are mentioned most often in connection with liver health. You must have plenty of them every day. They are abundant in fresh, unprocessed, unrefined foods. The best sources are liver and other organ meats, fish, whole grains, wheat germ, eggs, soybeans and brewer's yeast. All of these are excellent sources of protein, as well.

3. *POISONS.* Poisons will harm your liver. What about the new, deadly insecticides like DDT, and the even more poisonous newer ones? There is every reason to believe that exposure to these will harm your liver. They are all cumulative and you may not know for years what harm they have done. Avoid them. Avoid drugs and industrial substances like the white lead used in paints, carbon tetrachloride (used in many solvents), sleeping pills. What about chemicals and dyes used in processed foods? We do not know how poisonous many of them are for no research has been done on them, yet they are allowed in food. Avoid foods that contain chemicals. Eat fresh, unprocessed foods.

4. *DISEASES.* What if you suffer from one of the disorders like ulcerative colitis, or lack of appetite which may contribute to the depleted state of your liver? The wisest precaution against such diseases is the very diet outlined above, which is also the one that is best for your liver—a diet high in protein and fresh foods with no refined carbohydrates.

5. *SYNTHETIC VITAMINS.* They're dangerous, especially as you may get overdoses of some which will throw the level of others out of balance. Get your vitamins from natural food sources, like brewer's yeast, desiccated liver, fish liver oils, rose hips and so forth.

6. *EXERCISE.* Finally, a sedentary life may contribute to liver disorders. No one who is able to walk need live a sedentary life. For as long as you can walk, the very finest exercise in the world is available to you—walking in the open air.

60. How Close Are You to Hepatitis?

It is interesting and frightening to us to find that diseases we barely knew existed, except through articles in medical journals or textbooks, have suddenly become A#1 problems for almost everyone. Is there anyone today who hasn't a friend or acquaintance who is the victim of cancer or heart disease? An even rarer problem, before World War II, was hepatitis, a liver infection presumed to be caused by a virus which has yet to be isolated. A disease once largely confined to the armed forces, it is now, according to the Metropolitan Life Insurance Company (*Science News Letter*, June 11, 1955), "A relative newcomer among diseases (which) has rapidly reached into the top ranks among the leading communicable, or catching diseases. . . ." One after another headlines have popped up in 1960-61 such as this one from the *New York Times* (February 11, 1961) "Hepatitis in City Shows Sharp Rise." Same thing in St. Paul, Minnesota, Chicago, Illinois and cities in the Northeast and the Far West. The United States Public Health Service reported 5,171 cases in the first 4 weeks of January, 1961. Most publications pointed out that the figures do not, of course, include many cases that are known to have gone unrecognized.

Hepatitis is one of those cyclical diseases which are on the rise for a few years, then subside for a while, only to flare up again. (Polio is also recognized as one of these, and it was the periodic downtrend in 1955-57 which confused parents who were sure the Salk vaccine was responsible.) However, even in its wildest rampages, hepatitis never made a showing such as this current one! Those who study such things are puzzled by the hepatitis virus. They can only guess at how the virus is transmitted, how long it will stay, what damage it will do and if the disease will recur.

Two Types of Virus

These are two types of hepatitis: infectious and serum. Infectious hepatitis is thought to come to the victim through food, water, bodily contact, etc. The serum hepatitis virus is conveyed by way of transfusions and injections given directly into the blood stream. When hepatitis does occur, the virus can remain in the blood stream for as long as 5 years before making itself known by its classic symptoms. (*Wall Street Journal*, October 11, 1960.) When it does take hold, hepatitis is first characterized by a gradually increasing weakness and dizziness which appears to many to be the first stages of grippe or a bad cold. Soon utter and complete fatigue occurs along with nausea, pains in the stomach, tenderness in the liver area and an unconquerable loss of appetite. The urine is noticeably darker in color, the virus acts to destroy the tissue of the liver, and interferes with the liver's ability to process waste materials of the body. The skin and the whites of the eyes take on a yellowish tinge due to the escape of bile pigments into the blood and tissues. The seriousness of this attack on the liver can be gauged by the fact that this organ is responsible for the manufacture of important blood components, and the storage and processing of certain vitamins. It must eliminate poisons which come to the body through polluted air, insecticides and pesticides sprayed on foods, chemicals in processed foods and drugs. If it is not functioning, all of these elements pile up in the body and can poison the entire system.

Fortunately, the liver is able to restore itself, if given the proper nourishment. The trouble is that hepatitis victims are always short on appetite, and find it difficult, if not impossible, to eat the food they need so that the liver has something to work with in its repair operations. Injections of B vitamins are sometimes given to aid in nourishing the liver.

No Definite Treatment

No definite treatment for hepatitis seems to have been devised. For many years it was believed that prolonged bedrest was essential. Current thinking has the patient up and about as soon after the initial attack as he feels able, since comparison has shown that neither course has any effect on the length of the illness. *Newsweek* (March 28, 1960) tells us that standard therapy for hepatitis includes a diet high in protein, low in fats, supplemented with B_{12} injections and absolute avoidance of liquor. In the first month of illness the hepatitis patient should be kept in strict isolation. The article asserts that 20 to 30 per cent of hepatitis victims develop permanent liver damage and two per cent end up with cirrhosis, or hardening, of the liver tissue. There is a strong possibility of recurrence or relapse. The *Journal of the American Medical Association* (November 21, 1959) agreed on the diet, warning especially against chocolate, which, because it contains 30 to 50 per cent cocoa butter, is a concentrated source of fat. Also, the liquor ban is set by this article at two years.

Then we come across a complete about-face in another article which appeared in the *Journal of the American Medical Association* (November 30, 1957). This author, Franklin M. Hanger, M.D., with complete assurance, asserts that, "It is regrettable that so many physicians still entertain the impression that fats are injurious in viral hepatitis, there is no contra-indication for eggs and fresh dairy products in the presence of uncomplicated infection. Indeed, these foodstuffs, when well tolerated, are believed to be of value in maintaining the strength and nutrition of the patient . . . Vitamin supplements are indicated only in those in whom previous malnutrition is suspected."

Natural as Opposed to Hydrogenated Fats

Perhaps the reconciliation of the two views lies in Dr. Hanger's mention of natural fats, as opposed to hydrogenated fats and fried foods. Eggs, for example, while high in cholesterol, are rich in lecithin which helps the body to use the cholesterol properly. They are also rich in the B vitamins which are essential to the liver's good health. We do not understand Dr. Hanger's lack of enthusiasm for food supplements. He suggests them only for patients in whom previous malnutrition is suspected. Surely he is aware that with sufficient nutrition the liver would never have been susceptible to such a violent attack in the first place.

Dr. Hanger writes that the use of steroids as a treatment is not indicated. Aside from the risks of gastro-intestinal bleeding and the activation of latent infection induced by cortisone and its like, there is the added possibility of spreading the virus in the system before a sound immunity has developed. The *Medical Journal of Australia* (January 25, 1958) warns that if cortisone is started as a therapy, it must be continued until recovery is assured. Steroid therapy cannot simply be shut off, for the reaction could be serious. Sulphonamides may actually be harmful in hepatitis cases. We say they can be harmful in any cases. *Good Housekeeping* (February, 1957) states that an attempt in Germany to use aureomycin against hepatitis also proved useless.

How the Disease Is Transmitted

Hepatitis virus of the infectious type is largely propagated by unsanitary conditions, according to some experts. In the *Wall Street Journal* (October 11, 1960) we are told that hepatitis can be spread through polluted water systems and through contaminated foods. The Director of the Bucks County (Pennsylvania) Department of Health, Dr. Joseph W. Still, linked the more than threefold increase in hepatitis cases in his county to overflowing cesspools. (*Philadelphia Inquirer,* January 30, 1960.) We are reminded in this article that this virus is known to survive sewage, and flies can carry and spread the virus. Dr. Still suggests that hepatitis is probably one of the hidden costs of not having adequate sewage systems in many populous areas. In *Parents* magazine (February, 1958), an article on this subject stated that nothing short of boiling water vigorously for 10 minutes or longer is certain to kill the hepatitis virus. It is not enough to rely upon the chemicals used to purify our water. *Chemical Week,* as long ago as October 20, 1956, stated that epidemiological evidence was definite at that time, that conventionally treated drinking water supplies are a major factor in the transmission of hepatitis. This was the cause of an outbreak in North Carolina, according to *Good Housekeeping* (November, 1957), while that issue also told of 629 cases in Sweden that were traced to contaminated oysters which could have come from polluted oyster beds.

The problem of improperly guarded and cleansed municipal water supplies has been plaguing the United States for years now. Population booms have quickly made existing water supplies obsolete in many cities. This condition is aggravated even more by the dumping of industrial and sewage wastes into rivers and streams used for drinking purposes. Finally many states have little legislation to protect citizens against polluted water sources, and some that do are reluctant to enforce them, in the face of the powerful industries who are often the parties responsible for such pollution of streams.

The more sensational type of hepatitis, serum hepatitis, has really made the headlines in recent years. It is indeed alarming to know that a visit to a doctor or dentist for treatment of an illness or for some preventive measure might result in infection with an even worse illness, hepatitis.

The Doctors Tell the Story

In the *Illinois Medical Journal* (February, 1957) an article states that 30 per cent of the cases of hepatitis in the author's hospital could have been serum hepatitis. Over a two-year period, 68 per cent of the serum hepatitis cases he saw were due to exposure at the dentist's office. The article said that, for prevention of such occurrences, chemical sterilization of implements should be abandoned; the surer method of boiling for one-half an hour substituted.

In a Dutch journal (*Nederlands tijdschrift v. geneeskunde,* Amsterdam, August 13, 1960) we read of experiments with guinea pigs which convinced the researchers that hepatitis is easily transmitted in injections, even if platinum needles are used and flamed after each injection. *The only way, the article continues, to eliminate the risk of inducing hepatitis by inoculation is to use a newly sterilized needle and syringe for each injection.*

Injections are so common these days that the patient seldom asks why he is getting one. The doctor is so used to giving them that he has convinced himself of their harmlessness, and his precautions become less and less rigid. That a disease such as hepatitis can be conveyed so easily is enough to make one careful about how one's doctor prepares for giving injections. Disposable needles are one answer, but complete sterilization of all of the implements he uses, especially those which puncture the skin, should be the rule—that is, sterilization by boiling, not merely by chemical immersion. Apparently disinfectants are not enough. Protect yourself by insisting that your doctor follow this procedure. Better still, avoid any injections if possible.

Are You a Likely Victim?

If you are wondering how likely it is that you will be a victim of hepatitis, there is no direct answer. Many experts report that the disease is most likely to hit crowded, low income groups whose environment is likely to be less sanitary than that of other groups. But in the face of that, we read in *Scope* (August 17, 1960) of an English internist, Dr. Sheila Sherlock, Professor of Medicine, London Medical School's Royal Free Hospital, who describes an increasingly common hepatitis condition in London which she calls the "executive variety" of hepatitis. It strikes with greatest frequency those who are in the higher income brackets. In two years she says she has treated 60 patients in the executive class for this disease. Dr. Sherlock believes that it is "the man with the means to vary his dining habitat who seems most susceptible." This is due, she says, to the fact that there are probably different strains of the virus, and the person who can carry one strain without developing the disease, will come down with hepatitis when exposed to a different strain. These men travel in Paris, London, New York, with possible exposure at each place. That is why they are likely victims.

Science News Letter (June 11, 1955) says that the greatest incidence of the disease is among school age children. This is not surprising, since children eat what is probably the worst diet of all. They load up on sodas, cokes, candies and other sweets, and are aghast at the thought of a food that has some B vitamins in it. The sweets they eat rob their systems of the very B vitamins the liver needs to maintain its health, yet they eat nothing—eggs, brewer's yeast, desiccated liver, yogurt, wheat germ, liver, kidneys, heart—that will serve to replace these nutrients. Can anyone be surprised that children are most susceptible to hepatitis, a liver infection?

Effective Defenses Against Hepatitis

The *Medical Journal of Australia* (July 25, 1953) warns that in large families the possibility of infection being transmitted from one member to the other is great. Families, it says, may be regarded as epidemiological units, and more than one case per house is not uncommon. Extreme care in sanitation must be observed here. Concentration on vitamin-rich foods and avoidance of any others which might induce a weakness in the liver is certainly in order—this warning especially applies to liquor. Be sure of your water source. Bottled spring water is safest. Aside from these, effective precautions against hepatitis are scarce. In *Newsweek* (February 27, 1961), Dr. Alexander Langmuir, of the United States Public Health Service, wailed, "All we can do is to give gamma globulin injections to those who we think have been exposed. We have no new progress to report on a hepatitis vaccine."

The gamma globulin of which Dr. Langmuir speaks is a serum rich in antibodies which is believed to help the body fight infectious viruses when they attack. Unfortunately any protection that might come with this serum is temporary. Also, one who is injected with this preventive should be certain that all precautions against serum hepatitis have been taken, lest one be injected with the disease rather than the preventive.

You can die from hepatitis—about one in a hundred die or are permanently injured. This is the figure given in the *Boston* (Massachusetts) *Globe* (July 16, 1961) article, and it is intended to cover only healthy children and young adults. In persons who suffer from other diseases or from malnutrition the figure is 5 per 100. We wonder what category the average youngster would fit into, with his viruses and colds, and sores that are really staph infections, his poor eyes and bad teeth. Kids such as this are not healthy, even though they do play, go to school and don't have to stay in bed. If such a child were yours and were to contract hepatitis, could you be sure he'd survive? Could you be sure your diet would help you to pull through a bout with hepatitis? Dr. Langmuir in the *Newsweek* piece, says, "We are in the midst of a national hepatitis outbreak." We urge you to do your best, through good diet, to fortify yourself and your family against such an infection. Apparently this is the only defense.

~~~~~~

SECTION 13: THE PROSTATE GLAND

~~~~~~

61. Enlarged Prostate

A successful non-surgical treatment for enlarged prostate gland is cause for rejoicing among the thousands of mature men who yearly face the possibility of becoming a victim of this painful and dangerous affliction. Such a treatment is reported on in the *Journal of the Maine Medical Association* (March, 1958). Of almost equal importance is the fact that the medication used is not a drug to dull the pain or mask other symptoms, but a nutrient which exists naturally in food and attacks the problem at its source, curing completely in many cases. Its effectiveness in treating prostate was discovered quite by accident, but this fortunate accident can result in relief and cure for thousands of men whose only other recourse might have been an operation.

The Location and Function of the Prostate Gland

Before going into a detailed description of the treatment and its results, it might be well to concern ourselves with an understanding of the prostate gland and its function, as well as an idea of the symptoms which makes its enlargement painful and seriously dangerous. The prostate gland is located near the mouth of the male bladder. The gland itself functions as an auxiliary sex gland. It manufactures the liquid which acts as a vehicle for the sperm cells of the male. Without this important fluid there is no way of transferring the sperm into the female vagina for the purpose of fertilizing the female egg, and hence no way of carrying out the normal process of reproduction. Without the prostate gland to manufacture this essential fluid, the male becomes sterile.

[264]

When the prostate becomes swollen or enlarged, it invades the area occupied by the urethra. This is a tube through which the urine is expelled from the bladder, and the swollen prostate gland pressing upon the urethra interferes with the normal flow. As can be imagined, the complications which result can be frightening and almost unendurably painful.

Symptoms of Prostate Trouble

In the early stages, the symptoms of enlarged prostate are rather vague—a feeling of congestion and discomfort in the pubic area. There follows a constant feeling of fullness of the bladder, with frequent, urgent trips to the bathroom. Once there, however, there is often difficulty in starting a stream, and sometimes no urination at all. The recurring need to void during the night is also common. Eventually, a residue of urine that has not been expelled is collected in the bladder and dribbling occurs. This is the unconscious release of urine, in small amounts, forced out by a full bladder. When the urethra is interfered with to the extent that very little or no urine can escape from the bladder, the serious problem of possible uremic poisoning arises. This can occur when such large amounts of fluid accumulate that the bladder can hold no more. With the normal avenue of release through the urethra shut off, the urine floods back into the kidneys, presenting a grave danger of poison to the system.

Common Treatments Now in Use

What is the general procedure for dealing with prostate problems? There are several courses of treatment. For immediate relief of a full bladder, a catheter is employed. Usually it consists simply of a sterile rubber tube which is inserted into the opening of the urethra and gently pushed along its length to the mouth of the bladder. The bladder empties through the tube quickly and with ease. Of course, this method is excellent for emergency treatment, but not for constant repetition. For one thing, it is extremely painful, and the chance for infection as well as damage to delicate tissues is very real. For another, the bladder fills quickly, and catheterization would have to be almost a daily affair if relief were to be maintained. Finally, this is no more a solution to the cause of the problem than to give a man standing on hot coals injections of morphine to kill the pain instead of making him get off the coals!

Another means of relieving the symptoms of swollen prostate is to massage the gland. This can be accomplished by a physician, and is often effective in reducing the swelling. But the treatment must be repeated about once a week. So-called sitz baths in which one soaks only the lower portion of the trunk, have a soothing effect and often reduce the swelling, but are obviously inconvenient.

The average doctor's final opinion on what to do about prostate trouble is "have it removed." The operation has come to be reasonably safe (less than 2 per cent mortality) and relief is sure. Of course, sterility is an inescapable aftermath of the operation, though this does not mean that there is any lessening in the patient's desire for sexual activity. The person who has had his prostate gland removed is perfectly normal in this respect, but for the fact that he can't father a child. It is understandable, however, that men are anxious to find some other way to solve the prostate problem.

A word should be said here about cancer of the prostate. For some unknown reason this gland is extremely susceptible to malignancy. When prostatic difficulties do occur, it is wise, therefore, to make certain through a medical examination by your doctor that no cancer is present, before embarking on a system of self-cure. Sometimes surgery is the only recourse in such cases.

A Happy Accident that Opened a Door

If the prostate swelling is simply a benign condition of enlargement, then the non-surgical treatment mentioned above should be of great interest and help. As we said, the discovery of this treatment was a happy accident. It happened this way: Two physicians were treating a group of allergic patients with a mixture of 3 amino acids (kinds of protein)—glycine, alanine and glutamic acid. One of the patients thus treated volunteered the information that his urinary symptoms had disappeared while he took the amino acid mixture. This led to a trial of the same compound on non-allergic patients with urinary symptoms. Patients with enlarged prostates and associated urinary symptoms experienced prompt and rather spectacular relief. They remained free of the symptoms while taking the compound, but soon after discontinuing the medication, the symptoms returned.

A Controlled Experiment

A controlled experiment was set up. A series of 40 cases of prostatic enlargement, previously ascertained to be benign, or noncancerous, were included. Symptoms of discomfort were present in 35 of the patients; 39 complained of the urge to void often during the night; 23 experienced delayed urination; 29 suffered with excess frequency of urination; and 27 complained of extreme urgency to void which felt uncontrollable. The average age of the patients was 60 years, however their age range was from 37 to 75 years. The average duration of their complaints was 4 years.

The 40 men were divided into two groups. The odd-numbered cases were given glycine-alanine-glutamic acid in dosages of two capsules after each meal for two weeks. Then one capsule after each meal for 3 months thereafter. The second group, or even-numbered patients, were also given capsules on the same schedule, except that their capsules did not contain the amino acids, nor any other active ingredient.

Of the men who were treated with the amino acids, 92 per cent saw the size of the swollen prostate diminish, and in 32 per cent it shrank to normal size. The need to get up during the night to void unusually often was relieved in 95 per cent of the cases and completely eliminated in 72 per cent. Urgent urination was relieved in 81 per cent of the cases, frequency of urination was lowered in 73 per cent, discomfort was lessened in 71 per cent and delayed urination was remedied in 70 per cent of the patients. There was no comparable improvement in any of the patients who did not receive the amino acids until, after two months, they were switched from the inactive capsules to the amino acid compound.

There were no ill effects whatsoever in any of the patients as a result of the amino acid therapy. It was also noticed that edema, or swelling, of other parts of the body disappeared during treatment. Edema is known to be one of the most important symptoms of protein (source of amino acids) deficiency. Edema is also the result of too much salt, which retains water in the tissues. It follows then that a diet low in salt and high in protein would be an excellent protection against the problems presented by a swollen prostate gland.

Unsaturated Fatty Acids Seen Effective

Other nutritional elements have been employed in recent years to relieve enlarged prostate. One of the most effective of these is vitamin F, or the unsaturated fatty acids, according to the testimony of two researchers whose findings were published in a pamphlet by the Lee Foundation for Nutritional Research, 2023 West Wisconsin Avenue, Milwaukee, Wisconsin. These men reported that they gave unsaturated fatty acids and no other treatment to 19 patients suffering with symptoms of enlarged prostate. The results showed a more complete emptying of the bladder in 12 of the 19 cases. Thirteen of the 19 stopped getting up at night to void. There was shown to be an increase in sex urge and a lessening of fatigue and leg pains. Dribblings stopped in 18 of the 19 patients, and each of the men showed a reduction in the size of the prostate gland.

Though there are no formal experiments on record, there are two vitamins which should have a beneficial effect in the prevention and treatment of prostatic disorders—vitamin A and vitamin E. It is known that a deficiency of vitamin A shows up first in a sloughing off of the cells which line the digestive, respiratory and reproductive tracts. This indicates a weakness of the cells which make up the structure of these important organs, and serves as a warning that nutrition to these parts is lacking. Weakness such as this serves as an excellent breeding ground for trouble. Your vitamin A supply should be carefully maintained.

Aside from its demonstrated effectiveness in treating heart conditions and other illnesses, vitamin E is generally accepted as an effective agent in maintaining the health of the reproductive tract. Wheat germ oil, high in vitamin E, is considered to be effective in preventing reproductive disorders. Scientists hazard the guess that natural hormones which occur in wheat germ oil are partly responsible for its good effect.

TABLE 3: FOODS HIGH IN THESE AMINO ACIDS

Food	Alanine (Grams)	Glutamic Acid (Grams)	Glycine (Grams)
Brewer's yeast	3.456	6.334	2.427
Milk, non-fat, dry	1.228	8.320	.703
Casein (milk protein)	3.354	23.052	1.987
Eggs	——	1.583	.543
Egg yolks	——*	1.951	.571
Beef, lean	1.086	2.846	1.164
Lamb, lean	.955	2.594	.999
Veal, lean	1.169	3.073	.942
Chicken	——	2.309	1.378
Fish—haddock	——	2.318	1.005
Liver, beef	1.261	2.679	1.198
Liver, calves	1.216	2.584	1.155
Liver, chicken	1.414	3.006	1.344
Beans, kidney	1.316	3.696	.392
Lentils	.888	3.700	1.080
Peanuts	1.094	5.932	1.710
Soybeans	1.571	7.010	1.595
Filberts	——	3.079	1.421
Cottonseed flour and meal	2.155	9.122	2.322
Corn	.995	1.765	.399
Whole wheat flour	.465	4.156	.812

These elements should be in one's diet at all times. For a man faced with the danger of prostate trouble to chance being short of vitamins A, E and F (unsaturated fatty acids) and the amino acids found in protein foods, would really be tempting fate.

Foods high in these 3 amino acids are, as you would expect, those foods which are richest in protein. We think you will be surprised, as we were, to find the large figures for such foods as soybeans and peanuts. We should make it a practice to eat more of these foods. Table 3 gives the number of grams of each amino acid in 100 grams of food. One hundred grams is about one-quarter of a pound—an average serving.

62. A New Theory on Prostate Gland Disorders

We are told that most American men over the age of 50 have some difficulty with their prostate glands. During and after middle age it may swell (hypertrophy, as the doctors say). Because of its position, close to the mouth of the urinary bladder, this swelling may cause great difficulty with urination. Because of pressure on the bladder, urination may eventually become almost impossible with the result that urine accumulates in the bladder and may cause infection.

Operations and massages are the treatments most often suggested by doctors. In operations the entire gland is removed. This probably will not result in any change in sex life except for sterility. Most men past middle age are not especially concerned with fathering children these days, so the operation does not seem too objectionable on this score. However, the prostate does grow back sometimes, as tonsils and adenoids do. And, of course, anyone who can avoid an operation should do so.

A German doctor has recently announced a new theory concerning pumpkin seeds in regard to prostate gland troubles. Dr. W. Devrient of Berlin in an article entitled *Androgen-Hormonal Curative Influence of a Neglected Plant,* tells us that enlargement of the prostate gland is caused by the functionally weakened organ trying to make up for the loss of the male sex hormones which, of course, decline with advancing age. Just as women experience menopause due to a lessening of their production of female sex hormones, so men go through a period during which production of male sex hormones slackens.

Says Dr. Devrient, "Its presence (enlarged prostate, that is) can be demonstrated in every fourth American once he has reached the age of 52. It is maintained that the number of impotent males in the United States amounts to some two million. This, too, is related to the hormone production of the prostate, although all these processes are centrally regulated. In Berlin two large specializing urological hospitals had to be founded, because the surgical divisions of the existing hospitals were not sufficient. The causes of this trouble are to be sought in false methods of living. The poisoning of the glands with tobacco plays the most important role among them."

Giving hormone substances to make up for the deficiency in them does not meet with Dr. Devrient's approval. He says, "One gains the impression that artificial hormones favor the evolution of cancer rather than preventing it. We biological physicians, therefore, reject this treatment, basing our opinions on the conviction that an artificial hormone, though chemically identical, still does not for long have the same effect as a natural one.

"In view of the fact that, with the exception of operative urology (highly dangerous prostatectomy) and biophysical therapy, modern medicine has not been able to find any successful weapon against the early attrition and deterioration of the prostate gland, we have no other recourse than to seek prevention in the realm of healing plants." He goes on to say that in certain countries where pumpkin seeds are eaten in great quantity throughout life, there is almost no incidence of enlarged prostate or other prostate disorders.

Seed Nutriments Essential for Reproductive Functions

Dr. Devrient believes that the seeds contain materials which are the building stones for the male hormones. Thus they are actually supplying the body indirectly with the means of carrying on the work of the male hormones.

"Only the plain people knew the open secret of pumpkin seeds, a secret which was handed down from father to son for countless generations without any ado. No matter whether it was the Hungarian gypsy, the mountain-dwelling Bulgarian, the Anatolian Turk, the Ukranian or the Transylvanian German—they all knew that pumpkin seeds preserve the prostate gland and, thereby, also male potency. In these countries people eat pumpkin seeds the way they eat sunflower seeds in Russia: as an inexhaustible source of vigor offered by Nature.

"Investigations by G. Klein at the Vienna University revealed the noteworthy fact that in Transylvania prostatic hypertrophy is almost unknown. Painstaking researches result in the disclosure that the people there have a special liking for pumpkin seeds. A physician from the Szekler group in the Transylvanian mountains confirmed this connection as an ancient healing method among the people. Dr. Bela Pater, of Klausenburg, later published these associations and his own experiences in the Journal, *Healing and Seasoning Plants*.

"My assertion of the androgen-hormonal (the male hormone) influence of pumpkin seeds is based on the positive judgment of old-time doctors, but also no less on my own personal observations throughout the years. This plant has scientifically determined effects on intermediary metabolism and diuresis (urination), but these latter are of secondary importance in relation to its regenerative, invigorative and vitalizing influences. There is involved herein a native plant hormone which affects our own hormone production in part by substitution, in part by direct proliferation.

"Anyone who has studied this influence among peasant peoples has been again and again astonished over the effect of this plant in putting off the advent of old age. My own personal observations in the course of the last 8 years, however, have been decisive for me. At my own age of 70 years I am well able to be satisfied with the condition of my own prostate, on the basis of daily ingestion of pumpkin seeds, and with that of my health in general. This beneficial result can also be found among city patients who are prudent enough to eat pumpkin seeds every day and throughout their life. But one must continue proving this to the city dweller. The peasants of the Balkans and of Eastern Europe knew of the healing effect of these seeds already from their forefathers."

What Is the Powerful Substance in Pumpkin Seeds?

Dr. Devrient goes on to tell us that a number of different substances have been found to be contained in pumpkin seeds, but no one has ventured a guess as to which it may be that brings about the good results on the sex organs. We have been able to find out some facts about the makeup of pumpkin seeds. They are extremely high in phosphorus and low in calcium (as are most seeds). Their iron content appears to be higher than that of any other seed. The B vitamins are plentiful, as they are in other seeds, and there is a small vitamin A content. They contain about 30 per cent protein and about 40 per cent fat.

The fat is, of course, rich in unsaturated fatty acids, as are most vegetable fats. The unsaturated fatty acids are essential for the health of the prostate gland. Perhaps these are the responsible agents in pumpkin seeds. Recently we have come across information about the relationship of the mineral zinc to the health of the prostate gland. It seems that the healthy gland contains far more zinc than the swollen, sick one. Perhaps a deficiency of zinc in the diet may be partly to blame—and perhaps the pumpkin seed may supply much of this needed substance.

And what about the protein content of pumpkin seeds? It seems quite possible that the protein content of pumpkin seeds, along with the unsaturated fatty acid content, may be responsible for the seed's reputation as a regulator of sex organs.

Perhaps the best recommendation of all for the pumpkin seeds may at the same time be the explanation for the lack of prostate disorders in parts of the world where the seed is widely eaten. Pumpkin seeds are a completely natural food. Their fat and proteins are unchanged and untampered with. They provide in good measure all the rich nutriment that the plant needs to germinate and to grow.

Compare This with the Average American Diet

The average American man's food for a day goes somthing like this: processed cereal (little nutriment—most protein and all the valuable unsaturated fatty acids have been removed); doughnuts and coffee at midmorning (the fats in fried foods have been ruined and made dangerous for human health); lunch may involve a sandwich and a piece of pie (dangerous hydrogenated fats in the pastry); for dinner, unless he has a salad with plenty of dressing, there will once again be no unprocessed fats. Protein will be limited to a serving of meat.

Doesn't it seem possible that the freedom from prostate trouble among the groups mentioned by Dr. Devrient may result from the fact that they

[271]

are getting fresh unspoiled natural fats and proteins of the highest quality in their pumpkin seeds, and they are not getting all the unhealthful foods the average man in "advanced" countries is getting?

Why should folk lore and folk medicine prescribe the pumpkin seed as the specific prevention for prostate difficulty and the specific guarantee for male potency as Dr. Devrient states? Certainly the function of seeds in carrying the life spark from one generation to the next approximates the function of the reproductive organs in human beings. There seems little doubt that the actual chemical substances that enable the seed to germinate and to produce another plant with the characteristics of the parent are present in reproductive organs of animals—the same hormones, the same enzymes, the same vitamins and minerals.

Primitive agricultural people observe, of course, how seeds reproduce, and without any knowledge of chemistry, of vitamins, hormones and all the rest, are able to apply the same natural laws to their own health. If you want to be the father of many children, they believe, eat that part of the plant that is responsible for producing more plants. Nothing could be simpler or more obvious.

We think pumpkin seeds would make an excellent addition to your between-meal snacks. Eat some every day. They're delicious, crunchy, easy to eat and—best of all—completely satisfying due to their high protein and fat content.

63. The Prostate Gland and Zinc

The normal prostate gland contains more zinc than any other organ in the body. Sperm cells, processed by the prostate gland, contain more zinc than any other part of the gland. These facts were turned up rather recently and several researchers have been doing further study on them. What do they mean from the point of view of the health of the prostate gland? Is it possible that a deficiency of zinc in the diet might be at least partly responsible for trouble with the prostate gland?

Zinc is a trace mineral—that is, a mineral which exists in very small amounts that can just barely be "traced." It has been found to be an important part of a body enzyme, "carbonic anhydrase." This enzyme takes an essential part in conveying carbon dioxide in the blood and is also concerned in some way with the body's acid-alkaline balance. All of these mechanisms would be considerably hindered if the body lacked zinc.

In laboratory experiments, it has been found that a diet lacking in zinc causes some of these changes in animals: decrease in growth, hair that does not grow properly, spots around the mouth like those of patients suffering from vitamin B deficiency, changes in the eyes that suggest vitamin B deficiency. In the complete absence of zinc, reproduction is seriously affected. The association with vitamin B deficiency symptoms suggests, says Monier-Williams in *Trace Elements in Food* (Wiley) that zinc may somehow be related to the body's absorption of vitamins. Perhaps, if sufficient zinc is lacking, the body cannot properly absorb B vitamins and this leads to a deficiency in these as well.

Zinc and the Pancreas

In addition to the prostate gland, zinc is concentrated in the human body mostly in the liver and spleen, although the pancreas contains considerable amounts. Diabetics know that the insulin they take is generally "protomine zinc insulin."

The necessity of zinc for the pancreas can best be explained from the point of view of the diabetic. The pancreas of the diabetic does not secrete enough insulin to regulate the blood sugar level properly. So insulin is given by injection. It is desirable to spread this insulin out in the blood stream as slowly as possible so that it will be some time before more insulin is needed. It has been found that the addition of zinc to the insulin prolongs its effect on blood sugar. Thus we see how powerful an infinitely small amount of this mineral is in the working of one organ of the body. It seems quite possible that the relation of zinc to the prostate gland may be just as important.

One further fact about zinc and the pancreas. The pancreas of the diabetic person contains only about half as much zinc as the normal one. This certainly suggests that zinc may play a very big part in the normal functioning of the pancreas and lack of it may be partly responsible for trouble here.

It has been discovered that the same thing is true of the prostate gland. The sick one contains far less zinc than the normal one. According to one group of investigators, concentrations of zinc in the normal prostate tissue and in the swollen gland are about the same. But cancer of the prostate and infection of the prostate result in considerably less zinc in the gland. Other investigators have found that the zinc content of the prostate is lowered in any disorder of the gland. So it seems that zinc may be just as important to the functioning of this gland as it is to the pancreas.

Furthermore, it has been found that the semen itself is extremely rich in zinc. Three researchers, George R. Prout, M.D., Michael Sierp, M.D., and Willet F. Whitmore, M.D., who performed experiments with radioactive zinc and wrote about them in the *Journal of the American Medical Association* for April 11, 1959, conclude their article on zinc and the prostate with this paragraph: "Still unanswered is the major question regarding genital zinc. What is its function? As pointed out elsewhere, sperm are richer in zinc than any human tissue studied, yet the testis is relatively poor in this element. From this observation alone, it would seem that zinc is related to spermatic physiology. It is conceivable that the prostate acts as nothing more than a purveyor and receptacle for zinc

[273]

until ejaculation occurs and at this time zinc is incorporated in the sperm in a perhaps essential capacity. Certainly, under the conditions of the experiments, the unfailing appearance of Zn 65 (that is, radioactive zinc) in prostatic fluid and the prostate suggests that prostatic fluid without zinc would no longer be prostatic fluid."

Are We Getting Enough Zinc in Our Diets?

All of the researchers insist that zinc is plentiful in the diets of Americans and there couldn't possibly be a deficiency. However, we are always skeptical of conclusions like this. First of all, do we know how much zinc is needed by the average person on a day-to-day basis?

Trace Elements in Food by Monier-Williams tells us that human requirements for zinc have been given tentatively by one authority as .3 milligrams per kilogram for a child. Another decided from his calculations that the average person may get about 12 milligrams daily. On the other hand, it has been found that children who were getting as much as 15 to 16 milligrams daily have retained most of it, suggesting that the requirement for it may be quite high. So we don't really know how much we need of this mineral and whether even a good diet contains an unneeded abundance.

We must remember, too, that there may be a relationship between zinc and the B vitamins. Sufferers from beriberi (a B vitamin-deficiency disease) showed a lack of zinc in their tissues. Hair, nails and skin of beriberi sufferers contain only half that found in healthy persons. So perhaps individuals who are short on B vitamins may also be short on zinc. We do not as yet fully understand the relationship here.

We do know, however, that millions of Americans are not getting enough vitamin B in their daily meals. This fact keeps turning up time after time in nutrition surveys.

So we would conclude that quite possibly many Americans *are* short on zinc, for one reason or another.

The person who eats a good diet, nutritionally speaking, will certainly not suffer from a zinc deficiency. Eggs, wheat germ, liver, legumes and poultry should furnish him with plenty of zinc, along with fresh fruits and green vegetables which are somewhat lower in their zinc content. But what about the average American (male especially) who has coffee for breakfast, a white-bread sandwich, a piece of pie and more coffee for lunch, and for dinner spaghetti or pizza pie or meat with white bread and a bakery dessert? With the exception of the bit of meat at lunch and at dinner, such a day's menu contains nothing of any account in the way of minerals, least of all zinc which occurs in minute quantities even in those foods in which it is most plentiful.

Consider for a moment the difference in zinc content of a diet like the kind that we recommend. Breakfast consisting of fruit, eggs and wheat germ; lunch and dinner consisting of meat or fish with fresh raw vegetables and fruits and nuts. Sunflower seeds for dessert. Liver once a week or oftener and varied food supplements like yeast, rich in zinc. Bone meal and kelp—two other food supplements recommended highly for their mineral content—also contain zinc. Do you see the difference such a diet can make in the intake of a mineral so scanty and so little-known as zinc? Do you agree that the wide incidence of prostate disorders in civilized countries today may be closely related to a lack of zinc in diet?

Foods Rich in Zinc

Which foods are richest in it? Here is a list showing the approximate zinc content of a number of foods.

.25 to 2 P.P.M. (*parts per million*)—*apples, oranges, lemons, figs, grapes, chestnuts, pulpy fruits generally, blanched green vegetables, mineral waters, honey.*

2 to 8 P.P.M.—*raspberries, loganberries, dates, unblanched green vegetables, most sea fish, lean beef, milk, polished rice, beets, bananas, celery, tomatoes, asparagus, carrots, radishes, potatoes, mushrooms, coffee.*

8 to 20 P.P.M.—*some cereals, yeast, onions, brown rice, whole eggs, almonds.*

20 to 50 P.P.M.—*oatmeal, barleymeal, cocoa, molasses, egg yolk, rabbit, chicken, nuts, peas, beans, lentils, tea, dried yeast, mussels.*

Over 50 P.P.M.—*wheat germ* (140), *wheat bran* (75 to 140), *oysters* (270 *to* 600), *beef liver* (30 *to* 85), *gelatin.*

SECTION 14: THE SKIN

64. Skin Problems on Contact

The dialing of a telephone results in a ring of blisters around one victim's index finger; another finds that turning his car key and zipping his brief case have caused the itchy blisters that are so bothersome. The patient suffers from contact dermatitis, or, more simply, skin disease from the touch of an object. In recent years, tracking down the cause of dermatitis conditions has become highly specialized, and sometimes the search may go on for months. Success depends on many factors, including the ingenuity of the doctor in interpreting the shape and type of skin disturbance as well as the patient's powers of recall. The doctor must puzzle out, from just where the sores appear and how they develop, what object one would contact only in these spots, and whether it is liquid or solid, round or flat, rod or rope, etc. Then, to cooperate, the patient must try to record his every contact throughout the day, he must try to remember any changes that might have occurred in his daily schedule—any clue he can offer might carry in it the key to his problem. Imagine, of the thousands of things one touches in a day, narrowing the suspects down to the dial of a telephone! This dermatology business is tricky.

Women Suffer More Than Men

We are told in Dr. George Waldbott's book, *Contact Dermatitis* (published by Charles C. Thomas, Springfield, Illinois), that all age groups are subject to contact dermatitis. Even infants of a few weeks of age have been known to be sensitive to their mothers' lipstick. Incidence is shown, however, to be more prevalent in later life than in the early years. Also, women are known to be more susceptible than men—the percentage of women who suffer from contact dermatitis is almost double that of men. Though it has not been proven, it is supposed that the large variety of cosmetics, hair dyes and perfumes employed by women account for this difference.

Substances Break Through the Skin's Barriers

The normal skin has built-in defenses against the invasion of foreign elements. These are two important barriers, the horny layer of epidermis and the oily secretion of the sebaceous glands. Substances which are capable of destroying either of these defenses are those which are most likely to reach the living cells beneath the skin in sufficient quantities to cause sensitivity which shows itself in the form of itchy or painful blistering and scabbing.

The materials which are most likely to penetrate the skin are usually oily in character—plant oils or certain lubricating oils cling to the fatty covering of the skin and dissolve more readily than water soluble materials. Certain dyes have the ability to become fixed in the horny layer of the skin. During their prolonged stay, the elements of the dyes come into intimate contact with the sensitive cells, and eruption of tiny blisters often results. Other common offenders are metallic salts and local anesthetics.

All of these sources are easily contacted in an ordinary day's activities. The plants which give off oils which cause dermatitis are common enough; ivy, oak, sumac, chrysanthemums, ragweed, certain bulbs, etc. The dyes are everywhere: leather shoes, wallets, belts, colored clothing, furs, gloves and many more objects that are dyed, including soaps, fingernail polishes, hair rinses, toilet tissues, powders and lipsticks. Among the metals nickel and aluminum are the worst offenders, but can one get through a day without contacting one of these somewhere in his normal activities?

Cosmetics—A Chief Offender

Perhaps it is well here to discuss more specific causes of dermatitis which can and should be avoided in anticipation of the trouble they can cause. Chief among these is cosmetics. The general use of cosmetic products among women and men in the United States has boomed the sales to well over a billion and a half dollars per year. And some of these are actually dangerous in every sense of the word!

Hair dyes, for example, contain metallic salts, such as lead, copper, silver and iron, as well as aniline dyes which are especially harmful. Even the vegetable dyes used in these preparations (henna, indigo and walnut) contain damaging components. Infections are not uncommon and even death from the use of hair dyes has been reported in extremely sensitive cases.

Dr. Waldbott warns that no one should permit her hair to be dyed without careful preliminary testing. Even if the dye has been used before without ill effects, subsequent applications might still be dangerous since the skin could have become sensitized in the interim. We say, stay away from hair dye entirely. It makes the hair coarse and robs it of any body and resiliency it might possess. Besides, nothing is more attractive than hair, no matter what its color, which is kept well-brushed and neatly arranged, and which is healthy due to proper nutrition. The health-minded person will always avoid hair dye of any kind.

How Can You Get Clean Without Soap?

One of the questions which keeps recurring in our mail is this: How can one get clean without using soap? Critics of our stand against the use of soap will be interested in the opinion of Dr. Waldbott, one of the country's outstanding allergists, concerning this matter: "A patient can take his daily baths without soaps and cleanse his body sufficiently by gently rubbing the skin with a dry towel after the bath." It is well known that soaps can cause dermatitis in sensitive persons, and in those not so sensitive, who are frequently exposed. Further, the use of soap is likely to aggravate any existing skin problem no matter what its original cause. Sensitivity to soap is usually attributed to coloring matter, or the medications and perfumes included in various kinds. But the basic composition of soap makes it a natural troublemaker. The soap molecule includes an oil soluble fatty acid and a water soluble alkali. The alkali softens and dissolves the protective layers of the skin, and both it and the fatty acid are likely to produce skin irritation. Since we know that soap isn't essential in cleansing the body, why invite the problems of soap dermatitis by using it?

You can pick up a dandy skin problem from the use of drugs, too. Dr. Waldbott tells us that, "Any allergic disease as well as practically every known dermatological break in the skin may result from sensitivity to drugs." There is no drug whatsover that is free from sensitizing properties. These two facts alone should serve as sufficient caution against the indiscriminate use of drugs. And remember, aspirin is a drug; pep pills and tranquilizers are drugs. Avoid them. Substitute good diet for them, and you'll soon see a pleasing difference in yourself.

[277]

Pruritus Ani Often Due to Contact

Under the general topic of dermatitis we must also mention a condition commonly experienced but generally neglected in medical magazines for the public—pruritus ani, or itching of the rectum. It seems that the rectum is a very likely location for contact dermatitis. Not only are the sources of contact more numerous than one would imagine (soap, clothing, toilet tissue, enema nozzles, suppositories, orally administered antibiotics which have passed through the digestive system and laxatives), but the area is moist and covered, so that germs and fungi have an excellent breeding ground. The foods we eat which pass out of the body undigested, in fecal matter, might also cause a reaction with the tender skin of the rectum. This is especially true of such foods as mustard, horseradish and hot peppers.

Moisture, which is always aggravating to skin rashes, is constantly present in the rectal area due to a system of sweat glands which are part of the sexual glandular system. These glands are highly responsive to emotion or sexual tension, so that a person in a highly emotional state or one who is excited sexually exudes large amounts of perspiration in this region. The perspiration which is released here is high in proteins and carbohydrates, two elements which favor the growth of bacteria. This increased moisture also leads to the release of dyes from clothing worn in this region, and these dyes can initiate or aggravate a condition of pruritus ani. Once the condition exists, the itching is more severe than in most areas of the body, due perhaps to the abundant nerve supply and the delicacy of the skin. Few victims can resist scratching, and the added irritation only causes a worsening of the condition.

Diet and Pruritus Ani

It is known that pruritus ani is sometimes coupled with a lack of certain dietary constituents. Vitamin A and the B complex, as well as iron, are often mentioned in this connection. Diabetes is frequently accompanied by a fungus infection of the rectum, due to the high sugar content of the skin, which favors the growth of fungi. Good diet would be the very first thing to check—is one getting sufficient B vitamin foods (liver, brewer's yeast, wheat germ, sunflower seeds) and those rich in vitamin A (carrots, squash, dark green vegetables) and iron (grapes and raisins, celery, liver). Editor Rodale found that excessive use of citrus juices could cause an irritation of this area. There appears to be considerable evidence that such a relationship is not rare.

Effective treatment of this condition is based on these general principles: keep the area clean by careful removal of all fecal matter, but do not use soap or toilet tissue, for both of these should be avoided. The use of clear tap water is best. Then dry with cotton or a soft, clean cloth. Do not scratch through clothing, as harmful dyes are readily introduced in this way. White underclothes should be worn to lessen this possibility. The area should be kept as dry as possible, and no ointments or greasy salves should be used.

Food and Contact Dermatitis

Dr. Waldbott brought out an interesting point in his book with regard to food sensitivity. He says that contact with the food itself is not always the cause of a reaction, but the disinfectants and insect sprays that are on it might be. Not to be forgotten are the toxic colorings on citrus fruits and those chemicals used in wrapping and packaging the food (e.g. colored papers, plastics) for they often contain sensitizing agents.

Consider the possibilities of contact dermatitis in daily life, and try to avoid having possible causes of this uncomfortable disease around you. Avoid cosmetics especially for they are great offenders. Above all, keep your nutrition at a good level, for a healthy body can help greatly in minimizing the effects of harsh irritants to the skin.

65. Detergent Dermatitis

The most effective claim a detergent can make—even more important than whether or not it is an effective cleaner—is that it is kinder to hands. Along with the advertised quick efficiency of modern detergents has come the almost universal complaint that they literally eat into the skin.

One of the most common points of attack is the tender portion under the fingernails. In the *Journal of the American Medical Association* (November, 1958) Dr. Peter I. Long gives histories of 3 patients who experienced great pain and severe hemorrhages under the fingernails as a result of the irritant factor in detergents. An interesting sidelight to each of these cases is that the victims actually wore heavy rubber gloves to protect their hands. Some of the water got into the gloves and collected in the fingers, thereby serving as a constant irritant to the wearer's finger tips. Further, through some reaction with the rubber, the acidity of the water in the gloves was actually higher than that which was in the dishpan. As surer protection against detergent irritation, we have seen a suggestion that one wear cotton gloves under rubber gloves when exposing the hands to detergent water.

Skin Irritation Almost Certain

There is no doubt that detergents are hard on the skin. In the *Journal of the American Medical Association* (June 22, 1957), Dr. Matthew J. Brunner told of experiments in which dermatitis (skin irritation) was produced by repeated hand-soaking in detergent water. He stated that women engaged in housework suffer from hand dermatitis more frequently

[279]

than those engaged in occupations in which contact with detergents doesn't occur. The *Southern Medical Journal* (January, 1954) concurs, saying that "the number of cases of housewives' eczema has increased many times," since the advent of soapless detergents.

The explanation for this unprecedented irritation of the skin, according to *Consumers Research Bulletin* (January, 1954), is that contact with detergent solutions damages keratin, a fibrous protein that forms the outer coating of the skin. When the harsh chemicals contained in detergents eat away this protective substance, the tender underlayers of the skin are defenseless against a similar attack.

A Suit Results

An indication of how serious detergent dermatitis can be is seen in a case brought to the district court of Winona, Minnesota, involving a Mrs. Bruce Miller and the Proctor and Gamble Distributing Company. (*Golden Valley News,* Beach, North Dakota, January 27, 1955). The plaintiff asserted that she had suffered severe burns due to the use of that firm's detergent products, Tide and Joy. The resultant infection had Mrs. Miller hospitalized for several weeks. Several specialists were called in to help rid the lady of the stubborn infection, and one of them, Dr. John J. Sevents, of La Crosse, Wisconsin, testified that the condition was certainly due to Mrs. Miller's contact with Tide. He added that his experience had shown that detergents are a common cause of such infections of the hands. With that, Proctor and Gamble settled out of court.

Chemical Week (July 24, 1954) gives an interesting list of statistics on the way detergents act. For example, they are more likely to irritate the skins of blondes than brunettes; men are more susceptible to irritation than females; Negroes are least susceptible. The condition of the skin is important; oily skins are less easily affected than dry skins, and excess perspiration increases chances of contracting dermatitis and makes existing dermatitis worse.

Cost to Industry

In industry, soaps and alkalis are rated among the leading causes of occupational disease which cost employers about one hundred million dollars per year. Skin diseases constitute 60 per cent of the total types of disability, and the aforementioned soaps and alkalis are responsible for the largest proportion of these cases.

If one must be exposed to detergent solutions, the suggestions carried in the *Medical Journal of Australia* (November 24, 1956) might help: (1.) avoid making unnecessarily strong solutions (the ads boast about the relatively small amounts needed); (2.) rinse and dry the hands after exposure (the longer the solution, or any residue of it, remains in contact with the skin, the more chance of irritation developing).

66. Skin Health and Soaps

An inquiry from an attorney representing a client who believed she had contracted a dermatitis from using a detergent caused us to search for material on the subject. We found two very enlightening articles dealing with detergents, soaps and other cleansers in their relation to skin health.

Joseph V. Klauder, M.D., of Philadelphia, writing in the *Archives of Dermatology and Syphilology*, Vol. 63, 1951, tells us that a total of 3,709 cases of skin diseases have been presented for claims for compensation under the Pennsylvania law since this law went into effect. Of these, 1,673 were occupational in origin; 2,036 were non-occupational. Of the occupational dermatoses, 13.1 per cent were the result of "wet work"—that is, working in water, water and soap or water and detergents.

Dr. Klauder reviews standard tests of the ability of the skin to withstand such substances. The normal pH (acidity) of the skin on the hands ranges from 4.5 to 6.5, so normal skin is acid. When the skin is bathed in sweat, its acidity increases. Exposing the hands to alkali increases the alkalinity of their skin in proportion to the length of time they are exposed and the frequency, and the degree of alkalinity. The two persons in Dr. Klauder's article whose hands required the longest time to return to normal were two dishwashers whose hands, of course, were in soapy water most of their working time. It was discovered that not until 20 hours after their hands had been exposed to soap and water did the pH of their skin return to normal. This means that during their daily work their hands were constantly in an abnormal, alkaline condition, for the pH did not ever have time to return to normal on those days. On their days off they might expect a normal condition of the skin on their hands just as they were ready to go back to work!

Dr. Klauder studied the effects of many commercial detergents and reported on them: 7 nonsoap detergents advised for dermatitic hands, 103 hand cleaners for industrial workers and 19 nonsoap detergents for kitchen and household purposes. Of the 103 hand cleaners, 94 were alkaline and 57 were gritty powders which contained one or more alkaline salt detergents.

The Normal Skin Is Acid

A. L. Hudson, M.D., of Toronto, Canada, writing in the *Canadian Medical Association Journal* for January, 1951, tells us more about the effect of soaps and detergents as well as different drugs, shampoos and ointments on the skin. We have somehow come to think of alkalinity as something to be highly desired. But when speaking of the skin, it is well to remember that alkalinity is not normal. Dr. Hudson tells us that normal skin has a pH from 4 to 6, depending on the location of the skin and when it was last washed with an alkaline substance. In parts of the body where a great deal of perspiration is excreted, the acidity is greater. And, naturally, in hot weather this *p*H goes even lower, for then there is more perspiration. This normally acid condition of the skin is spoken of as "the acid mantle." If one can maintain a constantly acid condition of the skin, one can prevent the development of contact dermatitis since the skin is much more susceptible to disease when alkaline.

Tests have shown that a skin area with a normal *p*H of 4 shows a *p*H of 7 one minute after it is washed with soap and may require 70 minutes before the skin returns to its normal *p*H. When washing with some soaps it has been shown that this increased alkalinity may be present for as long as 3½ hours. We should keep in mind that when we talk of alkalinity in connection with soap, we mean all soap, because alkali is set free in water as soon as soap is put into it and the alkalinity of the solution may rise to as high as 10 or 11.

When there are certain kinds of disorder present in the skin, this change to alkalinity is more marked and more prolonged in the diseased area and the skin directly around it. In summer, when the skin is normally more acid, it takes less time to return to the normal *p*H after using the soap. This may be the reason, says Dr. Hudson, why so many more people complain of dermatitis and eczema on their hands in winter. Variations in normal skin acidity occur according to: the character and quantity of perspiration, the prevention of evaporation of this perspiration, the amount of secretion of the oily glands of the skin which becomes alkaline as it is evaporating. So the acidity of the skin and, to a certain extent, the health of the skin, depend on the composition of sweat and how much of it is left unevaporated on the skin. Other conditions aside from washing with soap make the skin alkaline—dust, disintegrated sweat glands, seborrhea, psoriasis, tuberculosis and several other skin diseases.

It seems obvious that medicines, ointments or soaps applied to any part of the body where the alkalinity is already high should, if possible, be acid, so that they may bring that part back to normal acidity rather than increasing the alkalinity. Especially in the case of fungus growths, such as cause athlete's foot, any medication used should make the skin more, rather than less, acid. Of course, soap on athlete's foot is bound to increase the alkalinity still further and make the condition worse.

In testing soaps and shampoos, Dr. Hudson reports on Canadian products with which we are not familiar, but mentions several American products as well: Ivory soap has a *p*H of 7.5 which means that it is quite alkaline. French castile is somewhat better with a *p*H of 6. Tide, the detergent, has a *p*H of 9.5—extremely alkaline. Drene shampoo has a *p*H of 6.5 and Halo a *p*H of 4.

Dr. Hudson's Conclusions

Dr. Hudson summarizes by telling us that the *p*H of the skin is the result of the physiological functions of the skin and is changed by certain environmental conditions and/or agents and by disease. Soaps increase the *p*H for relatively long periods and thus may make the skin much more susceptible to irritants or allergenic material. Once a dermatitis has been contracted, the use of soap will prolong it by keeping the skin alkaline rather than allowing it to return to its normal pH. So using soap or alkaline detergents is the most harmful thing you can do under these conditions.

If you have one of the skin conditions mentioned, you are probably being treated by a physician, so there is no further precaution you should take except to avoid soaps and detergents like the very plague. If your hands, feet and legs suffer in cold weather (and what housewife can honestly say she never has trouble with rough, painful hands in winter?), you would do well to take every precaution against exposure to soaps and detergents. It's awkward to use gloves for every kind of household task, but it's worth it in the end. So when you are doing laundry, washing dishes, cleaning and especially if you are using water outside in the winter, make certain that you do wear gloves, for you will be protecting your hands against painful roughness and possible skin disease.

Too many of us are likely to dismiss rough winter hands as "a bad case of chapping" and rub on some lotion which we hope will make them smooth again. Alkaline soaps and detergents, as we have seen, produce a definite unhealthy state of skin by the chemical action of changing the pH of the skin. And many kinds of disorders may result. You can buy lined rubber gloves these days which are much easier to work in, as well as to put on and remove. You can buy gloves with ridged fingers so that wet, slippery dishes will not slip out of your hands.

67. Skin Trouble from the Linings of Shoes

Among the many tormenting disorders of the feet are dermatoses—that is, afflictions of the skin of the feet. We understand from doctors that these conditions are rather common and may often be wrongly diagnosed due to the similarity of symptoms among the various ailments—the fungi, the bacterial infections and the inflammations that may occur from other causes. It seems that allergies to the various materials used in shoe manufacture frequently cause foot skin troubles, often serious enough to warrant an immediate trip to the doctor; sometimes not so serious, so that the patient tries to cure the condition himself and does not go to the doctor until his home remedies have failed. Apparently the doctor quite frequently diagnoses wrongly, for often what appear to be fungus infections may turn out to be allergies to shoe material.

Two researchers, Irvin H. Blank, Ph.D., and Owen G. Miller, M.D., did a study of 24 cases of dermatitis of the feet which seemed to be caused by shoes. In the *Journal of the American Medical Association* for August 9, 1952, they described their search for the possible causes. They studied the different linings of the shoes and found that the patients appeared to be sensitive not to the linings themselves but to the adhesive with which they were glued together. They then collected from shoe manufacturers samples of as many as possible of these different adhesives and patch-tested their patients with the material.

Ten representative "antioxidants" and 17 "accelerators" used in making the adhesives were tested on the patients. Apparently none of these was responsible for the dermatoses. But, of course, the doctors did not know which of these substances, if any, had been used in any of the shoes their patients had worn. So they went to a manufacturer of shoe linings and got all the separate ingredients and combinations of ingredients used in linings. These included: various kinds of rubber, an antioxidant, a tackifier, a plasticizer, a peptizing agent and two accelerators. Now we are not in the business of manufacturing shoe linings and we do not know what all these various chemicals are or why their use should be necessary. However, judging from the chemical names of these substances, we'd say they are all made from coal tar. "It soon became apparent" the authors tell us, "that the patients reacted violently to the antioxidant and to any combination of ingredients containing the antioxidant." Other patients were recalled and found to react violently, too.

Sleuthing for Chemicals in Shoe Lining Adhesives

Then linings were made up and put into shoes. The offending antioxidant was included in the lining of one shoe and not in the other. The patient was not told which shoe contained which lining. Every patient showed blisters on the foot which had been in contact with the antioxidant. The blisters occurred 12 to 24 hours after the shoes had been worn for 30 minutes.

The report suggests that allergy should be considered as a possible cause of mysterious dermatoses of the feet. But furthermore, if you were a doctor trying earnestly to diagnose a patient's complaint, wouldn't you become awfully impatient with having to wade through all this time-consuming research just to find out what might or might not be present in the linings of shoes? Some doctors will, of course, read this article in the *Journal* and will be alerted to the dangers of sensitivity to shoe lining adhesive. But even when they decide that this may be what is causing their patient's trouble, they, too, will have to spend many hours or possibly days or weeks trying to find out what is in the offending shoe linings and then trying to locate for their patients some shoes in which this same substance is not used.

Would it be too much to ask, do you think, that shoe manufacturers list on the label or the box all the chemical ingredients that go into the make-up of their shoes? How else will physicians be equipped to deal with foot dermatoses caused by sensitivity to chemicals used in the shoes?

68. The Mystery of Psoriasis

"The cause of psoriasis is unknown." "Psoriasis is a disease of healthy persons." "Psoriasis is a constitutional disorder." "This skin disease has stubbornly defied all attempts to conquer it for almost 350 years."

This is the kind of statement we found when we worked our way back through 50 years of medical and scientific literature looking carefully for all available material on psoriasis. We started our search because the number of letters we receive asking for information on this subject convinced us that this must be one of the most widespread disorders of modern life. Indeed it is one of the 4 most prevalent skin disorders. And it currently affects about 4 per cent of all individuals with skin ailments.

Yet medical science says its cause is unknown. Recommendations for treatment consist largely of salves, ointments, compresses. Yet throughout all the articles we read, there was a pattern which indicated to us that psoriasis must be a disease involving chiefly incorrect diet. Hence it should be easily preventable and perhaps easily cured by proper diet.

Psoriasis seems to run in families, we are told. (So do bad eating habits.) Psoriasis is unknown among primitive peoples in tropical countries. (Possibly climate explains this, but what about civilized diet versus natural diet?) Psoriasis may be related to arthritic conditions. (These certainly are caused by wrong diet.) Complaints of psoriasis always increase during fall and winter months and decrease during spring and summer. (Cold weather and dry heat in our homes? Possibly, but what about the kind of food we eat in winter?) Overweight patients report that their psoriasis improves when they diet carefully and lose weight. (Doesn't this suggest that wrong diet created both the psoriasis and the overweight?)

Time and again we come back to the positive suggestion that psoriasis is a disease involving incorrect use of fatty foods by the body. Those researchers who have achieved any measure of success treating the disease have concerned themselves chiefly with elements of diet involved in fat metabolism.

What are these elements of diet? First, of course, the fat soluble vitamins—that is, the vitamins which exist and are soluble in fats and oils, rather than those that are soluble in water. The fat soluble vitamins are vitamins A, D, E, K and those fairly mysterious substances we are just now investigating which some researchers call vitamin F—the essential unsaturated fatty acids.

In addition, we must not forget that certain of the B vitamins are necessary in the diet if the body is going to use fatty substances properly. Pyridoxine, a B vitamin, must be present in the digestive tract if we are going to digest and use properly the unsaturated fatty acids. It is believed that inositol, another B vitamin, is concerned in the metabolism of fats.

[285]

Choline, still another B vitamin, is necessary for fats to be transported in the body from the liver to their proper destination.

No One Or Two Things Are Responsible

So obviously no one thing is concerned in psoriasis or any other disorder involving fats in food. Many things are concerned. And we believe that this is the reason medical science has failed to find a cure or preventive for psoriasis. Researchers are specialists; they deal in one thing or one set of things. Someone who is studying vitamin A and patiently goes through experiment after experiment observing the results of lack of vitamin A, or medium or large doses of vitamin A may not be getting the answer because, for significant results, he may have to employ some or all of the vitamins we mentioned above.

However, it is interesting to note that research on psoriasis has involved almost exclusively the fat soluble vitamins and vitamin B, which seems to indicate that we are on the right track when we talk of these substances in relation to this pesky chronic disease.

Nowhere could we find any evidence of what we think would be an ideal way to run down the cause or causes of the disease—a survey of, say, several hundred psoriatics which would include in great detail everything they eat over the course of several months. Comparing this to the day-by-day diet of several hundred individuals who are free from psoriasis should certainly indicate what items of diet might be involved in the disease.

However, we must depend instead on reports of scattered trials with vitamins, like the following: A diet low in protein was tried by one physician who believed that too much nitrogen (which occurs in protein) might be responsible. Such a diet could be administered only in a hospital. Results were confusing, because local treatment was used as well. And, of course, on this basis it is impossible to explain the occurrence of psoriasis in vegetarians whose diet naturally contains less nitrogen than diets containing meat.

A low salt diet appeared to benefit several cases. A low fat diet (20 grams of fat per day) seemed to bring improvement. In young people two or three weeks might be necessary to show this improvement; on older folks 6 weeks or longer might be necessary. In stubborn cases as long as 6 or 8 months might be needed. Hospitalization seemed to be necessary.

A Recommended Diet

The diet that interested us most was tried by Gross and Kesten and reported in the *New York State Journal of Medicine*, Vol. 50, p. 2683, 1950. In this diet eggs, fat meats, poultry, fish, cheese and excessive amounts of butter and cream were eliminated. And soybean lecithin was given freely along with vitamins A and D and the following B vitamins: thiamin, pyridoxine, riboflavin and pantothenic acid. Of 235 patients treated, 23 remained well after one year of therapy and two and one half years of observation.

This may not seem like a very large percentage of cures. However the cures were accomplished by diet alone and, judging from the length of time the patients remained well, the cure seemed to be permanent. Had brewer's yeast been used and a diet of completely natural foods, perhaps the rate of cure would have been much higher.

It is interesting to note that Carroll S. Wright in the chapter on skin diseases in the book by Wohl and Goodhart, *Modern Nutrition in Health and Disease* (Lea and Febiger, 1955) comments, after reporting on the diet outlined above, "The present writer has often seen psoriatics enter the hospital for various gastro-intestinal disorders which interfered with normal eating and improve remarkably without benefit of any particular vitamin or local therapy. . . . One cannot help concluding that it is restriction of food that is primarily important in the treatment of psoriasis. . . ."

An article in *Your Health* for fall, 1949, titled "New Hope in Psoriasis" is written by Herman Goodman, M.D., one of our country's best-known dermatologists. He describes a new medicine which had been successfully tried on a small number of patients. The name of it is unimportant—we could find no other mention of it anywhere in medical literature. But, "it is one of a group of lipids—fatlike chemicals—which include lecithin and vitamin A," says Dr. Goodman. Lecithin is a substance rich in unsaturated fatty acids, other important fats and the B vitamins we mentioned above —those the body must have to use fats properly.

We know that the skin is a most sensitive indicator of mistakes in diet. Certain skin disorders are a sure sign of vitamin A deficiency. Skin eruptions are always present in several diseases that spring from vitamin B deficiency. Vitamin D is manufactured in the skin when the ultraviolet rays of the sun fall on it. Eczema in children has been known to disappear almost miraculously when fats containing lecithin or the unsaturated fatty acids were added to the child's diet. In fact Adelle Davis in her book, *Let's Eat Right to Keep Fit* (Harcourt Brace and Company, New York, New York), says, "Even the stubborn eczema-like condition known as psoriasis usually disappears rapidly when salad oils and lecithin are added to the diet."

The Kind of Fat You Eat Is the Important Thing

If indeed the answer to psoriasis lies in those elements in diet which concern fats, how is it possible that the disease should affect so many present-day Americans? Don't we have plenty of fairly inexpensive fats available for anyone to eat? However, the important thing is not the quantity of fat you eat. It's the kind of fat you eat that is important. Fats occur naturally in many foods of animal and vegetable origin. Seeds are our chief source in the vegetable kingdom—grains, nuts, sunflower seeds, etc. Butter, milk, eggs and fat meats are sources in food of animal origin.

From the vegetable fats our refining processes have removed much that is of value nutritionally speaking—especially lecithin and the B vitamins that go along with it in nature. White flour, for instance, contains none of these valuable substances. Doesn't it seem to you that anyone who has eaten white bread and other foods made from white flour would be bound to suffer from deficiencies in these substances? Wheat germ contains lecithin and all the B vitamins. But wheat germ is a "fad food," we are told.

Many vegetable fats such as corn oil, peanut oil and so forth are hydrogenated these days. This means that hydrogen is forced through them during a chemical process which destroys the unsaturated fatty acids—those essential fatty substances which we must have to be healthy. Hydrogenated shortenings are the thick, white ones, used for frying and baking. Margarine is hydrogenated, and commercial peanut butter. And, speaking of frying, did you know that the nutritious elements in fats are destroyed when you fry foods and there is abundant evidence that extremely harmful substances are formed in their place?

Finally, of course, our present-day refined and processed diets almost completely eliminate the B vitamins, for they are destroyed ruthlessly when food is processed.

Some Healthful Suggestions

What, then, are our recommendations if you would avoid psoriasis? Watch your diet with the eye of a hawk. And we mean be conscious of every mouthful of food you eat. Eat little fatty food of any kind. Those you do eat should be all natural fats—eggs, for instance contain lots of lecithin—they are good for you. Salad oils and fats from other vegetable sources (not hydrogenated, processed or fried) such as sunflower seeds, avocados, raw nuts—these are healthful fats.

Shun the "hidden fats" which you are bound to encounter if you buy any packaged foods at all or if you eat in restaurants. Crackers are crisp because of the hydrogenated shortening they contain—these are not for you. Cake mixes, baked goods, anything fried, gravies, sauces are taboo.

Eat your meats, poultry and fish broiled or roasted, without gravy. Eat plenty of fruits and vegetables, as many raw as possible. Ignore desserts as if they did not exist—any and all desserts except fresh raw fruits. Sugar and white flour rob your body of B vitamins. Put your sugar bowl up on the shelf with the other antiques. It's out of date if you would be healthy.

Baker's bread (any kind of bread made in a factory) may contain a variety of unhealthful fats, even including synthetic ones made of chemicals with no relation to food at all—fats the human body has never encountered up until 10 or 15 years ago.

Surely years from now we will discover to our shame what harm we have been doing ourselves with these synthetic fats. We suggest doing without bread altogether unless you have the facilities and the time to make your own out of nothing but the finest ingredients including real whole grain flour.

[288]

Then, make certain you are getting in your food supplements enough of all the food elements we mentioned above—vitamins A and D (plentiful in fish liver oils), the B vitamins (wheat germ, brewer's yeast or desiccated liver are your best sources), lecithin and/or the unsaturated fatty acids, available in flakes or in capsules.

Probably your best source of unsaturated fatty acids is sunflower seeds. They're tasty food. Eat them with fruits for dessert. Eat them instead of coffee and sweet snacks between meals.

69. Vitiligo

Almost every day inquiries come to us pleading for specific information concerning vitiligo, a painless skin disease which is characterized by the disappearance of natural color, or pigment, from patches on the skin. Even the fairest skins have some color, and when it goes, these patches of absolute white are very definitely visible and can be most embarrassing. In a darker skin the problem is emphasized.

Unfortunately, our searches through medical literature led us nowhere. There was plenty of talk about vitiligo, but we couldn't seem to find anything definite on how it can be prevented or has been treated. Now at last we have found something we can pass on. The article by Benjamin Sieve, M.D., at that time instructor in medicine, Tufts Medical School, appeared in the *Virginia Medical Monthly* (January, 1945), and it gives a comprehensive history of the other treatments in use for the 15 years before that date as well as the then-current thinking on the subject. It is our guess that very little has been accomplished in the treatment of vitiligo since then, so that Dr. Sieve's findings are still worth investigation and application.

Among some of the earlier treatments for vitiligo is that of H. W. Francis, M.D. He considered the cause to be an absence of free hydrochloric acid in the stomach because he had vitiligo and found an absence of the acid in himself. He took hydrochloric acid in 15 cubic centimeter doses at each meal for 2 years and noted that the vitiligo areas had completely disappeared. He used the same therapy on 3 other patients and reported similar results. Dr. Sieve suggests that the hydrochloric acid might help in the body's processing and absorption of necessary B vitamin factors in food.

In 1931 a paper appeared describing a Negro who suffered from vitiligo patches on his face, but was originally hospitalized for 16 weeks for treatment of a fracture. Though no specific remedy for the vitiligo was attempted, the patches regained their natural color during this time. It was assumed by the writers that the hospital diet was so far superior to that which the patient usually had, that the nutrients in it were partly responsible, along with the bedrest and absence of direct sunlight for the return of proper skin color. The theory of nutrition and pigment was followed up by an article in the *Archives of Dermatology and Syphilology* (March, 1937) on the use of vitamin C to restore skin color. The following year a German medical journal carried another article on the same subject, again recommending vitamin C as a treatment, though we do not know the dosages used.

Para-amino-benzoic acid (PABA), a B vitamin, has been mentioned repeatedly in connection with the treatment of vitiligo. M. J. Costello, in the *Archives of Dermatology and Syphilology* (February, 1943) told of success in treating vitiligo of the eyelids in a two-year-old child with the daily administration of 100 milligrams of PABA. Two others who tried this treatment did not find it so effective. Dr. Sieve was still impressed with the potential of PABA, and decided to set up an experiment to observe its effect on 48 cases of vitiligo.

Other Problems in the Group

The group consisted of 25 females and 23 males, ranging in age from 10 to 70 years. The duration of the vitiligo condition had varied from 2 to 28 years. In most of the patients evidence of a poor diet for from months to years and a history of gland imbalance was obtained. Fatigue, irritability and emotional instability were almost constant. Constipation, weight gain and various types of headaches were frequent. Arthritis was not uncommon. Physical examinations in general revealed varying types of deficiencies, of which many presented classic findings consistent with an underactive thyroid condition. Along with these came a preponderance of brittle nails, coarse and thickened skin and varying degrees of hypertension (high blood pressure).

An accurate history of each patient was obtained, including blood counts, smears, urine tests, blood sugar, basal metabolism, etc. The gland balance was established through the use of hormones. Then all patients were given a patent combination of B complex vitamins—more than the recommended daily dosage. In addition, PABA was administered in the form of 100 milligram tablets 3 or 4 times daily. This treatment continued for a period of 10 months.

The rate of improvement in the skin using oral PABA was found to be slow. Some patients followed the described regime for 18 weeks with no results. The author instituted injections of the vitamin coupled with monoethanolamine (to help the vitamin remain in the blood longer) twice daily—evening and morning—and a 100 milligram tablet of PABA to be taken at noon and at bedtime. It was soon observed by the author and by the patients themselves that new pigmentation in the depigmented areas occurred. Within 4 to 8 weeks the milk white areas of vitiligo turned pinkish. In 6 to 16 weeks after therapy was started, small islands of brown pigment were usually noted within the areas of vitiligo. Soon streaks were thrown from these islands and the streaks reached out to join other islands. Eventually the islands disappeared or the repigmentation became complete. The results of the therapy in all 48 patients were termed "striking" after 6 or 7 months.

Young Woman A Classic Case

One of Dr. Sieve's most impressive cases involved a young woman of 26 years who, when first seen, complained of irregular menstrual periods, lack of appetite, dry skin and brittle nails. She had vitiligo of the entire body, but especially both legs; now slight graying of the hair was occurring. It had all begun 13 years previously after a bruising accident. Except for mild typhoid fever at 17, and a fairly common aversion to sunlight, her history gave no special clues as to the origin of the vitiligo. She ate practically no meat or fish.

Examination showed definite gland and vitamin imbalance. The entire torso had tiny areas of pigment loss and the legs from foot to knees had large areas in which the pigment was completely gone. A growth of white hair was noted through the areas of vitiligo, and the line of demarcation between the normal skin areas and those affected was clearly defined.

The treatment instituted by Dr. Sieve consisted of two PABA tablets of 100 milligrams each and two intramuscular injections of 144 milligrams per cubic centimeter of monoethanolamine para-amino-benzoic acid (PABA) given every day. An elixir of B complex (5 cubic centimeters) was taken 3 times daily. After 4 months the number of injections was reduced to one daily, until a total of 214 had been received.

Marked improvement in the vitiligo condition was noted within 10 weeks after treatment was begun. Each successive examination showed additional improvement. After 9 months of treatment, the vitiligo throughout the body and torso was completely repigmented to such an extent that there was difficulty in distinguishing any of the areas. The hands and arms were almost entirely filled in, and the legs showed great improvement. Improvement continued through the next 6 months while the medication was taken spasmodically and there were no injections. At no time were any toxic manifestations from the medical treatment observed.

A Combination of Elements

Dr. Sieve asserts, time and again, the important part diet plays in vitiligo. He also believes that hormonal imbalance can cause the disease. Contributory factors can also be wounds, infection, pressure points and light rays. Dr. Sieve says that the problem of vitiligo is more complex than the simple lack of the B vitamin PABA. He insists that dietary deficiencies must be corrected, hormonal imbalances righted and local infections cleared up before a single specific vitamin can be expected to have any effect. He also emphasizes that the injections to supplement the tablets are essential,

[291]

because the vitamin alone, taken orally, does not remain in the blood stream for a sufficient length of time to act effectively.

The B complex, as it appears in brewer's yeast, desiccated liver, wheat germ and the organ meats, would seem to be essential in preventing the occurrence of vitiligo. This, of course, coupled with a diet complete in other essentials, will act to avoid most diseases. For those who are plagued with vitiligo, we think Dr. Sieve's article on his experience with his treatment is a godsend. At least it is something to be rid of this distressing problem—and apparently without danger of side effects. Talk to your doctor about it. Ask him if he can think of even one reason for ignoring the opportunity presented here. We feel sure he will want you to try Dr. Sieve's treatment. Incidentally, we cannot refer any inquiries to Dr. Sieve as he died several years ago. However, your doctor can, of course, send for a copy of the original article we refer to.

SECTION 15: THE TEETH

70. Tooth Decay and Diet

In a report entitled *Control of Tooth Decay,* the National Research Council discusses our present knowledge of tooth decay and suggests rather hesitantly that diet may have something to do with it. Fluoridation, of course, is safe, cheap, simple and sure, they say, giving the impression that fluoridation is probably the best answer, according to them. But they do mention diet and they do suggest a proper diet for reducing tooth decay. As usual, they give only about half of the picture.

In their suggested diet you are to be sure to get protein, green leafy and yellow vegetables, citrus fruits or tomatoes and berries, and whole or enriched cereals. Now, with such a limited recommendation as this, any school child would eat almost precisely what he is eating now—the same diet that is ravishing his teeth and making him a dental cripple by the time he is grown. He could live on white bread sandwiches, cokes, cake, candy, ice cream and all the other refined carbohydrates with a piece of carrot or fruit from time to time. We wonder why such a diet continues to be recommended. Mothers read it, check on their family's diet, and then go happily on, convinced that diet has nothing to do with decay, for this diet is just what their children are eating!

As a matter of fact, there is a great deal of literature available showing exactly what kind of diet *does* decrease tooth decay. We wonder why this kind of diet is not recommended by organizations and institutions who want to be helpful. In the *Medical Journal of Australia* for June 20, 1953, there is the story of a group of children who live on such a diet. They range in age from 4 to 9 years. The majority of them have been living in the institution, Hopewood House, since the earliest months of life. In general, their surroundings are "healthful"—that is, they have regular meals, good clothing, supervised exercise. They live as much as possible as though they were in their own homes, rather than an institution. The home is located on a 750-acre estate in the southern highlands of New South Wales.

The diet the children eat consists of: wholemeal bread, wholemeal biscuits, wholemeal porridge, wheat germ, fruits, fresh and dried vegetables (cooked and raw), a small amount of meat, butter, eggs, cheese, milk and fruit juices. Every child takes vitamins and is allowed a little honey or molasses, and occasionally nuts.

We quote from the *Journal,* "As far as possible, food was taken uncooked and/or with a minimum of preparation, the idea being to present the food in its natural state. Notable for their absence from the diet were such items as sugar (white and brown), white flour products (including cakes and sweet biscuits) and any combination of these items. No tea was used. The water was drawn from the town supply. *This water has been examined for the presence of fluoride but none was detected."* (Italics are ours.)

Tests and examinations were made of all the children for a period of about 5 years. It was found that, of 81 children, 63 had no tooth decay. This proportion of children without decay is far in excess of those in other groups throughout Australia, Canada and New Zealand. The teeth of the group as a whole were remarkable for the very small number of decay spots. No child had more than 6 teeth needing care. The rates of decay beginning and proceeding in the mouths of these children were very far below those of the population in general. Say the authors, B. Lilienthal and his associates, "The outstanding difference in the environment as between this group of children and groups living in the population at large is the nature of the diet. Foods containing refined carbohydrates (for example, sugar, white flour) are either excluded from the diet or eaten in very small amounts." We suppose that the refined foods "eaten in very small amounts" are simply those the children may get at school or from visitors. Their noonday lunch is provided by the home, however, so 3 meals a day are good, unrefined foods.

How To Get Such a Diet for Us All

In a later issue of the *Journal* (July 24, 1954) we were interested in reading a discussion of this article by H. R. Sullivan and N. E. Goldsworthy of the Institute of Dental Research of the United Dental Hospital, Sydney.

They say, "This desirable state of freedom from caries presumably can be attained by any person who is prepared to adjust his dietetic habits or those of persons in his charge so that the carbohydrate intake satisfies nutritional requirements but does not greatly exceed them and is obtained from the products of wholemeal flour and other cereals and carbohydrates, *in their natural state.* (That is, not refined or processed.) Under the conditions of western civilization the use of refined carbohydrates, including white flour products has become an accepted, almost basic, part of the dietary pattern. Therefore, in order to satisfy nutritional requirements and to prevent caries, a sustained effort is needed if we are to establish a new dietary pattern."

The rest of the article is an attempt to outline how we might go about attempting to revise present-day diets to bring them nearer to the kind of diet the children ate at the Hopewood House. By the end of the article the authors have just about convinced themselves that it cannot be done. And here are some of the reasons:

1. The disease of dental decay is neither fatal nor crippling so people don't get very upset about it.

2. People in different social strata have fixed ideas about food which are difficult to change.

3. Cultural patterns in different national groups are hard to change (those who *had* to eat black bread in the old country are determined to eat white bread in America, etc.). Then, too, there are such insurmountable difficulties in supply at local and world level, that foods simply must be refined so that they can be cheaply distributed to the consumer.

We do not believe these reasons are sound. It is our firm conviction that if our food processors could be persuaded to give us unrefined food (regardless of how many changes had to be made in production, marketing and transportation facilities), if all our mighty magazines, newspapers, radio and television networks took up the message and promoted unrefined food, within a year, practically everybody in the country would have changed over. It wouldn't be any harder than that. But so long as the merits of refined, degerminated, worthless, lifeless foods are preached day and night in every piece of reading material we pick up and every commercial we hear on the air, then just so long will it be impossible to revise our diets into healthful ones.

Why Not Tax Sugar?

We found what we believe is an excellent suggestion in the *Journal of the American Medical Association* for October 16, 1954. In a report from Sweden, we learn that the Ministry of Health in that country has outlined many voluntary measures that could be taken to reduce tooth decay there. The medical and dental professions were invited to cooperate in promoting health education on the radio and in the press.

The Ministry went on to recommend discouraging the use of candy, and other sweets and producing sugarless bread which could be easily recognized by the consumer. It was also suggested that taxation might prove effective in reducing the consumption of sugar. It might even be a good idea, says the report, to select for very high taxes those products that contain most sugar—such as candy.

Could this possibly be the solution we have been looking for? Tobacco and alcohol are taxed and this does not seem to reduce their consumption. In fact, it has been suggested that the vast income from taxation on to-bacco and alcohol is one reason why government agencies appear to be loath to make statements on the possible harm these two categories of poisons can do. No, people who want to drink and smoke will continue to do so, were the taxes even higher than they are.

But taxing sugar seems to us a little different. Especially if we make it clear why the tax is there. We are sure that thousands of mothers do not know the harm that sugar is doing their children. It is cheap and ac-cessible, so why shouldn't they have as much of it as they wish? If sugar is taxed and the price of everything made from sugar goes up as a result, won't it bring home to people as nothing else could the danger that lies in our present high consumption of this white drug? We believe that Sweden may have something there and we hope the project of taxing sugar goes through so that other countries can study the results. This will be one step on the road to doing away with all refined foods!

71. Sugar, Candy and Caries

Some months ago, in our usual coverage of medical and dental jour-nals, we came across an exciting concept in relation to the control of dental caries in children. A public health nurse, Mary Cantrell, had written in the *Journal of School Health* (December, 1959) of a "Health Snacks" pro-gram initiated in her district that was meeting with great success. The idea is so simple that one wonders how it escaped discovery for so long.

It all began when Miss Cantrell began to notice the cakes, cookies and jelly sandwiches brought to school by the children for the midmorning snack most schools allow to tide the smaller children over until lunchtime. Why not make these snacks pay off in better teeth and better health? Why not encourage the children to bring healthful foods that would satisfy their hunger without taking the edge off their luncheon appetite?

It was decided to begin with the kindergarten group. In this way one could initiate good nutritional practices early and set a pattern that might be followed through all the school years and adult life as well. Besides, children at this age are susceptible to new experiences and enjoy teamwork.

Explain to the Parents

A meeting was held with the parents, explaining the importance of having a health snack rather than a sweet, both to maintain the appetite and to help prevent dental caries. The parents cooperated beautifully, so that a rather special program was soon in force. Each day one child would bring a treat for the entire class, and serve it himself. The date was, of course, pre-arranged with the parents. These treats consisted of carrot or celery strips, apple or orange wedges, dried prunes, raisins, dried apricots, peaches or fresh fruits in season. When the children were finished with their snacks they were urged to get a drink of water and "swish and swallow," thereby cleansing most of the food from their mouths.

Once these habits become routine, the children are less and less apt to bring sweets to school for a snack. They accept the idea of good nutrition readily. When a new child transfers to the kindergarten class, he soon learns from the group that sweets are not acceptable snacks. What more effective way could there be to implant the idea of the desirability of eating healthful foods?

Continue in Upper Grades

Of course, Miss Cantrell's district doesn't stop with kindergarten instruction of good eating. A program of parental information and continued opportunities for the children in the upper grades to eat well is maintained. All the high schools have health snack machines that dispense apples, oranges, peanuts and fruit juices.

Such a program would be a worthwhile project for any PTA to support. It is a wonderful opportunity for antifluoridationists to offer a positive program for reduction of dental caries, when they are asked for an alternative plan. And even if fluoridation is not an issue in your community, the answer to healthy teeth lies in avoidance of sweets in and out of school. You can do your best to see that candy and soda aren't everywhere in the corridors and cafeterias of the school your child attends.

As if to corroborate Miss Cantrell's position against sweets, Dr. James J. Macmillan, writing in *Dental Digest* (April, 1955), told of his own experiments with the patients who come to him. For many years he made it a policy to advise all of his patients who were parents to feed their children plenty of milk, unrefined foods, meat, eggs, fresh fruit and vegetables. Sugar, pastries, candy and soft drinks were to be taken in moderation. This was known as *Method I,* and Dr. Macmillan hoped by use of nutritious foods and a warning against excessive sweets, to cause a decrease in the number of cavities present in the teeth of his patients. *Method I* was a complete failure. There was little if any lowering of decay rates. Questioning of parents as to sugar consumption proved futile. Even where caries was classed as rampant, parents always maintained that the child had not had "much" candy or "much" soda.

[296]

The Trouble with Method I

Dr. Macmillan decided that the fault lay in his recommendation concerning sweets. They were not definite enough. Keeping the sweets down could mean that a child would be eating 8 candy bars a day instead of the 10 he was used to, or that he would drink 6 sodas instead of the 10 he drank every day. This kind of restriction is certainly not enough to eliminate the problem of caries. Also it was discovered that the child who could have 6 sodas could coax his parents into getting a seventh.

This led to the inauguration of *Method II*, which has been operating with much greater success in keeping the cavity count down. The new system called for the child to eat the regular family meals, with desserts at the proper place, but not to be eaten until the preceding food has been eaten. *"At no time are the children to be allowed any candy or soft drink."*

Dr. Macmillan's edict had some interesting effects. First of all, the parents cooperated much better in keeping sweets away from their children. This was attributed to the definite character of the order: no candy or soft drinks. Parents knew exactly what to do. There was no time at which the question of how much was in doubt. There was a solid rule.

The Effect on the Children

Another interesting thing happened with the children. The ones on this regime did not particularly care for desserts. It was more common for them to refuse dessert than to eat it. Dr. Macmillan was led by this to wonder if eating sweets is not actually an acquired taste—a training to eat a type of food which is actually unpleasant at first. The children raised on *Method II* had no desire for soda and candy because the taste had not been created.

The neighbors and relatives were more likely than the parents to tempt the children with sweets. Once parents took a firm stand and had their wishes understood, outside interference was eliminated. The children gradually became sweets-resistant. They actually enjoyed attracting attention by refusing candy and soda at parties, etc. Most children like to be the center of attention, and in this case the reason for the attention is praiseworthy. Clinically, the result was that one cavity in a 9 year old child was the only incidence of caries in the teeth of all the children following *Method II*. Could fluoridation accomplish as much? Even its strongest supporters don't make such a claim.

Whatever the type of diet one eats, the food remaining on the teeth can be a serious threat to freedom from decay. Toothbrushing after meals is one solution, but few youngsters are concerned enough about their teeth to make this effort. Two British scientists, Geoffrey L. Stack, D.D.S., of the School of Dental Surgery, University of Liverpool, England, and W. J. Martin of the London School of Hygiene and Tropical Medicine, University of London, set up a study to test the value of apples in preventing dental caries. Children of varying ages up to 15 years were chosen at random and divided into Apple Group and Control Group, to be studied for two years. Each child was carefully examined for cavities before the experiment began. It was found that the apples used had to be firm and crisp with a skin that was not too tough.

The apples were served at the end of each meal, and after eating anything between meals. The unpeeled apples were cored and sliced horizontally to give apple rings of about ½ inch thick. This allowed the smallest number of apples to be used freshly cut for each serving. Serving of whole apples would have been wasteful. Also the shape of the rings made it likelier that the children would take a large enough bite to bring the back teeth into action.

The results were impressive. The percentage of gum disease in apple eaters, which had been about the same at the start of the experiment, dropped considerably; the improvement is termed a "large increase" by the observers. Of those who had primary teeth, at every age the caries incidence was greater among those not eating apples. The older children who had their secondary teeth throughout the experiment showed a significant benefit from the apple diet, in that their caries rate was definitely below the control group, even though the apple group began the experiment with slightly more caries than the controls.

The beneficial action of the apples is twofold: first, the low acidity of the apples stimulates the flow of saliva, which is also increased with the chewing; second, the mechanical cleansing action of the fibrous apple fragments sweeping over the teeth and gums in the presence of increased saliva flow, removes debris and stimulates gum tissues.

Why not introduce a post-meal apple slice or two into the regular routine at your house? It's a lot cheaper and pleasanter than a call on the dentist.

These are some uncomplicated and effective ways for stopping tooth decay among your children. It's hard to think of a reason for anyone's refusing to take advantage of these suggestions. We also think they are worth introducing to the people who are determined that fluoridation is the only answer to dental caries. There are other, better, cheaper and safer answers. A year or two under any of these plans would prove the point. Why should pro-fluoridationists object to such a test; it won't cost anybody any money. Of course, every reader should be following these worthwhile projects among his own children. The results are bound to be gratifying.

72. Vitamin B₆ Fights Tooth Decay

Fluoridationists push on, trying to convince the country that there is no measure other than fluoridation that will bring to a halt the problem of tooth decay. However, with almost every publicity blurb we see the same old song and dance that gets pro-fluoridationists off the hook: "Of course fluoridation cannot eliminate all dental bills or all dental ills. Nor can it remove the necessity for such additional dental health practices as good diet, conscientious brushing and regular visits to the dentists."

Now you see, from all the other publicity we read, we got the impression that every child eating the usual quota of candy bars, drinking the regular number of sodas and licking the average number of ice cream cones could expect to see a big drop in dental decay. Apparently this is not the case. The child must eat a good diet to make fluoridation work. Cut the sodas, candy, ice cream; get calcium from milk or some milk substitute, eat vegetables and meats, etc.

Then there is brushing. We thought the fluoridationists were promising healthy teeth to kids who brush or don't brush. Not so. You've got to brush them regularly, buddy, if your teeth are to be free from decay in a fluoridated community.

Good Diet Works Without Fluoridation

Let's see now: good diet, careful brushing, regular dental consultation —it adds up to healthy teeth without fluorides, especially without fluorides. Why should we have trouble with our teeth if we eliminate decay-causing foods and eat foods which reinforce good, strong teeth? If we brush these strong teeth to eliminate food deposits, and if we visit the dentist to be sure no decay is beginning, there is nothing fluorides can do to make us safer.

There is no doubt that diet is of great value in preventing tooth decay. The value of the various nutrients that go to make up good diet has been established by scientists. We were interested to see the work that has been done on vitamin B₆ (pyridoxine) in relation to protection from dental caries. In the *New York State Dental Journal* (August-September, 1956) there appeared an article by L. P. Strean, Ph.D., D.D.S., Elizabeth W. Gilfillan, B.S., and Gladys A. Emerson, Ph.D., in which the suppressive effect of pyridoxine on dental caries of hamsters was noted.

Five male hamsters (the males usually developed 3 times as many caries as females) were placed on each of two dietary regimens, average in their content of caries-causing foods. They each drank a 5 per cent sucrose solution in place of water. One of the groups had a supplement of 50 milligrams per 100 grams of ration. The other had 20 times as much, or 1000 milligrams of pyridoxine per 100 grams of ration. The study lasted 10 months to permit maximum development of caries. The average weights of both sets of animals were about the same throughout the test. A numerical scoring system, considering the 5 surfaces of each molar, was set up. A possible value of 240 was declared to mean that all tooth surfaces were destroyed. The better the state of the teeth, at the end of the experiment, the lower the number.

The results were astonishing even to the researchers, we are sure. The 5 hamsters which were fed the low B_6 rations showed an average of 26.1 per cent loss of tooth structure. Their combined score was 313. The group which was given the large pyridoxine dosage in the ration showed an average tooth structure loss of 4.2 per cent. The total score for this group was 50.

Said the authors: "The 6-fold difference in the total score between the two groups appears to be more than coincidental. The fact that weights of the two groups were substantially the same would rule out any effect of inanition. The difference between the two groups would be that one received an intake of B_6 barely sufficient for maintenance while the other was supplied with an optimal amount (in fact, an excess) of this vitamin . . . The results observed in this preliminary study on a small group of hamsters are sufficiently encouraging to warrant further investigations. Mishett and Emerson have consistently observed dental abnormalities in monkeys and dogs deprived of vitamin B_6."

Why did the pyridoxine, or vitamin B_6, have this remarkable effect on the teeth of the hamsters? One guess was that the vitamin was able to maintain a climate of bacterial flora which is beneficial to the proper development and good health of the teeth. Dr. Lyon P. Strean decided to undertake further investigation of this possibility. His findings were published in the *New York State Dental Journal* (February, 1957).

The Theory Behind Vitamin B_6 Activity

Dr. Strean theorized that some type of friendly bacteria, a lactobacilli, which would need vitamin B_6 as an essential nutrient, was multiplying rapidly with the extra vitamin B_6 dosage. Its growth worked to ease out and eliminate certain bacteria which are detrimental to the health of the teeth.

Dr. Strean found that, in pregnant women, notorious for their dental problems, there is a larger amount of cortisone secreted from the adrenals. The cortisone interferes with the body's ability to use vitamin B_6. Therefore, pregnant women should make an especial effort to increase their B vitamin intake to offset this known interference.

In another study involving a large number of hospitalized children being treated for rheumatic fever, massive doses of cortisone were used. It was observed that these children developed rampant dental decay. It may be presumed, says Strean, that the stress of the crippling disease, plus the large amounts of cortisone administered, interfered with the availability of the pyridoxine to the tissues of the children.

It has been seen that children who chew sugar cane, as it is used particularly in the Caribbean Islands, show resistance to dental caries, even though their hygienic practices are at a minimum. When Dr. Strean saw this, he analyzed the sugar cane for its vitamin B_6 content, and found it to be very high in this nutrient. Also the molasses prepared from the sugar cane and eaten by these children is high in vitamin B_6.

Dr. Strean then tells of a report by the Food and Drug Administration (Public Health Report 71, May, 1956). There had been a series of cases of convulsions in infants that had been maintained on an infant milk formula which was found to be deficient in B_6. When the formula was changed to provide adequate quantities of this vitamin, complete recovery from the convulsions followed at once. The investigators concluded that the pyridoxine had effected a substantial and beneficial change in the intestinal flora. The action approximates the action of pyridoxine in the mouth.

An interesting observation on the values of pyridoxine was made in connection with a clinical trial involving the use of specially-prepared pyridoxine lozenges (3 milligrams) for the control of dental caries in children. Some of the mothers decided to take the lozenges for the protection of their own teeth. Two of the mothers who had suffered from a form of mucous colitis, passing loose stool several times daily for 3 to 5 years without remission, reported that within 72 hours following the use of the lozenges the stool was well-formed. Relief was maintained for a period of one month, when the mothers were requested to stop taking the lozenge. Two days later the stool reverted to its previous loose consistency. When the lozenges were reinstituted, well-formed stools resulted.

How Pyridoxine Worked for the Children

The story of the mothers is interesting and informative, but one wonders about the effect of the lozenges upon the children's teeth for whom it was originated. Abram Cohen, D.D.S., and Carl Rubin, D.D.S., made that report in the Bulletin of the Philadelphia Dental Society (January, 1958). This is what they reported: "Of greater importance is the fact that the children receiving supplementary amounts of pyridoxine showed a lower DMF (Decayed, Missing, Filled—a measure used to evaluate teeth in oral examinations) rating when compared with the control group receiving placebo ("dummy") lozenges . . . This study suggests that pyridoxine supplementation may be an aid in the suppression of dental caries even in areas where the water is fluoridated . . ."

It is interesting to know that such an evaluation can be made about fluoridated areas. One wonders if, so long as the health authorities insisted on adding something to the water, pyridoxine wouldn't have made a better showing than fluorides. It should also be pointed out that the authors seemed to feel that if the children had been more consistent in the use of their supplementary lozenges, the results would have been even better.

A test, using similar lozenges, was done by Strean and others in a nonfluoridated area, and reported in the *New York State Dental Journal* (March, 1958). The study involved 28 children between the ages of 10 and 15 years. When the children who took pyridoxine lozenges for a period of one year were compared with a control group taking placebo lozenges, they showed a 40 per cent reduction in tooth decay over the control group.

In our opinion, the use of individual B vitamins is not wise. It is believed that serious imbalances occur in the body when the B complex is not taken as it occurs in nature. Therefore, we advocate the frequent inclusion in the diet of B-rich foods such as wheat germ and brewer's yeast, as well as the organ meats of all animals (desiccated liver tablets are an easy way to get these complete nutrients).

73. A Review of the Theories of Tooth Decay

Prevention of dental caries in children—what an encouraging ring the words have! We were interested in this article by N. J. Ainsworth, M.C., MRCS, LRCP, FDS, RCS, in the *British Medical Press* for April 23, 1952, mostly because of the word "prevention" used in the title. We found the article was a review of all the various theories that have been advanced on the cause and prevention of tooth decay.

Our modern thinking on tooth decay seems to start with W. D. Miller who in 1882 carried out many experiments and wrote many articles on his theory that decay is caused by mouth acids produced by bacteria living on carbohydrates. First, he believed, the enamel is destroyed by decalcification, then the dentine and the underlying parts of the tooth are attacked by the acids. For many years proponents of this theory worked hard, isolating bacteria from saliva and trying to find ways of neutralizing the acid formed in the mouth.

In 1918 May Mellanby, working with laboratory animals, published the results of her experiments which showed that adequate calcium, phosphorus, vitamin A and especially vitamin D in the diet were all necessary for creating good structure of teeth. She also showed that a diet lacking in vitamin D caused a defective structure which later on would yield readily to decay. So Mellanby concluded that structure is the main deterrent to decay and that, if teeth are well formed, they will have few caries. She also discovered—and this, we think, is immensely important—that "a diet of high calcifying properties, given *after* the eruption of teeth whatever their structure, could prevent or retard the onset of caries, or if the disease had already developed, bring about the deposition of well-calcified secondary dentine and ultimately the arrest of the carious process." In other words, Mellanby's research shows us without any doubt that good diet will stop tooth decay—no matter how late in life this diet is resorted to. Mellanby also showed in her experiments the ravages caused by a diet high in cereal products and low in vitamin D and calcium. Cereal foods contain a substance which is antagonistic to calcium, so a diet very high in cereals will not be a healthy one, unless plenty of calcium and vitamin D are included as well.

The Toothbrush Era

Early in the century a researcher named Leon Williams invented the slogan "clean teeth do not decay," thereby ushering in the era of the toothbrush and toothpaste, along with all the extravagant and wholly irresponsible claims that go with them. Dr. Ainsworth tells us this slogan was shouted from the rooftops of all the dental hospitals in England and America for a generation and "echoed rather half-heartedly (by the children) for children are realists and the retort that no amount of brushing seemed to reduce the number of holes found each holiday was difficult to answer." While it is possible, of course, to remove particles of food from around and between teeth, using a toothbrush or dental floss, we cannot possibly make our teeth bacteriologically clean, so long as they are in our mouths, washed by saliva.

Later experiments showed that saliva that has been mixed with sugar for six hours, reaches an acidity capable of dissolving tooth enamel. Eating a cube of sugar will increase the acidity of the saliva within a matter of minutes. Eating soft sweets will raise the acidity within 20 minutes.

So the recommendation then became to eliminate carbohydrates in general and sugar in particular or to remove them rapidly from the mouth after they are chewed, or to eradicate the acid-forming bacteria of the mouth.

Mouth Washes and Toothpastes

Working on this latter proposition, one researcher tested all the various substances that might be used in mouth washes and found of course, that nothing will guard the mouth against bacteria for longer than a few hours. Hydrogen peroxide, formaldehyde and such substances are the ones found most effective for bacteria-slaughter, understandably enough, since these are also quite dangerous substances for human beings.

Then two investigators found that there appeared to be less decay in mouths where the ammonium concentration was high. As a result of later experiments several researchers suggested the addition of ammonium phosphate to dentifrices, warning that one should not depend on this sub-

[303]

stance alone to prevent decay but that dietary measures also might be necessary.

Although tests have shown reduced decay in some persons using ammoniated toothpastes, the investigators themselves often suggest that this may be the result of the increased attention to toothbrushing encouraged by the experiment. Dr. Ainsworth also points out that, in spite of anything accomplished by an ammonium toothpaste, the acidity of the mouth is still raised to a decay-producing level within two minutes after rinsing the mouth with glucose (a sugar solution). So even if you use an ammoniated toothpaste, immediately after a meal, this might be too late to prevent decay, if you have eaten foods containing glucose or sugar at the meal.

"To sum up the conflicting evidence, the case for ammoniated dentifrices seems 'not proven'," says Dr. Ainsworth. Penicillin in toothpaste has been shown to produce some reduction in decay in an experiment by H. A. Zander in 1950. However, since the use of penicillin results in the production of strains of bacteria resistant to penicillin, there seems to be little point to its use in toothpastes, for any protection would surely be very temporary.

The Use of Fluorides

Dr. Ainsworth then discusses the prevention of decay by the use of fluorides, painting them on the teeth, or putting them in drinking water. Many readers are familiar with the controversy over water fluoridation in which more and more evidence is piling up to indicate that, while fluoridation of water may reduce or delay dental decay in very young children, its effects on the health of older people, infants and ill people have not been studied sufficiently to warrant taking a chance on artificial fluoridation of water. Dr. Ainsworth believes that applying fluorides directly to the teeth, while it is a tedious process for the child, may bring reduction in decay.

Finally he takes up the subject of soil and tooth decay. The organic farming theory, he says, "has a few enthusiastic advocates but no general support because it is difficult to devise proofs and impossible, under present conditions, to apply the principle generally." We believe there is ample proof right now of the wonderful results in good health obtained by eating organically grown food and Dr. Ainsworth himself quotes Sir Albert Howard and several other experts as to the effects of organically grown food on animals and people. Farming organically means returning to the soil all those elements taken from the soil, but returning them in the natural, slowly soluble forms in which they occur in nature. That is, using ground phosphate rock rather than a phosphate fertilizer, using compost (decayed leaves, grasses and manures) rather than a commercially prepared fertilizer that acts too quickly on the soil and may not offer the soil nutriments in the proper proportion.

It is our opinion, supported by numerous observations, as well as experiments reported in books that an individual living entirely on organically raised foods will have little or no difficulty with dental decay.

Dr. Ainsworth concludes his article with a quote from Weston Price, that famous dentist who made a trip around the world about 25 years ago, reported on the many nations of the world living on natural foods, to whom tooth decay is all but unknown. Dr. Price says: "We have accordingly today supporters of a variety of viewpoints. There are those who say that caries are of bacterial origin; others consider them to be all or partly nutritional, and there are others who would say that food has little or nothing to do with it. Some would expect to accomplish control of caries by prophylaxis procedures; others believe that prophylaxis cannot prevent dental caries or at least that it is not adequate alone. Some would persuade the public that particular brands of washes and dentifrices can accomplish the desired results. Others would put primary emphasis upon the mechanical phases, such as the method of using the brush, the coarseness or hardness of foods eaten, etc. As in all health problems we get our standards from Nature. When we study Nature, we find that animals throughout the passing periods have been largely immune to dental caries, that many races of humans have been immune, and that limited groups are today immune. These immune peoples, whether of the past or present, have had very little knowledge of the tooth brush, mouth washes, or dentifrices.

"From the above it is suggested that progress when it is made, must be through a better understanding of the natural laws as involved in nutrition and external environment of the teeth, as these vary with susceptibility and immunity to dental caries."

74. Official Statement on the Causes of Tooth Decay

In the current hubbub over water fluoridation, we frequently encounter an argument that goes something like this: "we must have water fluoridation because, since we do not know what causes that terrible scourge, tooth decay, we must snatch at any straw to prevent it. Since fluoridation apparently prevents it, we must fluoridate, regardless of the risk!"

What actually is known about the causes of tooth decay? We have come across many theories in the past—and very interesting ones, stimulating to thought. A large segment of our information has come from an informative and most convincing book, *Nutrition and Physical Degeneration* by Weston Price, D.D.S., available from the Lee Foundation For Nutritional Research (2023 West Wisconsin Avenue, Milwaukee, Wisconsin). Dr.

Price satisfied his intense interest in nutrition as it relates to health by traveling around the world, studying the teeth, jaw and facial bone structure of individuals in many countries, eating many different diets.

He found, without exception, every place he went, that people who ate diets free from refined foods suffered little if at all from tooth decay. In addition, their bone structure, jaws and nasal arches were superlatively formed for efficient chewing, breathing, singing and speaking. Hundreds of excellent photographs in the book attest to the impact of Dr. Price's words.

He also found that, within so short a time as one generation, eating refined foodstuffs could result in narrow nasal and dental arches, mouth breathing, malocclusion and rampant tooth decay. The book contains pictures of these conditions, too. You will find pictures of members of the same family, one with broken snags for teeth, the other with a set of perfect choppers unmarred by decay. The first individual ate the new kind of food from the store—chiefly refined cereals and white sugar products, the second liked his traditional diet of rough unrefined foods, unprocessed and unspoiled except for cooking.

Quote the conclusions, unmistakable and well-documented, drawn by Dr. Price in his book, and you will be named faddist and crank by your friends. You will be deluged with stories about Cousin Jim who pays such strict attention to what he eats and has such terrible teeth and cousin Mary who "lives on" cake and pie and has perfect teeth. Well, almost perfect. And, well, maybe she doesn't actually live on cake and pie but she does eat desserts.

Probably the most conservative group of researchers and reporters on health anywhere in the world is represented by the reports from the Council on Foods and Nutrition of the American Medical Association. You could not by any stretch of the imagination call these reports faddist. They are the careful result of years of study in university laboratories. They represent opinions from Harvard, from Yale, from the American Association for the Advancement of Science, and so forth.

The Official Statement Appears

So we were very happy to find in the *Journal of the American Medical Association* for February 8, 1958, a new report, authorized officially for publication by the Secretary of the Council on Foods and Nutrition, devoted to the subject of *Nutrition and Dental Caries* (that is, decay). The author, James H. Shaw, Ph.D., of the Harvard School of Dental Medicine, tells us first that there are undoubtedly several interrelated causes of tooth decay. But, regardless of the background, the heredity and the health of the individual involved, we know for certain that, in order to produce decay, food particles must be present in the mouth and must become entrapped on the surface of the teeth. We know further that these food particles must contain carbohydrates—that is, starches and sugars—which will be attacked by the bacteria in the mouth.

We know, too, says Dr. Shaw, that vitamins A, C and D must be present in sufficent quantity to prevent malformation of the teeth when they are forming. We believe, he says, that only vitamin D is involved in preventing decay, but we have not sufficently tested vitamins A and C. They may be involved, too.

During the war, Dr. Shaw tells us, there was a great reduction in tooth decay in many countries where food restrictions were severe. "Careful study of these data indicates that the nutritional influences imposed on the teeth during development and calcification through the consumption of coarse, unrefined diets of natural foodstuffs resulted in teeth that were more caries-resistant (decay-resistant) than those formed during the prewar days." Dr. Shaw is speaking, not Dr. Price the "faddist," but what he is saying sounds remarkably like what Dr. Price and other so-called "faddists" say.

Experiments on Decay Prevention

Dr. Shaw goes on to tell us of highly significant experiments carried on in various countries. For instance, one was conducted in an institution where the diet was noticeably poor. Fairly large amounts of sugar and candy were added to the diet. Result? Increases in the amount of decay. In another experiment—in an institution where a good, nutritious diet was being fed—sticky candy, the kind that clings to your teeth, was added. Result? In spite of the excellent diet there was increased decay. In another group of children on the same good diet sugar was fed in breads and in less sticky candy. Less decay, but it was still there. Feeding candy and sticky, sweet foods *with* meals resulted in less decay than feeding such foods *between* meals.

In other words, says Dr. Shaw, "It is not just a matter of the total amount of . . . carbohydrate consumed by the individual; of infinitely greater importance are the form of carbohydrates and the circumstances that lead to clearance from or retention in the oral cavity."

Then he tells us of experiments in which diabetic children were fed on carefully controlled and highly nutritious diets which resulted in practically no tooth decay, even in these sick children. "In addition to the highly desirable diets, the carbohydrate content was much lower than that usually found in diets of American children." The researchers feel that the excellence of the diet was responsible for keeping the teeth in good shape, systemically—that is, the food elements in such a diet sustain teeth in good health. The vitamins, minerals, proteins, enzymes of a good diet render the body so healthy that the teeth are resistant to decay. But could the results have been due just to the lack of carbohydrates, in the diet? It is almost impossible to tell, says Dr. Shaw, because it is impossible to design a good, nutritious diet that is high in refined carbohydrates! If you are testing a good diet, it will be bound to be a diet low in refined starches and sugars, so how can you tell whether the excellence of the diet or the lack of carbohydrates is responsible for the results?

[307]

Quality of Food Is Important

Here is one other angle from the AMA report on possible reasons for tooth decay. Hamsters fed a diet of corn grown in New England and whole milk powder prepared from milk produced in New England had a high incidence of decay. In contrast, hamsters fed a diet of corn and whole milk powder grown and prepared in Texas had a "significantly lower" incidence of decay. Here, of course, the carbohydrate content of the diet was much the same. Dr. Shaw does not comment on what was different about the Texas food, but any thinking person will agree that there is but one explanation for what happened in this experiment. The Texas soil is rich in minerals. The New England soil, worn-out, over-cropped, demineralized, is deficient in those elements that are necessary to protect teeth from decay.

In still another experiment, laboratory animals fed "cariogenic" diets—that is, diets known to produce decay, were then given mineral supplements, containing calcium, phosphorus and other valuable minerals. Tooth decay was retarded.

In conclusion, says Dr. Shaw, "For optimal results, the diet during this developmental period (that is, childhood) should be composed of a generous selection of foods from all the basic food categories with a minimum use of highly refined foodstuffs and with careful attention to cooking procedures to preserve original nutrient values. . . . After the teeth are fully formed and have erupted into the oral cavity, the same attention should be paid to the nutritional quality of the diet. In addition, there should be a strong emphasis on the restriction of sticky, high-carbohydrate foods that are cleared slowly from the oral cavity. As snacks and desserts in place of such foodstuffs, fresh fruits, vegetables, fruit juices or milk are much to be preferred from the standpoint of dental health."

In this same report, Dr. Shaw, for some reason that is not immediately obvious, feels that he must pay a two-paragraph tribute to water fluoridation. Says he, "A highly desirable factor in the over-all planning for the attainment of maximum caries-resistance is the availability of a fluoridated water supply." He makes no effort to answer any of the available arguments against fluoridation, including that of the Massachusetts engineer who has proved conclusively, using the official figures, that artificial fluoridation does not prevent tooth decay, but only postpones it for a few years. Neither does Dr. Shaw explain how it happens that perfect teeth, untouched by decay, exist in many localities in the world where there is not a trace of fluorine in the water. Instead he implies by his use of the words "diet-planning" that fluorine is an element necessary for good nutrition. There is not a single word of evidence to support this viewpoint throughout all of scientific literature.

All the rest of the information in the report strengthens what the "food faddists" have been saying for many years—our present-day refined and processed diets are responsible for our tooth decay. These diets are two-edged swords. On the one hand, their soft, sticky, highly concentrated sugars and starches remain in the mouth, clinging around the teeth, thus producing decay. On the other hand, a diet of which more than one-half consists of refined carbohydrate products (the diet eaten by most Americans) leaves no room for the good foods which should make up the bulk of one's diet. Dr. Fred Miller, D.D.S., of Altoona, Pennsylvania, has proven conclusively that eating an apple after each meal will cleanse the mouth of food particles left around the teeth. But what child, stuffed with soft drinks, candy, white bread and desserts is going to have room for apples?

Our answer to preventing tooth decay in your own family is, of course, avoiding all the white sugar and white flour products, which will leave plenty of room at your meals for the healthful foods—meat, fish, eggs, nuts and fresh raw, fruits and vegetables. In addition, of course, you must supply the minerals and vitamins and we heartily recommended using natural food supplements daily—bone meal for minerals, fish liver oils for vitamins A and D, rose hips for vitamin C, wheat germ oil and/or vitamin E and kelp for iodine and other minerals.

The next time someone in your community brings up the question of water fluoridation and tries to promote it by saying that we do not know how to prevent tooth decay in any other way, refer him to the report on the Council on Foods and Nutrition of the American Medical Association. Title—*Nutrition and Dental Caries*, by James H. Shaw. Available from The American Medical Association, 535 North Dearborn Street, Chicago, Illinois.

75. Can Malocclusion of the Teeth Be Prevented?

The science of orthodontics is today, in this country, a flourishing branch of dentistry devoted to the prevention and correction of malocclusion of the teeth and "such other deformities and abnormalities as may be associated therewith." Orthodontists are patient, painstaking men who spend their days correcting, mostly by mechanical means, the serious defects in structure which result in malocclusion—common in American mouths, especially the mouths of children.

Malocclusion is defined in the medical dictionary as "occlusion of teeth in positions not conformable to anatomical rule." In other words, if your teeth do not meet in such a way as to give you a fully functioning "bite" as well as good appearance, you have malocclusion. When your "bite" is ineffective, when your teeth are growing so far out of line with one another and with the plane in which they function that you cannot use your teeth as you should—that is malocclusion.

It is not a rare condition in America today. J. A. Salzmann, D.D.S., of New York City, writing in the *American Journal of Orthodontics*, Vol. 34, 1948, states that "there are approximately 40 million children under the age of 16 years in the United States of whom 7 or 8 million need major orthodontic care and of whom less than 4 out of every 100 who need it are actually receiving treatment."

The Meaning of "Normal"

There is a lot of debate among orthodontists as to what constitutes "normal" occlusion. Wendell Wylie, D.D.S., M.S., of San Francisco gives us the example of two players on a ball team—one the shortest on the team, the other the tallest. "Which of the players is normal, or is either of them abnormal?" asks Dr. Wylie in *Angle Orthodontist* for January, 1949. Does not the very wide difference existing anatomically among all men explain the fact that you cannot set standards for the shape of a mouth, any more than you can decide how tall everybody should be? Whether or not you will have malocclusion is determined before you are born and the best that can be done is to correct the malocclusion with mechanical means. "What then is malocclusion?" asks Dr. Wylie. "A view which has not been considered seriously enough and one which has an abundance of evidence in its favor is that the majority of our problems arise through the chance combination of component parts of the face in such a way that a truly harmonious relationship between them is the exception rather than the rule." We do not agree with Dr. Wylie's use of the phrase "chance combination" as you will see later on, but meanwhile surely no one can object to a definition which contends that teeth too far out of line for proper chewing constitute malocclusion, teeth erupting at odd places in the mouth rather than where they are supposed to be, extra teeth which have no place and no excuse for being—all these constitute malocclusion, no matter what the so-called "normal" mouth and face should look like.

Orthodontic magazines tell us, and we agree with them, that malocclusion should be treated by orthodontists rather than regular dentists who have not been specially trained. Dr. Salzmann says that many dentists have been known to examine the mouth without once asking the child patient to bring his teeth into occlusion (that is, close his mouth in a bite) or to move the jaw through its various possible movements to determine whether possibly there has been some injury or malalignment. "Today the advice most frequently given parents by the family dentist, often without examining the mouth of the child and occasionally in reply to a telephone call is that it is 'too early' for their young child to receive orthodontic care. This advice is only too frequently followed sometime later by the observation that it is already 'too late' to prevent and frequently also to treat the malocclusion which has now fully established itself."

Anatomical Causes of Malocclusion

What are some possible causes of malocclusion which we can recognize in our own children, so that we will know whether or not they may need the services of a trained expert? The condition of "baby" teeth is apparently of utmost importance. Not so many years ago it was generally believed that baby teeth were not too important and many parents paid little attention to cavities, missing teeth or teeth which came out, for "you'll soon get your permanent teeth and we'll take you to the dentist then."

Youngsters of 5 or 6 with missing teeth were proverbially cute and appealing. Such a viewpoint demonstrated a complete misunderstanding of what the role of "baby" teeth is. They are not there just so that Junior can have something to chew with until his permanent teeth arrive. They are there to reserve space for the permanent teeth in Junior's rapidly growing jaw. If Junior loses a baby tooth in a particularly rough cowboy game some day, his jaw begins to close very rapidly around the space left by that tooth and, especially if a molar has been lost, there is every possibility that the permanent molar may not be able to erupt properly. It may come in crooked, it may interfere with teeth on either or both sides or it may not erupt at all. In any case, there is a shortening of the arch of the jaw on that side which is bound to result in a disharmony in Junior's bite in later years.

So the first rule for preventing malocclusion is to take a child to the orthodontist if any one of his baby teeth has been lost prematurely. The orthodontist has a mechanism called a "space maintainer" which will provide and maintain room for the later tooth.

The second warning of possible malocclusion is the prolonged retention of baby teeth. If they stay in too long, the permanent teeth trying to erupt beneath them may be deflected out of their proper course or may not erupt at all. This is particularly true in the case of the cuspids which, if unable to erupt at the proper time, may not grow out at all. Generally the permanent teeth begin to replace the baby teeth at about the age of 7. Since the time varies with individual children, there may be doubt as to whether or not the permanent teeth are ready to erupt. X-rays are the most dependable way of knowing for sure.

A third hazard is the loss of a permanent tooth before the entire set of permanent teeth has grown in, for here again the space will tend to close rapidly, throwing out of line the teeth in that side of the jaw which are still coming through the gums. Of course, when any permanent tooth is lost, at any age, and not replaced, there may be resulting malocclusion, for the shape of the jaw is bound to change.

Another good reason for keeping baby teeth in good order is that if there should be unfilled cavities which are painful, the child may favor one side when he chews. This is certain to disturb the alignment of his jaws.

Extra teeth occasionally develop—that is, teeth which erupt where some other tooth should be. Even if they do not erupt they may be present in the jaw and an X-ray will reveal them. If such a tooth is interfering with the normal teeth, it should be removed. If there are teeth which fail to come in at all, these too are likely to cause malocclusion and restorations should take their place.

Habits Which May Cause Malocclusion

Among habits which lead to malocclusion are these: mouth breathing, lip biting, thumb or finger sucking, incorrect swallowing, tongue biting or thrusting, pencil biting or nail biting. Bottle-feeding continued for too long a time can also result in serious malocclusion. Dr. Salzmann mentions that improper selection of a nipple for the baby's bottle and improper position of both the baby and the bottle during feeding may also be important factors. He suggests that a nipple long enough to rest on the first third of the tongue be used and that small openings be punched in the side of the bulb of the nipple instead of at the end only, to prevent the infant from squirting the milk directly into the pharynx.

Richard C. Thometz, D.D.S., Instructor of Orthodontics at Loyola University, speaking on malocclusion at a meeting of the Chicago Dental Society March 7, 1949, described the results of mouth breathing. If the child cannot breathe through his nose because of adenoids, continued colds or some other reason, the muscles of his mouth structure do not properly do their job of supporting the teeth in their normal arches, resulting in malocclusion, difficulty in swallowing and speech.

Lip biting, says Dr. Thometz, is most frequently seen in girls, although it may be a habit acquired by anyone and it is believed to be a nervous habit. He suggests patient re-education of the lip-biter, perhaps having him stand before a mirror so that he can observe how deformed and unattractive he looks while he is biting his lips. Tongue biting and thrusting are not uncommon, he says, and if the patient persists in these, he should be referred to an orthodontist. Chewing on a pencil or some other object can be extremely detrimental to tooth enamel as well as a perfectly good cause of malocclusion.

Dr. Salzmann gives us some details on nail biting. In a survey of 100 nail-biting children, it was found that 13 per cent had suffered from early convulsions, 9 per cent from premature eruption of teeth, 20 per cent from bed wetting, 34 per cent from slight mental deficiency and 26 per cent from serious mental deficiency. It has been long suspected by psychologists that nail biting is a manifestation of rather serious personality difficulty and once this is discovered and overcome the nail biting will stop. In the meanwhile it can be most detrimental to teeth.

By some means or other orthodontists have discovered that many people do not swallow correctly. In correct swallowing, the jaws and teeth are brought together and the tongue thrust against the sides of the teeth and palate. The tongue functions best during swallowing when its tip and sides are braced against the hard palate and teeth. In incorrect swallowing the tongue is braced against the lips, which eventually produces malocclusion.

Poor Nutrition Basic Cause of Malocclusion

The most interesting controversy among orthodontists is the question of whether malocclusion is caused by heredity or environment. Granted that bad habits may wreak havoc on tooth-alignment, what about those youngsters who do not bite their lips, breathe through their mouths and so forth —why do they have teeth that do not meet in a perfect "bite"? Because one parent or both had this same trouble, says one school of orthodontists, and facial structure is hereditary. If I have a jaw so narrow that my full quota of teeth cannot erupt without crowding one another, then my children may possibly have just such jaws, too. The other school of orthodontic thinking declares that heredity is not the whole answer, but that other factors in environment must be important, too. They are bent on finding out what these other factors are.

It seems strange that none of the articles on malocclusion that we read mentioned a book called *Nutrition and Physical Degeneration* by Weston Price, D.D.S., M.S., F.A.C.D., published by the author in 1939. This is the story of a scientist in search of the cause of malocclusion and tooth decay. Dr. Price visited Canada, Australia, Europe, South America and the South Sea islands, studying primitive peoples in all these places who had never eaten modern, "civilized" foods. In some cases he also studied the children of these same people who had been eating store-bought food.

Dr. Price quotes Dr. Ernest A. Hooton of Harvard: "I firmly believe that the health of humanity is at stake and that, unless steps are taken to discover preventives of tooth infection and correctives of deformation, the course of human evolution will lead downward to extinction . . . The facts we must face are, in brief, that human teeth and the human mouth have become, possibly under the influence of civilization, the foci of infection that undermine the entire bodily health of the species and that degenerative tendencies in evolution have manifested themselves in modern man to such an extent that our jaws are too small for the teeth which they are supposed to accommodate, and that, as a consequence, these teeth erupt so irregularly that their fundamental efficiency is often entirely or nearly destroyed. . . . The dental practitioner should equip himself to become the agent of an intelligent control of human evolution, insofar as it is affected by diet. Let us go to the ignorant savage, consider his ways of eating, and be wise. Let us cease pretending that toothbrushes and toothpaste are any more important than shoe brushes and shoe polish. It is store food which has given us store teeth."

Dr. Price Blames Our Modern Foods

Dr. Price goes on to say that orthodontists have ascribed malocclusion to the blending of racial stocks. Crowded teeth have been said to be due to the inheritance of the large teeth of one parent and the small bone formation of the other. But Dr. Price has studied and photographed for

[313]

his book hundreds of examples of young people whose diet is "store-bought" while that of their parents was primitive. In the course of this one generation, the bony structure of the children has degenerated to such a degree that cases of malocclusion are commonplace and of course dental decay is rampant among these young folks, who live in the same houses with their parents and grandparents whose jaw structures are flawless and whose teeth have never known decay, simply because their diet has always been the same natural, unrefined food their ancestors ate.

Dr. Price also shows you in his book, pictures of whole families of children of which one brother may eat refined foods and suffer from malocclusion and faulty dental arches. Another brother in the same family eats unrefined foods and has perfect occlusion and perfect teeth.

In many of these countries where he visited, the available food was quite scarce and monotonous. The year-round diet may have consisted of oats and fish, or rye bread, milk and cheese with no fruits and few vegetables—an unvaried diet which according to our modern nutritionists does not give nearly enough proper nourishment. But, in these lands at the time Dr. Price investigated, no refined or processed foods of any kind had *ever* been available. But in places where white man's civilized food had made its way, there was tooth decay and malocclusion in *every single individual who ate the new food.*

Now considering the millions of dollars spent every year in this country for orthodontic work, dental bills and now fluoridated water, how does it happen, do you suppose, that Dr. Price's book fully documented and representing years of research, has never been made widely accessible in public libraries all over the land? Why is it not being studied by Parent-Teacher Associations? Why do not local and national health authorities recommend it when they admit themselves that dental decay and malocclusion are two of our most pressing health problems?

Preventing Malocclusion

How do you prevent malocclusion? If the malocclusion is threatening in an individual already alive, we would certainly recommend the suggestions above for preventing it. But if you are speaking in terms of planning a family of children who would not be subject to malocclusion, then we would certainly recommend a healthful diet, for mother and father both, long before their children are born and the same healthful diet for the children from the very day of their birth. You cannot in today's America eat a primitive diet. The very seeds you put into your garden bear the mark of civilization on them. But you can plan your meals so that a very minimum of processed food appears on your table. You can learn how to preserve most food value by cooking methods. You can serve quantities of raw food. You can decide that good health, sound teeth and strong, functioning bone structure are the most important things for you and your family and are worth all the money, extra effort and possible ridicule of your underfed and unbelieving neighbors.

76. Causes and Remedies for Malocclusion

As long ago as 1944 our Secretary of the Navy announced that half of the men of our country who were of military age were rejected as unfit for service. According to J. Minez, D.D.S., writing in *Dental Items of Interest* for December, 1951, this fact is just another way of saying that the people of this country are rapidly deteriorating, both mentally and physically. As a dentist, he is primarily concerned with the problem of malocclusion which, he says, has been constantly increasing so that today it presents a major problem. Malocclusion, as we have seen, means that the teeth do not come together as they should to form the proper biting surface.

Mouth Breathing and Lip Biting Major Causes

Mouth breathing is one of the causes of malocclusion and Dr. Minez tells us that 80 per cent of the children born today are mouth-breathers. He believes it is caused largely by parental malnutrition. It is quite general, he says, among first-born children. Because of the stress and overwork involved these days in preparing for a marriage ceremony, the prospective bride and groom are physically run-down by the time they are married. When their second child arrives, they are adjusted to one another and this child is likely to be stronger.

Mouth breathing is frequently associated with colds, headaches, bleeding at the nose and sinusitis. If it is continued, the child is likely to become flat-chested, round-shouldered, anemic, pale and subject to respiratory diseases. The nose acts as an air-conditioning system to prepare the air for entry into the lungs. In mouth breathing, the air is not properly conditioned, so that every other process connected with breathing and oxidation is thrown out of line.

Lip biting is another cause of malocclusion. Dr. Minez believes that practically all children born these days are lip-biters. It is an unconscious habit and difficult to control, except in cases where patients can concentrate and deliberately break themselves of the habit.

Other causes of malocclusion, according to Dr. Minez, are: (1.) Children born of weak parents. (2.) Improper diet—that is, plain undernourishment even in families whose income is high. The following diet is typical: white bread, white rice, potatoes without their skins and an insufficient amount of raw fruits and vegetables. (3.) The enormous increase in the consumption of white sugar. The per capita consumption of sugar in this country in 1860 was 4 pounds per year. In 1940, it was 120 pounds per year. Taking into account diabetics and many people who do not eat sugar, this means that the average consumption of sugar per year for those who do eat it is higher than 120 pounds. (4.) Smoking at an early age. The amount of nicotine young boys and girls take into their systems undoubtedly affects their children, Dr. Minez believes. In 1900 the total number of cigarettes smoked in this country amounted to 34.9 for every man, woman and child each year. This figure has now increased to 170 packs or 3400 cigarettes per year, for every adult in the country! (5.) Pressure at home and at school and the many over-stimulating radio and television programs which result in not enough sleep and rest. (6.) Carbon monoxide poisoning from autos and unnecessary noise. Traffic-jammed streets produce both. (7.) Competitive games. It is interesting to note that Dr. Minez believes that competitive games—basketball, football and so forth—are definitely harmful to young physiques. Women seldom die of heart trouble at an early age, possibly because they do not engage in these games to the extent that men do.

Dr. Minez's Solution

As a solution for the problem of malocclusion, Dr. Minez suggests the correction of diet and an attempt to lessen the evils of over-stimulation, noise, insufficient rest and so forth.

From our research on the dental equipment of primitive tribes who suffer from none of the environmental conditions listed above, it would seem that malocclusion is another disorder of civilized people, caused mostly by their "civilized" diet, we think. In our opinion, boys and girls who eat correctly will be far better equipped to withstand the other health-destroying aspects of civilized life.

BOOK TWO

GENERAL DISORDERS
OF THE BODY

77. The Disease of Alcoholism

"It is our opinion that the disease of alcoholism is *essentially a disease of one's appetite* and insofar as this is true, it probably can be consistently prevented by the application of nutritional knowledge. The role of individuality in body chemistry must be recognized, as well as the fact that no individual person can be sure, in advance, that he does not have the potentiality of becoming an alcoholic. Any young person who finds himself or herself liking alcohol or its effects very much, or who has any tendency to become intoxicated, should be on his guard, always, at all times.

"Alcoholism is such a devastating disease—so real and so prevalent— that it should be possible to educate young people and their parents in the direction of its avoidance. There are few diseases that can bring as much distress into the lives of the victims and their families as can alcoholism, and anyone educated to its perils should, as a matter of course, be willing to put forth some effort to avoid it, especially when there is a special threat."

We are quoting from an extraordinary and stimulating book written by an extraordinary man who is Professor of Chemistry and Director of the Clayton Foundation Biochemical Institute at the University of Texas—Dr. Roger J. Williams. The 111 pages of this vastly absorbing and easily understood book contain more wisdom on the subject of alcoholism than any other one piece of literature we have ever seen. For years, Dr. Williams has been studying alcoholism as a nutritional disorder. He has experimented extensively with rats and mice in an effort to find out why people drink to excess and whether supplying something that they may lack, nutritionally speaking, may bring about such a complete adjustment of their difficulties that the appetite, the desire, for alcohol may leave.

In his laboratory he has placed rats on the average laboratory diet and given them the choice of two liquids to drink—water or a 10 per cent alcoholic beverage. Some of the rats drink the water exclusively and will not touch the alcohol. Others may drink a little alcohol—a very little, every day regularly. Others may drink a little at first, then increase to a quite high level; others may arrive at a high level of consumption within a few weeks. Some may drink heavily for short periods, then abstain. Many, many such experiments with rats demonstrated that in regard to drinking alcohol they behave just about the same as a similar number of human beings might behave. There are some alcoholics right from the start; there are some teetotalers and there is a wide range of difference in between.

It is obvious that the alcoholic rats did not become alcoholic because of the stress of business worries, or the anxieties and maladjustments of family life, or the burden of making important ethical and moral decisions, for none of these things exist in rat communities. Dr. Williams did find, however, that he could change the pattern of alcoholism by subjecting the rats to stress—in this case, flashing lights and jangling bells. Some of the teetotaler rats were induced to drink when they were subjected to these stresses.

The Nutritional Deficiency Creates the Craving

By making sure of one or another of the rats being deficient in certain vitamins, Dr. Williams was able to increase its appetite for alcohol. He says, "Rats that drank heavily on a standard stock ration, which, however, is not necessarily perfect, may stop drinking overnight when the ration is fortified with needed extra vitamins. Repeatedly rats have been made deficient with respect to a certain vitamin (e.g. thiamin, riboflavin, pantothenic acid, pyridoxine) with the result that their alcohol consumption climbs up to 5, 10, or 20 times the original level. Immediately on supplying the missing vitamin the alcohol consumption drops again to the original level or even below. In one experiment of nearly 8 months' duration, a rat was made deficient 3 separate times. Its alcohol consumption rose to about 30 times its minimum consumption, then dropped in a few days to almost nothing when it was given a single dose of missing vitamins as before. There is no question whatever that the tendency of experimental animals to drink alcohol is influenced most remarkably by the composition of the food that they get."

Dr. Williams believes that the rats' response to alcohol takes this form because the malnutrition they suffer as a result of vitamin deficiency brings out a disorder in the body's appetite mechanism. "Body wisdom becomes body foolishness" he says, and instead of the rat's craving good food (which is the natural response to the body's needs) the disordered appetite mechanism causes the rat to crave alcohol instead. Alcohol, containing as it does large amounts of carbohydrates and no vitamins to help the body use the carbohydrates, only makes the rat more deficient and the cycle goes on. The urge to drink alcohol is just as strong and just as uncontrollable, Dr. Williams believes, as the urge to drink water when we are dehydrated and thirsty.

It is well known, he says, that in the field of nutrition, a chain is only as strong as its weakest link. There are about 40 elements in food that are essential. If one of these 40 is present in the diet at too low a level, the result is deficiency, just as surely as if you were deficient in 10 or more items!

Furthermore, Dr. Williams believes that one can be predisposed to alcoholism by inheritance—not that one inherits the "craving for drink" but that *one's inheritance may control the amount of the various nutriments one needs to be healthy.* Let's say one person has inherited from his parents a need for 20 times more thiamin than another person. It is obvious that such a person will be deficient in thiamin even if he eats exactly the same good diet as someone else whose need for thiamin is not so great.

Preventing Alcoholism Before It Begins Is Best

Now, the person whose nutritional needs are high is vulnerable—he should be especially careful to avoid alcohol. Once he starts to drink, for social or other reasons, the deficiency is made worse because the alcohol crowds out of the diet the nutritious foods he should have—dilutes the diet, as Dr. Williams says. So his deficiency grows worse and as it grows worse his craving for alcohol is increased, because the deficiency has somehow disrupted his appetite mechanism so that he craves the very thing that is worst for him.

No one can say, therefore, that someone is an alcoholic because he simply won't "pull himself together" and stop drinking. He can't stop, any more than he can live without water or air. He has a definite physiological appetite for alcohol created by deficiency in his diet. It is not right to say that by seeing that such a person has "a good, all-around diet" he can be cured of his disease. *This is the diet he was eating when he became an alcoholic.* If his alcoholism indicates that he has extraordinarily high requirements for vitamins and other nutriments, then he must be given far larger amounts of these than normal people. We do not know why his requirements are so high. We just know that they are.

Working on theories using laboratory rats is one thing. Trying out the theories on human beings is quite another. The diet and diet supplements of mice can be controlled completely. Their environment can be controlled completely. If you want them to have certain vitamins, you inject them. If you want to remove the stress from their lives, you turn off the glaring lights and jangling bells. It's not so easy to remove stress from human situations. And it's practically impossible, Dr. Williams found, to get human beings (even desperately ill ones) to follow a program of good nutrition with food supplements taken regularly every day. It's also unfortunately true that, while there is plenty of money available to provide for feeding rats in a laboratory, a nourishing diet is expensive and the kind of food supplement Dr. Williams devised is almost prohibitively expensive—more reasons why testing his theories on human alcoholics were difficult.

It is also true that an alcoholic completely cured of his craving may decide, as a laboratory rat would not, that he can now experiment with a little social drinking without any harm. Overcoming the nutritional deficiency will not permit the alcoholic to drink safely; it will simply keep him from craving alcohol. Dr. Williams outlined for alcoholics a diet high in protein, fresh fruits and vegetables in which refined carbohydrates (white sugar and white flour products) are sharply curtailed or forbidden. Then he gave food supplements which contain, according to our reckoning, almost astronomical amounts of certain synthetic vitamins—amounts which

[321]

are not present in any of the synthetic all-in-one tablets we have ever seen and of course couldn't possibly exist in the natural kind which are more in the nature of food, rather than medicine.

The results he got from some people who followed the prescribed diet and took the food supplement as directed are almost unbelievable. Confirmed alcoholics lost their craving for alcohol within a matter of weeks or months. Dr. Williams quotes from many letters he has received from alcoholics and their families. Unfortunately, he says, such good results cannot be obtained with regularity. This is because, he thinks, there is lack of persistence in following the diet and taking the supplements; there is the danger of experimenting with social drinking. There is the cost involved.

Inability to Follow Program Defeats Us

Of course, the fact that alcoholics and their families are desperate does not make them any less susceptible to human frailty than the rest of us—but rather more so. It is hard to follow the kind of diet required; it is hard to remember to take a given number of pills at every meal, without fail. In addition, Dr. Williams reports that some of his patients suffered mild upsets when they began their massive doses of vitamins. Apparently something about their body chemistries demanded that they take in such large quantities of vitamins gradually. However, he says, "I seriously doubt if any except the most extraordinary case would resist treatment if it were begun early rather than late."

Dr. Williams is a firm believer in prevention of alcoholism. He stands strongly in favor of the moral, ethical, religious and social reasons for avoiding it. He thinks that homes, schools and churches should do everything they can to build strong character which will help one to withstand the many pressures which lead to drinking. But, he says, "good nutrition is a powerful adjunct which is too often taken for granted and overlooked as an essential factor."

Finally, he pleads for understanding on the part of the others. "People in general, potential alcoholics and others, need to recognize the importance of being individuals. This individuality which is so important socially and politically must be generally recognized so that no one will be placed in an embarrassing position because his liquor consumption does not follow a prescribed pattern set by the majority of his associates."

We think all readers would be extremely interested in Dr. Williams' book, *Alcoholism: The nutritional approach*, which is available from the University of Texas Press for $2.50. It will make you understand much more about your own individual requirements where diet and food supplements are concerned. It will make you realize that you cannot determine your nutritional requirements according to those of your neighbor, or even a close relative, or someone who has written a book or an article on the subject. Nor can you, least of all, depend on the official recommendation for the "optimum amount" of each vitamin that you should be getting.

What may be right for someone else may be 10 or 20 times less than you need. You must work out your own requirements, knowing your own conditions and the kind of diet you eat, the amount of stress in your daily life and so forth.

If you have an alcoholic in your family, Dr. Williams' book is even more important. He tells you where you can buy the supplements he has been using and makes other very practical and easy-to-follow recommendations for treating an alcoholic. If possible, get a copy, too, for your doctor, your minister, your public library.

78. Is Alcoholism a Disease of Starvation?

Within the past 30 years perhaps no change in thinking in this country has been so great as the change in our thinking about alcoholism. In the last century the "drunk" was a figure of fun, abuse or contempt. Popular songs spoke righteously of the disgrace he brought on his family, the poverty, broken homes, deaths, illness and misery. Ministers railed in their pulpits against the evils of the demon rum. Temperance workers steadied the steps of confirmed alcoholics as they tottered forward to take the pledge. Wives nagged, children wept, doctors scolded, saloon keepers got rich, and through it all the agonized and helpless alcoholic suffered more shame, pain and bewilderment than anyone involved.

In those days apparently no one suspected that an alcoholic was ill, just as ill as respectable people who contracted tuberculosis, scarlet fever or diabetes. In those days it was believed that the alcoholic was the result of pure cussedness and that he could give up drinking if he would just pull himself together. Somewhat the same theories had prevailed earlier about mental disease. Mental patients were beaten, chained and exposed to all kinds of outrages in the belief that this would cast out the devils that possessed them.

Who Is the Alcoholic?

What kind of people are alcoholics? Do personality and physical make-up give us any clue as to which people can "take it or leave it alone" and which people have a compulsive need to drink to excess? Many studies have been done on this aspect of the problem. Dr. James T. Smith of Bellevue Hospital in New York in a General Electric Science Forum radio program on January 9, 1952, said that "an alcoholic is a person who becomes socially or financially irresponsible because of drinking. . . . The alcoholic is the person who gets an excessive effect from alcohol. . . . If the alcoholic takes alcohol, he has lit a fuse which will inevitably lead on to the explosion of acute intoxication. . . . In a detailed study of over 2,000 male alcoholics we have found, for example, that they show physical characteristics differing from the average healthy male. It is striking that baldness is rare among alcoholics; they usually have a full head of hair, often prematurely gray. In general they do not have much body hair. Acne, so common in adolescent boys, occurs seldom in the history of alcoholics. Such physical characteristics are dependent on the chemical functioning of the body. . . ."

Another investigator, Jackson T. Smith, M.D., of Houston, Texas, has this to say in an article in the *American Practitioner and Digest of Treatment* for July, 1953: "More often than not the alcoholic is from a 'broken home,' either there has been a separation or divorce by the time he reached his teens or else one or both parents will have died. The alcoholic may be very labile emotionally, tending to express his moods without average restraint. There may be a continuously vacillating attitude toward whatever authority he is faced with; at one time he is openly defiant (particularly when drinking) and at another time totally dependent. It would appear that the individual's confidence in himself varies from time to time, but is always increased by his taking a drink. . . . Intellectually he may be above average, but may have repeatedly failed to utilize his innate abilities to achieve any particular goal . . . he is apt to be more self-conscious than average. . . ."

The Adrenocortical Deficiency

Harold W. Lovell, M.D., and John W. Tintera, M.D., of New York, writing in *Modern Medicine,* for May 15, 1951, say, "Two distinct groups of alcoholics are recognized. One group comprises the constitutionally hypoadrenocortic (suffering from diminished activity of the adrenal glands). Such individuals are tall, asthenic (inclined to be weak physically) men who usually report low tolerance for alcohol from the outset. These men are predisposed to alcoholism from an early age.

"In the second group are those with acquired adrenocortical insufficiency. Initially, these individuals have good tolerance for alcohol, but prolonged over-indulgence damages the adrenal cortex and reduces cortical function. Consequently alcohol tolerance is lowered and addiction results."

In an earlier issue of *Modern Medicine,* Dr. Tintera had this to say: "For many years we have maintained that an adrenocortical deficiency is as much of a genetic factor as the well-established diabetic hereditary factor. Individuals manifesting this genetic influence . . . usually show a decreased metabolism, marked hypotension (low blood pressure) and orthostatic (caused by standing upright) changes in blood pressure, a characteristic hair distribution and a fondness or even a real craving for salt and carbohydrates. . . . It is so often found that the offspring of alcoholic parents either become alcoholics themselves or teetotalers because they realize their inability to handle or tolerate alcohol. These same individuals are the ones who retain their leanness and asthenia' throughout life since they are not able to metabolize carbohydrates properly. Like their teetotaler forbears they may expect to have longevity much beyond the average with the assurance that senility due to arteriosclerotic changes will not usually ensue."

What do all these statements and big words boil down to? Well, the typical alcoholic seems to be a thin, not-very-energetic person, who is insecure and self-conscious. He may be above average in intelligence; he probably thinks of himself as a failure whether he is or not. His body seems to have a chronic inability to handle carbohydrates properly and this is the reason why alcohol spells his downfall. This is what is involved in hypoadrenocortical function. And we will explain later on just how this mechanism for regulating the digestion of carbohydrates seems to work.

What Alcohol Does in the Body

First let us investigate how alcohol behaves in the body—what it does and what it does not do. Alcohol is a carbohydrate—that is it is made of carbon, hydrogen and oxygen with a certain proportion and arrangement of molecules that differentiate it from other carbohydrates. Says John J. O'Neill in the *New York Herald-Tribune* for June 10, 1951, "alcohol acts in the body the way gasoline acts in an automobile engine. The gasoline is burned to provide heat and power but it contributes nothing to the maintenance and growth of the engine. Alcohol acts as a fuel, not as a food." Dr. Lovell in his book, *Hope and Help for the Alcoholic* (Doubleday and Company, 1951), says that alcohol is a depressant. The impression of a stimulating effect after a few drinks is the result of the temporary lift in blood sugar. But this is followed by a sharp decline if drinking is continued. A drink dilates the tiny blood vessels at the surface of the skin, bringing with the increased amount of blood a sensation of warmth. But if the skin is exposed to cold while these vessels are dilated, body heat is lost and the whole body temperature goes down. "Alcohol is not directly responsible for any disease except alcoholism," says Dr. Lovell. "Alcoholics and other excessive drinkers may impair their resistance to many diseases by allowing themselves to become undernourished, but it is the bad nutrition and not the alcohol which is the direct cause."

Alcoholism Is a Glandular Disorder

Perhaps one reason why we keep coming back to the comparison of alcoholism with diabetes is this—diabetes is also a disease of those who cannot properly metabolize carbohydrates. In the case of diabetics, not enough insulin is produced by the pancreatic gland which has this function, so the patient suffers from high blood sugar. This is why he must be given insulin to reduce his blood sugar. In the case of alcoholics, there is *too much insulin* rather than too little, with the result that the alcoholic has low blood sugar. Now the answer would be simple if it were possible

[325]

just to drain off this extra insulin, but we find it is much more complicated than that. What causes the extra insulin that causes the low blood sugar? Apparently the function of at least two glands is involved—the *adrenals* (and it is the *cortex* or covering of these glands that is involved) and the *pituitary* (which regulates adrenals).

Says E. M. Abrahamson, M.D., in his book, *Body, Mind and Sugar,* "Alcoholism is caused by a deficiency in the adrenal cortical hormones— those hormones whose action is antithetical to insulin. The trouble may not be in the adrenal cortical itself, however, but in the master gland, the pituitary, which for some reason fails to stimulate the adrenal cortical glands as it does in normal operation of the endocrine system. It is believed, moreover, that this disability of the pituitary is not caused by the alcoholism itself but antedates its development." Dr. Abrahamson goes on to tell us that physicians have achieved almost miraculous results by giving injections of ACTH and cortisone to alcoholics in their very worst condition of delirium tremens or hangovers. ACTH and cortisone are the gland extracts of the adrenal glands, in which the alcoholic is deficient. "These spectacular 'cures' are a great step forward," says Dr. Abrahamson, "and they provide evidence in reverse for the theory which the medical and the lay members of this collaboration arrived at independently; that hyper-insulinism, with its chronic partial blood sugar starvation, is an essential underlying condition of alcoholism."

It all sounds almost impossibly complicated, doesn't it? And yet the answer, as Dr. Abrahamson gives it, is so remarkably simple that we feel it should be blasted from loud speakers in every metropolis in the country and headlined in newspapers and magazines. The answer is a diet which regulates the blood sugar so that it does not fall below safe levels. This is a diet high in fat and protein and low in carbohydrates which will result —and *has* resulted in many cases treated by Dr. Abrahamson—in a complete lack of desire for alcohol. The alcohol was needed to raise the low blood sugar level which is responsible for the "jitters," the uneasiness, the lack of confidence, the restlessness of the alcoholic, which caused him to crave alcohol.

We then arrive at the question—did the alcoholic become an alcoholic because of his low blood sugar, or did the use of alcohol bring about the low blood sugar to begin with? The answer seems, at present, to be that both these suppositions are correct. That is, the individual who has a tendency (perhaps inherited), toward an improper functioning of the glands that regulate blood sugar may take to alcohol because it raises his blood sugar and thus relieves his jitters and nervousness. On the other hand, an individual who begins to drink early in life simply because of the exhilarating effect of liquor, may so damage the functioning of these glands (by drinking to excess) that he eventually gets a bad case of low blood sugar in which case, of course, he feels an overpowering compulsion to go on drinking to keep his blood sugar high.

[326]

Stress and the Alcoholic

One other factor enters in to which many researchers have devoted a lot of time. Says George N. Thompson, M.D., of the University of Southern California, writing in *Industrial Medicine and Surgery* for June, 1951, "The alcoholic is a person who, because he cannot stand the strain and tension of life without developing strong anxieties, escapes from responsibilities into oblivion . . . we are quick to state that the human organism can tolerate just so much stress. *But in spite of this knowledge, and in spite of the realization that our mental hospitals are filled with those who have fallen under the stress of their environments, under working situations intolerable to them . . . we continue to place workers in jobs for which they are unsuited, to enforce factors of stress to which we would not subject a mechanical contrivance and to expect performance beyond the capacity of the emotionally handicapped person.*"

Such a statement arouses another question in our minds—is the alcoholic a person who cannot stand stress because of his glandular make-up, or does his constant anxiety and nervousness disorder his glands? And if so, what causes the original anxiety? Could it not be lack of those vitamins whose chief function is to safeguard the health of the nervous system? One of the chief treatments for alcoholism is, and for some time has been, psychotherapy and drugs which will make alcohol repugnant to him. The question in our minds is: is it possible to rehabilitate an alcoholic by removing the frustrations and stresses in his life, without at the same time repairing the functions of his glands that affect and are affected by these emotions? Quite apart from this, of course, is the question of how many of us can afford psychotherapy, even if it is available in our home town. And how many of us can afford hospitalization which the taking of Antabuse and other drugs necessitates?

The Value of Alcoholics Anonymous

It is noteworthy that practically all writers on alcoholism mention Alcoholics Anonymous. It appears to be one organization to which unanimous approval and support is given. But it has been pointed out that the word *Alcoholic* is always used by a member when he introduces himself. He does not qualify himself as a "cured alcoholic." For he knows that, unless and until he corrects the body disorder that creates his craving for alcohol, he must remain a teetotaler—at whatever cost to his peace of mind —and can never again touch alcohol. We are in agreement that, for the confirmed alcoholic, this organization offers much in the way of psychotherapy. Socializing with people who are in the same boat and who are dedicated with fanatic fervor to helping other alcoholics appears to us to be a healthful and sound step to take.

We are convinced, moreover, that an alcoholic can be returned to health by diet, and vitamin and mineral supplements, administered at home without expense and without upsetting the family's way of life. The diet

[327]

we outline at the end of this chapter is our version of the one Dr. Abrahamson publishes in his book which, incidentally you can buy at your local bookstore or direct from the publishers—*Body, Mind and Sugar,* published by Henry Holt and Co. Two other books on alcoholism we want to recommend are *Hope and Help for the Alcoholic* by Harold W. Lovell, published by Doubleday and Company, Garden City, New York and *Alcoholism: The nutritional approach* by Roger J. Williams, published by the University of Texas Press, Austin 12, Texas.

For those of you who may have had alcoholics in the family or who, for some reason, fear that some member of the family may have inclinations this way, we would say don't try to prevent alcoholism by scolding, lecturing and forbidding alcohol in the house. Liquor is easily available at almost any corner of the street these days. Instead, try putting the whole family on a high protein diet with as few sweet and starchy foods as possible. This means meat, eggs, nuts, fresh vegetables and fruits, supplemented by brewer's yeast or desiccated liver for vitamin B, rose hips or some other natural food supplement for vitamin C, fish liver oil for vitamins A and D, bone meal for calcium and other minerals and wheat germ for vitamin E. Sunflower seeds are high-protein snacks.

Diet To Prevent Low Blood Sugar

The diet which is found in Dr. Abrahamson's book includes such items as bacon, ham, bread, milk, butter, cheese, soft drinks and distilled liquors. We, of course, do not approve of these foods and beverages. Naturally, alcoholic beverages do not belong on a diet list for an alcoholic, but we contend that he will soon not want them. Also note that we do not recommend using citrus fruits as freely as Dr. Abrahamson suggests and we do not approve of drinking citrus fruit juice. Any lack of vitamin C can be made up by taking rose hips.

Here is our version of the diet. Get the whole family accustomed to eating this way:

On arising: fruit or vegetable juice.

Breakfast: fruit or vegetable juice; one helping of protein food such as eggs, nuts, etc.

Two hours after breakfast: Vegetable or fruit juice or fruit.

Lunch: Meat, fish, poultry or eggs; salad of fresh raw vegetables and greens, cooked vegetables, if desired; dessert (see below which desserts are allowed); beverage.

Three hours after lunch: high protein snack—seeds, nuts, etc.

One hour before dinner: fruit or vegetable juice or fruit.

Dinner: Vegetables, salad, meat, fish or poultry, dessert; beverage.

Two or three hours after dinner: Protein snack.

Every two hours until bedtime: fruit or fruit juice, nuts or other high protein food.

Allowable vegetables: all except potatoes.

Allowable juice: Any unsweetened fruit or vegetable juice, except grape juice or prune juice.

Allowable fruit: all except grapes, raisins, prunes, figs, dates, cherries.

Allowable beverages: weak tea (teabag, not brewed), Postum.

Allowable desserts: fruit; unsweetened gelatine; junket (made from tablets, not the mix).

Avoid absolutely: sugar, honey, rice, candy, cake, pie, pastries, custards, puddings, ice cream, caffeine (ordinary coffee, strong brewed tea, cola beverages), spaghetti, macaroni, noodles, alcoholic drinks, and of course such starchy products as pretzels, doughnuts, crackers, and so forth.

Lettuce, mushrooms and nuts may be taken as freely as desired.

~~~~~~

SECTION 17: APPENDICITIS

~~~~~~

79. Appendicitis Is Still a Problem

We don't hear much about appendicitis anymore. Most people have much more exciting operations to talk about. With hearts being stitched up and kidneys removed or transplanted, an appendicitis sounds pretty tame. But it is sobering to note that *Parade* magazine for January 2, 1955, reported over 5,000 deaths in the United States during the preceding year due to appendicitis complications. Medical men will point out, as does *Physicians Bulletin* (September, 1955) that the present mortality rate for appendicitis is less than one-seventh what it was in 1900.

The *Canadian Medical Association Journal* (72: 175-178, 1955) has even more comforting figures: it reports only two deaths in 1,000 cases, as opposed to 26 deaths per 1,000 cases only 15 years ago. Quite a reduction. But such figures tend to obscure the unpleasant fact that, while it is true that fewer people are dying from appendicitis, the number of people who suffer from the disease is the same as ever. The *Pfizer Spectrum* (no date), a drug trade magazine, reports that appendectomies are still the most frequently performed operations in general hospitals. Ten to 15 per cent of major operations are appendectomies.

How An Appendicitis Acts

Acute appendicitis attacks are sudden and give little forewarning. Typically, a case will follow this pattern: the patient will quite suddenly find that he has a terrible stomach ache. The pain will be generalized throughout the entire abdominal area. Gradually it will concentrate in the lower right portion of the abdomen. Though the pain is usually much more intense, the distress the patient suffers is much like constipation. (It is for this reason that the dangerous temptation to use a laxative presents itself.) Strangely, in spite of the pain and general stress on the body, a high fever is not one of the early symptoms of appendicitis.

When a doctor sees the patient, he will check for tenderness at the expected site of the pain by touching the abdomen. He will note that the abdominal muscles are rigid. A blood count will usually show a high majority of white blood cells, which have been called out by the body to fight the illness. These are the usual warnings of appendicitis, but doctors agree that the presence of these signs is no guarantee that the appendix is really the problem, nor does the absence of several of them mean that appendicitis can be ruled out. A doctor writing in *New York Medicine* (January 5, 1955) said, ". . . . there is no one single test that we can rely on absolutely."

Problems of Diagnosis

One of the complicating factors in the diagnosis of appendicitis is the type of person it happens to. Children under 14 accounted for ¼ of a total of 3,229 cases in one report carried by the *Journal of the American Medical Association* (January 23, 1954). The symptoms of appendicitis—bellyaches, nausea, vomiting, constipated feeling—are rather common in children. And trying to get any definite information out of a frightened and crying child who is in some kind of pain is pretty nearly impossible.

When the appendix of an elderly person acts up, the problem of diagnosis is complicated once more. They are often inclined to disregard even severe pain, their stomach muscles are often so weak that the characteristic rigidity is not apparent, or the symptoms are masked by any number of other old age disease conditions. Because of this unfortunate resistance to accurate diagnosis, almost all suspected appendicitis cases are operated on as soon as possible.

Just what the function of the appendix is in the human body is not known. Many physiologists suggest that it might be left over from some evolutionary process. One experimenter whose work was written up in *Time* magazine (June 5, 1950) was convinced that the appendix is a blood-forming organ. He had been studying the effects of radiation on living things and found that radiation victims are likely to die of anemia because the blood-building powers of the bone marrow are damaged. However, experiments with rabbits showed that when the spleen and appendix of the animal were protected with a lead shield, the animal survived what would normally be a fatal overdose of X-ray. It was deduced from this that the spleen and appendix make enough blood to enable the damaged tissues to recover. But remember, this is only a theory; the opportunity to try it on man has not yet presented itself. Aside from this theory, the positive reason for the existence of the appendix in the body has eluded science up to this time.

The reason that a seemingly insignificant organ, little bigger than the index finger and similar in shape, can cause such misery is that it sometimes becomes blocked by foreign matter or infected. The infection grows until the entire organ is a cylinder of infection, and then the symptoms begin. When laxatives are taken as a means of relieving the distress which follows, they encourage peristaltic action (that wave-like motion of the intestines which pushes fecal matter through and out of the body) and this causes a pressure on the full and rigid appendix, often forcing it to burst.

Why Do We Get Appendicitis?

The question of why some appendices last a lifetime without giving any trouble, while others don't even hold up to adulthood has been the subject of much guesswork and experiment. An article in the *British Medical Journal* (April 16, 1955) seeks to place the blame largely on psychological factors. The author suggests that since activities of the colon and small intestines are generally believed to be influenced by stress and emotion, why not those of the appendix, since it is also a part of that network? In 1948, J. W. Paulley tried using appendicitis cases as controls in an experiment. It was found that appendicitis usually occurred in tense individuals with unduly rigid outlooks. Also it was noted that the attack of appendicitis was closely related in time to some family disaster or period of emotional strain.

Dr. A. L. Ribeiro, practicing in Kenya, South Africa, wrote a similar report. He was convinced that fear or anxiety could cause appendicitis. Dr. Ribeiro described 4 cases of Negro women who had been seriously threatened in various ways and had developed appendicitis soon after the incident.

We are inclined to go along with the observation of A. Rendle Short, M.D., who states in his book, *The Causation of Appendicitis*, that the appendix is a part of the alimentary canal, and is therefore directly affected by diet. This viewpoint would seem to be backed up by the following evidence which points to the fact that appendicitis is extremely rare among those people who live on a simple diet, unencumbered by modern refined foods.

Diet—A Causal Factor

The *Medical Journal of Australia* (September 14, 1957) carries an article which asserts that appendicitis is unknown among the natives of New Guinea and the Territory of Papua who live in their natural environment and eat traditional foods. However, the Europeans living in the same area have a good deal of the disease. The writer found too that those natives who, through work or schooling, came under the influence of the European diet, are open to the disease. To illustrate, the author cites these figures for the city of Port Morseby. The European population there is 4300, while the natives number 10,000; the Europeans had 54 appendicitis cases listed, and the natives had 8. Every one of the 8 natives showed a history of eating a European diet, including preserved foodstuffs.

H. M. Karn, in the *British Medical Journal* (September 6, 1952) writes that he was impressed by the absence of acute appendicitis among the native troops of West Africa, Sudan and Egypt and attached native civilians. Yet the disease was as prevalent as ever in European troops. Karn notes further that the natives so immune to appendicitis were affected by the disease when they were transferred to active duty and forced to eat European rations.

A Dutch physician, Dr. L. W. Van Ouwerkerk, writing in *Science Digest* (March, 1950), also notes that natives of Asia and Africa where diet is simple showed a rarity of appendicitis. However, when natives eat the diets of Europeans living there, a rise in incidence is seen.

The Value of Natural Foods

In *The Causation of Appendicitis*, Dr. Short remarks that vegetarians are relatively immune to appendicitis. Several of our other sources suggest too that the meat in the diet might be responsible for appendicitis. This idea probably finds its root in statistics which show wartime figures of appendicitis incidence to be below those of other times. Of course, meat was scarce during World War II, but so were sugar, canned goods and other refinements of modern diet. We are more inclined to believe that the scarcity of the many really harmful foods was responsible for the downgrade of appendix problems, rather than the lack of meat. Further, if meat-eating were responsible, how does one explain the disease-free record of the primitive natives everywhere whose diets sometimes consist of meat exclusively?

Sluggish elimination, and the lack of fresh, unprocessed foods which can cause it, appear to be the most likely causes of appendicitis. Eating foods that are as close to nature as possible is your best defense against this disease of civilization. Keeping a high percentage of cellulose, or "roughage," foods in your daily intake will keep your alimentary channels open. Such foods as cabbage, asparagus, apples, cauliflower, carrots, peas and onions are excellent for this purpose.

A healthy well-nourished body functions with ease. If the foods we eat are worthwhile, and free of ingredients which can undermine the body's supply of nutrients, the body automatically takes from them what it needs and effortlessly discards the rest. There is no pile-up of waste which might seep through to clog the appendix and cause the serious discomfort of appendicitis.

Give your body what it needs through healthful foods and food supplements, and it will do the rest.

[332]

80. Arthritis and Arthritic and Rheumatic Diseases

Rheumatism is a disease older than man. Prehistoric man suffered from rheumatism, and the animals who lived on the earth for millions of years before man suffered from rheumatism. Evidence of rheumatism has been found in the skeletons of dinosaurs. Animals, either in captivity or in their natural, wild state, may develop rheumatism; it is common to both meat-eating and vegetarian animals. In America it is estimated that approximately 7,500,000 individuals have one form or another of rheumatism. Of these, 147,000 are considered permanently invalided!

Rheumatism is not a dramatic quick killer like heart disease. It has not the slow but certain malignancy of cancer. Patients with rheumatism may live to a great age, and in fact, seldom die of this disease. It is a "chronic" disease, but considering that it afflicts more people than any of the other chronic diseases and that its one common symptom is excruciating pain, it seems strange that medical science has not come any nearer to finding a cure. Most of us think of rheumatism as a disease of later life. While it is quite true that most elderly people suffer to a certain degree from rheumatic symptoms, it is also true that 50 per cent of the disability incidental to rheumatism is found among persons under 45.

Since symptoms may come and go without any apparent cause, some physicians believe that rheumatism may have a psychosomatic origin. This means that the disease itself is real enough, but that the reasons for it lie in some unresolved conflict in the patient's life. According to *Time* magazine for June 13, 1949, Dr. Edward Weiss of Philadelphia theorizes that the patient may be troubled with "chronic resentment"—an unhappy marriage, some bitter disappointment in his career, some frustration against which he subconsciously battles every day.

Physicians are certain by now that there is a definite relationship between hormones (gland secretions) and rheumatism. The emotions affect the glands that manufacture hormones; in turn the hormones affect the emotions. While we do not minimize the importance to health of a happy adjustment to one's life environment, we are inclined to take hold of it the other way around. We believe that healthy people don't meet with as many conflicts and frustrations or, if they do, they find ways to overcome them. We have a notion that most frustrations and conflicts exist in sick

[333]

minds, and sick minds are at least partly caused by sick bodies, in which, for instance, hormones may not be functioning properly for some very sound physical reason. Animals as well as men suffer from psychosomatic illness, true, but honestly now, isn't it just a bit far-fetched to imagine a dinosaur wasting away with rheumatism just because of some unbearable frustration in his life with the other dinosaurs?

It seems to us that rheumatism must have certain definite physical reasons for being. In clinics, rest homes, hospitals, spas and laboratories, here and abroad, noted scientists have devoted themselves to the study of rheumatism. Why is it that, over all these centuries, no answer has been found? We believe it may be because each investigator is looking for some one answer—which he *has* to do in order to be scientifically accurate. But perhaps one answer will not solve the problem—more things may be involved.

The Different Kinds of Rheumatism

There are many kinds of rheumatism, all of them related. In the *Medical Clinics of North America* for November, 1940, rheumatic diseases are classified as follows: atrophic (rheumatoid or proliferative) arthritis, and hypertrophic (osteo- or degenerative) arthritis. Those patients who show symptoms of both are said to have "mixed arthritis." Then there are types of arthritis caused by definite, known poisoning, such as tuberculous, pneumococcal and so forth. Rheumatic fever, muscular rheumatism (fibrositis) and menopausal neuralgia are other related diseases in which actual joint involvement is not so great.

In atrophic or rheumatoid arthritis there is evidence of "atrophic" or "wasting" manifestations in the bone and muscle system of the body as well as disorder in other body tissues. Victims of rheumatoid arthritis are usually individuals from 30 to 50, more women than men. Exhaustion, anemia, nervous disturbances, digestive disorders and sometimes liver trouble are accompanying symptoms, aside from the swelling and pain in the joints. Osteoarthritis is generally considered a degenerative disease— that is, a disease of old age, resulting from wear and tear on the body generally, and strain or injury in some particular part of the body. For instance, the hands of farmers, craftsmen and housewives are particularly susceptible to osteoarthritis, because they have worked so hard and gotten so many knocks and bumps.

Experiments with Cures for Rheumatism

In 1950, Dr. Granirer of Queens General Hospital, Jamaica, Long Island, reported on a new therapy involving the injection of blood drawn from women 48 hours after childbirth. It is known that rheumatism often disappears completely during pregnancy. It also disappears when the patient contracts jaundice. So physicians reasoned that some substance present in the blood of pregnant women, or in jaundice patients, might be antagonistic to rheumatism. According to the one report we read, all arthritis patients treated with the new substance showed great improvement in symptoms, half of them maintaining their gains after treatment had been discontinued for a year. One patient had no symptoms of arthritis 22 months after the injections were stopped.

A year or so later, a new remedy for osteoarthritis was announced by Dr. W. S. Collins and his associate of Maimonides Hospital, Brooklyn. This consisted of an extract derived from the livers of pregnant cows. In many cases, this substance brought relief from pain and joint stiffness.

Among the various cures experimented with through the years, most have been aimed at alleviating the symptoms of the disease—that is, stopping or lessening the pain, improving the stiffness and preventing deformities. Shock treatment, ozone therapy, massage, percussion therapy, sulfur baths, thermal therapy, injections of sulfur have been used. Counter-irritants have been tested, injections of proteins, bee and cobra venom have been tried. Gold salts have been given orally and injected.

In preventing deformities from the twisting and crippling of the disease, physicians have used surgery, splints, plaster casts, exercise, massage, heat treatments, underwater exercise, various kinds of baths—the list is almost endless.

How Much Have We Learned About Rheumatism?

Under the heading of possible preventives of rheumatism, there seem to be two aspects of living that might be involved—diet and posture. What do we know up to now of the relation of diet to rheumatism? Arthritis does not seem to be a disease in which there is a gross deficiency of vitamin A, yet certainly some deficiency is suggested by the frequency of respiratory tract infections in conjunction with rheumatism—colds, bronchitis, laryngitis, etc. Could these not result from a lack of vitamin A to strengthen these delicate tissues against bacterial invaders? The frequency of liver disorder in arthritics suggests that the liver might be unable to do its work of transforming carotene into vitamin A, so that a greater quantity of vitamin A would be necessary in the patient's diet.

Most arthritics have difficulty assimilating carbohydrates—that is, starches and sugars. This suggests a deficiency of vitamin B which is the vitamin necessary to accompany these substances on their way through the digestive tract. There also may be lack of appetite, another symptom of vitamin B deficiency. There may be neuritis or edema (swelling), both of which may indicate need for vitamin B. Digestive disorders point to deficiency of niacin, one of the B vitamins; anemia and nervousness both indicate need for niacin. The B vitamins will also relieve the frequent constipation of arthritics. In the early part of 1952, the *American Practitioner* reported remarkable results in the treatment of osteoarthritis and osteoporosis with vitamin B_{12}—the fabulous vitamin occurring most abundantly in liver. Of 33 cases of arthritis, 20 patients benefited from the treatment within the first week, 7 of whom obtained complete relief. By the end of the third

[335]

week, all but 3 of the patients showed some benefit. Three cases of rheumatoid arthritis did not react at all to the vitamin.

Vitamin C is found to be abnormally low in the blood of arthritics. Charles W. Buckley, M.D., F.R.C.P., writing in the *Practitioner* for September, 1938, has this to say about the importance of vitamin C in the diet of arthritics: "From available evidence, this deficiency (of vitamin C) is the result rather than the cause of the infection, and it has been found that the amount of vitamin C required to raise the level in a normal individual to saturation point is much below what is required to produce the same effect in one suffering from acute rheumatism or rheumatoid arthritis. It seems probable that there is an increased destruction of this vitamin owing to a greater metabolic demand. There is, however, no definite evidence as yet that vitamin C has any curative effect on the disease." Dr. C. Wesler Scull, writing in the *Medical Clinics of North America*, tells us that placing animals on a diet low in vitamin C results in conditions similar to human arthritis. Although vitamin C will not apparently cure these symptoms after they have appeared, does it not seem possible that they may be brought on by lack of vitamin C?

In osteoarthritis, a demineralization of the bones takes place which is similar to that occurring in rickets, a disease due entirely to vitamin D deficiency. So it is considered good clinical practice generally, to give ample vitamin D to all arthritic patients.

Vitamin E Is Important in Rheumatic Diseases

Considerable investigation has been carried out on the subject of vitamin E and rheumatism. C. L. Steinberg, physician in charge of the Arthritis Clinic, Rochester General Hospital, tells us in the *Annals of the New York Academy of Science* for October 3, 1949, of his success in giving vitamin E to rheumatic patients. Treating fibrositis (muscular rheumatism) in 300 patients with vitamin E, he found that relief was obtained in the vast majority of cases. He cautions that the patient should keep on taking a "maintenance" dose, after the symptoms have disappeared.

He also treated rheumatic fever with vitamin E. He relates 5 case histories of young people whose rheumatic fever symptoms were relieved by vitamin E. It is interesting to note that he gave natural (not synthetic) vitamin E throughout the experiment.

Dr. Morris Ant of Kings County Hospital, Brooklyn, treated muscle diseases and industrial injuries with wheat germ oil directly applied to the painful spot. Reporting on his experiences in *Industrial Medicine* for June, 1946, he tells us he used a 55 per cent ointment of wheat germ oil and food supplementation by wheat germ oil, as well as a diet rich in vitamin E foods. Out of 20 cases treated successfully, he reports in detail on 4— one, a housewife whose hands were swollen and stiff. Local application of wheat germ oil soon returned the hands to their normal condition. A physician with swelling of his knees and back so painful that he could not walk was given wheat germ oil locally and internally, and was soon able to resume his practice once more. An elevator operator who had had a serious fall developed pain and stiff muscles in his chest and legs, along with bronchial asthma. After several months of wheat germ oil therapy, both locally and internally, he went back to work free from all symptoms except for an occasional slight limp. Incidentally, the asthma disappeared, too. A clerk who had fallen against the sharp corner of a desk suffered from a long-standing pain over her ribs, so violent that she was unable to sleep. Wheat germ oil locally and internally left her symptom-free within several months.

In a later article in the *Annals of the New York Academy of Science,* Dr. Ant, along with Erwin DiCyan, describes the use of vitamin E in rheumatic diseases—this time given orally, intramuscularly and locally. In a series of 100 patients, there was relief from pain, improvement or disappearance of physical symptoms and increased mobility of joints. In addition to the therapy which these patients received at the doctor's office, they were placed on diets high in vitamin E—for instance, a tablespoon of wheat germ was taken at breakfast; one-fourth head of lettuce with peanut oil dressing and one banana were added to the lunch menu; at dinner, lean beef, spinach and lettuce with peanut oil dressing contributed to the vitamin E content of the day's meals.

The Raw Food Diet for Rheumatism

Dorothy C. Hare, C.B.E., M.D., writing in the British journal, *Proceedings of the Royal Society of Medicine,* Vol. 30, 1936, contributes what seems to us the most convincing piece of evidence on diet influencing the course of chronic rheumatism. Dr. Hare describes an experiment at the Royal Free Hospital, in which rheumatic patients received a diet of raw fruits and vegetables with results that were, it seems to us, spectacular. Dr. Hare is apparently a conservative physician who indicates that she does not advise this diet to replace other forms of medical therapy, nor does she advise it in all cases. She simply reports on it and suggests that further research would be valuable.

Twelve patients were selected for the experiment—all were sent to the hospital for this purpose. They represented the main types of rheumatic disorders—muscular, osteoarthritis and rheumatoid arthritis. No other treatment was given them aside from the diet; they were encouraged to be up and around, whenever the severity of their ailment allowed. Some of them were bedridden.

After they became accustomed to the hospital life, eating the diet usually served in the wards for one week, they were placed for two weeks on a diet consisting of nothing but fresh, raw fruits and vegetables, nuts, cream, salad oil, milk and raw oatmeal.

A day's menu went like this:

BREAKFAST—apple porridge made of grated apple, soaked raw oatmeal, grated nuts, cream, fresh orange, tea with milk and cream.

[337]

MID-MORNING—tomato puree with lemon.

DINNER—salad of lettuce, cabbage, tomato, root vegetables; salad dressing with oil, mixed fruit salad and cream.

TEA—dried fruits, nuts and tea with milk and cream.

SUPPER—fruit porridge, prune, apricot or apple; salad dish with dressing.

BEDTIME—lemon and orange juice with hot water.

After two weeks, the following cooked foods were added to this diet:

vegetable soup	two ounces of bacon
one egg	two ounces of bread
two ounces of meat	butter, cheese and milk

At no time during the weeks of the diet was any salt added to either the raw or cooked foods. The dried fruits and raw oatmeal were soaked in water, the vegetables were shredded, nuts crushed or whole. All food was prepared fresh for every meal and was served attractively.

Eight of the patients began to feel better in one to four weeks on this diet. Two improved up to 5 or 6 weeks, then relapsed. Two showed no improvement at all. In the follow-up, after the patients who improved had gone home, it was found that 7 of them continued to improve to a marked degree. For example, one patient aged 46 had suffered for 4 years with occasional pain and swelling of the knees, but for the 3 months before she was admitted to the hospital, she had general pain and stiffness in shoulders, arms, hands, knees and legs. She had been in bed for 10 weeks. There was fluid in both knee joints, swelling and pain in other joints. She was discharged from the hospital after being on the diet for 3 weeks. Later, after continuing with the diet for 7 more weeks, she was free from all pain and able to do her housework.

All of the patients lost considerable weight during the first week on the diet, but those who continued to lose in the following weeks lost much less, and in every case, except very obese patients, weight was properly maintained on the diet. For the obese patients, of course, losing weight was extremely helpful, as overweight adds greatly to the problems of an arthritic.

In commenting on her diet and its success, Dr. Hare remarks on the fact that the rawness of the food seemed to be the one outstanding factor that brought about results. The fact that the food was raw made a great impression on the patients themselves and on observers. She tells us that a Zurich physician, who used raw diets similar to this in treating rheumatism, claimed that the diet was successful "because of the absorption of the unaltered solar energy of plant life." Says Dr. Hare "science has so far revealed nothing . . . of this occult solar energy, as something apart from vitamin and chemical constituents (of food)."

We have made no study of "occult solar energy," but it seems that science will soon have to be convinced of the healthfulness of raw foods, for every day we are finding out more and more about the vitamins and enzymes destroyed by heating foods. May there not be many other elements in food, unknown as yet to science, that we destroy when the food is heated above body temperature?

Then says Dr. Hare, such a diet contains a lot of vitamins C and B (as well as vitamin A, we can add). Protein and fat are lacking in the vegetables and fruits. This deficiency is partly made up for by the nuts, and salad oil, later by the meat and eggs. Finally, Dr. Hare remarks, we must consider how much of the effectiveness of the diet depends on the fact that it was low in sodium. Vegetables contain little sodium and considerable potassium. No salt (sodium chloride) was added at any time during the diet, so that, even though bacon and other foods were added later on, the diet was still extremely low in sodium, compared to the usual diet.

Raw Foods and Vitamins and Very Little Salt

As we found in reviewing symptoms of vitamin deficiency in rheumatic patients, many vitamins appear to be in short supply. Vitamin C (found in fresh fruits and vegetables) is most abundant in its natural form in rose hips, which also contain vitamins A and E and several of the B vitamins. Vitamin A is in the yellow foods—carrots, sweet potatoes—and most abundant in fish liver oil. Vitamin B_{12} has produced almost miraculous results in cases of osteoarthritis. Vitamin B_{12} is found most abundantly in liver along with the other members of the B complex of vitamins. Desiccated liver tablets or capsules are the one sure way of getting enough vitamin B_{12} every day. We hardly need to add that all of us—adults and children alike—must have ample vitamin D, the sunshine vitamin, which is also plentiful in fish liver oil.

Dr. Hare's success in treating rheumatic patients with raw foods does not surprise us at all, and we are firmly convinced that the results would have been even better had these been organically raised foods, brought fresh from the garden to the trays of these patients. We do not advise going on such a diet on your own, as an experiment. Undoubtedly your need for animal protein (meat, eggs, and especially organ meats like liver) is great, and some of these foods are not palatable eaten raw. But we urge you to include raw foods as part of the menu at every meal. Eat fruits raw, always. Don't cook any vegetable that you can eat raw. At breakfast, be certain you have raw fruit. Make sure that lunch includes salad, raw carrots, celery, cauliflower or tomato, etc. For dinner, serve as many vegetables raw as you can and develop your skill in combining them and seasoning them with herbs and dressing, so that your family will ask for more.

Remember, too, that the low-sodium diet appears to be helpful in treating rheumatism. As you know, we believe that most of us use far, far too much salt and advise cutting it down to a minimum. Try leaving the salt shaker off the table for a week. Then, the next week, begin to omit salt from some dishes as you prepare them in the kitchen. You'll soon find how easy it is to do without salt altogether. You'll discover, too, how much better the food tastes when you're tasting *it,* instead of the salt.

[339]

81. Stress

One of the most persistent and interesting theories concerning the cause of arthritis is that which connects arthritis with psychological or emotional problems. This idea is not a new one, for there are studies on the subject that were conducted as early as 1935. Just about all of these researchers agree that arthritis is the result of many physiological factors, but the evidence we've seen is significant enough, we think, to make emotional upsets a part of the list. We believe that poor diet is the essential and underlying cause of most diseases. However, it is possible that the causes often mentioned with arthritis, such as local infections, dampness, heredity, etc., are triggers that can activate arthritis symptoms in a body run down by unhealthful eating habits. In this sense, the emotions, too, must be seriously considered.

An article in the *Canadian Medical Association Journal* (September 15, 1957) says rheumatoid arthritis is a "stress disease and represents a maladaptation of psychobiological stress." Or, more simply, a severe emotional problem can lead you right into a case of swollen joints and arthritic misery.

A Summary of Previous Research

The authors discuss previous research and study along these lines, and summarize the findings of the past 20 years. It is emphasized that these conclusions can only be classed as generalized, due to the many uncontrollable factors involved in dealing with individual emotions and attitudes that have been shaped by a million impressions over a lifetime. It is amazing, though, to see the similarity of personality development in the arthritic individuals studied. Briefly, here are the findings up to now: In 1935, a study showed that arthritics seemed to try to escape from emotional conflicts through physical function. A study involving 32 patients, in 1935, led the observer to note that "a fairly severe emotional disturbance of one kind or another had been present before any sign of rheumatoid arthritis." This doctor (Thomas) also remarked that, in general, he had found that sexual adjustment of rheumatoid arthritics was inadequate.

A very common emotional mark in rheumatoid arthritics was noted by Halliday in 1937 and 1942: rheumatoid arthritics show a definite restriction of emotional expression, as well as strong elements of self-sacrifice. This impression is backed up by a 1954 study which concluded that rheumatoid arthritis seems to follow events which upset the balance between aggressive impulses and their control. For example, let's say a man is unhappy in his job, but knows that he must keep it for the sake of his family's welfare. His resentment against his circumstances might never be spoken outright, but repressing it might lead to arthritis. This is the kind of circumstance we mean.

[340]

It seems to be of major significance in supporting the emotional stress and arthritis theory to note that there is a relative absence of arthritis among those who are actually adjudged insane. It would seem that these people have given up the struggle to control the repressions and frustrations which are believed to manifest themselves in arthritis.

A Detailed Psychological Study of 18 Patients

These brief summaries are contained in the above-mentioned Canadian journal as a preface to the detailed description of a similar study. Eighteen arthritis patients were studied. The problem was to get 18 non-arthritics whose background was as similar as possible, to act as controls. The solution lay in using the brother or sister of the patient, as close in age as possible, and of the same sex if that were possible. This procedure also would eliminate hereditary differences. The age of the subjects ranged from 20 to 60 years.

All of the people, both arthritics and non-arthritics, used in the study were interviewed by a social worker, to determine their physical environmental background, both in the past and at present. They each spent from 3 to 10 hours with a psychiatrist, who attempted to acquire an accurate picture of their individual personalities and mental attitudes. And finally, all were given objective psychological tests.

The general findings of the examinations were these: In childhood, the arthritic patients had shown impulsiveness and love of strenuous activity—sports and games, etc. The brothers and sisters of these people showed an opposite tendency in childhood; they were quiet, shy and obedient to the point of envying the boisterousness of their brother or sister.

As adults, these characteristics reversed themselves in the people observed. The arthritics had restrained their activity in games and sports (not necessarily due to invalidism), as though answering some inner compulsion. They were obsessed with the need to be tidy and punctual, etc. Any aggression they'd shown as children was now replaced with self-sacrifice and forgiving attitudes.

And what of the non-arthritic brothers and sisters? Of course you've guessed it: they became aggressive, full of self-confidence and free of shyness as adults.

In the interviews, an interesting physiological fact was revealed. Many of the arthritis patients had experienced other psychosomatic ailments, such as eczema and migraine headaches, preceding the onset of the disease.

Another study on the same subject is outlined in the August 15, 1957, issue of the same periodical, the *Canadian Medical Association Journal*. The author in this case states at the outset that emotional or psychological factors are usually listed among the causes of rheumatoid arthritis in standard textbooks dealing with this disease. Also, it is said to be common that flare-ups and relapses of the disease often follow emotional stress from various sources.

Studies of 43 chronic rheumatoid arthritis patients yielded some interesting generalizations. For example, a majority of the patients associated the onset of the disease with the death of a spouse, separation from a spouse, prolonged separation from a family or leaving home to become established—all situations which carried in them the elements which could be woven into great emotional stress. Add to this the traits of immaturity, dependence, concealed hostility and excessively insistent cooperation in everything, and you have a picture of the average arthritic in this study.

This information does not imply that any person to whom such unfortunate things happen will end as a rheumatoid arthritic. Most persons who lose parents, who end an unhappy marriage in divorce or separation, or who meet with frustration in beginning a career do not find themselves victims of this disease. Somehow or other they must have accumulated inner resources to battle against such a breakdown. Even though the trigger of stress was pulled, it did not bring on a physiological breakdown. No one can be sure he is possessed of such resources, but we can all do our best to see that our bodies have the raw material to manufacture the nutritional blocks against arthritis.

Dr. Hans Selye, an expert on stress and its consequences, has found that even the slightest strain on the body, mental or physical, will cause it to use vitamins and minerals in excess of its normal needs. A sudden scare, an argument, a slight cut or bruise—any one of these happenings will call on special reserves in the body. Now people who live under a constant, day-in, day-out strain, such as dangerous or unpleasant working conditions, unending financial worries, miserable family life or broken homes, etc.— these people are using excessive amounts of nutritional reserves every day. Without increased use of supplements and careful selection of foods, there is no way for them to avoid some kind of physical breakdown—arthritis being a common one.

It all goes back to diet, whether the immediate cause seems to be mental stress, dampness, any one of a hundred other things. The body must have fighting equipment, and if the enemy is strong, the body must be made equal to the task by extra ammunition in the form of food supplements, especially the B vitamins and vitamin C. If you think you are under undue stress, increase your vitamin intake. You may be warding off a lifetime of arthritis misery.

82. Rheumatism and Eggs

May G. Wilson in a book, *Rheumatic Fever,* published by Oxford University Press, 1940, speculates on the fact that cases of rheumatic fever reach their peak in April, and then decline during the summer months. Eggs are plentiful and, hence, cheap during spring and summer, scarce and, hence, expensive during winter. Could the eating of eggs be related, therefore, to the incidence of rheumatic fever?

The reasoning goes like this: eggs are rich in a B vitamin, choline. (Notice we did not say *chlorine,* but *choline.*) This vitamin is extremely important for the health of the liver. It helps to manufacture a substance called phospholipid, a fatty substance, for the blood. This substance is one of the elements that fights against streptococcus infection. Rheumatic fever is associated with streptococcus infection. Therefore, rheumatic fever may be conditioned partly at least by egg intake.

Wallis, writing in the *American Journal of Medical Science,* Vol. 227, p. 167, 1954, states that he did a survey among 184 adult and adolescent patients with rheumatic heart disease and a group of normal subjects. Forty-one per cent of the rheumatic heart patients said they thought they ate few eggs in childhood. Only 16 per cent of the normal people claimed they did not eat eggs as children. Ten per cent of the rheumatic patients said they still did not like eggs; only 5 per cent of the healthy folks had this food prejudice.

You may say that such a survey could not be significant enough to base a theory on, since it depends on the patients' memories of what they ate as children. However, rather elaborate precautions were taken during the survey to eliminate any biased answers.

Two other researchers, Coburn and Moore, reporting in the *American Journal of Diseases of Children,* Vol. 65, p. 744, 1943, state that the diet of rheumatic heart children appeared to be lacking in eggs, as well as other valuable nutritional elements. So they supplemented the diet of 30 convalescent children with the equivalent of 4 egg yolks a day (the yolk of the eggs is the part highest in choline and other fats). The rheumatic fever recurred in only 7 per cent of these children, compared with a recurrence of 38 per cent in children whose diets were not so supplemented. Later, in 1950, Dr. Coburn reported in the *Journal of the American Dietetic Association,* Vol. 26, p. 345, that 8 to 10 egg yolks daily given to children who had previously had rheumatic fever prevented relapses, even when the children were later subjected to streptococcal infection.

Now we have uncovered another piece of evidence implicating egg-less diets as possible predisposing causes of rheumatic fever. Dr. Coburn and two colleagues, writing in the *Journal of Experimental Medicine,* Vol. 100, p. 425, 1954, tell us of experiments in which they induced rheumatism in laboratory animals by eliminating eggs, and prevented it by giving egg yolks. Here, surely, is another link in the chain of evidence that will one day lead to the complete elimination of this disease.

The authors tell us their experiments show that, under certain conditions, "some lipid substance" (that is, some fatty substance) of egg yolk will prevent the animal from getting rheumatic symptoms when a substance is given him that would otherwise produce them. Now, note carefully the following further observations: it did no good to give the egg yolk daily to adult animals which were at the same time subjected to the rheumatism-producing substance. But animals born and bred throughout their lifetimes on diets which included egg yolk received a high degree of protection when they were later subjected to conditions that would have caused rheumatism. Supplementing the diet with egg yolk even two to four weeks before inducing the disease gave some protection.

The authors go on to say, "Attention is called to the possibility that these experimental findings (on arthritis) . . . may be pertinent to the genesis of the rheumatic state." The factors among "less privileged" persons which favor the development of rheumatic fever are not well defined. In other words, we do not know exactly what kind of diet is eaten generally by children who later come down with rheumatic fever. But there seems to be no doubt that it is lacking in natural fatty substances. Rheumatic fever does not occur in patients who have a high level of fat in the blood (diabetics, for instance), but it does occur in cases of Graves' disease where the blood level of fat is low.

The Fat in Egg Yolk Is Important

What was the substance in egg yolk that gave the protection? The authors do not know. But they do know that it was a fatty substance. And they found, too, that breaking down crude lecithin gave them a substance which protected the animals against the rheumatism.

We hear a lot of frightening facts about fats in the diet these days. Headlines in newspapers and magazines caution us against eating eggs, because, we are told, eggs contain cholesterol and cholesterol seems to be responsible for the fatty deposits that cause hardening of the arteries. Sure eggs contain cholesterol, but they also contain lecithin which, scientific research indicates, emulsifies cholesterol, so that it does not collect where it is not wanted. Hence, the cholesterol content of eggs cannot harm you, because it comes equipped with the one substance that (in nature) controls and directs it.

Do the children in your family like eggs? If the adults not only eat eggs, but exclaim about how delicious they are, chances are the young ones will do the same. An egg a day is a passport to vitamins A, D and E, lots of good minerals, especially iron to prevent anemia, and plenty of all the B vitamins, even the most obscure ones. As we have seen above, eggs also contain some kind of fatty substance (can it be lecithin or something else?) that protects against rheumatic tendencies.

[344]

Let's say you or your children prefer packaged cold cereal to eggs for breakfast. Are the cold cereals just as good? No matter how many enticing premium offers come on the boxtops, cold cereal offers you absolutely nothing in the way of nutrition. Most of the vitamins and minerals were removed in the processing. A couple of synthetic B vitamins and a dab of iron are sometimes added, synthetically of course. Responsible scientists question whether such "enrichment" is positively harmful, since it may result in a state of imbalance among the vitamins. Could the tragic rise in the incidence of rheumatic fever in this country be at least partly caused by the gradual substitution of worthless cold cereal for health-giving eggs in the diets of our children? *There is no food that can be substituted for eggs.* Use more of them!

83. Drugs for Arthritis?

"There is but one miracle in the treatment of rheumatoid arthritis. And that is the skill of the physician in selecting from the wide range of available drugs and procedures that which is best for the patient. Except for this, there is no miracle drug and no miracle cure for this crippling and devastating disease. The cause of rheumatoid arthritis may never be known."

We are quoting a press release from the Arthritis and Rheumatism Foundation.

Considering the fact that hardly a month goes by without publicity about some new "miracle" drug for arthritis, it may seem surprising that the foundation established for arthritics should take such a negative point of view about the usefulness of drugs in rheumatic diseases. But a glance through medical literature on this subject will indeed justify pessimism.

One in a long series of drugs hailed as wonder-workers is *chloroquine,* which started out as an antimalaria drug. A report given in *Chemical Week* for September 7, 1957, describes the work of a Canadian physician who used the drug on 125 arthritic patients over a 4-year period and got, he says, good results in 71 per cent of the cases. Even though half of his test patients were still enjoying remission of the disease, Dr. Bagnall considers chloroquine only an agent to control arthritis—a "major step forward"—a drug to be used perhaps in conjunction with the so-called steroid drugs like cortisone. Needless to say, it is only a matter of time until the side effects begin to show up and this drug, too, will be discarded.

One of these side effects has been noticed by some users of this drug—it bleaches the hair. One writer in the *British Medical Journal* for August 4, 1956, had come across two such cases within 6 months of starting the drug. Both ladies became universally blond, even to the eyebrows. Luckily, the change in pigmentation did not disturb either of the women emotionally, but what the drug did to the rest of their systems, if it could bleach hair, is something we may never know. If an arthritis compound can be invented that will bleach the hair, perhaps researchers should reverse their field and begin the search for a bleaching agent that will work against arthritis. And if all else fails, maybe someone will discover that diet is the most effective treatment for arthritis.

Cortisone and ACTH, Outmoded "Wonder" Drugs

What, then, of cortisone, the miracle drug that preceded chloroquine? Cortisone is a substance derived from the adrenal glands, which have a lot to do with maintaining resistance to disease. Human beings, and animals as well, have these glands. ACTH (now being used as a drug, too) is a substance made from the pituitary, or master gland of the body. When ACTH is injected, it stimulates the adrenal glands to produce cortisone. When cortisone was first tried out on arthritis patients, results were astonishing. Pain disappeared, a sense of well-being and a good appetite returned. However, it was soon admitted that improvement stopped as soon as treatment stopped, so cortisone was no cure. In addition, it was found that, in many cases, extremely serious aftereffects ensued.

Patients might be disturbed mentally. They might develop abnormally round faces and abnormal growths of hair. ACTH might bring about diabetes or high blood pressure. Then, too, any slight infection becomes a menace to the patient taking these drugs, for he is not aware of the infection. If it should be tuberculosis or something equally serious, it can develop into a fatal disease rapidly, while the patient, delighted that he feels so well, overexerts himself and courts disaster.

No one knows exactly how these side effects come about, but we do know that glands are powerful influences, governing all the activities of the body. Taking a hormone, any hormone, is bound to disturb the delicate balance among the glands and bring abnormalities. Cortisone and ACTH, as well as any other drugs affecting glands, should never be taken except under strictest supervision, so that side effects can be detected early.

It is understandable why arthritis patients, suddenly relieved from long years of agonized pain, are reluctant to give up drugs which make them feel so well, even though they know that they bring no lasting cure. In the case of drugs like cortisone, however, one can use the secretions of one's own glands, rather than depending on a drug. We know that healthful exercise causes the adrenal glands to produce their own cortisone. That is one reason for the wonderful feeling of well-being you get from a stimulating walk in the open air.

So we recommend walking as one of the finest preventives of arthritis. And, of course, it is doubly important for folks who have arthritis and fear the deformity and stiffness that it brings. Activity keeps the joints mobile. Exercise, especially walking, provides a natural source of cortisone

[346]

which cannot possibly bring with it any of the ill effects of an injection of cortisone, because your own glands are manufacturing it.

An earlier treatment for arthritis was "gold therapy." This consists of injections of a preparation of gold salts. Says Dr. Walter C. Alvarez of the Mayo Foundation in his book, *How to Live With Your Arthritis* (Wilcox and Follett Company), "The drug works best in the early stages of the disease before the joints are badly damaged. The big difficulty is that the medicine can do much harm to some persons and it can even cause death. Hence, it should be given only by a physician who has had enough experience with it so that he can quickly recognize the danger signals and stop."

The old story. A drug so dangerous that, in careless hands, it may be far worse than the disease it is being given to cure.

Aspirin Is the Most Popular Drug

Aspirin is the drug which has been used longest to relieve the pain of arthritis. Most of us think of aspirin as just about the least harmful of all drugs. But medical literature is full of warnings about aspirin and dire tales of what happened to people who took too much or took it too long.

Of course, when we talk about aspirin, we mean as well practically all the pain-killing drugs, for it forms the base of many of them. Many people are allergic to aspirin and will suffer reactions to even the smallest dosage. Aspirin is an irritant to the stomach lining, so severe an irritant that it is not advised for ulcer patients, or indeed, anyone with any kind of stomach disorder. Taking aspirin for rheumatic pains over a long period of time may cause any or all of the following: nausea, heartburn, stomach pain, deafness, dizziness, ringing in the ears. Doctors generally wait for their arthritic patients who are taking aspirin to tell them that their ears are ringing before they decide to cut the dosage. That is the sign that you've had enough.

Aspirin may cause intestinal bleeding or hemorrhages in other parts of the body, for it destroys vitamin K, which aids in coagulation of the blood. It may cause albumin, red blood cells or stones in the urine. It may bring serious trouble to patients susceptible to coronary thrombosis.

We mention all these symptoms to warn against the casual and prolonged taking of aspirin. The effects of the newer drugs, like cortisone, are usually closely watched by physicians. But we can buy aspirin at the drug store and take as much as we want without any advice from a physician. And we do buy 10 billion aspirin tablets a year in this country, donating a total of close to $200,000,000 to the drug companies for this one item alone.

Of course, no one pretends that aspirin does anything for arthritis or any other disease except to relieve pain temporarily.

This brings us back to where we began this chapter. There is no miracle drug for arthritics, and there probably never will be. We believe, however, that arthritis can be prevented and that its severity can be greatly lessened by following the proper diet. The pathway to arthritic disease is lined with desserts, candy, soft drinks, heaping spoons of sugar in coffee or tea, jelly, white bread. The surest preventive is a diet high in protein, and fresh fruits and vegetables, a diet in which refined carbohydrates are completely lacking and vitamins and minerals are provided in abundance by natural food supplements.

84. Cherries for Gout and Arthritis

Ludwig W. Blau, M.D., writing on "Cherry Diet Control for Gout and Arthritis" in the *Texas Reports on Biology and Medicine,* Vol. 8, fall, 1950, proposed a large cherry intake as effective in the treatment of these diseases. Though he adds that "apologies are offered for unsatisfactory clinical and laboratory data and control," he feels, nonetheless, that the discovery merits the "propriety of publishing the information available."

Twelve cases of gout responded so favorably to this food that the blood uric acid of the sufferers dropped to its usual average and "no attacks of gouty arthritis have occurred on a non-restricted diet in all 12 cases, *as a result of eating about one-half pound of fresh or canned cherries per day."* Supporting his evidence with details concerning 3 of these cases, Dr. Blau demonstrates the relief brought by the eating of either canned cherries, sour, black or Royal Anne, or fresh Black Bing varieties. In one case, the juice only was drunk, and this proved to be about equally effective.

Eight years later, in *Food Field Reporter* for November 10, 1958, appeared an article on canned cherry juice relieving arthritis. Says the *Reporter:* New evidence that canned cherry juice may relieve gout, gouty arthritis and similar ailments is reported by Reynolds Brothers, Incorporated at Sturgeon Bay, Wisconsin. According to the article, a number of residents of Sturgeon Bay cooperated in testing the cherry juice daily. "Outstanding results were reported," said the president of the firm who sold the cherry juice. He says further that sales of his product have increased considerably in Texas since the article appeared there linking cherry juice to arthritic cure. He also disclosed that several local dentists have been suggesting cherry juice to their patients and one of them found it useful for the treatment of pyorrhea.

"To date," says *Food Field Reporter,* "there is no definite scientific data on just how the juice aids in relieving pain caused by diseases where improper balance of calcium is evident. However, it is believed that it may be the pigment in the cherries that brings relief."

Morris B. Jacobs' book, *Food and Food Products,* tells us that cherries contain several pigments. They also contain quite a concentration of malic acid and a surprising amount of pectin. That is the substance in fruits that is used to make jelly harden and "jell." There are also small amounts of citric acid, oxalic acid, succinic acid and lactic acid in cherries. The oxalic acid exists in only trace amounts, fortunately, for this is a substance very destructive of one's calcium supply. Surprisingly enough, there is also a small amount of linoleic acid in cherries. That is the unsaturated fatty acid which apparently has such a powerful effect on the body's use of the fatty substance, cholesterol.

In this information, there seems to be no clue as to what may be effective against gouty arthritis. It would certainly be a challenging experiment for scientists to work on. And we are sure that any of the thousands of gout sufferers would be more than willing to act as guinea pigs for such an experiment, if there was the slightest possible chance that they might be relieved of their symptoms.

Meanwhile, what can readers who are suffering from gouty arthritis do about this information? Canned cherries are, of course, available in grocery stores everywhere. Most brands are loaded with sugar, probably also artificial coloring matter and other chemicals. The cherries themselves were, of course, sprayed with insecticides, and on a small fruit like this which is not peeled, these insecticides can mount up to a frightening total.

If you have cherry trees or know anyone who does, by all means freeze or can some this spring for your own use. If you get very sour cherries, you can use honey for the processing. Remember that honey has almost twice the sweetening power of sugar, so judge the amount you use accordingly.

85. Sugar and Arthritis

Diet as a weapon against arthritis occurs in a book called *Degeneration-Regeneration* by Melvin Page, D.D.S. (published by Biochemical Research Foundation, 2810 First Street, North, St. Petersburg, Florida). In Dr. Page's view, the whole source of arthritic problems lies in the occurrence of an imbalance in the calcium-phosphorus ratio of the blood. The ideal proportions, says Dr. Page, are a level of 10 for calcium against a level of 4 for phosphorus in a blood test reading. Any alteration of these proportions can lead to trouble.

The body chemistry can be affected by several types of conditions. Mental stress can cause an upset in the chemistry and bring on strong arthritic symptoms, via aching joints, that will disappear with the relief of the worry. Certain mechanical conditions can be the cause. If, for example, normal blood flow is impeded by bad sleeping habits or posture faults, arthritis can result in the affected area. This theory was proven in experiments with animals in which circulation was deliberately impeded in a certain limb, resulting in arthritic conditions in that limb. Many readers are, of course, familiar with Editor Rodale's work on arthritis and the way you sleep.

The calcium-phosphorus proportion is normally agitated by infection. Dr. Page found that many cases of arthritis could be arrested by eliminating a source of infection. One of the chief sites for infection was found to be the stumps of tonsils which had not been completely removed. The infected part that was left was overgrown with scar tissue, cutting off the chance for drainage. However, Dr. Page cautions against the automatic diagnosis of infection in every case of arthritis. Many good teeth, as well as gall bladders, tonsils and other possible seats of infection have been needlessly removed by doctors who acted on suspicion rather than evidence. Strangely enough, almost every operation leaves the patient greatly relieved of the arthritis symptoms, because, says Dr. Page, the healing process following the operation serves to raise the phosphorus level to a balance with the calcium. This relief is short-lived if the operation was not founded on an actual need, and the arthritis is soon back again.

Another common cause of upset in the proper balance of calcium and phosphorus in the body is menopause. The glandular changes that take place at this time are often enough to upset the body chemistry to the extent that any incipient arthritic condition is aggravated into showing its symptoms. Though we do not approve of Dr. Page's treatment, in this instance, we think it only fair to report that he suggests that female sex hormones and insulin be ingested for relief of pain. Also, a tablespoonful of molasses or honey after each meal may be used to raise the phosphorus level and ease the pain, in the early stages of arthritis. (We believe that following a proper diet with plenty of vitamins and minerals will minimize or eliminate entirely the unpleasantness of menopause symptoms.)

Dr. Page says sugar will have the same effect. However, the food values in honey and molasses make them much more desirable in this case. Our readers are well aware that sweets of any kind are to be avoided, but if a reader feels that one of the above treatments must be had to relieve the pain of acute arthritis, it would seem that using the natural products, molasses or honey, would be least likely to cause any further harm.

Diet Is of Great Importance to Arthritis Sufferers

The best cure for arthritis of all kinds is a diet that will reverse the depleted efficiency of body chemistry. Dr. Page calls it "Biologic Diet," but it's the same horse-sense type of diet that we advocate—complete elimination of refined foods.

In his work with arthritis, Dr. Page found that most sufferers from the disease eat similar diets. Usually they consist of high amounts of carbohydrates, low trace mineral intake and low consumption of foods rich in vitamin B. The large amount of white sugar ingested displaces, by its large calorie count, an equal amount of calories from foods that contain the elements the body needs. Sugar is the surest means of knocking the calcium-phosphorus balance out of kilter. It always boosts the calcium count while lowering the phosphorus; then, when the effect has worn off, the reverse occurs, with the phosphorus shooting up and calcium becoming depressed. The elimination of sugar, along with white flour and alcohol, both of which have a similar effect, is the most important step in the cure of arthritis. That alone should put the arthritic on the road to cure, but further insurance lies in abandoning completely the use of refined and processed foods. These foods seem to contain many elements which adversely affect the calcium-phosphorus ratio in the blood.

A case cited in the book describes a woman of 52 who became arthritic. She ate a typical American diet, laced with 6 cups of coffee (one tablespoonful of sugar in each), plus two cocktails and a highball every day. Besides this, she ate candy, cookies and canned fruits—all of which contain white sugar. After 3 months on the Biologic Diet, the proper level for the calcium and phosphorus had been reached, and best of all, the arthritis had disappeared.

Dr. Page warns that response to this treatment may take more time in some individuals than in others. Usually those whose family is relatively new to American diet have faster results than those whose family tree is American from way back, and has been steeped in bad dietary habits for generations.

When one considers the expensive treatments that most arthritics bargain for, and the poor results they get, Dr. Page's suggested treatment seems worthy of careful attention. Can intelligent diet be such an impossible assignment that arthritis victims would rather suffer the crippling pain than change their bad food habits? If so, then America has a bleak future, for degenerative diseases are bound to climb as long as these suicidal dietary trends persist.

86. A Proposed New Diet for Arthritics?

A new system of dieting for relief of arthritis is proposed in an article by two physicians from Cambridge, Massachusetts, published in the *Journal of the National Medical Association* for July, 1959.

A summary of the article, written for inclusion in scientific books, tells us that the diet produced major clinical and hematological (blood) improvement in arthritis and rheumatism. According to the summary, the main points in this new system are the taking of cod liver oil on an empty stomach and the restriction of all water intake to a single portion taken one hour before breakfast.

We read the article with great interest. It is well written and thorough in the detail with which the authors have cared for their patients and followed through, during the 6-month treatment, to check on their welfare. One hundred and forty arthritic patients were originally scheduled for the test, but some had to drop out, so final facts are given on the 98 who could follow the suggested diet that was being tested over this period.

The results were excellent. Dr. Charles A. Brusch, M.D., and Edward T. Johnson, M.D., the authors, tell us that 92 of the patients showed major improvement in their arthritic symptoms and favorable changes in their blood chemistry. The blood sedimentation rate dropped to normal. Cholesterol levels dropped or could be controlled, even though eggs, butter, milk and cod liver oil were everyday items of diet. Blood sugar levels "turned to the lower side of normal," say our authors. One diabetic patient was compelled to give up taking insulin. Blood pressure levels were found to be lower at the end of the experiment.

Doesn't all this sound just wonderful from the point of view of health? Doesn't it sound as though our authors have uncovered a veritable treasure of information and a simple-as-can-be system for guaranteeing good health to most of us, just with a few small rules about drinking water and taking cod liver oil?

Why Is Test Successful?

But wait a moment! Although the summary of the article states just "a special dietary regimen" and implies that water drinking and cod liver oil were the main items in that regimen, the article states clearly, "there was complete curtailment of soft drinks, candy, cake, ice cream or any food made up of white sugar . . . Those who felt that the sacrifice of coffee was too great were allowed black coffee—15 minutes before breakfast."

So we have a group of 98 arthritics starting on a 6-month diet, in which they are allowed nothing that contains white sugar and, most of them, no coffee. It's not hard for us to believe that such a diet produced almost miraculous improvement in their physical condition, but it is hard to believe that the cod liver oil and the pattern of water drinking were the main reasons for the improvement.

Here are the diet rules which the arthritic patients observed. (1.) All daily intake of water was consumed upon arising, preferably at warm temperatures and about one hour before breakfast. (2.) Room temperature milk or warm soup (not creamed) were the only liquids permitted with meals. These were allowed any time. (3.) Cod liver oil, mixed either with two tablespoonfuls of fresh, strained orange juice or two tablespoonfuls of cool milk, was taken on a fasting stomach at least 4, but preferably 5 or more, hours after the evening meal and before retiring, or one or more hours before breakfast, upon arising, and at least one-half hour after water intake. Diabetics and people with heart disease took the oil only twice a week. The cod liver oil mixtures were shaken well in a screw-top glass before taking. (4.) Tablets, pills or supplements of any kind were allowed either with water upon rising, with milk or soup at mealtime or with milk or soup at any time. (5.) No sugar or any food made with sugar. (6.) No coffee except before breakfast.

Several Other Tests Necessary To Convince Us

It is our belief that such an experiment is not really a proof of any of the various things involved—the oil, the water, the food supplements which were allowed or the restriction of sugar. It is a test of all these. We would have something worthwhile in the way of scientific research if the two Massachusetts physicians would follow this up with a 6-month experiment in which the patients eat exactly as they had been eating before, but take cod liver oil as directed and regulate their fluid intake as directed. Then, we want to see another 6-month experiment in which mixtures of cod liver oil and water drinking are ignored, and patients are put on a sugar-free diet *with no other restrictions*—and are permitted to take food supplements. Until someone proves us wrong, we are expecting to see improvement on *this* kind of a diet.

We have nothing against the taking of cod liver oil. As a matter of fact, we urge readers to assure their proper intake of vitamins A and D by taking fish liver oil every day. We think it matters not at all whether it is cod liver or some other kind of fish, and we think that perles are just as effective and certainly much more convenient and pleasant than taking the straight oil.

It seems to us a harmless enough thing to experiment with different patterns of water drinking. We know perfectly healthy people who never drink water at all, but depend entirely on the ample fluid in their fruits and vegetables to keep themselves from drying out. We know other people —healthy, too—who drink water any time they feel thirsty.

Sugar is a highly concentrated carbohydrate, remember, from which all the water has been removed. This is why it cakes so easily in a damp climate and absorbs water thirstily. So, of course, anyone who includes in his meals lots of food made with white sugar will want water, and will probably want it while he is eating, because the sugar is absorbing water from his tissues which must be replaced. Start him on a sugar-free diet and see his thirst decline!

Here are some other interesting comments from this very provocative article by Drs. Brusch and Johnson in the medical journal. They state that cholesterol levels dropped or could be controlled, even with the introduction of milk, eggs, butter and cod liver oil. *"For many patients in the study, these were new foods,"* they say.

Such a comment shows clearly that these fatty foods (all fats from animal origin) did not cause a rise in cholesterol content of the blood. On the contrary, the cholesterol content of the patients' blood had become high while they were not eating these foods, and was lowered when these foods were given to them on this special diet. We know that fish liver oils, although they are animal rather than vegetable in origin, contain the valuable unsaturated fatty acids, which apparently help to emulsify cholesterol so that it does not collect in the blood. For further information about eggs, see chapter 82, dealing with eggs and rheumatism.

Another significant remark from the medical article. In quoting an earlier experiment done in 1920, our authors tell us a Doctor Pemberton found, in treating 400 cases of arthritis in the army, that there was improvement on cod liver oil therapy, "provided the patients were kept away from 'inferior type' starches." Of course, the most inferior type of starch known is white sugar.

A national best-seller, *Arthritis and Common Sense* by Dan Dale Alexander (published by Witkower Press), advances many of these same ideas on water drinking and cod liver oil. The book also warns against eating sweets and desserts. Menus printed in the book ignore desserts as if they did not exist. This is praiseworthy. We are in general agreement with the diet suggestions made in the book, although we believe that the theories about water drinking and the order of eating foods are overemphasized. But we see no possible harm anyone could come to by following Mr. Alexander's suggestions—and indeed, they might find great improvement. Just being on a strict diet in which sweets are nonexistent will surely do a lot for one's arthritis.

Our thoughts on the Cambridge experiment are about the same. If you want to try the suggested water drinking program and cod liver oil taking, by all means go ahead. It couldn't possibly do you any harm. But please do consider the most important recommendation of Drs. Brusch and Johnson to be their positive prohibition of any foods made with white sugar, and their strong recommendation to give up coffee.

87. More on a New Diet for Arthritics

We said in the preceding chapter that we believed the excellent improvement obtained was the result of the "no-sugar" part of the diet, whereas the authors emphasized the cod liver oil-water drinking aspects of the treatment. We wrote to one of the authors, telling him what we intended to say and asking him if he had any comments. We received a letter from him which we reprint below. We think it is a fine letter, honest and generous. The author admits that our theory has merit, while defending his own. This is surely the best way to deal with a problem as complex as this one.

We reprint below the letter we received and invite our readers to make their own decisions as to just what use they want to make of this information.

"Dear Editor:

"Thank you for your letter of September 30, 1959; I felt that your inquiry merited a considered answer, hence the delayed response. In answer to your questions:

"1. *Your view is partially true.* Complete abstinence from white sugar plus a wholesome diet (which we believe you have in mind) would perhaps automatically give 25 to 50 per cent of the results noted in our paper. This is based on the observation of noticeable skin improvement, hair and scalp improvement, degree of cerumen correction and diminishing of inflammatory ear condition to name a few of the objective changes. In addition, of course, we noted favorable blood chemistry and urine changes.

"We felt these (*rapid*) improvements were due primarily to the Cod Liver Oil and unusual arrangements for liquid intake. While it is true that these favorable objective and laboratory findings would eventually appear with a favorable diet (*alone*)—'*the relativity of time' to obtain these more or less same results—would differ.* We obtained our results in 3 to 6 month's time. A wholesome diet alone would perhaps take 6 to 36 months to produce 50 to 75 per cent of our results, at best.

"2. In our opinion, there is a difference between water taken per se and the water content taken in the form of fruits and vegetables. We agree with you that water is water, regardless of its source and that the digestive tract cannot tell the difference; but their surface tensions are considerably different; tap water having the highest surface tension level and fruit and vegetable water content being of the low range of surface tension levels.

"More important, however, one must remember that water delivered into the digestive tract from an apple or a carrot *would take* 1 to 4 hours, depending on the rate of digestion—if it or they were singular foods or combined in a meal. This water (from fruits and vegetables) would appear in the blood stream *at a very slow rate.*

"On the other hand, a glass of water, taken on an empty stomach, as suggested in our paper, would be delivered in the system in a matter of *minutes; not hours.*

"In the need for the matter of unusual arrangement for water intake, we felt it important to our sedimentation rates, for one laboratory finding, let alone others. The sedimentation rate levels were erratic unless water was thus controlled.

"At this time, we might cite that water, taken upon arising, will literally 'flush the kidneys'—the urine at this time being frequently crystal clear in the second voiding. Water taken with, or immediately after a meal was seldom found crystal clear in the first voiding after a meal. We found an unusual arrangement for water intake plays a significant role in many areas.

"3. Your question three concerns the absence of control groups on Cod Liver Oil taken without regard to the empty stomach routine and/or Cod Liver Oil perles taken in place of liquid Cod Liver Oil.

"Medical literature indicates the use of both of these measures with indifferent success in the past.

"When other clinical studies, such as you note, were carried out, they did not differentiate between a natural wholesome diet and a refined diet, nor did they account for the great varieties of liquids of choice and their temperatures.

"We feel that it is the *combination* of several factors that we were striving to coordinate:

"a. A wholesome diet, free from refined foods.

"b. Control of water and liquid intake—so that the 'rates' at which *all food and liquid* 'entered the blood stream' were more or less constant. The average person's rate of assimilation of their diet varies widely.

"c. We were trying to gain maximum help from the organic iodine in Cod Liver Oil. Medical history notes that this is best done on an empty stomach. Liquid form of Cod Liver Oil was used intentionally, not perles. Organic iodine per se, as found associated in the conventional Cod Liver Oil molecular structure, was more in line with what we wanted to get into the system with the hope of improving body metabolism. We also found it had a beneficial effect on blood serum cholesterol. We do not believe Cod Liver Oil perles would have had a fraction of the success.

"In relatively quick time we found results in connecting skin luster, hair and scalp conditions. We found this working with ordinary Cod Liver Oil.

"We agree with you—further testing of the points you raise would be worthwhile.

"We hope that the above will serve to clarify the questions and we again thank you for your interest.

"Yours truly,

"Charles A. Brusch, M.D.
Medical Director,
Brusch Medical Center,
831 Massachusetts Avenue,
Cambridge 39, Massachusetts"

[356]

88. Vitamin P and Vitamin C for Arthritis

"There is a tendency to pay exclusive attention to the heart and the blood vessels. It is often forgotten that the sole function of the heart, the arteries and the veins is to maintain an adequate rate of blood flow through the capillaries. It is in the capillaries that the essential business of the circulatory system is carried on."

At first glance, these words seem astonishing. Capillaries are the tiny blood vessels that crisscross all our tissues, through the walls of which food and oxygen are carried to cells and waste material is carried away. Is it possible that we have missed the point in concerning ourselves exclusively with the heart and blood vessels and largely ignoring the health of tiny capillaries?

Still, come to think of it, the function of the heartbeat and the pulsations of the arteries is to circulate the blood to every cell of the body. Getting it there is important, but what happens after it gets there is just as important. And this happens in the capillaries!

The words we quoted above are from an article in *Clinical Medicine,* Vol. 52, p. 157, 1945. We found them in an article on the treatment of arthritis with vitamin P and vitamin C. Four researchers studied 42 patients with rheumatoid arthritis and 17 patients with osteoarthritis over a period of 7 years to discover how their health could be improved if they took quite large doses of these two vitamins every day. The story of their findings, as reported in the *Journal of American Geriatrics* for June, 1956, is amazing. We think we owe a debt of gratitude to the authors for their work in following up 59 patients over such a long time. The authors are Peter J. Warter, M.D., and Henry L. Drezner, M.D., of McKinley Hospital, Trenton, New Jersey, Dominic A. Donio, M.D., of Sacred Heart Hospital, Allentown, Pennsylvania and Steven Horoschak, B.S., of the National Drug Company.

The authors remind us that all of us are troubled with minor injuries during every day. We bump our ankles, pinch our fingers, stumble over cracks in the sidewalk, hit our heads on the cellar stairs and so on. Usually we pay no attention to these knocks except for a casual, "Oh, I wonder where I got that bruise." "That bruise" means that capillaries have hemorrhaged. You are bleeding internally, even if ever so slightly. Our authors tell us that these bleedings might well develop into something serious in a defective capillary system, made so by poisons of various kinds—drugs, for instance, or tobacco.

Furthermore, they tell us that rheumatic fever is believed to be a disease of the blood vessels, involving fragility of these small capillaries so that they burst easily. High blood pressure, or hypertension, is another disease in which the stability of the capillaries is of utmost importance. Patients who have fragile capillaries often have strokes, hemorrhages in the retina of the eye and other serious disorders. So it seems certain that disorders of the capillary system are at the bottom of many chronic diseases.

Vitamin C, Vitamin P and Capillaries

What are the capillaries made of? Cells and intercellular material. We know positively that the intercellular material is kept in repair by vitamin C. In scurvy, the disease of vitamin C deficiency, there is a breakdown of this intercellular material which can be reversed almost magically by giving vitamin C. Walter H. Eddy in his book, *What are the Vitamins?* (Reinhold, 1941), says he thinks that "country rheumatism" which develops at the end of a long winter is nothing more or less than hemorrhaging capillaries in the joints, as a result of vitamin C deficiency.

Later researchers have shown that vitamin C cannot function well in the absence of vitamin P or the bioflavonoids, as they are sometimes called. Then, too, vitamin P does not take its part in body processes without vitamin C being present. So, in testing the effect of vitamin C on arthritic patients, the authors felt it necessary to add vitamin P as well.

They tested the rheumatoid arthritis patients for capillary fragility and found that it was almost universal. In other words, pressure on the capillaries caused them to burst. These folks consistently have bruised themselves from everyday bumps. Blood pressure was low in these patients; the heartbeat was rapid. The 17 osteoarthritis patients were obese and had high blood pressure. In the most severe cases of the rheumatoid arthritis patients, as much as 600 to 1000 milligrams of vitamin P-vitamin C (in equal amounts) were given daily in divided doses. Gradually, the dose was reduced to 300 milligrams daily. For milder cases, 400 to 600 milligrams were given at the beginning and these were then reduced to 300 for a "maintenance dose." In the osteoarthritic patients, the treatment was begun and maintained with 300 milligram doses. The reason given for the larger doses in rheumatoid arthritis is that there is inflammation in this disease which taxes the capillary resistance to a greater degree.

What were the results obtained? In the rheumatoid group, normal capillary resistance was established in 6 to 8 weeks. That means no more bruises for them. These patients apparently utilized their food better, too, for protein and vitamin B supplements brought a gain in weight and an increase in red blood, to combat anemia. This did not happen in patients who were not taking the vitamins. The blood pressure in most patients soon came to normal range. Some of the patients who had been subject to colds voluntarily reported that they had much more resistance to cold, even though the researchers were not testing for this angle. The arthritis, which improved steadily, flared up again when the vitamins were discontinued for several months in the case of a few patients. There were no strokes or other blood vessel disorders.

[358]

In the osteoarthritic group, those who bruised easily developed resistance to bruising within 6 weeks. Six patients with high blood pressure brought their pressure down to normal. The authors admit that rest and diet may have played some part in this, but they believe the vitamins should get some credit. The arthritic symptoms improved. Even though damage to joints could not, of course, be repaired, the patients had less fatigue, less discomfort in the joints and general improvement.

The conclusions of the authors are that the combination of vitamin P and vitamin C has the capacity to correct abnormal capillary fragility and permeability, and thus enhances the effectiveness of therapy directed against the rheumatic diseases.

It seems apparent that anyone who wants to prevent conditions of this kind will see that he gets ample amounts of these two vitamins. Where can you get them? Actually the substance used in the rheumatism experiment was a combination of hesperidin and ascorbic acid—just these two. Now vitamin P is a conglomeration of "elements," as the chemists call them, all of which are apparently important. Hesperidin is one of these elements.

The only way to get all of the elements—both vitamin P and vitamin C—is to eat foods that contain them all and to take natural food supplements rich in them all. The foods you should be sure to get in ample quantity are mostly raw fruits. Grapes, plums, black currants, apricots, cherries and blackberries are good sources of vitamin P. And the citrus fruits, which we think should be eaten sparingly, due to their citric acid content. Other foods rich in vitamin C are broccoli, Brussels sprouts, cabbage, dandelion greens, melons, cantaloupes, tomatoes, mustard greens, green peppers.

Finally, the easiest way to make certain you are getting plenty of both of these vitamins is to take a natural food supplement—made of rose hips or green peppers. Rutin, too, is part of vitamin P. Taking synthetic vitamin C is not the answer. Natural vitamin C supplements contain all of the "elements" that go along with vitamin C in food. These are for you!

89. Arthritis and Vitamin C

Arthritis—tormentor of millions of Americans and crippler of millions more—can it be caused by something we do or do not eat?

Certainly it is not the result of eating or not eating any one food. But it has seemed to us for a long time that arthritis and all the other rheumatic diseases must be related to patterns of eating—habits that lead one into all the wrong paths, dietetically speaking.

Confirmation of our belief comes in an article by W. J. McCormick,

M.D., of Toronto—"The Rheumatic Diseases," in the *Archives of Pediatrics* for April, 1955. Dr. McCormick tells us that only recently have we classified these diseases according to the way they manifest themselves—rheumatic fever, rheumatoid arthritis, primary osteoarthritis, rheumatoid spondylitis, bursitis, synovitis and so forth. The one thing all these diseases appear to have in common, says he, is that the cartilages involved in joints and the connective tissue surrounding them disintegrate. So it seems that, if one could explain this one symptom, one could get to the bottom of the matter.

Dr. McCormick believes that the early writers on scurvy gave the most significant clues to the cause and cure of arthritis. Scurvy? How is it possible? Scurvy is a disease of long ago, before we knew the value of fresh raw foods in the diet. Nobody in our enlightened era ever has scurvy! Or do they? Listen to Dr. McCormick's reasoning and make up your own mind.

He quotes James Lind, who wrote medical treatises in 1753, as saying that in scurvy the muscles are so lax and tender that they readily fall apart during autopsies. He said, too, that scurvy affected the cartilages of the ribs so decidedly as to sometimes separate them entirely from the breast bone. He had no explanation for the fact that "scurvy seats itself so commonly in the joint of the knee."

Lind reviewed the findings of earlier writers on scurvy, who had observed that the bones of the scurvy patient cracked when he moved, "in some we perceived a small low noise when they breathed. . . . The ligaments of the joints were corroded and loose. Instead of finding in the cavities of the joints the usual sweet oily mucilage, there was only a greenish liquor. . . . gout is known to proceed from scurvy."

It is well to remember that 200 or 300 years ago medical students had ample opportunity to study scurvy. It was nearly as common as colds are today. So, from many autopsies, they knew the symptoms of this disease, then so puzzling, which as we know today, is the result of a deficiency in vitamin C.

"The most definitely established function of vitamin C is that of assisting in the formation of collagen for the maintenance of integrity and stability of the connective tissues generally, and this would include the bones, cartilages, muscles and vascular tissue," says Dr. McCormick. Collagen is the substance that is so important in all connective tissue— the material that makes gelatin when you boil bones and cartilages. "In a deficiency of this vitamin (C)," Dr. McCormick continues, "instability and fragility of all such tissues is believed to be caused by the breakdown of intercellular cement substance, resulting in easy rupture of any and all of these connective tissues," which would include the discs of the back-bone, the ligaments and small sacs in the interior of the joints and the cartilage which helps in the movement of joints. The vulnerability of these joints may be, then, the common cause for the rheumatic diseases, says Dr. McCormick.

Rheumatism in Animals

Coming up to modern times, we find two researchers, Rinehart and Mettier, who correlated deficiency of vitamin C with rheumatic disease. In an article in the *American Journal of Pathology,* Vol. 10, p. 61, 1934, they relate that they found impairment of the joints in animals deprived of vitamin C. When the animals were subject to some infection, the joint symptoms became worse. Those animals which were subjected to the same infection while on a diet rich in vitamin C did not develop the joint disorders.

Extending these researches further, Rinehart found that the amount of vitamin C in the blood of arthritic and rheumatic fever patients is extremely low. He believes that the important basic cause of rheumatic disease is infection, superimposed on a vitamin C deficiency. Dr. Mc-Cormick believes that both the infection and the rheumatism are direct results of vitamin C deficiency.

Infection and lack of vitamin C do go hand-in-hand. In this article, we find reference to many different examples—a mouth infection associated with rheumatic fever, which was shown to be due to vitamin C deficiency; a streptococcus and pneumonia epidemic in a naval training school which did not affect students who were taking liberal doses of vitamin C; a report on a less-than-usual excretion of vitamin C in rheumatoid arthritis patients who were getting plenty of the vitamin in their diets, seeming to indicate that the vitamin was being used at a faster than normal rate.

Rinehart, in a paper read before the California Heart Association, May 6, 1944, told of his findings that vitamin P (the flavonoids), used in conjunction with vitamin C, had a favorable influence on the condition of the blood vessels in infections. It seems to us that Rinehart may have the answer right here—that is, that natural vitamin C, which occurs along with vitamin P in foods, may be what the rheumatic tissues lack—not just vitamin C as it appears in synthetic preparations, unaccompanied by any of the other food elements.

Dr. McCormick, a great believer in the use of vitamins for prevention and for cure, tells us that he has given massive doses of vitamin C in injections and orally in a number of cases of rheumatic fever. "The patients made rapid and complete recovery in 3 or 4 weeks without cardiac complication." The usual hospital treatment may go on for 3 or 4 months, with cortisone or aspirin being given and a high rate of heart complications. Dr. McCormick has also given massive doses of vitamin C in cases of "incipient arthritis"—that is, arthritis which is just beginning—with "similarly favorable results."

What does he mean by "massive doses"? From one to ten grams daily; that is, in terms in which one buys natural vitamin C products, from 1,000 milligrams to 10,000 milligrams a day. Is it necessary for the average person on an average diet to take this much vitamin C in order to prevent arthritis? We believe not. These are curative doses for patients who already have the symptoms of disease. However, we do not think it is possible to get too much vitamin C in your diet these days, and it is likely that most of us are getting far too little.

How does this happen in an age when fresh vegetables and fresh fruits are available the year round? Too many other foods are available, too—worthless foods—soft drinks, pastries, candies, cakes, etc. Every mouthful of these foods that your family eats means that they can eat less of fresh foods. Just in the case of children, how much of their diet consists of worthless foods compared to their daily intake of fresh, raw foods?

Why We Lack Vitamin C

An article from the *Journal of the American Dietetic Association* for May, 1954, gives us part of the answer. In a survey of 131 children with rheumatic fever, compared with 131 carefully paired children who did not have the disease, it was found that the rheumatic fever children were eating less of vitamin C-rich foods than the healthy children. The sick children did not get even one serving per day of foods that contain even moderate amounts of vitamin C.

In another survey, 35 per cent of the children of one parish in Louisiana ate *no fruits or raw vegetables at all!* In another survey, it was found on autopsies of infants dying at Johns Hopkins that 6 per cent of them suffered from scurvy. In another survey, reported in the *Journal of the American Dietetic Association,* it was shown that of a group of school children studied, 47 per cent had a low intake of vitamin C, 53 per cent had a low blood level of the vitamin. College students eating at dining halls were found to be eating meals, 62 per cent of which were deficient in vitamin C.

In another survey of institutional inmates over the age of 50, it was found that *87 per cent were deficient in vitamin C.* Dr. McCormick tells us that he has examined more than 500 patients with particular reference to their vitamin C status, and has found that less than 10 per cent of them have had the optimum amount of vitamin C in their blood at any time.

Remember, too, that vitamin C is most perishable, so that even today, with our wonderful methods of transportation and marketing, the fruits and vegetables you buy may have lost much of their vitamin C by the time you buy them. Storing and cooking destroy much more of it. The poisonous substances to which you are exposed day after day use it up. Cigarette smoke is an enemy of vitamin C in your tissues, for example.

If, indeed, lack of vitamin C is responsible for initiating rheumatic troubles of all kinds, is it any wonder that the medical journals report dolefully that practically everybody over the age of 40 has or shortly will have arthritic symptoms?

Some time ago, we received a letter from a reader who had just begun to notice arthritic stiffness and pain. On the advice of a doctor friend, she began to take massive doses of vitamin C—synthetic vitamin

C bought at the drug store. It helped a little, but not much. She switched to natural vitamin C. The arthritis was gone within a few weeks. Incidentally, she still takes smaller amounts of the natural vitamin C and, after more than a year, she has had no more trouble with arthritis. It's just one instance, of course, that happened to be reported to us. If you have a tendency toward arthritis, you may be able to prevent it entirely.

90. Vitamin D for Arthritis Patients

Vitamin D for arthritis seems to be a treatment that carries little, if any, risk and one which can be applied with a good chance of success as a preventive measure.

We found, in a 1935 medical journal, the account of the treatment of a number of patients with vitamin D. Two physicans, Dr. Irving Dreyer and Dr. C. I. Reed of the University of Illinois Department of Medicine, writing in the *Archives of Physical Therapy*, Vol. 16, p. 537, 1935, have this to say, "In general, the results suggest that this material may prove an efficient form of therapy, as well as a valuable aid in the study of the fundamental nature of arthritis."

They treated 67 patients, who were suffering from a variety of arthritic afflictions. Forty-four of these showed clinical improvement, 13 showed none and 10 cases were uncertain. About 200 other cases being treated privately showed approximately the same results. The doctors gave massive doses of synthetic vitamin D. We have written often about the unlikeliness of readers getting too much of any of the vitamins when they take natural supplements in doses not too much greater than those recommended on the labels of the containers in which the supplements come.

Since vitamin D is one of the two vitamins (vitamin A is the other) which has been known to produce toxic results if taken in too large a dosage over a long period of time, it is interesting to know that these arthritic patients were started on a daily dosage of 200,000 units of synthetic vitamin D. This dosage was given daily for a month. If there were no improvement and no indication that any harm had been done by this quite large dose, it was increased by 50,000 to 60,000 units each week, until there was some improvement or indication of overdosage. In some stubborn cases, it was found necessary to increase to 600,000 units or even to 1,000,000 for a few days and then reduce again to 200,000. "Most of our results have been obtained with daily doses of 300,000 to 500,000 units," say the authors.

Are Massive Doses Dangerous?

They tell us that they do not believe vitamin D in such enormous doses poses any greater risk than many preparations used daily by physicians. And, they say, one knows within a few weeks if symptoms of over-dosage are present. When the vitamin is discontinued, the symptoms disappear.

It is interesting, too, to note that some patients who could not take massive doses of vitamin D found that they could manage perfectly well if large doses of brewer's yeast were given at the same time. This is not successful in every case, they say, but they tell us of one woman patient who, on 3 successive occasions, with intervals of 2 to 3 weeks between, took 300,000 units daily for 10 days, but became nauseated on the eleventh day. Nausea is one of the first symptoms that too much vitamin D is being taken. When she took 6 grams of brewer's yeast 3 times daily, she was able to take up to 600,000 units of vitamin D daily for 3 weeks without becoming nauseated, or suffering from other unpleasant symptoms.

"The total number of human subjects to whom large doses of viosterol (synthetic vitamin D) have been administered for all conditions now numbers approximately 700," say our authors. They continue, "Of these, 63 have, at some time, manifested evidence of toxicity. The actual size of the dose producing toxicity varies in different individuals. Human subjects have received as high as 3,000,000 units daily for 5 days. Single large doses have been given by others. It is apparent, however, that toxicity is more likely to occur after prolonged administration of moderate amounts than as a result of brief administration of large amounts."

Let us compare the amounts the investigators are talking about to some of the all natural vitamin D supplements. The all-in-one combination food supplements average between 1200 to 3200 units of vitamin D. Individual vitamin A and D preparations from fish liver oil provide around 1,000 units of vitamin D per capsule. The labels of such products carefully state what the recommended dosage is and give also the daily minimum requirement of each of the two vitamins.

Vitamin A is suggested in amounts of 5,000 units daily for adults. No daily minimum has been set for vitamin D for adults, as the official board which decides these things does not believe that adults in general need additional vitamin D. It's a vitamin for children, they say, whose bones are growing and who must have vitamin D so that the calcium and phosphorus can be used properly for bone growth.

It seems unlikely, then, that anyone could possibly get too much vitamin D taking natural food supplements where the source of the vitamin is fish liver oil. It would be foolish, we believe, for anyone to try to give himself massive doses of this vitamin by taking natural food supplements, because he would be bound to get too much vitamin A at the same time, since the two are both present in fish liver oil. Of course, we do not recommend using synthetic vitamins at all.

[364]

Adults Benefit from Taking Vitamin D

So what lessons can we learn from the work that was reported on vitamin D for arthritis cases? It seems to us that we should learn that vitamin D is indeed essential for adults and, perhaps, lack of it may be a definite factor in the cause of arthritis. No one knows apparently why the vitamin brings relief in those cases where it does. Couldn't it be simply that there was a lack of the vitamin? Vitamin D is almost completely lacking in food. Our chief source of it is sunlight which, falling on our bare skin, produces a substance which the body then changes into vitamin D. Doesn't it seem quite likely that people who spend most of their time indoors could very definitely be lacking in vitamin D, especially in the winter months when sunlight is weak and infrequent?

We had never heard before of any relationship between the taking of brewer's yeast (rich chiefly in vitamin B and minerals) and protection against the possible toxicity of large doses of vitamin D. But it seems to indicate again that one is safest to take whole foods and to take all the important vitamins and minerals in natural food supplements, like brewer's yeast. Who knows? There may be many more important functions performed by brewer's yeast that we do not know anything about as yet. If it protects against toxicity of large doses of vitamin D, perhaps it also acts to protect us against many other unknown poisons in our environment.

We would not suggest that readers attempt to cure arthritic conditions by using massive doses of vitamin D as the doctors at the university hospital did, unless they are taking these doses under the supervision of a capable doctor who understands just what the symptoms of overdosage may be. We do think everyone should take vitamin D in their daily diet by taking food supplements as a possible preventive of arthritis and other disorders. And, along with the fish liver oil, which is the natural source of vitamin D, take other food supplements as well—brewer's yeast or desiccated liver chiefly for vitamin B content, kelp and bone meal for a rich supply of minerals, rose hips or other natural preparations for vitamin C.

91. Arthritis and Foot Disability

By SIMON J. WIKLER, Doctor of Surgical Chiropody

Arthritis is the term applied to many different diseases affecting the joints of the body. It is irritation and inflammation of the bony joints. The most common types are called degenerative arthritis and rheumatoid arthritis. Of these two, rheumatoid arthritis is the more dangerous and deforming, but it is less common. Degenerative arthritis is less severely crippling, but it is a leading cause of chronic illness.

It is the purpose of this chapter to demonstrate that modern foot disability may be the commonest cause of rheumatoid and degenerative arthritis. Foot trouble, of course, is not an exclusive cause. Stressful occupations, injuries and aging processes are important predisposing factors. Arthritis has been found in the bones of Egyptian mummies and the joints of wild animals where, naturally, influence of the modern shoe is no factor.

Rheumatoid Arthritis

The cause of rheumatoid arthritis is still unknown. It is uncommon where people go barefoot or wear non-deforming footgear. In most cases, a postural factor can be demonstrated before the onset of this disease. In its later stages, it causes permanent damage and contraction of the various joints, making any movement difficult and free use of the hands and feet often impossible.

Women outnumber men in the ratio of three to one in contracting the disease. It may be pointed out that, in considering foot disability as a cause, we find that also more common among women. The typical person contracting rheumatoid is between the ages of 20 and 40, inclined to be asthenic, chronically fatigue-ridden, with poor posture and imbalance, strained feet. The usual history then reveals that such an individual is subjected to a physically stressful period when joint coverings become actively inflamed and the disease first manifests. If the strain continues, the disease progresses at a rapid rate. However, in the cases which this author has reviewed, if the patient recognized the postural source of the illness and avoided undue stress or use of the feet, the progress of rheumatoid arthritis became subdued. Sufferers of this disease are less prone to cancer, as though their difficulty in movement protects their tissues from further injury.

Undoubtedly, previous illnesses, nutritional factors and emotional crises all play a role in the contraction of rheumatoid arthritis. The success of cortisone in ameliorating the symptoms strongly indicates that the disease is essentially one of unusual physical stress and, as previous arguments have shown, extensive use of disabled feet is the most important and malignant source of stress today.

In an asthenic (weak) individual, the most important preventive measure as considered here is avoidance of strain and the rehabilitation of disabled feet. In the case histories here presented, it will be also seen that, once the process of rheumatoid arthritis has begun, care of the feet is an important aspect of treatment.

Degenerative Arthritis

Degenerative arthritis is very common in modern shoe-wearing societies, and it is estimated to affect over 75 per cent of the population over 40 years of age. It is characterized by a chronic destruction of the joint cartilages, and by excessive growth of bone around the joint. These changes are not necessarily painful, but they limit movement.

The constant pulling of joint ligaments in an imbalanced foot acts as a perpetuating agent of inflammation to the edges of the joint surface, which eventually take on a lipped and irregular appearance. The pulling of tendons and larger ligaments can be so intense with imbalanced feet, that bone can be pulled away from the normal outline in the form of an osteophyte (bony outgrowth). Joints in the center of the foot (which are tighter and have a smaller range of movement) are the first to show evidence of these injuries. When the metatarsal and toe joints are affected, however, complete dislocations of the toes commonly take place, thus destroying irretrievably the balance of the foot.

Degenerative arthritis of the foot may have a serious secondary influence on degenerative arthritis changes in other parts of the body. If we should assume that the injuries from foot disabilities are a direct cause of arthritis in the feet and lower limbs, it is still difficult to account for the concurrent appearance of arthritis processes in the joints of the fingers, elbows and shoulders, which obviously are not influenced by any direct postural factors originating in the feet. It can be speculated that the syndrome of chronic stress and fatigue that disabled feet originate, can cause humoral (fluid) imbalance and tissue irregularities throughout the body; that in such individuals, minor injuries of the joints of the upper limbs will develop into arthritic degeneration. This author has found on a number of occasions that an individual, upon being relieved of arthritic severity in the feet, after rehabilitation, likewise experienced relief of arthritis in the fingers upon which no local therapeutic measures had been taken.

In the usual case of osteoarthritis in the lower limbs, not enough attention has been paid to the contributing factors of foot disability. The following case is offered.in illustration.

When this patient consulted me, she complained of painful feet. Previously there was X-rayed and diagnosed arthritis in the feet, that made walking only barely possible. Activity caused muscular pain throughout the body. Chronic fatigue, after the slightest activity, became more intense. The feet were grossly deformed with the toes extended 30 degrees beyond a horizontal line, with movement impossible. The joints throughout the foot had little mobility and pained on palpation. The feet were somewhat swollen and painful to the touch; deep calluses were present on the ball; a sparse musculature on the plantar (sole of the foot) surface permitted the cuneiform bones (3 wedge shaped bones in inner center of the foot) to be readily palpable. Steel arch supports were being worn, with a heavy corrective shoe having a heel an inch and a half high. Marked stooped shoulders were also observed.

Past history of the patient revealed that she had suffered with unusual foot discomfort since early adolescence. At the age of 13, she found walking difficult, especially because of pain in the ball of the foot. The toes had been deformed at an early age; probably due to the fact that the family income did not permit frequent replacement of shoes for growing children, together with the radical styles and disinterest in foot prophylaxis. At 18, she began work as a salesgirl. Her feet commenced to ache continuously and became worse than ever. Arch supports were secured and they gave some relief.

Marriage at 19 released the patient from the necessity of being continuously on her feet, and, while she still suffered from moderate foot pains and chronic fatigue, gross symptoms were largely quiescent for a period of 10 years. At the age of 30, the patient resumed her occupation as a salesperson, and her feet shortly became sore once more. For a period of 20 years, subsequently, all sorts of arch supports and corrective shoes were tried, with only moderate relief. One Christmas season the patient had a particularly strenuous time on her feet, pursuing her vocation. The pains became intolerable and finally she was unable to walk at all. Joints and muscles throughout the body were stiff and acutely painful, with the result that complete bed rest became obligatory. She remained in bed for 14 weeks, including 4 in a hospital, during which time, thorough examinations left the attending physicians with the opinion that the patient suffered from some form of acute degenerative arthritis. However, no definite diagnosis was reached. On becoming ambulatory, she began taking physical therapy and corrective exercises, but they seemed to exaggerate the symptoms.

Treatment consisted of first making it plain to her that her feet were woefully inadequate to meet her daily physical need, and that she must immediately cut down all activity that required her to stand or walk up steps. She was permitted walks of short duration. The arch supports were discarded and the feet were bandaged with adhesive tape with a view toward limiting lateral motion, by firmly holding the foot in approximation of a normal attitude. The calluses were pared on each visit and felt pads were inserted behind them. Moderate manipulative therapy was used in an attempt to produce a progressively greater range of movement in the feet. In preparation for the future use of flat-heeled shoes, she was given stretching exercises which would lengthen the shortened calf muscles. At first, she wore flat shoes for only a few minutes each day, and within two months, flat shoes could be worn the entire day with perfect comfort.

Her feet slowly achieved greater mobility until, within 6 months, her toes had almost a complete range of movement. The toes were still extended considerably, but had become flexible. The calluses had decreased, so that a metatarsal pad was no longer necessary. The patient began taking on some weight, and symptoms progressively reduced until, another two months later, all symptoms of chronic fatigue, nervousness and pain in the feet had disappeared entirely. The subject now spoke of being able to walk free of pain and fatigue for the first time in her adult life, and of experiencing a well-being she had never known before. She was cautioned against subjecting herself to any activity that her feet could not endure comfortably, since it is felt that the results of extensive damage to foot tissues over a period of 40 years will leave a limitation to capacity. However, she resumed her saleswoman's position with ease.

Degenerative Arthritis in the Knee

This, when caused by imbalanced feet, is usually seen in middle-aged and elderly women who have habitually worn heeled and pointed shoes. In the typical foot posture, with weight thrust on the inner side of the foot, the leg is compensatingly turned out in a degree of genuvalgum (knock-knee). This causes unusual pressure to be exerted against the soft tissues. The fact that this condition becomes relieved by balancing of the foot, indicates that its precipitating cause may be foot imbalance.

An older woman patient, who came regularly to have her corns treated, complained of a chronic aching in the knees which, within the past year, had become so acute that she was hardly able to climb steps or rise from a chair. She was no longer able to stoop in order to take care of her garden, which had been her greatest source of pleasure.

This woman had been in the custom of wearing 3-inch heel pumps. Various arthritic changes had taken place in her feet, which became stiffer with the combination of constant effects of injury from such footwear and advancing age. Finally, her feet had become so limited in movement that, in order to sustain her weight, they had to turn outward more than ever. This created strain and irritation to the inner part of the knee. She had consulted various specialists and had even tried whirlpool-bath treatment, diathermy, massage and some cortisone, only to find no relief. I advised her that the pain in her knees could be relieved, but not completely removed, since it was part of the wear and tear of growing old with disabled feet.

I applied an adhesive bandage to the foot and leg, to hold the inner side of the foot and ankle firm, thus permitting the weight on the foot to be placed in such a manner that no straining leverage action had to take place on the inner side of the knee. The patient walked around my office and exclaimed "Eureka! It no longer hurts!" Because of the age and degree of arthritic changes that were present in her feet, no hope was held out that the condition could be permanently relieved. However, as in other similar cases, when the strain to the knee is temporarily relieved, elements of inflammation disappeared and the knee was somewhat improved, even after the bandages were removed.

One day, when the patient called at my office, she reported that the past week had been her best in over a year. She had even been able to start her spring garden. I did not like the flushed look to her face, and I feared her blood pressure might mount.

I communicated with her daughter to ask if her mother was being moderate. The daughter admitted that the patient had attacked the garden work too vigorously and we agreed that no further correction to the knee would be attempted. Such a pronouncement was a keen disappointment to the patient, because of the relief she experienced when bandaged, but she could see the wisdom of our decision. Six months later her knees were still better than they had formerly been—evidently because they had not been overused—and her general physical condition was good—evidently because she had not overtaxed her strength.

Limited Movement in the Hip Joints

Limited movement in the hip joints affects the use of the entire limb and inclines the body to a strained, waddling gait. When stiff hip joints are induced by imbalanced feet (and they commonly are), they are caused by chronic attitudes of the limbs rotated outward, with the weight thrown on the inner side of the foot. In this chronic posture of the hip, non-exercise forces the joint to become incapable of full inward rotation. Unless too many degenerative changes have already taken place, restoration of foot balance will dramatically help restore normal movement in the hip joints.

One woman, on hearing that I had been able to relieve a friend of hers from backache, by means of foot treatment, consulted me about her chronic backache. Just a gross examination revealed a definite curvature of the spine, for which her physician had ordered a corset that gave her much relief and without which her usual activities were impossible. Attempted inward rotation of both limbs showed that the left hip joint was turned outward and was so stiff that inward rotation of the limb was impossible.

The patient had sprained her ankle 7 years earlier and had more or less forgotten it. The ankle was still swollen, however, and the torn ligaments were still tender. It was conjectured that, because of chronic pain to the outer side of the ankle, she had habitually turned that foot outward to avoid strain. This limited the range of movements of the hip joint, and stiffening resulted. Walking in this manner, with one side of her body tilted downward, had in turn caused a number of the joints in the spine to become irritated. As a matter of fact, her physician had diagnosed a herniated disc of the spine.

The author's first but mistaken impression was that the condition was of too long duration to lend itself to ready correction by foot treatment. It seemed that the causative lesion had been the sprained ankle, but the focus of the problem at that time was the fact that her left hip was stiff and did not permit her to walk properly or keep her back straight. At any rate, the foot and leg were bandaged in such a manner as to bring the foot forcibly inward, so that the inward rotation of the hip would have to be used.

After two weeks of such bandaging, the author was pleasantly shocked to find that the left hip was now entirely free to rotate inward, the difference in the height of her hip bones having been corrected. Besides, the formerly obvious curvature to the spine was no longer present. With a return of function to the hip joint, blood circulation increased so markedly that the skin under the adhesive broke out in a rash, and further adhesive bandaging was out of the question. The patient spoke of feeling better than at any time for years, and the ache in her back, which had always been present, had now disappeared entirely.

Low Back Pains

With shifting of the pelvis and spine necessary to compensate for imbalanced feet, the muscles and joints in the small of the back are placed in an unnatural and disadvantageous position. The heavy muscles and large sacroiliac joint, which support the upper part of the body, must now support them in a strained attitude. Any unusual demand or exertion on this region in its unbalanced condition may rupture part of the muscle or tear a ligament, or strain some of the nerves so abundantly close to the spine. Of course, one of a variety of backaches could ensue. Low back pain is common in this country, because of widespread foot trouble.

A man whom I had been treating for painful corns under his toenails complained of a chronic low back pain. He had suffered for a number of years and had experimented with various treatments, finally receiving relief from osteopathic treatment. The pain, however, always returned after a period of time and, therefore, the patient found it rewarding to go to his osteopath once a week.

He was a traveling salesman and, besides driving long hours in his car, he frequently had to carry heavy sample cases. He was not a robust person; this part of his work was strenuous for him, and may have precipitated the chronic backache.

His toes were not particularly deformed, but he customarily wore fashionable, pointed-toe shoes which caused the corners of his great toenails to become pressed against his flesh. When his toenails hurt, he found it more comfortable to walk with his feet pointed outward, so as to keep his large toe away from the side of the shoe. On examination of the movements of the joints in the mid-portion of his foot, it was found that they were locked in that position and could not be moved very far inward. A gross examination of his back showed that he had a pronounced hollowing at the lower portion so that his buttocks protruded.

The mechanical source of his backache seemed to be influenced by his feet. By not being able to bend his foot joints to manage a heel-to-toe gait, he was forced to rely on the inner side of his foot for support. To compensate for that chronic disadvantageous position, his pelvis tilted forward. In his case, this meant that the ligaments connecting the spine and the pelvis had the weight of the upper body on them in an awkwardly forward position. If he carried heavy suitcases in this condition, he might further strain that joint and ligament.

It was decided to try to loosen up the joints in the center of his foot by means of manipulation, and then gradually to force the feet, by means of adhesive tape, to be used more in a heel-to-toe movement. Much wider

[371]

and broader-toed shoes were prescribed, and a weekly treatment of the above nature was given, with the agreement of his osteopath.

It was some months before any appreciable increase in range of movement to the mid-joints of the foot was achieved. However, the adhesive bandaging to the foot was always an immediate comfort to the patient and the backache commenced to disappear. At the end of 6 months, the patient reported that the backache was no longer present, that he felt stronger and secure in that region of his body. The hollow back (lordosis) deformity had disappeared. His toes had become much stronger and the mid-portion of his foot was so much more flexible that the assumption of his former gait was no longer likely. He had gained weight, looked healthier, and spoke of generally feeling heartier.

Foot Disorders and Spine Curvatures

Acquired postural spinal abnormalities are commonly started in early life, while the bones are still soft and pliable. (If a child must twist the feet in an abnormal position in order to stay upright, compensating changes take place throughout the body, including the spine.) The usual deformities are swayback and stooped shoulders. When one foot is less adequate than the other, the child will place more weight on the better foot, with a tilting of the hips and a lateral curvature of the spine as a compensation for the uneven distribution of weight.

Should foot imbalance become acute in adult life, when the bones have already hardened and formed, the spine cannot be easily twisted to the new posture and irritation to the spinal joints results, perhaps explaining the causes of many of the cases chiropractors and osteopaths are called upon to deal with.

Men have certain spinal diseases more frequently than women, because their lower heels do not require gravitational adjustment until the higher levels of the body are reached. In women with grosser feet imbalance, compensatory deformities more often occur at the lower level of the ankles, knees and pelvis.

This case will demonstrate how foot deformation may influence spinal deformities in a child. A mother accompanied her 22-year-old daughter, who came to my office for the treatment of a painful corn. The corn was satisfactorily removed, but I observed a curvature of the spine, together with toes that appeared to have been deformed early in life. The mother said that the girl at birth had appeared normal in every way and it had not been until her fourth year that she noticed a curvature. The deformity was not of a gross nature, but obvious. The mother then recounted how she had taken her daughter to a hospital clinic, where she was advised to get a brace and to admonish the child to stand straight. This therapy was followed for a period of years, but did no good whatsoever. As a matter of fact, the daughter finally rebelled, and the family became resigned to her deformity.

[372]

The mother had not been aware of the condition of the girl's toes until I drew her attention to them. The toes had been bent in a manner that could only have been created by a short shoe, and the mother could recall that in the third and fourth year the girl had complained of growing pains in the legs, and that some difficulty had been encountered in forcing her to wear shoes. Vividly, now, the mother recalled that it was afterward that the deformity to the spine was first noticed.

The great toe of the left foot had been forced back in a hammer-toe arrangement, but some use to that toe was still possible, because the forward joint could be bent and the toe could thus make contact with the ground at each step. On the right foot, the great toe had been pushed toward the inside of the foot, so that its normal function was largely lost. Here the girl walked more on the inner side of her foot. The right foot extended downward one-half to three-quarters of an inch further than the left foot, with the hips and pelvis tilted to match. The spine was curved in the other direction, so as to gravitationally line up the body, and the head was cocked on the other side.

The girl had no pain in her back, but did tire rather easily and suffered from menstrual cramps that none of the doctors she had consulted were able to relieve. In my estimation, they were due to the disadvantageous position of the uterus as a result of postural factors.

It seemed that a deforming shoe had been the initial provocative factor in the deformation to the foot and, consequently, to the spine. No corrective foot treatment was recommended, however, because the compensatory changes to the deformity seemed gross and permanent. Because of the disadvantagous position of the body, it was recommended that occupations requiring the girl to be on her feet constantly should be avoided, and that she should wear the least deforming shoe possible.

It was pathetic in this case that a closer study of the influences of the feet had not been made in time.

Imbalanced Feet and the Head and Neck

Imbalanced feet often cause the head and neck to assume abnormal attitudes. The neck is bent forward and, if one foot is worse than the other (which is usually the case), the neck is also inclined to one side. Holding the neck constantly in this abnormal attitude (which in the case of badly deformed feet is often necessary), can cause a partial dislocation between the spinal vertebrae of the neck.

A farm wife who had worked physically hard her entire life came to me for treatment of imbalanced feet. After rehabilitory treatment, her feet became more functionable and she experienced relief to other aches throughout her body. Of particular interest was the fact that, at the time she consulted me, she was also receiving therapeutic adjustments to her spine from a chiropractor. That the woman's condition improved there could be no question. Exactly which of the treatments had contributed to

[373]

her recovery was difficult to calculate. The chiropractor, who had an excellent reputation, agreed to make a comparison of our notes.

The New Professions and Modern Shoes

I explained the weakness in the former condition of the woman's toes, which had been compressed and made useless by the habitual wearing of a pointed shoe, the manner in which her weight formerly had to be borne on the inner side of the foot, with the attendant pelvis-tilting and excessive spine-curving to compensate for such a posture. Now that the woman was using her toes and feet more effectively, her gross postural influence was alleviated.

The lesion which had most interested the chiropractor was a partial dislocation of the joint of the first two vertebrae of the spine, which he demonstrated by an X-ray picture before the treatment and a recent picture showing the subluxation (partial dislocation) corrected. He maintained that, when this joint became affected, it further affected all the other joints of the spine, and in addition, so interfered with the nerve and blood supply to the lower limbs that such a lesion was capable of causing incapacities and symptoms in the feet.

However, he did agree that foot deformation could be, and probably was, a gross cause of many of the lesions he encountered in the spine. I pointed out that, in habitually barefoot peoples, postures were unusually good; the spine was held straight; that in such peoples chiropractors and chiropodists would find very few cases to treat.

Chiropodists, osteopaths, chiropractors and others are all doing heroic and valuable work in relieving the sufferings of our crippled population. The ultimate goal of these expanded professions should be the elimination of the causes of newly increased diseases. I predict that, with the dissemination of information such as is contained in this book, the need for many such services will be diminished.

Overweight, Underweight and Ungainly Figures

With the feet in an imbalanced position, muscles thereby uncoordinated must be strained in order to keep the body upright and capable of walking. Thus, the leg, thigh and back muscles must do extra duty. In robust people, the unusual activity of these muscles causes them to become larger and stronger, giving a bulging and ungraceful appearance.

Together with muscular overdevelopment, excessive fat will also accumulate in robust but weakfooted people. The constant misery of uncomfortable feet makes these people crave pleasures and energy to compensate. Indulgence in the pleasures of the palate seems to fill a void in their uncomfortable existence, and of course, excessive fat is the result.

Additional weight for the feet to carry will strain them to a further point. Aggravation of foot symptoms with overweight is to be expected. People who start to reduce in weight because of painful feet would do better first, or simultaneously, to have their feet corrected.

[374]

Asthenically constituted people react to imbalanced feet in an opposite manner to that of robust individuals. They proceed to get more frail and underweight with the advance of foot disorders. The constant fatigue seems to impair their appetites, and the food they do eat appears not to be absorbed by abdominal organs that are in strained positions from poor posture. Many such people gain weight only after the foot is trained in less stress-inducing attitudes.

92. Preventing Stiff Shoulder

Pain and stiffness in the shoulder have become so commonplace that quite a considerable number of articles in medical journals are devoted these days to the causes and possible cures of these disorders.

There are several reasons why our shoulders appear to be especially susceptible to strain and injury. First of all, is our upright posture. Animals walk on 4 legs, but man walks on two, with the result that he has problems of posture which animals do not have. The whole construction of a shoulder seems to make it that part of us that can most easily be strained or hurt by our daily activity. Because man uses his hands almost constantly all day long, the shoulder has a lot of work to do. Then, too, much of today's kind of activity requires monotonous and often difficult use of the shoulder. We will discuss some of these circumstances later on.

Meanwhile, there is the curious "syndrome," as doctors say, called variously painful shoulder, frozen shoulder, periarthritis (inflammation of the tissues around the joints), the shoulder-hand syndrome and so forth. Generally, this kind of disorder appears first after the age of 40 or so. It is common to both men and women. Sometimes it is serious enough to result in complete disuse of the shoulder, which means a serious crippling of the individual's activity. The *Medical Journal of Australia* devoted several articles and a long discussion to this problem. Selwyn Nelson, M.D., of Sydney tells his physician readers that, if pain is present only in the shoulder and in no other joints, no one should suspect rheumatoid arthritis, for it definitely is not that. He also describes a condition which, he says, is quite common among women at the time of menopause. It consists of a tingling sensation in the hand, occurring most often at night, which may be combined with pain in the upper arm and shoulder. There may be blanching and a feeling of coldness in the hands, too. He suggests relieving this condition by exercise that will improve posture. He also advises against the carrying of heavy shopping bags or anything heavy.

Richard Hodgkinson, M.D., also of Sydney, tells us that all the many modern activities we engage in often demand an "extended and abducted" position of the arm to which the shoulder joint has not become accustomed.

[375]

He tells us, too, that shoulder pain in later years is often caused simply by degeneration of the tendons. They are growing old. If an examination shows that there is no physical injury in the joint, he advises rest, pain pills and heat treatments as the best form of therapy. He concludes by saying, "It is obvious, however, that there are many other causes of this condition which are not understood and much work is still required."

Causes of Painful Shoulder

Mark B. Coventry, M.D., of Rochester, Minnesota, discusses painful shoulder in an article in the *Journal of the American Medical Association,* January 17, 1953. He says there are 4 possible causes: (1) muscular—which may mean overuse, fractures, dislocations, bad posture, tumors or calcification of joints; (2) nervous—caused by inflammation of nerves; (3) visceral—that is, the shoulder pain may actually originate in a gall bladder, heart or pancreas disorder; and (4) vascular—when there is a disorder of the blood vessels.

He discusses the possibility of occupational causes for shoulder pain. One patient of his worked in an overall factory and, when he had finished his particular operation on a pair of heavy overalls, he had to throw them over his shoulder onto a pile. Shoulder pain is also common among farmers after a session of especially heavy work, such as silo-filling. But some occupational hazards are less obvious. One of Dr. Coventry's patients was a retired school teacher who had taken a job as a typist. The extended position of her arms as she typed all day was the cause of her painful shoulder. Another patient was a baker who decorated cakes. Apparently he stooped over a table, with his muscles tense, all day as he worked away at this very fine and intricate work.

Disuse can cause a painful or stiff shoulder, says Dr. Coventry. When a joint has been immobilized in a cast, of course, there is pain when you begin to use it again. On the other hand, when there is pain, you have a tendency not to use the shoulder, so that it becomes stiff. Then when you try to use it again, those creaking unused muscles give you such a twinge that you decide not to try to use them, thus leading to more stiffness.

Finally, says Dr. Coventry, there is the factor of the "periarthritis personality." A painful shoulder becomes stiff only if the patient does not use it and if the patient has a personality which makes him susceptible to this kind of disorder.

The "Periarthritis Personality"

Three physicians of Madison, Wisconsin, discuss this kind of personality in greater detail in an article in the *American Practitioner* for May, 1953. They examined 300 patients who seemed to have psychosomatic illnesses and found that 60 of them suffered from pain and stiffness in the shoulder. Their ages ranged from 25 to 55 years; most of them were in their forties. The majority of them had other complaints along with their bad shoulders: headaches, some kind of chronic nose trouble, weakness and fatigue, dizzy spells, stomach trouble, heart trouble or some muscular discomfort, such as muscular aches, cramps in the legs and so forth. All of them, say our physicians, were tense and likely to overreact to physical stimulus—the kind of people who jump nervously at a hand laid on the shoulder or a leaf dropped on the hand. In most of these folks, an X-ray showed no physical injury or disorder in the shoulder.

Questioning elicited the discovery that, in almost all cases, the pain and stiffness had begun at a time of particular stress and heightened emotion. This does not mean necessarily some grave emergency. These people were the perfectionist kind who thought of themselves as self-sufficient, independent and energetic. They were all overly conscientious. They lived well-planned lives, following rigid patterns of activity and any interruption of their well-laid plans brought frustration. But, gritting their teeth, they "carried on" bravely, all the time unconsciously resenting the fact that their responsibilities were too heavy.

In their daily work, they did not use their hands or arms more than the average person, but they did everything with their muscles under tension which created a lot of resistance in the voluntary muscles which were working along at their usual speed and tension. "The protracted co-existence of these two opposing forces, plus the vulnerability of the shoulder joint might explain why this structure is so frequently the site of this type of musculoskeletal disability," say the authors.

So these patients were given psychotherapy. We do not know of what this consisted, but we suppose that the psychiatrist or psychologist, simply by talking to them, managed to convince them that there was absolutely no need to be so tense, hurried and conscientious about the things they were doing. Actually, no matter how hard we try, none of us can be perfect. So if we plan to get something done by noon, let's try working at it in a relaxed fashion. If we succeed, fine. If not, then let's not get worried, tense and upset about it. Let's postpone it for the next day, without any regrets or self-blame. This is not a plea for laziness. But those folks who work (or play) at too intense a pitch are well aware of what they are doing. And if they wish to avoid ill health, they simply must learn to relax and not try so hard for perfection. In the case of the 60 patients, the psychotherapy worked wonders. They learned to take things much easier and, as their muscles relaxed, their shoulder pain disappeared.

All the articles in our file on painful shoulder mention the factor of personality. Whether you take it from the point of view of a psychosomatic personality—that is, someone who unconsciously interprets frustration or insecurity in terms of actual physical illness—or whether you decide that the muscular strain of such overly conscientious people results in stiffness and pain in the shoulder, it boils down to the same thing—a defect in personality that somehow brings about a quite serious and common disorder.

Preventing Stiff Shoulder

Common methods of cure include various pain-killing drugs, deep X-ray, diathermy, injections of novocaine and posture exercises. Of these, we can only recommend posture exercises. Our field is not cure, but it seems to us that painful shoulder might be prevented by sensible rules of good health. We all know surely when we are overworking some particular part of us, and we should know enough to stop before this overwork results in pain or stiffness. Yes, even if it means changing jobs, it would certainly be worth it.

Our research has shown us, too, that vitamin B and calcium are preventatives of muscle stiffness. The diets of most of us are deficient in these two food elements. Brewer's yeast and bone meal are good sources.

Editor Rodale discovered something helpful in his own experience with shoulder pain. Several years ago, he noticed that his right shoulder was painful. He thought it might come from doing so much writing with a pencil gripped hard in his hand. He switched to a typewriter and the pain disappeared. But he did not like to type, so he had to find some other solution. He began to use his left hand, rather than his right, whenever he could—in opening doors, putting on his hat, eating, brushing his hair and so forth. As he gradually began to make his left hand do more of the inconsequential manual work, his right shoulder improved. Furthermore, he did a little research and found that the theory of using one side to rest the other side has long been known to primitive people. The American Indians practiced it in their long journeys by land. They marched part of the way using the right foot harder than the left, then shifted and made the left foot do more work. When you are eating dinner tonight, check and see if you are naturally chewing on just one side. You can bring on a fine case of malocclusion that way. So make a conscious effort to use both sides of your mouth in chewing—or chew first on one side, then on the other.

Interestingly enough, time and motion study experts, whose profession it is to get industrial jobs done with the least effort, the most production and the greatest saving of time, have found that one of their most important principles is to get both hands to share the work, so that neither of them becomes overly tired. Time and again, by proper planning, these experts have arranged a given piece of work so that both hands work at once or so that each hand works equally with the other, thus saving time, motion, money—and incidentally, making the job faster, easier and not so tiring for the worker.

One final caution. It seems to us quite possible that an explanation of many of the cases of stiff shoulder which become worse at night might very well be incorrect sleeping positions assumed. As Editor Rodale has shown in his book, *Sleep and Rheumatism,* no one knows exactly what is the best or healthiest position in which to sleep. But he has discovered a number of very significant things about ways *not* to sleep.

93. Sleep and Rheumatism

By J. I. RODALE

I would like to tell you the story of how I stumbled upon an interesting fact about neuritis.

Around 1940, I began to experience neuritic pains in the hands, arms and shoulders. There would be dull twinges and pains, and I found it extremely difficult to don my overcoat. If I raised my arms above a certain level, the pain would increase. I couldn't turn my head without experiencing pain in the neck and shoulders. I would get up in the morning with a feeling in the shoulders and neck as if someone had sat on me all night, and my fingers had a numbness which made it difficult for me to tie my shoelaces.

The doctor diagnosed it as neuritis, but its cause had him baffled and, in spite of months of medical treatments of all kinds, including osteopathy, the painful condition persisted. As I look back now, I can see that in this doctor's practice, he specialized in finding cures, but never spent any time in seeking causes. He asked me no questions about my daily life and habits in order to come upon some clue that might lead to the answer. I just kept coming and he kept treating it, mainly with diathermy, but nothing happened.

A friend of mine had about the same symptoms that I did and every time we would meet we would swap talk about our condition.

The Cause Discovered

One night I discovered the cause of my trouble. It was about 3:00 A.M. when I suddenly awoke from a disturbed sleep. My entire arm was numb from shoulder to finger tips. In fact, it was practically paralyzed. I tried to think quickly and noticed that I had been sleeping with my head on the paralyzed arm. I became convinced that this habit was at the bottom of all my trouble. My own hard head had been digging down on my arm for hours.

I stayed awake for a long time, thinking and observing the actions of my arms and head. I would catch my arm attempting to move upward so that it could be a pillow to my head, but I fought against it. It took about a week to win complete control over them, and after that, the habit was completely mastered. Never again did I sleep with my head on my arms and, miracle of miracles, the neuritis in my arms completely vanished.

I then went to see my friend who had the same condition I did, and when I related my experience to him, a light came into his eyes. He did not sleep with his head on his arms. In his case, it was a way he had of folding back his left arm in a v-shape and sleeping with his body pressing on it. He now cured himself of this habit, sleeping with his arm spread

[379]

out in a relaxed way, and within a week his neuritic pains completely disappeared.

When I saw how simple it was to cure these two cases, I began to think of the hundreds of thousands of people who must be suffering from the same thing, and since, in questioning people, I found that a majority of them did sleep with their head pressing on *their* arms, I figured that I had a job to do. I had to share my knowledge with as many persons as possible. So I wrote a book on the subject in 1940, as well as several articles which appeared at that time in *Fact Digest* and *True Health Stories,* two magazines which I edited and owned. As a result, hundreds of people have been cured of what I call pressure neuritis.

Medical Recognition of the Idea

A doctor friend of mine, a phlebitis specialist in New York, was incensed when he received a copy of my book, and said to me at our next meeting, "Why do you meddle in such things? You are not a doctor."

To give you another reaction from a doctor, may I quote from a letter received from Mrs. Susan Snyder, 135 Eastern Parkway, Brooklyn, New York (October 29, 1953):

"The doctor tells me that I have osteoarthritis. The pains I complained about—terrific headaches and pains from the back of the neck up and down to lower back as well as between shoulders—completely disappeared after I arose and walked about for about a half hour. I asked my doctor (an M.D.) if it wasn't pressure pains. I suspected what your book confirmed. The doctor gave me some 'double talk' and said that the pain was due to adhesions, and he suggested 'radar' treatments. I went 3 times a week until your book opened my eyes. I was mad clean through. Why wasn't my doctor honest enough to tell me the pains were due to pressure exerted in sleep?

"I sent him your book and told him 'I know and so does Mr. Rodale that osteoarthritis is incurable (degenerated bones cannot be restored), but I am glad to have been corroborated in my suspicion that my pains were pressure pains and I didn't need a doctor for that.' "

Mrs. Snyder turned over to me the answer from her physician. He said, "Proper sleeping habits are helpful in these conditions—but by no means curative—since they do not remove the, as yet, unknown cause or causes. Mr. Rodale oversimplifies the entire matter, principally through ignorance of the basic sciences relating to the human body. Improvement by any method of treatment may be only apparent, concurrent and coincident with a period of natural remission of symptoms—which usually recur in spite of the continuance of the temporarily 'miraculous cure.' "

I make no comment except to say that my own cure has so far been in effect for over 16 years. Many others have had similar experiences. I have had hundreds of letters testifying to my method's efficaciousness in completely clearing up pressure neuritis.

Here is a typical case: One day I was in a broker's office and overheard the bookkeeper complaining to a customer's man that she had been having terrible pains in her arms and shoulders. "I have to go to my doctor this afternoon for vitamin B injections and I dread going," she said, "and tomorrow I am supposed to go to my dentist to have my teeth X-rayed. The doctor thinks that it might be infected teeth, and I might have to have all of them extracted."

I walked over to her and related my own experience. When I explained that possibly head pressure could be the cause of her own trouble, she was delighted to find an excuse for not going to the doctor or dentist. She at once admitted that she slept with her head on her arms. In about a week, that girl was as free of pain as a new-born baby, without the benefit of any vitamin B injections. Of course, not everyone who has pains in the arms and shoulders gets them from sleep pressures, but it is surprising how many cases do arise from this cause.

Some Letters

Here are a few letters received from readers who have benefited from my book on the subject. They are only a few chosen from hundreds:

Here is one from Bernard Singer, 16 Shanley Avenue, Newark, New Jersey:

"I had been experiencing sharp pains across the back occasionally. After reading your pamphlet, I became aware of two faulty sleeping habits. I was resting my head on my right arm and my wife frequently threw one leg over my back as I slept. By avoiding these two faulty habits, I have found that my backaches disappeared."

James M. Moore, Route 4, Greenville, Ohio, writes:

"I had found my two big toes were becoming numb, with almost no feeling in them. By breaking myself of lying so that one leg was under the other, this situation has cleared up also. Now these toes have a normal feeling."

Mrs. C. C. Wacker, Wilton Junction, Iowa, writes:

"I used to wake up more tired than when I went to bed, and so full of aches and pains that I was miserable—until I read your book *Sleep and Rheumatism*. Now I wake up refreshed. It's almost like a miracle. Others have been helped by your method through my telling them, including my husband who has been greatly benefited. So we decided to give 4 of these books as Christmas presents."

John H. Stevenson, 26 Southbridge Street, Worcester, Massachusetts, writes:

"Your book *Sleep and Rheumatism* has taught me how to get more rest in my sleeping hours. Now I get up in the morning without that swollen feeling in my hands, which our family doctor says is a sign of arthritis. We are hearing too much about that dreadful trouble, and I believe you have told me how to stop it."

Hugo Mayerhoefer, Salem, Oregon:

"My dear Mr. Rodale: Your book *Sleep and Rheumatism* told me exactly where 90 per cent of my rheumatism came from. However, none of the positions you illustrated (see figure 10) fit my case and so it did me no good for about a year or so until I finally discovered that my collarbone, in sleeping on my side, pressed against some nerve and choked off the 'supply line,' and a few weeks after, noticed a change for the better. Twenty years' suffering because my doctors didn't find the cause of my trouble. A million thanks to you."

Some Additional Facts

The sleep neuritis comes from pressure on nerves, which damages them, and from blood congestions caused by pressure on veins, but the amazing thing is how quickly the condition clears up when the sleep pressures are eliminated. You might ask: but how can I prevent myself from doing these things during sleep? The answer is that you begin by trying, and pretty soon your subconscious mind has learned a new set of sleeping habits. All you need do is to draw an imaginary line along your shoulders, and in sleep never let your arms go above that line. Keep your arms down at the sides and as relaxed as possible. (See figure 11.)

In Germany, a survey showed that practically 100 per cent of the population aged between 40 and 50 were afflicted with some form of arthritis or neuritis, but this, of course, included very mild cases. Ask any person over 60 and you will find that they are suffering from vague bodily pains and twinges. Many of these cases are due to pressures exerted in sleep, although I have also found that some of it is due to sleeping on soft mattresses, which cause the spine to curve downward. Most of these people continue to suffer because cures are usually attempted with medication, whereas the cause is purely a mechanical one.

Dr. Emanuel Josephson of New York City, who wrote a commentary on my book, said that pressures on the arm and shoulder during sleep can lead to bursitis. The cause is injury to the lubricating system of the shoulder. There is a delicate sac in the shoulder joint which is moistened by an oily fluid. Pressure on the shoulder muscle during sleep can in some cases cause a breakdown of its lubricating system, giving rise to a case of sub-deltoid bursitis. Many of these cases are usually operated on.

Many a drunkard has fallen asleep in a hallway and, because there are no pillows handy, used his arm for that purpose. But when one is drunk, the circulation and forces of the body are at even a lower ebb than in ordinary sleep, so that when the man is suddenly awakened, his arm is so paralyzed that he can hardly move it. Such cases sometimes have to be hospitalized, and in the big cities, so many of them are brought into hospitals that this condition has been called Drunkard's Neuritis. It has also been called Saturday Night Neuritis, from the fact that so many workers are paid at the end of the week, indulging in wild bouts of drinking and sleeping it off under tables, etc.

Yet, though the doctors have handled so many of these drunkards, and knew that it came from sleeping on their arms, they did not think to associate it with other cases of arm neuritis. You can search high and low in the medical profession and nary a word will you find that the head pressing on the arm in sleep is the cause of these thousands of cases of pressure neuritis. Patients come to doctors with symptoms of waking up in sleep with arms paralyzed, and the doctors call it *Brachialgia Statica Paresthetica,* which means numbness in the arm during sleep, but always, in their writing about it, they state that it comes upon the person suddenly and that the cause is not known. I am wondering if what I have discovered is really *Brachialgia Statica Paresthetica.*

Spontaneous Numbness During Sleep

In the November 5, 1955, issue of the *Journal of the American Medical Association,* a physician asks a question of the editor. A patient of his, a 30-year-old plumber, complains of his hands becoming numb every night during sleep. Upon awakening, he has to shake his hands vigorously to do away with the numbness. There seems to be no evidence of disease that could be at the bottom of it. What could be the cause?

The editor replies. It is possible that this could be a scalenus anticus syndrome, the background for which could be a cervical rib and enlarged transverse process of the cervical spine, or even a hypertrophy of the scalenus anticus muscles. The editor advises an X-ray, and an injection of procaine solution into the affected muscles. The trouble could also be in the thyroid, says the editor, and advises quite a complicated and expensive procedure, including complete studies of the spine.

Then, he says, that sometimes such a condition has been vaguely diagnosed as *idiopathic nocturnal paresthesia.* This means a nighttime numbness of spontaneous origin, which I will discuss in a little while. Sometimes patients with this condition have what is called arterio-spasm, and for this, priscoline is given 3 or 4 times a day, as well as barbiturates. Also, treatments with mecholyl every second day, 10 times in all, have helped.

Now, with all due respect to this editor's medical gobbledegook, which I have attempted to simplify, all that is probably the matter with this plumber is that he is sleeping with his head on his arms, causing pressures on nerves and the circulatory system. Sometimes people sleep with their arms curled up in positions which also cause stagnation in the circulation. All that is needed is about 3 nights of relaxed sleeping, with the arms down at the sides, and presto, no more *nocturnal paresthesia.* (Now he's got *me* talking that way.)

Now what is this *idiopathic nocturnal paresthesia* that the editor mentioned? Years ago, when I was doing a thorough research of the medical literature, I made it my business to read as many articles on the subject as possible. It seems that *idiopathic nocturnal paresthesia* is a form of numbness in the arms which comes on during the night for no reason at all. It just as suddenly disappears and nobody seems to die from it. But

[383]

FIGURE 10. SLEEPING POSTURES TO AVOID.

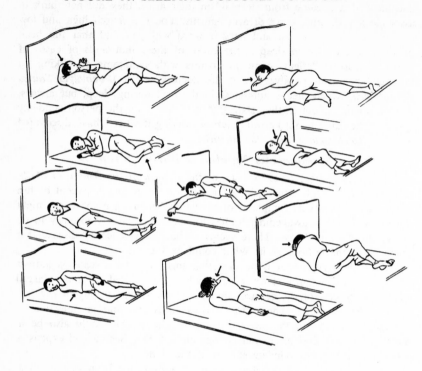

FIGURE 11. SAFE POSITIONS IN SLEEP.

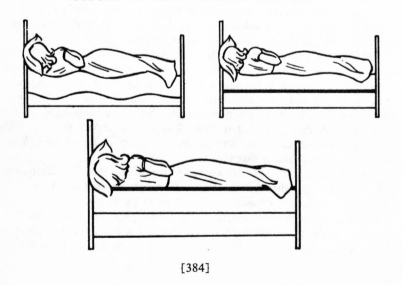

the medical profession seems to be baffled as to its cause. The medical profession is so easily baffled, and then goes on to create elaborate, expensive cure procedures which pay them handsome premiums for their lack of desire, or energy, or what-have-you, in looking for causes. But from the experience that I have had in this field, my opinion is that there is no such thing as spontaneous paresthesia. The numbness must be caused by a pressure of one part of the body on the other. It can't be otherwise.

Just about that time, I was invited to speak to a health group in Cincinnati, and part of my talk was to be devoted to pressure neuritis in the arms. In going over my papers the night before at the hotel, I found an article that had appeared in the May, 1944, *Journal of Nervous and Mental Diseases,* entitled *"Brachialgia Statica Paresthetica." Brachialgia* means pain in the arms, *statica,* at rest and *paresthetica,* an abnormal sensation, as burning, prickling, etc. This article was practically a complete review of what was known in this field. The author, Robert Wartenberg, M.D., even said in it, "Under the titles: 'Sleep and Rheumatism,' 'How I Cured Neuritis,' and 'Pain in the Finger,' etc., a layman, J. I. Rodale, wrote a book and magazine articles on this subject."

Again it was stressed that arm numbness could come about during the night spontaneously, without pressure being applied, and again I questioned it. Evidently my subconscious mind was reading the article along with me and differed with me, for during that night I had the most beautiful case of *idiopathic nocturnal paresthesia* you would ever want to see, and I am sure that it was my subconscious which did it, purely to teach me a lesson.

Now, I must tell you that, a few years before, I had cured myself of a severe case of *pressure neuritis* in my arms by learning not to sleep with my head on them. I had learned this so thoroughly that it had become automatic. I suppose that that little imp which is my subconscious, stood watch for me while I was asleep, to see that my arms did not go above my shoulder line. Thus my head would not be able to reach them.

But on this night of which I speak, I know that I had a case of arm numbness brought about without any pressure. It was purely psychosomatic. It did not last very long, but there it was. The next morning I took my subconscious to task and spoke to it in no uncertain terms. "Subconscious," I said, "you and I are going to go through life together. We are going to read many medical journals and articles. We are going to have lots of fun, but don't take it personally or be too serious about it. Be objective! Remember what I tell you, now, because I don't want to have any more trouble with you. I don't want to insult you by telling you who is the master, but let us each know our place and function. I need you to remember things for me. Remember them well, but don't try any more experiments on my body."

That was about 10 years ago, and I have not had any similar trouble since. My subconscious and I have been the best of friends.

94. Good Posture Prevents Rheumatism

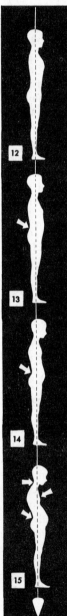

What is the importance of posture in the prevention of rheumatism? Good posture is essential for good health, and it is especially important in any disorder in which bones, joints and muscles are involved, for these are the parts of the body which suffer most from bad posture.

Dr. Ben T. Bell of Abington Memorial Hospital, writing on "The Diagnosis and Treatment of Low Back Pain" in the *Medical Clinics of North America* for November, 1940, says that the assumption of upright posture by man, with the resulting angulation, the systems of balance and leverage necessary to hold this upright posture, is one of the main reasons why the lower back is so susceptible to strain. The muscles of the lower back also seem to be insufficient to perform their work in the anatomy of mankind.

Says Dr. Bell, "Sedentary occupations or manual occupations in which the worker remains seated all day, together with poor habits of posture, result in a back which is barely compensating. A strain of lifting, or a fall, an excessive increase in weight or even increased weight-bearing will increase the load so that the symptoms of strain or more serious injury result. An illness resulting in further loss of muscle power may be the cause of insufficiency in the muscles and strain. In the back subjected to continued mild strain, chronic irritation increases the changes which appear as osteoarthritis in later life. . . . Often the patient with postural defects of flat feet, lumbar lordosis (swayback), sagging abdomen and obesity, is symptom-free until some trauma (injury) is literally the last straw on the camel's back."

Fig. 12. Perfect posture . . . head, shoulders and feet in perfect alignment. Plumb line divides boy in half indicating body is in balance.

Fig. 13. Good posture . . . even though body is not quite in perfect balance. Pelvic structure has slight forward tilt as indicated by arrow.

Fig. 14. Posture becomes poorer as the forward tilt of the pelvic structure increases. Curve in boy's back starts to deepen and other adjustments follow.

Fig. 15. Bad posture . . . pelvic structure tilted completely out of line, curve in back deepens . . . chest hollows out . . . head thrusts forward at ugly angle.

Doctors agree on the importance of good posture. They also agree that the individual determination to achieve good posture can work wonders, even though there are some postural handicaps that cannot be overcome without the aid of professional therapy. Perfect posture is so simple that there can be no disagreement as to what it means. It means keeping one's body in balance so that there is as little strain as possible on muscles, bones and nerves, when one stands, walks, sits or works.

The base of support for one's body is the pelvic structure—that is, the bony basin to which one's legs are attached, and which contains the abdominal organs. Figure 12 shows perfect posture, with the head, shoulders, knees and feet in perfect alignment with pelvic structure. A plumb line dropped from this boy's ear to his ankle would be straight and would divide him in half—that is, half of his body weight would be found to be on each side of the line.

What Is Bad Posture?

In figure 13, something has happened. Perhaps fatigue, perhaps injury, perhaps just carelessness and lack of exercise have thrown him a little off balance. His pelvic structure has been titled forward slightly, with the result that the rest of his body must adjust itself somehow so that it can remain upright. By the time of figure 15, his pelvic structure had tilted completely out of line, the curve in his back had deepened, pushing his stomach out. Since the upper part of his body must compensate for this bad balance in the lower part, his chest is hollow, his shoulders rounded and his head thrust forward at an ugly angle. The sagging muscles of his abdomen must still support his abdominal organs. Since these muscles are attached to his spine, the added strain on them deepens the curve in his back and weakens it still further.

The next time you are standing on a street corner waiting for someone, look at the people who pass. You will be amazed to find that most of them have posture like figure 15. You will notice that bad posture can completely ruin an otherwise attractive appearance; you will see that tasteful and expensive clothes look like rags when the framework beneath them is sagging and out of balance. If you wait on your corner long enough, perhaps someone may come along who has good posture. He will look relaxed, rested, healthy. There will be a spring to his step and a buoyancy in his appearance that will make you feel good just to look at him.

When you get home, take a look at yourself in a full-length mirror. Just stand naturally, as you usually stand. How do you look? Like figure 15 or perhaps figure 14? Be honest with yourself. Then decide to do something to improve your posture. It won't be easy. If your body has accustomed itself to the frightfully bad posture of figure 15, you will have to do a lot of coaxing to regain good posture, for by this time, bones, muscles and nerves have gotten "set" in this bad pattern. Incidentally, looking at figure

15, do you agree with us that here is a perfect setting for rheumatism, or, for that matter, any other bone, muscle or joint affliction that might be around? Every bone, small or large, is out of place in this body. Every muscle is strained. Every nerve is pinched and crowded.

Correcting Bad Posture

The first and, yes, we might say, the only exercise necessary to begin correcting this sad off-balance posture, is to pull in on the muscles of your abdomen. It's just as simple as that. Look at figure 15 and imagine (if you could change it all at once) what would be the result of pulling in those stomach muscles. The curve in the back would straighten out, which in turn would correct the flat chest and rounded shoulders. As these fall into line, the legs and feet would assume their rightful positions and the posture of figure 12 would be a reality again!

However, if your posture is really like figure 15, you'll find that it's not easy to pull in your stomach muscles. They're flabby and soft from disuse. Try again the second day and the third. It may take weeks before you notice the slightest improvement in the trimness of your figure. You don't have to set aside any time for exercise if you want to have good posture. Just fit it into your daily regime. You can practice good posture while you are waiting for a trolley, standing in an elevator, talking on the telephone.

Housework involves a large percentage of us, so let's discuss posture in terms of housework. While you're getting breakfast in the morning, waiting for the eggs to boil, check on your posture. Pull in your tummy and tuck your lower back under where it belongs. Now see how you can improve posture and ward off fatigue while you're working. When you bend to pick something up, to reach something or to do some particular kind of work, bend at your knees or hips—don't bend your back (Fig. 16). No matter how you manage to do it, see that your sink, stove, laundry tubs and other working spaces are at ex-

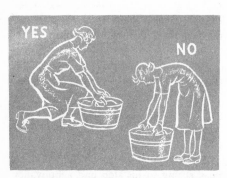

FIG. 16. Use leg and shoulder muscles to lift. Back-bending is back-breaking and can cause unnecessary posture-wrecking fatigue.

actly the right height for you—not so high that you must stretch to reach them, not so low that you must bend or stoop (Fig. 17). Sitting is better than standing at any job where it can possibly be managed (Fig. 18). Until you've tried sitting while you iron, you won't realize how much energy you can save this way. Sit down in the kitchen while you're preparing vegetables, sit down to wash the dishes. Make sure your chair is comfortable and that you are sitting with your back straight, your stomach muscles pulled in. Be certain you have support for your feet, check from time to time to make sure your shoulders are back, but relaxed, so that you are not "humped" tensely over your work.

You can exercise for good posture while you are making a bed, sweeping a floor, setting a table, running a sewing machine. If you remember only one basic commandment—keep your stomach muscles pulled in—the rest of your body will align itself prop-

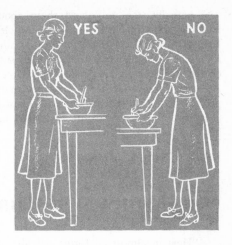

Fig. 17. Height of table affects posture. Stand erect, have working surface at correct height. Make sure you do not have to stoop or bend over your work.

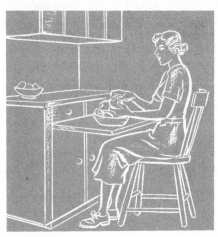

Fig. 18. Sitting saves energy . . . sit at your job whenever possible. Use comfortable chair and keep back straight, stomach muscles in.

erly. Have you ever estimated how much time you spend each week walking to and from stores carrying packages? Have you ever stopped to think how important to your posture the way in which you carry those packages is? At your dressing table mirror, you can check on your shoulders. When you are standing as you normally do, one is probably higher than the other, for no other reason but that, since you were in school, you have become accustomed to carrying books, purse, umbrella, packages, always in the same arm. In most people, this practice results in carrying the shoulder of that arm as much as several inches higher than the other shoulder —bad posture. This throws the whole upper part of your body out of line and somewhere, your bones and muscles must compensate, resulting in a lot of wear and tear, which you might easily avoid by simply remembering to carry equal weights in both arms or by shifting the weight from side to side.

Actually, the only hard thing about regaining good posture is reminding yourself of it. Once the muscles have been strengthened, you'll have good posture without giving it another thought. But meanwhile, make a habit of studying your reflection in shop windows when you're walking on the street. One glance will remind you to pull those stomach muscles in. At home or at work decide on some one object—a calendar, a window, a piece of furniture that will be your constant reminder, every time you look at it, to correct your posture. You may be saving yourself years of agonizing pain with arthritis later on in life.

95. Mineral Baths for Arthritics

"Heat in almost all forms is highly desirable. The types of heat may vary with each case . . . hot water bottles, heating pads, hot packs or compresses, warm baths . . . give a lot of help." So says the Arthritis and Rheumatism Foundation in a leaflet, *What You Should Know About Arthritis*.

Comments Walter S. McClellan, M.D., writing in the *Cyclopedia of Medicine, Surgery, Specialties,* "The treatment of a patient with rheumatoid arthritis with physical medicine, including heat, massage and exercise, stands out as one of the most universally valuable forms of therapy. Hydrotherapy (baths) offers a valuable adjunct both for the provision of heat and a medium for exercise."

Since the beginning of history, people have used mineral baths to treat diseases. Mineral springs, you know, are springs in which considerable amounts of minerals occur naturally; the springs in Yellowstone Park are examples. And, of course, there are many natural mineral spring spas in various parts of the country which were popular health resorts not so long ago. You went to the spa to "take the cure" or to "take the waters." You drank or bathed in it, or both.

The popularity of the spa has declined in this country. The main reason for this seems to be that wealthy people (the only ones who could afford to "take the waters") began to look elsewhere for treatment of their diseases, as well as the elaborately organized social life that went along with "taking the waters." The fancy hotels began to crumble, there was not enough business to pay for repairs and eventually, the whole idea of a healthful vacation at a mineral spring became passé.

Besides, during the past 15 or 20 years, we had the wonder drugs, so the milder and less dramatic methods of treatment ceased to appeal. Who wants to spend a couple of months getting rid of the pain of arthritis, when he can get a shot of cortisone in 5 minutes?

But the wonder drugs have not been successful in treating the rheumatic diseases. True, some of them can control symptoms for brief periods, but the disease goes right on and may even become much more serious without giving the patient any warning that this is so (see Chapter 83).

In the case of the rheumatic diseases, then, it seems wise to reconsider one of the old, time-honored methods of treatment, which can certainly do no harm, and judging from the material we have read, may accomplish a lot of good. Hot baths relieve many kinds of pain. We all know this. We know that a hot bath can loosen tight muscles and relieve aching joints when we have overworked at some unusual activity. We are told by experts that moist heat is far more effective in relieving pain than dry heat. There are 3 reasons for this, Dr. McClellan tells us: (1.) increased elimination of waste products through the skin and the kidneys; (2.) improved circulation of the blood and other body fluids, because the heat expands the blood vessels; (3.) mechanical breaking down of adhesions and softening of any thickening in muscles and tissues.

The effectiveness of a hot bath depends on how much of the body is submerged, how hot the water is and how long the patient stays in the bath. Stiffness of joints is perhaps the most troublesome characteristic of the rheumatic diseases. Anything (such as moist heat) which will loosen these joints and permit freer motion is beneficial. Keeping the muscles inactive tends to cause them to become less and less usable; this leads to less and less activity, more and more pain and decreased mobility.

How Important Are the Minerals?

Is there any value in taking mineral baths rather than just plain water baths?

We think there is. Apparently the minerals are absorbed through the skin. In 1929, 3 researchers at the Mayo Clinic published in the *Archives of Dermatology and Syphilology,* Vol. 20, p. 158, their findings on the absorption of sulfur from sulfur baths. They found that all of the subjects had increased sulfur in their blood after the bath—some of them 4 times as much.

We know that sulfur is important for the efficient working of the human body. It is present in every plant and animal cell. In the body, the muscles contain about half the sulfur, while bones and skin contain most of the rest. Foods high in protein are also high in sulfur, for it is contained in several of the amino acids or forms of protein which are absolutely essential to human welfare.

Is it possible that the arthritis patient may be lacking in sulfur? And the sulfur supplied by the bath helps to make up this deficiency? We are told that, in a test conducted by two researchers and reported in the *Journal of Bone and Joint Surgery,* Vol. 16, p. 185, 1935, it was found that the cystine content of the fingernails of arthritic patients is far lower than that of normal subjects. Cystine is one of the forms of protein which contains a lot of sulfur. It has also been found that the cystine content of the fingernails increases after a sulfur bath.

Are the good effects of mineral baths perhaps just the result of the hot water and the relaxation that goes along with the bath? Apparently not, for researchers have tested patients with and without minerals in the baths, and have found that the mineral baths produce better results than plain water, even though they do not know what the reason is. A series of tests was done by several New York physicians. Sixty patients, all of whom were suffering from one form or another of rheumatic complaint, were given a mineral preparation, of which, the chief ingredient was sulfur, and were instructed to use it in a 20-minute hot bath every night just before going to bed. Another 60 patients were instructed to take hot baths consisting of plain tap water.

The results showed that, in the 60 cases treated with the sulfur preparation, there was relief from pain in 51 cases, no relief in 8 cases and an increase in pain in one. Relief of pain was complete in 27 cases. Among those who took the plain hot baths, there was relief of pain in 42 cases, no relief in 17 and aggravation of pain in one. Relief of pain was complete in 15 cases. In many cases, patients who had trouble sleeping found they could drop off to sleep with no trouble after a sulfur bath. In no case was there any difference in the amount of movement possible for the affected limbs.

Another interesting experiment was performed at a United States Veterans Hospital at Saratoga Springs where some 1000 veterans with arthritic symptoms were given mineral baths. Of these, 26.3 per cent were slightly improved, 52.2 per cent were moderately improved and 8.7 per cent were markedly improved. Only 7.8 per cent showed no improvement at all. Says Dr. McClellan, reporting on this experiment in *Rheumatic Diseases,* prepared under the auspices of the American Rheumatism Association, "the program built around mineral waters and associated treatments, particularly when occupational therapy and corrective exercise are included, can be of real benefit in the rehabilitation of many patients with arthritis. . . . The way in which mineral waters produce these effects must have further study before it can definitely be stated that any specific chemical or agent in the water is responsible for any particular response in pathologic physiology."

As our readers know, we do not prescribe treatments for diseases. It is our sincere wish to make available to everyone ways of preventing disease. We believe that arthritic conditions are mainly caused by wrong diet as we have pointed out many times. But there are other aspects of our life besides diet that undoubtedly have something to do with our tendency to become rheumatic, especially after middle age. The unnaturalness of walking on hard surfaces all our lives, the fact that we sit so much and travel so much in cars rather than on foot, the positions we take when we are sleeping and the beds we sleep on—all these and many more present-day stresses and strains put a burden on your bony and muscular structure that undoubtedly contributes to arthritis.

96. Physical Therapy Is Effective

Bernard Aschner, M.D., author of a book called *Arthritis Can Be Cured*, bulwarks his statement with many case histories from his own practice.

Dr. Aschner's methods are derived from the classical system of medicine. In fact, the entire last third of the book consists of notes on the history of medicine, covering the early Roman and Greek physicians, the Hindus, the Arabians, the Chinese, the American Indians. In every case, Dr. Aschner talks mostly of arthritis treatment, though, of course, other diseases are mentioned, too.

Astonishingly enough, Dr. Aschner does not give drugs or advise operations for arthritis. He believes, instead, in the ancient remedies. Purges, sweat baths and blistering poultices are his favorite treatment. The purges, or in some cases, emetics (to force one to vomit) are for the purpose of cleansing the body of waste products. The poultices are for counter-irritation. Dr. Aschner calls it "draining of the skin."

"Labeling these methods as old-fashioned may be the blind spot of laboratory medicine," he says. "My own everyday experience and that of my associates over a period of more than 40 years reveals the alarming fact that, all over the world, millions of people, stricken by arthritis, are suffering unnecessarily for months, for years, even for a lifetime. Why should simple and effective methods that were used successfully by the greatest masters among our medical predecessors and that are being used successfully today be 'labeled' and shoved aside?"

Among the blistering substances Dr. Aschner uses in his practice, are mustard plasters, liniment of ammonia, tincture of green soap, oil of chloroform, camphorated alcohol and so forth. He stresses the fact that the substance *must blister the skin* to be effective. No "mild" ointment will accomplish anything. The blister, he believes, drains the skin of harmful substances.

It seems incredible, in these days of wonder drugs, X-rays, cobalt bombs, serums, tranquilizers, hormones and all the other fantastic new medical treatments, that the head of a department for arthritis at a great hospital should go on record as endorsing only the ancient remedies, known for thousands of years. And that he should endorse them for the very reasons their originators did—to rid the body of poisons. This concept of disease has almost disappeared, along with the belief that disease is caused by demons which must be driven out.

However, we can find no fault with Dr. Aschner's methods of treating arthritis and rheumatism. Certainly poultices, hydrotherapy (treatment by water) and a sensible way of living are infinitely preferable to drugs. There can be no serious aftereffects. Even if it seems almost impossible that these methods should effect permanent cures, there is certainly no reason why one should not try them.

Poor Recommendations for Diet

The spot at which we depart from our admiration for Dr. Aschner's methods is the page on which he discusses diet. It seems to us inexcusable for him to ignore all the wealth of information scientists have accumulated, during the past 25 years or so, concerning diet and its importance for good health.

Yet, Dr. Aschner, who emphatically denounces smoking for arthritics and gives case histories to back up his opinion, says among other things, "Desserts are a problem for many. A greater concentration on farinaceous (bakery) foods will help. Farinaceous foods in great variety can be made from the same dough as noodles. They may be prepared with tasty ingredients, such as poppy seeds, nuts, marmalade, sweetened white cheese, etc. Fluffy pancakes are also easy to digest. Spaghetti and macaroni come next as a recommendation, but the quality in noodles is better. Farinaceous foods, including pastry of all kinds, deserve more attention than they are getting in this country. European nations have learned that such foods add to the pleasure of eating, are easily digestible and do not burden the metabolism as much as vegetables, fruits or a surplus of meats."

This is the most astounding statement we have ever encountered in modern medical writing. And we think that Dr. Aschner should be criticized severely for making it. If, indeed, he has not familiarized himself with the scientific literature which indicts such foods as one of the basic causes of disease, then he should not mention diet. He apparently does not know that more than one-half the food consumed in this country is made from white sugar and white flour.

He states that in any arthritic clinic "at least half of the patients and frequently far more are usually overweight." How do these folks put on this undesirable weight, Dr. Aschner? By eating protein foods, fruits and vegetables? Obviously not, for this is the very diet you put your patients on to "reduce them."

He says, "The principal nutrition in a reducing cure should consist of meat in moderate amounts, eggs, fish and other seafood, cheese, vegetables and fruit, the last not too sweet." How can anyone who knows enough about nutrition to prescribe such an excellent reducing diet as this go on to advise his arthritic-ridden patients that they should eat more pastry? Why does it not occur to Dr. Aschner that the very foods which made his patients fat also gave them arthritis? Why does he not understand that the very foods which will preserve their good figures will also preserve their good health?

Yet, ignoring all the nutritional facts that have come to light since our scientists began to study vitamins, minerals, blood sugar, healthful and unhealthful food fats and so on, he counsels those patients with chronic in-

[394]

digestion to begin breakfast with black coffee with sugar added. "It strengthens the stomach," he says. He suggests that you need very few vegetables and eat only certain fruits.

Our advice to readers who have arthritis is: if you buy the book, ignore every word in it about diet except the brief note on a suggested reducing diet. Stick to that diet faithfully while you are trying out any of Dr. Aschner's treatment and we daresay you will benefit more from the diet than from the treatment. And if you want to be doubly sure of success, take your food supplements regularly, particularly natural vitamin C.

97. Notes on Arthritis

Quotes from *Nutrition Reviews*, March, 1953: "Collagen is an albuminoid; that is, a protein made exclusively of amino acids. . . . It is widely distributed throughout most tissues and is found in large amounts in bone, cartilage, tendons and skin. It has been estimated that fully one-third of the total mass of the protein of the mammalian body consists of collagen. . . . Various disturbances of common occurrence, such as rheumatic diseases, have been shown to be characterized by degenerative changes in the collagen." Later on, the same article states that, in the animal with scurvy (the disease of vitamin C deficiency), no collagen is formed. When vitamin C is given, bundles of collagen are formed within 24 hours.

How can anyone doubt the utmost importance of vitamin C to the health of those body structures that become rheumatic, when we read that collagen, the substance of which they are largely made, depends for its very formation on a sufficiency of vitamin C! The collagen is actually made of protein—a good indication, too, that enough protein in the diet is necessary for preventing damage to the collagen which might eventually turn into rheumatism.

Osteoarthritis and Vitamin E

Chemical Week for July 21, 1956, reported that a new theory on osteoarthritis may herald important advances against the disease. Dr. Esther Tuttle, a New York physician, told the British Commonwealth Medical Congress that osteoarthritis is not simple wear and tear on the joint, as had long been thought. Rather, she said, it is brought about by an impaired mechanism that upsets the normal balance inside the body cell. It starts with a deficiency of oxygen in the cell and then goes on to destroy the cell.

The oxygen content of the cell is, of course, controlled by diet. Vitamin E is the most helpful element in food for assuring the cell of enough oxygen. It works in an indirect way—by making the cell need less oxygen than it did before. Are you getting enough vitamin E to keep all your cells well oxygenated? It's been largely removed from processed foods, remember, and you can't possibly get enough of it unless you take supplements rich in this particular vitamin.

Arthritis Victims among Farmers

A statistical study of arthritis victims shows that it is an occupational hazard for farmers, according to *Chemical Week* for July 21, 1956. About 23 per cent of America's farmers have arthritis, says the Arthritis and Rheumatism Foundation. Medical people believe it may be because of exposure to the elements, hard physical labor without letup and lack of relaxation. This strikes us as one of the least observant statements ever made. Surely farmers are no more exposed to the elements than any other individual who works outside all day. As for the "without letup" part of it, most farmers have little or nothing to do during winter months when the rest of us stick close to the old office or factory grind. And as for relaxation, surely these days a farmer has as much opportunity as anyone else for relaxation, with ball games, television, grange meetings, movies, church activities and everything else within easy reach of the family car.

We think the reason may be that farmers may be eating worse diets, generally speaking, than city folks. And we wish someone would do a survey on this. It's all very well to talk about how he raises his own food, but actually, in these days of specialized farming, how many farmers depend on their own gardens and fields for their daily food? In summer, the vegetable garden provides fresh food, but in winter, the farmer eats canned or frozen foods like the rest of us. Usually his flour, sugar and other staples come from the grocery store. And, in many cases, meat as well.

Hypoglycemia and Arthritis and Diet

Attacks of hypoglycemia are characteristic of rheumatoid arthritis, according to Dr. Howard L. Holley, writing in the *Annals of Internal Medicine* for September, 1956. He uses this as one stepping stone for developing an elaborate theory about the "disturbance of the ratio of mineralo- and glucocorticoid production by the adrenal cortex," which we suppose means something to other researchers.

We have a different theory—a theory so obvious that you, Dr. Holley, are likely to stumble over it while reaching for a hypodermic needle to inject your rheumatic patient. Hypoglycemia is low blood sugar, sir. It can be alleviated by a diet high in protein and fat and low in starches and sugar. Doesn't it seem possible that the same diet may alleviate the arthritis at the same time?

Bioflavonoids for Arthritis Sufferers

"Twenty-one patients with varying degrees of rheumatoid arthritis were given 3000 milligrams of bioflavonoids daily for 2 to 6 months. Here is a typical case. A 52-year-old woman with rheumatoid arthritis in both hands, wrists and elbows, and in the right shoulder, knees and ankles was given 3000 milligrams of bioflavonoid complex by Dr. James R. West of the Morrell Memorial Hospital, Lakeland, Florida.

"In 7 days she 'felt better'. In two weeks, the pain had practically gone, her digestion was improved and bowel action normal. Her blood pressure dropped from 190 to 176, and by the end of 5 weeks, she had more action in her joints and more endurance than she had known in several years. This was a very severe case with crippling changes in the joints. Her improvement was described as 'dramatic.'

"It is quite common today to hear people complain about 'bursitis.' Doctors Biskind and Martin have had 'rapid and complete relief' with this ailment when bioflavonoids were given. For instance, one 38-year-old man with severe sub-patellar (knee-joint) bursitis had extensive local swelling, local heat, extreme tenderness, severe pain and limitation of motion. With 200 milligrams of bioflavonoids 3 times a day—a total of 600—the swelling and pain were almost completely gone in 24 hours. In 72 hours, the lesion had subsided almost completely leaving only slight local tenderness." All these quotes are from *Feel Like a Million*, by Catharyn Elwood, published by Devin-Adair, 23 East 26th Street, New York 10, N. Y.

Tracking Down Rheumatism by the Noise It Makes

Ever listen to your joints crack? Normal joints move silently, except for those times when you bend or stoop and a joint will crack with a loud noise. But in arthritis and similar joint disorders, the joints squeak or make other noises. Not the kind you can hear without special equipment, however. According to a Science Service dispatch from San Francisco for May 4, 1955, scientists at the Canadian Department of Veterans' Affairs at Toronto are picking up the noises by amplifying them several thousand times.

The amplification is done by a standard electrocardiograph machine such as hospitals use for measuring the electric potential of the beating heart. It's not that the doctors like to listen to these peculiar noises, you understand, it's just that they can better locate, measure and record abnormalities of the joints when they have the noises to guide them.

98. Your Enemy, Asthma

Asthma is a disease which has been known from very ancient times. Hippocrates, who lived in the fifth century B. C. described it and warned that asthmatics should guard against anger, because it was well known that such a violent emotion increased the severity of asthmatic attacks.

Because of its close relation to emotional states of mind, asthma has been blamed on psychological reasons down through the years. Even medical dictionaries that are not very up-to-date define asthma as "a paroxysmal affection of the bronchial tubes characterized by difficulty in breathing, cough and a feeling of constriction and suffocation. *The disease is probably a neurosis.*" It is equally common in children and adults, but so are many neuroses these days. It is not fatal in itself. That is, people do not die from it as they might die from cancer or heart trouble. But they may die from other complications as a result of having asthma. For instance, someone with a desperately bad heart condition might die in the throes of an asthma attack, because of the extra strain imposed on his heart by the violent gasping and wheezing that go with an attack. Someone suffering from one disease or another might be seriously weakened by asthmatic attacks which would not permit him to sleep at night.

What does the conservative medical press say about asthma? A leading article in the *Journal of the American Medical Association* for October, 1952, by Leon Unger, M.D., and Albert Howard Unger, M.D., of Northwestern University Medical School deals first with preventive treatment for bronchial asthma. They tell us that children of allergic parents are quite likely to have allergic diseases. If therefore mother and father are hay fever or asthma sufferers, or demonstrate symptoms of distress at the sight, touch, taste or feel of some allergenic substances, it is best to provide the children with a home as protected as possible against any subtsance that might produce allergies.

Pets should be removed from the house, they tell us, for cat and dog hairs are allergy-producing to some people. The house should be kept free from dust. By this they do not mean that it should be dusted frequently— quite the opposite, for dusting with a dry dust cloth usually only creates more dust and spreads around whatever dust is there. Mattresses, pillows and furniture upholstery should be made of rubber or covered with plastic material tightly zippered so that dust cannot enter. Clean curtains, drapes and rugs collect dust very rapidly. They should be thoroughly cleaned with vacuum attachments or should be eliminated entirely. Linoleum makes an eminently satisfactory floor covering—non-allergenic. The usual stuffed toy may be filled with kapok to which some individuals are sensitive.

Since molds cause allergies, the house should be dry, and moisture should not be permitted to collect in the basement. Cosmetics made from orris root (your druggist can tell you which these are) should be forbidden in the house. Certain foods may produce symptoms of coughs, wheezing, "runny nose." Eggs, milk, wheat products, seafoods, nuts are some of the common allergenic foods. Your doctor can easily give you a diet in which each of these foods in turn has been omitted. Then by including each food once again you can easily find out which one it was that caused the symptoms.

Asthma and Pollen

Pollen is the villain we all think of first in terms of hay fever, asthma and related allergies. The best ways of avoiding pollen are unfortunately all very expensive, unless you happen to live in a pollen-free locality. There is not as much pollen in the city as in the country, although plots of ragweed and other allergenic growths are becoming more and more common even in cities. One hundred miles from the shore on an ocean liner one can breathe air practically free from pollen. High mountain slopes and certain parts of our country, such as Arizona, California and so forth, are almost free from pollen. You can have your home air-conditioned which will bring relief from wheezing at night. But it is certainly neither possible nor wise for anyone, adult or child, to stay all day in an air-conditioned house during the summer months when pollen is most abundant. Skin tests given by your doctor can reveal much about your sensitivity to allergenic substances and once you have decided what you are allergic to, you must see to it that as little contact as possible takes place between that substance and you, from then on.

Allergy specialists have also discovered ways of immunizing sensitive persons to the things that bring on their symptoms. You can now be injected with, at first, small and then ever-increasing amounts of prepared serums which will supposedly render you insensitive to your allergens eventually. Let's say you have an allergy to goldenrod pollen. You can take injections long before the goldenrod season. Your doctor will give you first a very little bit of goldenrod serum, then a little more and a little more. As the serum builds up in your body, your own immunity to it also builds up and by the time the goldenrod is golden you can walk through a field of it without the slightest discomfort.

The two doctors Unger, whose article is, of course, addressed to the other doctors who read the *Journal of the American Medical Association,* go on to relate the various kinds of medicine that can be given to asthmatics (and there are a lot of them) mostly concerned with expectorants, sleeping pills and sedatives. They also mention the fact that the psychological factor is extremely important in asthma. Over-sympathy on the part of the family may make symptoms much worse. Nervous tension due to fear, coughing and so forth can sometimes be relieved by a sympathetic doctor who encourages his patient to talk about the things that are bothering him.

The Psychological Side of Asthma

An article in the *Canadian Medical Journal* for August, 1952, deals with the psychological aspects of asthma in more detail. Peter G. Edgell, M.D., of the Department of Psychiatry of the Montreal General Hospital, tells us there are two kinds of asthma—extrinsic and intrinsic. Extrinsic asthma is quite clearly related to one or another of the various allergens. Intrinsic asthma may be the result of a number of different complicating causes; and both kinds may occur in the same person at the same time.

In a survey of 1129 asthmatic persons, 50 per cent showed definite and typical allergic reactions in skin tests with various substances. For 23 per cent of the 1129, no cause at all could be found for the asthma. In a further investigation 21 per cent appeared to have personality maladjustments which seemed to precipitate the asthma. At a round table conference in 1947, psychiatrists and allergenists agreed that a badly adjusted personality might not be the direct cause of asthma, but emotions might very well bring on attacks and aggravate the symptoms of susceptible persons.

Everyone agrees, says Dr. Edgell, that asthmatics have in common a "deep-seated emotional insecurity and an intense need for parental love and protection." One can see such traits more easily in children who have not as yet learned to disguise their emotions. They cling to their mothers, they are self-centered, usually of high intelligence, but often unable to perform well in school because of their continual anxiety that they may fail. The real or imagined rejection by parents is the cause of such behavior, says Dr. Edgell.

We have all heard stories of the psychological importance of asthma, such as the classic story of the man who suffered from an allergy to roses. The sight of a rose would set him to coughing, sneezing and weeping, *even if the rose happened to be made of paper.* And medical science contains some astounding stories of the relation of emotion to asthmatic attacks. A girl who fell two stories while she was cleaning a window had her first asthma attack immediately after she hit the ground. A man who identified himself strongly with his father became asthmatic after his father's death, apparently from being a witness to the gasping and choking of his father's losing battle with pneumonia. Repressed sex impulses can be a cause of asthma apparently. Repressed fears or anger that cannot be spoken out may turn into an asthmatic attack.

In addition, says Dr. Edgell, a feeling of depression may bring on an attack in some susceptible individuals. In others the asthma may alternate with the depression. A patient of a famous psychiatrist was cured of his asthma by a series of Coué treatments. (This, you will remember, was the system in which you cured yourself by auto-suggestion—"Every

[400]

day in every way, I'm getting better and better.") But the attacks of anxiety that came in their place distressed him so much that he asked the psychiatrist if he might not have the asthma back again! He preferred it to the anxiety!

But Is Asthma Psychological?

In an astonishing book called *Body, Mind and Sugar* by E. M. Abrahamson, M.D., and A. W. Pezet (published by Henry Holt and Company, 1951) we found an entirely different approach to the subject of asthma. We want to recommend to you Dr. Abrahamson's approach and his conclusions, for they sound remarkably sane and reasonable. The course of action he suggests for preventing or curing asthma involves no drugs, no travel, no psychiatry, no air conditioning, no expense.

Dr. Abrahamson tells us that there are about 3 million hay fever sufferers in this country. Including other allergenic conditions, he estimates that the total number of allergics must approach 5 million. Out of a vast number of possibly allergic substances, he lists fungus spores, the dander of animals, feathers, karaya gum (used in some wave set preparations) wheat and other flours, dusts (industrial and house), orris root, flax seed, kapok, insect scales, "practically any food,." poison ivy, primrose, sumac, many drugs, chemicals and dyes, many flavoring and preservative materials, toothpastes, mouth washes. In fact, according to Dr. Abrahamson, "it is probable that the length and list of allergens is limited only by what so far has been observed and recorded."

The fact that allergies appear to run in families and that they appear only in animals of "higher intelligence" has suggested that they have a psychological origin. One test of allergic children showed that 98.4 per cent of them were "rejected" by their mothers—that is, the children felt, whether consciously or unconsciously, whether justly or unjustly, that their mothers did not want or love them. In general, however, the allergy specialists refuse to recognize the opinions of the psychologists that asthma has psychological origins. "The medical profession, like other segments of humanity, is composed of a minority who believe in anything that is new and a majority who refuse to believe in anything that is new. Between them, the open-minded man of science, willing to pick up crumbs from the right and the left but unwilling to put them in his mouth until he has thoroughly tested them, has a difficult time of it," says Dr. Abrahamson.

Surprising Things about Asthmatics

The "anything that is new" referred to is a fairly recent investigation of the relationship of blood sugar to asthma, in which Dr. Abrahamson played a leading part. In general, this investigation went as follows: (1.) Tests showed that asthmatics have a consistently low blood sugar. Reasoning from this point it seemed to follow that diabetics (whose blood sugar is abnormally high) should not suffer from asthma. "Joslin the great authority on diabetes, had a few patients who had suffered from asthma but lost it

[401]

when they acquired diabetes." (2.) Asthmatics have an excessive amount of potassium in their blood. Diabetics have a low level of potassium. (3.) Asthmatics become worse when they eat excessive amounts of table salt. Diabetics can get along with less insulin when they take large amounts of salt. (4.) Asthmatic attacks are especially dreaded because they occur most frequently at night after the patient has been asleep for several hours. In these early hours of the morning, the blood sugar level is at its lowest. (5.) Injections of glucose are sometimes given to asthmatic patients to relieve their attacks. This of course raises their blood sugar, relieving the attack. But it does not permanently help the asthma for taking more and more glucose (or any other form of sugar) eventually results in a still further lowering of the blood sugar. (6.) The drugs used for asthma, such as morphine, amytal, ephedrine and adrenalin all raise blood sugar levels. Can this be merely coincidental or is this the reason for their temporary effectiveness?

Testing the theory that low blood sugar may make one susceptible to asthma, Dr. Abrahamson put 12 asthma patients on a diet designed to prevent low blood sugar. All of them improved considerably. How then could he explain a patient who was being treated for asthma at the allergy clinic and was also taking insulin for her diabetes? This patient's asthma grew so much worse that she carried a hypodermic needle of adrenalin always with her and could not get through a day without several injections. A 6-hour test of her blood sugar revealed that for the first two hours after she took the prescribed dose of glucose, her blood sugar level soared to the diabetic range. Had the test been stopped then, it would have revealed just diabetes, resulting from a high blood sugar. But during the next 4 hours it fell far below the normal range and at once her asthmatic wheezing began once again. In this unusual case the patient suffered from both high and low blood sugar at different times of day, depending on when and what she had last eaten. The medicine she took for her diabetes made her asthma worse. The adrenalin she took for her asthma made her diabetes worse. She was given a diet which would bring her blood sugar to normal levels and both the diabetes and the asthma finally disappeared.

How to Eliminate Low Blood Sugar

The answer to achieving a normal blood sugar level is to eliminate those foods which bring about a sudden, but short, rise in the blood sugar. In general, these are sugars and starches and, as Dr. Abrahamson discovered with all his patients, caffeine, which gives you a "lift" by stimulating the Islands of Langerhans (a part of your pancreas) to produce insulin. As a result the blood sugar level drops too far and all kinds of symptoms can result. This persistently low blood sugar which, according to Dr. Abrahamson, is responsible for asthma and other allergies, is called "hyperinsulinism" meaning, simply, too much insulin.

Dr. Abrahamson's remarkable book contains a great deal more information on hyperinsulinism and its relation to such diseases as peptic ulcer, rheumatic fever and even epilepsy, alcoholism and neuroses. We strongly advise you to read this book whether or not you are suffering from any of these disorders. Perhaps the information in it will help some friend, neighbor or member of your family. The book, *Body, Mind and Sugar*, is published by Henry Holt and Company, 383 Madison Ave., New York 17, New York.

The famous diet that worked wonders for the sufferers of hyperinsulinism appears at the end of chapter 78.

99. Asthma—Is Climate the Answer?

Anyone who has ever seen an asthmatic in the throes of an attack has no difficulty in understanding the lengths to which he will go to escape these dreadful symptoms. Jobs are abandoned, businesses liquidated, whole families transplanted to the arid West, or the crisp North in the hope that Dad or one of the kids can sleep at night or work a full day without the racking wheeze and cough that at once resembles choking and asphyxiation. It has become almost a cliché in medical movies or novels for the white-coated wise man to look kindly from behind his desk and say, "Young man, you need a change of climate. You must get away from here or I won't be responsible."

So many letters have come to us asking about the relationship between climate and asthma that we decided to search our files and gather what information we could as a concrete reference for our readers.

In offering the information below we are careful to point out that many medical authorities are doubtful as to climate's being able to work the miracles often attributed to it. In most cases of asthma they are convinced that allergy is the main culprit. A change of climate is suggested only as a last resort after patch tests and subcutaneous injections have failed to show a cause. We are certain that whatever the immediate cause, asthma would be eliminated or nonexistent if a healthful diet were universally observed. It is the weakening of the body's defenses, resulting from an undisciplined intake of foods that is responsible for such violent reactions to otherwise neutral objects such as woolen sweaters or feather pillows.

Possibly a check on the day's menu when a spell occurs would show an intake of a food processed beyond any usefulness, such as white sugar, bleached flour or some food impregnated with additives and preservatives that the body cannot and will not tolerate. To check on such a condition, an excellent method is to give oneself Dr. Coca's pulse test.

Keep a daily record of your pulse readings after each meal. Note any radical changes in the pulse rate and see if they recur whenever the food is repeatedly included in the diet. If you can see any connection between the bad asthma days and the days when the food is eaten, you may have a clue that will save you the complicated and costly process of relocation.

However, for those who have begun to eat a good diet and tried every medical suggestion to no avail, there is always the hope that a new location will have an atmosphere which is free from the offending irritant. This possibility alone will send thousands scurrying—some to the West to escape whatever it is that bothers them in Maine, others to the East Coast to escape Arizona's aridity.

The Effect of Barometric Pressure

Insofar as climate can affect asthma, barometric pressure is considered to be the most acute cause. As far back as 1698, Floyer wrote that a drop in barometric pressure, resulting in excessive humidity is injurious to the asthmatic. To ascertain just how much of an independent factor barometric pressure is, an experiment, reported in the *New York State Medical Journal* (January 15, 1957) was run. Seven asthmatics, known to be sensitive to pollen were confined in a room that had been made pollen-free. The following weather changes were then simulated: pressure fall, rise in humidity and heavy rain. By evening all 7 had asthma. A few days later the same group went into the room again. This time heavy rain was simulated, but no temperature variation or drop in pressure. None of the participants experienced any asthma symptoms. Pressure change was considered proven as the cause. As further evidence against barometric pressure changes, many allergists consider pre-storm weather, with its marked pressure fluctuations, to be adverse to many asthmatics. This is not to say that it is a sure thing that an asthmatic will suffer from a quick pressure change—for many asthmatics are entirely independent of the barometer for their attacks—but those whose chest becomes tight and breathing labored for no apparent reason may find that they can predict their distress periods by keeping an eye on the barometer.

If sudden pressure changes are a bother, then the solution would appear to be a change of locale to a place whose barometric pressure is fairly constant. A few minutes with a good atlas or almanac should supply that information, or a request to the United States Weather Bureau would probably bring one barometric data for any place in the world.

Consideration of Other Weather Factors

In the study of weather factors as they affect asthma, other elements such as wind, humidity, temperature and altitude were discussed as important considerations.

The individuality of asthmatic problems is emphasized by this same article's remarks on humidity. The author, Harry Swartz, M.D., says first that, generally speaking, marked increases in humidity are bad for asthmatics (foggy atmospheres are considered almost intolerable—pity the poor Londoner!). However, one can suffer just as dreadfully from a lack of humidity. In hot desert areas, many asthmatics suffer just as desperately as those in moist atmosphere regions. The reason is that the desert dusts are highly alkaline and may act as bronchial irritants, thereby causing attacks.

Those asthmatics who are easy prey to temperature are legion, too. Some asthmatic victims react to heat and cold as others react to pollen or dust. This does not mean that it takes a hot, hot summer day to make them wheeze, or a winter's morning that makes one's breath freeze. Any definite change in temperature—so long as it is noticeable—will bring on the symptoms. In this same category are those who are affected by the wind. Dr. Swartz tells of some people who suffer attacks merely by walking in a cold wind, even to the point of actually dying as a result. Though cold winds are most often named as dangerous, it has been noted that many asthmatics find that winds affect them if the wind comes from a certain direction! Of course, this phenomenon is partly explained by the fact that winds carry all types of potential irritants such as pollen, smoke, insects, dust particles, etc.

Sunlight—plain, simple sunlight—plagues many asthma sufferers so that bright, pleasant days actually force them to remain indoors.

Another test concerning asthma and atmosphere was reported in *New York State Medical Journal* for November 15, 1953. This time guinea pigs were used as subjects. A group of these animals was made highly sensitive to pollen. When the guinea pigs were injected with high concentrates of pollen, there was almost no reaction so long as the atmospheric pressure was kept rising, but when the barometer was allowed to fall the animals showed a response so severe that it was nearly always fatal. Again the point is made that the important factor was not any specific level to .which the pressure rose or fell, but the very fact that there was a change at all.

A more general recommendation was offered in *Munchener Medizinische Wochenschrift*, Vol. 81, p. 97, 1934. Evers and Schultz in their article stated that the average asthma patient feels better in the warm summer months than in the cold months of winter, or even the chill of spring or fall.

Other Dangers

It will be no comfort to those who have asthma and use aspirin or a similar compound to alleviate colds or headaches—though it might save them from serious consequences—to know that the *Journal of the American Medical Association* for October 11, 1952, carries a statement that acetylsalicylic acid (a component of all types of aspirin) may cause severe asthma. Asthma patients are warned to avoid all mixtures which contain this drug. Further, they're enjoined to keep asking any doctor who prescribes for them if his prescription contains any acetylsalicyclic acid, lest they be inviting a serious attack by taking prescribed medicines.

Appropriate to a discussion on the effect of travel on asthma conditions is a letter published in the *British Medical Journal* for June 6, 1953, which describes frequent asthma attacks among the passengers of ships sailing to Australia. It was found to occur on older ships for the most part, and was explained by the fact that these older ships held much dust from disintegrating paint, furniture, textiles, molds and more irritating sprays were used to combat cockroaches and other pests. The *Journal* suggests that if one is liable to asthma attacks, one should avoid older ships, no matter how well kept up, and should get the best accommodations one can afford.

Science News Letter for January 3, 1953, has a piece concerning the children at the National Home for Jewish Children which approaches the new location question from a different point of view. The asthma problem for these children is related to problems of pressure in the home environment. Once, they say, the child is removed from these stresses, the symptoms show a marked decrease almost immediately. So here is a theory that says asthma has a psychological basis and can be relieved merely by a change of scene. Presumably this could involve a change of climate, too, but the authors seem to think that a change to the next street or the next town without the family, eliminating thereby the stressful environment, will be effective as well.

An Ideal Spot For Asthmatics

Finally, from *Coronet* for October, 1952, we found out about a town in the foothills of the San Gabriel Mountains, Tujunga (Ta-hunga) California. The article by Victor Boesen told how 80 per cent of adults and virtually all children as well who go there suffering from asthma, find relief. There are enthusiastic quotations from people who have found relief during only a brief visit to this haven, who have moved themselves there forever, venturing out only in cases of dire necessity. And they are unanimous in their statements that they have never had a recurrence of the wheezes and coughs since. Dr. Frank Crandall, Jr., Director of Allergy Clinic at U.C.L.A. and special consultant in allergies to the Los Angeles City Health Department, is quoted as saying that he sends underprivileged asthmatic children to the area who are underweight, on restricted diets and are suffering constant attacks. In the short space of a few weeks, Dr. Crandall says, they have gained weight, are taking foods they could never eat before, and most of them are free from any further seizures. This is quite a recommendation, you must admit.

In none of our research could we find another statement, recommending a single location to all asthmatics. Even Tujunga, we are sure, has failed for some. If you think climate is what causes your asthma, try your best to recall or make note of the time of year it bothers you least, the type of day that allows you to be most comfortable. Do a little research and find out just where such a climate is general, then go there—for a visit. Stay a few weeks to see if it's the cure you hoped it would be. Wait until you're sure before you leave your house and job for a dream that may turn out to be the same nightmare you've been trying to get away from.

Though the effects of a lifetime of bad eating habits cannot be undone in a few weeks or even months, we are certain that a steady diet of healthful foods and food supplements can release anyone from the shadow of asthma attacks. They will eventually replace the sick cells that are susceptible to irritation with a whole network of healthy tissue, not given to easy irritation by climate, pollen, food or anything else. Before making a radical move, give nutrition a chance.

100. Bronchial Asthma

Bronchial asthma is due, in most cases, to food allergy or in combination with some irritating substance inhaled from the atmosphere. This is the contention of Albert H. Rowe, M.D., who is one of the country's, possibly the world's, leading experts on the treatment of bronchial asthma. In collaboration with his son, Albert Rowe, Jr., M.D., and E. James Young, M.D., Dr. Rowe has set forth his observations and theories in the *Journal of the American Medical Association* (March 11, 1959). The most important foods involved in causing asthma are cereals, says Rowe. When he is confronted with a new asthma patient, he immediately puts him on a trial diet which eliminates all cereal grains (wheat, corn, oats, rye, barley, etc.) in any form, and certain other common allergenic foods such as milk, eggs, chocolate, fish, etc. If these prohibitions do not reveal the cause of the asthma, then Dr. Rowe feels justified in trying other foods or considering objects, climates or infections. Dr. Rowe considers infections the least likely cause of bronchial asthma.

The course of recurrent bronchial asthma follows a pretty regular pattern and can usually be expected to act in the following manner: it acts up about every two to 6 weeks, with moderate to severe symptoms for one to 3 days, then diminishing within the next 5 days and disappearing until the next full scale attack.

What An Attack Is Like

These attacks are not easy to take, and it is no wonder that the prospect of their regular occurrence is enough to make the victim seek relief through injections, diet, change of locale or any other means that offers

[407]

hope. The inability of the patient to take a good breath of air is one of the most common and alarming characteristics of an asthma attack, but this is accompanied by coughing and wheezing and a fever that hovers between 100° and 104° F, for as long as 4 days. Couple this with loss of appetite, nausea and vomiting and you have some idea of the ordeal imposed by an attack of bronchial asthma.

The physiological reasons behind susceptibility to bronchial asthma are rather hazy. Dr. Rowe and his son, in *California Medicine* (October, 1948), attempted to explain attacks as due to reacting bodies, present in the systems of unlucky asthma victims, which gradually accumulate in the cells of the lungs. When a sufficient number of these bodies are present, they unite with the trigger elements in the food or pollen to which the patient is allergic, and react on the cells of the lungs which control our breathing. The reaction continues until, for some reason, the reacting bodies become exhausted. Then the symptoms disappear, even though the allergenic foods continue to be eaten or the allergenic air continues to be breathed by the patient. During this "quiet" period, the reacting bodies are again building up in the body and after a regular interval the attack can be expected again. Between attacks the patient may be partially or completely free of any hint of his asthma condition.

There is no age limit to consider in cases of asthma. It can occur at any time in life, though bronchial asthma usually makes itself known within the first 3 years. In a study of 411 children plagued by the disease, it was found that boys outnumbered the girls two to one, though this ratio generally tends to even out in later years. It is interesting to note that a disposition to bronchial asthma was shown in 50 per cent of the families of the children in this group. (Remember, families have the same eating habits.)

What of the patch tests that are widely used in cases of allergy for determining the cause of the irritation? Dr. Rowe contends that these tests, in which patches spread with the suspected allergen, are taped to the skin for possible reaction, are not conclusive in bronchial asthma conditions. He tells us that many patches of substances which were serious causes of asthma have shown little reaction when put in contact with the skin.

No Limit to Possible Allergens

It is obvious, from several instances quoted in the *Quarterly Review of Allergy* (September, 1954) by Rowe, that the possible causes of bronchial asthma among foods are limited only by the number of foods we know. One of Dr. Rowe's patients was found to be allergic to all foods, with equally intense severity, except beef, sugar, salt, water, and a tolerance for a few vegetables which are rotated every 3 to 7 days. She supplements her enforced diet with vitamins A, B, C and D, and remains well and free from the symptoms of her disease.

Another of Dr. Rowe's patients found himself similarly afflicted with allergies which caused him severe discomfort. As a result of tests he found that the only foods he could tolerate were fish, frogs' legs, tapioca, rice, potato and cottonseed oil.

The testing period is a complicated and exact one. The patient must exercise great patience, in the initial weeks especially. He must continue with his cereal-free diet without deviation until the doctor is sure it has been given a fair trial. It takes more than a few days for most food allergens to leave the body, and an even longer time for cellular changes to diminish or disappear. Only then can one expect the normal function of a body that is free from allergens. This whole process is so sensitive that Dr. Rowe does not even permit the patient to smell suspected foods, nor to touch them. He suggests that they be kept out of the house until they have been proven safe.

Difficult to Avoid

One can imagine the difficulty of avoiding certain foods used in the commercial preparation of others; e.g., wheat and milk in bakery products, citric acid in canned foods. For this reason allergic patients are wise to use foods that are fresh and unprocessed so that they can be assured of what they are eating.

It is noted that the persistence of attacks usually abates in the summer due to the seasonal influences on food allergy. It is not difficult to progress from that fact to the thought that vitamin C-rich foods are largely available in the summer months, and that this vitamin has often been mentioned in connection with allergies.

One of the more unusual types of sensitivity is that of some people to fruit. Dr. Rowe says that if one is allergic to one type of fruit, one is then likely to be allergic to most or all types of fruit, condiments, spices, flavorings and to fresh, though ·not to cooked, vegetables. When such a patient occurs, Dr. Rowe prescribes a daily supplementary dose of vitamin C. For that matter, whenever a patient is treated by him, Dr. Rowe insists that the patient's nutritional level be maintained during testing.

Drugs to Control Allergies

The use of drugs in treating bronchial asthma is scored by Dr. Rowe and his colleagues in the *Journal of the American Medical Association* (3-11-59) article in these words: "The control of bronchial asthma with corticosteroids (ACTH) and other new and old drugs without the adequate and persistent study of allergenic causes and especially of usually neglected food allergy is unscientific. It unfortunately ignores the responsibility of the profession to recognize and control atopic allergy which is causative in practically every patient." It would indeed be unfortunate to ignore food as a factor if one believes Dr. Rowe's estimate, in *California Medicine* (April, 1950), of food as the sole cause of bronchial asthma in 20 per cent of 970 cases and a major or secondary cause in an additional 53 per cent.

The popular psychosomatic causes of asthma are given short shrift in this same report. The author states that such influence was not recognized as the sole cause in any true case of bronchial asthma. If the disease is already present due to food or inhalants, at times it was shown to be activated or aggravated by excitement or nervousness. This situation did not occur when the allergenic causes were known and controlled.

The undesirable aspects of cereal foods, especially for some individuals are shown quite plainly in the attitude of Dr. Rowe. He eliminates them immediately, along with milk, eggs and chocolate, as the first and most likely suspects leading to bronchial asthma. Perhaps they are responsible for other diseases whose causes elude us, especially those which seem to affect one individual and pass by another for no apparent reason. Editor Rodale has written of his distrust of wheat and other grains. Could the elimination of these foods from your diet be the one thing you haven't tried in licking a persistent disease?

101. Asthmatics Might Try Exercise

A startling theory that asthma may be partly caused by a disorder of the adrenal glands is presented by Karl Schutz, M.D., in the pages of the *New York State Journal of Medicine* for March 1, 1955. This disorder may in turn be caused by modern man's relatively inactive life. The article shows clearly that exercises—especially of the lower part of the body—may be of considerable benefit to sufferers from bronchial asthma. Twenty-three patients are reported on.

We discovered during both world wars that the majority of the soldiers who were asthmatic were free from attacks while they were in active service under severe conditions, only to relapse again when they returned to civilian life. (We wish there were a fuller report on this angle—what the soldiers ate in active service as against what they ate in civilian life, for instance.) However, we know that the value of muscular exercise has been shown, especially in the reconditioning program of the armed forces of the last war.

Patients who took Dr. Schutz's exercises for asthma were requested to breathe only through their noses at all times. If there was some nasal obstruction it was removed by surgery. However, there is another condition in which no functional abnormality is involved. The nose seems to be obstructed, the reason being that certain parts of it are filled with an excess of blood. To get rid of this condition, the following exercises are suggested:

1. In an upright standing position, lift the heels as high as possible and lower them to the floor, both within one second. Repeat 50 to 60 times.

2. Draw in the abdominal wall and push it out again (the belly dance, he calls this one) all within the space of a second. Repeat 50 to 60 times.

3. In a sitting position the "sucking" in of air is to be done only after the patient has mastered the various breathing exercises.

Such exercises as these demonstrate the importance of the lower part of the trunk to the whole process of breathing. Says Dr. Schutz, when you exhale, the chest is lowered and becomes narrower. The muscles of the abdomen begin to contract. The abdominal contents are pressed against the diaphragm, elevating it from its position when you are exhaling. You should accompany this exhalation with a long-drawn "humming" sound. In the short pause after you have exhaled, the contracted abdominal muscles relax, the abdominal wall falls forward, the pressure inside the abdomen is lowered, thus making it possible for you to begin to inhale again. In cases of bronchial asthma, Dr. Schutz feels that the part the diaphragm plays in breathing is the important thing to remember—not how high you can lift your chest or how full you can fill your chest with air.

Breathing can be practiced sitting down with the elbows on the thighs near the knee and the chin supported by one hand. The other hand is laid on the abdomen. The best way to train the abdominal muscles is to do the "belly dance" often—pulling in on the abdominal muscles, then letting them relax, then pulling them in again.

Pressure breathing—a whistling expiration of air—through tightly pressed lips as if the patient were trying to blow out a candle held at arm's length—is used after the patient has been trained to breathe through his nose and using his diaphragm. After the patient has learned how to breathe, he is to time his breaths according to his activity. In walking the exhalation can be done during 4 normal steps, inhaling during two such steps.

Exercise According to Your Capacity

In addition to breathing exercises Dr. Schutz also recommends physical exercises for his patients—light, moderate or strenuous, according to the individual's point of view. Light exercise is lifting the heels in a standing position; drawing in the stomach and pushing it out; stretching the fingers and closing them into a fist; sitting up from a lying down position with the help of the arms (3 times); walking not farther than a half mile. Moderate exercise consists of: bending forward and straightening up in a standing position, sitting up from a lying down position without the help of the arms, walking for more than one-half to one and a half miles, uphill walking for not more than 100 feet (on an incline about like that of a steep stairway) short distance running. Strenuous exercise consists of calisthenics, athletics, walking and climbing, limited only by indications of overexertion.

Of Dr. Schutz's patients, 6 were put on light exercise, 15 on moderate and 2 on strenuous. Improvement was almost universal. In only 4 cases was it doubtful that the patient had improved. All the rest appeared to improve, ranging from "some improvement" to "very good improvement." One case history tells us that the patient (who had taken cortisone therapy before this treatment) said that he felt just as well after the exercise therapy as he did on the cortisone. And, of course, there were no bad aftereffects from the exercise as there might be from the cortisone.

Dr. Schutz stresses that the ill effects of mouth-breathing have to be emphasized. Although it is not generally known, these effects include insufficient ventilation of the lungs and deformities of the chest. Exercising the lower part of the body clears the nasal passages by redistributing the blood during the exercise. Doing exercises while standing erect causes the blood to flow from the head to the muscles that are being active. Perhaps most important of all is the business of learning to breathe from the diaphragm, keeping the hand on the stomach so that the rise and fall of the diaphragm can be felt.

Exercises should be performed when the patient is free from an asthmatic attack. Patients accustomed to physical work will probably learn the exercises faster than those who do not use their muscles so much. It is interesting to note that belts and any other constricting clothing should be avoided when the exercises are being done. "Humming" as the patient exhales is also important, for X-ray studies show that it markedly improves the act of exhalation.

Now we come to Dr. Schutz's theory about the modern inactive life and its relation to asthma.

The Part Played by the Adrenal Glands

Physicians know that cortisone (a product of the adrenal glands) relieves asthma. The world's greatest authority on the activity of the adrenal glands in relation to "stress," Dr. Hans Selye, believes that muscular exercise is different from all other known stimuli in that it produces large amounts of cortisone from the adrenal glands.

Says Dr. Schutz, another researcher has compared the adrenal glands of domesticated rats with those of wild rats and has found that the adrenal glands of the domesticated rats have undergone a marked atrophy—that is, they are gradually becoming less and less active. So they are less able to help the rat to protect itself from the effects of stress and fatigue. Man may have undergone parallel changes during his transition from a wild to a controlled environment. As he has become more civilized, his adrenals may have become less efficient, thus accounting for the high modern incidence of diseases that respond to treatment by cortisone.

We believe this is a startling and quite reasonable conclusion—that, as man's life becomes easier from the physical point of view, his adrenal glands (needed to combat stress, fatigue, fright and so forth) may be growing less and less active. And perhaps this is one of the main reasons for the very wide incidence of all different kinds of diseases for which cortisone provides a remedy. What will become of mankind if he finally loses the function of his adrenal glands entirely? When that time comes he will not be able to withstand any stress or fatigue! Dr. Schutz concludes: "Appropriately adapted muscular exercises are most suitable measures for training of atropic, inefficient adrenal glands." This theory certainly adds weight to Editor Rodale's point of view—that our lives have indeed become gradually less and less active. Rodale believes that our present-day lack of exercise may be partly responsible for our high incidence of heart and blood vessel disorders. Might not this, too, be related to the adrenal glands and the fact that they seem to be gradually wearing away from disuse?

We have one further comment to make which may be of value to asthma sufferers. This concerns the experience of a chest surgeon of Buenos Aires who was treating his young son for asthma. In operations on asthmatic patients, Dr. Ernesto Escudero found that they had not been breathing properly and were suffering from an excess of air rather than too little. Testing his theories on his son, Dr. Escudero persuaded the child to lie on his stomach at night, rather than on his back. He also played "human wheelbarrow" with the boy, walking him around the room on his hands while his father held his feet. He had the boy lie down for a few minutes each day, half in and half out of bed, with his head cradled in his arms on the floor. He also trained him to change his breathing habits and to inhale in short gasps instead of deep, slow breaths.

Today the doctor's son is free from all symptoms of asthma and has been for more than 5 years. Dr. Escudero tried the same therapy on more than 400 asthmatic patients. While he did not have complete cures in all cases, most patients were helped considerably. The reason why his treatment was so effective may have been the peculiar upside-down position recommended for the patients. But, on the other hand, perhaps it was partly because of the exercise involved—and the added cortisone which the exercise caused the patients' adrenal glands to produce.

102. A Doctor's Case of Asthma

A doctor with asthma describing his own experience with this disorder and the various remedies he has used throughout his life! What a chance for a layman to eavesdrop on doctors letting down their hair and revealing the whole story of how they treat themselves when they are ill!

The editors of the *Medical Press*, introducing this story in their September 26, 1956, issue, remind us that a doctor taking a remedy for an illness doesn't go at it in quite the same way a regular patient does. They say, "Faith, as we know, moves mountains, the patient confronted by a bottle from a doctor in whom he has every confidence will wash down its contents with a strong infusion of helpful suggestion, whereas only too often the doctor will embark on the same formula in a very skeptical frame of mind." So, gentlemen, "faith healing" isn't confined to us food faddists!

It doesn't surprise us that the M.D.'s have such little confidence in their bottled nostrums especially when we read this doctor's account of what the various asthma "remedies" have done to him. He has had asthma since the age of 10 and gets no relief except during and immediately after the several sieges of "flu" that he can expect regularly every year, says Dr. F. H. K. Green, who, incidentally, has several important positions in the medical world in London. Flying at high altitudes has also brought him relief, for he found that on a 70-day trip around the world he did not need to use any of the asthma remedies he had brought along.

What are these remedies which the doctor has tried over the years? Adrenalin (which usually brings him relief but may be responsible for his "mild to moderate" hypertension); isoprenaline (to which he becomes "resistant" very soon so that it does him little good after the first few days); ephedrine (which gives him insomnia and painful urination); Stramonium mixture (which brings on symptoms of iodine poisoning); Felsol (which has "objectionable side effects"); aspirin (which, he says, "induces severe asthma in some patients"); cortisone (which brings about no change whatsoever either in his asthma or his state of health in general); khellin (which brings on severe nausea, vomiting, insomnia and depression).

Now doesn't it seem to you a tragic thing that an M.D. with all the facilities at his finger tips for doing research in the subject of asthma, should not have discovered in 45 years any satisfactory remedy for the discomfort and misery this condition has brought him? Even if he gives cortisone and adrenalin and all the rest *to his patients* without hope of doing them much good, doesn't it seem to you that, for his own sake, he would try to find something better for *himself?*

Is it possible, do you suppose, that this M.D. has never heard of the relationship of diet to asthma? Doesn't he know that adrenalin is manufactured by the adrenal glands in the body and that the health of these glands is dependent on their nutrition? Hasn't he ever read in his medical publications that vitamin C is especially important for the adrenals? Doesn't he know that a New York doctor has done a lot of work on asthma which he has written up in the book *Body, Mind and Sugar?* In this book it is clearly shown that many cases of asthma are the result of low blood sugar caused by eating too many foods made from white flour and white sugar. Naturally if you eat a diet high in these starchy foods you can't begin to eat enough of the foods that are rich in vitamin C, so you are bound to have a shortage of it in your diet.

Wouldn't you think that, after a lifetime of suffering either the misery of asthma, or the torment of the side effects of the various drugs he takes for it, this gentleman would be willing to try something—*even diet?* It wouldn't be hard for him to find out about the relationship between diet and asthma. We are not doctors, not scientists, not even asthma sufferers, *but we found it out!*

103. The Asthmatic Ordeal of Marcel Proust

The suffering connected with asthma is dramatized every so often in the biography of a famous person who has been a victim of this disease. In the *Eye, Ear, Nose and Throat Monthly* (April, 1959) there appears an enlightening and entertaining biographical sketch of the famous French writer, Marcel Proust, author of the classic, *Remembrance of Things Past,* by Dr. Noah D. Fabricant. The main theme of the piece is the losing battle Proust fought against a series of severe asthmatic attacks which plagued him from the time he was 9 years old to his untimely death at 51.

His first attack occurred one spring day when he was out for a walk with some companions. He was suddenly seized with an attack of wheezing and breathlessness so severe that his friends were prepared to see him die before their eyes. His recovery seemed miraculous to them and to Proust, and he spent the rest of his life living in fear that the attack might happen again. He became obsessed with this fear and gradually gave up more and more of the normal activities of a young boy in order to avoid it. Spring became for him a time for the strictest avoidance of the outdoors. His allergies multiplied to include all flowers, any dust or pollen, perfume and cold temperatures. Any or all of these could trigger the gasping fight for air which held such terror for Proust.

The circle of allergies was ever widening and soon began to include emotional and psychological factors. It is no wonder, then, that we read of Proust's eventual decline into a state of semi-invalidism for the rest of his short life.

Born in a Time of Strife

Proust was born in 1871, at a time when France was in the process of tremendous internal upheaval, shortly after the abdication of Napoleon III. In the months before his birth, Proust's parents lived in Paris during a siege of that famous city which saw continuous shelling from the attackers' cannons and the most abject privation for the citizens in the way of food. Proust's father, a doctor, insisted upon staying in the city, though all who could do so had fled, and his new wife would be nowhere but at his side.

Finally, the fighting got so close that Dr. Proust narrowly missed being wounded by a stray bullet, and the experience so unnerved his wife that her condition made it imperative that she leave Paris. It was this circumstance that caused Marcel Proust to be born in a small suburb outside the capital city. In later years, Proust often credited his sickliness to the terror, anxiety and the privation, suffered by his mother during the time of her pregnancy. He might well have been correct in his assumption, since we know that prenatal diet and the mother's frame of mind are vital factors in the formation of a child in her womb.

Because Proust's family had some means, they were able to indulge him as a child, and his illness led his mother to lavish affection upon him. He became increasingly dependent upon her, and though they lived in the same house, mother and son would often write long letters to each other, he describing his latest symptoms and she sympathizing and consoling. Luckily Proust was not required to hold a job. His whole life was geared to keeping peace with his asthma, and this meant, for one thing, that night and day must be reversed. Proust would sleep all day and write all night. He would surprise his friends with social calls at two or three o'clock in the morning! All of this because he believed the night air was less oppressive to his breathing than the air of the daytime.

How Proust Treated Asthma

Proust's treatments for his ailment were bizarre-sounding by today's standards, but quite ordinary for his time. He would take what was known as "fumigations" to relieve attacks. This consisted of smoking anti-asthma cigarettes or burning anti-asthma powders. Some of the efforts of today's asthma victims are quite similar, even if they sound more sophisticated: mentholated cigarettes are suggested in place of anti-asthma cigarettes, and ultra-violet lamps have succeeded anti-asthma fumigations.

It is true, though, that we don't resort to the precautions Proust took to avoid chill. He had a habit of wadding his chest and neck with cotton wool to protect against sudden changes in temperature or a draught. Leaving the warm house to go out in the cold, he would try to prepare himself by a cooling off process. For him this meant that, after having dined at a party, and, wearing a fur-lined overcoat during the meal, he would undress before going out into the cold night air, and then don his steaming attire once again when he thought he had cooled off. He had such a penchant for dressing warmly that his clothes even prevented him from accomplishing his traditional duties as best man at his brother's wedding. It was the custom for the best man to pass among the wedding guests collecting for the poor. Marcel had to explain that he couldn't manage the collection, because the 3 overcoats and cotton wool padding he wore made it impossible for him to move between the pews.

Even in bed Marcel Proust was desperately concerned with avoiding chill. He slept fully clothed, and wore sweaters and mufflers as well as stockings, nightcap and gloves.

[416]

In spite of this great concern, Proust was eventually to fall victim to a chill which led to fatal bronchitis. Thus an end came to a life of genius and misery. In his last years Proust's eyesight failed badly, and he had become a slave to drugs—he depended upon sedatives to put him to sleep, then woke so dazed that he required adrenaline and caffeine to return him to reality.

Developments in Diet Since Proust's Death

We see little mention of diet in this biography, but it isn't much of a trick to imagine what Proust ate. In the Paris of his day gargantuan meals of the richest foods were in the highest style. Perhaps if he had lived in a later day, when the knowledge that grain products can often be a major cause of asthma attacks, or that sugar can bring on the wheezing and breathlessness, he might have survived into old age. Possibly you, or someone you know, suffer from asthma and have not been alerted to the power of diet in treating this disease. Talk to your doctor about it, and see if diet won't save you from discomfort and dependence on drugs.

SECTION 20: BAD BREATH

104. A Discussion of Bad Breath

One is almost forced to conclude, after reading the experts, that bad breath is an individual problem which cannot be solved by employing general measures. There is disagreement on what causes bad breath and more disagreement on how to treat it. Everyone does know that, while the condition itself is not harmful, it is a source of great embarrassment and concern to those who suffer with it—both the breather and the breathed-upon. In ancient Rome, orators and writers spent some well-chosen words talking about it—and in public! Cicero, in one of his speeches, said, "When I speak to him (L. Piso), I know what he has eaten and drunken today, yes—today and the day before that, because his mouth smells like his kitchen." The Roman playwright, Titus Maccius Plautus, excused his marital infidelity by saying, "My wife's breath smells awful. I would rather kiss a toad." Plutarch, in writing of a man told by his physician he had halitosis, reported that the man asked his wife, "Why didn't you tell me that my breath offends you whenever I kiss you?" She replied: "I thought that the breath of all men had this terrible odor."

Scientists have spent considerable time and effort in attempting to pinpoint the cause of bad breath and work out a remedy. We have searched the literature and offer here the most acceptable theories on the cause and cure of bad breath. Perhaps some of them will work for you. Certainly they're worth considering. Remember, however, this ccmment found in an article on the subject in the *Journal of the American Medical Association* (June 15, 1957): "There is no one very effective way of controlling this unpleasant condition."

Guesses and Contradictions

The article listed a number of possible causes of bad breath: certain incompatible bacterial flora in the mouth, constipation and infrequent bowel movements, gases absorbed from the intestinal tract and breathed out through the lungs. This last is considered the chief cause of this unpleasant problem. In overweight people, it is this problem that is more prevalent due to the additional number of blood vessels in which odorous debris can collect before being deposited in the lungs.

That same publication, in a later issue (March, 1960), carries the statement that constipation is usually not the cause of bad breath. The article stated that upper respiratory infections—colds—can be an important causal factor. A coated tongue, gum infections and dental cavities are mentioned as common causes; so are menstruation, pregnancy and nervous tension. And don't forget smoking as a well-recognized cause of bad breath.

Of course, the most obvious step to be taken if bad breath afflicts you is to be certain of the cleanliness of your mouth. If one does not brush one's teeth properly or frequently, the collection of debris that accumulates there will give off a foul odor.

It might be fitting here to include what is probably the first recipe for tooth powder, as introduced by Hippocrates, the prototype of the ideal physician. He asserted that, "there exists only one remedy—to burn at midnight a rabbit and 3 mice to ashes, mix the remains with the dust of marble in a stone mortar, and apply this mixture 3 times daily to the teeth." Actually this formula works out to a sort of bone meal (high in important minerals) laced with an abrasive. Perhaps something like this, using bone meal as a tooth powder, could be used today. It would certainly be safer and more effective than the toothpastes and powders being sold commercially. Sometimes the most careful brushing fails to catch foods lodged in tight places between or behind the teeth. If foods frequently become entangled in what seem to be traps formed by the teeth, it is wise to consult a dentist about grinding these formations to form a smoother, less vulnerable surface. Denture plates sometimes are responsible for caught foods. Do not buy dentures that cannot be removed for cleaning. Check them frequently and disinfect them with a cleansing solution daily. Meantime, one should employ dental floss to keep corners and crevices free of any odorous, decay-causing food remnants. Decayed teeth, themselves, are perhaps the most easily recognizable cause of bad breath.

Systemically Originated Bad Breath

Now suppose you have carefully checked on the likelihood of orally-induced bad breath, and are certain that neither accumulated food particles nor decay is responsible. That's when the problem becomes more difficult to deal with. A theory published in the *Journal of the American Medical Association* (December 27, 1941) might explain what happens in the system to cause bad breath. The author concluded that this condition is the result of the body's excretion of malodorous fats, fatty acids or volatile substances on the breath. These things are absorbed from the intestines and carried to the liver which somehow does an inefficient or ineffectual job of neutralization. Of course, if the liver is diseased, halitosis will be even worse. Some are then excreted by the bile, but more are picked up by the blood stream and carried to the lungs, where they are deposited. They are then exhaled with the breath which, of course, comes from the lungs. Oxygenation of the blood with vitamin E might help in clearing odorous factors. Long walks in fresh air could also be helpful in oxygenation.

Even as far back as 1935, the July 1 issue of *Time* magazine carried a denial from a medical source that the lungs could be the source of bad breath. The report insisted that the objectionable odors are due to nothing but particles of odorous foods such as garlic and onions retained in the mouth. This man is not alone in his opinion, for many scientists, even today, are convinced that bad breath originates in the mouth—period.

Rubbed Garlic on the Feet

This view does not explain the outcome of an interesting and amusing experiment, described in the *Ohio State Medical Journal* (December, 1936). The experiment concerned a 12-year old boy whose breath was judged to be free of any odor by several observers. A small clove of garlic was then rubbed on the bare soles of the boy's feet until it disappeared. The boy was then taken to another location in the building, more than 100 feet away from the original site of the garlic-rubbing episode. A team of observers were asked to determine if there were any trace of garlic on the boy's breath. Within one hour such odor was decidedly present. In an hour and a half the odor was described as strong. If the experiment is to be credited, it must be concluded that the volatile oils of the garlic bulb were absorbed by the skin and eventually deposited, by the blood stream, in the lungs, where they were expelled with the breath.

The Food We Eat May Be A Cause

In *Dental Abstracts* (August, 1960) there was a description of the work of a Japanese researcher who is convinced that the type of food one eats is responsible for the degree of odor on the breath.

Dr. Kawasaki used a group of female students, ranging in age from 20 to 22 years of age, to test his theory. He believes that, because the food one eats causes a change in the chemistry of one's saliva, a change in the odor of the breath is also due to this phenomenon. In the tests he conducted he found that, within 3 hours, the saliva is affected by the type of food eaten. The odor of the saliva is strongest after carbohydrates are eaten; it is somewhat less after protein foods are taken in; fat foods actually inhibit the odor.

According to Dr. Kawasaki, a component of saliva known as mucin is the cause of odor on the breath, and carbohydrates cause it to increase, while fats cause it to decrease. Another doctor holds that fats cause an increase in bad breath, and cites ulcer patients, who frequently suffer from bad breath while on the Sippy diet. This diet calls for plenty of milk and milk products—all rich in fat.

Both of these men do give the nod to protein foods as less likely to give breath problems. Protein foods are excellent for the health of the body in every way and should be heavily included in the diet of everyone, whether there is a problem of bad breath or not. Carbohydrates are the sugars which can cause tooth decay and serious body problems when taken in excess. Fats can rob good health, too, and are best taken in the form of unsaturated fatty acids contained in vegetable oils and fish liver oils, rather than fatty meats and hydrogenated shortenings.

Animals seldom have foul-smelling breaths, and when they do, it is cause for concern, because chances are very good that there is something physically wrong with them. In *Veterinary Medicine* (July, 1950) Dr. M. E. Serling wrote: "Lowered vitality, malnutrition, poor skin health and abnormal eliminations are sources of mouth odors in dogs and cats. Irregular diets resulting in poor digestion and faulty metabolism are contributing causes." We don't know why Dr. Serling's observations would not be valid for humans.

An interesting effect on the breath is caused by leukemia, says the *Journal of the American Medical Association* (February 15, 1958). "Over the last few years some patients have been seen in whom acute leukemia was accompanied by a peculiar sweet odor of breath resembling that of a freshly opened corpse. But not associated with clinical involvement of the gums, mouth or upper respiratory tract . . . In 6 out of 73 cases of leukemia, the peculiar sweet-smelling breath was of value in reaching a tentative diagnosis of acute leukemia, after a clinical examination only."

On another front we see that certain chemicals can cause bad breath when they are present in the body. Among these are arsenic, lead, bismuth and methane. They are all food additives and are likely to be present in some part of what you eat every day. If bad breath plagues you, perhaps the processed foods you eat are responsible.

Bad Breath Caused By Emotions

A sudden occurrence of offensive breath may be due to the emotions. One doctor tells of having come to examine a female patient of long standing after she was bitten by a pet dog. In the course of the examination he noticed that her breath was unusually foul. Because it was so unusual, the doctor asked the lady if she had eaten anything that could have caused such bad breath. She replied that she had been so emotionally upset by the experience that she had not been able to eat at all. It was the doctor's opinion that the bad breath was caused by the emotional strain setting up unusual reactions in the body, which were expressed by bad breath.

Similarly, in the *Journal of the American Medical Association* (January 5, 1952) a Los Angeles M.D. reported the case of a 33 year old woman who had bad breath for 10 years. She traced the onset to the time of her father's death in an automobile accident. She noted that the bad breath became even more foul two years previous to the report, when she was engaged to be married, and her fiance married another girl. The patient had no physical problems which could have been responsible.

Chances are that all of us are likely to have bad breath at one time or another. *Time* (July 1, 1935) announced that only one billionth of an ounce of onion oil can be detected on the breath by the sense of smell. Garlic travels in the blood stream with such determination that it can be demonstrated on the breath of a newborn baby if the mother has eaten it not too long before delivery. There are many other such pungent odors as well. Even pleasant ones sometimes take on a less desirable character when mixed with others. Aside from these, we all get foods stuck in our teeth, we all sometimes forget to—or can't—brush our teeth; we have coated tongues or sore throats; we suffer from indigestion or gas at some time. The only healthful way to disguise unpleasant odors at these unavoidable times is to chew parsley, long known for its power to neutralize breath odors, or pungently pleasant herbs such as mint, rosemary, basil or thyme. Chewing gum and lozenges, and other candy breath disguisers do more harm to the teeth and the system due to their artificial flavoring and sugar, than any help they might give the breath.

What good do mouth washes and toothpastes do for bad breath? Very little. *Dental Abstracts* (September, 1958) says, "Not only do mouthwashes fail to live up to the advertized claims, but some may be harmful if used continually. Some medicated mouthwashes are toxic, even in dilution; those which contain organic mercurials are potential kidney poisons; others containing antibiotics may lead to allergies, to the development of bacterial resistance and to the development of black, hairy tongue. All medicated mouthwashes are apt to disturb the healthy balance normally prevailing among the many types of oral microörganisms."

"The greatest psychological inducement to the use of mouth washes is the promise that they sweeten breath . . . The quality of the breath can be improved more effectively by mechanical procedures than by cosmetic preparation. The use of a toothbrush lessens mouth odors for at least two hours, whereas the masking aroma of a dentifrice lasts only a half hour."

If bad breath persists, see a dentist or physician to be certain that no serious physical disorder is the cause.

105. Enuresis at Teenage

By WILLIAM MOODIE, M.D., F.R.C.P., D.P.M.

Most people think of enuresis as the habit some children have of wetting the bed long after most are dry by night. As a matter of fact, the word means loss of control of the bladder by day, or by night, or both, and it is by no means limited to young children. Many adolescents and adults are afflicted in this way, either constantly, or in times of stress.

It is looked upon as a shameful thing, so much so that sufferers are often too shy even to consult their doctor about it.

This is quite understandable, but it really should not be thought something to be ashamed of.

It is a symptom, and as such is just like a cough, or a pain.

It is something that cannot be controlled at will, though usually it is thought of as something that ought to be overcome, and as childish.

If the loss of control occurs both by day and night, it is a sign of serious disturbance of the nervous system, and medical advice should be sought at once; but such cases are rare in comparison with those in which it happens only at night.

Usually the habit has existed from early life. It often results from overstrenuous toilet training. Perhaps a child has continued to be wet at night after the time that his mother thinks he "should know better" and so much pressure is brought to bear on the matter that it turns into a major issue, a cause of tension and anxiety in the household, or perhaps the child is blamed.

Anxiety in a child's mind is one of the surest ways of making the whole thing permanent. Of course, the child often does not show the anxiety, and adopts a "couldn't care less" attitude, but this is only his way of covering up his shame.

Boys and girls can both be enuretic and it is generally accepted that the age of 5 should be taken as the time when the average child is dry. Many are dry long before that, but it is as damaging to have a child dry too soon, as too late. If a child is over-trained and dry very soon, tension and anxiety too often appear in other disguises. Toilet training should be a steady and easy process. Then it is normal and leaves no ill effects.

The commonest form of enuresis is bed wetting, and in the simple case and the commonest, it happens according to a certain pattern. In this article we shall discuss the symptom as it occurs over the age of 10.

Between 5 and 10, psychological factors play the greatest part in perpetuating the trouble, and these must be sorted out in each particular case in a clinic where such matters are dealt with.

After 10 the psychological factors have usually become less important, though at all ages any causes of deep anxiety should be sought out and eliminated.

Any special strain associated with the trouble may be enough to keep it going. Even the popular "star charts" often do more harm than good. Punishment because it is called "just laziness" is quite hopeless, and so is the attitude that the child is doing it as a revenge. Children will often wet their beds after a family row, but it is the anxiety following the incident that causes it, not revenge.

As in all mental matters there are exceptions. There are parents who have "cured" the habit by punishment. There are some few children who do it deliberately. But in these cases skilled advice should be sought because there is something seriously wrong somewhere.

Now let us talk about the commonest form and some of the symptoms that are found frequently to accompany enuresis.

The wetting may happen every night, or only after a long and tiring day, or excitement, but, associated with it is *precipitancy,* which means that when the desire to pass water (or to micturate, in medical language) comes, it is sudden.

Often it is only just possible to get to the lavatory in time. This accentuates the anxiety. It often happens that the sufferer wakens from sleep when he begins to pass water, and can stop before passing much.

Usually it is noted that it does not matter much whether drinks are stopped for a time before going to bed, though drinking a lot of tea or coffee late at night may make wetting more likely.

Besides precipitancy by day there is often frequency. The desire to micturate comes on often, and the tendency is to visit the lavatory on any possible occasion, and to sit through a film or theatre performance is uncomfortable.

The cause behind the trouble, when it has been established for a long time, is that the bladder has become accustomed to hold much less than it normally should.

Every hollow organ in the body has in it a mechanism that makes it tend to empty when it is filled up to a certain extent. The bladder is no exception. Normally it fills up, and when it is getting nearly full, one becomes aware of the fact.

This signal, however, gives considerable latitude. It can fill up a good deal more before it empties automatically, and there is a point beyond which no effort of will can prevent this.

In people who have frequency, however, this emptying reflex happens before the bladder is full, because it has been so constantly emptied before it has fully filled, and, what is more important, before it is full enough to send the message up to the brain to tell of the need to empty. The message that comes then is often not from the bladder but from just beyond it, and is caused by the first drops coming away. This is what wakens the sleeper, or causes slight "leakage" in the daytime.

Enuretics are usually said to be heavy sleepers, and it is easy to see that these weak messages are often not strong enough to wake the sleeper. That is also why drugs which lighten sleep are sometimes helpful, while sedatives can make matters worse.

The first part of treatment must be, therefore, to accustom the bladder to hold more and more, until its content becomes normal. To do this control must be practiced during the day, gradually teaching it to hold back by not going to the lavatory so often. If this is persevered in, the frequency will decrease.

It is known that bladders that have become accustomed to too frequent emptying get atonic. The muscles are weak; therefore, after seemingly emptying, there will still be a certain amount of fluid left behind.

Therefore, it is very important that at each act of micturition the bladder must be emptied, and when the flow first stops that that must not be taken as indicating that there is no more to come. There we find the second part of the curative "drill."

When a person lies down, the kidneys secrete, so, when we go to bed, a slightly increased production of urine occurs. Therefore, on going to bed, one should go to the lavatory, and pass all the fluid that will pass, and then lie down for half an hour and read, and then go and pass what has since collected.

When a drink is taken, the kidneys become active for a short period, and so the enuretic subject should not drink for at least an hour before going to bed. Fluids, within reason, at any other time do not matter at all.

There is another "drill" that sometimes helps, and that is to increase control by voluntarily starting and stopping the flow say 3 times in each act of micturition.

In the majority of cases this "5 point drill," if really persevered in, will show effects within 6 weeks, and often the whole trouble will have gone in 3 or 4 months.

Sometimes certain drugs help, but they are usually quite useless without the bladder re-education.

Behind all this the importance of anxiety must always be kept in mind. There is nothing that upsets all reflex mechanisms so much as an uneasy mind.

It is therefore very important to concentrate on the removal of anxiety at every stage. Any drill must be carried out with a completely optimistic spirit, and failures must be overlooked and made light of. All the time the child must be kept in a hopeful mood and success continually kept in front of him.

106. Buerger's Disease

It is seldom that medical men have as clear-cut and final a cause and effect set-up in dealing with any disease as they have in the case of smoking and *Buerger's disease*. Not absolutely everyone who gets Buerger's disease smokes, but by far the largest majority of them do. Not absolutely every patient who stops smoking in time will be cured of Buerger's disease. But medical men everywhere are generally agreed that patients with Buerger's disease dare not smoke. If they stop smoking, symptoms generally improve, only to become worse again if the patient goes back to smoking.

Aside from the fact that smoking appears to have a great deal to do with it, no one knows what causes Buerger's disease. Its other name is thrombo-angiitis obliterans. Dr. Leo Buerger made an intensive study of the disease about 30 years ago, so it is called after him. It is a disease of the blood vessels, in which the inner linings of both arteries and veins become inflamed. There is also clogging of the blood vessels due to blood clots. In general, the disease affects the legs and feet. It may start with pain in the legs on exertion. As the blood vessels become more and more inflamed, the pain becomes more severe and continuous. In the acute stage, there is great pain after walking a short distance. As the disease progresses and becomes chronic, the pain becomes so severe that the patient is unable to sleep. Eventually a spot develops on a toe or under a toenail and gangrene is on the way. It may take a year or 10 years, but the epilogue to a case of Buerger's disease is generally amputation of a foot or leg to save the patient's life.

Relationship between Smoking and Buerger's Disease

Just in case there should be any doubt in the minds of smokers as to the relationship of tobacco to the disease, here are some quotes on the subject. An editor's answer to a reader's question in the *British Medical Journal* for December 22, 1951: "As a general rule, however, withholding cigarettes has a beneficial effect on Buerger's disease." In the *Journal of the American Medical Association* for May 18, 1946, appeared a warning about diabetics smoking: blood vessel disease of a kind that incapacitates the patient with pain and weakness in his feet and legs so that he cannot walk or that leads to ulcers and gangrene afflicted significantly more smokers than non-smokers in a group of 301 diabetic men. Smoking constricts the blood vessels. A patient whose vessels are constricted already may have them further constricted by using tobacco.

Another article in the *Journal of the American Medical Association* for June 12, 1954, indicates that filtered cigarettes will be just as bad for the Buerger's disease patient as the ordinary cigarette. Dr. Irving Wright of New York told of a patient with Buerger's disease who had not smoked since 1940. So long as he did not smoke and followed treatment, he was free from symptoms. In 1954, impressed with the ads for the new filter-tip cigarettes, he began to smoke them and almost immediately his disease appeared again and soon he was faced with the prospect of gangrene in his toes. Says Dr. Wright, no one has ever found a tobacco that does not have an effect on the blood vessels. And it is believed that the dangerous element in tobacco may not be the nicotine at all, but may be something else, at least for persons who are sensitive to tobacco, as Buerger's disease patients appear to be.

In *Risk Appraisal,* published by the National Underwriter Company, we find some appalling statistics on smoking and health. The smoking of one cigarette by a person who inhales produces a 5 to 20 increase in pulse, a rise of 10 to 25 in blood pressure, a drop of from 3 to 6 degrees Fahrenheit in the temperature of the fingers and toes. Twenty per cent of Buerger's disease patients have diabetes, too. Thirty-five per cent of them have hypertension or high blood pressure. There are many more males than females among the victims of this disease. And many more smokers than non-smokers.

In one series of 1000 patients studied by one physician, every patient was a smoker. In another series of 948 cases in which the average age was 42, there were only 68 who did not smoke. In 401 of these incidentally, the disease became so bad that amputation eventually was necessary.

Vitamin E for Buerger's Disease

Until recently practically nothing could be done for the Buerger's disease patient. If he could not stop smoking, and sometimes even if he did, he was a candidate for amputation. Since the disease is a disorder of the blood vessels, it seemed logical to try vitamin E in its treatment. In the large file of material from the medical journals on the subject of vitamin E, we find that, sure enough, it has been used with success in treating Buerger's disease. An article in the *Medical Record,* Vol. 161, p. 83-89, 1948, by A. B. Vogelsang, and the Shute brothers, tells us that symptoms of Buerger's disease have been relieved, as well as those of other vascular conditions where better circulation of oxygen can improve disease conditions. These researchers found that the dose of vitamin E was extremely important and might be different for each individual. Small doses were not effective. In general, doses of about 500 milligrams were used to begin with, then they were reduced to about 200 milligrams as a "maintenance dose" thereafter.

Dr. E. V. Shute in *Seminar,* Vol. 1, 1949, describes a series of 23 consecutive cases of Buerger's disease treated with vitamin E. Of these only 4 got no relief and two were doubtful. Seven patients were under treatment for a year or longer and all remained improved. In more recent medical literature we find an article by W. R. Cameron in the *Summary,* Vol. 3, 1951, describing 35 cases of Buerger's disease who had had it for an average of 6 years. They were treated with vitamin E and for 4 years the researchers kept in touch with them. Fourteen of these patients did not follow the directions. Of the others, 15 got good results, 5 got only fair results and 5 got poor results. Two received no benefit. Says Dr. Cameron, "thus alpha tocopherol therapy is the best, safest and simplest treatment for Buerger's disease and deserves an intensive trial before other medications are used or before surgical measures are attempted."

The *International Record of Medicine* for July, 1951, reports on the use of vitamin E for Buerger's disease. Of 18 patients treated with vitamin E, 17 were cured, only one was not. It was found that the medication had to be continued indefinitely.

In the *Journal of Bone and Joint Surgery,* Vol. 31B, 1949, there is an article by A. M. Boyd, A. H. Ratcliffe, R. P. Jepson and G. W. H. James on 3 different kinds of arterial disease of which Buerger's disease is one. The authors conclude that alpha tocopherol (vitamin E), 400 milligrams daily, is the only substance that has given consistently good results in treatment of these disorders. Of 72 patients, 27 were completely relieved and 32 were markedly improved. The consistency with which there is a lag period of 4 to 6 weeks before improvement was most striking. After a few months of treatment, there was obvious improvement in the appearance of the feet of the patients.

Advantages to the Use of Vitamin E

These are but a few of the many references given in medical literature on the treatment of Buerger's disease with vitamin E. Do these samples indicate that any and all cases of the disorder will respond to vitamin treatment? Not at all. They do show that in many cases it works. This is all that is expected of any treatment. The miracle drugs and all the various hormone, antibiotic and pain-killing treatments which are used by the medical profession today have no better record than this. Sometimes they work. Sometimes they don't. And most of them have serious aftereffects which means that the patient must be watched very closely to make sure that the cure is not worse than the disease. But there are no harmful aftereffects in the use of vitamin E, because it is a food substance. So its use is surely to be preferred to that of drugs. In addition, there are apparently no drugs that are the least bit effective in Buerger's disease!

Two further notes on Buerger's disease that came to our attention. Dr. Julius Kaunitz of New York, addressing the American Medical Association convention on June 24, 1954, presented the theory that eating too much rye bread might possibly lead to Buerger's disease. Ergot, a poisonous fungus that grows on rye, might be responsible, he said, for the symptoms of Buerger's disease. Even though grain in this country is closely watched for evidence of ergot, it is conceivable that just enough of the fungus escapes detection so that there is a small but fairly constant amount of it in rye bread. This wouldn't affect you, of course, if you eat rye bread only occasionally. But if you are a confirmed eater of rye bread, eat a lot of it every day and eat no other kind of bread, perhaps you would do well to cut down. (Editor Rodale recommends removing all bread from the diet.) Dr. Kaunitz mentioned that Buerger's disease has a high incidence among the Jewish people of New York who are known to be heavy consumers of rye bread.

Lung Cancer and Buerger's Disease

One final clipping on Buerger's disease. From *Newsweek* for December 17, 1951, comes the suggestion that Buerger's disease may be related in some way to lung cancer. Drs. Martin M. Fisher of New York and Lew A. Hochberg and Nathan D. Wilensky of Brooklyn report that they have a new method of detecting lung cancer. They watch for thrombophlebitis and check closely for lung cancer in anyone who has a recurring case of the blood vessel disorder. Apparently the idea occurred to them when the late King of England died, presumably from lung cancer, after he had suffered from a blood vessel disorder in his legs.

The investigators reported 4 cases of lung cancer in men, 3 of whom were suspected of having Buerger's disease and all of whom had had more than one attack of thrombophlebitis. The attacks of the blood vessel disorders preceded the diagnosis of lung cancer by one to 6 months. The physicians believe that early detection of a second attack of phlebitis or Buerger's disease should lead to a thorough examination for lung cancer. They offered no explanation as to the possible connection between the two.

We do not deal in cures for diseases. We are interested in preventing disease. It seems to us that Buerger's disease is surely an outgrowth of our modern way of life. It seems completely possible that lack of vitamin E in the diet may be responsible for predisposing individuals to the disease. Smoking increases this susceptibility.

How then to prevent the disease? First, decide to stop smoking if you are dedicated to that habit. Then take vitamin E as part of your daily food supplements. In former days, before food was refined, we used to get enough vitamin E in our meals. Nowadays we have to watch our diets closely to make certain we are getting any at all and in addition we should, all of us, take a protective, preventive amount of vitamin E each day—about 50 or 100 milligrams.

We know well that vitamin E in the diet confers other benefits as well. It is closely tied up with the health of all muscles and it seems to have a part in increasing their oxygen supply. It was first investigated because of its efficient way of dealing with disorders of the reproductive tract. Infertility, abortions and stillbirths are prevented in stock animals by including vitamin E in their chow. It is effective in preventing and curing menopause symptoms in women. It is being used internationally in treatment of heart and other circulatory disorders.

Can you get vitamin E in wheat germ oil? Yes, wheat germ oil is rich in vitamin E. But it contains other substances as well—all of these very good for you, too. If you take the vitamin E that has been abstracted from wheat germ oil, you are getting much more of the vitamin in a more highly concentrated state. It was alpha tocopherol, the most active form of pure vitamin E, that was used in the experiments we have outlined above.

~~~~~~

SECTION 23: CANCER

~~~~~~

107. What Is Raising the Cancer Rate?

The death rate due to cancer has increased 50 per cent in the last 10 years. And what are we doing about it? We are helping the rate to climb even higher. Why are we doing such a suicidal thing? Nobody really seems to know. It's not that we're not aware of what is happening, for respected scientists warn us about it every day. It isn't that we don't care, for we do care very much. When many of us read that more cases of cancer occur among children than any other disease, our emotions are certainly jolted. We are terrified at the thought of 11,000 new leukemia victims that materialize each year. But neither our knowledge and concern, nor our terror, seem capable of arousing any effective action on our part that would put a stop to this deadly game we play with such a consistent losing streak.

Once again from reliable, respectable sources, comes the warning that we'd better go slow on food additives, that we had better stop nuclear explosions until we know for certain that the consequences will not be tragically irreversible.

A Deadly Mix?

The *Journal of the American Medical Association* (April 11, 1959) calls our attention to the danger in which we place ourselves by manufacturing chemical substances outside of our biologic experience. By this is meant, for example, the unpredictable substance that results when a housewife adds fluoridated water to a cake mix, bakes it in an aluminum pan, ices the cake with a prepared icing mix and adds some coal tar coloring to top it off. Does the manufacturer of the cake mix, with its spoilage retardants and flavor controls, know for certain that artificial fluorides brought into contact with these ingredients in a stomach crammed with a hundred other chemical unknowns will not have a harmful effect? How could he? How could anyone who had not made careful and particular observations over a long period? Yet such cake mixes are sold—and bought—with not the slightest thought that such a product could be a main factor in our cancer record.

Radiation Might Penetrate Natural Barriers

Dr. M. Burnet, whose writings in the *South African Practitioner* (no date) are referred to in the article, warns that we might unknowingly be producing substances which are capable of penetrating protective barriers which normally keep internal organs from contact with chemical substances that are capable of causing undesirable changes—poor eyesight or hearing, greater susceptibility to cancer, etc., if not in us, in future generations. Dr. Burnet is referring, here, to radiation. This means radiation of all kinds— diagnostic X-ray, radioactive fallout, therapeutic X-rays, etc. We know full well that mutations, or changes like those Dr. Burnet mentions, can be caused to happen in animals by experimental procedures with radiation.

These irrefutable facts do exist: the cancer rate is rising; cancer can be caused by radiation; the nuclear explosions we are detonating have released more absorbable radiation in the years from 1945 to 1960, than was ever known in the world. Burnet says exposure to physical and chemical agents capable of causing mutations should be reduced as far as possible. Has any such thing been done? Is the thought of possible serious physical mutations due to radioactive fallout the main consideration in the so-called "bomb-talks?" No, it is far down on the list, after first and second rate powers, preparedness, scientific advances, etc.

Leukemia Rate Advances

The incidence of leukemia (cancer of the blood that is almost always fatal) has been rising all over the world in our present century. In the *Lancet* (October 24, 1959), T. Alun Phillips, M.D., tells us that, in Britain, the leukemia rate in 1957 was 5 times what it was in 1920—a 500 per cent increase! Dr. Phillips uncovered a few other statistical facts on leukemia: It is more prevalent in males than females; children and the aged are more affected than others; prosperous areas seem to be hit more frequently than lower standard of living areas. Dr. Phillips' most startling revelation came from his comparison of figures on leukemia incidence in England for two four-year periods: 1950-53 and 1954-57. In the second period the leukemia rate increased 13 per cent, and in some counties the increase was as high as 30 to 50 per cent. At that rate of increase, can it be long before leukemia is as common as colds?

In the 14 years since the first nuclear explosion in 1945, the leukemia count has increased in Britain by 150 per cent, says Paul Mammet (the *Lancet,* November 14, 1959). After the infamous Windcastle nuclear reactor accident which caused the release of radioactivity over the territory, the nearby town of Seascale showed, that year, a leukemia death rate *that was 36 times the national average.*

A Practical Suggestion

A letter in the *Lancet* (November 14, 1959) from S. Lewin conceded that there is indeed a basis for concern, but urged that the geographical calculations of leukemia incidence are not as vital as finding a means for removing the leukemia-causing radioactivity which we find contaminating everything. He wants our scientists to work on finding a way to remove strontium from the milk we are drinking, and from water, too, as well as from the grain and vegetables we eat every day. The problem is already with us and will be for many years, even if another nuclear explosion never occurs, so let's find a way to counteract it, says Mr. Lewin.

We think Mr. Lewin's view is an intelligent one. We think that some thought should be concentrated on dealing with the radioactivity we are already facing. We might be labeled prophets of doom to suggest that the radioactive elements in the atmosphere right now are enough to annihilate humanity over 100 or 200 years, but it is not impossible. Many scientists have said as much, after calculations which must, of necessity, be partly guesswork. But one guess is as good as another. We are dealing with a whole new entity. We can't predict what it will do to us, for we have no past experience for reference. Why not choose the safest course? We can do without atomic energy for a while longer. Let it be proven safe for living things, then everyone can relax while experiments go on. But this running at full speed in the dark, when at any moment one might plunge off a cliff, must seem the sheerest folly to any thinking person.

Why Continue Testing?

We must protest the testing of nuclear devices. Each major power already claims that its weapons are strong enough to wipe out humanity with a single thrust, so where is the need for more powerful weapons? As for peacetime nuclear power, let's do more work with the radioactive materials we already have. Let's find a way to counteract their harmful effect on the body before we take more chances on exposure.

When it comes to chemical substances we are being exposed to, let us petition our government for more careful consideration of the pure food laws. Support the public servants who uphold the food laws we have, as well as those who introduce newer ones for our protection. Such actions are taken in the face of strong pressure from very powerful lobbies. Finally, the consumer can show his disapproval of heavily processed and chemical-ized foods by simply refusing to buy them, and by writing to the manufac-turers to tell them why.

These are our immediate defenses against the rising cancer rate. These might be the means of saving future generations from physical disabilities not yet dreamed of.

108. Do We Know What Causes Cancer?

No one claims to have found all the causes of all the different kinds of cancer. No one knows or will know for many, many years to come, all the different combinations of circumstances, inheritance, injuries, expo-sures and deficiencies that finally produce a cancer in one person and possible not in another.

But we do know of many, many things in our present world that are potential cancer-causers. They have caused cancer in other human beings or in animals. Some of them, the more notorious ones, will cause cancer *every time* one is exposed to them under certain circumstances. Others have caused cancer sometimes, frequently or rarely. All of them involve foods and objects which we meet with every day.

Why then the to-do over cancer? Why search for clues and cures and nostrums and treatments? Why not just outlaw all these known cancer-causing things and bring our cancer rate down? The answer is apparent when you study the lists we present here. Outlawing these things would disrupt our entire economy. Great industries would go bankrupt. Things which we consider essential today for their usefulness, convenience or beauty would be unavailable.

One famous cancer researcher, Dr. André Berglas of the Pasteur Institute in France, has said that it is impossible and unthinkable for us to remove all the cancer-causing items from our environment. He believes that the only answer to the frightening yearly increase in cancer incidence is to find a cure. We disagree, partly because we do not see what benefit one will have from a cure, if one goes right back into the same polluted environment and gets another cancer!

Dr. W. C. Hueper of the National Cancer Institute has published a list entitled "Environmental Cancer Hazards—a List of Causal Agents, their Occurrence in Industrial Operations and Products." A subhead states that these substances have "demonstrated cancer hazards."

[432]

Only A Few Substances Are Listed Here as Examples

We reproduce only a few of the things listed. There seemed to be no reason to list them all, for they cover just about every field of activity and everything with which most Americans come into contact every day.

CHEMICAL	HAZARDOUS IN OR TO THE FOLLOWING:
CHROMIUM NICKEL	*utensils and tableware.*
ARSENIC	*wallpaper, paints, insecticides.*
8-HYDROXYQUINOLINE	*(see later comments).*
CELLOPHANE POLYETHYLENE POLYVINYL CHLORIDE POLYACRYLIC PLASTICS POLYSTYRENE POLYAMIDES	*medical and dental protheses, surgical implants, cosmetic, sanitary and medical preparations, wrappings.*
SODIUM CARBOXYME- THYL CELLULOSE POLYVINYL PYRROLIDONE POLYVINYL ALCOHOL	*detergents, emulsifiers in foods, hair sprays, cosmetics, drugs.*
CARBON TETRACHLORIDE CHLOROFORM DDT ARAMITE CHLORINATED NAPHTHALENES	*paint removers, dry cleaners, fire extinguishers, insecticides, machinery grease, lumber preservatives.*
BERYLLIUM	*exposure to broken fluorescent tubes, air pollution from beryllium plants.*
THIOUREA THIOURACIL THIOACETAMIDE ACETAMIDE	*food and medicine.*
DIETHYLENE GLYCOL	*tobacco.*

What substances from this list might one come into contact with every day? Let's take chromium, for instance. Here is a partial list of the operations and processes in which workers come into contact with chromium: tanning, photography, paint, ink, textile, rubber, plastic, glass, petroleum, pyrotechnical, pottery, printing, wood preserving, electroplating, aviation, railroad and shipbuilding industries, dye manufacture, chemical and pharmaceutical industries, explosives, matches, wax, oils and fats, fiberglas, cement,

[433]

blue prints, metal wares and machinery, electrical appliances, anti-rust industry, dry cleaning fluids, paint pigments, bleaching agents in fats and oils—shall we go on? The list is a long one.

Who, not employed in such industries, might be exposed daily to the possible cancer-causing threat of chromium? Residents in the vicinity of chromate plants, airplane manufacturing and maintenance establishments, railroad yards, ship building plants, scrap metal smelters, oil refineries. And people who use at home paints containing chrome pigments and chrome-containing anti-rust agents, consumers of drinking water polluted with industrial waste which contains chrome and *consumers of fats bleached with sodium dichromate.* Which fats are these? We do not know.

Let's take another chemical substance—this time, one with a long name no one is likely to remember—8-hydroxyquinoline. This chemical (cancer-causing) might present a hazard to any of the following people: users of cosmetics, rectal suppositories, contraceptives, fungicidal powders and ointments, amebacidal drugs, baby powders (yes, that's right—baby powders), processed foods containing additives with this substance, or packaged in containers using this chemical in adhesive, smokers of tobacco treated with it.

In the report of the International Union Against Cancer meeting in Rome, August, 1956, a number of anti-oxidants were listed as being "probably not carcinogenic, but, because of other undesired properties, not considered suitable for human use." This list includes butylated hydroxyanisol, a regular ingredient of many processed breakfast cereals. Does your breakfast cereal contain it?

In the following chapter we print an article by Dr. Hueper, revealing what has happened to him and his career as a result of his insistence on publicizing widely information like the above. Every effort has been made to remove him from his position as Chief of the Environmental Cancer Section of the National Cancer Institute—a governmental institution supported by your tax money.

We have, in our library, a 600-page book entitled *Bibliography of Cancer Produced by Pure Chemical Compounds* (published by Oxford University Press). This book lists articles in scientific journals from all over

SUBSTANCE	HAZARDOUS IN OR TO THE FOLLOWING:
COAL TAR AND PITCH	*residents living near tarred roads, steel plants, gas houses, railroad yards, power houses, users of insecticide bombs containing methylated naphthalenes, cosmetics, medicines.*
SOOT	*charcoal-broiled food, liquor aged in charred kegs, eyebrow pencil containing carbon black.*
MINERAL OILS	*insecticides, laxatives, ointments, sprays, etc., fuel oil dumped in bodies of water, diesel and automobile exhaust in polluted air.*
PARAFFIN AND PETROLEUM WAXES	*food coated with wax, drinking cups, lipsticks, milk cartons, depilatories, impregnation for sanitary napkins, chewing gum, etc. etc., the list is long.*
CARBAMATES	*insecticides and medicines, cosmetics containing urethane, foods in which carbamates are used for flavoring.*
AROMATIC AMINES	*dangerous to repair and maintenance men, airplane pilots; dangerous in baked goods, margarine, butter, cosmetics, textiles, plastic, citrus dyes, soft drinks, detergents, rubber goods, the chemical sweetener, dulcin.*
DETERGENTS	*household detergents, foods containing emulsifiers, fat substitutes and stabilizers, dentifrices.*
BENZOL	*rubber cement, paint, lacquer and varnish removers, spot removers, dry cleaning fluids, drugs, polishes.*

[435]

the world dealing *only* with cancer-causing chemicals. The index includes 4,960 articles on this subject.

We do not know, of course, what has caused every individual case of cancer in this country—but, with a list like the one above to guide us, can we any longer say that we do not know, in general, the cause of cancer? Take the things listed above to which most of us are exposed every day, add to this the deadly impoverishment of our food which leaves all of us deficient in the necessary protective agents, add to this the lack of exercise, the pollution of air and water, the physical ease of our lives, the insult of drugs and operations which most of us suffer at one time or another—isn't it strange that we don't all have cancer?

109. Information on Environmental Cancer Hazards

By W. C. HUEPER, M.D., Chief, Environmental Cancer Section, National Cancer Institute, Bethesda, Maryland

Present efforts toward a control of cancer are heavily loaded with salvage measures against cancers in being. Doubtlessly to cure cancer victims is more exciting, more tangible, more glamorous and more immediately rewarding than prevention even if failures of cancer therapy are still frequent. Prevention of cancers from being formed by eliminating or containing cancer producing agents is obviously less spectacular and less attractive. However, primary cancer prevention is definitely more humane and can be made not infrequently, even with the limited existing knowledge of cancer causes, much more effective than cancer cures.

Since a considerable amount of reliable information is available on chemical and physical carcinogens (cancer-causers) being constituents of our natural and artificial and mainly industrial environment and on their distribution in the human environment, a sound factual foundation exists for instituting a practicable and economically feasible cancer control program by applying preventive measures. Exposure to environmental carcinogens is not limited to a few small population groups, but is present to varying degrees for the population at large. Preventive cancer control therefore should be everybody's concern for purely selfish reasons.

A principal step in launching such a program consists of a comprehensive educational campaign by disseminating through all means of communication the available facts on environmental cancer hazards not only to a few specially interested parties but especially to the general public which will furnish the cancer victims. The general public must be alerted to the health hazards which are associated with the development of modern industrialism. Mankind has to be made aware of the introduction of new man-made disease producing agents which have become superimposed on the natural environmental pathogenic spectrum. Preventive medicine properly applied against these new industry-related health hazards can become as effective as it has been in the past against communicable diseases.

It is gratifying to know that Dr. A. Lanza recently expressed in a foreword to a monograph on industrial carcinogens by Dr. Eckardt similar sentiments when he stated that "knowledge made as widely available as possible is still the major weapon in this attack." There can be little doubt that a part of the confusion and controversy which surrounds the present public and legislative discussion concerning control measures of cancer hazards associated with additives and contaminants of foods, cosmetics and drugs is the result of highly defective or totally lacking recording of experiences made on man with carcinogenic substances produced, processed and used in industry, which are reaching the general population through the medium of industrial waste products and consumer goods in a usually mitigated form. It may therefore be appropriate to list some of the sins and omissions of the past so that we may benefit from them in the future.

The American dye and rubber industries have been manufacturing and using in preceding decades carcinogenically highly potent aromatic amines, i.e. naphthylamines, benzidine and 4-aminodiphenyl, which were employed in the production of dyes including food and cosmetic dyes and of rubber antioxidants. These chemicals were made in millions of pounds and can elicit cancers of the bladder upon contact to microgram quantities. Except for a brief report on the occurrence of some bladder cancer among 4-aminodiphenyl producers published a few years ago, the American literature contains no information on the occurrence and number of such cancers and the type of workers involved for the last 25 years. Quite complete and thorough studies on this subject, on the other hand, were published during recent years from English industrial investigators.

Not only is the scope of the aromatic cancer hazard for workers, users and consumers of these chemicals and the products made with such carcinogens an unknown quantity, but the medical director of one of these chemical companies has gone out of his way also to block the presentation of such evidence before an International Cancer Congress in 1929 by threatening me with legal prosecution of divulging company's secrets. In 1948, he declared in a letter to the Public Health Service that my publications revealed communistic leanings and that for this reason I would never be allowed to enter any plant of his company. Somehow he was not successful in his attempted character and professional assassination. Occupational bladder cancer among several hundred dye workers is on record in files of chemical companies. Representatives of the dye industry refused at two occasions to divulge the number of bladder cancers among the employees of their companies.

Coal tar cancer of the skin and of the lung is, as far as American

[437]

workmen are concerned, an almost nonexisting occupational disease. The unpleasant fact is that their occurrence has merely not been reported. After I had some years ago an opportunity to study the cancer records of workers employed in a coal tar distillery I followed this experience by visiting one of their customers. However, as a matter of precaution I stopped first at the State Health Department to consult there the official cancer records kept regarding the occurrence of skin cancers among workers of this large paper mill. Its management first denied the existence of a cancer hazard and conceded it only when I confronted them with the official evidence of their State Health Department. Similar observations were subsequently made in another paper mill located in another state. Some 15 manufacturers and processors of coal tar banded together some 10 years ago to sponsor experimental studies on cancer hazards. These investigations for which I devised the plans and which were executed by a private research organization have been carried out during the past decade. Nothing has ever been published about the results obtained in studies on man and animals.

A similar situation prevails in connection with published records on carcinogenic properties of products of the petroleum industry. Although the occurrence of skin cancer among paraffin pressers of American oil refineries belongs to the oldest observations on occupational cancers, there elapsed thirty years between 1930 and 1960 before the continued existence of such cancers was again placed on record. Nevertheless, one must appreciate the relative broadmindedness of this particular company, because it is the only one during the last decades which has seen fit to make some of its clinical and experimental observations on oil cancers public property. In recent litigations on cancers of the skin from contact with cutting oil the confession was made by the chief investigator of prolonged and extensive experimental studies on various products of the petroleum industry sponsored by the American Petroleum Institute that none of the results concerning carcinogenic properties of such materials made during the last 12 years have been published and have therefore been made available to the medical profession at large for analysis and application.

Experiences of similar nature are available for other industrial carcinogens, such as asbestos, arsenic, chromates, nickel, isopropyl oil, and others. Some of the recently published statistical investigations on lung cancer among asbestos workers and railroad employees are of peculiarly colored quality and contain most dubious statistical data.

There remains the question whether governmental agencies facing similar problems are immune against such manipulations. Apparently they are not, according to my own experiences during the past 12 years. When in 1948 I advocated a thorough survey of our uranium miners in the Rocky Mountains for evidence of lung cancer hazards, a high medical official of AEC declared such an undertaking as nonsense and tried to block it, although unsuccessfully. When in 1951 I had been invited by the Colorado State Medical Society to address its annual meeting in Denver on cancer hazards in Colorado and had included in my communication a description of the circumstances accounting for the highly excessive lung cancer incidence among radioactive ore miners in Saxony and Bohemia observed and published since 1879, I was requested to omit these references as being "not in the public interest" and not sufficiently confirmed and applicable. The delivery of my paper was made dependent on complying with this demand. Since I refused to be made a scientific liar by omission, I cancelled my talk as being censored. I have been told that someone in AEC asked then that I should be dismissed for using allegedly "bad judgment." Since about that time Dr. Sebrell, former Director of NIH had objected to my appearance as a private citizen for giving testimony before the Delaney Committee in matters of cancer hazards from food additives, my punishment consisted of having my promotion to a higher grade rescinded and of being removed from all further field of work on occupational cancer; i.e., I was forbidden to contact State Health departments and industry. This arbitrary order almost killed also my experimental work on environmental cancer hazards, although it was quite effective in obliterating almost the entire epidemiologic work on occupational cancer hazards at the National Cancer Institute since 1952.

My most recent experience on this line came from the Food Protection Board of the National Research Council. After I had been instrumental as a member of an *ad hoc* committee to establish the scope and nature of cancer hazards from food additives, I was excluded from becoming a member of the permanent committee because of objections raised against me by some members of the Board.

After exchanging some personal correspondence with the chairman of the committee on this point, one member of the Board, Dr. King, executive director of the Nutrition Foundation, addressed a letter to Mr. Larrick, Commissioner of FDA, in which he bitterly complained about my activities in declaring irresponsibly in papers and speeches that carcinogens were getting into our food supply, that I had criticized allegedly competent scientists and members of the National Academy of Sciences on that account. He seemed to consider them apparently as some sort of infallible and untouchable scientific holy cows. Finally he suggested that his denunciation might be submitted to Mr. Folsom, at that time Secretary of the Department, apparently in the hope that my further services might be dispensed with by the USPHS. Well, a copy of his letter drifted down through channels and seems to rest peacefully now in some file cabinet.

This is the record of some types of present day efforts to disseminate information on environmental cancer hazards and to support cancer prevention.

Through such a distortion of occupational cancer epidemiology, the seriousness of this problem for modern industry is conveniently minimized. Attention is thereby, moreover, diverted from investigating and assessing properly the role that industrial and industry related carcinogens play in the present day cancer panorama.

110. Cancer-Causing Chemicals in Food

The question of cancer-causing substances in food was one of the most significant topics taken up at the Seventh International Cancer Congress held in London in July, 1958.

William E. Smith, M.D., Director of Nutrition Research at Fairleigh-Dickinson University, brought the matter squarely to a head when he said, in his prepared address before the Congress: "Increasing knowledge of the ability of many different chemicals to incite cancer has, however, pointed to the need for tests extending over much longer periods of time, preferably over the full life-spans of test animals. It is, of course, now well known that a few doses, or even a single dose, of a carcinogenic (cancer-causing) chemical administered to a young animal can lead to development of cancer in middle life or in old age."

Does it surprise you to know that just one exposure to a cancer-causing substance early in life can produce cancer 20 or 30 years later?

Dr. Smith goes on to say that the peculiar long-delayed effect of these substances sets them apart from other chemicals which are just ordinary poisons. In the case of the latter substances, symptoms of poisoning appear rapidly and, if the person lives, he recovers from the experience with few ill effects. But with cancer-causing substances, there are usually no warning symptoms, yet the changes that occur in cells are irreversible and lead to cancer possibly many years later.

In 1939, Dr. Smith tells us, the International Union Against Cancer suggested that governments revise legislation regulating the toxicity of chemical food additives in the light of the fact that they might be cancer-causing. Later this Union established a committee on cancer prevention which, meeting in 1954, stated again that cancer-causing substances must be considered in a different category from other poisons. For substances that poison temporarily we can set "tolerances"—that is, we can allow small amounts of these substances in food, assuming that, in such small quantity, they will be harmless. But, said the statement of the cancer congress, "No substance which in tests at any dose level induces any type of malignant tumor in any species of animal can be considered innocuous (harmless) to human health."

Another symposium of the International Union was held in Rome in 1956. At this meeting, Dr. W. C. Hueper of our National Cancer Institute made some very strong statements on the subject of chemicals in food and their possible relation to the increasing incidence of cancer in our country. The *New York Times* published a story about Dr. Hueper's speech in which he listed 20 groups of suspect food additives and 17 groups of suspect food contaminants. Many of these, he said, have not been ade-

[440]

quately investigated for their possible cancer-causing qualities. These include dyes, thickeners, synthetic sweeteners and flavors, preservatives, shortenings, bleaches, oils and fats, antibiotics, estrogen (a hormone used for fattening animals), insecticide residues, soot, chemical sterilizers, anti-sprouting agents, wrapping materials, radiation.

Such a frightening report did not go unnoticed by the American people and such was the clamor that the Food and Drug Administration was forced to make a statement. They said that the people of this country are "well protected" against possible harm from food additives and that Dr. Hueper had been an alarmist.

Meanwhile, the Congressional committee to investigate chemicals in food held some hearings. Astonishing revelations were made before this committee as to the possible harm chemicals in food might be doing our people, especially in relation to cancer. Congressman Delaney, chairman of the committee, introduced a bill in Congress which includes provisions to (1.) require testing of chemical food additives for their cancer-causing potential, and (2.) forbid for use in food any additives that are found to be cancer-causing.

This seems to be a simple solution to the problem, doesn't it? And surely one on which everyone would agree! There cannot be an American food processor alive today so unfeeling as to knowingly cause cancer in any of his customers. Why then has the legislation been shelved? Why then do the years drag on with no regulations on cancer-causing chemicals in food, while at the same time the number of food chemicals is increasing every day? And the number of cancer deaths.

Complications Are Ever Present

Dr. Smith gives part of the answer in his statement before the Cancer Congress. Tests for possible cancer-causers are complex in the extreme. Certain substances may cause cancer under certain circumstances and may be highly beneficial foods under other circumstances. For instance, sesame oil which had been heated to 350 degrees centigrade caused cancer in laboratory animals. Unheated oil did not.

Other aspects of the tests must be considered. Injecting certain substances may cause cancer, while giving them by mouth may not. Substances which occur naturally may cause cancer when they are used out of context—that is, in other than natural ways.

Dr. Smith tells us that estrogen, a female sex hormone, is a powerful cancer-causer. Now obviously estrogen exists naturally in all females and does not cause cancer when it is performing its perfectly natural function of stimulating and regulating the various sex processes. But when estrogenic material from an animal is injected or given to a human being or another animal, it becomes cancer-causing. "The fact that some carcinogenic (cancer-causing) substances appear in nature is hardly a justification for extracting them and adding them to food," says Dr. Smith.

[441]

Finally—just what is a "safe" dose of anything which can produce cancer? Several years ago an insecticide was tested and it was found that laboratory rats got tumors when they ate this substance in relatively high doses. So a ruling went out that such and such a residue of this insecticide might appear legally in food. Later, further tests revealed that cancer might be caused *at much lower levels* than the first experiment had shown. So the ruling was changed and no residue of that substance is now permitted in food.

How many people died of cancer because of that earlier erroneous ruling, do you suppose?

Dr. Smith tells us that Congressman Delaney, under whose direction the hearings on chemicals were held several years ago, made a speech in Congress in which he drew attention to the irreversible actions of cancer-causing substances on cells. He stated that, when such substances are used in food, their later withdrawal affords no assurance that cancer will not develop years later in persons who ate them during the period when they were in use. Mr. Delaney's bill submitted to Congress specifically requires that all food additives must be tested as possible cancer-causers *before* they are used in food.

In closing, Dr. Smith tells us the unhappy news that what may cause cancer in one kind of animal may not do so in another kind. So tests with animals may show possible hazards for man, but cannot afford complete assurance of safety.

What Can We Do?

What is the answer for those of us who want to avoid cancer—and surely this means every one of us? Dr. Smith believes that, "In legislation to assure safety of chemicals in food, a conservative position would therefore be to limit artificial food additives to as small a list as possible sufficing to meet actual needs for production and distribution of foods." This is a very general statement, of course, and we wonder who is going to be the judge of what will "suffice to meet actual needs for production and distribution of food."

A certain dye was forbidden on Florida oranges because it had been found to be cancer-causing. But the citrus growers convinced the authorities that this dye was necessary "for production and distribution" of their product. It would be the ruin of the citrus industry if they could not dye their oranges, they said, so the dye is still being used. If this is the kind of decision such legislation will produce, then it will be meaningless indeed.

We believe that legislation should be passed *outlawing all chemicals in food.* Certainly with today's provisions for refrigeration preservatives are never necessary. Dyes, thickeners, emulsifiers, bleaches, flavoring—all of these should be outlawed for good. Processed food will look and taste a little different, true. Will the food companies lose money? Of course not, for the millions of dollars they are spending now promoting all these fantastic chemicals in foods they could spend in a grand, concerted publicity campaign to explain to the public just why and how such changes were made and what they will mean in increased health.

Don't you think everyone in this country would be delighted with such a prospect?

When you write to your congressman, senator, state health department and state legislature, ask for legislation outlawing all chemicals in food. Only then can we talk meaningfully of safety from cancer-causing substances.

111. Statistics Reveal Some Probable Cancer Causes

While scientists all over the world are studying cancer cells under the microscope, trying to determine how they grow and how they can be stopped, others are fighting cancer from a different angle. They use a science known as epidemiology. The experts in this field study large groups of people who have the same particular disease, and try to find a common denominator which might be significant.

Semmelweiss Established Importance of Sanitation

For example, Dr. Semmelweiss used this technique in solving the puzzle of frequent deaths in childbirth due to childbed fever. He observed that in each case of death, the officiating doctor had performed the delivery without first washing his hands. Dr. Semmelweiss then concluded that the contaminated hands of the doctors might be introducing the disease, whatever its form, into the new mothers. Once the rule for careful sanitation was adopted, childbirth mortality rates fell. The important point of this example is that it was not necessary to identify the exact microbe or virus that caused these deaths, but rather the need was to discover how it got into the body and a means of eliminating its entry. This was done by observation. The common denominator was correctly found to be the unclean hands of the doctors.

As we have seen many times in medical history, this approach can be very effective. It has been applied to the problem of cancer. Some of the results are already well known, some are new and seem to becloud rather than clarify the situation. However, as you will see, certain types of cancer show similar backgrounds, whether it be type of work or geographic location, type of food or preference in liquor.

Similarities Have Been Discovered

In an article in the *Practitioner* (June, 1959), Percy Stocks, C.M.G., M.D., F.R.C.P., former Senior Research Fellow of the British Empire

[443]

Cancer Campaign, has outlined what similarities have been discovered about the victims of various types of cancer. We believe that this information is at present the most tangible and effective means we, as individuals, can use to protect ourselves. You will note that certain elements, particularly polluted air and smoking, appear time and again as causes of cancer in various parts of the body. Such repetition is certainly significant and should lead to our avoidance of these elements whenever possible.

Skin cancer has been found to be associated mainly with occupational exposure to, and direct contact with, soot, tar and certain crude oils. Where protective measures have been taken, the rate has been lowered. It is an interesting footnote to industrial cancer hazards that Dr. Stocks found bladder cancer a common occurrence in men who handle certain chemicals in their work. He does not specify which chemicals these are, however, working in close proximity to any chemicals strikes us as a dangerous way to make a living.

City Men Most Susceptible To Cancer of the Larynx

Cancer of the larynx occurs more often in men than in women; and men who live in the city are victims more often than men in rural areas. The risk of this type of cancer is statistically greater in men addicted to heavy smoking and drinking. An area of occupation which shows up rather strongly in cancer of the larynx and esophagus is the making and serving of alcoholic beverages. Is it possible that the fumes from these liquids could be enough to irritate the tissues of the throat, or are men in such jobs more likely to develop strong drinking habits? Then, too, it must be remembered that the smoky, closed atmosphere in which such work is done could have bearing on the problem.

Geographical Location Important

Cancer of the stomach shows marked geographical prevalence. Its incidence in Japan, parts of Wales, England and Switzerland is very high. In the United States, for some unexplained reason, the number of deaths from stomach cancer is falling. In relation to occupation, dock workers, furnacemen and metal workers are the most likely candidates. The wives of these men do not show any such weakness, leading to the conclusion that some factor of the men's jobs must hold the cause.

In the course of their observations, Dr. Stock tells us that epidemiologists found the content of the soil to be a factor in the incidence of stomach cancer. Mortality tends to be low where underlying chalk and limestone are in the ground, and high where coal is close to the surface.

Pipe Smokers and Rectal Cancer

Rectal cancer is higher in the city than the country, and shows an affinity for pipe smokers, whose rate of incidence is higher even than cigarette smokers and consumers of large amounts of fried foods. Beer drinkers in North Wales are highly susceptible to this form of cancer, though the wine drinkers of France, who consume greater amounts of alcohol, showed no such connection. Could the answer lie in an ingredient of beer, aside from its alcoholic content? Again in this type of cancer, those who make and serve alcoholic beverages are found to be likely victims.

Virgins, and single or infertile married women, have the best chance of escaping cancer of the uterus. The death rate from this cancer rises in direct proportion to the number of children a woman has borne. An important causative factor appears to be frequent sexual intercourse at an early age. Women in communities where male circumcision and ritual marital hygiene are practiced tend to have lower death rates from cancer of the uterus.

Lung Cancer Offers Best Data

As would be expected, the data on lung cancer are the most complete. Surprisingly enough, the United States is not mentioned as having a very high lung cancer rate. Britain and Finland are listed as having a very high incidence, and Holland and Switzerland as only slightly less. The low-incidence countries are Norway, Sweden and Iceland, while Japan is singled out as having a very low rate of death from lung cancer.

Occupations which seem to increase chances of acquiring this disease are those concerned directly with coal gas, tar, asbestos, oil, varnish, certain hot metals and metallic dusts. The rare work of diamond cutting shows a connection with lung cancer, due to the inhaled dust, we imagine, as does merely selling tobacco and, once again, serving alcoholic beverages. Air pollution is also considered an important cause of lung cancer.

Of course, the connection between smoking and lung cancer is discussed by Dr. Stocks. He writes that more than 20 investigations in 8 countries have shown that a larger proportion of lung cancer victims occurs among those who smoke heavily than those who do not. Studies have shown that the rate goes down as the number of cigarettes smoked decreases, and lowers even among heavy smokers who have stopped the habit altogether.

How Much Do Statistics Prove?

Regarding those who refuse to accept the statistical evidence which links smoking and lung cancer, saying that statistics cannot actually "prove" anything, Dr. Stocks quotes Sir Julian Huxley, from his book, *Biological Aspects of Cancer:* "The conclusion to be drawn from the evidence is definite; increased smoking increases the probability of developing lung cancer . . ." Dr. Stocks remarks that many persons insist on proof from actual experiments with human beings which will show lung cancer to develop from smoking. A well-known British authority, Sir Ernest Kennaway, has predicted that such evidence is a long way off, and that until then we shall have to rely on statistical evidence. Dr. Stocks goes on from there. "In my opinion the inescapable answer to all this is that in the face of rapidly rising mortality from lung cancer and the strength of the evidence jointly incriminating cigarettes and atmospheric smoke, everything possible should be done to remove or prevent production of carcinogens already known to be present, to educate people as to the risks and discourage boys and girls from acquiring the cigarette habit, and to reduce the pollution of the air in towns by potentially carcinogenic substances."

We think Dr. Stocks says it all in this statement. While we might not have control over the country in which we live, and we might not be able to change our jobs, we can change our habits of drinking and smoking, and we can insist on laws which will prohibit the release of industrial wastes into the air which are a recognized cancer hazard. These are the ways we can act to protect ourselves in some measure from the threat of cancer.

112. Lung Cancer and Tobacco

"That befogged, wooly sensation reaching from the forehead to the occiput, that haziness of memory, that cold, fish-like eye, that furred tongue and last week's taste in the mouth—too many of you know them—I know them—they come from too much tobacco." These words are from the renowned Dr. William Osler's address to Yale students, quoted in the March, 1952, issue of the *Medical Comment*. If you smoke, you are familiar with the sensations Dr. Osler describes. If you don't smoke, there is undoubtedly someone in your family or close circle of friends who does and who would also recognize these symptoms.

It has always seemed irrelevant to us to rail against smoking as a vice, an immorality. Probably each of us is addicted to some personal habit no more immoral than smoking. If I smoke 10 cigarettes a day and you drink 10 cups of coffee, which of us can call the other's habit a vice? If you puff constantly on a pipe and I carry with me a package of chewy candy for all-day munching, let's face the fact that we are both addicted to dangerous habits we'd do well to break. But let's not discuss them on a plane of righteousness or morality. Let's discuss them on the basis of health.

Most people who smoke realize that smoking is bad for them. They know it because of their own physical sensations while they are smoking, the aftereffects so graphically described by Dr. Osler and the warnings they read constantly in newspapers and magazines. They know it in spite of the lilting jingles and the "scientific tests" of the cigarette ads. Most people who smoke regularly have tried once or many times to stop smoking, for social, health or economic reasons. Most of them have been appalled at how difficult it is to stop.

Evidence of the Harm Tobacco Does

Physicians generally seem to regard smoking with a lenient eye; many of them smoke. Yet medical literature teems with evidence of the harmful effect of tobacco. For instance, the *American Heart Journal* in Vol. 42, 1951, shows the result of cigarette smoking on the action of the heart. The subjects in this experiment each smoked a single cigarette after not smoking for two hours. Out of 31 persons, 18 showed a difference in heart action after the cigarette. All of them had an increased range of pulse beat.

The *British Medical Journal*, Vol. 2, p. 1007, 1951, describes an experiment on the effect of smoking on blood flow through the hand. When smoke is inhaled every 20 seconds, there is a steady decrease in the flow of blood through the hand during the period of smoking. An article in *Modern Medicine* for March 1, 1952, reports on smoking and hyperthyroid (goiter) patients. The conclusion of the two authors, Elmer C. Bartels, M.D., and James J. Coll, M.D., is that smoking should be completely forbidden to the hyperthyroid patient because of the rise in rate of basal metabolism, blood pressure and pulse rate in the patients studied. The *Journal of the American Medical Association* has warned confirmed smokers of the danger of tumors of the vocal cords resulting from too much smoking. This warning issued from a study made of 143 persons suffering from injuries to the vocal cords due to over-smoking. The patients had smoked from 20 to 120 cigarettes daily.

Most significant—and most frightening—of all the articles in our file on tobacco is a study of lung cancer in relation to smoking. This was an address delivered by Ernest L. Wynder, M.D., at a meeting of the Cancer Prevention Committee in New York on December 21, 1949, and reprinted in *Industrial Hygiene and Occupational Medicine* for March, 1952.

The author notes the fact that lung cancer has greatly increased in recent years. Although it affects a younger group than cancer of the stomach, yet the increase noted in lung cancer has not been paralleled by a similar increase in stomach cancer. In addition, lung cancer at present selects 12 men as victims for every one woman. While more and more women take up smoking as time goes on, it is true that, historically, men as a group have been smoking longer than women.

Cancer and the Amount You Smoke

Dr. Wynder's study was done mostly in a large city hospital whose patients were an average cross section of American city people. In interviews he discovered whether or not patients smoked, how long they had smoked, whether they smoked pipes, cigars or cigarettes and how many. Consistently, the lung cancer patients turned out to be those who smoked most and those who had smoked longest. Here are some of Dr. Wynder's statistics.

Among the non-cancer patients in the hospital, 14.6 per cent were non-smokers. Among the lung cancer patients, only 1.5 per cent were non-smokers. Eleven and a half per cent of the regular patients were light smokers, while 2.6 per cent of the lung cancer patients were light smokers. Of moderately heavy smokers, there were 19.0 per cent among the regular patients, 10.3 among the lung cancer patients. You will notice that, as the figures of cigarette consumption go up, so do the percentages of lung cancer patients. Of heavy smokers, 35.6 per cent of the patients classified themselves in this bracket, while 35.2 per cent of the lung cancer patients were heavy smokers. Eleven and a half per cent of the regular patients called themselves excessive smokers, while 30.3 per cent—almost 3 times as many—lung cancer patients fell in this group. There were only 7.6 per cent of chain smokers among the general patients, while 20.1 per cent of the lung cancer patients were in this category.

"This indicates," says Dr. Wynder, "that the greater the amount smoked, the greater the chance of incurring primary cancer of the lungs." In case you're worried about where your own smoking classifies you in this grim index, here is Dr. Wynder's interpretation: "light" smoking means 1-9 cigarettes daily; moderate—10-14; heavy—15-20; excessive—21-34; chain—more than 34 cigarettes per day. Pipe and cigar smokers are included by figuring one cigar as five cigarettes and one pipe as two and one-half cigarettes.

This is how the different kinds of tobacco stacked up. In the general hospital population, 7.8 per cent of the patients smoked cigars, while 3.6 per cent of the lung cancer patients smoked cigars; 12.4 per cent of the general patients smoked pipes and 4.0 per cent of the lung cancer patients smoked pipes. Now 65.2 per cent of the general patients used cigarettes and —hold onto your seats!—90.9 per cent of the lung cancer patients smoked cigarettes. "The percentage of cigarette smokers in the lung-cancer group is greater than can be expected from the general use of cigarettes in the normal hospital population," says Dr. Wynder.

Cancer and How Long You Have Smoked

Here are more facts and figures, frightful enough to scare you out of even listening to cigarette commercials: more than 95 per cent of the lung cancer group had smoked for more than 20 years. About 85 per cent of them had smoked for more than 30 years. Among the regular patients a number of men had smoked for about the same length of time, but had not smoked nearly so much each day. Among the women patients, there were very few in the non-cancer group who had smoked for as many years as this. "The difference in long-term smoking habits of the two sexes is believed to explain the present ratio in lung cancer," says Dr. Wynder.

Then he discusses surveys made by other scientists in which, for instance, two British researchers found (in 1950) only two non-smokers among 649 males with lung cancer. These two scientists concluded that "tobacco plays an important part in (causing) lung cancer and the risk of developing lung cancer increases with the amount of tobacco smoked."

Not nearly so much work has been done in studying the possible cancer-inducing substances in tobacco as has been done on coal tar products, Dr. Wynder believes, although there are two substances inhaled by smokers which should be studied in relation to lung cancer—the tobacco tars themselves and the arsenic residue present in tobacco. As Dr. Wynder points out, it is difficult to determine in animal experiments whether constant smoking produces cancer, since we obviously can't persuade animals to smoke. (And isn't it interesting that all animals intensely dislike the odor of tobacco smoke?) Also, it may be that animals are not susceptible to the same kinds of lung cancer that afflict mankind.

There may be a question in your mind about the 1.5 per cent of the lung cancer patients who were non-smokers and the 2.6 per cent who were light smokers. Dr. Wynder gives no further information about them. Evidence in our files makes us wish that a further investigation had been made into the occupations of these lung cancer patients who smoked not at all or very little. We're willing to wager that a large percentage of them work in plants where they must inhale the dust or fumes from such substances as silica, pitchblende, arsenic, asphalt, beryllium, asbestos, nickel or some of the many petroleum products. Although not all of these have been proven to produce cancer, yet all these and many more substances present a constant hazard to workers exposed to them day after day.

Some of Dr. Wynder's conclusions are:

1. The great increase in city living, though it may expose us to cancer-causing substances, cannot account for the recent increase in lung cancer.

2. Tobacco smoking and particularly cigarette smoking is believed to be the main cause for this increase.

3. Cigarette smoking is more prevalent than other kinds among all smokers. Cigarette smoke is more commonly inhaled than are pipe and cigar smoke, naturally exposing the lungs to more smoke.

4. Lung cancer is now one of the commonest cancers among men. Preventive measures, including a study of the possible cancer-inducing substances in tobacco, should be taken.

Arsenic in Tobacco

During the discussion that followed Dr. Wynder's remarks, Dr. Kanematsu Sugiura reported on tobacco tar and arsenic. He related how he heated tobacco and collected the tar which the heat distilled from the tobacco. This material "induced tumors when painted on mice" said Dr. Sugiura. He added that, in addition to these tars, the other substance in tobacco is known to produce cancer. This is arsenic, residue from the insecticides used on the tobacco leaves. He referred to a table printed in the *American Journal of Public Health* and the *Journal of Industrial Hygiene and Toxicology* showing the arsenic content of tobacco:

	Milligrams per pound	Milligrams per cubic meter of puffed smoke
Cigar tobaccos	5.3 to 12.1	0.6 to 1.9
Pipe tobaccos	14.1 to 20.5	1.7 to 3.3
Cigarette tobaccos	5.3 to 15.1	3.3 to 10.5
Maximum permissible in food	0.7	

It will be noted, said Dr. Sugiura, that the arsenic content of samples of tobacco products ranged up to 30 times the amount permissible by federal law in marketed foods!

How pleasant it would be if, we could propose a simple remedy that would forever "cure" tobacco addicts, one and all. It doesn't seem to be that simple. Some of the most sensible suggestions we have found come from Dr. Gelolo McHugh, Psychologist of Duke University, reported in the *New York Times* for March 13, 1952. Dr. McHugh declares that swearing off cigarettes entirely is not to be advised, for if you fail, the next try will be harder. If you limit your cigarettes to 8 or 10 a day, chances are you'll spend much of that day thinking about the longed-for-cigarette, wondering if it's time for another.

Instead, he suggests: set aside a certain time at the beginning of the day when you will not smoke at all. Do not take a chance on failure by deciding on too long a time. Perhaps two hours is long enough, perhaps you can hold out for three. The rest of the day smoke as much as you wish. Based on research collected over 5 years and covering the smoking history of some 600 people, Dr. McHugh's idea is that you will at least *cut down* on smoking by this method, for, he claims, you will not smoke more than usual during the free part of the day. In fact, he says, you will find yourself lighting cigarettes less and less frequently after you have once accustomed yourself to not smoking at all during part of the day. This idea sounds reasonable to us. At any rate, considering the statistics on lung cancer, it seems eminently worth a try.

113. A New Theory on the Cause of Cancer

The theory that cancer may be a deficiency disease is explored by Dr. L. A. Erf and Dr. B. J. Miller of Jefferson Medical College and Hospital, Philadelphia, in an article that appeared in *GP*, published by the American Academy of General Practice, for April, 1957.

The fascinating theory put forward by these two researchers is that cancerous cells are cells that have not matured. If the proper materials are present, every human cell will mature as its nature demands to perform whatever its function is. But if the "maturant" substances are not present, the cells will continue to grow and divide, except that they will be immature cells, incapable of doing what they are supposed to do.

The authors tell us that, in the disease pernicious anemia, many, many red blood cells are found—all of them immature, that is, incapable of doing what red blood cells are supposed to do. So the patient may die from lack of mature red blood cells. In fact, the patient who dies of pernicious anemia does so from lack of mature red blood cells, even though he has far too many such cells that are immature in his body.

Recently it was discovered that vitamin B_{12} cures pernicious anemia. This, then, is the "maturant" substance—the material that goes into the cells and causes them to mature so that they can do what they are supposed to do. And the patient gets well. How did he get sick? Obviously from a lack of vitamin B_{12} which caused the whole process of red-blood-cell making to go awry. Since there was not enough vitamin B_{12}, cells began to divide as they are supposed to, but did not then develop into true red blood cells. They stayed babies.

This situation, say our authors, is similar to cancer, especially to leukemia and myeloma, two forms of cancer. In both these diseases, too, there is an abnormal production of immature red blood cells invading the bone marrow, the liver, the lymph, the lungs, the kidneys, etc.—taking up room, but doing nothing that a red blood cell is supposed to do because they are immature.

Scientists can tell (using microscopes, we suppose) whether cells are mature or not. And they have found that as a vitamin B_{12} deficiency grows worse in pernicious anemia, the red blood cells become more and more immature in appearance and character. In cancer, too, as the disease progresses, the cancerous cells become more and more immature, seeming to indicate that less and less of some important "maturant" substance is present as the disease goes on.

What Is The Maturing Substance?

Now, in pernicious anemia, we are told that vitamin B_{12} matures the red blood cells up to a certain point and after that protein, iron, vitamin C, thyroxin (from the thyroid gland), folic acid (another B vitamin) and several other "maturants" are necessary to finish the development of the cells so that they are completely mature once again. And the patient then recovers.

The authors believe that this maturing process may be one reason why X-ray may be helpful in cancer. It breaks up cancerous cells and they may release whatever they contain of the "maturant" substance. New cells, then, can take it up and become mature, healthy cells rather than cancerous ones. "One can go a step further and believe that many humans have 'cured' many cancers by overcoming maturant deficiencies," say the authors.

They point out that the substance responsible for maturing cells to prevent cancer may be enzymes (they exist in raw food), hormones (they are made by the body's glands), vitamins, catalysts (trace minerals, perhaps?) or certain kinds of protein. In the case of pernicious anemia we have seen that several vitamins, proteins, minerals and hormones are concerned.

[451]

The main effort in years past has been to "kill" cancer cells rather than maturing them so that they would be harmless. In this way, X-ray and the deadly poisons used in orthodox cancer therapy to "kill" the cancer cells may indirectly result in more of the "maturant" substance, as we showed above. For this reason, it seems, say our authors, that treatment which uses both a substance to kill off immature cells and a substance that may help cells to mature would be most effective.

Cancer may be more prevalent in the older age groups because there is more chance of deficiency of the maturant substance in older persons. Why? Because there is continual damage to cells throughout life—repeated infections, allergies, hardening of the arteries and poisons to which they are subjected. All of these together can produce changes in the cells. Perhaps they also result in a deficiency of the material that is necessary for maturing cells.

Dr. Erf and Dr. Miller tell us that researchers of the future, working with normal fresh human blood and body fluids, may be able to isolate and identify in that blood what the substance is whose job it is to cause cells to mature normally. When that time comes we may have the cure for cancer.

Why Not Prevent Cancer?

A conclusion like this, to an article describing such an exciting new theory, seems to us to ignore the most important facts brought out in the article itself. Using pernicious anemia as an example, the authors showed how certain substances *that occur naturally in food*—food present in a good diet, that is—cure this deadly disease. If the vitamin B_{12}, the protein, the iron, the vitamin C and the folic acid had been present in the patient's diet in ample quantity and if the patient's thyroid gland had been functioning properly, there would never have been any pernicious anemia, would there?

At least two forms of cancer, leukemia and myeloma, seem to show many of the same characteristics as pernicious anemia. Doesn't it seem that the authors of the article could have urged that researchers do tests to determine whether the same battery of vitamins and minerals and hormones might not have the same beneficial effects in these diseases, too? All of these substances mentioned (except for the thyroid hormone) occur in food. They are *not* obscure, expensive drugs developed in a laboratory. They are the natural elements in a good diet. They are practically nonexistent in the diets of many Americans, who live on refined foods, canned goods, soft drinks, coffee and bakery products.

Why not point out, Dr. Erf and Dr. Miller, that the same thing may be true of cancer as of pernicious anemia? In other words, the mysterious "maturant" substance you are searching for in the blood is bound to be something taken in with food—right? Any researcher knows that food, air and water are the only things the body has with which to conduct all

[452]

its processes. Therefore, the "maturant" substance is bound to be something in which the food of cancer patients is deficient, is it not?

What Can We Do Now?

All you have to do, gentlemen, is look around you and read some statistics on the proven deficiencies in modern diets. One or 10 or 15 or more of the elements that have been removed from our diets during the last hundred years or so by improper farming methods, by refining and processing of foods, by enriching of foods, by eating foods that have been weeks, months or years away from the fresh earth in which they grew— somewhere along the line, the "maturant" substances disappeared.

Must we wait for years while hundreds of thousands die of cancer, while researchers painstakingly test in laboratories substance after substance, then test them in combinations and more combinations until we find which combination of vitamins, minerals, proteins, hormones will cure cancer as the other combination cures pernicious anemia! Why not, instead, by education, by advertising, if you will, present the true facts about nutrition, so that everyone in this country will know how to eat a diet so rich in all the important food elements that no "maturing" substance or combination of substances can possibly be missing from it?

114. Our Poisoned World and Cancer

A Welsh physician, Dr. R. A. Holman, believes he has the answer to the cause of cancer—and a stimulating and convincing theory it is, too. Dr. Holman, a bacteriologist, has spent the past 15 years studying cells —specifically the respiration of cells, how cells breathe. Although there is much that is still unknown in this field, it is apparent that there are at least 3 substances which are intimately involved in the process—oxygen, hydrogen peroxide and an enzyme called *catalase*.

Oxygen, as we all know, is important for every moment that we live. In fact, as Dr. Holman says in an article in *International Symposium of Medicine and Social Hygiene,* September, 1957, life *is* essentially respiration, or oxidation. Exactly how oxygen is involved in the process of energy making we do not know. But we do know that somewhere in the chain of events, oxygen reacts or combines with other substances to produce hydrogen peroxide.

Hydrogen peroxide is a poison to living tissue. So, obviously, if the process of life is to go on, something must be provided to counteract the possible harmful effects of hydrogen peroxide. A body substance, or enzyme, called catalase, has this function. It combines with the hydrogen peroxide, causing it to change into water and oxygen. So long as there is plenty of catalase in the cell to dispose of the hydrogen peroxide, all is well. But if something should cause more hydrogen peroxide to be present or if something should destroy the catalase in the cell, then we might expect trouble, for the hydrogen peroxide would be certain to do damage. As Dr. Holman puts it, "permanent changes may take place which will result in the genesis of malignancy."

If this theory is sound, it seems that those tissues which contain less catalase should be more susceptible to cancer than others. Investigators have found, sure enough, that those parts of the digestive tract where there is a smaller amount of catalase have a higher incidence of cancer than other parts of the digestive tract having a larger content of the enzyme. The liver, where there is more catalase than any other part of the body, is rarely the site of primary tumors among people who have adequate diets.

We know, too, that the level of catalase is reduced in the liver and tissues of individuals with cancer. The faster the cancers grow, the greater the loss of catalase. One might think, therefore, that, in cases of cancer, you could simply give a preparation of catalase and the progress of the cancer would be arrested. But this is not so, in the case of catalase. It seems that giving catalase once the cancer growth has started, causes the cancer cells to grow. The whole thing is, of course, another lesson in leaving well enough alone. We should not tamper with the delicate balance maintained at all times in the healthy cell. Naturally harmful substances can be handled by the body. It is only when we bombard it with man-made poisons that we run into difficulties.

What Substances Destroy Catalase in Our Bodies?

Dr. Holman tells us that barbiturates (sleeping pills) and various drugs for bringing down fevers (he does not mention these by name) have been cited as possible cancer-causers because of their action on this balance of hydrogen peroxide and catalase. The sulfa drugs also destroy catalase, thus adding to the risk of cancer. "During the past 15 years," he goes on, "millions of people have been subjected to the action of antibiotics. Most of these are very potent respiratory poisons, the exact nature of their action being, as yet, unknown."

Antibiotics are excreted rapidly from the body so perhaps they may not be as dangerous as they might be, but, he adds, no one knows how dangerous they may be when they are given in the form of long acting preparations and over long periods of time. We think it is important to remember, in this connection, that much of our food contains antibiotics— milk, cheese, butter and meat because the animals involved have been fed antibiotics, whereas fresh produce and poultry are soaked in antibiotics to preserve them. What other substances reduce the amount of catalase available to body cells, with disastrous results? Says Dr. Holman in the October, 1960, issue of *Mother Earth,* the Journal of the Soil Association in England: "During the past 50 years many diverse chemical agents have been added to food and drink in order to kill bacteria, resulting in a longer shelf life. Most of these agents are potent catalase poisons. One of the main arguments in favor of adding chemicals is that this prevents much bacterial food poisoning in the consumers. This attitude, in my opinion, is overstressed. It is not only the catalase content of the bacteria which is destroyed but also that of the food! This latter is an enzyme which is all-important for the prevention of cancer.

"In my opinion," Dr. Holman continues, "most of the chemicals added to food and drink for preservation or coloring could and should be abolished. The obvious way to preserve food is to make use of the energy provided by atomic power for deep-freeze transportation and storage. This would ensure a non-toxic food supply with many vital enzyme systems intact (assuming, of course, that the foodstuffs are not covered or impregnated with toxic chemicals as a result of spraying. etc.)."

It is also extremely important, Dr. Holman believes, that we take in as much catalase as possible in our food. This means eating as much raw food as possible, for enzymes (and catalase is an enzyme) are destroyed by heat. This fact alone must have a long-term effect on our health. "Cancer of the stomach is perhaps the commonest of our cancers," he says, "and yet we continue to ingest very hot materials coupled with catalase destroying chemicals. No other species of animal has such a diet. It would be to everyone's great advantage if the consumption of fresh, uncooked fruit and vegetables were markedly increased, thus ensuring a far greater catalase intake than hitherto in civilized populations."

Polluted Air Is Part of the Problem

We inhale many substances which destroy catalase, he goes on. The vast amounts of various forms of sulfur which pollute our air are catalase poisons. The fumes from our industries and our home heating units and incinerators, the deadly exhaust from trucks and cars which pollutes our highways, as well as the ever-present haze of cigarette and cigar smoke to which most of us are constantly exposed—all these are destructive of the important enzyme, catalase.

Dr. Holman mentions as extremely important, too, the aerosols containing insecticides, fungicides, antibiotics and so forth, which we use so extensively. We would add the many hair sprays used by women. The continued use of these over the years is what is dangerous, for there is no doubt of the adverse effect they have on our cells, especially those of the respiratory tract.

This is what Dr. Holman has to say about oxygen: "A good oxygen intake is essential for good health. Totney would go so far as to explain the high incidence of cancer in the human race on the basis of poor or diminished oxygen consumption, and in a sense he is right. Oxygen is essential for the removal and destruction of many toxic agents present on or in our cells, and it is, therefore, quite obvious that the more actively oxygenated our bodies the better we shall be able to combat the toxic agents which help to influence adversely our normal cells."

Finally, Dr. Holman warns us of the dangers of radiation. He protests particularly against the indiscriminate use of X-rays. At last, he says, we are just beginning to realize that we do not know where the threshold of safety lies in this regard or if indeed there is any level below which one can feel safe. No one can predict what will be the effect on the incidence of cancer 20 years from now of all the forms of radiation to which we are at present being exposed, he believes.

We think Dr. Holman's ideas, which have received wide and favorable notice from cancer researchers, are of the utmost importance. They provide yet another urgent reason for us to be ever alert to the dangers that surround us and eager to eliminate as many as we possibly can. Most of us cannot eat only food that has been organically grown and hence is free from all the poisons which are cancer-causing. But we can, certainly, buy food as fresh as possible and eat as much of it raw as possible. Dr. Holman's findings should add impetus to our letter-writing on the subject of chemicals in food—our protests to congressmen, to the newspaper editors, to boards of health.

Vitamin E Is Important

We can avoid air pollution to some extent by living in the country, if possible, and taking time for plenty of exercise in the open air. We can avoid using aerosols for any purpose whatsoever. We can avoid suspect household materials like detergents, highly chemicalized cleansers and solvents.

And we can do much to increase our body's supply of oxygen by taking vitamin E, whose main job is to aid the tissues in getting along healthfully with lessened oxygen. We can take, too, other food supplements which protect against chemicals—especially vitamin C and vitamin B which are mentioned most often in this regard.

115. A New Approach to the Cancer Problem

Among the many trails that have been followed by researchers seeking the cause, prevention and treatment of cancer is a fascinating one involving the nature of the first cell of a human being—that tiny center of life which divides into two cells. One of the theories which developed is called today by Howard H. Beard, Ph.D., the "trophoblastic theory of malignancy."

Dr. Beard bases his ideas on the original ideas of Dr. John Beard (who is no relation to him)—a Professor of Embryology at the University of Edinburgh—"the only individual who was destined to solve the riddle of cancer" according to the present Dr. Beard. The embryologist discovered the nature of cancer, according to Dr. Beard, in 1902, and suggested the use of pancreatic enzymes in treating it. He published a book on the treatment of cancer in 1911.

Dr. Howard Beard, who lives and works in Texas, published a book in 1958 on this theory and treatment of cancer which is called *A New Approach to the Conquest of Cancer, Rheumatic and Heart Diseases* (Pageant Press, New York). Dr. Beard tells us that the earlier book formed the basis of treatment at the John Beard Research Institute in San Francisco. He later developed tests for cancer which have proved, he says, to be 95 per cent reliable. He tells us, further, that 10 different groups of doctors in this country, in England, Italy, Belgium, Japan and the Philippines are using his ideas and his treatment for cancer.

Dr. Beard says, in the introduction to his book, "The conquest of cancer will only be accomplished by the cooperation of the public and the clinicians. The clinicians cannot treat cancer without documented proof of the effect of any new therapy of cancer and the public doesn't know the cancer story. So it is hoped that if the layman gets bored with reading so many case histories, just let him put himself in that patient's shoes and then the story will be entirely different. The greatest mistake made today is that almost 100 per cent of the population believes that the other fellow will get cancer but he will never get it himself. Cancer is no respecter of persons; it can attack anyone at any time. Hence, the only way to convince the doctor and the public that the cancer problem is solved is to cite many case histories where recoveries have occurred under chymotrypsin and laetrile therapy."

These are the two substances used by Dr. Beard in treating cancer. He also has developed a test which, he says, will show the presence of malignancy long before it could be detected by biopsy; giving injections of laetrile can prevent the discovered cancer or tendency to cancer from developing into malignancy.

[457]

Dr. Beard's explanation of the trophoblast theory of cancer is, to a layman, extremely complex and difficult to understand. Perhaps to an embryologist (one who studies the very beginnings of life—the embryo) it would be clear. But the combination of unfamiliar and extremely technical terms and the assumption that the reader knows far more than most laymen know about cell structure and the actual process of cell division with which life begins makes it an almost frustrating experience for one who reads the book.

What Is the Theory?

As we understand it, the basis of the theory is this: a certain kind of cell produced in the pregnant female is the same kind of cell that becomes the cancer cell. It is simply a question of where the cells develop, says Dr. Beard. Pregnancy and malignancy are analogous—that is, the same, in some aspects. Pregnancy is physiological and sexual. Malignancy is asexual and, from the clinical point of view, pathological or diseased. "The development of a malignant tumor is simply an attempt of the asexual life to take over the sexual life of the individual," states Dr. Beard.

To put it another way, you might say that a cancerous cell is a cell that might have developed into a child. Instead, it is found in another part of the body, but it has the ability to divide and reproduce rapidly, as we know cancer cells do.

These potentially dangerous cells are controlled in the healthy individual by an enzyme, chymotrypsin, which, says Dr. Beard, prevents cancer just as insulin prevents diabetes. Insulin is, of course, a hormone, and chymotrypsin is an enzyme.

It seems reasonable, then, if one could predict the development of cancer in an individual, he could administer the enzyme mentioned above and prevent the cancer from developing, just as insulin prevents diabetic symptoms in persons to whom it is administered. And Dr. Beard tells us that he has developed such a test. In this test, which Dr. Beard calls the Anthrone test, a certain substance is revealed which is present only in the urine of pregnant women and those who have a malignant or cancerous condition. Its amount is directly proportional to the degree of malignancy present.

The test has shown an amazing degree of accuracy. It will not work in the case of pregnant women, women recently delivered of babies, women who have a certain kind of mole, in cases of male or female acromegaly (a disease of the pituitary gland), in uncontrolled diabetes or in advanced liver disease. Aside from these exceptions, the test is practically 100 per cent certain, according to Dr. Beard.

The center portion of Dr. Beard's book is devoted to about 60 pages of case histories of cancer patients treated with laetrile. Dr. Beard believes that "cancer cures" claimed by orthodox medicine for X-ray or surgery cases are not "cures" at all. He says that the cancer patient suffers from a lack of the enzyme, chymotrypsin. "Once a cancer patient has developed a tumor, this patient is suffering from a chymotrypsin deficiency and this patient will always be a chymotrypsin deficient patient regardless of treatment or no treatment. A tumor may show up as long as 60 years after the patient has been pronounced cured."

Basic Nature of the Theory

Our interest in Dr. Beard's work stems partly from the very basic nature of the theory—relating cancer to the beginning of life, as well as his description of cancer as a deficiency disease. We were extremely interested in his test for potential cancer and we think such a test holds very great promise for conquering cancer, if indeed it will indicate the presence of malignancy early in the game when steps can be taken to reverse the state.

Finally, we were interested in Dr. Beard's story because, throughout his entire career, orthodox medicine has turned a stony ear to what he has to say. It does not recognize Dr. Beard's work with even so much as a nod. Dr. Beard has taught at several universities—Western Reserve, Louisiana State, Chicago Medical School. His employment has been hazardous, because it is dangerous, these days, to talk of your own work in cancer treatment.

The Role of The National Cancer Institute

Concerning his treatment and his test for cancer, we do not know whether or not he can do what he says he can do. His evidence sounds impressive and impelling. We are not cancer experts.

We believe it is the job of the experts—chiefly the National Cancer Institute, a government department established to deal with matters like this—to test any such claims and such treatments—to test them fairly, objectively and with the greatest good will. We, who pay the taxes, assume that the National Cancer Institute is there to find the answer to this terrible disease. They dare not—*they simply dare not*—neglect or slight or damn with faint praise any cancer treatment or test that shows promise, let alone one where the evidence is as convincing as Dr. Beard's. We urge readers to demand a congressional investigation which will bring to light all such work done in all parts of the country along with an explanation from our government bureau as to why they persist in repressing, discouraging and attacking such work. Can it be, as Dr. Beard says flatly, that the medical profession does not want to find a cure for cancer?

We cannot help but recall an article in the Pittsburgh *Post Gazette* for November 8, 1958, which quotes the Associated Press in a news item entitled, "Curing of Diseases Seen as Major Disaster." This was discussed at the 11th annual meeting of the Gerontological Society, at a banquet, in a speech by A. I. Lansing, M.D., the organization's outgoing president. He is certain that some day cancer and heart disease will be conquered and that will be too bad from the financial point of view. He said, "It is no exaggeration to point out that elimination of these degenerative diseases, which at first glance might appear to be a blessing, could easily constitute a major disaster." If these diseases are controlled, then the majority of the people will live 10 or 20 years more and since insurance, social security and annuities are based on a lower death level there would occur bankruptcy of insurance companies and difficulty in our Federal Government.

116. Is Cancer a Virus Disease?

Another theory about cancer, its cause and treatment is found in the book, *Pathogenesis of Cancer,* by John E. Gregory, M.D., published by the Fremont Foundation in Pasadena, California. Since 1946, Dr. Gregory has been studying a cancer virus which he photographed in the electron microscope. An electron microscope is one in which the illumination is given with electrons rather than ordinary light, with the result that infinitely small objects may be perceived.

Dr. Gregory reminds us first of the famous "milk-factor" that is involved in cancer. We know that there is apparently something in the milk of a cancerous mouse that is transmitted to the offspring of the mouse where it may produce cancer. In these experiments mice born to cancerous mice were nursed by cancer-resisting mice and did not develop cancer. Reversing the experiment, newly born cancer-resisting mice were allowed to feed from cancerous mothers. These mice developed as much cancer as they would, had they been offspring of cancerous mothers. So apparently some substance contained in the milk brought about the cancer.

It seems that it is not one specific type of cancer that may be transmitted from the cancerous mice to their offspring. Mothers with breast cancer do not transmit breast cancer necessarily. The cancer may be produced at any location depending upon the amount of irritation present at any one location or the working of the glands of the mouse.

Dr. Gregory tells us that, with the help of the electron microscope, he has isolated a virus from human cancerous tissue. He has found it in more than 1,000 malignant tissues tested. He has not been able to find it in tissues from benign tumors—that is, tumors which are not cancerous. He has made this virus grow in his laboratory and has injected it into animals, thereby producing cancer. He has also found that specific antibodies have developed in the blood of these animals. A virus, incidentally, is a bacteria infinitely smaller than most. An antibody is a certain substance manufactured in the body to fight against a given bacteria. Dr. Gregory has also destroyed the cancer virus by heating it to a high temperature. At any rate it appears to be destroyed, since it will not, after being heated, produce cancer in animals into which it is injected. We know that other bacteria and viruses can also be destroyed by heat. This is one reason for the pasteurization of milk and the boiling of water that is suspected of being impure.

Working on the theory that cancer is caused by a virus, Dr. Gregory then proceeded to develop 4 different antibiotics which appear to be powerful against the cancer virus. The two earlier ones Tracin and Magnesium Tracinate were developed from bacteria. The third Gregomycin comes from the streptomycetes. The fourth, Gregocin, comes from a mold. This last-discovered antibiotic has given such good results that he is using it now instead of any of the 3 that were discovered earlier. In his own words, "having 4 antibiotics that give satisfactory results in the treatment of cancer is extremely strong evidence that cancer is a virus disease." He says further that the degree of malignancy is in direct proportion to the amount of the virus present. Cancer virus is a living organism, as are other bacteria.

How the Cancer Virus Works

He tells us then that normal cells which are stimulated to grow cannot become cancerous unless the cancer virus is present. For example there might be a certain part of the body that had been subjected to blows or other mistreatment that would cause it to become very sore. If the cancer virus was not present the wound would heal after a period of time.

Here are samples from the many case histories given in the book. One, a woman of 65, had had cancer of both breasts for 18 months. Both breasts were amputated, she was given X-ray and Magnesium Tracinate daily for one year. After 3 years there was no recurrence of the cancer. A woman with primary cancer of the liver suffered from severe jaundice, loss of appetite, weakness and rapidly enlarging liver. After taking Magnesium Tracinate for one year, she had gained back most of her weight, her appetite and strength were good and she was up and around. Many, many other similar case histories are given in the book, along with pictures of the patients and microscopic studies of the cancerous tissues.

Other Aspects of Dr. Gregory's Research

Discussing the public health aspects of the virus theory of cancer, Dr. Gregory has this to say: "Cancer in mice has been proved to be transmitted through their milk. The physiology of milk formation in the various animals is essentially the same. Pasteurization of milk should be considered of value in preventing the spread of cancer from milk sources. Steps should be taken to make appropriate cancer tests in cows similar to the tuberculin test. This will be of value in protecting the purity of grade A raw milk. There is an important point in the transmission of cancer which has apparently not been a factor in tuberculosis. This is the finding of cancer virus in eggs. Up to 70 per cent of some eggs have been found to contain cancer virus, but in eggs from carefully cared-for hens eating only greens and grain, I have never found the virus."

Other interesting facts brought to light by Dr. Gregory are these:

"Calcium given intravenously daily to cancer patients has been found to retard some tumors." "Animals with a cancer tendency have been fed coconut and none developed cancer." It is believed, he says, that the lauric acid in the coconut was responsible.

"If butter yellow is fed to animals it will be deposited in the liver and cause cirrhosis and tumors of the liver. However, if riboflavin (one of the B vitamins) is first fed in large quantities, it will take up all the loose bonds of the protein, so that when the butter yellow arrives at the liver there will be no place for it to attach itself. Thus the butter yellow will pass through the liver without disturbing it."

"Another important physiological factor is that all the B vitamins will improve the action of the liver and cause it to destroy the excess estrogenic and androgenic hormones faster, thus cutting down the excess stimulation to breast cancer or cancer of the prostate."

Dr. Gregory's comments on the subject of nutrition in relation to cancer are interesting. He tells us that a diet low in calories will reduce by 10 per cent both the rate of growth of cancer and its occurrence among laboratory animals. He also tells us that there are many excellent natural antibiotics in vegetables, fruits, nuts and grains. Although these may not be the exact antibiotic that will kill the cancer virus, still almost any antibiotic will enhance the activity of any other antibiotics. We wonder if by any chance the antibiotic content of fruits and vegetables is related to their content of vitamin C which is powerful in preventing infectious diseases.

Diet and Cancer

Finally, Dr. Gregory says, "Also vegetables grown with organic fertilizer will keep longer than other vegetables, which indicates that their antibiotic activity is greater. These vegetables have a higher mineral content and thus naturally will keep a person's tissues from being demineralized, which apparently occurs before cancer develops."

As we were reading Dr. Gregory's book, we were reminded strongly of the work of another cancer investigator, Dr. John R. Davidson of Winnipeg, Canada, who declared throughout his long and devoted research on cancer: "Cancer is a nutritional deficiency disease." Quoting from a story in *Saturday Night*, a Canadian publication, "This conclusion was derived from experiments on mice. Davidson found that the regular experimental forms of cancer could be produced easier in mice that had been raised on food lacking in vitamins. The opposite was also true. Mice fed special vitamin-rich diets were very resistant to cancer. Furthermore, after generations of mice were raised on vitamin-deficient diets, the offspring became more and more liable to cancer. In this Dr. Davidson believed that he had a clue to the puzzling fact that there are 'cancer susceptible' families, although the disease is definitely not hereditary.

"Linking the Davidson research with the virus theory, it could be said that the cancer virus, existing in bodies, passes over to the active, virulent form under certain definite chemical conditions brought about by prolonged lack of sufficient vitamins.

"Dr. Davidson was able to produce mice families susceptible to cancer. In 5 generations, by feeding with 'excess' vitamins and minerals, he bred from those susceptible mice a new generation quite free from any abnormal tendency towards cancer. This type of evidence—the reversible demonstration—is among the most powerful that can be provided by experimental science.

"What are the vitamins used in the Davidson research? Mainly those associated with chicken embryos and with wheat germ. Why? Because the doctor's work convinced him that the disease of cancer is related in some way to normal cell multiplication that takes place so rapidly in developing embryos, such as that of the fertilized hen's egg. Here again there is nothing that is scientifically unsound.

"But it is from his clinical work that Dr. Davidson has collected most convincing evidence. He has stopped human cancer from spreading. He has completely cured some cases. A child suffering from lymphosarcoma and given only a few months to live was gradually restored to health without surgery or radium. After 3 years the affected glands were cured and normal.

"In this case the treatment consisted of special feeding. The Davidson diet is adjusted to individual patients, but in general includes large amounts of fresh vegetable juice (carrot and lettuce), raw vegetables (carrots, spinach, lettuce, peas, beans), wheat germ and rare beef. In addition, the patient gets massive doses of vitamins in the form of cod liver oil, wheat germ oil, and brewer's yeast. Finally there is a preparation made from chick embryos."

Piecing all this information together it seems to us that we have clear evidence in support of our theory that diseases—even cancer—can be prevented by good nourishment. Vitamins A, B and C especially, and all of the important minerals as well, are involved in protecting the body from the ravages of the powerful virus diseases. We know, too, from many experiments, that the B vitamins, especially, prevent induced cancer in laboratory animals exposed to substances known to produce cancer. Perhaps Dr. Gregory's research will spark a whole new approach to the problem of preventing cancer by diet and curing cancer with antibiotics.

117. Your Emotional Make-Up

"Let me speak to you regarding the things of which you must most beware. To get angry and shout at times pleases me, for this will keep up your natural heat; but what displeases me is your being grieved and taking all matters to heart. For it is this, as the whole of physic teaches, which destroys our body more than any other cause."

The physician who wrote thus to his patient was Maestro Loranze Sassoli, and he inscribed this letter in the year 1402. He was revealing a common medical notion of the times that cancer, specifically, was related to one's temperament. Galen, the father of modern medicine, who lived in the second century A.D. believed that melancholic women were more prone to cancer than those whom we today would call happy-go-lucky.

By the eighteenth century, European physicians were noting in their medical articles that a severe emotional shock (usually the death of a loved one) contributed to a large extent to the onset and development of cancer. Physicians of that time had available none of the tests which modern researchers use to discover facts about personality and personality difficulties. So they could do nothing but record their observations about personality and cancer.

Here are some of the notes they made:

1822—Nunn described a woman who died of breast cancer shortly after the death of her husband.

1846—Walshe wrote in part as follows: "Much has been written on the influence of mental misery and habitual gloominess of temper on the deposition of carcinomatous (cancerous) matter. If systematic writers can be credited, these constitute the most powerful cause of the disease; and Lobstein, assuming the fact as established, exercised his ingenuity in tracing the connexion of cause and effect: moral emotions produce defective innervation, this perversion of nutrition which in turn caused the formation of carcinoma (cancer) . . . I have myself met with cases in which this connexion appeared so clear that I decided questioning its reality would have seemed a struggle against reason."

On the basis of this conviction Walshe advised patients with a family background of cancer to select their professions with great care. Avoid those which entail constant care and anxiety, he cautioned. Clearly, he believed that an inherited tendency to cancer plus a long-term period of psychological stress might result in cancer.

1885—Willard Parker, an American, studied 97 cases of breast cancer and reported that grief is undoubtedly associated with the disease. Cancer patients are not people who have been noted for cheerfulness before the disease struck them. Another physician, Cutter, remarked that mental depression is too often an element in cancer to be overlooked. He believed, furthermore, that the disease could be cured by diet and by stimulating the patient's will to live.

An English physician reported, "Great mental stress has been assigned as influential in hastening the development of cancer. Another said that cancer of the breast and uterus follow immediately upon depressing emotion, too often to be mere chance.

By 1921 Willy Meyer, who introduced radium therapy for cancer into America, wrote that he believed that cancer is often the result of social and emotional stress because of changes in the body produced by such stress—in other words, changes in the actual chemistry of the body necessitated by its reaction to severe stress.

As psychoanalysis became popular, as the ideas of Freud and Jung received wider acceptance, we find analysts stating that cancer is an "acting out of deep frustrations" by the body. Here are some other more modern viewpoints:

Physical Habits Influence Mental Condition

Hoffman, writing in 1915, "From dietary disorders to nervous disorders is but a step. The two are frequently interrelated and cause and effect are often hopelessly confused . . . This naturally brings me to the question of the interrelationship of cancer and worry, or the mental attitude of the patient toward the development, spread and curability of the disease." Another researcher, Foque, in 1931 spoke of the "role of sad emotions as activating and secondary causes in the activation of human cancers." His theory, important and well-conceived, we believe, was that the stress or emotion affects the nervous system which in turn affects the body's metabolism which acts on the glands in such a way as to make individual cells susceptible to the effects of a cancer-causing substance. He spoke of his patients thus, ". . . you can see in the patients prolonged and silent sorrow without the release of sobs and tears."

He and many other modern writers believed that the death of a child, a spouse or another loved one, plays an important part in the chain of events that result in cancer.

As statistical methods were developed for studying such theories, it was found that indeed this appeared to be the case. In different marital conditions among women it might be presumed, therefore, that there would be the largest incidence of cancer among widows, the next largest among those who had been divorced or separated, less among those who were legally married whether or not much remained of a happy relationship, and least cancer among single women. A survey of cancer statistics in 1956 showed that this was the case, where there were adequate statistics to work with. Other statistical studies seemed to show similar trends. Invariably widows in all age groups had a higher cancer mortality than happily married or single women.

[465]

The Cancer Personality

Psychiatrists delved deeper and found that apparently there was a relationship between incidence of cancer and unhappy relationship with other members of the family, especially, so it seems, an unresolved conflict with the mother of the family. Extensive studies have been done showing that there is apparently a very definite connection between certain kinds of personality and cancer incidence. Time and again, the "cancer personality" is described as a person who has a defensive attitude toward society, more anxieties than normal and less ability to reduce tension by some outward manifestation. That is, the person who broods silently rather than shouting when he is angry; the person who grieves and harbors silent fears and grudges, who cannot "work off" a feeling of depression, anger or frustration with exercise, singing, hard manual labor, or loud talking.

Then, too, there seemed to be a certain undoubted relationship between emotions and the state of a patient who had finally succumbed to cancer. We are told by Trunnell in a paper read at a cancer symposium in 1956 that almost without exception the cancer patient reacts with certain definite emotional and also physical changes to the degree of illness or the deaths of patients around him. The need for narcotics varies, there are chemical changes in the urine and so forth.

In *Cancer and Personality: A Critical Review,* by Lawrence LeShan, published in the January, 1959, issue of the *Journal of the National Cancer Institute,* the author tells us that such investigations as he reports in this article (which we have covered briefly above) do not give us a cure for cancer. Easing the emotional strains of the patient will not necessarily halt the disease. "One does not put out a forest fire by extinguishing the match that started it," he says. "It is nevertheless true that it may be necessary, after putting out the fire, with other means, (surgery, radiation or chemotherapy) to extinguish the match in order to prevent a new fire."

We would add—isn't it a better idea to warn against match-lighting and so prevent the forest fires from ever starting in the first place?

Dr. LeShan's conclusions—and we think they are important for all health seekers to know—are: that there seems to be a certain relation between some emotional states of mind, some kinds of personality, and cancer. The loss of a loved one seems to be one of the most common starting points for cancer. There also seems to be some relationship between the kind of personality one has and the time newly-discovered cancer results in death. And there seems to be some connection, little understood, between the kind of personality and the location of cancer.

What We Can Learn from This Research

It seems to us that there are some things crying to be said in regard to this very interesting theory. We know that diet and way of life have a great deal to do with one's adjustment to life and its inevitable sorrows and stresses. This is obvious from the fact that deficiencies in certain essen-

[466]

tial nutriments can produce within a short time depression, nervousness, anxiety, even in individuals who had previously been happy, strong and self-reliant. Depriving test volunteers of the B vitamins alone brings about results of this kind.

We know, too, that stress situations are wasteful of vitamins and minerals. Loss of a loved one is perhaps the most acute stress any of us is subjected to. There is no doubt that all the body changes that accompany such a shock use up one's supply of food elements. For those who do not immediately replace them, it seems only reasonable that a serious disease like cancer might get a strong foothold at such a time when all resistance is low.

Then, too, it seems obvious that prolonged stress over years of quarreling with one's family or associates or resenting the things they do, without showing open hostility, would be bound to take a serious toll in one's physical make-up, once again making one more susceptible to the onset of a disease.

On the other hand, doesn't it seem possible, too, that it is the ill, badly nourished people who are the ones most likely to have emotional difficulties? We all know families in which some are happy, easy to get along with and well adjusted to their jobs and their associates, while others in the same family are irritable, "difficult," nervous, depressed. Doesn't it seem that the same set of prenatal conditions, childhood and adolescence habits and diet which produced the unhappy personality may also, later on, produce the cancer?

Several months ago Editor Rodale reviewed the theory of a famous British physician who asked if the happy man ever gets cancer. He quoted Sir Heneage Ogilvie as saying, "The instances where the first recognizable onset of cancer has followed almost immediate on some disaster, a bereavement, the break-up of a relationship, a financial crisis, or an accident, are so numerous that they suggest that some controlling force that has hitherto kept this outbreak of cell communism in check has been removed."

While the thinking about the relationship between emotions and cancer remains in its present stimulating but unresolved state, it seems to us that the best idea is to do everything you can to avoid being the kind of person who seems to be most susceptible to cancer—depressed, silent, worrying, anxious, resentful or "all wrapped up in yourself."

Aside from a definite conscious effort to turn one's thoughts in a happier direction, there is the necessity to do everything possible to create a body so radiantly healthy that happiness is unavoidable. We are sure that following the program of a well-balanced diet, exercise, rest and good daily habits will bring about this state of mind. Isn't this, perhaps, one of the most important steps on the road to cancer prevention?

[467]

118. Hair Growth and Cancer

The suggestion that there might be a connection between cancer and the amount and color of one's head of hair would seem rather far-fetched. The possibility might never have been explored in these pages were it not for a series of letters which ran in the *British Medical Journal* in 1958. In a section of that magazine devoted to letters from subscribers on clinical subjects there developed a series of exchanges involving the amount of hair noticed in patients suffering from cancer.

On October 5, 1955, Dr. H. Grundmann wrote in to quote his medical school professor, Dr. H. Eppinger, holder of the Chair of Medicine at Frieburg, Germany, who said, "Beware of the middle aged male patient with hardly a grey hair on his head; he may quite likely have or develop a cancer of his stomach or elsewhere." Dr. Grundmann noted that his teacher had never done any scientific research to back up his statement, but that he made the statement as a result of his observations through his years of practice.

Hair Grew at a Phenomenal Rate

This prompted another letter to the *Journal* (October 29, 1955) from Dr. J. Nesfield. He told of his observations of a female patient, aged 54, suffering from a cancerous tumor of the lymph gland. The lady, when she first became ill had thin, greyish hair, however, during the 18 months of her illness, the patient's hair grew at a phenomenal rate and came in in its original color, dark chestnut, with no grey at all. In the end, the patient had such a luxuriant head of hair that the weight of it was almost too much for her weakened neck muscles to carry. Dr. Nesfield also remarked that his last 5 male cancer patients all had fine heads of hair, although they were grey.

Another interesting observation was recorded in the same issue. Dr. J. H. Bruce wrote of a male patient whom he treated for a year and a half for lung cancer. In the last weeks of illness Dr. Bruce became aware of an unmistakable increase in the length of the patient's eyelashes, an increase far in excess of normal. To attest to the fact that the doctor wasn't just imagining the change, the wife of the man, without any previous mention of the subject by Dr. Bruce, called the doctor's attention to the amazing growth of her husband's eyelashes.

In the February 4, 1956, issue of the *Journal*, G. A. Lista, M.D., quoted the authority, Strompell as saying, ". . . it is striking how frequently patients of over 50, with cancer of the stomach, hardly show a beginning of greying of their hair."

Survey Upholds Theory

Apparently this discussion piqued the curiosity of Cyril G. Eastwood, M.D., even more than it did ours, for he undertook to make a closer, more accurate survey of the relationship between cancer and hair growth. The doctor consulted health department records for the names of one hundred deceased male cancer victims, ranging in age from 30 to 90 years at the time of death. He then wrote to the attending doctors asking for their opinion as to the amount of hair the patient had at death, considering age. Was it more or less than average; did the patient have normally colored hair, or was it grey or white?

The answers bore out previous observations: 40 per cent of the patients had an above-average head of hair; 42 per cent were average, and only 18 per cent had lost their hair to any marked degree. It was concluded that cancer patients are more likely to keep their hair than to lose it.

The information on the color of hair was not very relevant: 70 per cent had hair which varied from grey to white, 20 per cent had retained the natural color of their hair and 10 per cent were characterized by their doctors as normal to grey.

Hormonal Activity

Doctor Eastwood explains the growth of hair as due to a hormonal activity. And this same activity might also be an underlying factor in the cause of cancer. We believe that it could be just as possible that the growth of hair is the result of the body's secretion of extra hormones to combat an invasion of cancer. Perhaps some of these hormones spill over and activate the body's mechanism for hair growth.

Certainly there is no reason to believe that everyone past middle age who has a good head of hair is a prospective cancer victim. As a matter of fact, most evidence we have seen points to the opposite: persons who have plenty of hair live longer, healthier lives. A full and healthy head of hair is obviously intended by nature, as is natural color instead of greyness.

We think that the main value of Dr. Eastwood's work is that it gives researchers another angle from which to attack the mystery of cancer. Is there some true connection between cancer and the growth of hair? Does some specific homonal factor come into play in the presence of cancer which causes hair growth? Perhaps the reason for unusually rapid growth of hair in a cancer patient is the reason for the growth of cancer itself. Doctors treating patients for undetermined disorders might find the relationship between cancer and hair growth a valuable clue. It might lead to needed tests for cancer that might not otherwise have been made.

How does this information affect the ordinary reader? It should help him to remember that the look of health does not always reflect the interior condition. The only way to be certain of one's health is to maintain a proper diet, fortified with necessary food supplements, and to get the proper amounts of rest and exercise. If an article such as this frightens the reader, it is meant to do exactly that. It is the man who complacently thinks of how well he feels, how well he eats or how rich and full his hair is, who could be the cancer victim. Are you eating the average diet that people tell themselves is adequate, or have you eliminated processed foods and added high protein foods with supplementary doses of all the vitamins and minerals you can? If so, you needn't worry about your hair and cancer. If you are scared into doing that by this article, its purpose is fulfilled.

119. Cancer: Possible Side Effect of Polio Vaccine?

A ticking bomb quietly appeared in one of the columns of the *New York Herald Tribune* (June 6, 1961). Earl Ubell, Science Editor for that paper, wrote a story that should have rattled the foundations of American medicine from sea to shining sea. But it didn't, for we saw little more about Mr. Ubell's jarring statement that polio vaccines have been shown to cause cancer in any other paper or journal.

Said he, ". . . the *New York Herald Tribune* reports the detection in the (Salk and Sabin vaccine) monkey broth of a virus that produces cancer in hamsters." (Editor's note: This "broth" is that which scientists use to grow the polio viruses for both live and killed polio vaccines. Some of the broth goes along with the vaccine virus when it is injected or swallowed, so if you or your family have been vaccinated, you have gotten some broth.)

Dr. Bernice Eddy, who, Mr. Ubell says, made the discovery in the course of her work at the United States Public Health Division of Biologic Standards and Control, refused discussion of her findings until a report is published in a scientific journal, as did her boss, Dr. Roderick Murray, who heads the division. However, it is termed by Mr. Ubell an "open secret" among those who work closely with polio virus. So everyone knows about it but us—the ones who get the shots.

One summary of the work tells of Dr. Eddy's taking monkey kidney broth and injecting it into newborn hamsters. In 100 out of 154 cases there were cancers at the site of injection. Three of the cancers were transplanted to other animals and continued to grow. Experiments established the cancer as real, and not a similar, less serious condition.

We're Alarmed—They're Not

When we read this news we were alarmed, as Mr. Ubell says some scientists are: "The central worry . . . arises over the question of cancer. Will any of these viruses, given to babies, now, cause cancer 20 years later?" But the Public Health Service is not worried. "Dr. Luther L. Terry, the Surgeon General of the United States Public Health Service cautioned against any cessation of polio vaccination because of the discovery of the peculiar viruses. Dr. Murray, Dr. Eddy's superior, told the *Herald Tribune* and Dr. Terry that "more research would have to be done to identify the 'cancer agent' but there was no concern at this time nor any reason to stop polio vaccination." They don't know what the virus is, or how serious it could be, but there is "no concern."

In addition to this presumed cancer virus in the monkey broth, scientists both in the United States and England have found other "viruses" in the broth made from the kidneys of apparently healthy monkeys. The chemical treatment used to kill the live viruses in the Salk vaccine does get some but not all of these mysterious viruses. How these viruses will act in the human system no one can say.

Surgeon General Terry has known for some time that certain lots of vaccine have this similar virus. It is known to change the cells in experimental tissue cultures, "but has not caused any disease in human beings even though it will grow in humans. Efforts are being made to eliminate the virus from all future Salk vaccine," says the Public Health Service.

The enormity of this story is difficult to reconcile with the off-handed way it is treated by this government department. Remember, the United States Public Health Service is largely responsible for the launching of the Salk vaccine, its supervision in manufacture and its effect on us as humans and as citizens. The laboratory in which Dr. Eddy made her discovery is supported by this Service, presumably for the very purpose of maintaining a check on just such Public Health projects as the Salk vaccine. Now when one of the scientists chosen to do this type of work comes up with the news that the government has been urging the public to have injections which can cause cancer, the Surgeon General's office is unimpressed. They say, in effect, "We are not sure that Dr. Eddy's findings are correct—not that we're sure she's wrong either, you understand—but don't let it worry you. We intend to do more work on the possibility of cancer caused by Salk shots. Meantime, rush out and get the shots, just in case they don't really cause cancer. And if they do . . . well, don't let that bother you."

Thousands of Possible Cancers

What can these people be thinking of! Thousands of children get polio shots every day. If Dr. Eddy is correct, each of them is freely taking an injection of a possible carcinogen! Is urged to do so by a government health agency! Is held still by a loving parent for what could be an injection of cancer! The Public Health Service doesn't know whether this is the case or not, but it is willing to risk cancer in these thousands of children while Dr. Eddy's work is checked.

This story follows close on the heels of the adverse comments on the Salk vaccine by Dr. Herbert Ratner in the *Journal of the American Medical Association* for February 25, 1961. Dr. Ratner questioned the value of the Salk vaccine on the grounds that the process of production is not

[471]

standardized and neither is the resultant vaccine. No one can be sure exactly what is in the vial of Salk vaccine your doctor uses, unless each is tested individually by him. Dr. Ratner stated then that this means no one who has been inoculated with the Salk vaccine can be sure he has received the shot that carries the proper amount of dead virus to immunize him. He said, further, that anyone hopeful of full immunity would have to be injected with a full series of a new, more potent vaccine whose production has been carefully supervised. Dr. Ratner did not say that such a polio vaccine was available at the time he wrote.

We cannot comprehend the reasoning that would prevent the Public Health Service from doing the logical thing: suspend further polio vaccination until this mess is cleared up! We wonder, too, at the humanity and judgment of science when Mr. Ubell writes: ". . . and the scientists agree, *regardless of their concern over the new development,* (italics ours) polio vaccination must go on. To stop now, they say, would produce catastrophic epidemic." How can anyone say, months before the traditional polio season begins, that a catastrophic epidemic is on its way? Even before the Salk vaccine we had very few polio epidemics, and never could they be forecast. This could be the mildest polio year we've ever had. It should be, if the Salk vaccine is as protective as we are led to believe it is. Americans have been getting shots since 1955, and each year more of us are supposed to be immunized. After 6 years of the immunizing program, surely the danger of a "catastrophic epidemic" should be at a minimum, even though some of us have not been vaccinated.

The question really is: should one take a shot, which has a very doubtful effect in protecting against paralytic polio (a disease whose incidence is one per 3,000) and could invite cancer (fatal in many cases) which is already striking one American in 4? It is difficult to imagine that anyone would chance cancer to prevent the remote possibility of contracting polio, if the choice were actually spelled out for him.

The choice is not to be ours, apparently. The Public Health Service is not telling the public that it must beware of polio shots because they carry a cancer threat. It is saying not a word about any danger. It is telling us to get our Salk shots at once—don't delay, don't hesitate, don't wait for anything!—because they're *safe and effective.*

We wonder how the *Journal of the American Medical Association* will reconcile its recent official preliminary statement in favor of the safety and effectiveness of the Salk vaccine with Dr. Eddy's work and the work of Dr. R. E. Merrill and Dr. R. Batson and D. Kinsman, M.A. These last 3 are the authors of a paper: "Vaccination Status of Patients in an Outbreak of Acute Poliomyelitis." It appeared in the *American Journal of Diseases of Children* (December, 1960, Vol. 100, pp. 857-60), which is a publication of the American Medical Association. It was the aim of these researchers to ascertain the amount of protection given by some or all of the recommended number of Salk injections. They were prompted by the fact that it is probable that "commercially prepared poliomyelitis vaccine is of inconstant potency and therefore produces inconstant degrees of protection." How much could the vaccine be depended upon to protect against paralytic polio?

A high incidence of acute poliomyelitis occurred in the mid-Tennessee area during the summer of 1959, making possible a study of the effects of vaccination with killed virus vaccine (Salk) on the characteristics of the disease.

Sixty-nine persons were seen during the acute phase of the disease, and are included in the study. In each patient the polio diagnosis was confirmed by the commonly accepted techniques. The ages of the patients were from 6 months to 41 years.

In order to evaluate the vaccination status, patients were divided into the following groups: Group A—those who had never received vaccine; Group B—those who had either one or two poliomyelitis vaccine injections at anytime prior to the onset of the disease; Group C—those who had Salk injections, but had received the third one a year or more prior to the onset of the disease; Group D—those who had received 3 or 4 injections of vaccine, the last within the year.

It Just Doesn't Work!

"The study resulted in the following observations" says the report: "(1.) Paralytic poliomyelitis does occur in patients vaccinated with commercially prepared killed virus vaccine, given according to a schedule which is considered acceptable; (2.) the paralysis in such patients, in our series, was comparable to that of the unvaccinated groups; (3.) partial or incomplete vaccination afforded no apparent protection in terms of degree of paralysis; (4.) a preponderance of preschool-age children was noted in this series; and (5.) most of the cases were due to Type I polio virus."

Say the authors, *"It may be concluded that neither partial nor complete vaccinations with commercially prepared vaccines according to presently acceptable schedules necessarily prevents significant paralysis in poliomyelitis."* (Italics ours.)

This commercially prepared vaccine is the stuff your children were given. It is the stuff which was hailed as having reduced paralytic polio more than 90 per cent in vaccinated persons. It is the same stuff the Surgeon General is urging us all to get, in spite of the cancer it might cause. This is the stuff without which the Public Health people say there would be a catastrophic epidemic, the very vaccine which, this test showed just does not work at all.

If you are not convinced of the uselessness of the Salk vaccine, and still intend to have your children injected, we urge you to wait at least until Dr. Eddy's work is confirmed or denied (with proof) officially. Write to the Public Health Service, as we did, demanding to know more about

[473]

Dr. Eddy's work right now. As a citizen, you paid in taxes to have the job done, you have a right to know immediately, and in detail, how it came out, and if you really are in danger in receiving Salk shots. We believe the Salk and Sabin vaccines should be frozen in supply until they are proven—not assumed, but proven—to be safe.

120. Experiments Show Heated Fats Can Cause Cancer

Have you ever passed the exhaust fan from the kitchen of a restaurant? When you do, it is easy to detect the dominating odor of frying fats. These fats bubble and spit in deep fryers for days on end, without even a slight decrease in temperatures, which are held at 350°C. to 400°C. When a customer orders fried chicken or fried shrimp or French-fried potatoes, with them he receives a free sample of the fat in which they were fried. This highly heated fat has been shown by some of our most prominent researchers to be a likely cause of cancer.

Are All Fats Dangerous?

The distinction between highly processed or heated fats and natural ones is important. It would be wrong and dangerous to eliminate all fats from our diet. Our bodies need fats, and we number them among our most important foods. They are one of our best energy sources, offering 9 times as much energy per gram as sugar does. Fats carry the B vitamin pyridoxine and the fat soluble vitamins A, D, E and K, which make fats vital to cell formation, especially cells of the brain and nerve tissues. Finally, the body absolutely needs the unsaturated fatty acids contained in fats. These are indispensable in some processes of metabolism and cell structure. In high heats, the vitamins A, E and K are utterly destroyed. This vitamin destruction is illustrated by an experiment conducted by Dr. Lane and reported in the publication, *Cancer,* Vol. 3, 1950. A group of rats were mated for 3 years into 7 generations. They were on a milk and white bread diet. After the second generation, a ration of lard heated to 350°C., then cooled, was included in the rats' diet. From then on it was found necessary to feed the rats wheat germ oil and fresh vegetables prior to mating, because of the deficiencies in vitamins A and E caused by the preheated fats.

Use of Heated Fats Common

The use of heated fats by Americans is an insidious habit, so automatic that many health-conscious housewives include them in their menus without even being aware of it. For example, the lady who is so concerned for the health of her family that she wouldn't dream of serving deep-fried foods, can be found making a sauce from the drippings of a roast, quite unconscious that half of this liquor is fat that has been heated to 350°C. or more for several hours! Such fat has been made as hot as that used in the deep fryer—and it can be just as damaging.

Some Experiments with Heated Fats

In the periodical, *Cancer*, Vol. 3, No. 6, November, 1950, gastric (i.e. stomach) cancer is noted to be the leading cause of all cancer deaths, according to statistics. Further, Dr. Geoffrey Hadfield, Dean of the Institute of Basic Medical Sciences, Royal College of Surgeons, has stated that cancer of the gastro-intestinal tract appears to be associated with a high fat diet. If this is the case, and if the body needs unprocessed fats as seen before, it is entirely logical that the processed, heated fats are the culprits in the case.

It is especially so when one reads that experiments with local applications of heated fats have shown tumors to develop at the site of the application. The *British Journal of Experimental Pathology* (Vol. 22, 1941) published data on experiments that resulted in cancerous lesions at the site of the injection in two out of twelve mice injected subcutaneously with cottonseed oil which had been preheated to temperatures of 340-360°C. When highly heated fats are brought into close connection with part of the body, apparently a weakness and predisposition toward cancer is introduced to that same part. It should be noted, too, that in the same experiment cottonseed oil heated to a lesser degree (200-220°C.) did not produce any cancerous tumors in any of the experimental mice when injected in the same manner, leading to the conclusion that the dangers in fats vary in proportion to the heat applied.

In searching for clues to this highly heated fat and cancer relationship, a theory has been advanced by Dr. A. C. Ivy in *Gastroenterology* (March, 1955) which holds that hot fats reheated again and again undoubtedly increase the chance of producing carcinogenic substances. Obviously Dr. Ivy feels that there is a dangerous change in the make-up of the fat each time it cools and is fired again, with the intensity of the heat of less importance. This should be a warning to housewives who save cooking fats for re-use.

A similar point of view shows up in the *Journal of Nutrition* (Vol. 55, 1955) in an article which discusses fats heated to relatively low temperatures (95°C.) and maintained at that heat for 200-300 hours. Refined cottonseed oil, heated thusly was included to make up 15 to 20 per cent of the diet of experimental rats. It was observed that rats on such a diet rapidly lost weight and died within 3 weeks. The loss of weight was accompanied by diarrhea and the occurrence of enlarged livers, kidneys, and adrenals and by shrunken spleens and thalami.

In spite of varying theories the strongest suspicion for cancerous ac-

[475]

tion of fats still seems to lie with fats that are preheated to a high degree, as witnessed by Lane and associates and reported in the *Journal of the American Medical Association,* February 17, 1951. In an experiment, 54 rats were given regular rations of brown lard heated for 30 minutes at 350°C. Papillomas (tumors) of the forestomach and malignant tumors of the glandular stomach occurred in 37 per cent of the rats, while similar symptoms were observed in only 5.7 per cent of a control group which was fed unheated lard (though the fat was, of course, heated to make the lard in the first place).

For further data Dr. Lane injected 31 experimental rats with heated lard or vegetable oil. Three cancers developed in these rats, while none developed in a control group of 150.

A definite relationship between preheated fats and cancer showed up in a test discussed in *Modern Nutrition* for August, 1953, the official publication of the American Nutrition Society. A healthful, normal diet was fed to a group of rats. Then the rats were separated into two groups, and the normal diet continued, but for one addition: one of the groups was fed a daily ration of heated, hydrogenated fats, while the other group received a like amount of unprocessed fats.

After the eating pattern of this diet had been well established, a known cancer-producing substance, butter yellow, was introduced into the diet of all the rats. Every one of the rats on the diet which included the preheated, hydrogenated fats developed tumorous growths, some of which proved to be malignant. The rats eating the unprocessed fats developed no tumors of any kind.

What Are Hydrogenated Fats?

Hydrogenated fats are everywhere. They come in cans and jars and cartons, looking as white and creamy as cold cream or yellow as the sun. They are guaranteed not to spoil, for there is nothing left in them that could spoil. And how did they get that way? They have been through about 18 different processes, including boiling, cooling and boiling again, agitation, straining, catalytic action, bleaching, coloring, etc. Every life-removing process imaginable is applied to these fats. Margarines are hydrogenated, too, and the false security bred by the idea that the margarines are not made from animal fats but from vegetable oils is banished in an instant by this fact. Hydrogenation is what makes them spreadable and unmelting in summer temperatures, etc. They are as damaging to health as the frying and baking shortenings that are white and lardy-looking. Nor does the yellow color they are given, and the merchandising technique of presenting margarines in brick-shaped cartons make them as safe for you as "that other spread."

As seen by the various experiments noted here, it is still not generally agreed upon which heated fats do the most damage. Some say the danger lies only in fats heated to very high temperatures, others say it lies in fats heated and reheated, still another impression has it that fats heated for very long periods, even at relatively low temperatures, are the ones to watch out for. But one thing on which all of the experts agree—preheated fats can and may cause cancer! The investigation of treated fats in this connection is still a largely unexplored area. The explanation as to why these fats are antagonistic to our system has yet to be discovered, but the evidence of danger is clear enough to act as a warning.

We are convinced that the body welcomes the vegetable fats much more readily than the fats from animals. If there were no other reason, it is undeniable that most animal fats go through some processing before we get them. This may consist of cooking them at high temperatures in a roasting pan or broiler.

Of course, the vegetable oils (especially those in unheated nuts, sunflower seeds and so forth) have not been thus exposed and they are able to give the body what it needs without the risk of cancer that is lurking in heated fats. But even vegetable and cereal fats, once they are heated, may be cancer-causing.

Some Practical Suggestions

How can you use this information practically in your kitchen? Does it mean that you should stop using fats altogether? Not at all. Here are some rules to follow if you would be absolutely certain you are not exposing your family to this particular risk so far as cancer is concerned.

First, never buy anything that has been fried. This means no potato chips, no roasted nuts, no frozen foods that have been fried or breaded and fried. Steer clear of anything fried in restaurants—fried clams, fish fillets, French-fried potatoes, fried eggplant, etc. Check closely with the waitress on any food where there is the slightest doubt.

By the same token, don't fry foods at home. This means don't do any frying at all, either in deep fat or in a frying pan. Any meat you would fry can be broiled just as successfully. And we advise removing the fat before cooking the meat, if you broil it and also discarding the fat from roasts. Let's say you want to sauté liver. A little vegetable oil—just enough to keep the meat from sticking to the pan—probably couldn't do harm if you keep the heat low at all times.

Finally, don't buy hydrogenated shortenings (the solid kind) and don't ever, ever use drippings or oils over and over again. There is the risk of such fats being rancid, and, of course, there is the additional risk that they may be cancer-causing.

121. Cancer and Antibiotics

In the United States, recorded deaths from lung cancer for the period 1935 to 1948 increased over 140 per cent. The mortality rate for all other forms of cancer increased by only 31 per cent. In England somewhat the same thing has happened and according to projections made by statisticians the rate will continue to increase at about the same speed. On the other hand, the primitive races in Asia and Africa show no increase in the incidence of cancer. Why should such a situation exist?

Many authorities have placed the blame for the terrible increase in lung cancer on air pollution and smoking. Indeed the evidence against these two villains is overwhelming. And it appears that the more we study the matter, the more information we discover leading us to the inescapable conclusion that these two factors have at least a large share of responsibility for the present frightening status of lung cancer incidence.

However, B. A. Meyer and J. D. Benjafield of London, writing in the *Medical Press* for August 31, 1955, say there has been no comparable increase in cancer of the larynx. If you are inhaling the smoke of a cancer-causing cigarette or a cancer-causing layer of smog, the concentrated strength of the deadly agent would seem to be brought to bear on the larynx or voice box. By the time this puff of whatever-it-is reaches the lungs, it has been somewhat diluted and furthermore it is then spread out over thousands of little cells in the lungs. How does it happen, then, that cancer of the larynx has not increased at the same rate as lung cancer?

Antibiotics Enter The Picture

In 1928, penicillin was discovered, say Doctors Meyer and Benjafield. In 1935, sulfanilamide therapy was born. Since then we have had all manner of antibiotics and the list grows almost daily. Sir Arthur Fleming, discoverer of penicillin, showed that it is a powerful killer of bacteria in concentrations that were harmless to the tissues of the body. "Antibiotics are by far the greatest life-saving discovery in the history of medicine, and most of the antibiotics are relatively innocuous when compared with antiseptics, but it seems that a minority of patients are sensitive or allergic to some of them. The impairment of their therapeutic value through reckless and indiscriminate use is a very serious matter, for they are too frequently given for mild infections, such as coughs, colds, coryza (sniffles), sinusitis and many respiratory infections, no matter how trivial they may be. Patients often demand penicillin injections from their doctors and many a doctor is forced to give them lest he should offend the patient and be thought not to be keeping abreast of modern methods," say Drs. Meyer and Benjafield.

Now antibiotics have no killing effect at all on viruses, so any disease caused by a virus will not be cured by a dose of antibiotic. But is it not possible, ask these thoughtful and probing writers, that, if cancer is due to a virus, the antibiotics may damage tissue in such a way that the body does not feel the need to bring into play the normal mechanism that protects against viruses—a mechanism that has been acquired over the many thousands of years that man has lived on the earth! Perhaps in addition the antibiotic may upset the virus-bacteria balance and so predispose the tissues to invasion by cancer cells.

Doesn't it seem to you that this theory may explain *in part* at least the seeming immunity of some individuals to cancer? Here is a man, let's say, who boasts that he has always smoked many cigarettes, yet he has no disposition toward cancer. Might not his apparent immunity stem from the fact that he has never been ill with the kind of disorder for which antibiotics are used? On the other hand, you can find additional evidence that seems to back up the theory in the fact that smokers in general *do* suffer from frequent colds and often chronic coughs—the very kind of thing for which the antibiotics are given. People who live in areas where there is air pollution may get more frequent colds. Might the antibiotics they take for the colds be partly responsible for their incidence of lung cancer?

To get back to the article in the *Medical Press,* our theorists remind us that town dwellers have more cancer of the lung than country dwellers. And the primitive countries show no increase in lung cancer such as the so-called "civilized" countries show. Town dwellers have more and closer doctors than rural folks. Since antibiotics are fashionable, they are freely given in cities where doctors are up-to-date and patients are demanding. In the country, with its few and far-between doctors and its complete lack of medical clinics, how many people insist on having antibiotics for slight colds? And in the primitive countries, of course, doctors and antibiotics are both so rare that there would be no such problem there.

We feel that this theory should be thoroughly investigated by research organizations. Perhaps it may reveal something very significant. And meanwhile, it certainly behooves all of us to keep our bodies so healthy that we will never have to take antibiotics for some serious illness. Certainly none of us should *ever* take them for a minor illness.

122. Rimless Eyeglasses and Skin Cancer

A most unusual and at the same time reasonable explanation for a currently very common kind of skin cancer is presented in an article by 4 Philadelphia and New Jersey physicians. The article illustrates well, we believe, the fact that explanations for serious conditions may often be so simple and obvious that we tend to overlook them.

Do you know anyone who wears rimless eyeglasses? Did you ever take a good look at this individual when he was sitting with his back to a window through which the sun was streaming? Did you notice that the lenses of his glasses reflect the sunlight onto two spots on his cheeks? If you have ever lighted a piece of paper by turning on it sunlight through a curved piece of glass, you know that the sun's rays, reflected in this manner, can produce considerable heat. So your friend with the rimless eyeglasses is probably exposed, every time he is in the sunlight, to a certain degree of solar heat, concentrated always on the same spot of his cheeks, below his eyeglasses.

This observation is what started the research done by Drs. Edward F. Corsan, George M. Knoll and Herbert A. Luscombe of Philadelphia and Dr. Henry B. Decker of Camden, New Jersey. They reported their findings in a paper read at a meeting of the American Dermatological Association April 27, 1948. They tell us that an important writer on skin disease, G. C. Andrews, in discussing cancers of the skin of the face, declares that over 40 per cent of them occur in this region of the face—just below the edge of the eyeglasses. This is the region, say our authors, where light from behind and overhead is focused directly on the cheek by certain types of spectacle lenses. It does not matter apparently whether the lenses are round or elliptical, or how the lens has been ground to correct the individual's eyesight. In every case they examined, there was a certain degree of refraction of light down onto the cheek. Testing to see how they might shut off this reflection, the doctors found that a substance called rim black could be applied around the upper or lower edge of the lenses and immediately the concentration of light disappeared.

Then the researchers decided to test the heat produced by these reflected rays. They placed the person to be tested first in sunlight, then in the light of a 500 watt photoflood lamp and a 100 watt electric light bulb. Thirteen tests of 3 different persons showed that the temperature in the area just below the glasses was from one to 3 degrees higher than the temperature outside this area. The photoflood lamp brought a temperature of 2 to 4 degrees higher to this area. An ordinary lamp bulb produced no difference in temperature.

They found, too, that rimless lenses which have a different shape (hexagonal) or a straight lower edge did not focus the light quite so directly and hence did not cause so great an increase in temperature.

Evidence from Cancer Patients

They then discuss 12 cases of skin cancer, which appeared to be related to the wearing of rimless glasses. In the first case, a man of 47 who had worn glasses since he was 18, the cancer appeared on his right cheek at exactly the spot where light rays were reflected. The second patient was 51 and, once again, a beam of light turned on over his head focused into a sharp, bright spot just below his glasses where the cancer had appeared. A woman, aged 49, who liked to garden in bright sunlight with no hat, showed a defined area of her face where light was reflected. And in this area the cancer was located. The same circumstances were true with each of the other 9 patients. In no case did the spectacles actually touch the skin of the cheek, so the lump or spot could not possibly have been caused by the glass rubbing against the cheek and irritating it.

Rimless glasses are not as popular as they once were. But many people still wear them, especially middle-aged or older folks who are, of course, the most likely victims for cancer to strike.

If you know anyone who wears rimless glasses, you might suggest that he get his family to observe him standing in bright sunlight, to see whether or not the light is concentrated to one spot below his glasses. In fact, it might be wise for all of us who wear glasses to check on whether or not our "specs" are refracting light on our cheeks. In case you find that your own glasses are doing just this, you won't necessarily have to buy a new pair, incidentally. The optician can paint the rims with rim black or he can change the rims, giving you a pair made of some of the new light plastics or metal. Apparently, any rim around the edge of the lens breaks the rays of light and guarantees against damage.

123. Is Cancer Related to Nutrition?

Would you say that how much you eat has anything to do with whether or not you will get cancer? Would you say that someone who eats processed foods might be more, or less, susceptible to cancer than someone who eats foods in their natural state? Would you say that there are any vitamins which might protect you against some forms of cancer?

The answers to questions like these and many more that are intriguing to readers are to be found in a little book, *Cancer, New Approaches, New*

Hope, by Boris Sokoloff, M.D., Ph.D., of Florida Southern College, published by Devin-Adair, New York. Dr. Sokoloff is a cancer researcher and in this book, he tries to present and help the layman to understand more about cancer research and also help him to live so that he can possibly avoid cancer.

It is, of course, in this last matter that we are interested. And Dr. Sokoloff has done such a good job, as far as he goes, that we wish he had gone further. For instance, in his chapter on nutrition and cancer, Sokoloff relates the stories of how brewer's yeast and desiccated liver prevented liver tumors in laboratory animals who were given a cancer-causing substance.

All of the animals were kept on a diet low in protein and containing a substance called "butter yellow" which is a coal tar dye known to produce liver tumors or cancer. Adding dried liver in a proportion of about 10 per cent to the cancer-causing diet brought about a distinct decrease in the number of cancers among the animals. Adding brewer's yeast (3 to 5 per cent of the original diet) to the animals' food also brought down the incidence of liver cancer. The investigators then began to search for what particular element in yeast and liver might be responsible. It turned out to be riboflavin, one of the B vitamins. Adding riboflavin alone, together with a protein, casein, reduced the incidence of cancer to 3 per cent. According to Dr. Sokoloff, this fact is well known by physicians who now regularly give riboflavin for cases of cirrhosis of the liver (which might, of course, precede cancer).

But what kind of an approach is this? Would it not be a little more helpful to discover whether or not riboflavin added to the diet of human beings helps prevent cancer? Do you know any human being who would not willingly be a subject for such an experiment?—taking a B vitamin which could not possibly do him any harm and would almost certainly benefit him in many ways aside from the probability that it would protect him from cancer of the liver? It is well known among nutritionists, incidentally, and has been shown in many surveys that the American people are woefully short on riboflavin. Could this be one of the main reasons why cancer incidence is increasing by leaps and bounds in our country?

Natural Versus Processed Food

Sokoloff tells us that "when rats and mice are kept on natural (stock) diet, they are less predisposed to develop cancer than are animals kept on purified feed." What does he mean by that? He means that animals which get natural food in as nearly its natural state as possible are less likely to get cancer than are animals which get food that has been processed until the natural food elements are gone from it. In other words, the kind of diet many Americans live on exclusively. A diet consisting of sucrose (purified sugar), casein (a protein), degerminated corn (the kind you get in cornmeal) gave 90 per cent of the rats in one experiment breast cancer and they died from 6 to 7 months sooner than rats given "natural" foodstuffs—that is, we suppose, whole corn, meat or eggs rather than casein, fruits and vegetables rather than refined sugar.

Sokoloff says, "Why the animals kept on a purified diet are more susceptible to cancer-producing substances is not known." The fat, vitamin and mineral content was the same in both diets. Is it possible, he asks, that something happens to the food during processing which causes it to become cancer-causing? It remains an open question which deserves the full attention of investigators, says Sokoloff.

Indeed it does, sir, and there is apparently no one in this country who is willing to admit, even, that such an experiment has already been carried out.

Did you ever hear of any such experiment from the National Cancer Society which is supposedly dedicated to the prevention and cure of cancer? Did your national magazines ever carry stories about these experiments indicating that it might be wise to avoid processed food, *just in case,* even though the full laboratory proof of their effect on human beings is not available?

Why do you suppose material like this is not widely publicized? The experiments were reported in the professional magazine *Cancer Research* in 1952.

Overeating and Overweight are Dangerous

Has your Cancer Society ever warned you that overeating may be a cause of cancer? In an experiment on overeating reported as long ago as 1940, two groups of mice were used, both from a strain of mice developed purposely to be very susceptible to breast cancer. Both groups were kept on the same diet. But one group was allowed to eat all they wanted, which turned out to be about 3 grams a day. The other group was restricted as to diet, being allowed only 2 grams a day. The mice of the group whose diet was restricted *had no cancerous growths at all,* even though they came from a strain of mice highly susceptible to breast cancer. Of the mice which ate an unrestricted diet, more than half developed cancer after 90 weeks. In later experiments the same general idea was proven again and again with liver cancer, lung cancer, skin cancer. All types of tumors investigated were prevented by a restricted diet and *"as yet no tumor has been found that does not respond in this way."*

Even a slight restriction in diet affects the incidence of cancer in mice. One group given 3.2 grams of food daily developed 54 per cent cancer growth, while another group given 2.3 grams of the same food developed 22 per cent and the third group given only 2 grams developed no tumors at all.

Does this mean that you should starve yourself to a shadow? Not at all. The mice who ate less appeared to be much healthier than those who overate. Did they have to eat the restricted diet all their lives in order to be protected from cancer? No. It seems that the important time is when the mouse is approaching middle age—the time when the cancer

[483]

is most likely to appear. Restricting the diet for a time just before this period will prevent the cancer and allow the rat to live to a healthy old age. But in every experiment, the more the diet is restricted in calories, the less is the incidence of cancerous growth.

In further experiments it was found that the *kind* of diet was also important. Increasing the protein and decreasing the carbohydrates *in every case* brought less cancer. What kind of lesson is this for us in modern America where more than 50 per cent of our diet is made up of refined sugar and white flour and products made from them? Why is it that our government agencies, the nutrition departments of our great universities and the private agencies that exist for preventing cancer have not broadcast this news the length and breadth of the land—a land in which overweight from overeating is the most widespread disease of all?

In *Look* magazine for June 12, 1956, there is a big hullabaloo about a new diet for reducing—a diet on which you can eat all the goodies you supposedly long for—a diet low in protein and high in carbohydrate. Such a diet is likely to become very popular. Refined white sugar is unrestricted in this diet—you can eat as much as you want of it! What will be the toll in cancer incidence over the next decade among weak-willed followers of this so-called scientific diet, which breaks every law of nutrition we have painfully learned over the years? Do you hear the American Cancer Society protest against the publication of this diet, considering the facts they know about the experiments described above?

Chemical Poisons and Vitamin C

There are many chemical substances in daily use all about us which are known to cause cancer. Arsenic is one of these. It is used on tobacco leaves which are later smoked. And, of course, all of the arsenic cannot possibly be removed. It is used as an insecticide on fruits and vegetables which we eat. Listen to what happens to a normal healthy mouse when its skin is painted with a substance known to cause cancer. Dr. Sokoloff is speaking, "long before this growth is detected, noticeable changes in the tissue of the mouse might be observed. The intercellular substance, which binds together the cells, undergoes peculiar changes. It loses some of its binding properties. The binding factor which holds the cells together and makes from thousands of cells an organized unit is less effective. The cells are less adhesive each to the other, more free to move and to live independently."

Researchers on vitamin C have told us that this is the vitamin which is responsible for the substance that holds cells together. Unless you have enough vitamin C, this intercellular cement will disintegrate gradually and the cells will fall apart.

We know, too, that vitamin C fights against poisons introduced into our bodies. And that it is used up in the battle. Could it not be that the vitamin C of a tissue painted with a cancer-causing substance is used up in a vain effort to counteract the poison, and from that point on the cells begin their disintegration which eventually leads to cancer? If so, what of us, surrounded as we are with poisons—breathing them, drinking them, eating them, every day? And, incidentally, getting less and less vitamin C every day as our food preserving, transporting and processing facilities get ever more efficient! Who would eat a piece of fresh fruit, when orange juice is available at the store in a carton, or grape juice in a can? Of course, there isn't a chance that there's much vitamin C in the juice by the time it reaches you, but never mind! The important thing is to save time, and show how up-to-date you are by buying what the ads tell you to buy.

Incidentally, along with riboflavin, which we mentioned earlier, vitamin C is the element most likely to be lacking in American diet, according to nutrition surveys. Is it coincidence that pre-cancerous cells show breakdown in the substance vitamin C helps to manufacture?

We have another note on cancer prevention which is not mentioned in Sokoloff's book but which we consider vitally important—a piece of research done by Ehrenfried E. Pfeiffer at his laboratory at Threefold Farms, Spring Valley, New York in 1948-49, which was financed by the Soil and Health Foundation. Two groups of mice were fed—one with food raised with chemical fertilizer and the other with organic fertilizer. The experiment proved that the group of mice fed with the organically raised food was much healthier than the other. In a strain of mice chosen for their susceptibility to cancer, the survival rate was 64 per cent in the organically-fed mice and only 35 per cent in those fed commercially-raised food.

Heeding Dr. Sokoloff's Advice

Is there any conceivable reason why we do not hear, in ringing, confident, challenging words, in every publication put out by the government and the cancer agencies, the astonishing facts about the relation of nutrition and cancer, presented so casually but nevertheless with scrupulous scientific accuracy by the respectable cancer researcher, Dr. Boris Sokoloff?

We do not go along with the theory that telling these facts about nutrition and cancer will "raise false hopes" in the minds of readers. We do not, of course, have positive proof that these same facts hold good for human beings. But we believe that every scrap of information about nutrition that might possibly be helpful in the fight against disease should be broadcast. How can readers use the facts we have presented here?

1. Overeating is deadly. One reason we overeat is that our food does not nourish us. Getting plenty of vitamins and minerals in our meals and in food supplements will help us to establish normal eating habits again.

2. Diets high in carbohydrates may be conducive to cancer. From the other information in the book, we would say this indicates eliminating from your diet the refined carbohydrates, not good natural foods like potatoes and beans, because . . .

[485]

3. Refined and processed diets create more cancer than completely natural ones.

4. The B vitamins (of which riboflavin is a most important member) are instrumental in preventing some kinds of cancer. Most of us are deficient in B vitamins and it is almost impossible to get enough of them in modern diets without supplementing your meals with brewer's yeast, wheat germ or desiccated liver.

5. Vitamin C, so essential to help the body fight against poisons, may be a preventive of cancer. Eat fresh raw fruits and vegetables and take natural rose-hip vitamin C supplements to make sure you are getting enough.

124. Cancer and Poor Nutrition

"If man would keep himself fit instead of fat, the chances are that cancer would be less of a menace to the human race than it is. There is evidence from animal experiments that caloric restriction reduces the incidence of several types of tumors; there is statistical evidence, from various insurance companies, that overweight persons have a distinctly greater tendency for developing cancer."

These words are from *The Challenge of Cancer,* published by the National Cancer Institute, a department of the Public Health Service. So even the most conservative sources of information recognize that cancer is definitely related to diet. Yet the average M. D., asked if cancer has anything to do with diet, will tell you that such ideas are the disproved notions of food faddists and cranks.

There is much material available showing that diet influences the incidence of cancer. We will simply list some of the articles we have on it and comment briefly. First, some evidence we collected from a Spanish medical magazine, *Revista clinica espanola* for October 15, 1956. It describes an experiment in which 120 people living in a residential home for the aged were divided into two groups, an experimental group and a control group. The experimental group received a diet amounting to 2300 calories on alternate days. On the other day, they received only about a quart of milk and a pound of fresh fruit. The control group received the 2300 calorie diet every day.

At the end of 3 years the number of days in which persons in either group had reported to the hospital department of the home was twice as great for persons in the control group as for those who got a so-called starvation diet every other day. The incidence of heart and blood vessel disease, cancer and bronchitis was twice as high in those in the control group. The results of the experiment showed, the authors feel, that the hunger diet on alternate days maintains a feeling of well-being in the elderly and prolongs the health and life span. Chalk up point one for a sensible, moderate diet, high in natural foods.

2. As long ago as 1946, D. H. Copeland and W. D. Salmon at the Alabama Polytechnic Institute published in the *American Journal of Pathology* for September, 1946, the results of their experiments with rats in which they showed that a deficiency in just one of the B vitamins, choline, resulted in an incidence of 58 per cent cancer in laboratory rats, whereas the second group of rats, fed exactly the same diet, with added choline, had no cancers at all. In 1950, E. R. Jaffe, R. W. Wisser and E. P. Benditt reported in the *American Journal of Pathology* for September, 1950, that rats given high amounts of choline and two of the amino acids (forms of protein), methionine and cystine, had far less cirrhosis of the liver than those which received less. This disease is closely related to cancer of the liver.

3. The *Denver Post* for December 12, 1954, told of the findings of Dr. Clarence G. Salsbury, Arizona's Public Health Commissioner, who found that the Navajo Indians, ravaged by disease for centuries, were very infrequently victims of cancer. Of 60,000 hospital admissions among Navajos, only 208 cancer cases had ever been seen. Among 118 female cases only 3 breast cancers had ever been recorded. "The typical primitive Navajo diet does not include highly refined foods," Salsbury said. "It consists mainly of meat, corn, squash, some fruits and nuts, herbs, native tea and 'squaw bread'—a type of crisp panbread. That simple diet may be the key to the comparative lack of cancer. But just why or how we don't yet know."

4. *Nutrition Reviews* for March, 1956, reviewed the subject of overweight and cancer and showed that restricting the diets of laboratory animals "markedly delayed" the appearance of both spontaneous and experimentally induced cancers.

5. An article by Associated Press Science Editor, Howard Blakeslee, tells of the theory of Dr. F. E. Chidester, author of a book, *Nutrition and Glands in Relation to Cancer*. Dr. Chidester believes that in the early stages of vitamin deficiency the human glands are overactive. This extra activity causes the body to lose enormous amounts of calcium, iodine and iron and, he claims, leads to goiter, anemia, diabetes, nerve degeneration, rickets, ulcers and so forth. In the later stages of vitamin deficiency, when the glands have become exhausted, a form of fat accumulates which leads to gallstones, cataracts, hardening of the arteries and the most malignant cancers. Dr. Chidester says vitamins are extremely important for keeping the glands working properly. He says that vitamins A, B and E have been tested in experimental cancers of animals with good results and that they have also been beneficial in some cases of human cancer.

6. Dr. W. C. Hueper of the National Cancer Institute, the gentleman who speaks so forcefully against chemicals in foods as possible cancer-causers, said that some dietary factors that affected the incidence of cancer were well established, according to an article in the *Milwaukee*

Journal for October 11, 1956. Obesity is one. The amount of protein in the diet appears to be another, since liver cancer is much more common in nations in Asia and Africa where there is little protein in the diet. There are many substances added to our food today which may be found some day soon to be cancer-causers, he said. The finding of gastrointestinal cancers mostly at sites where the stomach or intestines narrow, slowing the passage of food so that it is in contact longer there, was additional evidence that what we eat might influence the production of cancers. He predicted that, when more is learned about dietary factors in cancer, the disease would be controlled.

7. Seymour J. Kreshover, D.D.S., and John J. Salley, D.D.S., writing in the *Journal of the American Dental Association* for April, 1957, tell us that deficiency in vitamins A and B are definitely known to be responsible for some mouth cancers. Cancer of the female reproductive organs can result from lack of vitamin A—in many cases caused by faulty absorption of the vitamin due to lack of hydrochloric acid in the stomach.

8. A high consumption of salt may be responsible for a predisposition to cancer. There is a low incidence of the disease among peoples who use little salt. It is true, that too much salt in the diet may produce a mineral imbalance, since the sodium of table salt is the chemical enemy of potassium—a mineral in which we are likely to be deficient.

9. In Editor Rodale's book, *Cancer, Can It Be Prevented?* (sorry, out of print) he describes the possible threat of sulfur in foods in relation to cancer. Earlier in the book he talked of the Green theory of cancer—that sulfur-containing smoke from chimneys may have a great deal to do with cancer incidence. If sulfur in smoke can cause cancer, what about sulfur in food? Sulfur is used almost universally in dried foods, such as prunes, raisins and so forth; it is also used in the processing of many, many other foods. Alum, for instance, widely used in food and in drinking water, is made by treating bauxite with sulfuric acid.

10. *Newsweek* for November 28, 1949, told of experiments performed at the Medical Research Department of the University of Toronto. For 6 weeks researchers fed one group of rats on alcohol instead of drinking water and another group of rats the same amount of sugar as that contained in the alcohol. Both sets of rats lost their appetite for food containing choline, that most important B vitamin which protects the liver from harm. Another indication of the deadly nature of sugar. Isn't it pathetic to think of all the fine, earnest American mothers, horrified at the thought of giving alcohol to their children, but who regularly feed them a substance that is just as harmful from the point of view of good health—white sugar! The liver, as we know, is one of the most important organs in the body and its health is essential for preventing cancer.

11. Another link in the chain tying cancer to poor nutrition comes from an article in *Science* for April 12, 1946, by Drs. J. Ernest Ayre and W. A. G. Bauld of the Royal Victoria Hospital and McGill University,

Montreal. These researchers believe that the lack of a B vitamin, thiamin, may be the first link in a chain leading by way of the liver and female hormones to cancer of the uterus. "If tests show a dangerous precancerous linkage between low vitamin and high female hormone concentration, prevention of cancer might be possible through corrective treatment."

The doctors suggest that the vitamin lack might begin to operate by damaging the liver. This damage might be slight, so slight that it could not be perceived by any known tests of liver function. But even so, it might be enough to keep the liver from inactivating female hormones which is one of its functions. This material might, then, accumulate in the body and cause cancer of the uterus.

Studies of 23 patients as well as various laboratory experiments give, say the scientists, "excellent circumstantial evidence that the nutritional deficiency may have been a primary factor leading to the malignancy." Has your cancer society or your doctor ever told you of such a theory? And if not, why not? The B vitamins are practically nonexistent for many modern women, in whose diets coffee, soft drinks, bakery products, packaged desserts and sweets play a big part. Doesn't it seem likely that present-day food habits have a lot to do with cancer of the uterus, in the light of this theory?

125. Nature-Conforming Nutrition and Cancer Prevention

(*Some observations on the problem of Cancer, the civilization disease, from an article by P. G. Seeger, M.D., in the medical magazine* Hippokrates, *Vol. 13, 1951, translated from the German.*)

In a lecture on the principles of oncology (the study of tumors) and the crisis of cancer research, A. Greil, at the first Austrian Cancer Congress, 1949, emphasized that "primitive forest-nomads living from hand to mouth with completely natural habits of eating and propagating are utterly incapable of producing abnormal cancerous tissues." During a 10-year residence in East Asia, J. Pick proved the fact that cancer is a rare disease among natural peoples who also do not eat meat. An English physician confirmed this observation during a 9-year stay in Tibet where he was able to establish the existence of only 3 cancer cases. The disease is also said to be rarer in Russia than in other European countries and statistics show it to be more prevalent in cities rather than in the countryside and to occur in higher economic brackets rather than in poorer sections. These differences seem to rest on the more nature-conforming and simple diet of poorer people and farmers.

In 1932 Schrumpf-Pierron found that malignant cancers were 10 times more common in Europe and America than in Egypt and that the degree of malignancy—when they did occur—was far less among Egyptians. The native peasants of Egypt rarely sicken with cancer. However, as they adopt European customs and collect in cities, abandoning their ancestral ways of diet, just to such an extent does their immunity to cancer disappear. According to statistics from South Africa, cancer is extremely rare among the natural-living African peoples there. However, with the adoption of the white man's way of life, including white bread, white sugar and cooked food, the cancer rate rises proportionately and is highest among those sections of the population who have intermarried with the whites. With truth does A. Waerland state: "Civilized man is the only living creature on the earth who defiles his food before he devours it." In this one sentence he touches on the most basic fact of the entire cancer problem, Dr. Seeger believes.

Oxidation—Enzymes

The separation from nature that begins with city-dwelling, in association with civilization-dictated ways of living, requires that civilized man adopt a diet consisting almost exclusively of cooked, therefore denatured, substances. The cooking results in a deficiency of chlorophyll (the substance that makes plants green) and consequently a deficiency in all the products which chlorophyll assists in manufacturing in the body. All living things require oxygen which, by the process of oxidation, changes food into energy and growth. This process is aided by the presence of chlorophyll. If little or no chlorophyll is present, all the other substances created or influenced by it in this very complex process are also deficient. These substances are called oxidation-enzymes. The result, therefore, is an impoverishment of the organism in the vital oxidation-enzymes and in the vitamins, especially vitamin C. Cancer cells always show a complete absence of vitamin C.

After 15 years of research, Dr. Seeger's theory on the origin of cancer is (greatly simplified): the cancer virus passes into the cells of a new born child through the placenta or in mother's milk. Up to a certain age the cells of young organisms contain enough oxidation-enzymes to provide for the oxidation process, so that viruses and bacteria are checked and remain in the cells without producing disease. But when, as a result of age and improper nourishment, a deficiency of these enzymes occurs, the virus grows and propagates, unchecked, along with malignant degeneration of the cells. It has been proved that cancer cells do not contain 3 of the enzymes which are active in the process of oxidation. Cancer cells have also been found to be deficient in cytochromes, another substance important in oxidation. These discoveries suggest that deficiency of these substances in the human body may cause, or partially cause, the growth of cancer.

Enzyme Deficiency Traced to Devitalized Food

A condition of deficient oxygen often exists not only in cancer cells but in pre-cancerous ones and in the total organism as well. As a result of this, the molecules of protein in the cells regroup themselves and become instead giant virus molecules. So even without an actual virus infection, a formation of a virus is possible simply because of a deficiency of the various oxidation-enzymes. There follows in Dr. Seeger's article the description of other very complex changes that take place in the structure of the cells under these circumstances, including the release of several substances found in cancer cells. This entire breaking-down process in the cell appears to be the result of deficiency in the oxidation-enzymes, because of the denatured and devitalized food which forms "civilized" diet.

Vitamins

In addition to the oxidation-enzymes, the vitamins have a great significance in the origin of cancer. Cancer cells lack vitamins C, B, and A. Cancerous and even pre-cancerous organisms have a terrific deficiency in them. Through a continued deficiency of vitamin A, an idleness in vitamin C supply occurs and the vitamin C is not replaced quickly enough. Hence a deficiency in vitamin C will always exist. The presence of vitamin C is of utmost importance in the entire oxidation process that takes place in the cells. Vitamin A is also important, for the presence of vitamin A brings about the decomposition of certain fatty acids. Through a deficiency in vitamin A the increase of these fatty acids in cancer cells can be explained.

Greatest attention should be paid to the vitamin B_1 deficiency caused by the use of white flour and white bread. On the other hand, vitamin B_1, along with vitamin C, may increase twice and even threefold the oxidation-enzymes in the blood, which are so important to the whole oxidation process.

Contrary to the opinion held by the majority of doctors, the cause of cancer has nevertheless something to do with a natural diet and a healthy way of living. Anyone who for a period of 10 years nourishes himself falsely and has an intake of denatured food (that is, a man who omits the items of raw diet and chlorophyll that are needed as suppliers of oxidation-enzymes and vitamins) is on the best way to kill himself with his diet; he has good reason to be fearful of death by cancer. Complete vegetarianism will not be necessary to prevent this, but there is a need for the liver and muscles, for example, to contain considerable quantities of oxidation-enzymes found only in green, leafy vegetables.

The respiratory system consists of systems for the oxidation of the cells and of the smallest blood vessels, the capillaries. The cells are violently disturbed in a cancerous condition. But the capillaries, too, are damaged by denatured diet, the result of which is impaired blood and oxygen supply. Certainly fruits and vegetables rich in enzymes and vitamins are necessary for a healthy, efficient circulatory system, filled with easily flowing blood.

[491]

Disturbance of the inner respiratory system is not the only basis for the cause of cancer, but it is the chief factor, claims Dr. Seeger. The basis of the disturbance is unnatural, denatured diet.

In addition, Dr. Seeger believes that most persons breathe superficially, with only about one-fourth to one-third of their lung capacity. He says that the farmer working in fresh air breathes better than the city dweller seated at an office desk. One consequence of improper breathing is, of course, a decreased supply of oxygen which creates the danger of the oxygen-deficient disturbances we have described. We suggest that the farmer who certainly gets more oxygen in his fresh-air job also needs more oxygen to carry on his heavy physical work, while the city dweller does little hard physical work sitting at a desk, hence needs less oxygen.

Salt, civilization's poison, dare not be forgotten. Salt causes not only increased cramping of the capillaries, but it has also been shown to be concentrated in body cells becoming increasingly cancerous, in reaction to which its biological opponent, potassium, fails. Under the influence of 10 milligrams of salt the activity of one of the oxidation-enzymes in human blood falls to one-half and even one-third of its normal value. As a result of this, cooking salt has a direct effect in stimulating cancer, says Dr. Seeger.

Also to be mentioned are the cancer-producing artificial coloring matters used in food processing, whose effect is to impair and destroy oxidation-enzymes. Although the use of butter yellow (one of these deadly coloring matters) has been prohibited by law, there are many other coloring matters now being used in candy, ice cream, etc., which are looked at with grave suspicion by many cancer experts.

The editors of this book are not convinced of the value of vegetarianism, for we favor a diet high in protein and feel certain that some portion of this protein must be eaten in meats. Nor do we favor eating all vegetables raw. Waterless cooking at low heat, or cooking with as little water as possible preserves nearly all of the vitamins and minerals.

126. Does Gardening Prevent Cancer?

By J. I. RODALE

In the early part of 1955, while reading the January 22 issue of the *Medical Journal of Australia,* I was jounced out of a state of tranquillity by a letter which appeared in the correspondence column of that journal. As I read it, I could not believe my eyes, for it had astounding implications. Here it is:

"Sir: It is my clinical impression that patients who are active gardeners have a much greater host resistance to internal carcinoma (cancer) than do non-gardeners. Their survival period appears to be far greater in my experience. Whether this assumption is coincidental and false could be ascertained by practitioners working in city, suburban and country districts. May I, with respect, suggest this observation be made, and if established, submitted to the biochemists.

Yours, etc.

ERIC GOULSTON, M.D.,

Sydney, December 20, 1954."

You can well imagine my excitement at the discovery of this item and I lost no time in getting off a letter to Dr. Goulston, as follows:

"Dear Dr. Goulston:

"I read your letter in the January 22, 1955, issue of the *Medical Journal of Australia* and I am wondering if you could give me more information about cancer and gardeners. We publish the magazine ORGANIC GARDENING AND FARMING, which represents Sir Albert Howard's idea of farming or gardening with non-chemical fertilizers.

Sincerely yours,

J. I. RODALE, *Editor.*"

Under date of April 4, 1955, I received the following reply from Dr. Goulston:

"Dear Mr. Rodale,

"Thank you for your letter concerning cancer and gardeners. All I can say is that I have noticed over the years that there seems to be a greater host resistance against cancer in patients who are suffering from this disease and who delve in the garden, than is the case with complete non-gardeners. This may be due to some anti-carcinogenic agent ingested from soils or from plants. We are trying to investigate this problem biochemically but haven't got very far, so that at present, it is only a clinical impression.

"I would be very interested to learn if any similar work is being done in the States. Your idea of not farming with chemical fertilizers, would make an interesting study for a surgeon in your district to investigate and compare the incidence of cancer there as with other centres.

"I would like to hear from you again. I hope to visit the States next year, and if in Pennsylvania, I should like to make your acquaintance."

Here is a doctor after my own heart, and it would be a pleasure to meet him.

Logic would seem to tell us that the good doctor is on the right track, for gardeners grow their own vegetables, thus eating fresh foods. Gardeners live more of an outdoor life, breathing the fresh air, exercising more, bending over as they weed, which improves the tone of the stomach muscles. I recall seeing some cancer figures which showed that rural folk get less cancer than city people, which could be because they garden more. But yet, I was not satisfied. I felt vaguely that these factors somehow were only a part of the whole picture and I therefore kept probing and seeking over the next few days. Then an idea struck me!

It is a known fact that the earth contains electricity and magnetism, and gives them off in a steady stream. In fact, it has been said that the world is one big magnet. We know also that the body is an electrical power station, every cell being charged with electricity. Could it not be possible, therefore, that in placing the hands in the soil, an electric circuit between the body and earth is completed, and that some of the ground electricity gently begins to course through the body, invigorating the latter? In other words, if a person gardens every day, is he or she receiving a healthful daily electrical treatment?

How the Body Functions Electrically

Let us go a little further into this realm of thinking and see if we can find examples of the way the body functions electrically. That there is electricity in the body was proven by Nobel prize winner, Dr. Pauling, of the California University of Technology, who found enough electricity in the blood to light a 25 watt bulb for 5 minutes. This may sound like a small amount of electricity, but in terms of the body's electrical economy it could be more than enough. Dr. Frederick Golla, former professor of Pathology of Mental Diseases at the University of London, showed that the brain, like a condenser, stores up electricity in its nerve cells which is being constantly accumulated and discharged. In fact, all living matter, from the lowliest bacteria to the body of man, gives off a steady current of electricity. All matter, in fact, *is* electricity. It is by an electrical process that viruses attach themselves to the walls of bacteria before they invade them. The atoms which make up the molecule consist of a positively electrified nucleus called the *proton*, surrounded by fast moving *electrons* which are charged with negative electricity. Every cell in the human body has an electrical basis of operation. Each cell is a little electrical world, a

[494]

miniature factory, where it would be very cold and inactive without electricity.

Dr. Crile, the famous medical scientist, has said that "the primary function of the cell is to fabricate electrical charges." This is no doubt true, but a strong factor in this fabrication process could be a stimulation from outside electricity that comes into the cell by sundry means, one of which could be earth electricity that could enter the body by means of the hand or foot in gardening.

Being somewhat acquainted with the operation of machinery, I know that there is an ideal set of conditions which is conducive to its ideal performance. And so it must be with the body and the cells of which it is composed. Too little or too much electricity might play havoc with it. I can conceive of an electrical threshold below which the cell could go berserk and multiply wildly. That would be cancer! There might be trouble also if the life of the cell is speeded up by too much electricity.

While we are on this subject we cannot overlook atomic fallout and its effect on the cell's electrical integrity. The intrusion of such powerful radiations cannot do it any good. It may push it in a direction harmful to the life processes of the body. In the same way, there are certain chemicals called *carcinogens,* usually coal tar products such as benzol, certain coloring chemicals, coke, illuminating gas, etc., which are known to cause cancer. Is it possible that the end-products of body chemical combinations in which they are a part invade the cell, and affect its electrical system? Does it in some way depress or increase too much the store of cell electricity, which touches off the forces that could lead to cancer?

Electric Machines Used in Medicine

In the days before the advent of the wonder drugs many orthodox physicians used electric machines in their practice. These are devices which send a gentle electric current into the body, and in many cases with good results. Today the practice is still resorted to, but only in emergency situations and with the use of more powerful charges of electricity. In the *New England Journal of Medicine* (November 1952), there is described a situation where a person was kept alive by electricity. His heart began to fail but by means of electricity his life was saved. Dr. Paul M. Zoll, Associate in Medicine at the Harvard Medical School, who wrote the article said, "Whenever the electric stimulator was stopped, the heart beat failed. During a period of 52 hours not a single natural heart beat of the ventricle muscles was observed when the electrical stimulator was turned off. After 52 hours, the heart started beating slowly by itself . . . Eight days after the treatment began, the patient's heart was pumping adequately on its own."

In the May, 1955, issue of *Today's Health* (an American Medical Association publication) there is described a case where, after continued attacks of unconsciousness and convulsions, a man's heart began to miss some beats. He went into a coma. But when electric currents were sent into his chest, the man awoke, but became unconscious again when the electricity was shut off. After 7 days of electrical treatment his heart returned to normal.

A news event which brings home the fact of how important electricity is in the cell, is a piece of research discribed in the *Science News Letter* for June 26, 1954. It is a new method for testing whether women have cancer of the uterus and is done by measuring the electrical difference between the inside and outside of cells cast off from the birth canal. If the electrical reading is slightly negative there is no cancer. If it is positive by a moderate amount there is some kind of cancer in the uterus.

Many years ago a process was developed by Dr. James Homer Burgan, of Hollywood, for reducing high blood pressure by passing a weak direct electric current directly through the human blood stream for half an hour. In the case of several hundred patients, the blood pressure was reduced by a single treatment. It was thought at the time that the current in some manner dislodged certain chemical deposits that interfered with the free passage of blood, but it could be that the reduction occurred for more basic reasons. High blood pressure could be caused by some interference with the body's electric-distribution system, which in turn could have a chemical or dietary basis, such as too much salt or sugar in the diet.

In some instances, Dr. Burgan reports the electrical treatment has resulted in a rather surprising increased growth of the patient's blood cells. "The fact must be recorded," he says, "that the treatment results frequently in the building up of the body's defense mechanism. We have observed changes in the blood vessel walls in the eye which indicate some reduction of calcium deposits that play at least some part in the cause of high blood pressure tension."

The day-to-day contact with the earth by an active gardener which means the absorption of a good deal of earth electricity, could be the equivalent of electrical treatments which would set the electricity of each one of the body's cells into perfect order, thus being the means of helping all functions of the body attain normalcy. Add to this the beneficial effect of actively working in the outdoors, and you could have a double insurance against many conditions of disease.

Does any kind of physical exercise improve conditions for the better electrical functioning of the body? When my heart used to undergo symptoms, sometime ago, when I would go for a walk, it would show them usually only the first 15 minutes. After that, the exercise seemed to have the effect of opening up the big arteries leading to the heart, the coronaries, usually eliminating all further symptoms, even in climbing hills during the latter part of the walk. But how are the arteries dilated? It could be that the exercise generates electric current, as the wheels of a moving auto cause its generator to make electrical current. It could be that this manufactured electricity, produced by the steady movement of the body's parts, could open up plugged arteries. Of course, there is the oxygenating effect of the blood produced by the forced breathing occurring in exercise, but can oxygen move in the blood without electricity? The active gardener, who keeps moving about, could also be making electricity by such action. A little research on this aspect of electricity in the human body could reveal interesting things.

Tissue Repair and Electricity

In *Principles of Human Physiology* (Lea and Febiger) appears the statement: "Every beat of the heart, every twitch of a muscle, every state of secretion of a gland is associated . . . with electrical changes." Again he says, ". . . every functional change in a tissue has been shown to be associated with the production of differences of electrical potential. Thus, all parts of an uninjured muscle are iso-potential," which means that, "any two points may be led off to a galvanometer without any current being observed. If, however, one part of the muscle be strongly excited, as for instance by injury, so that it is brought into a state of lasting excitation, it will be found that, on leading off from this point, and a point on the uninjured surface to a galvanometer, a current flows through the latter from the uninjured to the injured surface." This would seem to indicate that a repair process has begun, and that electricity takes a part in that process.

In this regard, Dr. Roy M. Keller, writing in the September, 1953, issue of the *Journal of Medical-Physical Research* said, "Repair of wounds is no doubt brought about by the change in the electrical potential of the traumatized (damaged) cells. Injury breaks the cell covering and allows the electrons to escape more freely, as in cutting or mashing a comb of honey, the contents escape."

Whichever way you look at the performance of the various parts of the body you come smack up against electricity, and yet, 99.999 per cent of medical researches confine themselves exclusively to a purely chemical basis of bodily operation. Should we not begin to think of checking on a sick person's body electricity? Should this not become routine practice, along with the determination of metabolism, blood counts, heart check-up, etc.? Would not accumulated, averaged data relating to the body electricity of sick and well persons tend to teach interesting facts that might lead to methods of correcting distortions or weaknesses in body electricity, thus also in its health?

Electricity and Food

In cancer we cannot rule out the effects of the foods that a body ingests and in handling that food, electricity takes a big part. To put it in popular language, electricity sparks the food elements to combine properly in various chemical combinations. Electricity is part of the combination process just as electricity is necessary in an oil furnace to break down the oil to a combustible form. Vitamins, I am sure, could not do their work without electricity entering into the picture. Vitamins have been referred to as sparks in relation to the other food elements which they activate.

All the elements of which foods are composed give off electrical radiations. Carbon, hydrogen, nitrogen, phosphorus, potassium and all the other minerals, together form the integral parts of an electric battery in the body. Some of these food elements in the digestive process absorb electrons—others release electrons. It would be a very profitable field of research to study the electrical effects of each type of food and its elements on the body, in relation to states of health and disease, and to particular kinds of disease, including cancer.

In this respect the effect of table salt should be closely researched insofar as its effect on the body's operation is concerned. In *Principles of Human Physiology,* previously mentioned, appears the following statement, ". . . the smallest trace of salt, acid or alkali added to distilled water enormously improves its conducting power." The question is, whether such an enormous increase in electrical conductivity is desirable. In the case of the earth, there is given off a gentle electrical stream. Actually salt is not a food but an inorganic chemical. It is the only item of our diet that does not come either from an animal or a plant. It is a strong stimulant to cell metabolism—too strong and no doubt interferes with its electrical operation.

L. Duncan Bulkley, M.D., writing in the July, 1927, issue of *Cancer,* has a great deal to say on the effect of salt in cancer. He quotes Frederick Marwood as follows, "What would happen to electrical storage batteries if we added sulphuric acid greatly in excess of the necessary formulas, seems to me, will happen in another degree to our internal storage batteries, if we ingest a powerful corrosive chemical, sodium chloride (table salt), to the extent of 10, 20, 30 times, or even more, than nature has prescribed."

Nature has worked out the formula for the body's storage battery, in the blood which feeds every cell in the body. Nature wants the blood components in certain amounts. Calcium should be two and one-half times the phosphorus. There should be a definite relationship between the blood's sodium and potassium, but if too much salt is taken, its sodium content (salt being sodium chloride) adds greatly to the blood's sodium, thus distorting the sodium-potassium relationship.

So, the next time you grab hold of the salt shaker, pause for a moment and think of what you have just read, and do not throw unnecessary clinkers into the furnace. Think of the fact that by taking in salt, you are dangerously altering the formula of the medium through which the body's electricity flows—the blood.

Diagnosing Disease With Electricity

A few years ago something interesting occurred which forcefully brought home to me the fact that our body is a storehouse of electricity. A representative of the telephone company called to describe a new service, the use of a device which a person places in his pocket to keep him in touch with his office. If his secretary desires to contact him when he is away from the office, she calls the telephone company where a record is kept of the wave-length for each subscriber. By the mere push of the button they reach the man. The device in his pocket begins to buzz which is a signal for him to call his office. I asked the telephone man whether I could keep this device on the seat of my auto, but he replied in the negative. "Your body is an aerial for it. You must keep it on your person." So our body is an electrical aerial! That is interesting—isn't it? Actually Dr. Otto Rahn of Cornell has shown that there are continuous electrical radiations from people's finger tips, noses and eyes strong enough to kill certain micro-organisms.

In September, 1953, I visited the Delawarr Laboratory in the city of Oxford, England, where a new electronic method for diagnosing disease is being developed. There I saw photographs of radiations from various elements such as chlorine, potassium, etc. It seems that each element has its own lines of radiation and no two are alike. Mr. George Delawarr told me that their work has shown that, similarly, each person has a certain wave force emanating from his body, the design of which never changes basically, although there may be slight variations with change in character.

I would like to pause here and quote a news release issued by the *American Institute of Electrical Engineers* of New York, which said, "The possibility of electricity playing an even greater role as an aid in the diagnosis of disease was forecast today.

"The possibility, contingent on new contributions by electrical engineers, was raised by Clyde A. Dubbs, of the Veterans Administration Center, Los Angeles, in a paper entitled, *Electrophoretic Techniques; Some Applications and Problems,* presented during a medical radiation instruments session at the Summer and Pacific General Meeting of the American Institute of Electrical Engineers at the Hotel Biltmore.

"Electrophoresis, the study of movement of proteins in an electrically charged fluid field, is valuable in medical practice for evaluating responses to therapy and for providing diagnostic information, the author said, pointing out that normal blood plasmas give typical normal electrophoretic patterns, and abnormal plasma give abnormal patterns, although rarely specified for a given disease.

"These patterns," he said "can provide more helpful information to the physician than any empirical clinical test often performed today. In certain diseases of the liver, kidney and bone marrow, and in general infectious states, patterns are quite characteristic; and for diseases distinguished by a deficiency or lack of a major protein fraction (as gammaglobulin or fibrinogen), the patterns are decisive. Moreover, proof that certain diseases can be diagnosed by the presence of specific protein components, (Itano's recent work on hemoglobin proteins in some hereditary anemia) possibly forecasts a greater role for electrophoresis as a *specific* diagnostic tool.

"Citing the difficulty of using only a small amount of electrical energy for electrophoresis, which produces unwanted heat, necessitating more electrical energy for refrigeration to dissipate the heat to prevent the proteins from denaturing, the author said, 'If new contributions from electrical engineers can solve such problems more efficiently and economically the advantages of electrophoresis can be given many more laboratories'."

This news release was issued in 1955, but in 1953, the Delawarrs were already telling me all about this method in their Oxford city laboratory. Already they had many years of experience in this field of research. With their specially developed camera which costs in the thousands of dollars, they are able to diagnose a person's disease from a tiny specimen of blood taken by pricking the finger.

Letter from the Delawarrs

When I came across the item in the Australian medical journal regarding the average gardener's host resistance to internal cancer, I immediately thought of the Delawarrs and wrote to George. Here is part of his answer, from his letter dated March 21, 1955:

"It was originally supposed that by walking barefoot on dewy ground one's body was 'earthed' in some way, but it is now known that more than this goes on—there is a contact with that basic life force that is being evoked in the living soil. Just take a brass pot, suspend on 3 brass wires, and fill it with moist soil and hang it on to a spot galvanometer and see the 'current' it produces. It is wired by suspending the 3 wires from one terminal of the galvanometer and then connecting the other terminal to a central electrode in the soil in the pot. In this way, all the electrical energy passes through the galvanometer. Precaution must be taken to keep the moisture content constant so that any variation in potential must be from causes other than those due to moisture variation.

"The shattering thing is that potentials of 192 micro.V. can be recorded during the summer, and 2½ hours later they will have fallen to 60 M.V.I., although the rainfall and sun have not varied at all. The meter used had an internal resistance of 500 ohms. Pundits will try and say 'Electrolysis, old boy.' If that is so, it cannot be due to the difference of the material forming the pot and the electrode because each are brass. 'Internal chemical action' is probably nearer the mark, but what sort of chemical action and what makes it vary so?

"This experiment shows us the presence of 'vital force' even in a pot of soil with no plants or seeds in it. The so-called 'current' is really the aggregation of a series of electrostatic charges that are the end result of 'life' in progress. Here is the factor in health that has been overlooked by the scientist because it does not record on a Geiger counter. Here is a flow of energy charges, each one having its own complex *energy pattern*. It is these energy patterns that we detect photographically. Radionics deal only with this basic energy.

"Yes, put your hands in the soil as much as you can; handle living plants and drain their health-giving electrical charges into your body."

The medical profession would do well to hot-foot it out to the Delawarr's laboratory in the city of Oxford. There they would see things that would astonish them.

Father Kneipp's Cure

Mr. Delawarr in his letter, mentioned that in the handling of living plants one could drain their health-giving electrical charges into one's body, which should remind us that the gardener in weeding does exactly that. In pulling out an undesired plant, he touches it while it is alive, and thus he drains its health-giving electrical charges into his own body. He, therefore, gets electricity both from placing his hands in the soil and also upon the plant. Mr. Delawarr in his letter touches upon another aspect of how one can absorb earth electricity and that is by walking barefoot on dewy ground. This prompted me to think of Father Kneipp, who in 1886 wrote his book, *My Water Cure,* which gave him great fame and attracted patients from all over Europe. The basis of Father Kneipp's treatments was to walk barefooted in the dewy grass in the early morning. Let me quote from his book:

"I knew a priest who went every year to stay for a few days with a friend who owned a large garden, and there his morning walk was always taken barefooted in the wet grass. He has many times spoken in glowing terms of the excellent effects of this kind of promenade; and I could name a number of persons of the highest ranks of society, who did not despise his well-meant advice, but tried to harden themselves in the better season, by going barefooted during their morning walks in the solitary woods, or on a remote meadow.

"One of this comparatively still small number has owned to me that in former times he seldom spent a week without a catarrh, if it were only a slight one, but this simple practice had entirely cured him of this susceptibility."

Further on he says: "I can highly recommend it to young and old, healthy and sick. . . . The wetter the grass, the longer one perseveres in the exercise, and the oftener it is repeated, the more perfect will be the success. This exercise is generally taken for 15 to 45 minutes. After the promenade, all the improper adherents, such as leaves, or sand, must be quickly wiped off the feet; yet the feet are not to be dried, but must be left as wet as they are. Dry stockings and shoes have to be put on, however, without delay. The walking in the grass has to be followed by walking with covered feet on a dry path, at first briskly, by and by in the ordinary measure. The time of so walking depends on how long it takes the feet to get dry and warm, but should not be less than 15 minutes. I urgently call attention to the words 'dry stockings and shoes,' for wet or damp stockings must never be worn after an application. The consequences would soon be felt in

[501]

head and neck . . . . This exercise, likewise the walking barefooted generally, may be taken even when the feet are cold."

Father Kneipp's work should be re-evaluated based on the possibility that in walking on the dewy grass one absorbs liberal charges of earth electricity.

Modern Primitives

On May 2, 1955, Mr. and Mrs. Emory L. Harrison and their 13 boys posed barefoot for the New York *Herald Tribune* photographer. They had come up from Tennessee because Mrs. Harrison had been named *Honor Mother* of 1955. Mr. Harrison did not care for New York. "New York is all right," he said, "but I like the country best. In the country we can put a big barrel of milk on the table for the boys, and it won't cost us a thing!"

I'll wager that the milk is not pasteurized.

"In the country," he went on, "we can put up 1,000 cans of fruit and put six hogs in the smokehouse and cure them—and it won't cost us a cent." I'll wager they don't use the speed-up chemicals for smoking as is the practice in modern smoke-house methods.

"I don't spend more than 13 to 14 dollars a week for food for all of us. Our 72 acre farm gives us everything the family needs except sugar, coffee, and cereals." I'll wager that the Harrisons use very little chemical fertilizer on their farm.

"And what's more," continued Mr. Harrison, "I'd like to show these city folks how to bring up their boys. Ours can go barefoot, summer and winter, and they've never been sick."

The Harrisons, in their barefootedness, were following unconsciously the teachings of Father Kneipp. And their "primitive" diet did not hurt any either.

Today the farmer has been mechanized. He sits on a tractor so that even his shoes do not touch the ground. He has lost that health-giving contact with the good earth. Over the hundreds of centuries man went barefoot. Shoes are only a recent innovation. Man does not thrive in paved cities. He should live where he can take his shoes off occasionally and walk barefoot.

Geographical Incidence of Cancer

It is a known fact that cancer is far less prevalent in the South than in the North. Here are some of the figures of cancer deaths per 100,000 of population for 1947:

Alabama	83.6	Mississippi	86.5
Arizona	80.9	New Mexico	77.9
Arkansas	85.5	North Carolina	74.8
Georgia	86.3	South Carolina	72.2
	Tennessee	95.4	

And here are some for a few of the northern states for the same year:

Colorado	141.1	Massachusetts	173.3
Connecticut	157.3	New York	174.9
Illinois	161.2	Pennsylvania	141.6
Maine	160.5	Washington	127.4
	Wisconsin	149.6	

In my booklet, *Cancer: Can it be Prevented?*, it was shown that this disease increases in frequency with remoteness from the equator. I stated that it could be due to less coal smoke in the air and I still think that that is an important factor, but isn't it possible also that there is more working in gardens in the South? The people there are not stopped by winter weather. And there is more going barefoot, especially when one gets closer to the equator, where the cancer figures are the lowest of them all.

I have shown that the Hunzas, a northern Indian race, do not get cancer. Sir Robert McCarrison, the famous English research physician who was with them for more than 10 years and did not come across a single case of cancer, attributed it to the unusual care these people exercise in the raising of their food. But could it not also be the fact that they go about barefooted? And the fact that they spend so much time in gardening and farming?

Organic Versus Chemicalized Soil

That there is electricity issuing from the soil there can be no doubt, but is there a difference in this electricity as between a soil farmed or gardened by the organic method as against one operated with chemical fertilizers? We saw how salt could be a factor in doing something to the body's electricity. Chemical fertilizers are strong, soluble chemicals, some of which are salts, that enter in the soil's water solution, and may in some way affect the pattern, or quality, or amount of electricity coming from it. In the breakdown of organic matter, electricity must take a part. But it is a gentle, natural process and, therefore, it may cause a gentle stream of beneficial electricity to issue from it.

The organic gardener, working his hands in his composted soil, treading barefoot over the earth of his organically-treated garden, should have a feeling that he is receiving natural waves of electricity from the earth and not stepped-up or in some way artificialized gusts of electric waves which could throw the metabolism of his body off balance. Of course, what I am suggesting here is rank speculation, but here is a simple subject for research, one that is purely mechanical with all the equipment available. Who will do it?

The situation with regard to cancer is becoming worse each year. Here is a charted forecast of cancer deaths issued in 1950 by the American Cancer Society (fig. 19):

[503]

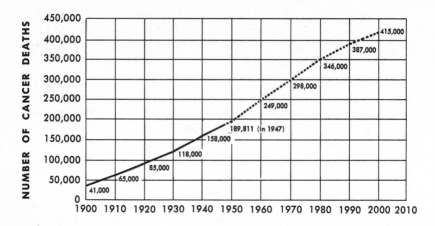

FIGURE 19: FORECAST OF CANCER DEATHS

(*If recent trends continue*)

Evidently the American Cancer Society is throwing up its hands, for up to the year 2010 its chart shows no place where cancer is checked. They expect it to go on and on and on, and it *will*, unless there comes a different mentality, one which does not fear to grasp at straws, one which does not fear to research in the primitive, one which does not fear to walk barefooted so to speak, midst the test tubes.

The Lesson We Must Learn

What is the lesson? We must go back to nature if we wish to live long. We must garden and go barefooted. If we live in New York we must go searching for four-leaf clovers in Central Park, and no policeman will arrest you if you do it barefooted. We do not have to stop the trend of industrialization. We do not have to stop the advances of technology, but we have to learn to live with these forces. We must not permit them to overwhelm us. We must not industrialize or technologize our own bodies.

The medical profession in its researches must become aware of, and not ignore, this electrical phenomenon. They must not in observing sick people, keep on saying, we see results but we do not know causes, for some of these causes assuredly are in the realm of the electrical.

The idea that it might be earth electricity which aids the body to combat cancer might be used to help cancer cases in the hospital and in the home. An electrical connection could be made between the patient's body and the earth which would establish a circuit of earth electricity into the body. Of course, this must be preceded by a thorough series of researches to establish a scientific basis for the general principle of applying earth electricity to aid the body. But, after principles are established, electrical treatment centers might be opened in every town and city in the country. Perhaps every home could own an electrical device, which would cost less than a television set and which could give the body a daily electrical charge, to counteract the effects of our citified, sedentary, artificialized way of living.

More power to Dr. Eric Goulston of Sydney, Australia, who touched off this discussion. May it be the beginning of scientific studies that will lead not only to the conquering of cancer, but to diseases of all kinds.

127. Some Facts on Cervical Cancer

Cancer of the uterine cervix (that is, the neck or opening of the uterus) is the second most prevalent kind of cancer among women in this country and Europe. An interesting article in the German medical publication, *Deutsche Medizinische Wochenschrift,* Vol. 81, 1956, p. 1560, comments on the fact that apparently certain things in the daily environment have a lot to do with this high incidence of such a dreaded disease. In other words, cancer here is not a mysterious process striking blindly at certain individuals and not at others. Even though, as the author says, the primary cause of cancer of the cervix is unknown, still investigations have disclosed a number of environmental factors which seem to have a lot to do with who gets this particular kind of cancer and why. If this is so, indeed, then prevention should be easier.

Cancer of the cervix is extremely rare among nuns. One researcher reported that in examinations of 13,000 nuns over a period of 35 years, he had not found a single case of cancer of the cervix. Records at a university in Munich show that, among 8,000 women with cervical cancer during the past 20 years, only 4 were virgins.

These observations seem to indicate that pregnancy, childbirth and sexual intercourse are precipitating factors in this kind of cancer. Women who are married are far more likely to get it. Women who have had children are more susceptible than childless women. And it seems, too, that the more children a woman has the more likely she is to suffer from this kind of cancer. Another investigation involving several thousand women patients indicates that having children before the age of 25 predisposes to this kind of cancer.

Statistics Prove A Point

Checking these statistics against those for cancer of the male reproductive organs, we find that cancer of the penis is unknown among nations whose boy children are circumcised at birth, as Jewish children are. Moslems, who circumcise their children between the ages of 7 and 12 rarely suffer from cancer of the penis. It is noteworthy that Jewish and Moslem women suffer from cervical cancer less (in the proportion of 1 to 7 and 1 to 10) in comparison to other women. Apparently, then, circumcision of the husband, effecting as it may his sexual hygiene, has a great deal to do with the possibility of his wife's becoming a victim of cervical cancer.

Several other sets of statistics bring out unusual aspects of this problem. Caesarian births and miscarriages do not seem to have any bearing on the incidence of the disease. But it does seem to occur more widely among populations where early marriages and large families are the rule. The risk is twice as great among women who have had 5 or more children as among those who have had one to 3 children.

Cervical cancer occurs 50 per cent more frequently in the poorer section of the population, seeming to indicate that poor sexual hygiene, lack of cleanliness chiefly, may be partly responsible. The actual physiological changes that a woman experiences during pregnancy and childbirth seem to retard the development of cervical cancer in some respects while they are known to favor it in others. "It is very much more likely," we are told, "that frequent lacerations of the cervix during labor and consequent inflammatory processes play a predominant role."

Precautionary Measures

What is there to learn from all these statistics? That one should not marry or have children? That one should limit families to one, two or 3 children? That one should have children only after the age of 25? Certainly not. There is a lesson to be learned, however. There seems to be no doubt that this increasingly frequent kind of cancer could be largely prevented by following certain precautionary measures.

First. All women married or unmarried should make certain that they do not suffer from any chronic inflammation of the reproductive organs, the cervix especially. A good diet is essential for the health of these tissues— vitamin A being especially important. But, if you already have such a condition, don't delay in getting your doctor's help for correcting it, while at the same time you improve your diet and add plenty of vitamin A.

During pregnancy do your utmost to assure yourself of an easy and safe labor and childbirth. Here again diet counts more than anything else. Most physicians these days regulate the diet of expectant mothers carefully, but we think that most of them do not begin to recommend large enough quantities of the vitamins and minerals. Take plenty of natural food supplements.

Finally, if, during labor, there are lacerations or other damage to the reproductive passages, by all means don't delay in having them repaired. Here, too, good nutrition will help in the healing process. Vitamin C assures quick wound-healing.

128. Experiments with Garlic and Cancer

Research on the effectiveness of garlic against disease has not been so popular of late as it has been during the past 50 years or so. This is one reason why we were especially pleased to find in *Science*, Vol. 126, November 29, 1957, p. 1112, an account of research that seems to show that garlic is powerful against tumor-formation. And that means, of course, cancer, too.

Working with laboratory mice, Austin S. Weisberger and Jack Pensky of Western Reserve University found that by injecting cancerous cells into mice they could produce rapid growth of cancer and death within 16 days. They could produce the same result even when they treated the cancerous cells with an enzyme they had isolated from garlic. The enzyme by itself did not protect from cancer. But when they treated the cancerous cells with an equal amount of the garlic enzyme and the substrate which is also present in garlic (that is, the substance with which the enzyme is naturally associated in foods), and then injected mice with the treated cells, no cancer grew and there was no mortality among the animals for a period of 6 months (equal to about a fourth of a lifetime in a human being).

Thus we see that the cancer cells were prevented from doing any damage by treating them with the preparation from garlic. But our researchers went further than that. They inoculated mice with the virulent cancer cells and then gave them injections of the garlic preparation. The garlic delayed the onset of the malignant tumor and in some instances completely prevented its formation and saved the lives of the mice. However, in all cases it was necessary to keep giving the garlic preparation, for tumors developed very rapidly if it was discontinued.

Details of The Experiment

Such findings, which link the humble, smelly garlic bulb with the prevention of cancer, the greatest modern plague, are spectacular. But, in addition, note some of the details of this experiment. Scientists have known for a long time that there is a certain enzyme in garlic that is powerful against disease bacteria. But when they used just this enzyme, you will notice, the Western Reserve scientists got no results. They had to use both the enzyme and the substrate from garlic to attain success in preventing cancer. The word *substrate* refers to the substance which works with the enzyme to bring about chemical changes. Every enzyme has its substrate; indeed, every enzyme takes its name from its substrate. Thus the enzyme name *lipase* reacts chemically with fats or lipids. Proteinases react chemically with proteins, and so forth.

In the case of garlic, the enzyme alliinase is liberated when the garlic bulb is crushed. It immediately reacts with its substrate to form a new chemical compound, which is the powerful anti-bacterial compound for which garlic is noted.

Using the enzyme alone or using the substrate alone produces no effect. The researchers found that they must use them together. They do not of course know why they obtained these results and they suggest in the article several possible ways in which the garlic enzyme and substrate may bring about the desired result.

So we learn two lessons from such an article—first, that the simple garlic bulb is indeed a powerful agent against disease and secondly, that wholeness is best where health is concerned. The less we separate, divide and fragmentize where food is involved, the better off we are. Whole foods, containing everything that occurs naturally in them, are best.

129. Vitamin B Deficiency and Cancer

Many readers write to us about troubles with their mouths, tongue, lips, gums. They have burning sensations, they have ulcers, boils or patches of inflammation on their gums; white spots may have appeared on the gums or insides of cheeks, their tongues are smooth and shiny or swollen and deeply fissured, the corners of their mouths have cracks or sores.

Experts have found that many such symptoms are what they term "precancerous." This does not mean that cancer is caused by these disorders. It means simply that often the bodily condition that produces such disorders in the mouth may later produce cancer. It was thought for a long time that such conditions were caused by irritation of some kind. And it is believed that cancer is often the result of irritation superimposed on just the right combination of ill-health factors to make the body susceptible to cancer.

We can report some conclusive work which seems to show that a deficiency in vitamin B is responsible for most such mouth disorders. Readers who suffer from them can take heart, for not only is there a good possibility that plenty of vitamin B will bring back good health, but the fear of cancer can be permanently disposed of. Such mouth conditions need not be precancerous if you get plenty of vitamin B.

"In most cases of intra-oral cancer, there are in addition to the primary lesions, definite degenerative changes in the oral mucous membranes which obviously have antedated the malignant growth. It has long been

[508]

noted that such degenerative tissue changes are found in a majority of patients with mouth cancer, and, therefore, they are commonly referred to as precancerous," says Hayes Martin, M.D., and Everett Koop, M.D., in an article in the *American Journal of Surgery* for August, 1942. Here are the medical names for some of the changes they are talking about: leukoplakia, subacute or chronic inflammation, vascular infection, atrophy or hypertrophy of the papillae, erosion of the epithelium. Most of them can be produced by chronic forms of irritation—from tobacco, venereal disease, badly fitting dentures and so forth.

It is well known, these authors say, that the B vitamins are important for mouth health. In studying 300 patients at Memorial Hospital, New York, they found that those who were suffering from mouth disorders, ranging all the way from the slightest irritation to full-blown advanced cancer of the mouth, were short on vitamin B. They found, too, that, in general, other symptoms of vitamin B deficiency accompanied the mouth symptoms in these patients. Depression and malnutrition went hand-in-hand with constipation and other digestive disorders. Interestingly enough, Drs. Martin and Koop mention fragility of fingernails as one of the most easily recognized symptoms of vitamin B deficiency. A tendency for nails to break easily, and ridges that extend lengthwise or horizontally are further indications of lack of vitamin B.

Some Actual Conditions

Here are some of the actual mouth conditions that prevailed: *glossodynia* (a burning sensation of the tongue), chronic inflammation of the mucous membrane lining of the mouth, ulceration of the tongue, cheeks or gums, atrophy and hypertrophy of the papillae of the tongue (this means a decrease or increase in the size of the little knobs on the surface of the tongue, so that the tongue may be partly or wholly bald), fissure folding (this is a condition in which the tongue has become too large and is compressed into folds which look like crevices or fissures in its surface), *leukoplakia*, consisting of white spots on the inside of the mouth (incidentally, our authors tell us that about 50 per cent of all men and about 10 per cent of all women over the age of 45 have some degree of leukoplakia), *gingivitis* (bleeding from the gums), salivary changes (the mouth becomes dry and the scanty saliva becomes sticky and thick), Plummer-Vinson disease (inflammation of the esophagus, anemia, inflammation of the tongue).

Since these are the visible changes in the lining of the mouth, our authors state that undoubtedly, farther along in the digestive tract where we cannot see them, similar disorders are prevalent. "The evidence is plain," they state, "for at least a tentative diagnosis of lack of vitamin B when an inflammatory oral mucosal lesion is associated with one or more of the following symptoms: malnutrition, mental depression, dermatoses (skin trouble), nervousness, insomnia, constipation and irregularities of the fingernails."

[509]

Which of Us Is Deficient in Vitamin B?

What is a vitamin B deficiency? Can you pick one person out of a crowd and say that he is deficient in vitamin B and pick out another and say that he is not? According to our authors, "It would be impossible to separate a group of individuals into two definite classes, one with conclusive evidences of vitamin B deficiency and the other with no evidences whatsoever. No laboratory test has been devised which furnishes an accurate basis for this determination. For this reason, there is as yet no method of determining the absolute incidence of lack of vitamin B in mouth cancer or precancer. The proof of such dietary inadequacy is found in the fact that a large percentage of patients with mouth cancer do manifest one or more of the general and local abnormalities. And that these are almost always improved by administration of vitamin B."

Then, too, there is the complicating factor that people who start out with some mouth disorder generally end up with rather serious vitamin deficiencies as well as other forms of malnutrition for the simple reason that it is so hard for them to eat. In spite of any encouragement, they avoid most carefully those foods which would contribute most to curing their deficiency—fresh raw foods—fruits and vegetables.

Drs. Martin and Koop took careful dietary surveys of hundreds of patients while they were collecting material for this article. It is, of course, difficult to find out exactly what people eat unless they are under constant and very close supervision. But the several case histories they give in the article show extremely bad dietary habits. For instance, there was one woman who lived almost completely on gin. And, although she eventually died of "alcoholism," they say they are quite sure that her main difficulty was a lack of vitamin B, and she could have been saved, had she been given massive doses of the B vitamins.

Wide Survey Made by Physicians

Giving brewer's yeast as the best source of the B vitamins was done uniformly throughout the experimental period. And we mean large doses of brewer's yeast. The average dose was 3 tablespoons a day. In one case a man who was being treated for cancer of the tongue was given liver and yeast. Within two months he had gained a badly needed 25 pounds in weight. About a year and a half after treatment was begun he appeared to be losing ground even though he continued to take the yeast and to eat large quantities of vitamin B-rich food. So the daily intake of yeast was increased to 8 tablespoonfuls daily, "a dose which few patients can tolerate without marked nausea and diarrhea." There was tremendous improvement in his condition almost at once. From then on, so long as he maintained this enormous daily intake of yeast he remained healthy and the condition of his mouth remained good.

"These cases in which massive doses of vitamin B must be taken in order to maintain health can be explained on the basis of marked individual variations in ability, either to absorb or utilize ingested vitamins," say the authors. Among patients they studied whose diets contained apparently enough B vitamins to keep them in fairly good health, there were some who were definitely suffering from deficiency. Although their intake of B vitamins was not far below normal, their requirement was abnormally high. It is well to remember in this connection the theories of Dr. Roger Williams of the University of Texas, who believes that alcoholism is a disease of persons who require far more vitamin B than the average person and just don't get it, no matter how good a diet they eat.

"Fad" Diets Actually Worsened Conditions

How did people fall into the practice of eating the diets that were notoriously bad? According to Drs. Martin and Koop some of these diets were prescribed by doctors for such diverse conditions as ulcer, gall bladder disease, obesity, colitis and so forth. Some patients had blindly followed completely inadequate diets for many years firmly believing that some disorder of theirs could be cured by "dieting." Instead, they had brought on a worse condition than the one they had started out to cure. In some cases, a deficient diet brought about such loss of appetite and interest in food that the patient progressively restricted his diet still further to "those substances most easily and cheaply obtained, mainly pure carbohydrates." For instance, there was a wealthy eccentric who ate only breakfast and then took beer and onions whenever he got hungry during the rest of the day. A woman voluntarily went on an "ulcer diet" along with her husband who actually had an ulcer. A beer salesman drank beer when hungry. A traveling salesman ate only sandwiches because he was afraid of dirty food in restaurants. A woman avoided pork, fruit and eggs because certain members of her family were allergic to these foods.

Dietary Prejudices Can Harm Health

The most frequent underlying cause of an inadequate vitamin intake lies in personality factors such as peculiar dietary prejudices based on family customs. Often deficient diets are encountered because of fear of overweight. "In most city dwellers," say our authors, "there is a tendency to eat at 'quick lunches' and drug store counters, where green vegetables and fresh meats are replaced by carbohydrates in the form of sandwiches, ice cream, malted milk and pastry."

According to these researchers, there is little storage of excess vitamin B in the body and deficiency symptoms occur *within a few days* after withdrawal of the vitamin source. For this reason, correcting such a deficiency must be done on a daily basis. "We have found it advisable," they go on, "when using natural concentrates such as yeast and liver, to provide from 5 to 10 times the normal minimum requirement of thiamin and riboflavin or 30 to 45 grams (two to three tablespoonfuls) daily of granular yeast. In exceptional cases the maximum relief cannot be obtained unless inordinately high therapeutic doses are consumed, as for instance, one of our patients who ingests about 240 grams (two teacups) of brewer's yeast a day and who insists that unless this amount is taken, marked asthenia and mental depression occur."

It is noteworthy that these doctors do not give synthetic vitamins for treatment of vitamin B deficiency. They say, "In some instances the administration of a single fraction of the vitamin B complex (thiamin, riboflavin, niacin, etc.) may cause marked improvement, but combinations of the known fractions almost always give better results." Discussing the kind of yeast to take, they deplore the use of brewer's yeast *tablets* for, they say, it is almost impossible to get enough brewer's yeast for a good big dose when you take tablets. It would require about 70 ten-grain tablets to make up the equivalent of 3 tablespoons of yeast.

Vitamin Intake Must Be Increased and Maintained

"It would be easier to impress both physicians and the laity," say our authors, "if it could be maintained that there is one sole cause for cancer and precancer, and that there is one simple remedy which, taken in pill form, so many times a day for a few weeks, would effect a lasting cure and a preventive of the basic abnormality. *In order to relieve avitaminosis (deficiency in B), however, the mode of life must be permanently modified, that is, the intake of vitamins must be increased and maintained as long as the patient lives.* Such a permanent regime will, in many cases, become tedious since it is not supported by the emotional stimulus which accompanies a shorter, more intense course of therapy."

The italics are ours. We put them there because this seems to us to be the key sentence for readers in all this discussion. There is no quick and easy way to good health. There is no pill you can take to relieve any physical condition or any vitamin deficiency. Being healthy is a way of life. And if you have allowed yourself to fall into a state of diet deficiency—and most of us have—you must make a permanent change in your way of life —nothing less than this will accomplish what you want. Vitamins are something you need every day and, if you would cure a deficiency, you must decide to take vitamin supplements permanently.

Drs. Martin and Koop tell us in their summary that degenerative changes are found in the lining of the mouth in most cases of mouth cancer. The most frequent reason for these changes is a deficiency in vitamin B. Most patients are already suffering from a marked deficiency when they go to their doctor. This is aggravated by the necessarily restricted diet during the painful stage of any mouth disorder. Supplementary vitamin therapy is one of the most important factors in the successful treatment of mouth cancer or conditions that are called "precancerous." There is much evidence suggesting that the mouth symptoms are repeated farther down in the digestive tract, so it seems logical that what we say here about mouth cancer applies equally to stomach and intestinal cancer as well.

Remember We Need B Vitamins

Finally, we believe you will gather, from what we have said above, a slightly different idea about how to go about taking your B vitamins. Most of us are deficient in B vitamins. Many of us may need extremely large amounts of them to stay in good health. The evidence above illustrates well the reasons for taking brewer's yeast or some other purely natural food supplement rather than synthetic vitamins. Since Drs. Martin and Koop wrote their article, several more B vitamins have been discovered. They could not have been put into synthetic vitamin preparations at the time this article appeared, for their existence was unknown. But they were already in the brewer's yeast and the liver preparations, and these patients benefited from them, even though they had not been discovered.

Don't be afraid to take large quantities of brewer's yeast and other completely natural food supplements rich in B vitamins, like desiccated liver and wheat germ, especially if you have distressing symptoms in mouth or digestive tract. And eat a diet high in B vitamins, too. Meat, fish, eggs, wheat germ and fresh vegetables and fruits are the best source.

130. Is Vitamin C Deficiency Related to Cancer?

Several years ago an article on the possible relationship between a deficiency in vitamin C and suceptibility to cancer was written by W. J. McCormick, M.D., which appeared in *Archives of Pediatrics*, October, 1954. Now Dr. McCormick has written another article in the same magazine, enlarged on his theory and brought it up to date with new research.

It is such a simple and easily understood theory that we marvel that it has not achieved more prominence among medical researchers. Perhaps it is too simple. Perhaps the solution to our cancer problem by a change in diet and environment that would bring all of us ample supplies of vitamin C, is just such a simple everyday thing that the majority of our learned researchers will not even consider it.

Dr. McCormick tells us that the injury that precedes cancer (whether it is an actual physical injury or a chemical injury) produces a certain condition resulting in the formation of what some researchers call "pseudo-elastic tissue." He quotes Dr. T. Gillman and colleagues, writing in the *British Journal of Cancer*, Vol. 9, pp. 272-283, 1955, as saying that such tissue is regularly encountered in sites of chronic injury to connective tissue in the skin as well as in other parts of the body—arteries and gall bladder, for example.

This tissue, which is preceded by and associated with an invasion of dermal cells by epidermal cells, can consistently be produced in human beings who have injuries. The British researchers go on to say, "It is shown that similar elastotic degeneration of collagen (tissue) is invariably present in the dermis in many degenerative skin conditions which may and frequently do become precancerous." They believe that such a degeneration of this layer of cells may play an important part in causing cancer.

Dr. McCormick then quotes a researcher who wrote in 1908 (long before vitamin C was discovered) that precancerous tissues always show a loss of connective tissue. The edges of the cells in the epithelium (the lining of all parts of the body) are frayed. Yellow elastic tissue disappears. *And it is in this de-elasticized area where connective tissue has disappeared that the first beginnings of cancer occur.*

How Vitamin C Protects Intercellular Cement

We know that the cement holding cells together can be manufactured only if vitamin C is present in ample quantity. This cement becomes watery in an individual suffering from scurvy which is the disease of vitamin C deficiency. The protein contained normally in this cement disappears into the blood. In cancer patients, recent tests have shown that there is an increase of this particular protein in the blood. When vitamin C is given, almost immediately the intercellular cement begins to reform in its normal consistency.

More evidence. Several researchers have found that there is a pronounced deficiency of vitamin C in the blood of cancer patients, compared to that of healthy persons. It has been found that guinea pigs suffering from scurvy and given just enough vitamin C to be kept alive are far more susceptible to cancer and get it sooner than healthy guinea pigs.

Dr. McCormick believes that all this evidence shows definitely that the degree of malignancy of an illness is determined inversely by the degree of connective tissue resistance. And this, in turn, is dependent on the adequacy of vitamin C intake. In other words, the less resistant the connective tissue is, the more serious the trouble is likely to be. And lack of vitamin C is perhaps the basic cause of lack of resistance.

Hard Cancer Spreads Slowly

To illustrate this point, he tells us that the scirrhus or hard cancer of the breast is slow to metastasize or spread throughout the body. It may remain just as it is, completely inactive for years. On the other hand, soft cancer of the breast is "extremely invasive." That is, it spreads rapidly to other parts of the body. In the former there is plenty of connective tissue which binds the cells together more effectively. In the second kind of cancer, there are mostly only cells and the connective tissue is lacking.

It may be, says Dr. McCormick, that cancer cells, which are known to move around in the body, may do so because of an inherent propensity which becomes manifest solely because they have lost their connective

[514]

tissue anchorage as a direct result of vitamin C deficiency. The teeth become loose in an individual suffering from scurvy—the disease of vitamin C deficiency. This is because the cementing substance holding them in has liquefied because there is not enough vitamin C to keep this cementing substance in good repair.

So cancer may not be a "malignant" disease, striking its victims like a bolt of lightning out of the blue, but rather, says Dr. McCormick, it may be an ailment that we cultivate all during our lifetime by our habits.

Preventing Cancer Is the Important Thing

We should, then, direct our attention to preventing the cause of cellular disarrangement—that is, the breakdown of connective tissue. What about sores or fissures that fail to heal? What about unusual and easily produced hemorrhages—not necessarily with visible blood as in a nosebleed, but the bruises so many of us take for granted?

Dr. McCormick tells us he has found that fully 90 per cent of our adult female population show bruises or "black and blue marks," yet little or nothing is ever done about it. No one should ever show bruises unless he is in an extremely serious accident. The bumps and knocks we get in everyday living should never produce bruises. They are as easy to prevent as the nearest vitamin C tablet and a glass of water.

Easy Bruising a Symptom of Vitamin C Deficiency

Easy bruising is one of the earliest—hence one of the most important —symptoms of vitamin C deficiency. And, make no mistake about it, bruising is a serious symptom. As Dr. McCormick has suggested, it may be your first and most valuable warning of a predisposition to cancer.

Dr. McCormick believes that one reason we moderns are so likely to be deficient in vitamin C is the almost universal habit of smoking. Smoking destroys or neutralizes to a large extent what little vitamin C is taken in food. The smoking of one cigarette, as ordinarily inhaled, tends to neutralize in the body about 25 milligrams of vitamin C, or the vitamin C content of an average orange. This fact alone would do much to explain the terrible increase in lung cancer in recent years.

But poisons other than nicotine are counteracted by vitamin C in the body. And the vitamin C is used up in the process. We know of many. Could it be that all physical and chemical carcinogens (causes of cancer) may act by using up the body's supply of vitamin C, thereby destroying the connective tissue and leading the way to cancer that spreads rapidly through the body?

Who is Susceptible to Cancer?

The Sloan-Kettering Institute recently conducted a test, using live, virulent cancer cells. These were transplanted under the skin of the forearm of 15 advanced cancer cases. In every case the transplanted cancer tissues grew vigorously and spread for from 6 weeks to 6 months before they were removed by surgery. On the other hand, the same cells transplanted to the forearms of normally healthy and cancer-free volunteers, were destroyed by an overwhelming defense reaction on the part of these individuals.

No study was made, unfortunately, of the nutritional background or living habits of the subjects. Such a study would certainly have thrown a lot of light on the subject of susceptibility to cancer. However, the test surely shows that cancer is a disease of the whole body. Therefore, it seems reasonable to suppose that it can be prevented by keeping the body healthy.

Vitamin Status Study Advised for Middle-Aged

Dr. McCormick suggests that all persons of middle age or over should have a study made of their vitamin C status. Your doctor should be able to do it.

Or, as a general overall test, ask yourself these questions: Do your gums bleed or do you have some loose teeth? Do you bruise easily? Do you get colds easily? Do open sores heal slowly? Are you exposed to tobacco regularly, or smoke, or fumes of some materials like solvents, fresh paint, etc.? If you answer yes to any of these questions, better get concerned about your vitamin C status. Now, before there is any possible chance of a serious deficiency that might mean a predisposition to cancer.

A natural vitamin C food supplement is your best assurance that you won't be short. In addition, concentrate on getting as many fresh raw foods as possible in your diet every day.

131. Does Breast Feeding Prevent Cancer of the Breast?

By WILLIAM PERRIN NICOLSON, JR., M.D.

Every intelligent woman is interested in the subject of cancer. Since cancer of the breast and uterus are the two most frequent sites affected in a woman, she naturally centers her interest in these more than any others. She is taught the signs of early cancer and told how she should have periodic health examinations, but too little is said about the possibility of preventing cancer.

Lactation is the normal desire of most women. Those who do not nurse their babies fail to do so for various reasons. She may have heard of the so called "milk factor," which some feel may be transmitted from the mother to the infant, and she may be afraid to nurse her baby because of the possibility of transferring this potential disease to her child. There

[516]

may be economic reasons such as one who has to return to her work. There are numerous others, so that the answer to the question of whether or not lactation might help prevent cancer of the breast is a very important one to her.

Unfortunately, it is practically impossible to say with any degree of certainty that lactation does or will prevent cancer of the breast. Contrariwise, it is equally as impossible to state that it does not prevent cancer of the breast. It is hard to prove either statement. Statistics may be juggled to prove what is wished proven, but the burden of the evidence seems to be that the answer is definitely in the affirmative.

In the first place, the breasts are undoubtedly provided an individual for the purpose of secreting milk. They are not there as ornaments to attract the opposite sex, though they are all too frequently used for that purpose. And it's frequently the fear that one will lose the shapeliness of her mammary glands that prevents a mother from nursing her child. The females of all mammalian species are endowed with mammary glands for the purpose of suckling their young. This not only transmits to the offspring needed nutrition, but also aids in developing immunity and stabilization of the nervous system so that the individual will later be "well adjusted."

In the second place, lactation prevents stagnation. The late Dr. James Ewing said that if stagnation in the breast could be prevented, there would be no cancer of the breast. He probably did not mean this literally, but wished to emphasize the irritating effects that the stagnant fluids in the breast have on the duct cells. To further establish the relationship between stagnation and cancer, Bagg, many years ago, at Memorial Hospital in New York, carried out some interesting experiments. He ligated (cut) the mammary ducts on one side of a mouse or rat and allowed these animals to continue to breed. Carcinomas (cancers) developed invariably on the ligated side, and not on the other side, whereas, in control animals from the same litters, the malignant lesions manifested no choice between the right and left sides. Obviously it is impossible to carry out such an experiment in a human being and equally as obvious that one human case proves nothing by itself, but considered in conjunction with the animal experimentation, the following case is most interesting.

A 47 year old, white female was admitted to St. Joseph's Infirmary Tumor Clinic giving a history of having borne 13 children. All of these were nursed on one breast but none nursed the other. The breast which had lactated was perfectly normal, the one which did not lactate was filled with what appeared to be an inflammatory type carcinoma. She died in less than 3 months in spite of large doses of X-ray and androgens (sex hormones).

According to Dr. James C. Moloney, the neonatal mortality in India is extremely high (40 per cent or more), and it is said that breast cancer occurs at least 8 times more frequently in India than in this country. Could the fact that the baby dies and therefore cannot nurse the breast be one of the reasons why this high instance of mammary cancer is found?

According to the same authority, on Okinawa all mothers nurse their babies whenever they are hungry until the time they are two years of age. In 1945, of a population of 375,000 persons, only 3 cancers were discovered by teams of civilians and pathologists, and none of these were breast cases. Could this be because all women nurse their babies over a long period of time?

Statistics are of necessity boring, but when no other means are available to determine a fact, one scrutinizes pertinent figures, always remembering that a juggling of these may sometimes lead to false conclusions. Dr. Ralph W. Murphy of the Georgia State Board of Health furnished the following information. It seems to be statistically significant.

It is a well known fact that the Negro is much more likely to nurse her offspring than is the white person. If this is true, the death rates in these two races are of material interest. In the state of Georgia in 1948, the death rate from all causes was almost twice as large among Negroes as among whites (1012.1 vs. 662.0), whereas death from cancer of the breast occurred more frequently among white women (18 vs. 14). Practically the same difference in the death rates existed from 1930 through 1948, in these two races in Georgia. If we consider the United States as a whole, it is found that the average death rate from cancer of the breast among white women from 1930 through 1947, was 23.7 and for the colored races 13.5. This is an even more striking difference than existed in the state of Georgia.

Another angle from which one can view this problem is the difference between the urban and rural dweller. In the 5 year period from 1945 through 1949, the rural death rate in Georgia showed that there were 6.3 white deaths to every 4.2 colored deaths from cancer of the breast, whereas, the opposite is true when we consider the cases of cancer of the uterus (8.7 White vs. 13 Colored). Here, too, we know that the rural infant is more likely to be breast fed.

A consideration of the urban statistics shows that the death rate for whites for the same period in the state of Georgia was 11.4 against 10.1 for Negroes. Whereas, the uterine carcinomas showed 13.8 for the whites and 23.8 for the Negroes. This same study carried out through 5 states selected at random shows practically the same thing, namely, from cancer of the breast 15.2 for the white and 14.7 for the colored, and the uterine carcinomas 23 for the whites against 41.7 for the colored in the rural areas, whereas, in the urban areas the whites had a death rate from breast carcinomas of 21.3 against 17.6 for the Negroes and the uterine carcinoma were just the opposite with 14.3 for the whites against 31.1 for the Negroes.

One final argument in favor of the affirmative answer to the original question is the fact that cows practically never, if ever, have cancer of the udder. A study carried out by an Australian veterinarian many years ago, in which thousands of udders were examined, found not a single carcinoma except in a few of the teats. The additional fact that the cow goes on 4 legs helps prevent carcinoma, also, because the circulation in the breast is not interfered with, but undoubtedly the frequent lactations are the principal factors in preventing this dread disease.

Reed has just published his findings in a *Survey of the Breast Cancer Patient in the Tumor Clinic of the University of Minnesota,* and among his conclusions was the fact that cancer of the breast occurs more frequently in childless women (married or single) than among those who have children. He didn't unfortunately, separate those which had bottle babies from those who nursed their babies.

The cancer education of the layman has stressed mainly the early detection of a lesion while it is still a localized disease. This is being accomplished by frequent self-examinations, and periodic check-ups, and has resulted in more so called "cured" cases. Unfortunately, too little has been said of *prevention*—what, if anything, can a woman do to prevent cancer of the breast? There are 3 things: (1.) Proper support; (2.) Prevent stagnation; (3.) Lactation. And of these, lactation is the most important one.

If then, these conclusions are correct, it behooves each doctor, especially the obstetrician and the pediatrician, to urge his patients to do their best to nurse their infants. A girl should be psychologically prepared for lactation. "As a man thinketh, so is he." If she anticipates the pleasures that she will derive, she will be building up her supply of milk before the baby arrives, then if the surroundings in her home are adequate and she has the cooperation of her pediatrician she will usually be able to nurse the baby, and if she does, she will be less likely to have cancer of the breast.

Reprinted from *Child-Family Digest* Vol. 10, No. 6, June, 1954.

132. Krebiozen—The History of a Tragedy

You will read Herbert Bailey's book, *A Matter of Life or Death, The Incredible Story of Krebiozen* (published by G. P. Putnam's Sons, 210 Madison Avenue, New York, New York, $4.95), with certainly two emotions, indignation and outrage. If you have known someone who suffered with cancer, you are likely to become bitter as you read of a cure for this disease whose release, Mr. Bailey says, has been thwarted and suppressed by the American Medical Association since 1951.

The story began with the experiments of Dr. Stevan Durovic, a former assistant professor at the University of Belgrade. He came to the United States after several years of experimentation in South America, with a drug which he had discovered and which he believed to be a cure for cancer. Once in the United States, he was brought to the attention of Dr. Andrew C. Ivy, a medical researcher of unassailable reputation and gigantic stature in his profession. Dr. Ivy was, at the time, vice president of the University of Illinois, and head of its huge Medical School. His efforts in cancer research had led to his appointment as Executive Director of the National Advisory Cancer Council and he was also a director of the American Cancer Society. An important, a respected, an honored man.

Early Results Show Promise

Dr. Ivy became interested in the theory and possibilities shown in Dr. Durovic's substance, Krebiozen, and he decided to test it in the scientific manner his experience had taught him was necessary for an accurate picture of the drug's potential. From the very beginning the results were astounding in their positiveness. Though Krebiozen was used only on persons who had been diagnosed as hopeless and close to death, its remarkable characteristics showed themselves almost at once. There was a lessening or complete disappearance of pain, and in many cases tumors were dissolved and replaced with healthy tissue. Physicians who were trying it all over the country reported like results. It began to look as though science had finally come up with a weapon against cancer that had a chance to win the fight.

With such a product as a cancer cure, scientific and humanitarian considerations are joined by a third consideration—commercialism. Without a doubt, a cancer cure is worth a lot of money. What victim would not offer all he owns, or all he can borrow for even a chance that he might be cured? Large drug companies have made millions on substances designed to treat diseases far less urgent and wide-spread than cancer. This then is why two Chicago businessmen tried to get control of the distribution rights to Krebiozen. When they were refused, they threatened to ruin Krebiozen and everyone connected with it. One of the men who made this threat was the friend of J. J. Moore, then treasurer of the American Medical Association.

The promise shown in the early tests of Krebiozen seemed to be emphasized with each new experiment. The excitement and relief provided by such apparent success left little room for worry over the threat that had been made. How could so proud and secure a venture as a scientifically proven cancer cure be scuttled by the influence of commercial interests?

Dr. Ivy Pays the Price

The answer to that question came with devastating swiftness. In rapid succession Dr. Ivy was suspended from membership in the Chicago Medical Society, removed from the vice presidency of the University of Illinois, and had his resignation accepted by both national cancer societies noted above. But worst of all, his work with Krebiozen was assailed as inaccurate and unscientific. His conclusions were dismissed or so interpreted as to discredit his research methods, methods which had been good enough to earn him a world-wide reputation, methods which till then had been regarded as the ultimate in scientific detachment and objectivity. Suddenly the approach was wrong, the conclusions untrue, the impression was fostered that Dr. Ivy was no longer capable of reliable scientific observation. It was even suggested that Dr. Ivy had become senile and was loyal to Krebiozen only because his mind was failing.

How Krebiozen Fared

The fate of Krebiozen itself was similar. Within a few short months after Dr. Ivy made known some observations on 26 patients whose history showed Krebiozen to be of "promise," the *Journal of the American Medical Association* published a Status Report on Krebiozen. It dealt with 100 case histories, a project which top scientists would have difficulty in completing properly in two years, not 6 weeks, even working at top speed! The report was extremely damaging, and the temper of the average observer after reading it is reflected in a *Chicago Tribune* editorial which said, "Medically speaking, Krebiozen is dead. Let it be buried without ceremony." These people, among them thousands of doctors who rely on the *Journal of the American Medical Association* for all of their current medical information, never knew that the core of the report was faked. Mr. Bailey shows that the doctor who wrote the article made so many omissions of factual and favorable results and so altered the findings that were at his disposal that even the most naive researcher would have discredited his conclusions at once as thoroughly unscientific and worthless. These and other facts showing that the AMA acted in a biased and arbitrary fashion concerning Krebiozen were sworn to under oath at a subsequent investigation of the whole situation by the Illinois State Legislature. But still the smudges on the reputation of Krebiozen could not be erased. When anyone powerful enough to effect a change became interested, he would contact a doctor, perhaps a cancer specialist, who had seen and believed the AMA report, and the doctor could only say he'd seen a report proving Krebiozen worthless. How could the doctor be aware that the article, not Krebiozen, was a fraud? How could he know that 5 patients examined by the author of the report (but deliberately omitted from it) were free from any detectable cancer after 5 years, due to treatment with Krebiozen?

Bailey Names Names

The intrigue involved in this story is of melodramatic proportions. There are monitored phone calls, South American undercover agents, falsified medical reports, threats of deportation and suggestions of influence by the Vatican. The story is all written out, and every word is documented by

Mr. Bailey. The villains are painted with certainty and positively identified. No innuendo or veiled references are employed to shield the author from possible libel or slander, yet in spite of Mr. Bailey's invitations, no single action of this kind has ever been instituted. To illustrate: a reporter on the staff of the *New York Post,* after reading the indictment contained in Mr. Bailey's first book on the subject: *K-Krebiozen—Key to Cancer?,* called the AMA for specific answers to specific questions, such as, "Does J. J. Moore deny that he formed a conspiracy to gain control of Krebiozen?" or, "Does the AMA deny that its official report against Krebiozen was falsified?" and was met with this stock answer: "The AMA will not answer specific questions concerning Krebiozen." The reporter's comment: ". . . it sounds a bit like the AMA is pleading the Fifth Amendment."

A Book Is Buried

The negative attitude of the AMA toward Krebiozen showed itself in the fate of Mr. Bailey's first book on the subject. The *New York Times* accepted one advertisement for the book, then refused subsequent ads on the recommendations of its medical advisors. A favorable review of the book was written by the same paper's science editor, but it never appeared in print. An unfortunate review followed. The New York Public Library, one of the world's largest, kept the book off its shelves until nearly a year after its publication, because of its "controversial" content. To underline the precariousness of being connected with such a book, the records will show that the publishers of *K-Krebiozen—Key to Cancer?* were out of business within a year of publishing it.

Dr. Ivy was having similar problems in publishing a monograph in which he reported on 687 patients over a 6 year period who had been treated with Krebiozen. The work showed observable benefits in 70 per cent of the cases, and directly objectively beneficial results in 50 per cent of the cases. Dr. Ivy sent an article based on this monograph to one medical journal after another—remember this was news on an effective treatment for cancer!—only to have it returned with apologies and excuses for not being able to publish it. The monograph was finally published by a small general publisher, Henry Regnery, Chicago. Instead of headlines and excitement over the proven claim that Krebiozen had destroyed cancer cells in half of the patients treated with it, the monograph was greeted with apathy and indifference. The American Cancer Society officially announced that it would stand by the AMA verdict of 1951 in the matter, as did others whose opinion could have helped foster interest or general acceptance.

Misrepresentations Detailed

The stories of Krebiozen's fight for acceptance against organized medicine are catalogued in *A Matter of Life or Death* up to 1957. They are too numerous for even a brief mention of all of them here, however the details of a correspondence between 3 Sloan-Kettering cancer specialists and a Mrs. Dorothea Seeber on behalf of a friend in the last stages of cancer are typical. Mrs. Seeber wrote a letter asking Sloan-Kettering doctors their opinion of Krebiozen and whether it would be advisable to use it on a "hopeless case." One doctor, whose signature is printed with his letter, as are the others, answers that "We tried it (Krebiozen) on 100 patients and I regret to say that we could not substantiate any of the claims ascribed to its use." Another answer said, "I have had only a few patients who have been tried on Krebiozen, and there was no improvement in their condition." A third wrote: "A considerable amount of work has been done on this drug and we found it is absolutely worthless." An affidavit by Dr. Ivy is printed in the same chapter in which he swears that these three doctors never asked for nor received any Krebiozen for use on cancer patients and could not, therefore, have come to any first-hand findings concerning it. Until 1956, the date of the affidavit, not a single ampule of Krebiozen had ever been sent to the Sloan-Kettering Institute!

As this book was written, Dr. Ivy was making every worthwhile effort to get the AMA to run a blind experiment on Krebiozen, the type in which neither the doctor nor the patient is aware of whether or not the injection he gives contains the substance being tested. The experiment would be set up by AMA experts; they could choose the doctors and the patients, and the results would be published for all the world to see if Krebiozen is a miracle or a fraud. As yet, the AMA refuses to have any part of such an objective test. Why?

The last chapter of the heroic Krebiozen story is yet to be written. When it is, it will be a humiliating admission to the American people that the most powerful medical authority in the world saw fit to deprive of a proper investigation a promising, now-proven, nontoxic cure for cancer, due to personal motives of one of its highest officials. It will also tell the glorious story of selfless men who sacrificed everything—money, security, position and reputation—in the attempt to get Krebiozen to those who need it. These and other heroes and villains will be brought to light. When this story is told openly, and to the world, the indignation and scorn that will be heaped upon those responsible for holding back Krebiozen defies the imagination.

133. Cancer and Drosnes-Lazenby Treatment

"The battle against death is too important to condemn a single weapon without exploring its possibilities," so said Frank Edwards, news commentator for the Mutual Broadcasting System, in a broadcast on April 18, 1950. He was speaking about a clinic in Pittsburgh, Pennsylvania, where a substance developed from a mold was being used successfully to treat cancer. Edwards made a study of the clinic and its file of case histories. He gave it nation-wide publicity. Various newspapers and magazines around Pittsburgh have taken up the story.

Two lay people founded the clinic—two people who had worked for years conducting experiments with a mold substance they grew. Excited about the possibilities of using the mold for cancer treatment, they went to the Director of the National Cancer Institute who listened to them carefully and encouraged them to go ahead. Six years of hard work went by—years in which Philip Drosnes and Lillian Lazenby spent their own time and money buying laboratory equipment and working almost around the clock on experiments to prove that cancer tissue could be broken down and destroyed by the substrate of their mold. (A substrate is the liquid that drips from the mold—the extract of the mold.)

They had gotten something started that they couldn't stop. What if this were the long-sought key to the problem of cancer? Or what if it might throw some light—even if ever so little—on that problem?

This was the thought that kept them going through one discouragement after another. Finally they were convinced that they had found an organism under their microscope which existed in cancerous tissue and also existed in the mold they had grown. By injecting the substrate from their mold they could stop cancerous growth in their laboratory animals. And the organism no longer appeared in the formerly cancerous tissues.

Analysis of the mold product made by the National Institute of Health showed that it contained two substances called Rhizopus and Mucor as well as various strains of penicillium. The name of the substance— Mucorhicin—is derived from the names of these various elements. Sending in a report of this to Mrs. Lazenby, the National Institute suggested that she interest some local physician in giving the antibiotic (as it could now be called) to cancer patients and make careful studies of results over a long period of time. Paul A. Murray, M.D., of Pittsburgh, who was already using the antibiotic, proceeded enthusiastically to give it to cancer patients and to work closely with the discoverers to keep records of his patients.

Working Against Opposition

For two people who are not medical practitioners or researchers, the path to recognition is fraught with perils. One of the easiest ways to discredit any cancer "cure" is to claim that the patients treated did not have cancer at all. At the Drosnes-Lazenby Clinic a rule was made to take only "terminal" cases of cancer, that is, patients whose cases had been declared hopeless by their physicians and who had been sent home to die. They must present at the clinic a statement from their physician or hospital giving the diagnosis of cancer.

This sounds watertight. But there are always angles and loopholes. For instance, in the files of the clinic are photostats of a hospital record of Jimmy M. which was changed (in a different handwriting) *after the patient was cured at the clinic.* His diagnosis had been sarcoma—cancer of the jaw. His parents had been told that he had only a short time to live. What possible objection could there be to his coming to the clinic to see if Mucorhicin might ease the pain of his dying days? When, a month or so later, he was discharged as cured, the draining hole in his cheek grown over with new skin, the story got around. A friend of the clinic looked up Jimmy's record in the hospital file. The diagnosis of "sarcoma" had been crossed out and a diagnosis of Fibro Hemangloma, a "non-malignant tumor" had been written in.

We have in our files a series of case histories of clinic patients written by Dr. Murray and his associate Dr. Joseph W. Wilson, another Pittsburgh M.D. Jimmy's case is not isolated. As soon as word began to get around that there might be a cancer cure over at the Drosnes-Lazenby Clinic, it became increasingly difficult to get records from hospitals and family physicians. The clinic does not diagnose.

Perhaps it is understandable that diagnosticians do not want to become involved in any action around a highly controversial cancer treatment. Certainly it would be unpleasant for a physician to diagnose a case of cancer, tell the patient he could do nothing for him and then have the patient cured by a mold preparation developed by two people who are not even physicians.

But are physicians today interested in curing cancer or are they not? If they are, then should they not seize upon any treatment that holds out even the faintest hope of a cure? Especially when, as in the case of Mucorhicin, there has never been a single toxic or harmful reaction of any kind on the part of anyone taking the substance! If the National Cancer Institute is interested in curing cancer, should they not send an immediate investigating committee, if there is the slightest chance that Mucorhicin may be effective?

But the Drosnes-Lazenby Clinic did not claim to have a cancer cure. They believed whole-heartedly that they had discovered something of great value to humanity and they wanted the chance to try it out on people already given up for dead. Sounds as though it would be simple enough, doesn't it? Especially with an ever-growing file of case histories of patients who were treated without fees up to 1950. But it is not so simple as it sounds, and what happened to these two folks is a nightmare of run-arounds, evasions, misrepresentations and arrest. Yes, Mr. Drosnes and Mrs. Lazenby were arrested on the grounds of practicing medicine without a license.

A Case History

We spoke to the father of one patient—Karen G. who was given up as a hopeless brain tumor case, when she was 8. *Intramedullary Glioma of the brain stem and cerebellum*—that was the diagnosis her physicians made. After a series of operations, she was taken home to die. She was in a coma, unconscious, paralyzed, and toes and hands twisted backward, when her parents came to the clinic. Karen was given Mucorhicin first through a tube in her nose. Her second dose was given orally. She began to improve at once and slowly, gradually she came back to life until about 8 months later, she could sit in a wheel chair and the paralysis affected only one arm which continued to improve.

Today Karen is blind, for the cancer had destroyed her sight before Mucorhicin therapy. But she is happy and well. Dr. Murray, in his written case history of Karen says, "Progress of this patient can only be described as amazing."

The same can be said for other patients who have been treated with Mucorhicin. While we were talking to Karen's father, he mentioned two friends of his whose cancers had also disappeared when they got the Drosnes-Lazenby treatment. Can we prove that they had cancer? This becomes increasingly difficult. For instance, Karen's hospital records have disappeared from the files at the hospital. We were told that the clinic doctors could not get them; her lawyer could not get them.

The blistering, searing campaign of ridicule, persecution and scorn that has met Mr. Drosnes and Mrs. Lazenby at every turn is more comprehensible if you think of it in terms of what might happen to you or any other lay person under similar circumstances. They had worked for many years developing their mold substrate and treating cancerous animals successfully with it before they used it on human cancers. They took only patients who had been told by their doctors that they could not be cured. There were only two of them at the clinic. There was no money except for their own personal contributions, for they treated everyone free of charge in the early years.

Growing and processing the mold substance, getting the medicine to a widely scattered group of patients, contacting hospitals and doctors to get case histories on their patients so that they would know that the diagnosis had been cancer, following up on patients over the years to check on how long death was postponed or finally outwitted—the amount of work involved in all this staggers the imagination, when you think of two people undertaking it alone for no purpose other than to use their dis-

[526]

covery to benefit desperately sick people. Obviously these are the kinds of jobs that should be done by a full hospital staff.

What Can You Do About It?

If you inquire, you will probably be told that the Drosnes-Lazenby treatment for cancer has been thoroughly investigated and found to be worthless. This is not the case. No bona fide investigation has ever been done. No official representative of the Cancer Society, the Public Health Service, the Medical Association, or any other professional group, has ever gone over the case histories, interviewed patients or studied the formula and processing of Mucorhicin, the mold substance which is used at the Drosnes-Lazenby Clinic. There is no secret about the mold. It is grown on a mixture of various food substances. Mr. Drosnes and Mrs. Lazenby are not only willing, but eager, to turn over the formula, the processing and the treating of patients to any reputable school or organization which will carry on their work. However, they will not turn anything over to individuals who want to make a profit from it, or to those who may want to buy it and hide it away.

If you are as indignant as we feel you should be after reading this story, what can you do to see that this kind of injustice and blind disregard for human life does not continue? Your congressman should be interested in the Drosnes-Lazenby story. We suggest that you write to him, urging him to ask for a Congressional investigation of this and all the other cancer treatments which are at present unrecognized by organized medicine. If you want more material on the Drosnes-Lazenby Clinic treatment, there is plenty available. Write to the Drosnes-Lazenby Clinic, 4774 Liberty Avenue, Pittsburgh 24, Pennsylvania.

134. Can Cancer Be Prevented?

By MAX GERSON, M.D.

Up to the present, the cancer research all over the world has been unable to find anything certain about the underlying cause of cancer and even less about the problems of curing it. Two examples may be quoted here: Jesse P. Greenstein, Chief of Laboratory of Biochemistry, National Cancer Institute, Bethesda, Maryland, says in his book, *Biochemistry of Cancer*, 1954, p. 598, "cancer is a phenomenon coexistent with the living process, that it will be present for some time to come, and that emphasis must be laid on a direct study on the site of malignancy itself." Greenstein is very skeptical about my cancer therapy, but he has the feeling that:

"cancer cell is not a system isolated from the living universe. . . ." C. Chester Stock of The Experimental Chemo-therapy, Sloan-Kettering Institute, New York writes in *Advances in Cancer Research,* 1954, p. 478: "No human cancer cures are available. . . . There appears no strong basis at present for prediction of the discovery of a cancer cure within the next few years. . . . However, the next few years will bring advances in experimental chemo-therapy . . . to be the *few feeble* steps which they are." That means: the scientific outlook is very pessimistic.

In the dietary field, Tannenbaum studied the effect of reduced caloric intake and found reduced incidence of tumor growths. King investigated the effect of other dietary restrictions, especially the vitamin C content in hypernephromas and Jensen rat sarcomas (two kinds of cancer). The increased vitamin C content of these neoplasms (cancers) could not be confirmed by other authors. More studies about that problem can be found in my article "Cancer, a Problem of Metabolism," June 25, 1954. Freund and Kaminer studied the avoidance of all animal fats and substituted oil for them in so-called inoperable patients. These restrictions and several others had little or no lasting success. All these experiments and studies did not prove to be of much value for the cancer therapy, as they took separately only one or another item of our nutrition into account. Much more is necessary. The combined effect of most of them in the whole metabolism is decisive.

To understand my favorable clinical results by treating the whole metabolism of the cancer patient, I have to go back to the old cancer experiments of Dr. J. L. Alibert, a famous surgeon living in Paris at the time of Napoleon. He was the first who inoculated cancerous material to himself and 3 of his students. The result was a violent inflammatory reaction lasting a few days, but no cancerous growth appeared in any of the human guinea pigs. These experiments were repeated by Dr. Alibert himself and other colleagues and showed always a negative result. The failure to transplant cancer into normal human beings was long regarded, scientifically, as uncertain, as the description of the experiments did not show sufficient scientific accuracy. However, many experiments in the following 150 years did reveal that transplantation of tumors is very difficult, even impossible in healthy animals of the same type but can be made successfully in the animals living under domestic conditions or damaged by abnormal feeding, virus infections or inbreeding, or weakened by inferior inheritance. These conditions increase the susceptibility, but decrease defense and resistance. Therefore, cancer patients often show secondary infections, an abnormal intestinal flora, osteoarthritis, chronic sinus trouble, different types of anemia and other disorders along with the cancer.

Modern civilization first damages the soil by artificial fertilizers, spraying, etc., correspondingly our nutrition is denaturalized and partly poisoned (see Wickenden, *Our Daily Poison* and other authors), while our bodies

[528]

are adapted, through millions of generations, to the natural food. Where there is no modern civilization, there is no cancer (see the Hunzas, Ethiopian people and others) but where civilization starts to change nutrition, cancer starts (see Albert Schweitzer's *Briefe aus Lambarene,* Central Africa, October, 1954, p. 18/19, and the reports of Eskimos after they accepted canned foods). In addition to the damages to the soil, the food is further damaged by preservation processes as it is refined, dried, powdered, bottled, color added. frozen. until it finally becomes a partly poisoned and entirely dead mass.

This transformation of the food affects the liver of the person eating it to the highest degree. This organ is, in regard to the cancer problem, the most important organ for two reasons. First, for our essential detoxification for which processes the liver uses oxidation; reduction (that is, depriving of oxygen), methylation (that is, mixing it with chemical radicals) or it may conjugate (or mix) the poisons with some amino acids and make them ready for the elimination with the bile. Second, the liver activates and reactivates the hormones, vitamins and oxidizing enzymes, thus regulating and protecting the most vital processes of our life. It is the largest organ in our body and has the strange property of not presenting any characteristic symptoms or pain for a long time, even years. This is most probably the reason why cancer remains a hidden disease till symptoms of one or several growths appear and can be diagnosed. No wonder that many leading surgeons come, at the end of their career, to the conclusion that surgery is not the answer to cancer, while I found in more than 25 years of clinical cancer work, that the diseased condition of the liver in connection with that of the intestinal tract is the underlying cause for cancer development. The correctness of this theory is proven among other findings by the statistical increase in cancer incidence corresponding with the increase in liver diseases, which is astonishing just in the last few years. Bateman reports in the *Journal of the American Medical Association,* October 20, 1956, that according to cancer statistics there is: "an increase in incidence, morbidity, and mortality in spite of improved X-ray techniques, increasingly extensive operative procedures, and education regarding early detection. It appears that the problem of the so-called hopeless case will remain large for some time to come."

The question of whether cancer can be prevented has to be generally answered as "no." To really wipe out cancer, it would be necessary to change our agriculture by avoiding artificial fertilizers and all types of sprays. In addition, it would be necessary to change the ways of preservation and distribution of foods and to avoid depriving them of their natural, vital values. That means: not to can, bottle, refine, or subject food to other damaging methods. I think that only some individuals will be able to accomplish the difficult task of avoiding or reducing to a minimum all methods which modern civilization has brought upon us. On the other hand, great revolutionary transformations would be necessary, pressed by the strongest demand of a great part of the population to accomplish this vital task for the well-being of our future offspring.

As long as all the historical observations and those of our present time remain "paper warnings" only, we cannot speak about prevention of cancer. Such paper warnings, even given in the strongest and most convincing way did not save old Persia, the ancient Egyptian people, the culture of Greece, and the people of the Roman Empire (Roma eterna). All these and many more had to go down after "their modern civilization" ruined the simple habits of life and nutrition, but increased degenerative diseases.

In the United States, our upward rise went quicker than in all other ancient countries and degenerative diseases with cancer and mental sicknesses, have increased much faster too. In the last years degenerative diseases appear in our babies and children, especially in the form of leukemias. It is an illusion that the clinical attempt to detect early symptoms means prevention of cancer. Prevention is possible *only* if we know the cause of cancer. In my opinion, it is based upon the degeneration of the liver and I repeat: the beginning degenerative changes in the liver do not show any symptoms for a long period. For that reason the removal of one or several cancer symptoms (growths) by operation, or X-ray or radium does not remove the underlying cause, therefore the tumors, regrow sooner or later.

The other question of whether we can cure cancer has been answered in a number of articles that I have published since 1946. I have shown that cancer can be cured even in so-called inoperable or far advanced, given-up cases. Four such examples of unpublished cases may be described here.

The treatment (a combined totality regime) has to make good what modern civilization and other methods and occurrences have ruined before, in the liver and whole digestive tract. In short: The treatment consists of a saltless, fruit and vegetable diet, excluding all refined, canned, bottled, powdered, frozen, etc., foods. The patient gets plenty of salads and, every hour on the hour, freshly prepared juices of apples and carrots, green leaves, one orange juice, and 3 calf's liver juices. In addition, vegetables, baked potatoes, and stewed fruit. Preferred are fruits and vegetables with high potassium and low sodium content, like apples, potatoes, apricots, etc. As the content of fruits and vegetables of modern farming shows potassium increasingly diminished by the years, we are forced to use more of them grown by organic gardening methods. Seventy-five per cent of the food we serve is raw, a living substance, finely grated or in the form of juices. All are easily digestible. The rest is cooked. After 6 weeks, saltless and creamless pot-cheese, buttermilk, and yogurt can be added. The medication used is a potassium compound, iodine in the form of thyroid and lugol, niacin and liver injections with vitamin B_{12}. Numerous cases published before and the following 4 unpublished cases show the effectiveness of this method.

Case No. 1. Mrs. M. A. K.

Diagnosis confirmed by biopsies: Neurofibroma with rapid growth and development of sarcoma.

1. Operation: February, 1941. Removal of tumor on the lower part of nose.
2. Operation: 1943. Removal of recurrent tumor mass (nose).
3. Operation: 1945. Again, removal of recurrent tumor. (Upper lip and gum).
4. Operation: June, 1949. Two tumors removed, one from forehead, one from top of head.
5. Operation: February, 1950. A large tumor, like a potato, removed together with the middle lobe of the right lung.

Condition when first seen on June 20, 1950:

There were 12 smaller tumors all over the body: one at the middle part of the left upper jaw bone; one at the right upper lateral eye bone (orbita) pressing on the eyelid; one at the right temporal part of the head; one at the left upper arm; two at the right lower arm; two on the left hip bone—abdominal wall, etc.; hearing of the right ear reduced; right eye partly closed by inborn cataract.

Treatment started immediately.

Within one month most of the tumors were no longer palpable. After two months all tumors disappeared. In the following months most of the scars were absorbed but the liver tests showed that this organ could not be entirely restored; therefore, she was advised to continue the treatment partly.

After her marriage she was, against my advice, off the diet for two years. All was good till December, 1955, when she noticed that the right arm became shaky and she could not write. She was dizzy and when going down stairs, she felt as though she were going to fall down. In the following months, her vision became reduced, especially in the right eye where she felt tightness and pressure. The eye specialist found the symptoms of a brain tumor and on May 15, 1956, recommended immediate operation for decompression to avoid blindness. She returned here on May 19, 1956. On May 22, 1956, the eye specialist here found "this is a serious case and deserves the utmost and immediate care," (decompression). However, with the agreement of the mother, we decided against the operation, but to apply the strongest treatment. On June 22, 1956 the same eye specialist found "a phenomenal improvement." In a corresponding way, the whole body, her walking, writing, etc., improved and continued to do so up to the present time according to her letters.

Case No. 2. Mrs. D. J.

1923 Diagnosis: Myosarcoma (according to biopsies).

Operations and Treatment:

1923—Growth on left upper femur removed.

1923—Removal of recidives (recurrences) from same spot.

1924—Removal of recidives from same spot. X-ray treatments begun.

1925—Removal of the whole mass of scars again at the same place. Since that time wound has remained open.

1928—Skin grafted on open wound.

1929—Removal of piece of bone at same place. Wound healed and remained closed until 1940.

1940—The scar mass-ulcerated again. Bone inflammation and destruction set in.

1941—All scar masses removed and skin grafted. Treatment with penicillin and antibiotics until 1944.

1944—Small bone splinters removed.

1945—More small bone splinters eliminated.

1946—Another skin graft attempted. Wound remained in status quo until May 25, 1951, when patient fractured leg.

1951—Long metal plate, 2/3 of entire length of femur, was inserted and nailed to bone with silver screws at Medical College of Virginia. The muscle and skin would not heal.

1952—Removal of necrotic masses.

September, 1952. First seen here and treatment started. Patient was bedridden. There was a large extended ulcer-opening, nearly the entire length of the left thigh. In the depth of the large defect, a greater part of the metal plate could be seen. There was abundant secretion of pus. Severe pain. Bursitis in left hip joint. Could hardly walk on crutches.

March, 1953. Entire ulcerous wound closed and healed. Growth of new bone has broken two of the metal screws causing slight pain while walking. Bone, surrounding muscle and tissues have been almost completely restored. Plate can now be removed to restore normal use of limb.

May 19, 1956. An orthopedic surgeon removed the metal sheet which had kept the separated parts of the left femur together. At the operation, he found that 4 of the screws were broken, one he could not remove. The healing power in the bone was so strong that the pressure against the metal broke 4 screws in pressing the sheet upwards and outwards.

Note: While the duration of the case of Mrs. J. under this treatment covers a period of only 4½ years, the case is one of the most interesting because of the long series of treatments and operations prior to this treatment, and due to the fact that the treatment has restored the use of a limb which was apparently destined to be lost.

Case No. 3. Mr. L. W.

Clinical Diagnosis: Cancer of the prostate with several bone metastases; arteriosclerosis and high blood pressure.

Previous History: Five to 6 years ago he was examined for prevention, in Memorial Hospital for Cancer, all was negative. Next year he was examined in Life Extension Institute where again all was negative. But from 1950-1951 he observed severe pain in the lower back, loss of weight, frequent urination, especially at night, and was examined by two urologists. His wife was informed that there was an enlarged prostate condition with metastatic findings (several) in the lower spine and pelvis. Therefore, no operation possible and no confirmation by biopsy necessary (medical report).

Condition when first seen in my Cancer Clinic, May 20, 1952: Patient complained about prostate condition of 15 years' duration. He had to urinate at night 3 to 4 times, in the morning it was very difficult for him to urinate but during the daytime the stream was mostly a little stronger. In the previous years he also observed some dizziness and eye trouble. The treatment before had consisted of several types of female hormones which enlarged his breasts, but did not help him otherwise. The blood pressure was 182/94. He had 64 not quite regular pulses. Rectal examination revealed a very large prostate, with some nodular surface on the left side. The heart was enlarged about one finger to the right and one finger to the left side. Both second vessel-sounds were accentuated.

The findings of the radiologist, Dr. Ziegler, on the X-rays taken on June 5, 1952, read as follows: "The upper two-thirds of the sacroiliac joints, especially the left one, are partly obliterated. In the surroundings there are a number of irregular areas of translucency extending also into the sacral regions. In addition, there are also several areas of osteosclerosis. At the lower portion of the spinal processes of the second, third and fifth lumbar vertebrae there are osseous defects with irregular and hazy borders. These alterations point to metastases of an osteolytic and osteoplastic character."

The urine showed, in the beginning, albumin plus two, trace of sugar, leucocytes 20 to 25 per H.P.F., and few red blood cells. Some of the specimen showed also hyaline casts and a few granulated casts.

The combined dietary regime was immediately applied, May 20, 1952.

In the months that followed, the X-ray examinations showed an increase in the osteoplastic process, especially in both sacroiliac joints.

On July 10, 1953, re-examination of X-rays revealed the following: "The previously seen osteoplastic process in the region of both sacroiliac joints has decreased. The joints themselves are again better outlined. No signs of metastases are revealed."

In the following years, the urination became more difficult. A urologist had to dilate the urethra several times and this did not help enough. He recommended a prostatectomy. The operation was performed on November 1, 1955, as a so-called suprapubic prostatectomy, one stage, with bilateral scrotal vasectomy.

The pathological diagnosis: "No malignant changes noted."

In the last year we were able to clear the urine and reduce the frequency of urination to a minimum. Remarkable in this case is that we were also able to reduce his uric acid condition in serum from 6.8 per cent

[533]

to a normal condition of 4 milligrams per cent. His arthritic pains were reduced to a minimum. He is free of dizziness and the blood pressure the last few years is around 140/84.

His present age (1957) is 81. The eye specialist writes on January 27, 1956: "The remarkable thing is that the whole vascular picture is very moderate compared to the patient's age." (After 4 years of treatment.)

Case No. 4. Mr. E. B.

Previous History: April, 1955. It started with a small lump in right testicle.

August, 1955. The right testicle was removed and a radical periaortic gland dissection was made, by a cut around the abdomen up to the right kidney.

Clinical and Pathological Report Reads: "In August of 1955 the right testicle was removed and a periodic node dissection was done for an embryonal cell carcinoma of the testicle. All the nodes along the aortic chain were involved with metastatic cancer. Following the surgery he had extensive X-ray therapy to the back, chest and mediastinum.

"In March of 1956 an X-ray revealed the presence of metastatic nodules in the chest. At the time of his departure from here he was receiving additional X-ray therapy to the metastatic nodules in the lung, 82 altogether. It is our feeling that this is a hopeless problem and any further treatment other than symptomatic relief as symptoms develop is unnecessary."

Despite the fact that Mr. B. had had the extensive surgery and extensive X-ray therapy, new lumps and glands appeared in the right pubic and pelvic area and metastatic nodules were noticed in both lungs. Hopeless prognosis was given to his wife, despite the fact that she was expecting a new baby in the next few weeks.

April 13, 1956. Patient was first seen here at the cancer clinic and treatment started. Patient looks pale, anemic, depressed, puffy. Weight 184 pounds. Blood pressure 107/70. Pulses regular 84. The abdomen is distended and shows, in the middle part, some resistance. The liver seems to be only somewhat enlarged, and somewhat harder. The lungs do not show any clinical symptoms. The right pubic and groin area is extremely enlarged from infiltration of tumors and glands, also the penis.

May 12, 1956. X-ray specialist's report: "The previously seen shadows in the left lung have decreased in number. The shadow in the right lung has nearly disappeared."

May 26, 1956. "The previously described shadows in the left lower lung field are partly smaller and are partly no more visible. On the right side they are scarcely recognizable any more."

The later reports in June and August, 1956, show that the patient feels well and hopeful, but the blood counts present an exceptionally slow recovery, most probably due to the many X-ray treatments (82). He is working now for 7 hours a day, feels well, and is continuing the reduced treatment. The last X-rays are free of shadows.

Readers who were saddened to hear of the death of Dr. Gerson will be glad to know that the foundation organized during his lifetime will carry on their work of keeping the public informed about the treatment. Write for further information to: Foundation for Cancer Treatment, Incorporated, 80-24 Austin Street, Kew Gardens 15, New York.

135. Cancer Cures

Everyone has his own idea of just what a "quack" can be. To most of us it means a crackpot who peddles useless products at exhorbitant prices. In recent years the term has been widened to include anyone who promotes a treatment which is not in complete accord with the policies or attitudes of organized medicine. People who are against fluoridation, no matter what their background, are classified as quacks; those who are interested in the power of vitamin E are quacks; an advocate of natural food in the diet is a quack, etc. But the term, in its most damning sense, is reserved for those who would presume to treat cancer by means of anything but surgery or radiation. It can be an untrained country boy who has treated his local neighbors with a homemade remedy, or a famous researcher who has tested his treatment in a hundred scientific ways, if the medical fraternity frowns on the treatment—often really because it was not perfected under their professional auspices—the treatment is finished. The developer and his associates are labeled quacks. Your doctor will be told it is a worthless treatment. He might run into serious professional trouble if he uses it.

Actually how good is the treatment? Medical authorities say it is no good. The researcher says it is beneficial. He has lists of patients who are willing to testify that they were helped, even completely cured, by the treatment. But nobody of any influence or authority will listen, or look at the evidence.

This is a story we can rattle off by heart. It has happened to Koch, Ivy, Hoxsey, Drosnes-Lazenby and many others. Several times a month our mail contains a letter from someone who claims to have found an effective treatment for cancer. We have no way of knowing whether the claims are true or not. The point is that they *might* be! The very thing that hundreds of scientists spend millions of hours and dollars to find, could nave passed across our editorial desks undetected. We are not equipped to investigate and those who are refuse to do so.

Beg for Impartial Investigation

In spite of the public picture organized medicine has succeeded in painting of these men, they all have one thing in common: they invite, they beg for objective evaluation of their work. That is all they ask, and it is the one thing they cannot seem to get. If the medical profession sees fit to pay any attention at all, it is to send a committee whose judgment has been colored by the opinions of colleagues. They will look at the evidence with no great interest and will report that the biopsies were fakes, that cures must be attributed to spontaneous remission or previous treatments, that the patients never really had cancer, or a hundred other accusations and qualifications that would never be applied to a recognized treatment. Of course, with such evaluation the treatment is doomed. The developer cries foul, and the medical men point to the committee report, arguing that an evaluation was asked for and given.

Why is an objective evaluation so difficult to achieve? Why can't ground rules be worked out before the inspection begins so that both parties can agree to a plan of procedure and then compare the actual activity to it to see if the rules were obeyed? Then the results would have to be accepted by both parties unless it could be shown that one or the other had deviated from the prescribed plan. Apparently such a situation is difficult to arrange. Backers of Krebiozen have been attempting such an arrangement for several years. Can't Congress formulate reliable ground rules that all would have to obey, so that we could have an accurate picture of the cancer situation and our resources to fight it? We spend millions of dollars yearly on cancer research. Why couldn't some of it be spent, at the insistence of Congress, to investigate claims that an unorthodox cancer cure has been found? The evidence is pretty convincing in some cases. It doesn't seem fair or wise simply to ignore it.

A Non-Conformist

All of this has come out of reading about still another of those hearty, fearless and dedicated men who claims to be able to treat cancer successfully, and has laid his reputation and career on the line to prove it. This time it is Dr. I. N. Frost of Raymondville, Texas. Dr. Frost characterizes himself as a "non-conformist so far as organized medicine is concerned."

It is Dr. Frost's theory that cancer and all other degenerative diseases (ulcer, arthritis, hepatitis, heart disease) are manifestations of a virus infection. His treatment begins with a complete reorganization of the diet to include only organically grown food. Then specially developed vaccines are employed, a vaccine made from the patients own fluids, and one made from the staphylococcus aureus. Along with these, certain antibiotics are used. Dr. Frost, and several of his patients, who have written to us, say the treatment has brought wonderful results.

With this good news to tell, Dr. Frost contacted the local medical societies, inviting them to inspect his formula, his patients and his records.

He wrote to 100 local doctors telling them he would like to make a formal report on his results. No reply. He later wrote to the same group volunteering his formula and its schedule of administration. Again no takers. He held two public meetings—5 came to one meeting, and none to the other. He wrote a pamphlet describing his work and sent it to the same doctors, but got no response.

That is the way Dr. Frost fought the old accusation that these cancer treatments are secret, but he couldn't even get anyone to listen to him talk about it. Lest he be accused of perfecting a get-rich-quick scheme, Dr. Frost also signed a contract giving all of the money he might collect in the course of treating cancer to a fund for a cancer hospital. He still has no takers.

Aside from his own treatment, he uses the Koch treatment, Krebiozen and Mucorhicin, the Drosnes-Lazenby treatment. He has seen beneficial results from all of these, he says. We presume that the favored treatment varies according to the type of cancer.

It is Dr. Frost's dream to treat 1,000 cancer patients, just after they have gone to the doctor for a checkup and learned they have the disease, and who have had no medication, no radiation or surgery, only a proveable diagnosis by biopsy. It is his opinion that he could completely cure at least 800 of the cases, and improve the others in some way.

Do we know if Dr. Frost is truthful and accurate in his claims? We have only his word, and that of some patients who know his work. But, you see, we have no evidence that he is wrong either. Nor has anyone else. We think Dr. Frost and people like him deserve a fair hearing. Why not give him a chance to prove what he says? Why not look at his records, talk to his patients, read their case histories? What is there to be lost?

If the medical profession is sincere in its desire to find a cancer cure, why is it not willing to look for it wherever it might be? Are we to miss it because it occurs in a small laboratory in the southwest instead of the stainless steel and stone skyscraper of a multi-million dollar research center? It is as though we had refused to use electricity because it was discovered by a publisher instead of a scientist, or refused to enjoy the Mona Lisa because it was painted by an inventor, instead of a bona fide artist.

We all know that the good things of this world are rare. It takes talent and courage to produce them. It takes insight, objectivity and courage to find and recognize them. Can we say we are civilized and yet be unwilling to apply these criteria to finding a cure for mankind's most terrible disease?

136. The High Risk of Finding a Cancer Cure

Have you ever dreamed of how wonderful it would be if, through some lucky chance, *you* could be the one to discover a cure for cancer? In your dream you are receiving the thanks of the world; governments give you medals, medical societies honor you with citations and testimonials, your respect and honor mount daily in proportion to the gratitude of the world for what you've accomplished. Your final years are spent in golden retirement, surrounded with expressions of the thanks of thousands you've saved from the horrors of cancer.

The alarm that will jolt you out of this reverie is sounded in the book by Maurice Natenberg entitled, *The Cancer Blackout.* (Published by Regent House, 4554 Broadway, Chicago 40, Illinois.) Chances are that after you've read this book you will add a line to your evening prayers, begging that you be left out when inspirations for discovering a cancer cure are dispensed. Mr. Natenberg serves up a history which shows that the only governmental recognition likely to come to any one who announces that he has found an effective treatment for cancer is a warning poster on post office billboards; from organized medicine he is likely to see testimonials turned into testimony which will have him disciplined and his discovery discredited; any respect and honor he might have had before he let his findings be known will be swallowed up in bad publicity and vilification; his old age will probably be iron with remorse and bitterness at the thought of having stuck his neck out and ruined his life for nothing, plus the awful frustration of watching deaths mount from a disease he knows he could alleviate. This is the fate that awaits the man who tries to conquer cancer, if past performance is any indication.

That there are men who are willing to face such a prospect is the saving grace of our society. How many more of such men we can hope to see is something else again. Will somebody be successful in introducing an accepted cancer treatment before the hopelessness of it all discourages even the bravest of men? We can only hope so.

Who Are the Discoverers?

In spite of the publicity that would lead one to believe so, the men who have discovered or sponsored treatments for cancer are not all illiterate bumpkins who have a secret poultice to promote, nor are they slickers who would bilk cancer sufferers of their savings to get rich quick. Most are careful scientists whose credits are indicative of the esteem in which they were held before they were seized with this "madness," the desire to do more for cancer victims than surgery and X-ray can do.

Prominent examples of such men are Dr. Walter B. Coffey, who was chief surgeon and director of Southern Pacific Railroad Hospital from 1926 to 1938, and was connected with a cancer treatment known as the Coffey-Humber extract, which was taken from the adrenal cortex of sheep; Dr. William F. Koch, discoverer of Glyoxylide, Professor of Physiology at Detroit Medical College, 1914-1918, and subject of a laudatory editorial in the *Journal of the American Medical Association* in 1913, heralding his work in endocrinology; Dr. A. C. Ivy, former vice-president of the University of Illinois, original organizer and director of the United States Naval Medical Research Institute, recommended by the American Medical Association to represent the Allied governments at the Nuremberg atrocity trials, former executive director of the National Advisory Cancer Society. Can men of such calibre suddenly be labeled crackpots? Can the intelligence which gained them the honor and influence they had be said to have deserted them the minute they began to sponsor a treatment for cancer? Is cancer so hopeless that society brands anyone who would attempt to treat it as demented? It would appear that such is the case.

Many Treatments Discussed

The stories of Krebiozen, Hoxsey, and Gerson have been told frequently. However, they are only a few in the long trail of frustrating instances in which a promising treatment for cancer was dismissed and its sponsor ruined. Mr. Natenberg's book discusses each of the major cancer treatments which have been introduced in the past century. He tells the story of the preparation used and the procedure employed by organized medicine for methodically destroying it. Much to Mr. Natenberg's credit is the method of presentation which is clear and all-inclusive without getting bogged down in such technical talk that the layman is left at the starting gate busily thumbing through a medical dictionary. And the excitement of these stories! You turn page after page convinced that the evidence you've just seen will *have* to draw official approval for this or that treatment. Of course, it never happens.

Mr. Natenberg Tells the Story of Glyoxylide

While each one of the stories is interesting, the individual reader is bound to be stirred by one more than another. One of the most arresting is the story of Dr. William Koch's Glyoxylide. This Glyoxylide was a substance designed by Koch to convert the poisons which he believed cause cancer into antitoxins which, by chain reaction, would eliminate the cancerous condition. He used this substance in connection with a rigid diet. Dr. Koch insisted that both must be used, since neither diet nor Glyoxylide would be effective separately.

Dr. Koch was outspoken in his criticism of surgery as a treatment for cancer, and was equally critical of those who promoted surgery in such cases. By public pressure the Wayne County Medical Society of Detroit, Michigan, was forced to initiate an investigation of the Koch treatment. The procedure devised was completely fair and thoroughly practical. The only trouble was that the agreed-upon procedure was utterly ignored by the investigators, leaving the result totally inconclusive.

How Dr. Koch's Treatment Was Tested

The plan was this: a group of 5 physicians would pick cases unknown to Koch to be treated by him. Seven advanced and hopeless cases of internal cancer were selected. So interested was the committee that for 3 weeks not one member of the committee could be persuaded to certify, officially, that the patients they had chosen had cancer. The patients were getting worse and the longer the delay the more difficult the cure. Dr. Koch then demanded that the head of the medical society direct the committee to perform its duty so that he could begin treatment. The committee examined one, and only one, of the 7 patients.

Dr. Koch finally instituted treatment on all 7 patients, in order to avoid criticism, without waiting for the committee's examination of the other 6. All responded exceedingly well after 3 weeks of treatment. The committee then called the tests off, saying that Koch had refused to cooperate, and they sent the patients home with a warning against continuing Koch's treatment.

The version of the story printed in the *AMA Journal* was in direct contradiction to this and included the accusation that Koch had given only one injection to the patients and simply hadn't bothered to return to continue treatment, so the patients left for home in disgust. Does it seem credible that Koch, after fighting for an investigation of his treatment, would abandon his one chance to prove its effectiveness?

Dr. Koch claims that he made every effort to trace the patients but could find only 3. All 3 were able to testify or submit affidavits to the effect that their cancers had been cured.

A Second Hearing

A second hearing was arranged with much difficulty, and in spite of opposition by the AMA, Dr. Koch presented a number of patients who had been diagnosed as hopeless and whom he had cured. The committee simply denied both the diagnoses and the cures. In one case a husband testified that his wife had been cured of Paget's disease after she had refused an operation to remove the cancer that had spread from her breast, because it might have meant the loss of her arm. Her surgeon who examined her during the course of her recovery acknowledged in the presence of her husband that she had been cured of cancer. When he was called before the committee, the surgeon testified that his original diagnosis had been falsified and that the woman's condition had really been a simple ulceration, and not cancer at all. He did not say why he had been willing to operate so radically on such a mild condition.

Dr. Koch received several letters of encouragement and expressions of confidence from influential men who sympathized with him because of the unfair treatment he had received at the hands of the committee. Professor W. A. Dewey of the Department of Medicine at the University of Michigan was present at the hearings. Of the committee he is quoted as saying, "For a studied intent to falsify, a premeditated determination to condemn everything, and an unscientific, un-American assumption to be judge, jury and prosecuting witness, the report of this so-called committee outstrips in bias, unfairness and mendacity anything that has ever been my lot to observe in a medical practice of 44 years. . . ."

A vicious campaign against Koch and his formula followed the hearings. Even those who employed Glyoxylide were in danger of losing their professional standing.

Meanwhile, still another cancer investigation was set up, this time in Ontario, Canada. The proceedings were conducted in a dignified and impartial manner. One witness, Dr. J. W. Kannel of Fort Wayne, Indiana, told of treating 72 patients in 14 years with Glyoxylide, due to their own pleadings, though he considered many of these too hopeless to treat in any way. He reported that 21 of these were still alive and 4 others had died of other causes. Dr. Kannel said that Glyoxylide was the only remedy that had offered him hope in treating cancer, in contrast to his poor results after 24 years of experience with X-ray or radium treatment and surgery. In spite of such impressive evidence, no formal report of this hearing was ever published. And that was how the AMA answered queries about its findings. Again an easy way out.

Dr. Koch Disposed Of

In 1942 Dr. Koch was arrested on a charge that his product was falsely labeled. A bail of 10,000 dollars was asked, though such a sum is customary only in murder cases. The district attorney admitted that he had asked for the bail on orders from Detroit, to keep Koch from returning to Brazil, where he was then doing research.

Dr. Koch was prosecuted in two more FDA trials concerning Glyoxylide which ended in a permanent injunction against Koch Laboratories. Dr. Koch finally gave up. He assigned the manufacturing process of Glyoxylide to a Detroit religious organization where the preparation was incompetently processed and was no longer effective. Dr. Koch is now living in Brazil and his discovery is no longer in use. Was Glyoxylide really a fraud, or was it an effective treatment for cancer which never got an even break? We will probably never know.

What Is So Outlandish About a Fair Test?

The pattern shown in this case is repeated time and again in every case of an independent cancer treatment that asked for recognition and approval. The authorities, instead of adhering to principles of investigation which could not be disputed whatever the results, resorted to tricks and vilification of personalities, to inconclusive tests which cast doubt on the outcome, and to hearings whose findings were preordained and whose judges

[541]

were undeniably biased. As Mr. Natenberg points out, if the medical authorities were as sure of the worthlessness of these treatments as they seemed to be, the fairest and most scrupulous tests by the many experts to whom they have access would only result in the swiftest and most economical proof that the discoverer was promoting a useless product. It is hard to understand why they didn't use that simple tactic, if honest inquiry was their motive.

Space does not permit us to discuss the other examples Mr. Natenberg offers to illustrate his point. In each of these discoverers there is a dedication and determination which make these people hang on, in spite of the obvious ruin to which they are heading. Surely, anyone in such a project for personal gain or enhanced reputation would cry "Enough!" while he could, and get back his practice and respectability before all was completely lost. None of these people seemed to give that possibility a thought; they fought just as long as there seemed to be something to fight with and fight for.

~~~~~~

SECTION 24: CELIAC DISEASE

~~~~~~

137. Celiac Disease and Whole Wheat

Constipation has been spoken of as the national disease of America. It is indeed widespread and is caused, we believe, chiefly by our American diet of refined foods from which not only most roughage but also most vitamins and minerals have been removed. Another disorder which appears to be relatively common is diarrhea, one form of which has been the subject of much research. This is the so-called "fatty diarrhea." The medical term for it is "steatorrhea." Two closely related disorders are sprue and celiac disease. Sprue is generally found in tropical countries. Celiac disease is chiefly a disease of infants. According to most medical authorities, we have no inkling as to the cause of any of these disorders.

However, it certainly seems reasonable to relate them to what we eat. In the case of fatty diarrhea, there seems to be an inability to digest either fats or starches. Apparently the undigested starch ferments in the intestines, causing bloating, gas and distention of the abdomen. These undigested carbohydrates are then excreted along with whatever fat has been in the stools. Stools of a patient with celiac disease are frothy, bulky, fatty and ill-smelling. In addition to the ever-present diarrhea, the patient is usually irritable and feverish. He suffers from lack of appetite and loss of weight. His abdomen is distended.

The Seriousness of Diarrhea

Why should diarrhea, especially this kind of diarrhea, be so serious an illness? Consider for a moment what happens to the whole mechanism of the body as a result of the diarrhea. Carbohydrates and fats are lost to it, so all the functions these food elements perform in the body are not performed. Calcium combines with the undigested fat in the abdomen and is carried away. So all the functions which calcium performs in the body go undone. This involves the nerves, the bone and tooth structure, the heart, the blood—all are affected by this loss of calcium. In infants, prolonged diarrhea of this kind can lead to rickets and in older persons, to osteomalacia or bone softening. Loss of calcium is one of the reasons for the irritability, lack of appetite and loss of weight as well. In addition to calcium other minerals are lost rapidly when the diarrhea continues for very long. No food, including minerals, stays in the digestive tract long enough to be absorbed. So potassium, iron, phosphorus and all the other important minerals are rapidly lost.

Equally important is the loss of the fat soluble vitamins. These are vitamins A, D, K and E. As the undigested fat is excreted, these vitamins go along with it and so they too are lost to the body. In the case of growing children this loss can mean the difference between straight strong bones and bones deformed with rickets. In adults and children, too, vitamin A is of the utmost importance in preventing infections and keeping the tissues healthy. Sure enough, in patients with celiac disease there is a high incidence of respiratory disorders—colds and so forth. And why not, considering that they are getting no benefit at all from all the many elements in their diets that prevent this kind of infection! We are told that one way of testing for celiac disease is to test for vitamin A in the blood. If it is far below normal then celiac disease is diagnosed.

Anemia will follow if iron continues to be lost. Anemia is another almost certain symptom of celiac disease, for it is bound to occur when iron is lost. It is interesting to note that the blood sugar level is low in these diarrheal diseases. Sugar in the blood must be kept at a certain level or all kinds of symptoms will appear—fatigue, weakness, blackouts, allergies, to name but a few. Apparently no one knows what the connection is between fatty diarrhea and blood sugar. But there seems to be no doubt that they are connected.

Treatments for Celiac Disease

There is obviously no "bug" involved in this kind of diarrhea. So the usual battery of antibiotics and sulfa drugs are not given. In general, physicians seem to agree that the disease is wholly one of nutrition and try to treat it on that basis. Some doctors report that they have had excellent results giving folic acid (one of the B vitamins) for celiac disease. Others found that they could not cure patients completely with folic acid, but that they got a good response when they gave the folic acid *along with brewer's yeast*. This strengthens our point of view that any and all of the vitamins should be taken in combination with the other vitamins and minerals that occur with it in foods.

Other physicians give diets low in carbohydrate and fat, high in protein, along with vitamins A and B and liver extract. In the case of patients who are infants taking nothing much but milk, the high-protein diet presents no problems. But in the case of older patients and adults there is a problem. What can these folks take for the carbohydrate part of their meals? It has been found that bananas (in spite of their high carbohydrate content) seem to be acceptable as food to most of these patients. Now this does not mean that the mere eating of the bananas works a cure. But they are a safe carbohydrate food, it seems, at a time when almost every other carbohydrate food causes digestive difficulty. So they are one of the first foods usually recommended when the celiac patient is gradually trying to get back to a normal diet. And they seldom cause trouble.

Wheat Incriminated

Recently a new aspect of celiac disease has been uncovered. Some Dutch investigators discovered that the glutenous part of wheat might be responsible for celiac disease in those who were susceptible. Other physicians began to put their patients on wheat-free diets with good results. In the *Lancet* for March 19, 1955, J. W. Gerrard and two co-workers wrote that the wheat-free diet is effective not only in the early and active phase of celiac disease which takes place usually in infancy, but also in the later stages extending on into later childhood. In some cases, it seemed to them, the diet should be continued right on into adulthood.

In a Norse medical journal, *Tideskrift for Den Norske Laegeforening* for September 15, 1953, investigators disclosed the harmful effect of wheat, rye and oats in celiac disease. They reported on good results in 12 cases of the disorder, when these 3 cereals were omitted from the diet. In a later issue of the *Lancet* (May 28, 1955) we are told of experiments in which 30 sick children were kept on diets free from wheat gluten. Twenty-eight of them recovered completely. The other two did not respond to the diet. One of these had a deficiency in bile salts and the other was apparently allergic to fat. But in the case of 28, it appeared that the gluten of the wheat was the sole thing causing the trouble. So now it appears that, for the kind of diarrhea caused by celiac disease, one of the first things the doctor will suggest is to leave cereal products out of the diet.

The peculiar thing about the story is that the *gluten* of the wheat seems to be responsible for the damage. Gluten is a protein substance that

[544]

occurs mostly in the germ part of the wheat, so it is not present in white flour in such large quantities. Gluten bread is eaten by diabetics—bread from which all the starch has been removed. In white bread, on the contrary, the germ part of the grain (containing much of the gluten) has been removed entirely. So what we are actually saying is that celiac patients get that way because their bodies cannot handle the protein of whole grain cereals! And, strangely enough, *eating just the starch from the cereals* does not bring on their symptoms. It's the gluten part of the grain that does it.

What does this prove—that all of us should stop eating whole grain cereals and eat nothing but starchy refined cereals? Of course not! We know that many food elements have been removed from whole grains when they are refined to make "white" flour. By "enriching" the flour, our millers put back two or three of the B vitamins and a little iron, without any regard for what this slicing up and re-combining is going to do to the wholeness of the food. So of course our story on celiac disease does not signify that you should immediately begin to eat breads made from refined flours rather than whole grains.

Testing Foods for Yourself

What it does mean is simply that there are foods which certain people simply cannot eat happily and healthfully—no matter what good foods they happen to be nutritionally. Wheat gluten is one of these—for people who are susceptible to celiac disease.

The other lesson we learn from this story is, we think, to experiment with your food, if you happen to be suffering from some disorder that does not respond to treatment. Whether or not you have celiac disease, perhaps you were not meant to eat bread at all. Perhaps something about bread just doesn't agree with you. How will you discover this unless you stop eating bread for a while (leaving everything else in your diet just as it was)? Perhaps milk is the cause of your trouble. Perhaps you just can't take citrus fruits. It won't do you a bit of harm to experiment. So long as you are eating a good diet and taking your food supplements you can leave almost any food out of your menus for 3 or 4 weeks without missing it. If your symptoms disappear, perhaps you should forget about this food permanently, so far as you personally are concerned. Just because everybody has always eaten bread is no reason why you should go on eating bread if it disagrees with you. (Editor Rodale does not eat bread.)

One caution though. You must be sure to replace, somehow, in your diet whatever food elements are plentiful in the food you decide to do without. Whole grain is rich in the B vitamins, vitamin E and iron. If you are going to stop eating it, you must make sure that you get enough of these precious substances from some other source in your food. Dried beans, lean meat, fish, liver—these are good sources of the B vitamins. Brewer's yeast is the richest source. Iron is plentiful in eggs.

We find ourselves wondering about the kind of bread the children in these experiments were fed. It seems almost impossible that it could have been real, whole grain bread, made from freshly ground grain. This is generally not available except in the home of some health-conscious person. Certainly it is not served in hospitals. Commercially processed whole grain flours must be treated with preservatives so they will keep on grocer's shelves. Do you suppose it might be the preservative in the flour that is responsible for cases of celiac disease?

~~~~~~

SECTION 25: THE CIRCULATION
~~~~~~

138. Intermittent Claudication

A disorder called by doctors "intermittent claudication" involves the legs chiefly. It becomes noticeable when one is walking and it consists of disagreeable sensations like "pins and needles" followed by pain, shaking and excessive perspiration. It is said to be caused by arteriosclerosis or, as we commonly call it, "hardening of the arteries."

From what we know of vitamin E and its benefits for heart and vascular conditions, it would seem that this might be helpful for such a condition. An article in the British *Lancet* for September 20, 1958, confirms this point of view. Written by Peter D. Livingstone and Clifford Jones, both of United Sheffield Hospitals, the article first reviews past experience with vitamin E for this condition. These reports are conflicting. Some researchers got good results and others claimed that they got none at all. But in most cases the treatment with vitamin E was continued for quite a short time.

Vitamin E Tested

The authors of the present article decided to test two groups of patients at their hospital, giving vitamin E to one group and a "dummy" tablet to the other group. Neither the patients nor the doctors themselves knew throughout the test which patient was getting the vitamin E, for a procedure was worked out whereby the patient was given his tablets according to a number system and the key to this system was not divulged until after the test was over. This, of course, was to make certain that no patient thought he felt better because he knew he was taking a medicine and the doctors did not diagnose any patient as being better because they wanted the test to succeed.

The 40 patients who took part in the test ranged in age from 40 to 57 and both groups of 20 were equally divided as to age. They were all men.

In all cases the symptoms had been noticed *for at least 5 years* and in all cases the pain was felt in the calf of the leg.

It was difficult to decide on a way of testing improvement in the patients since this is one of those conditions in which the symptoms are "subjective." That is, the doctor cannot tell whether there is improvement. The patient is the only one who knows. He must decide whether the pain and numbness are better or worse than they were the day before.

The doctors decided on an exercise tolerance test. This consisted of climbing up and down a series of steps 18 inches high and continuing to do this until pain made the patient stop. The number of steps taken by the patient were counted each time and also the length of time taken to recover from the pain and feel normal once again. By using this test the doctor had a measure of the patient's actual improvement apart from his own opinion as to whether he had improved or not.

It was decided to give large doses of vitamin E. Each tablet was 200 milligrams (or International Units) and the usual daily dosage was 600 milligrams. That is, each patient who was taking vitamin E took 3 tablets a day. We assume that he took one tablet in the morning, one at noon and one at night.

Those who were taking "dummy" tablets also took 3 a day, so that no one knew which group was getting the vitamin E.

Results of the Test

Thirteen of the 20 patients taking vitamin E thought they had improved, at the end of the test. In all these cases, the walking test on the steps indicated, too, that they had improved. In the 20 patients taking the "dummy" tablet, two thought they had improved and actually had. Two of the members of this group of 20 thought they had deteriorated.

Three patients dropped out of each group before the end of the test because of other ailments or death. The 4 patients who did not respond at all to vitamin E are described as follows: the first had very extensive disease of the arteries and both his legs were in grave danger of gangrene. The second had extremely high blood pressure. The third was grossly overweight, smoked heavily and refused to cooperate in any way so far as restrictions in diet or habit were concerned. In the fourth patient there seemed to be no reason for failure.

Of the patients who improved on vitamin E treatment, 7 were able to continue walking indefinitely at a slightly slower pace than usual. Four were able to walk any distance up to half a mile and do their full work. Two showed slight, but definite improvement and were quite certain that they were more active than they had been and that the pain was less severe.

Of the patients who took the dummy tablet, two recovered enough to walk a useful distance. One of these made a spontaneous and complete recovery after suffering severely for many years. All the other 15 members of this group had no relief.

The authors say in conclusion that there can be no doubt that vitamin E was responsible for improvement in 13 of the group of 17 patients. These patients are now carrying on their work with ease and enjoying their leisure. All of them had undergone certain forms of therapy before trying the vitamin E and had been disappointed. The fact that it took a number of months for them to improve seems to rule out the possibility that psychological factors played any part in their improvement.

The experiment seems to show definitely that large doses of vitamin E are necessary and that there is considerable delay before any response can be noted. The authors believe that treatment should be carried on for at least 3 months before being abandoned. Their test was conducted for 40 weeks or about 10 months.

There seems to be no doubt that vitamin E (alpha tocopherol) is vitally important for the health of our bodies. We do not know a great deal about how it works in the body. We know that it decreases the body's need for oxygen. If some part of the body is in trouble because its oxygen supply is low, vitamin E enables that particular part of the body to get along on less oxygen.

We know, too, that vitamin E is difficult to obtain in quantity in the average diet, especially since our foods these days are refined, processed and treated with hundreds of different chemicals, many of them destructive to vitamin E.

We think everyone should take vitamin E every day, along with his other food supplements, whether or not he is taking wheat germ or wheat germ oil. Wheat germ is only a fair source of vitamin E. It also contains many other substances, so it cannot contain a great deal of vitamin E, comparatively speaking. If you have a disorder of the blood vessels or heart you should be taking vitamin E in large amounts. If you want to make sure you are not ever subject to such disorders, then by all means include a certain amount of vitamin E with your daily supplements—from 100 milligrams up, every day.

And remember, if you suffer from intermittent claudication, the investigators in the article we talk about above found that large doses of vitamin E were required and there may be considerable delay before improvement is noted. So don't give up too soon if improvement is slow in coming.

139. Vascular Disorders

"This article deals with the problem of a possible causal management of all vascular diseases by systemic administration of high doses of vitamin B_{12}."

How would you feel if you came suddenly upon these words in a medical journal of the highest integrity? Wouldn't you be as surprised and excited as we were? Reading further in the English summary to this German article we found that the author believes that this same therapy with vitamin B_{12} may be useful in treating such things as diabetes, rheumatic diseases, ulcers, as well as certain disorders in neuropsychiatry, dermatology and others.

"The dramatic success following systemic administration of high and highest doses of vitamin B_{12}, as experienced by the author, necessarily led to the conclusion that vast fields of modern pathology (disease) must be subjected to a completely new way of thought with many consequences for therapy now and in the future," says Dr. H. Grabner in the October 31, 1958, issue of *Münchener Medizinische Wochenschrift* (*Munich Medical Weekly*). The patients he describes are only a few, but, says Dr. Grabner, "in full knowledge of the pitiable terminal conditions of those affiliated with vascular diseases I will not hesitate to make known my results."

Dr. Grabner tells us that no one knows for certain what causes heart and blood vessel diseases. He says that there are more than 100 different varieties of vascular diseases. But still we do not know, he says, "what damage of a chemical, physical and allergic nature is rather the actual result of the chronically progressive vascular diseases that finally lead to terminal stages." Anything that is done for heart and blood vessel diseases "helps" he says, that is, some of the symptoms disappear. But no one has claimed a cure for any of these diseases.

How Does Vitamin B_{12} Act to Cure?

He believes that such diseases come from an original damage to the blood vessel. Then the body, in a self-healing effort, "solders" the damaged areas with connective tissue, layers of fat and calcium. What kind of damage might cause this process to begin? Dr. Grabner believes that it may be a form of anemia and says that it may originate in a lack of tone in nerves. So, the whole disorder—or rather the whole series of disorders classified under this heading—may be due to a disturbed blood supply to the vessels.

He tells us that "in all the cases under treatment by me at the time there must be established as fact prevailing and absolutely improbable improvement in every respect." His successes in treatment show, he says, that a new concept of cause and treatment must be considered—not only

[549]

of the circulatory diseases, but all the degenerative diseases so common after middle age. The following disorders should be considered in a new light, he believes: diabetes, ulcers, rheumatic diseases and numerous neurological and psychiatric concepts including polio and muscular dystrophy, as well as epilepsy and schizophrenia.

Dr. Grabner makes no claims for curing these diseases. He says merely that massive doses of vitamin B_{12} should be tried by physicians treating such patients.

What a wonderful prospect it is—the thought that any or all of these plagues which disable, torment and kill millions of people might be caused basically by a lack of something that is triggered by vitamin B_{12}!

And perhaps the amount of vitamin B_{12} in the diet may not be the main consideration in this particular case, for it is well known that vitamin B_{12} is not absorbed easily by the body. Many people seem to lack the ability to absorb it at all.

Cases of Mental Confusion Improved

We feel that the most encouraging part of Dr. Grabner's article deals with the effects of vitamin B_{12} upon the mental confusion several of his patients were suffering from. This is perhaps the most distressing aspect of growing old. Families and friends are cut off from the mentally confused sufferer because he is unable to communicate normally with them. He imagines wrongs which have not been done; he is unable to conduct his affairs and becomes a burden on those around him. If injections of vitamin B_{12} can alleviate just this one condition which prevails among so many older folks—what a blessing it would be!

Here are some of the stories of Dr. Grabner's patients. First, a retired civil servant, aged 76. This gentleman had been under treatment for many ailments, all related to the wearing out of the system of blood vessels and heart. He suffered from intermittent claudication which is an inability to walk without extreme pain in the legs. His mind was affected, with alternating states of extreme depression and childish mirthfulness. A siege of pneumonia brought about a state of complete mental confusion necessitating the patient's hiring a housekeeper. When he came down with a siege of sciatica, Dr. Grabner prescribed injections of vitamin B_{12}. He gave 400 micrograms daily at first.

After the fourth injection the patient greeted the doctor at the door, fully dressed, fresh-shaven and wearing a tie. "An unprecedented turn of events," says Dr. Grabner, "when one recalls how helpless and utterly dependent his life had been in the last two years. But not only that—there was no trace of confusion. For the first time now it became clear to the patient that his wife had died of a stroke 5 months earlier. Mentally he appeared completely ordered and oriented and remains so today."

After two weeks of the 400 microgram injections daily, Dr. Grabner cut the amount to 200 micrograms daily, then cut that to every other day and finally was giving twice weekly injections of 200 micrograms. This is how he describes the patient's present condition: "He is in the best of health and completely normal mentally. He is fully able to leave the house daily, attends to his own purchases personally and even occasionally visits taverns. At the present time there is not the slightest trace of the coronary spasms and asthmatic attacks that occurred so frequently before, nor even of the ambulatory disorder of the kind described, apart from an occasional and extremely moderate spasm."

The second patient Dr. Grabner describes is 68 years old, in advanced emaciation, too weak to stand up. Has been bedfast for weeks. He suffers from difficulty in breathing, slow heartbeat (result of too much digitalis) and confusion to such an extent that his wife mentioned appointing a guardian for him.

He also suffered from acute vascular disorders of the lower limbs. In the past he had had arthritis with degeneration of the knee and hip joint; he had been given digitalis and anti-spasmodics until he lost appetite, lost weight, had spells of dizziness and also at times complete disorientation in time and space. He had been discharged from the hospital and sent home "to die in peace."

Dr. Grabner began with injections of 200 micrograms of vitamin B_{12} every second day, much against the wishes of the patient's wife, incidentally, for she had no faith in this treatment. There was an early return to orientation, an increase in appetite. By the end of 4 weeks the patient was able to leave his home for the first time in many months. He can now walk for two hours without the dreaded attacks of cramps in his legs which came upon him after as little as 20 minutes of walking in 1957.

Says Dr. Grabner, "The improvement in every respect has so continued that the patient and his wife were able to take . . . a vacation (this was 4 months after the treatment was started). He is completely and entirely the person he formerly was, able to fulfill all his social commitments in every way and to visit regularly with his cronies at their regular table for his evening half-pint of beer."

More Case Histories

The third patient was a pastry chef, 58 years old. Five years ago he began to have attacks of dizziness and ringing in the ears. Later he suffered from cramps in the legs and an infected spot on a toe. He had a latent diabetic condition, and a number of symptoms of vascular disease. For about two months Dr. Grabner gave him injections of vitamin B_{12} (200 micrograms daily).

The patient remained free of cramps and could work a full day. He said, "I could never in the past work at all the way I can today."

A 56-year-old nurse suffered from rheumatic pains, nightly cramps in the legs, difficulty in breathing, fatigue and diabetic symptoms. After the second injection of vitamin B_{12}, the pains ceased and the patient is now (about 6 months later) able to work full time.

[551]

The next patient was 63 years old and suffered from the condition called "intermittent claudication." He also had night cramps in the legs. Once again vitamin B_{12} injections resulted in a cessation of pain. The patient is planning to resume full-time work.

The next patient described is a woman, only 38 years old. Under treatment for lumbago, this woman was given every sedative and injection and physical therapy known, according to Dr. Grabner. A partial paralysis was diagnosed as a prolapsed disc. She became almost completely helpless and had to be assisted with even the simplest activities. Dr. Grabner gave her injections of 1000 micrograms of vitamin B_{12} daily. After the second injection her improvement was so striking that she drove her car to the doctor's office! Two weeks later she went off with her husband on a vacation to Italy—in perfect health!

There are two more case histories given in this extraordinary article. One of them was 76 years old and the victim of great mental confusion. The second, the same age, suffered from shingles as well as a serious vascular and heart condition. Dr. Grabner gave a combined antibiotic and vitamin B_{12} treatment for the shingles and says that he does not know which resulted in complete cure within about two weeks. He feels sure that the vitamin played a large part in the cure. The heart and vascular symptoms greatly improved meanwhile.

Although he does not review the case in detail, Dr. Grabner also tells about another patient who suffered for 18 months with an infectious acute inflammatory skin disease. After all this time in the hospital, the young man had attempted suicide, in complete hopeless desperation. After 8 injections daily of 200 micrograms of vitamin B_{12}, almost all eruptions disappeared, including infections in the throat, bladder and urethra.

Says Dr. Grabner in conclusion, "Cases of vascular diseases of most diversified nature were treated with massive, parenterally-administered injections of vitamin B_{12}. The dramatic results force us to a radically new concept of the origin and treatment of all vascular disease, and also other problems of the older persons." We should, he feels, at least test this therapy on diabetes, ulcers, rheumatism, polio, muscular dystrophy, epilepsy, schizophrenia and other mental health problems.

Can you think of any more important contribution that could be made to good health in America today than a thorough investigation of Dr. Grabner's methods and further case histories? Do you suppose anyone is going to take up his challenge and use his methods to prove that they will work for other practitioners, too?

140. Treatment of Vascular Disorders

One of the subjects for investigation in cases of hypertension (high blood pressure) has been rutin—a substance found most plentifully in buckwheat. Rutin is a part of vitamin P. Apparently vitamin P, like the other vitamins has many parts called "flavones." All of them are more or less related and have many of the same properties so far as human health is concerned, but some parts appear to be more effective in the treatment of certain disorders.

High blood pressure brings with it certain dangers, not the least of which is hemorrhage—including cerebral hemorrhage which we speak of as a "stroke." In cases of stroke, the small blood vessels or capillaries rupture, due to the pressure upon them and the hemorrhaging of the blood from this ruptured vessel brings about the unconsciousness and other symptoms of stroke. Doctors sometimes refer to strokes as "cerebral accident."

It would seem that more is involved in this rupturing of a blood vessel than just the pressure being put on it by the blood. Perhaps, researchers have reasoned, part of the fault may lie in the weakness of the actual walls of the blood vessels, or capillary fragility. Interest in rutin was aroused by the discovery that apparently it had a lot to do with maintaining the walls of the blood vessels so that they do not become fragile and hence are less likely to rupture and cause serious illness or death.

Immediately, a whole series of problems in research presented themselves. First of all, how can the fragility of the blood vessels be measured? It is relative to the blood pressure of course, and the higher the blood pressure goes, the more hardy the vessels must be not to rupture. In a patient suffering from stroke, one may assume that perhaps his blood vessels were indeed fragile, but how can one discover this *before* the accident takes place so that the patient can be treated for fragile blood vessels and so perhaps never have a stroke? The problem of measuring the fragility of blood vessels has never actually been solved satisfactorily and this is one reason for the doubt and confusion around the whole subject of rutin for high blood pressure patients.

Working with laboratory animals there are several methods of measuring fragility of capillaries and these have been used in experiments. H. K. Hellerstein, M.D., and his colleagues at several hospitals in Illinois and Ohio experimented by producing in animals blood pressure high enough to cause hemorrhaging from the blood vessels. To one group of animals they gave rutin 10 days before inducing the high blood pressure. Another group received no rutin. As reported in the *American Heart Journal* for August, 1951, all of the animals died as a result of the high blood pressure but those which received rutin did not show any evidence of hemorrhaging as the other animals did.

Vitamin P For Hemorrhagic Disease and Cancer

It is well known that patients exposed to X-ray may hemorrhage, supposedly because the X-ray has affected the walls of the tiny blood vessels. John Q. Griffith, M.D., and James F. Cough, Ph.D., writing in the magazine, *Blood,* for June, 1951, describe experiments in which they gave rutin to rats before they were exposed to X-ray. The rats which received the rutin did not hemorrhage, while those which did not receive rutin suffered the usual hemorrhagic disorders. Boris Sokoloff and his associates at the Florida Southern College in Lakeland, Florida, tested various vitamin P compounds on rats and found that the mortality from X-ray was reduced to 10 per cent in the group of rats receiving the vitamin P as against a mortality of 80 per cent in those rats which did not receive the vitamin. Say these authors, in commenting on their experiments in the *Journal of Clinical Investigation,* April, 1951, "capillary injury is by far the most frequent cause of clinical hemorrhagic disease," and this injury "may be due to infection, drugs, toxemia, allergy or nutritional disturbance." Increased capillary fragility appears to come, they say, from some defect in the intercellular cement—that is, the substance between the body cells which holds them together. They say, too, that vitamin P factors (rutin among them) appear to "affect the capillary system directly perhaps participating as a principal in the 'wear and tear' of a part or all of the capillary system, inhibiting its degeneration and taking part in its regeneration, specifically as far as the intercellular cement is concerned."

In another article in the *Archives of Pathology* for September, 1951, Dr. Sokoloff and his fellow-workers discuss the effect of vitamin P on experimental cancers. They note that many years ago researchers mentioned the possibility that the intercellular cement might be an important factor in the occurrence of cancer. In their experiment, they gave a vitamin P compound to animals with cancer and discovered that it had a moderate effect on the growths—that is, it decreased them. They also noted that the vitamin P had apparently no bad effects at all.

Bicknell and Prescott in their book, *Vitamins in Medicine* (Grune and Stratton, 1953), relate a number of experiments having to do with vitamin P in cases of high blood pressure. In one case rutin was given in a dose of 20 milligrams 3 times daily for periods up to 4 years. In 75 per cent of those tested, capillary fragility became normal. In the majority of cases the blood pressure was not reduced by the rutin. The authors are careful to point out that *rutin is not given to lower the blood pressure.* It is given to prevent accidents in which hemorrhages might occur in high blood pressure patients. In other words, it seems that rutin prevented the possibility of "stroke" in 75 per cent of these patients. It did not cure their high blood pressure.

Bicknell and Prescott give numerous other examples of vitamin P being used successfully in the treatment of cases involving hemorrhaging due to disease or due to drugs which the patient was taking for some disease. Hemorrhages due to drug poisoning, for instance, can be relieved by giving some vitamin P compounds.

Eye Disorders and Rutin

Rutin was also administered to a group of patients with glaucoma— the tragic eye disease in which the pressure inside the eyeball rises. Among 26 patients who received 20 milligrams of rutin 3 times a day, 17 noticed a fall in the pressure inside the eye, in 4 the results were not definite and 5 subjects noticed no change.

We found an extremely interesting article on the use of rutin in ophthalmology by L. B. Somerville-Large in the *Transactions of the Ophthalmological Society of the United Kingdom,* Vol. 69, pages 615-617, 1949-1950. Dr. Somerville-Large states that "in the eye we have what appears to be the only opportunity the human body affords of actually observing lesions (disorders) associated with capillary dysfunction. We must, therefore, forgive our medical colleagues for their caution in recognizing the value of rutin." He goes on to tell us that the tiny blood vessels in the eye can be studied by the ophthalmologist. It is actually the only place in the body where blood vessels can be directly observed. These tiny capillaries in the eye are packed closely together and they have a wider "bore" than other capillaries in the body.

He says that the commonest conditions in which the capillaries seem to be out of order are diabetes, toxic and inflammatory conditions, high blood pressure and hardening of the arteries. Although hypertension (high blood pressure) of itself has no relation to capillary fragility, he says, 6 to 10 per cent of those hypertensives who do have increased capillary fragility suffer from hemorrhages in the retina of the eye, and cerebral or brain hemorrhages. He gives doses of two 60-milligram tablets of rutin 3 times a day making a total dosage of 360 milligrams daily. "I find," says he, "that the larger doses give a more rapid and more complete negative result to capillary fragility tests." Incidentally he always combines the rutin with 200 milligrams of vitamin C daily.

It is interesting to note that throughout the discussion of vitamin P and rutin in medical literature, it is suggested that vitamin P and vitamin C work closely together and better results are always obtained when they are given together. Note, too, that Dr. Somerville-Large gives quite a large dose of vitamin C—200 milligrams. At the present time the official recommendation for the minimum daily intake of vitamin C is only 70 milligrams and it is believed that most of us don't even get that much! Does it not seem reasonable that two or three times this amount of vitamin C every day might do a lot to prevent the capillary fragility which is responsible for so much distress today? Remember that vitamin C is also involved in keeping the intercellular membranes healthy.

In conclusion, Dr. Somerville-Large states that in his experience he has not yet "met a case in which the capillary fragility skin test has not been reduced with rutin to well within normal limits." In speaking of the length of time it is necessary to continue taking the rutin, he says, "To me at the present time it looks like a life sentence. Whenever rutin has been discontinued the capillary fragility has again increased. Also, if the rutin is discontinued and the vitamin C alone persisted with, again the capillary fragility increases."

One last example of the use of rutin in treating capillary fragility. Bicknell and Prescott in *Vitamins in Medicine* tell of 12 children in a group of 100 allergic children who were treated with 100 to 150 milligrams of vitamin P daily for 6 months. At the end of this time their capillary resistance became normal.

How Much Vitamin P Are You Getting?

What application can we make of all these experiences to our daily life? First of all, if vitamin P (of which rutin is a part) is really a vitamin, how much of it do we perhaps need every day? The Federation of the American Societies for Experimental Biology have voted to discontinue the use of the term "vitamin" in relation to vitamin P. They declare that it has not been proved as yet that these substances (the flavones) are essential to good health and their absence in diet will cause any disorder that can be cured by administering them. However, it is interesting to note that people in other countries, and this country as well, go right on calling the flavones "vitamin P." Bicknell and Prescott state that the daily requirement may be not less than 33 units daily "and possibly considerably more."

Just like vitamin C, vitamin P is destroyed by cooking in an open vessel. So, much of the vitamin P value of food is lost in cooking. Once again we are faced with the absolute necessity for eating plenty of fresh raw fruits and vegetables, for it is in these that vitamin P is found in the largest amounts, along with vitamin C. The rutin concentrate used by doctors in treating hypertensive patients is made from buckwheat. Rutin occurs chiefly in the leaves of buckwheat which may contain as much as 7 or 8 per cent of rutin. It is rapidly destroyed when the leaves are dried slowly, so they must be processed with the greatest care. After the leaves are completely dried, there seems to be no further loss of rutin.

If you are suffering from high blood pressure and your doctor advises taking rutin to avoid any possibility of a stroke, we would certainly go along with his advice, on the basis of the evidence we have collected. If you are perfectly healthy and interested in preserving the state of your blood vessels so that you will not suffer from these disorders later on, then by all means see that you get, every day, plenty of the foods in which vitamin P (hence rutin) occurs, along with vitamin C. Of course, we always urge readers to get enough vitamin C, for we believe it to be one of the food elements most essential for good health. Now it appears that vitamin P, always associated with vitamin C in foods, may be of great value as well.

Here is a list of foods that are rich in vitamin P and we have given you their vitamin C content as well. We hope you notice that, just as rose hips are many, many times richer in vitamin C than any other food, so too they are especially rich in vitamin P.

TABLE 4: VITAMIN P CONTENT OF FOODS

	Vitamin P Content in Units	*Vitamin C Content in Milligrams*
Apricots	75-100 in 8 apricots	4
Blackberry	60-100 in ¾ cup	3
Black currant	200-500 in 1 cup	150
Cabbage (summer)	100 in 1 cup, raw	50
Cherry, black	60-100 in 12 large cherries	12
Grape, black	500-1000 in 1 small bunch	3
Grape, white	500-1000 in 1 small bunch	4
Grapefruit	100 in ½ grapefruit	45
Lemon juice	450-750 in 8 tablespoonfuls	25
Orange	300-500 in 1 medium orange	50
Parsley	130 in 1 cup	70
Plum	50-200 in 3 medium plums	5
Prune	300-400 in 8 medium prunes	4
Rose hips	240-680 in 100 grams	500 to 6000

141. Cleft Palate—Heredity or Nutrition?

The child talks through his nose; his upper lip is misshapen and stitched; he is shy with strangers because he is aware of being different. This description usually fits a child who was born with a cleft palate or harelip, that is, a lack of union between the two elements which normally meet to form the roof of the mouth or upper lip. This condition can now be surgically repaired, but the disfiguring element still remains.

Six thousand children are born with cleft palate every year in the United States—one in every eight hundred births. There is evidence to show that this number could be slashed to zero. The problem need not exist. The cause lies in the diet of the expectant mother.

More and more, the feeding of pregnant women is being accepted as *the* important factor in determining the physical and mental perfection of the new-born baby. All the drugs and advanced delivery techniques in the world will not erase the effects of a bad prenatal diet. Organized medicine is beginning to face this fact and now maybe we'll get somewhere in the struggle to insure our unborn babies against congenital malformations.

The Necessity of Vitamins A and B

In the case of cleft palate, there are several vitamins whose deficiencies could be the cause. Vitamin A found in large quantities in carrots, sweet potatoes, cod liver oil, calf and beef liver and greens is strongly identified with the basic vitamin needs of pregnancy, and cleft palate can be the result of a lack of it. As a matter of fact, this and other deformities such as horseshoe kidneys, hydrocephalus, heart and brain defects, could be induced at will in the litters of experimental sows simply by withholding vitamin A from the diet, according to an article in the *British Medical Journal* for June, 1956. To prove that vitamin A was the only cause, it was restored to the diet and perfect litters were born to the same sows! The same result, perfect or imperfect, could be induced every time.

Of the B vitamins, riboflavin and folic acid are called upon as the fetus develops to the point at which the palate would be formed. These vital elements must be on tap, so to speak, when the stage arrives at which they are needed. If they are not available, gestation proceeds, simply using what nourishment is available and leaving the job unfinished, if the supply

[558]

of nutrients is insufficient. To insure an adequate supply of all the B vitamins (for they are most effective when taken in combination as they occur in natural foods) brewer's yeast and/or desiccated liver should have a major place in the pregnant woman's diet.

All of the elements of good diet are important to the expectant mother, but the above-mentioned have been shown in animal experiments to have direct influence over the proper fusion of the palate.

Avoid Cortisone During Pregnancy

Another strong caution is voiced by the *British Medical Journal* against the use of cortisone during pregnancy. In animals, doses of cortisone have been proven responsible for the incidence of cleft palate in clinical experiments. That these animal experiments are indicative of human reactions is shown in an article in the *Lancet* (June 30, 1956) in which a detailed account of cortisone's effects on a pregnant woman and the subsequent stillbirth of her baby with a cleft palate is given. In this case cortisone was administered from what is judged to have been the 38th day of pregnancy to the 52nd day and a maintenance dose thereafter. The palate is calculated to begin forming on the 45th day and continue to the 12th week, so that the lady being discussed was receiving cortisone during the crucial period of palate formation. On the basis of animal experiments, a dose of 4 to 8 grams of cortisone would be considered dangerous enough to affect an unborn child. This patient was given 6 grams—4 of which were given at the time the palate was forming. The final outcome should have been no surprise to those attending the young mother. The dangers of cortisone during pregnancy, especially, cannot be overestimated.

In his book on diet, *Nutrition and Physical Degeneration,* Dr. Weston Price quotes veterinary reports stating that cleft palate, harelip and other facial deformities are often found among the litters of dogs that are pets and are lavishly coddled and given only what they like best to eat. Many women who are awaiting the birth of a baby expect to be treated in exactly the same manner. They expect to be pampered and catered to; they eat only what they "crave" with no regard for nutritional needs. It is a selfish way to have a baby, and worse, it is foolishly dangerous.

The psychological glow a mother can acquire in the knowledge that the baby she is carrying will be perfect is a priceless asset to her. Good eating habits for herself are her best assurance for her baby's health. Cleft palate and harelip can become as archaic as childbed fever if every mother-to-be will make sure she is getting enough A and B vitamins. It's that simple! Other vitamins and minerals are important, too, but if you are eating so that you get plenty of A and B, you will probably get enough of the rest.

We are convinced by our research and other scientific testimony that cleft palate is not a hereditary condition. Many stories come to us from

[559]

unhappy couples who would like to have children but are afraid to do so because the husband or the wife was born with a cleft palate or harelip. The experiments quoted above from the *British Medical Journal* were designed to prove just the opposite. With changes of diet—and only that—cleft palate could be induced into litters of rabbits or eliminated at will, though the same dam and sire were the parents in each case. The same effects are presumed in humans and this conclusion completely eliminates the hereditary elements in producing offspring afflicted with cleft palate.

SECTION 27: COLDS

142. Colds Are Everywhere

In our opinion, people are tired of reading about how many colds one can expect each year and how much colds cost in industrial money and man hours. When a person bothers to read an article about colds, he wants to find out what's to be done to protect himself against catching a cold or how best to get rid of the one he has now. These answers are hard to find. First of all, few people think seriously about protecting themselves against a cold until they see that everyone they meet is miserable with one, and by then it is often too late, for colds are extremely contagious.

Others don't think about colds until they have one, and then they want a pill or prescription that will rid them of their cold at once. This is another delusion, for there is no such panacea. The only sure protection against colds is good health through sound nutrition. The only way to speed the departure of a cold you already have is to give your body more ammunition to fight it through good food, food supplements and rest.

Colds and Carbohydrates

Colds invade when body resistance is too weak to keep them out. This resistance is not built overnight, and it can easily be undermined by even one or two types of unhealthful food eaten habitually. A perfect illustration of this point appeared in the *British Medical Journal* (April 29, 1933). In the article, it was contended that a high intake of carbohydrates (flour products, sweets, etc.) disposes one to upper respiratory problems, such as colds.

For one thing, high carbohydrate intake tends toward water retention in the body, as shown in experiments in which animals and human beings were fed diets high in sugar. Catarrhal persons are described as having an excess of water in the body. Of course, it follows that a restriction of carbohydrates results in "evident and permanent improvement" in the patient.

Cereals and Sugar

The *Journal* goes on to tell of a study of two East African tribes which demonstrated the role of carbohydrates where respiratory problems are involved. In one tribe, which was generally cereal-eating, the mortality from bronchitis and pneumonia was 10 times as great as that of the other tribe, which was primarily a meat-eating people.

The impression that cereal or grain products can influence the course of a cold is given added weight by a short article in the September, 1957, issue of the *American Journal of Digestive Diseases,* which said that the ingestion of wheat products, combined with high carbohydrate foods, is quite likely to alter nasal mucus and can be associated with the onset of a cold.

To get back to the article in the *British Medical Journal,* we were interested in a report on the consumption of the concentrated carbohydrate, sugar, among the pupils of a girls' boarding school, and their resultant colds. They consumed sugar at the alarming average of two pounds per week per girl. It was found, however, that in the dormitory which showed the lowest rate of sugar consumption, the percentage of catarrh cases was 19 per cent less than that of the dormitory with the highest rate of sugar consumption. This seems to be a pretty fair indication that a diet rich in sugar and pastry, dough, spaghetti, white bread, etc., increases the likelihood of a cold's finding its way into your system.

Dr. J. R. Jehl of Clifton, New Jersey, was quoted in *Consumer Reports* (no date) as saying that many colds are due to an allergy to certain foods and not to a virus at all. Frequently, says Dr. Jehl, infants' colds clear up when their formula is changed from milk to a soybean preparation. Does it not seem likely that this reaction could be carried into the grown-up years? How many teenagers and adults suffer from frequent colds that could be stopped by a change from milk to some other beverage?

The Serious Results of Colds

The consequence of frequent upper respiratory disease can be much more than congested breathing passages or loss of pep. The *British Medical Journal* (November 26, 1955) reported an obvious connection between bronchitis and lung cancer. This conclusion was reached on observing that there were approximately twice as many lung cancer deaths among 1,421 World War I pensioners, recorded as having bronchitis when pensioned, as would be expected among a similar group in the general population. Other men pensioned for injuries such as loss of limbs showed no excess of lung cancer. Bronchitis was considered to be the major difference between the two groups of men.

An article in the *Diuretic Review* (4:4, 1955) points to colds as a common, irritating and aggravating factor in congestive heart failure. A study of 300 cases of heart failure revealed that more than half began with some type of respiratory infection. The *Review* reports on another study, the results of which appeared in the *American Journal of Medical Science* (no date) which showed a direct relation between frequent occurrence of heart failures and the onset of "even minor colds." These respiratory infections may initiate heart failure by causing damage to the heart muscle.

The *Medical Journal of Australia* (January 11, 1958) sums up the whole situation in a concise and definite statement which leaves no room for misinterpretation: "Colds, in one form or another, probably cause more ill health and disability than any group of diseases." With this opinion, plus the evidence above, it is obvious that repeated colds can mean more than a day in bed or painful headaches and sniffling; they can mean your life.

What About Tonsils?

The idea is still prevalent that diseased tonsils in children lie at the root of the cold problem. However, tonsils have the function of channelling disease away from the system, not infecting it. In spite of the large number of tonsillectomies performed on children, the need for any of them can rarely be demonstrated. As for the effect of their removal on a disposition to future colds, consider your friends and acquaintances who no longer have their tonsils and ask yourself if they're immune. More convincing still is the note in an article on allergy and colds in the *Journal of the American Medical Association* (February 8, 1958), which mentioned that more people who had kept their tonsils were able to avoid colds than those who had had them removed. In a survey of London families, with regard to the problem of respiratory infections, it was reported (*British Medical Journal,* January 18, 1958) that comparisons showed a slightly greater tendency toward catching colds in children whose tonsils had been removed. The possibility seems to be growing that, in years to come, a good set of tonsils will be considered a strong asset in the avoidance of colds.

In the past year or two, the hope for a vaccine that will eliminate the common cold has been fanned to a blaze, only to be extinguished, several times. Actually the experts aren't sure just what a cold is, or how one gets it, so that a vaccine against colds would have to be a vaccine against everything. Don't be fooled by false claims.

"Contact" One of Many Avenues

It is the generally accepted theory that colds are largely "caught," by contact with a cold sufferer, and many studies have shown this to be a sound theory, but, undoubtedly, there are other factors. This was proven by a study of 8,000 volunteers in Holland in widely scattered areas (*British Medical Journal,* January 25, 1958). In spite of the distance that separated them, each section showed the appearance of colds at the same time as the others every year, and the rate of incidence in all widely separated areas was identical. It is hard to imagine that each case in each area could somehow transmit his cold to one person in another part of Holland. Therefore, these colds had to be due to something other than contact.

In a Wales cheese factory, a cold, humid room was found to be a source of protection against colds. Those who worked in this room found their susceptibility to colds cut in half, in comparison to the workers in the rest of the factory. How or why this was so no one seems to know.

Self-Help Suggestions

It's easy to see that the outside forces which harbor the beginnings of a cold are everywhere and practically unavoidable. Inner resistance is the only answer. A good diet of fresh foods, plus plenty of vitamins C and A, should be your foundation for avoiding a cold. Sugar and processed cereals should be high on your list of things to stay away from.

For best results with vitamin C, a campaign of massive dosage should be instituted the minute—the very minute—you have the first suggestion of a cold. From then on the routine should consist of about 250 milligrams of vitamin C or more every 4 hours. The vitamin must be taken at these frequent intervals for complete saturation of the body tissues with vitamin C. This state of saturation does not last longer than 4 hours and, by this time, whatever vitamin C is left has been excreted. In the process of fighting germs, vitamin C is oxidized or destroyed, so it must be constantly replaced. Vitamin C is the body's infection fighter, and steady doses of it will add up to more protection (and relief) than all the cold pills and throat sprays you can lay your hands on.

143. The History of My Colds

By J. I. RODALE

As a boy, I was not the hale and robust physical type. I was already taking Bromo-Seltzer at the age of 7, and can recall violent headaches as long back as I can remember. I was never laid up with any serious illness, but was continually plagued with those little recurring situations that had mostly nuisance value. There were dizzy spells at times, my swimming endurance was limited to about 8 strokes, there was a condition of almost continuous semi-catarrh and, whenever the wind blew the wrong way, I caught a cold. From about October to April I could expect to have them, one after another.

When I look back now, I can see clearly why I was not stronger and

[563]

able to resist colds, headaches, etc. It was mostly wrong diet—too much starch and sugar. I was imbibing sodas, candy, pastries, ice cream, bread, etc., in enormous doses. In those days (I was born in 1898), only the faintest glimmerings of nutrition were known. Had I known then what I know now, the story would have been entirely different.

At about 21, I began a systematic quest to discover ways and means to eradicate these colds. I took up tennis and went at it like a demon, but all it did was to give me a heart murmur. I then became a vegetarian, but that did not accomplish the task. Over the next 20 years, I experimented with M.D.'s, osteopaths, chiropractors, Turkish baths, Swedish massage, diathermy and everything else on the popular health agenda, but the colds continued to come with clock-like regularity. I will venture to say that I must have read 500 articles describing how to dodge catching a cold. In the main, the theme was—be sure to wear your rubbers when it rains and stay away from drafts. How ridiculous this now sounds! We shall see later how I mastered the cold bogey, but now I want to show you how important it is not to take any of the popular health concepts for granted. We must question every generally accepted health tenet or dogma, as rooted as it may be in the public's mind. You must observe the effect on your own bodily processes of your basic daily actions. Make your own interpretations.

This was beautifully expressed 700 years ago by Roger Bacon, who, in *Of Regimen of Health*, said, "A man's own observation, what he finds good of and what he finds hurt of, is the best physic to preserve health."

Colds Were Frequent and Certain

When I was about 40, I can remember that all I had to do was to take the two and one-half hour railroad trip from Allentown to New York in the winter and invariably a cold would come out of it. To sit at a football game meant a sure cold, and the same thing would occur after a Thanksgiving gorging. I distinctly recall that colds would occur after emotional upsets. At this time, I was beginning to make speeches in favor of the organic method of farming and gardening, and was so fearful of being on a platform, that the first 3 or 4 experiences resulted in a cold the next morning. I always had had an inferiority complex, but I am glad to admit that today I am more the extrovert, having given hundreds of talks, and recently even held an audience for about 10 minutes with a purely humorous speech, which, if I may be pardoned for my vanity, had them rolling in the aisles for the entire time. It is possible that the same thing that finally gave me an immunity to colds also chased away my inferiority complex.

Dr. E. W. Braithwaite, consulting psychiarist to the Ministry of Health of England, has the following to say about colds in the October 2, 1944, issue of the *British Medical Journal:*

"The following facts may be of interest to either sufferers from, or investigators of, the common cold. During the course of 25 years' practice of psychoanalysis for the treatment of psychoneurotics, I have observed

[564]

that in them (1.) a cold invariably occurred in a particular emotional state; (2.) the occurrence of a cold could be prognosticated whenever this state developed; (3.) the cold could be aborted if a different emotional state could be produced in the course of treatment or could be shortened if it had started; (4.) cold, wet, hunger, exhaustion and a source of infection do not result in the development of a cold in the absence of the appropriate emotional state; (5.) cold "proneness" disappears completely as a result of successful treatment and does not recur.

"Though these observations have little immediate practical value, my experience demonstrates to me, at least, that the solution of the problem of the common cold lies in the sphere of preventive psychological medicine. The specific factor is psychological; the microbic one secondary."

While this is interesting, I believe that the proper nutritional preparation will enable the mind to get into all kinds of emotional states without causing colds. What Dr. Braithwaite says is true of persons who are eating a devitalized diet and not fortifying it the way it should be.

Importance of Calcium in Cold Prevention

I would like to mention that the first relief in the reduction of the incidence of colds was given me by a New York City osteopath, Lucius Bush. Dr. Bush had developed a technique by which he placed his finger into the patient's nose, and gradually enlarged the passageways in it. He called it finger surgery, I believe. Dr. Bush claims that the habits of civilization are gradually reducing interior spaces of the nose, preventing oxygen from circulating and creating a wonderful breeding ground for cold-causing organisms. By a series of treatments, Dr. Bush gradually opened up the passageways in my nose and I experienced immediate benefits in having less colds, and milder ones. But I did not go long enough. It required 15 treatments, whereas I stopped at number 4. It is possible that, by Dr. Bush's method, one can get practically complete immunity to colds.

In this respect, may I mention another factor that may be responsible for the recent sharp increase in the number of colds experienced by the general public. In the nose, there are little, almost microscopic hair-like things called cilia, which cover the mucous membrane and which move back and forth like a field of wheat in a wind. They are as close together as the "hair" on a rug. They move the secretions of the nose into proper channels. They are easily affected and then either function poorly or not at all. One thing that can do this is medication, and secondly, a lack of calcium in the system. The cilia need calcium for "backbone," to stand up to their job, and, since a terrific percentage of the public is calcium deficient, we can see one place which courts trouble as far as colds are concerned. This shows one advantage of taking bone meal and staying away from nose drops.

At this period, namely about 1942, my condition had progressed to such a point that my colds were turning into asthma. The last phases of each cold, after about two weeks of severe suffering, would cause asthmatic wheezing, and when I would sneeze, it felt as if the top of my head was coming off. Thus, I was in deathly fear of an oncoming sneeze. I recall terribly sleepless nights, saturated with agonized worryings, and the future looked quite dark.

New or Badly Designed Houses Can Be Responsible

I would like to mention an experience we had that winter, which carries a valuable lesson. We moved into a new house on the organic experimental farm, and within a few days, the entire family, the 5 of us, were in bed with a bad case of the grippe. I attribute it to the fact that the new plaster of the walls was not yet dry. There was too much moisture in the house, and sleeping with our heads near a "wet" wall, was, I am sure, the causative factor which had brought about our condition. It is best not to be too anxious to move into a new house. Make sure first that the plaster is thoroughly dry. I wonder if this is why people hold "house warmings" in connection with moving into a new house. Incidentally, I once noted that when we built an addition to our printing plant, a linotype machine standing close to a brick wall suffered a bad case of rusting, due I am sure to the water still in the mortar.

Another thing I would like to mention is that we had a duct system of heating in our house, the kind of ducts used for air conditioning, and many of the ducts were at floor level. In that house, we all had had bad colds. In fact, this was where I began to get the attacks of asthma. An engineer friend of mine told me later that ducts should not be at floor level because from there they can set up currents of air or drafts which might bring on colds. He maintained that the ducts should be as high up on the wall as possible. This is a matter that should be discussed with heating engineers if you are in the process of building a house.

Investigations on Nasal Temperature

About this time, I read of some medical researches which changed my entire thinking along the lines of securing immunity from colds. The work, which took 3 years, was done by Doctors Irwin Spiesman and Lloyd Arnold of the University of Illinois. Sixty-three persons were used and they were of all types. Some of them rarely or never caught colds, while others were of that group that suffers one cold after another. It seems astonishing that the findings of Drs. Spiesman and Arnold have not received continuing publicity, since the project was done in cooperation with the research laboratories of the Illinois State Department of Public Health.

The scientists caused their 63 subjects to be seated, bare to the waist, for half hour periods, in a room 8 feet square, free of draughts and at a constant temperature. Ice-cups were clapped to their backs, and at the same time the temperature inside their noses was measured. Another portion of the experiments included the application of hot water to the bare backs of the subjects, along with the taking of their nasal temperature.

Drs. Spiesman and Arnold discovered that when the body was suddenly chilled by application of the ice-cups, the temperature of the mucous membrane of the nose dropped, as a result of the nasal veins becoming constricted. However, in normal persons, the nasal temperature soon rose to normal again, even though ice-cups were held continuously to the back. On the other hand, the nose temperature of chronic cold vicims remained for a fairly long period at a low level.

The experimenters discovered that these differences in nose temperature were more important in causing colds than infection from one person to another. It was while the nasal temperature was below normal that the bacteria, always present in the mucous membrane of the nose and throat, were able to become active and bring about the congested and inflamed condition we know as a common head cold.

Having discovered this, Drs. Spiesman and Arnold sought some means of causing the membranes of the nose to react normally when the individual was exposed to sudden changes of temperature. The doctors experimented with cold injections. These injections were given subcutaneously (under the skin) every other day over a period of 3 months. However, according to Drs. Spiesman and Arnold's report, "The frequency of cold was not affected by this treatment, nor was there any effect produced upon" the temperature reactions in the nasal veins of the subjects treated.

However, the doctors did discover a means of causing the membranes of the nose to react normally when the individual was exposed to sudden changes of temperature. The solution to the problem lay in giving the subject a treatment of baths and in having them follow a system of dieting.

A hot bath followed by a cold one in the morning, and repeated in the evening, before dinner, was decidedly beneficial in tuning up the circulation responses in the nose, so the arteries did not react too radically to sudden chill. Without sudden changes in nose temperature, cold germs were unable to gain a foothold. Drs. Spiesman and Arnold found that a few of the subjects showed marked improvement in ability to resist colds, as a result of these baths, but most of the individuals studied showed little benefit from bathing alone.

Wheat Products and Immunity to Colds

Far better than baths in keeping the nose temperature normal was the exclusion from the diet of bread and other carbohydrates, especially of the wheat-cereal variety. Time and again the doctors noticed that, after subjects were freed from the nuisance of head colds, because wheat foods and bread had been dropped from their diet, they returned to their former weakness in regard to colds the moment they started eating bread and other wheat products.

Regarding the diet used by Drs. Spiesman and Arnold for their subjects, the Spiesman-Arnold report says:

"All products made from wheat, i.e., white flour breads, pastries, pies, cookies, etc., were eliminated from the diet. The patients in this group were requested to abstain from the use of tea, coffee or alcoholic bever-

ages, and to smoke sparingly. They were instructed to eat two large vegetable portions, or a vegetable and fruit salad each day, and to make the
salad the main course of the meal. They were also asked to eat as much
fresh fruit as they could daily . . . and to drink 6 ounces of tomato juice
per adult per day. Eight glasses of water were prescribed a day. Fried
foods were prohibited. No condiments. Butter was to be added very freely
to all cooked vegetables and eaten generally very freely; two to four egg
yolks for each adult and one to two for a child per day. The patient was
not to hurry while eating, nor be tired or worried. He was to take a short
rest after every meal.

"The patients on this regime improved clinically. We found, in our
experience with dieting of these patients, that an overindulgence of carbohydrates, especially of the wheat-cereal variety, was most to be guarded
against. Time and again we observed, after excellent results were obtained,
that a return of the patient to an excess carbohydrate diet caused a recurrence of symptoms."

Drs. Spiesman and Arnold observed that persons unusually sensitive
in regard to cold-catching benefited most of all when they followed both the
bathing and the dieting systems. During the 3 years the patients were under
observation, the hypersensitive individuals were placed on the elimination-
of-bread diet alone, then given the bathing treatments without the dieting,
and finally given both dieting and bathing at the same time. It was found
that they benefited more from the bread elimination than from the bathing,
but showed most improvement of all when dieting and bathing were used
together.

The Effect of Worry and Apprehension

Drs. Spiesman and Arnold discovered that, curiously enough, the
benefits in avoiding colds brought about by wheat and cereal elimination,
as well as by the taking of baths, were completely offset by worry and
apprehension in the individuals studied. No matter how faithfully they
dieted or followed the rules in regard to bathing, if these subjects worried
about such things as the loss of job, the illness or death of a relative, etc.,
they immediately became susceptible to colds.

As long as a subject remained in a state of mental uneasiness, he
failed to benefit from either dieting or bathing. Drs. Spiesman and Arnold
noted specific cases of individuals who suffered great mental distress for
one reason or another; one suffered death in his family; another experienced
the harrowing ordeals of bankruptcy; another lost his job.

Drs. Spiesman and Arnold, in their report, mention physical exercise
as an important element in setting up resistance to colds. Twenty minutes
of setting-up exercises, in the nude, in a cool room, prior to taking a hot
and cold shower, are advocated. A brisk walk for one hour a day, either
in divided time or for an hour continuously, never hurrying, breathing
deeply, is excellent. A rest, even a brief one, after each meal, is recommended.

[568]

This experiment made sense to me, and the whole family decided to cut out the grain foods. We noticed an immediate effect, a great reduction in the number of colds that were "caught," but what was very important also, a reduction in the severity and duration in the fewer colds that did come. This family diet went on for about a year, but was then abandoned, as it seemed to be giving the lady of the house too much trouble in preparing school lunches for the children. As far as I am concerned, I went on and off a breadless diet over the last 15 years or so, and I find it excellent for keeping weight down. I will never forget the way my head catarrh vanished when first I began to cut out bread, and anyone so afflicted should give this diet a "try," but one should take wheat germ and vitamin E to replace those elements that are usually secured from the whole grain foods.

Poison Ivy Experiences

An interesting thing occured in the case of my son Robert during the year we went off the grain foods. He had always been extremely sensitive to poison ivy, and was attacked by it even if he did not come in direct physical contact with the plant. But he seemed to become completely immune to it during our breadless year. The only reason I can ascribe for this astonishing happening is that children usually stuff themselves with bread and cookies and therefore have little room or desire for vegetables. Lacking in the greenstuffs, he must have developed a subclinical case of scurvy, and it is possible that the ivy will easily burn a scorbutic skin. When Robert could not eat bread and cake, he had to eat the vegetables or go hungry.

This might be a good place to mention my own experience with poison ivy. When we moved out to the farm, I began to learn the ways of this plant, much to my own physical discomfort. Every summer I could expect to have it poison me once or twice. About 7 or 8 years later, I received a letter from one of our readers, in which the writer related that he had suddenly become immune to poison ivy, and believed it was due to cutting out sugar and taking bone meal as well as a few vitamins. Since I was on the same dietary program, I felt that the same thing must have happened to me also, as I suddenly came to a realization that for a year or two, I could not remember being afflicted with poison ivy trouble. As I related the contents of this letter to the family at the evening meal, I announced that I was going outside immediately, would find some poison ivy and rub it on my arms. To their horror, I did it, Nina, Ruth, Bob and Anna following me, thinking I was fooling. I rubbed the leaves on my arms vigorously and then washed my hands only, as I did not want to rub the stuff into my eyes. To my gratification, nothing happened. The vaccination did not take, which convinced me that the vitamins and minerals I was taking, and the cutting out of sugar, had fabricated a new healthier skin for me, and I have not been bothered with poison ivy since.

[569]

Diet and Colds

Today I am practically immune from colds and will get one perhaps only when I try some nutritional experiment. For example, a few years ago I cut eggs completely from my diet. Within a month, I had a cold. At another time, I decided to eliminate all fruits, just to see if anything would happen. This was the first time I ever caught a cold in the middle of July. Of course, at that time I was not taking halibut liver oil perles (vitamins A and D) and rose hips (vitamin C).

I must not forget to give credit to my organically produced diet, which began about 1941. On our 60-acre farm, beginning in that year, we began to grow crops without the aid of chemical fertilizers, and tests later showed that they had a higher vitamin and mineral content than average. Slowly I noticed a resistance developing against colds, and especially the complete disappearance of all asthmatic symptoms. It is difficult, however, to pin this down to any one thing as a complete and specific preventive. However, we know that the eating of organically grown foods has made the whole family healthier.

I must remark that in the old days, once I began to get the first sniffles of a cold, the cold always developed fully. Today I will sometimes experience a few sniffles, but rarely do they go further.

I believe one of the greatest aids in my preventive history of colds is the taking of vitamins A and C (halibut liver oil perles and rose hips). The advisability of this supplementation is covered thoroughly elsewhere in this book. But there can also be no question that my taking of bone meal, wheat germ and vitamin E, and cutting out the grain foods, sugar and salt, are also contributing factors. The body can be like a machine which does not get the proper fuels and other supplies required to run it. Then it may not function properly. I suppose that machines develop afflictions that may be compared to colds in human beings.

Good Nourishment Prevents Colds

Just a few words about the various fallacies that fly about regarding colds. Don't sit in a draft, they say. Keep your feet dry and warm. Gargle with X-brand of antiseptic—etc., etc., etc. These are all well and good for the badly nourished person, but one who is in top form—nutrition-wise—need not fear a draft or getting the feet wet. This is illustrated by an experience I had one January first. I called upon a friend who was suffering from an unusually severe cold, and when I proffered my hand in greeting, he said, "You had better not shake my hand. I have a very bad cold and you might catch it."

I surprised him by insisting that I shake his hand anyhow, and not only did I make sure to give it a thorough shake, but I amazed him by saying, "Now watch what I'm going to do!"

I took my hand and rubbed it into my nostrils!

His eyes bulged!

"Why do you want to have a cold?" he asked.

"I don't want to have a cold," I replied.

"Then why did you do this?"

"Because I have built my body up to the point where it does not catch colds from anyone, and I want to prove to you what good nutrition can do in warding off colds."

But the next morning I had a cold, albeit a mild one, which left in about 4 days.

Now, why did I catch my friend's germs? If you will recall, I stated above that the visit was on January first. The night before was New Year's Eve and I had been out celebrating. It is easy to follow diets and rules under ordinary conditions but it is much more difficult when you are out New Year's Eve-ing until 3 in the morning, and then get up 6 o'clock the same morning to work on an article you are writing. It was too stiff a test. I had also been cutting down somewhat on my eggs at that time.

On my farm, I have developed a flock of chickens that are practically disease-resistant. We feed them only on food we raise ourselves, without benefit of chemical fertilizers. Ordinarily a conservative farmer will not permit another farmer to enter into the chicken house for fear that on the bottom of his shoes he may be carrying disease germs from his own flock. A few years ago, a group of about 20 farmers visited my chicken house, and I asked them to rub their feet vigorously in the litter. They thought I was crazy, but I told them that my chickens were so healthy that no germ could do a thing to them. And I was right. Nothing happened, because my chickens do not go out New Year's Eve-ing.

Miscellaneous Facts

Taxi drivers get fewer colds than any other segment of our population. The next time you take a taxi, check up on this. It is due to the fact that the taxi driver sits in so many drafts that, even with his characteristically poor diet, he gains practical immunity. But your average taxi driver is more susceptible to kidney trouble. This organ cannot take the year-in-year-out shaking up that it gets in the course of a taxi driver's daily work. If I were a taxi driver, I would wear a kind of high belt worn by motor-cyclists, and if necessary, would spend my own money to equip the car with an extra set of, or stronger, springs or shock absorbers.

Benjamin Franklin, as part of his daily physical regimen designed to condition himself, sat at an open window in the nude for considerable lengths of time, every day, but, although he lived to be in his eighties, he finally succumbed to pneumonia which arose due to one of these window sitting sessions. Or so the legend goes! Franklin should have quit when he was ahead.

Dancing and Colds

About 25 years ago, I had a severe head cold which had settled in my throat. My vocal cords were on a sit-down strike and I could talk only in a whisper, and even then only with difficulty. Bob was only two years old then and he lay on a couch, the picture of melancholy gloom, for he also had a cold. A lively number was playing on the phonograph and, before I knew it, my feet began to move in rhythm with it. Since Bobby began to smile at what was passing for eccentric dancing, my feet gathered momentum. My body went into more active motion, contorting itself weirdly and defying the rules of gravity. I had to laugh myself and Bobby shrieked with delight. After all, he was only a baby and thus could not distinguish between his father and Fred Astaire. But the more he shrieked, the crazier I contorted my body, and after awhile, I practically collapsed in a corner.

I noticed that now my voice came 100 per cent easier. A complete transformation had occurred. The soreness had miraculously disappeared. I could talk with ease. The physical exertion had stimulated my breathing, and my uncontrolled laughter must have driven the accumulation of months of stale air out of my lungs. The quick change from the depths of melancholy to the pinnacle of joyous exhilaration, accomplished in about 10 minutes what would otherwise have required days of suffering.

Gustave Doré, the gifted Alsatian artist who illustrated the works of so many famous authors, was so fond of dancing that he could not go to sleep unless he first danced for his aged mother, who accompanied him on the piano. He was skilled in the hornpipe and Highland fling. He was especially adept in boleros, cracoviennes and cachuchas, but his specialty was the cancan. Those who had seen the sumptuous profusion of statues, pictures, busts and models which filled his apartments, and the fact that he never smashed a thing, marveled at his astonishing agility in executing these terpsichorean antics.

He claimed that this dancing animated his spirits and put him into the exciting moods that stimulated his creative genius. On going to bed after such a riotous orgy of prancing, he found that his aroused mind was enabled to plan the pictures which made him famous. Of course, this might be bad for insomniacs.

Dancing has a health-giving value and also acts as a stimulant to the mind. Since the beginning of time, man has danced. He has cast out devils in this manner. He danced to get rain, to make seeds germinate, to bring bountiful harvests, to have good luck in the chase, to increase fecundity and to praise God. He danced on joyous as well as sad occasions. He lived practically every aspect of his daily life through dancing. Primitive man did not dance for enjoyment, but as a means to master his daily problems, as a means to attain power. He may not have realized it, but it kept him in good health and spirits.

More than half the world today dances the traditional folk dances that have been handed down without change for thousands of years. This includes the American Indian, African savage tribes, Mexicans, Central and South Americans and practically all people of Asia. Dancing must

[572]

have great value, otherwise it would have died out in these places. Wherever urban civilization develops, it seems to disappear automatically, to be replaced by our modern jazz dancing, which has a purely sensual basis. In such cities many never dance. Our cities seem to breed tired people.

I believe that Henry Ford, in bringing back the square dances, was giving grim warning to the country of the dangers of going all-out in the direction of machine-age culture. It was his way of showing that people were not moving in the right direction in the ways of their daily life, that they had better keep one eye on the machine and the other on Old Mother Nature—that somewhere in between lies the happy medium.

144. Colds and Vitamin A

According to the *New York Herald Tribune,* business and industry lose nearly 4 billion dollars annually in production and services because of absenteeism caused by the common cold. Workers lose an estimated one billion dollars in wages and spend 400 million dollars annually on drugs and treatment. One-fourth of the people of the United States suffer from 4 or 5 colds annually. School children lose more school time because of colds than for any other reason.

These statistics are impressive, but the billions of dollars lost probably do not seem nearly so important to the average American as the actual misery he suffers when he comes down with a real good dose of cold, grippe, flu, virus or whatever his particular form of infection may be called. In our large file of material on the common cold, many of the articles impress us with their extreme lack of helpfulness, for they do not suggest any possible remedy or even the faint hope that some day we may conquer the common cold.

For example, *Newsweek* for January 28, 1952, quotes a famous British physician, Dr. Christopher H. Andrewes, who has discovered that school children are responsible for cold epidemics. He says that families where there are school children contract 3 times as many colds as families where the patter of little feet is not heard. The youngsters pick up the germ at school or in the playground and carry it home, where they spread it like wildfire, because "they are constantly blubbering, wiping and crawling all over adults," or, as *Newsweek* puts it a little more elegantly, "they lack well-developed habits of personal hygiene."

Dr. Andrewes gave a series of parties to prove his point, inviting only children who had bad colds and several hale and hearty adults who, we suppose, were encouraged to mingle with the young ones. The fact that none of the adults caught cold, Dr. Andrewes attributes to the fact that the parties didn't go on long enough. Granted that the small fry may do more than their share of spreading cold germs, it hardly seems practical to confine or quarantine the toddlers until they learn better habits of personal hygiene, if indeed they ever will. So what help does Dr. Andrewes give us?

Cold Weather and Infections

Another well-documented article, in the *Archives of Pediatrics* for December, 1951, discusses the factor of cold weather as an important aspect in the cause of colds. Louis S. Goldstein, M.D., of the Professional Hospital in Yonkers, kept careful records of a large number of children during the winter of 1951, and correlated the number of cold infections with the daily temperature. On 4 days that winter the thermometer went below zero. Approximately 9 to 12 days after each of these zero days, the index of colds rose, and increased again, to a lesser degree, 3 to 5 days after the first rise.

Discussing all possible explanations of this phenomenon, Dr. Goldstein concludes that extreme cold brings a "potent stress factor," which lowers the body's resistance and brings about a cold within 9 to 12 days, and may also bring about a secondary infection 5 days later. As person after person in the community gets the cold, they establish immunity and by the time the winter weather is over, the epidemic is also over. Dr. Goldstein's theory does not explain that pesky summer cold many of us are subject to nor, of course, does it give us any solution for our problem. So far as we know, there is nothing at all to do about a sub-zero day except to endure it.

An article in *New England Medicine* for August 9, 1951, describes the situation in a boy's school in Massachusetts, where almost half of the boys who developed polio during one school year had had colds, whereas only 19 per cent of the others in the school had had colds. The Harvard scientists who wrote the article point out that a disease of the upper respiratory tract may be a predisposing factor for polio. Of course, there are many other serious—sometimes fatal—diseases that get their start in a simple and uncared-for head cold. But here again, we have more statistics which make it evident that it is wise to avoid colds, but no shred of help as to *how* to avoid them!

Experiments with Vitamin A in Preventing Infections

When vitamin research was younger, a great deal of interest was aroused by the discovery that animals in a state of vitamin A deficiency were more susceptible to infections than animals on a well-rounded diet. A whole series of experiments followed, to determine just how and why this was true. An Italian physician, Di Salvatore Princi, wrote in *Bollettino della Societa Italiana di Biologia Sperimentale* for July, 1942, on the action of vitamin A on the influenza germ. Dr. Princi worked with two groups of mice on an identical diet, except that one group obtained, in addition, a daily quantity of vitamin A preparation. All the mice were injected with a lethal dose of influenza germs. All the animals in both groups died, but those who had received the vitamin A survived an average of 89.9 hours, while those who were deficient in vitamin A survived only 69.3 hours, showing that the vitamin resulted in a certain additional resistance to the disease.

Dr. Torsten Lindquist, in the German medical publication, *Klinische Wochenschrift* for September, 1937, announced the results of observation of the action of vitamin A in 45 cases of croupous and bronchial pneumonia. Dr. Lindquist found that the vitamin A content of the blood was drastically lowered during even the first 5 days of illness. When the patient began to convalesce, the level of vitamin A rose rapidly, even though no additional vitamin A was added to the diet. One week after the crisis of the disease passed, the level of vitamin A in the blood was 3 times as high as before the crisis. This evidence appears to indicate that the vitamin A was engaged in combatting the infection, in some way or other, until the crisis passed and hence, was used up rapidly, restoring itself when the patient began to get well.

Writing in *Romana Medicala,* two Romanian physicians, D. Hagiescu, M.D., and Gh. Bazan, M.D., discuss the use of vitamins A and D in pulmonary tuberculosis. We are encouraged by the fact that they used the two vitamins, rather than just one, for, as you know, we believe that all of the vitamins are necessary for health and that any one of them functions best when the others are also present. These two researchers remind us of the possible reasons for vitamin A deficiency—not enough food which contains this vitamin, an infectious disease which uses up the vitamin A, thus bringing about a deficiency, defective absorption of the vitamin or defective assimilation in the intestines, because of liver trouble or digestive disorders.

They also point out that calcium is important for the cure or prevention of many diseases and is especially important in the treatment of tuberculosis patients. As vitamin D is necessary for the assimilation of calcium, these doctors decided to administer to the tuberculosis patients both vitamin A and vitamin D together to see what results they would obtain. The vitamins were not used as a "cure" for the disease. Other regular treatment was going on at the same time and the vitamins were given simply to see what additional benefits might be noticed. As a special precaution, the vitamins were injected rather than being taken by mouth, for many of the patients suffered from indigestion and it was feared that this might interfere with proper absorption of the vitamins.

The results were (1.) all patients tolerated the injections perfectly; (2.) the weight of all patients showed an increase, which continued even after the injections were stopped; (3.) appetite increased in all patients; (4.) blood count improved in some patients; (5.) rate of sedimentation of blood improved; (6.) in children, even greater improvement was noted than with adults.

The authors believe this was because of the greater vitality and powers of resistance of children in general. The physicians also used vitamins A and D together in cases of anemia, loss of appetite and malnutrition, with excellent results.

Vitamin A and Disease-Resistant Powers

An article by H. J. Jusatz, M.D., in the German medical publication *Zeitschrift für Immunitatsforschung und experimentelle Therapie* for August 4, 1937, describes the results of feeding animals on a vitamin A deficient diet, then testing their blood to determine its power to form antibodies—that is, its power to fight off the germs of infectious diseases. It was found that, after a lengthy period of feeding the deficient diet, the germ-inhibiting power of the animals' blood became extinct. They could no longer resist disease, but would become ready prey for any germ that came along. Vitamin A was then added to their diet over an extended period of time and the tests were made again. There was no improvement in the formation of antibodies. Vitamin D in small amounts was then given with a resulting increase in the germ-inhibiting index of the blood. But when the vitamin D dose was increased to such an extent that the animals were receiving an overdose, the blood immediately reacted by a decreasing number of antibodies. This author concludes, then, that neither vitamin A nor vitamin D has the power of preventing infection by increasing the disease-fighting bodies of the blood.

From summarizing all these various articles, it seems we are safe in concluding that vitamin A, and to some extent vitamin D, makes the body more resistant to disease, but they do not accomplish this by changing the character of the blood. How then do they work?

We have not found the complete answer and we do not believe that the entire story has yet been told, but the following facts throw some light on the matter. A French physician, Henri Bourgeois, M.D., reporting in *Le Progres Médical* for February 26, 1938, tells us that he uses vitamin A successfully for local application during colds, sinusitis and so forth. He instills halibut liver oil directly into an infected sinus; he drops it several times a day into a runny nose. And with excellent results, except, he reports sadly, the oil smelled so bad that his adult patients refused to use it. The children, he says, did not mind. Whatever is the role of vitamin A, says Dr. Bourgeois, it produces only good results on the cells of the body tissues.

An article in the *American Journal of Diseases of Children* for March, 1939, recounts the results of autopsies on a number of patients who had died from a certain kind of pneumonia. In each of these patients, Dr. Bruce Chown found evidence of serious vitamin A deficiency and their case histories revealed that either they had not obtained enough vitamin A in their diets or, because of some digestive disorder, such as liver trouble or diarrhea, they had not assimilated whatever vitamin A they obtained.

[576]

So the evidence appears to be conflicting as to just how vitamin A prevents infection and lack of vitamin A leaves one open to disease. In most of the many medical articles we studied on this subject, we found experiments that directly contradicted one another. We found earnest advocates of vitamin A therapy and we found other writers sincerely puzzled as to how it works. Apparently the methods used in the different experiments created certain conditions, which caused varying reactions.

How Vitamin A Does Prevent Infection

Curiously enough, we found what appears to be the most logical and reasonable interpretation and solution of the controversy in—of all places —*Veterinary Medicine* for September, 1944. J. Lavere Davidson, Lt. Col., V. C., of the Sioux Falls Army Air Field tells us how he believes vitamin A works in the human body to prevent infection. Of course, the vitamin itself does not kill germs (cold, flu or distemper germs, for example), says Davidson. Instead, "by direct action, vitamin A preserves the normal physiological functions and anatomical structure of the mucous membranes, and also aids in the regeneration and restoration of these membranes in the event they become injured or destroyed." The surface of the normal mouth, nose and bronchial membrane is covered with cilia, which, under a miscroscope, look like tiny hairs, constantly in motion, waving in one direction. With this waving motion, the cilia sweep foreign matter, including germs, toward the pharynx where it can be expectorated or swallowed. In addition, these various mucous membranes secrete a substance called lysozyme, which is powerful against bacteria. In an individual who is not getting, or absorbing, enough vitamin A, a change takes place in the mucous membrane. The cells with cilia gradually disappear and are replaced by scaly, hard cells which do not have cilia. The substances secreted by the membranes are cut off and the dryness increases. So this individual now has two counts against him—the cilia are no longer wafting germs out of his respiratory passages and the antiseptic secretions of his nose and throat are no longer functioning. When the germ comes along, there is no defense against it.

Hence, says Lt. Col. Davidson, the action of vitamin A against colds is an indirect one. This vitamin preserves the strength and health of the cells of the mucous membranes. It also rejuvenates and replenishes these cells when they have been destroyed or injured by attacks of germs. In children, there is a two-fold demand for vitamin A—they need it for growing and they need it to safeguard the health of their tissues. Might not a deficiency of vitamin A be the reason for so many colds among school children? Lacking the vitamin A which they use up in their growing process, they do not take even the few precautions adults take against sudden chilling, drafts, dry air in overheated rooms and other factors which affect the mucous membranes of the respiratory passages.

A survey conducted among the school children of New York City revealed that a slight vitamin A deficiency was the most common diet deficiency found among all the children.

Recommendations for a Cold-Free Winter

Our conclusions and recommendations, then, are as follows:

1. Vitamin A is protective against infections—not directly by killing off the disease germs, but indirectly by providing for the health of the mucous membranes which the germs attack. Ample amounts of vitamin A should be provided in one's diet and, in addition, one should make certain that the supply of vitamin A is not being lost through lack of assimilation due to digestive disorders.

2. Since the evidence showing that vitamin A preserves the health of the mucous membranes is positive and emphatic, do not wait until you have a cold or an attack of grippe before making sure of your vitamin A supply. By this time, the susceptible tissues of your nose and throat will be weakened and much more likely to succumb to a secondary, or even chronic, infection. Begin now to build up your store of vitamin A against the rigors of the cold weather. Remember that food containing vitamin A (greens, sweet potatoes and so forth) contains much less vitamin A in the winter than in the spring and summer, for it has lost the vitamin in storage and the animals or plants who supply the food in winter lack the sunshine and warmth from which to provide it. So count on using food supplements of natural vitamin A in addition to the vitamin A foods you eat at every day's meals.

3. Some foods containing large amounts of vitamin A are carrots, beet greens, cantaloupe, collards, dandelion greens, whole eggs, endive, kale, lettuce, fresh calf and beef liver, mustard greens, parsley, alfalfa leaf meal, dried peaches, green peppers, spinach, winter squash, sweet potatoes, tomato juice, turnip greens, water cress and, of course, fish liver oils, which contain many times more vitamin A than any other food. In general, you can be guided by the yellow color of foods. This yellow comes from carotene which changes to vitamin A after it is eaten. So it's best to include at least one yellow vegetable in each day's menu, along with plenty of greens and eggs.

4. In spite of the best intentions, however, it is often impossible, especially during winter months, to obtain enough vitamin A. This is why we believe that adults and children alike should use natural vitamin A as a food supplement every day. Natural vitamin A is easiest to obtain in fish liver oil capsules, which also contain vitamin D, another vitamin that is scarce in wintertime when the sun's rays are short. As you have seen from the facts above, we are just beginning to realize how important the whole family of vitamins is to the proper functioning of any one of them. In treating the tuberculous patients, the doctors used vitamin D along with vitamin A. Other researchers have found that vitamin C is also important for the proper use of vitamin A in the body.

So we recommend that the very best preventive of sniffles, colds, grippe and other troublesome respiratory infections during the winter months is to eat a diet ample in all the vitamins, and to supplement this diet with fish liver oil capsules for vitamins A and D, brewer's yeast for vitamin B, desiccated liver for vitamins A and B, rose hip powder for vitamins A and C and wheat germ oil for vitamin E.

One last note of caution. In medical literature, a small number of cases of vitamin A poisoning have been reported, caused, usually in children, by the administration of enormous doses of fish liver oils. Usually someone in the family misunderstood the dose that was advised for a child and gave him 10 or 20 times more than he should have received. Because vitamin A is valuable for your health, it does not follow that the more you take the healthier you become. It is hardly possible to think of anyone getting too much vitamin A from sweet potatoes or carrots, but fish liver oils are highly concentrated foods. Take, or give to members of your family, the amount suggested on the bottle of the product you buy.

145. Ample B Vitamins Protect Against Colds

Vitamin B has been shown to be effective against invading germs. Dr. A. E. Axelrod of Western Reserve University, speaking at a meeting of the National Vitamin Foundation on April 4, 1952, described an experiment in which he deprived rats of 3 of the B vitamins, and found that the animals were severely impaired in their ability to build up antibodies with which to fight disease. Another experiment reported at the same meeting involved human beings.

Young men, on an ordinary diet, were immersed in cold water for 8 minutes, and this stress, although brief, produced chemical changes in the blood and urine, as well as in the temperature, blood pressure and heart rate. There was a significant increase in two substances in the blood— the granular red blood cells and the circulating white blood cells, which are the disease-germ fighters of the body.

Then, for 6 weeks, the men were built up with large doses of a member of the vitamin B group and again given the cold-water experience. Tests identical with the former showed that the changes in the blood and urinary components were less than before, and that this occurred because the vitamins had strengthened the effectiveness with which the adrenal glands produced various hormones, possibly including cortisone. These adrenal outpourings help the body to overcome physical strains and thus, the B vitamins increase the bodily capacity for resistance.

Two articles from the *Proceedings of the Society of Experimental*

Biology and Medicine (Vol. 67, 1948 and Vol. 62, 1946), describe experiments on animals made deficient in pyridoxine, thiamin and biotin—all B vitamins. In all cases, the rats who were deficient in the vitamins were able to produce fewer antibodies in their blood, for fighting off germs.

Experiments with Multiple Deficiencies

Finally, let us examine an article in the *Journal of Laboratory and Clinical Medicine*, Vol. 30, 1945, in which L. J. Berry, J. Davis and T. D. Spies discuss the influence of the B vitamins on the resistance of rats to infection. These researchers tell us that "single vitamin deficiency studies are important in elucidating the metabolic function of the vitamins, but single deficiencies seldom occur naturally." That is, in terms of human nutrition, a person who suffers from a lack of one B vitamin is certain to lack the others, too, for they occur mostly in the same foods. And they react with one another in the body. Someone who lacks vitamin B will probably lack vitamin C as well. If a person does not get enough vitamin A in his food, he almost certainly will not get enough of the other fat soluble vitamins—D and E—for they occur in many of the same foods.

In their experiment, these nutritionists decided to place one group of rats on the diet commonly eaten by many of the patients who visit their clinic in Birmingham, Alabama. They divided the rats into 10 groups— two of which received only the basic diet as eaten by families in the neighborhood. Two other groups received the basic diet plus casein (a protein). Two other groups received the basic diet plus casein and minerals. Two other groups ate the basic diet plus casein and B vitamins. The final two groups received the basic diet plus casein, minerals and B vitamins.

The basic diet consisted of corn meal, white flour, pork fat and cane sugar. Yes, this was the diet the researchers had discovered their clinic patients were eating every day. The animals were permitted to remain on the diets for two months before they were checked. The pictures taken at that time indicate more clearly than any words what condition the rats were in by then. Those on the basic diet were small, scrawny, weak. Their coats were rough and ugly. As the various elements were added to diets, the appearance of the rats improved. The final picture shows a handsome, sleek, healthy-looking rat who was, of course, eating the minerals, vitamins and proteins, as well as the basic diet.

Laboratory tests showed that the leucocytes (disease-fighting blood corpuscles) *decreased steadily in the rats on the deficient diets.* As the diets became progressively better, the number of leucocytes increased, and the total number of leucocytes was normal only in the rats on the best diets. "These studies support the working hypothesis that resistance to bacterial invasion may be depressed by inadequate nutrition," say these investigators. "Their importance is enhanced by the fact that the animals were eating the same diet that gives rise to the mixed deficiencies seen in patients in the clinic. . . . Therefore, in mixed deficiencies, the importance of restoring the organism to a balanced nutritional regime becomes apparent if that organism is to be able to defend itself against the onslaughts of bacterial invasion."

Now how can we use the information from these experiments to prevent colds? To us they seem to indicate that an abundance of vitamin B in the diet, as well as vitamins A and C, will help the body's defenses against germs. So, when you feel a cold coming on, what should you do— go to your doctor and ask for an injection? We think not. We believe you should use vitamin B, along with other vitamins, every day, as protection, so that you simply do not contract colds.

Our recommendations would go something like this: Meat or fish in your diet every day (organ meats like liver at least once a week), fresh vegetables and fruits in abundance, especially during the winter (and be sure to include green leafy vegetables and yellow vegetables every day). Omit all foods made from white flour or white sugar, for they rob your body of B vitamins. And finally, just to make certain, take desiccated liver and/or brewer's yeast every day for B vitamins. It's simple, really, to adjust your diet along these lines—and less expensive, too.

146. Vitamin C Is a Natural Cold Preventive

Cold weather may mean you need more vitamin C! Yes, it's true, at any rate for guinea pigs, who are the only creatures, aside from apes and human beings, who cannot manufacture their own vitamin C inside their bodies. Jolliffe, Tisdall and Cannon, in their monumental book, *Clinical Nutrition* (Paul B. Hoeber, Incorporated, 1950), tell us that rats exposed to cold weather develop more vitamin C inside their bodies, to protect them from this stress of cold. Those rats who, for some reason, cannot produce the required amount of vitamin C, may begin to show a decrease of vitamin C in their tissues, which may indicate that the cold actually uses up their store of vitamin C. Guinea pigs, who, like man, cannot make their own vitamin C, must depend on an increased intake in their food if they are to be able to survive cold weather. The lower the temperature, the more vitamin C is required.

An amount of vitamin C that is perfectly adequate for a guinea pig at room temperature is reported to be completely inadequate at a temperature of freezing or 32 degrees Fahrenheit. The small animals can adapt themselves to cold and manage to live healthfully only if their supply of vitamin C is increased. In studying the guinea pigs, it was found that this vitamin C supply was in the tissues of the bodies, especially the adrenal glands, of those which managed to survive. And when their supply of vitamin C was discontinued, those who had taken a large supply of the vitamin previously were found to survive longer than those who had not.

In our file on colds we found a letter from the *British Medical Journal* for April 21, 1951, written by John M. Fletcher and Isabel C. Fletcher, expressing surprise that more material does not appear in medical journals on the potency of vitamin C in protecting against cold germs. These two physicians state that, in their own practice, they have found vitamin C an excellent preventive of colds. Perhaps, they say, the general disregard of the vitamin as a cold preventive results from the difficulty among the experts in reaching agreements as to what actually is the daily requirement of vitamin C. With adults, they say, the disease of scurvy will occur when the adult is getting less than 10 milligrams of vitamin C daily. But, they continue, this represents far, far less than "saturation level." By this they mean that, to soak all the tissues of the body in vitamin C, a much larger amount than 10 milligrams a day is necessary. In cases of fever or hard physical exertion, the body uses up vitamin C much faster than usual. So it is not ever possible to set one figure as the absolute daily requirement for all people under all circumstances.

We agree wholeheartedly with the Fletchers, only, as usual, we would carry their argument a little farther. Aside from fever and exertion, modern adults are subjected to countless other hazards that deplete their vitamin C—sleeping pills, for instance, tobacco smoking, exposure to lead, benzene and other industrial poisons. And since no one has ever suffered from too much natural vitamin C, why in the world should we limit ourselves to a daily minimum when, apparently, the more we take, the better we will feel in every way? We know from laboratory experiments that animals suffering from infections have a very small amount of vitamin C in their blood streams. We know, too, that animals deliberately kept on diets low in vitamin C develop more infections than those who are getting enough. These two facts alone are sufficient indication that vitamin C in large quantities is necessary in the fight against any infection—including, of course, cold infections.

Preventing Infections with Vitamin C

The Fletchers go on to tell of a number of experiments in Holland, Germany and Australia in which colds were prevented by the administration of vitamin C. In the German experiment, there was a marked fall in the amount of illness over a period of 8 months among factory workers given 100 to 300 milligrams of vitamin C a day, a benefit not found when they were given 20 to 50 milligrams. N. W. Markwell, writing in the *Medical Journal of Australia,* Vol. 2, p. 777, 1947, describes the technique of giving vitamin C in cases where cold symptoms have just begun to appear. The colds were frequently, but not always, dispersed within a few hours and the aftereffects and complications which often accompany common colds were nonexistent. The Fletchers conclude: "We believe that, unlike the outcome of the antihistamine trials, the results may show considerable benefits can arise from ascorbic acid (vitamin C) treatment given in sufficient quantities at the right time."

In the *British Medical Journal*, Vol. 2, p. 617, 1942, Drs. A. J. Glazebrook and S. J. Thompson report an experiment in an institution in England caring for boys. At this institution, the handling of food—that is, the way it was stored, prepared, served and so forth—had resulted in a vitamin C intake of 15 milligrams per boy per day—just barely enough to prevent symptoms of scurvy. Part of the boys were given vitamin C for 6 months. The other boys went on eating their regular diet. During the brief period of 6 months, there was no appreciable difference in the incidence of colds in the two groups, *but* the boys who had the vitamin spent only an average of 2½ days in the infirmary, whereas those who had received no vitamin C spent an average of 5 days being sick. So the additional vitamin C, even for this brief period, apparently strengthened the children's resistance to germs so much that they were able to throw off the effects in half the time it took the untreated children.

H. W. Holmes, M.D., writing in *Science,* Vol. 96, p. 497, 1942, describes his own experiences in relieving hay fever, food allergies and asthma with vitamin C. He gave it in large doses—200 to 500 milligrams every day for a week. Does this perhaps demonstrate that the usual daily minimum we casually accept as correct for adults (about 75 milligrams per day) may be far too low?

Discussing vitamin C in relation to infections, Rhinehart, Connor and Mettier, in *International Clinician,* Vol. 2, 1937, and the *Journal of Experimental Medicine,* Vol. 59, 1934, tell us they found that guinea pigs suffering from scurvy (vitamin C deficiency) who were infected with a streptococcus germ, developed a condition similar to rheumatic fever and rheumatoid arthritis in human beings. They suggest that a "subclinical" degree of scurvy may make up the rheumatic tendency which, with an added factor of infection, causes the development of rheumatic fever. This means, simply, that infections develop more readily in animals (and why not also in persons?) who lack vitamin C—not to the extent of producing scurvy, but just to the extent that most of us lack it—a "subclinical deficiency."

It has been found that diphtheria susceptibility is greater in guinea pigs who lack vitamin C. And children with scurvy are more susceptible to diphtheria. Lawrynowicz, in the *Journal de Physiologie et de Pathologie Génerale,* Vol. 29, 1931, suggests the scurvy may so reduce the resistance, that a diphtheria carrier may become the victim of the bacteria which it previously carried without any ill effects. Three investigators showed that added amounts of vitamin C assist animals on normal diets in their reactions against tuberculosis.

Vitamin C—A "Super Antibiotic"

An experiment in a tuberculosis sanitarium showed the potency of even small amounts of the vitamin against tuberculosis symptoms. The patients were grouped in pairs. One patient was given a daily orange, while his control, in the other group, received a pastry. It seemed that the addition of vitamin C, even in such small amounts, assisted in healing the tuberculosis symptoms.

S. W. Clausen, writing in the *Physiological Review,* Vol. 14, 1934, throws light on the subject from the point of view of natural products supplying the vitamin. In testing guinea pigs, several researchers have found that an abundance of fresh, green fodder, which contains, of course, natural vitamin C, has protected against infections. In a study of 400 animals, one scientist (Wamoscher in *Zeitschrift für Hygiene und Infektionskrankheiten,* Vol. 107, 1937) showed that subacute scurvy—that is just a slight case of scurvy—predisposes to spontaneous pneumonia. Cure sometimes followed the administration of vitamin C in orange juice.

W. J. McCormick, M.D., of Canada uses vitamin C in enormous doses for curing disease. He tells us, in an article in the *Archives of Pediatrics* for April, 1952, that vitamin C is important for the healing of wounds, the prevention of hemorrhaging and the building of a barrier against germ invasion. It contributes to building up disease fighters or antibodies in the blood stream; it neutralizes toxins in the blood—that is, it helps to build a natural immunity to infectious diseases and poisons. In the rapidity with which it stops the course of some diseases, it compares favorably with the sulfa drugs, says Dr. McCormick, and it does not have aftereffects that may be unpleasant or dangerous. Dr. McCormick uses injections of vitamin C to saturate completely his patient's tissues. Any excess is carried away by the kidneys. Dr. McCormick has used vitamin C successfully in treating tuberculosis, scarlet fever, pelvic infection, septicemia and so forth.

F. R. Klenner, M.D., of Reidsville, North Carolina, has used vitamin C successfuly in the treatment of many serious diseases. He describes his point of view in a paper presented before the Annual Meeting of the Tri-State Medical Association of the Carolinas and Virginia, February 19 and 20, 1951. He compares the action of vitamin C with the antibiotics. "It has been reported," he says, "that one of the mold-derived drugs (antibiotics) is a super-vitamin. Conversely, we argue that vitamin C, besides being an essential vitamin, is a super-antibiotic." Dr. Klenner believes that it is the capacity of the vitamin as an aid to oxidation that makes it valuable against germs. Apparently it unites with the toxin or virus in the body.

He describes the case of a patient with chills, fever and head cold for 14 days and severe headache for 3 days. She had been given sulfa, penicillin and streptomycin without effect. Vitamin C injections were given. Within 72 hours, she was "clinically well of her pneumonia." In 3 other cases of pulmonary virus infection, results were equally good, using vitamin C injections.

In a person suffering from a virus infection, says Dr. Klenner, vitamin C is not only absent from the urine, but is also missing from the blood. So it seems that, as the infection gets worse, the patient's need for vitamin C becomes greater, for his body tissues are depleted, and what vitamin C he obtains from his food is rapidly used up in fighting against the virus. This is why Dr. Klenner gives massive doses of the vitamin in cases of serious illness. "Hippocrates declared the highest duty of medicine to be to get the patient well. He further declared that, of several remedies, physicians should choose the least sensational. Vitamin C would seem to meet both these requirements," says Dr. Klenner.

Why We Suffer from Colds

Perhaps many of us suffer from frequent colds for two reasons: first, we are not careful enough to choose foods that contain vitamin C and second, we may not know how to preserve the vitamin C in foods until the time we eat them. Vitamin C is the most perishable vitamin there is. It is lost when foods are stored or cooked. It seeps away into the water when foods are soaked.

So choose vitamin C rich foods the year 'round. In general, this means fresh fruits and vegetables. Frozen foods generally contain more vitamins than canned. Buy your fruits and vegetables as fresh as you can get them, never buy wilted or soggy produce. Wash it quickly as soon as you get home and put it immediately in the refrigerator. Prepare it just before you eat it, as quickly as possible; most of the vitamin C will be lost if you leave fruits or vegetables for even a half hour at room temperature. Eat as many fruits and vegetables raw as possible. Those you must cook place directly into a very small amount of boiling water. As soon as the water boils again, turn down the heat and cook slowly just until tender— no longer. Save the liquid left in the pot for soup.

And finally, in the wintertime especially, make sure of enough vitamin C by taking rose hips or one of the other natural vitamin C food supplements. If you should feel the symptoms of a cold coming on, double or triple the amount of natural vitamin C you take daily. It can't possibly harm you. Any excess which your body does not need will be excreted harmlessly.

147. Vitamin C and Bioflavonoids

Early in 1955, at a meeting in New York City, certain scientific researchers got together to talk about the merits of a certain element called "bioflavonoids." This is a substance that appears in many fresh foods along with vitamin C. It is closely related to rutin, which has recently gained fame in the treatment of high blood pressure. At the meeting, it was brought out that the bioflavonoids, given with vitamin C, help the body to use the vitamin C properly. It was also announced that the two together had been found to be powerful against the common cold.

We were delighted with this news, because we believe that natural vitamins are far superior to synthetic ones. In natural vitamin preparations, the bioflavonoids naturally accompany vitamin C, since they occur along with the vitamin in foods—fruits, rose hips, etc.

Remember, we have already mentioned the fact that colds can be prevented if, at the first sign of a sniffle, you begin to take massive doses of natural vitamin C. We also think that colds are shortened and made much less serious and troublesome if you take natural vitamin C preparations straight through the course of the cold. But we firmly believe that you should make every effort to prevent colds rather than trying to cure them after they get started. And preventing colds is easy—with plenty of vitamin C in natural form, which means that it will be accompanied by the bioflavonoids. So much for bioflavonoids and colds, then.

In the November 24, 1956, issue of the *Journal of the American Medical Association* appeared two articles written by medical researchers, declaring that all the hullabaloo over the usefulness of the bioflavonoids in treating colds is nothing but hullabaloo. These gentlemen say in essence that the bioflavonoids have no effect at all on the incidence of colds or the course they may take in the body. And they produce an astonishing array of evidence to back up their claims. A total of almost 2000 persons were involved in one of the studies. "The overwhelming impression gained," says the *Journal,* "is that there is a singular lack of effect in altering the course of the common cold, by either the bioflavonoids or vitamin C."

These articles set off a veritable furor of claims and counterclaims in the magazines of the drug industry. *Advertising Age* put it this way: "Grove Laboratories, Incorporated, leading maker of bioflavonoid cold tablets and the American Medical Association aimed squarely for the whites of each other's bleary eyes today" when the article was published. Grove declared that the research was paid for by a competitor of theirs who, we presume, didn't want to see the bioflavonoids cutting in on his profits from another cold remedy. The competitor, who manufactures Anahist, answered with a blast, and the battle was on.

Should We Become Concerned?

Our advice would be, relax, folks, and let the drug companies fight it out. If or when they come to any conclusions not arrived at by counting dollar signs, there may be reason to look further into the matter. But not until then. What are our reasons for this point of view?

First of all, the battle is drawn between two opposing drug companies. We have nothing but suspicion for drugs, no matter what kind of drugs. Synthetic vitamin C and bioflavonoids extracted from their natural base and put into tablets are certainly not what *we* are talking about when we advise taking natural vitamin C to prevent colds. Furthermore, the tests were not tests of anything, to our way of thinking, for the amounts of vitamin C and flavonoids used were certainly not large enough to signify anything at all.

And, since no check was made on daily habits of the people who took the pills, we have no way of knowing how much of the small amount of vitamin C they took could actually be used by the body to ward off colds. Did they take sleeping pills? Did they smoke or were they exposed to lots of tobacco smoke? Were they exposed to any of the other common industrial substances which destroy vitamin C in the body? Did they make any effort to get fresh, living raw foods in which natural vitamin C is present? All these questions were not considered important enough by the investigators to necessitate any consideration at all in the tests. So far as we are concerned, they are the most important factors of all.

How Much Vitamin C for Colds?

The several thousand subjects tested were given 200 milligrams of synthetic vitamin C every day during the test, with or without bioflavonoids. To our way of thinking, this amount of vitamin C (if it were natural vitamin C) might conceivably be enough for reasonably good health if one were exposed to none of the possible destroyers of vitamin C that are ever-present in our modern civilized life. But it is the function of vitamin C to be destroyed, to be oxidized or burned up in the performance of its task, which is, to a large extent, the neutralizing of poisons. The number and extent of poisonous substances to which you are subjected each day determine largely how much vitamin C you need for good health.

But in the case of a cold, or for that matter, any other illness of an infectious nature, vitamin C and bioflavonoids in massive doses will nip the infective process in the bud and the cold will be a thing of the past before it ever gets started. How much vitamin C and bioflavonoids do we mean when we say "massive doses"? To a certain extent, this depends on you and your need for this particular vitamin. But in general, it means far, far more than you take every day for good health, and it means taking the vitamin in large amounts at frequent intervals during the day—at least every 4 hours.

148. Stop That Cold With Garlic!

Have you ever tried garlic as a treatment for a cold? For centuries it has been a European remedy for many types of infectious disease, including clogged and running nose, cough and sore throat. Nobody who used it then could tell you just why it was effective, but they knew that a good dose of garlic, held the cure for many an illness that would respond to few other things.

Now such remedies have long been discarded as products of an old-fashioned era. How could those ignorant peasants find a cure for diseases the modern laboratories have not been able to conquer? And how could a common and odorous bulb hold the answer?

Curiosity Led to the Answer

Someone finally got curious enough to find out why garlic could do what antibiotics and sulfa drugs had been unable to do. The man was Dr. J. Klosa, and he reported his findings in the March, 1950, issue of a German magazine entitled *Medical Monthly*.

Dr. Klosa found that garlic oil had that elusive ability to kill dangerous organisms without attacking organisms vital to the body's health. It is this danger to bodily health that rules out (or should rule out) the use of many proposed compounds as medications, even though they are effective germ killers. For example, formaldehyde inactivates all viruses, but it also reacts unfavorably with the body's own protein, and is, therefore, a deadly poison to the body. (Unfortunately, many of the drugs actually being used today have shown themselves to be antagonistic to body processes, but because the reaction is not as immediate nor obviously violent as with formaldehyde, they continue to be used.) Oil of garlic is composed in part of sulfides and disulfides. These unite with virus matter in such a way that the virus organisms are inactivated, so their harmful effects cease, and they are prevented from any future activity. All of this is done without any harm to healthful organisms in the body.

Dr. Klosa experimented with a solution of garlic oil (obtained under specially engineered conditions) and water, and he administered this preparation in doses of 10 to 25 drops, every 4 hours. It was found that the desired effect was enhanced by the inclusion of fresh extract of onion juice in the dosage. The vitamin C content of the onion juice was believed responsible for this result.

Results Treating Grippe and Sore Throat

The paper by Dr. Klosa reports results with grippe, sore throat and rhinitis (clogged and running nose) patients. Of 13 cases of grippe treated, fever and catarrhal symptoms were cut short in every case. All patients showed a distinct lessening of the period of convalescence required. No patient suffered from any of the common post-grippe complaints such as chronic inflammation of the lungs, swelling of the lymph glands, jaundice, pains in muscles and joints, etc. Even the cough that often accompanies grippe was considerably suppressed.

In 28 cases of sore throat, the oil had a prompt and salutary effect. The burning and tickling abated to the point of disappearance in 24 hours. It was found that, if caught in its first stages, the further development of sore throat could be completely stopped by about 30 drops—or about two doses—of the garlic oil solution.

There were 71 cases of clogged and running nose treated in this manner. The oil was taken partly by mouth and part directly into the nostrils.

The congestion of the nostrils was completely cleared up in 13 to 20 minutes in all cases. There were no further complications.

Use Fresh Garlic or Garlic Perles

The oil of garlic spoken of by Dr. Klosa was probably distilled through a complicated technical procedure which would be impossible to duplicate in the average home. Nor have we heard of the availability of such an oil. However, the oil he describes does come from natural garlic cloves and these are certainly available to all of us. We can see no reason why a regular intake of garlic would not give the same protection from the cold symptoms described here as Dr. Klosa's preparation. If garlic has properties that will inactivate harmful viruses, why not include this tasty bulb in your diet. Good cooks use it in preparing meats to superb effect.

If you do not enjoy the flavor of garlic, or if you do not feel that you can include enough of it in your normal diet to be effective, you will find that there are natural concentrates of garlic available in capsules, or perles, as they are called.

Instead of using the aspirins and nose drops that sell by the thousands during the "cold season," why not give garlic a chance? You will be using a natural remedy whose properties have been proven to affect favorably many unhealthful conditions aside from colds, and a remedy you can be sure will do you no harm.

149. No Salt for Chronic Cold Sufferers

In his excellent book, *Diet in Sinus Infections and Colds* (Macmillan Company, 1942), Egon V. Ullmann, M.D., advises, among other things, the use of a salt-poor diet for chronic cold sufferers. We have long recommended giving up the use of salt in cooking or at the table, regardless of whether or not one is suffering from any disease. Dr. Ullmann is very emphatic about not using salt if you would be free from colds.

Part of his explanation is this: The chemical content of table salt is sodium and chloride. The chloride serves no purpose in our bodies except that it may go to form hydrochloric acid in the stomach, a certain amount of which is necessary for digestion of proteins. An excess of salt in the diet can result in too much hydrochloric acid in the stomach, which will surely produce stomach ulcers.

The sodium part of table salt is the part most of us have been warned against. It seems that, to a certain extent, sodium cancels out the excellent and necessary functions of calcium. "If large amounts of sodium chloride are taken," says Dr. Ullmann, "a good deal of it will be stored in the skin, mucous membrane and other tissues, and calcium will be liberated. Therefore each sodium molecule retained in the tissues will diminish the calcium effect. . . . On the other hand, with a reduction of sodium chloride in the diet, the calcium action will prevail and lead up toward an anti-inflammatory effect. . . . To sum it up, it can be said that the secret of calcium action lies in the relation of calcium taken with food to the other minerals, especially sodium, magnesium and phosphorus. If any of those are taken in too large amounts, the calcium effect may be impaired."

In the diet Dr. Ullmann outlines for chronic cold patients, he specifically recommends that no salt be added either in cooking the food or at the table. He suggests ways of making food tasty with herbs and seasonings other than salt. He also advises against the use of non-sodium salt substitutes. They are generally not liked by patients, he has found, they may leave an aftertaste, are hard to get used to and are expensive. He advises instead, and we agree completely, that the best way to learn to get along without salt is simply to stop using it. Within a few weeks, you will be used to the taste of food without salt and will, in fact, for the first time in years, begin to appreciate the real taste of food, for you will be tasting the food itself rather than the salt you used to douse it with.

Must We Salt Our Food?

He covers in his chapter on salt all the old arguments offered against the practice of doing without it. People will tell you, "But animals have to have salt. Human beings cannot get along without salt. Throughout history salt has been a valuable commodity and wars have been fought for possession of it." Spices have also been a valuable commodity down through the ages—so valuable that the voyages of explorers like Columbus were undertaken to find new sources of spices or shorter ways of reaching the old sources. But surely no one would claim that man cannot live without spices! There are whole nations of people whose languages do not contain a word for salt. There are many parts of the world where salt has never been eaten and where just the taste of it sickens the people. Animals who do not get enough sodium chloride in their food frequent salt "licks" because they have a need for the sodium and the chloride. But we human beings get plenty of both in our daily food. The only reason why we add more salt is the same reason why we add sugar—we like the taste of it.

It is generally agreed among authorities that we do not need more than 5 grams of sodium chloride per day. Adding up the sodium chloride in the foods eaten by the average American for a week, Dr. Ullmann lists the sodium chloride content of meat, milk, eggs, rice, wheat, peas, cream, bread, potatoes, fruits and vegetables and finds that we get, from a diet like this, without salting the food, 5 grams of salt per day. "The trouble is," he says, "that most of us consume about 15 grams or more per day, an amount which is in excess of what the body really requires. There is hardly a dish to which the cook does not add just 'a pinch of salt' and at the table, salt is frequently added in amounts which remind one of the salt licks of the animals."

Here is a chart showing the amount of sodium chloride in a number of common foods. Study it and you will agree with us that you do not need any more salt than your food naturally contains.

TABLE 5: MILLIGRAMS OF SODIUM IN 100 GRAMS (¼ POUND) OF SOME COMMON FOODS

ITEM	MILLIGRAMS	ITEM	MILLIGRAMS
Nuts		Navy beans, dry	.9
Almonds	2.0	Fresh peas	.9
Brazil nuts	.8	*Green leafy vegetables*	
Filberts	.8	Broccoli	16
Peanuts (unsalted)	.8	Cabbage	5
Walnuts	2.0	Cauliflower	24
Fruits		Lettuce	12
Apples	.1	Spinach	190
Apricots	.5	Celery	110
Bananas	.1	*Root vegetables*	
Cherries	1.0	Beets	110
Lemons	.6	Carrots	31
Oranges	.2	Potatoes	.6
Peaches	.1	Turnips	5
Plums	.1	*Eggs, whole*	140
Strawberries	.7	*Milk*	51
Cereals		*Butter, unsalted*	5
Barley	3.0	*Meat and fish*	
Corn	.4	Beef	53
Oats	2.0	Chicken	110
Rice	.8	Codfish	60
Wheat	2.0	Liver, calf	110
Legumes		Lamb	110
Beans in pod	.8	Turkey	92
Lima beans, fresh	1.0		

150. Dry Heat and Chilling Are Conducive to Colds

Aside from diet, are there other important considerations in the prevention of colds? We think there are and we are glad to present here some suggestions other than diet for preventing colds. In the past, cold preventives and remedies have been many and some of them, colorful. Remember the red flannel underwear, high shoes, flannel petticoats, hot bricks between the sheets, shawls for frustrating drafts and mustard plasters for chests? In days when houses were heated with a single wood or coal cooking stove and venturing into any other room than the kitchen meant a trip to near-Arctic conditions, such devices were useful and probably prevented many a chill that might have been lethal.

But today, we get colds rather because our houses are too hot instead of too cold. Central heating has turned most American homes into modified bakehouses where the air is so dry that floor boards shrink. Imagine, then, what becomes of the delicate tissues of noses and throats that must have moisture to be healthy. The problem of humidifying our homes in winter is one of the most pressing for all of us and no especially satisfactory answer has been developed by engineers.

Here is what the problem boils down to. In summer, spring and fall, when windows can be opened, the air inside any home contains ample moisture, for the earth, grass, leaves, flowers give off moisture all the time. On reasonably cool days, when windows are closed, there is still enough moisture in the air, for the house continues to hold moisture. But once the furnace is lighted, down goes the humidity! And it's comfortable, of course, to step into a warm dry house from a raging sleet or snow storm and you're grateful for the dryness. But the house gets drier and drier as winter moves along. The air you breathe inside the house does not contain enough moisture to keep nose and throat membranes moist. As they dry out, the thirsty tissues are more and more susceptible to cold germs. Those of us who do not go to work or to school every day may spend the entire 24 hours, day after day, in this unhealthful, dry atmosphere.

Then, too, it is not healthful to have rooms too warm. Sixty-eight degrees on your room thermometer should keep you comfortably warm. And it will, provided there is enough humidity in the air, for the moisture in the air makes you warmer. If the air in the room is completely dry, you may not be comfortable until you have turned the thermostat up to 75 degrees, for dry heat does not make you feel so warm as moist heat.

Enough Humidity Is Important

In the old days, the cookstove and the chimney, the cracks around the windows and between the floor boards let in enough outside air to keep room air moist. In addition, there was always a kettle steaming on the stove or wet clothes drying before the fireplace. On mild winter days, windows were steamy and on really cold days, the frost gathered in crystal designs on the inside of the windows. And this was healthy? Yes, it was. How many insulated houses do you see today where there is enough moisture in the inside air to permit steam or frost on windowpanes? Our efficient furnaces, that we can manage so well with a flick of the thermostat, bake the inside of our houses and the inside of our nose and throat passages with the dry, dry heat of an oven.

Those of you who keep filled pans of water beneath radiators know how rapidly these dry out and must be refilled. This gives you an indication of how dry the air is. It would be a good plan to keep large flat pans of water in every room of the house all the time the furnace is on. Some radiators are manufactured with a contraption that allows steam to escape into the room. This is beneficial. Yet still the air will probably be too dry. A doctor friend of ours, prescribing for a patient who lived in a house with a hot air furnace and who suffered from constant colds, advised buying a small spray gun and spraying the air with water every day. Boiling a kettle of water at low heat will release considerable moisture, as you can see by noticing how soon windows begin to steam. Keeping a lot of potted plants in the house helps raise the humidity, if you keep them well watered. The leaves of the plants give off moisture.

Chilling and Colds

Going from one extreme to the other—is chilling conducive to colds? The consensus seems to be that it is, but only under certain circumstances. On that basis, you might say, Arctic explorers probably suffer from continuous colds. As a matter of fact, they don't. A survey done in Spitsbergen, which our atlas tells us is in the Arctic Ocean 375 miles north of Norway, showed that this isolated community experienced a wave of colds only after the first ship came in, bringing cold germs with it. Trappers who fell through the ice and suffered acute chills did not come down with colds unless they had spent a lot of time "in town" the summer and fall before, where, presumably, they had come into contact with germs. It seemed, from this survey, that sudden chilling may bring on an attack in someone who has recently been exposed to infection.

Now obviously anybody who moves around at all in present-day American society is exposed to cold germs all winter long, so it does seem best to avoid sudden chilling, if you possibly can. This doesn't mean staying indoors all winter. It does mean not watching a football game until your hands and feet are stiff with cold, or driving in an unheated automobile, or staying outside for any reason after you have begun to feel cold. It also means not sitting up to read or watch television long after the heat is turned off in your apartment. Children are probably more likely to be exposed to sudden chilling than adults, for if they are enthralled with their play, they will stay out until the cold reaches the very marrow of their bones.

A valuable survey made at the University of California is reported by Marshall C. Cheney, M.D., in the *Practitioner* for December, 1952. His comments cover approximately 60,000 students at the University who were observed during a period of 15 years. Dr. Cheney found that there were students who were resistant to colds, those who were partially resistant and those who appeared to have little or no resistance. Just a word on their diet. "As measured by recognized standards for quality, freshness and completeness of diet, not one of the students could be said to have a perfect diet. All had given up foraging for food; living in the city, they depended upon canned, preserved, refrigerated, not-fresh foods. Many were on very incomplete diets, whilst some, working their way on one meal a day, displayed extremes of poor condition with emaciation, anemia and even scurvy and beriberi. Execrable physical condition made little difference in regard to colds if the individual was in the good natural resistance group. The average and poor natural resistance group, however, suffered more colds when on a deficient diet, and had better resistance when the diet was improved." High quality proteins included in the diets incidentally, gave the greatest improvement in colds.

This is what Dr. Cheney found about chilling. "Of no importance when agents of infectious colds are absent from the nose and throat, and in those who can 'take it,' chilling becomes a life and death matter for susceptibles in crowded city areas . . ."

Avoid Stuffy Rooms, Fatigue and Emotional Upsets

In his survey at the University of California, Dr. Cheney lists deficient, infected and poisonous air as another important predisposing factor in catching colds. Although carbon monoxide, dust and other air contaminants are important, it seems that the stale, stuffy air of classrooms, social rooms and business establishments produced the most colds. Here is a lesson to be learned by all of us. Winter is the time for social activity. School, work, movies, concerts, lectures, church, club meetings, parties— how many such activities do you and your family engage in week after week in winter? And how often do you stop to consider the air in the rooms where these activities are held? Windows and doors can and should be opened periodically when any group of people is gathered together in winter, to bring in oxygen and to drive out the poisonous mixture of carbon dioxide and germs that has accumulated. "Lethal for the susceptible, bringing the cold of the moment to the average group and occasionally dragging down the good natural resistance individual, classroom and similar air has much to do with colds," says Dr. Cheney. He adds that anyone who is especially susceptible to colds should avoid public gatherings, stay out of restaurants and spend much time out in the open.

A third villain in many of the colds studied at the University was fatigue. This is the scoundrel responsible, we think, for the epidemic of colds that sets in after the winter holidays. Shopping for gifts, decorating homes, cooking all kinds of elaborate dishes and going to late parties are an accepted part of Christmas celebrations. Which of us has not staggered into work on January second in a state of near-collapse and, sure enough, come down with a cold a few days later? Dr. Cheney tells us that examination time, big game or big party week ends at college always result in chronic fatigue and an outbreak of colds. "Many in the average natural resistance groups, and all in the poor natural resistance groups, reported colds after extra fatigue," he says. The lesson to be learned is simply to plan only what you know you can accomplish without fatigue. Just cancel out the rest or plan it for some later time.

Are Colds Partly Psychosomatic?

Recently some interesting experimental work has been done on the relation of emotions to colds. Thomas H. Holmes, M.D., Helen Goodell, A.B., Stewart Wolf, M.D., and Harold G. Wolff, M.D., report, in the *American Journal of the Medical Sciences* for July, 1949, on evidence that swelling of the nasal passages may predispose to colds and to other nasal disorders such as sinusitis. Then they relate a number of incidents which show the effect of emotion on these nasal passages. They tell us of a young physician whose home life had become unbearable because of a domineering mother-in-law. During all the time he was suppressing his feelings of frustration about this situation, he suffered from swelling of and secretion from the nasal passages. He lost his appetite and acquired a flushed face and a dull aching "sinus pain" under the bridge of his nose. A talk with his mother-in-law brought about a happier situation at home and a complete relief from all his symptoms.

In another case, a young man who felt unsuccessful and badly adjusted to his job experienced nasal discharge and swelling when he discussed his (imagined) unhappy plight. In another case, a young woman suffered from almost continual nasal symptoms because of her feelings of insecurity. Family arguments brought on such discomfort that she actually had an operation on her nose. After she married a man who gave her devotion and security, she was free from symptoms and became the happy and healthy mother of a child. During her second pregnancy, her physician told her that she had heart trouble and so could not have an anesthetic during delivery. At about the same time, her husband enlisted in the navy. All her nasal symptoms returned, the birth of her second child was extremely difficult and eventually her nasal symptoms "became incapacitating." During visits to the clinic, she managed to discuss all her fears and insecurity, came to understand them and soon was completely healthy once again.

The authors of this medical article interpret these reactions as an "attempt on the part of the organism to protect itself by shutting out, neutralizing and washing away an environment that is literally or symbolically noxious." Regardless of how one interprets it, all of us can agree, we believe, that emotional upsets and especially long-continued situations involving frustration and hidden resentment can wreak havoc with good health, and may very possibly be responsible for all kinds of symptoms. If you have frequent colds, why not try keeping track of them and see, just for your own satisfaction, whether or not they are related to emotional upsets, "scenes," arguments or times when the frustrations of your life seem particularly acute.

Final Suggestions

Here are some final miscellaneous suggestions on colds:

1. Get out of the habit of using handkerchiefs for anything except decoration. Use disposable tissues at all times, but especially when you or the people about you have colds. And dispose of the tissues promptly after each use.

2. Don't dress too heavily indoors in the cold weather. If the room is comfortably warm (and remember to keep it at 70 degrees or less), you don't need sweaters, jackets or heavy underwear. All they do is to make you perspire, and perspiration makes you an easy victim to chilling when you go out or stand in a draft.

3. Do wear warm enough clothes outdoors, and this precaution is directed mostly to the ladies. A suit simply won't keep you warm enough outside in winter, no matter how mild the air may seem to be. At any rate, take a coat along if you plan to be out any length of time.

4. Avoid buses, subways and streetcars if you can. Ventilation is nonexistent, dust is everywhere and a goodly percentage of the folks around you have colds. Walking is good exercise in the winter as well as other times of the year.

5. Cough and talk as little as possible if you do get a cold. Any extra talking or unnecessary coughing puts an added strain on the membranes of your throat and nose.

6. A letter from a reader tells us that her doctor prevents colds in himself by one easy precaution. As soon as he feels the slightest dryness or tickle in his throat, he gargles with hot water—as hot as he can comfortably stand. He claims that the heat stirs up circulation which carries away the infection. Gargling every 10 minutes or so until the warning symptoms have passed is his rule.

151. Breathing

A little book came to us recently which has some thought-provoking theories on colds and how to avoid them. We thought these ideas might be of interest to our readers. The title of the book is *Breathe Deeply and Avoid Colds,* by Emanuel M. Josephson, M.D., published by Chedney Press, 230 East 61st Street, New York, New York, $3.00. In the very first line of the book, Dr. Josephson makes the intriguing statement that "Nine out of ten colds can be prevented, or can be cleared up in their early stages, by simple breathing exercises."

Whether or not you think yours is a special case and that the cause of your cold is too deep-seated to have anything to do with the way you are breathing, Dr. Josephson offers theories which show a relationship between clear nasal passages and the proper functioning of most other parts of the anatomy. The good doctor tells how he became aware of the importance of unobstructed nasal corridors and how he educated himself to a system of corrective breathing. He simply made up his mind once, when a cold had been causing him a great amount of discomfort, to force himself to breathe easily through his nose. He was able to inhale only through the mouth, but could exhale through the nose with some effort.

He continued to do this, making the effort, with each exhalation, to clear the nasal passages. In time, he found his breathing easy through the nose in both directions. He also discovered that, so long as he continued to breathe carefully and with purpose, his nose remained unobstructed, but if he reverted to breathing carelessly, the nasal obstruction was evident once more. Obviously, the thing to do was to continue breathing with care until it became a habit (found to be a period of six weeks to two months). As a bonus, Dr. Josephson found that the type of breathing he practiced to clear his nose resulted in better health for every other part of his body.

The Nose Is an Air Conditioner

Probably the most fascinating parts of *Breathe Deeply and Avoid Colds* are those chapters in which the physiological functions of the nose are described. Dr. Josephson sees the nose and its passages as a kind of air conditioner for the body. As the air is inhaled through the nose, it is prepared for the inner system by being heated or cooled, as the case may be. For example, if the air is cold, it is heated to body temperature by contact with the mucous membranes of the nasal cavities and the sinuses, which are kept warm by the blood flowing through the veins next to them. When the air is very warm, the body automatically varies the amount and density of mucus secreted and increases the water content of it. The inspired air is afforded only a minimal contact with the mucosal vessels that contain the warming blood. The air conditioner comparison is carried further in characterizing the heart as the motor, the diaphragm and lungs as the circulating fan, the blood as the heating element, the mucus as the refrigerant as well as the humidifying element, etc. So you see what wonderful machinery your body has.

It is Dr. Josephson's belief that colds are caused by this air-conditioning system's breaking down, caused by changes in temperature that are so sudden as to give the body no chance to make the necessary adjustments. Accordingly, overheating as well as chilling can be the cause of a cold. "Roughly, it can be said that only one in a dozen colds begins as an infection. The balance start as disturbances in the body's thermostatic control," says Dr. Josephson.

Tension and Colds

Tension is advanced as another indirect cause of colds. Any state of anxiety or stress is known to cause shallowness of breathing, which, in the author's opinion, is the most frequent cause of nasal congestion. How often does one hear the expression, "I'm so excited that I am holding my breath." And it's true! Excitement and tenseness make correct breathing difficult. However, correct breathing will relax the body's tenseness. One must make an effort to breathe well when one is suffering from tension. "When you are nervous and tense, breathe slowly and deeply. You will generally find that you will relax and keep calm. You will find that it is well nigh impossible to breathe deeply and 'be on edge,' provided that your nose is not too badly blocked. Consciously deep breathing also relieves anxiety."

Signposts of Good Breathing

Dr. Josephson offers these signposts for good breathing exercises: (1.) Breathing must be as deep as possible without undue strain. (2.) Breathing must be through the nose only, unless the nose is so completely blocked as to preclude the passage of air. In this event, inhale through the mouth and exhale through the nose, until the nose is clear enough to permit inhaling through it. (3.) Breathing must be at a pace slow enough to avoid tiring. (4.) Breathing for the purpose of opening each side of the nose must be persevered in until it is completely open. (5.) Head posturing (that is, placing the head, during the breathing exercises, in positions that will favor the drainage of the sinuses under the force of gravity—usually reclining) should be resorted to from the start.

Perseverance is important to success in these exercises. Dr. Josephson advises that "Every hour, each side of the nose must be checked to make sure that it remains open. If either side has become blocked, the exercises must be resumed and continued until the nose is completely opened again, no matter how long it takes."

For those readers who wish to do what they can to avoid heart trouble, this statement will be of interest: "Nasal obstruction, especially of the left side of the nose, ranks high among the trigger mechanisms that precipitate angina pectoris, coronary thrombosis and other serious and fatal diseases of the heart. For older persons and for those with impaired hearts, relief of nasal obstruction by deep breathing may be a life-prolonging or life-saving measure. For everyone, it is a heart-sparing device."

Colds and Civilized Overdressing

There is an amusing and sensible chapter in which Dr. Josephson takes up the difficulty imposed on civilized men (not women) by the conventions of dress. By means of some clever cartoons and basic reasoning, he calls our attention to the sweltering male who, in winter, is bundled up in tweeds in a house kept warm enough for women's low cut dresses and chiffons, and, in summer, must wear jackets and ties in public, when the weather dictates the loosest and lightest of minimal attire. He states that a body thus prohibited from ridding itself of excess heat, and even adding extra warmth, is leaving itself wide open to colds and sickness. The doctor can be sure of plenty of support in these sentiments from other men who have suffered the discomfort of clothing that is impractical, no matter how socially correct it might be.

We suspect that the best inducement for investigating Dr. Josephson's theories on maintaining clear nasal passages is contained in the author's own words: "When finally you do open your nose completely, you will experience a startlingly new and pleasurable sense of well-being. It is characterized by a clarity of mind, and by freedom from the vague tension that marks nasal obstruction. Fatigability is replaced by endurance. Sinus pains and post-nasal drips disappear. Cold extremities, sensitivity to chilling and resultant intolerance of air conditioning are replaced by a healthy glow of skin and ready adaptation to temperature change and to air conditioning."

152. Should You Take an Aspirin for Colds?

Cold remedies have been with us since the time of the first cold. And lucky indeed is the man who can meet a friend, tell him he has a cold and not be greeted with this most cheerless and ubiquitous counsel, "I'll tell you exactly what to do for it. Clear it up in a matter of hours!" He then proceeds to describe one or another of the hoary remedies that have long since proved utterly useless—it's either baking soda in water or hot lemon juice and whiskey or hot milk with pepper in it. Or he may be from the modern school, in which case he will drag you off to the nearest drug store and exhort you to buy one or several of the new remedies attractively displayed with a great deal of advertising meant to prove that such and such a tablet will rid you of your cold within a matter of hours.

Remember, please, it's all just advertising. Ten thousand cold remedies have been patented in this country, and the only result has been an axiom famous in medical circles—*with a remedy,* you can get rid of cold in 7 days; *without any remedy at all,* it will take one week. We read in *Chemical Week* for September 26, 1953, that the people who make Four-Way Cold Tablets are suing the people who make Seven-Way Cold Tablets for deceiving the public (into thinking that 7 ways to cure a cold are better than 4 ways, we guess). Most horrifying angle to the story is the fact that the Four-Way Cold Tablet people have sold 20 million dollars worth of their product during the past 5 years! Their advertising expenses have been about $700,000 per year. Are any of your dollars among that 20 million? We hope not.

Foremost among so-called cold "cures" these days are aspirin, the antibiotics and the antihistamines. We have extensive files on all these preparations. It is now commonly accepted in medical journals that not one of the 3 "cures" a cold. Any of them may relieve symptoms temporarily. Aspirin may lessen the pain of that throbbing headache, antihistamines may make you so groggy that you won't realize how your bones ache. But as "cold cures" they are all completely discredited.

Why then should we warn against them? Because you may be tempted to nip into a drug store and pick up one of these inexpensive boxes of pills, just to relieve symptoms. And your cold may go on and on and even develop into pneumonia while you are apparently feeling better because your symptoms have lessened. Then, too, all of these drugs have side effects that—let's face it—may be fatal!

Aspirin Is Not a Harmless Home Remedy

Introduced into this country from Germany some 43 years ago, the original Bayer patent expired in 1917, but continues, even today, to harvest rich financial rewards from a product that now is being manufactured by many other laboratories over fundamentally the same prescription. Nowadays, advertising of the chemical ingredients of most of these aspirin-containing derivatives is given second place to their more easily pronounced trade names. Doctors often prescribe aspirin (or acetylsalicylic acid) in a variety of forms, without a patient's knowledge, acting on the assumption that, in moderate and regulated dosage, it can do no harm in its twofold general action of fever-reducer and pain-soother.

Bruce's *Materia Medica,* an authoritative teaching manual recognized by leading American medical schools, has this to say about aspirin: "Salicylic acid is rapidly absorbed and circulates as sodium salicylate . . . a moderate dose causes a more rapid heart beat, a rise in blood pressure, flushing and warmth of the surface, perspiration, fullness in the head, tinnitus (ringing in the ears), deafness, impairment of vision and possibly a slight fall in temperature. Larger doses may cause delirium, especially with visual hallucinations; respiration is disturbed; the heart is slowed and weakened; the vessels are relaxed and the blood pressure falls; and perspiration is increased. . . . Occasionally it induces an . . . eruption . . . sometimes (albumin or blood in the urine)."

As long ago as October 5, 1940, an editorial in the *Journal of the American Medical Association* reasoned that the main safeguard against overdose lay in a ringing sensation in the ears of aspirin users, "so that the drug may be discontinued before these persons become seriously poisoned." The editorial admitted that "No doubt much harm indirectly has probably followed its indiscriminate use, in that conditions for which it was used were not remedied. . . . Many reports have appeared on the adverse effects which may follow its unwise use. These have included depression of the heart, habit formation, miscarriage in pregnancy, and idiosyncrasy (allergic reaction) causing such alarming symptoms as urticaria (hives), pruritis (itching), erythema (redness of skin) and generalized angioneurotic edema (swelling of the skin due to a blood vessel disorder) . . . even ulceration and gangrene have been attributed to its use."

The editorial goes on to quote figures from the *Lancet* on a wave of fatalities that occurred in England from the use of aspirin. "According to this source, in England and Wales in 1938, the number of deaths due to poison was reported to be 735 of which 591 were suicides, 92 accidental and the remaining doubtful. The agent responsible for 43 of the suicides, for 8 of the accidental deaths and for 14 of the doubtful group of deaths was said to be aspirin; thus, aspirin was reported as the cause of death in 65 of the 735 fatal poisonings."

The list of undesirable aftereffects of aspirin also includes asthmatic attacks, as related in an article entitled *Allergy to Aspirin* by C. H. A. Walton, M.D., and H. W. Bottomley, M.D., of Winnipeg in the *Canadian Medical Association Journal* for March, 1951. Stating that "in relation to its very wide use the number of cases of aspirin sensitivity is small, but the effects are so striking and often dangerous, that physicians should be familiar with its character," the authors include hives and skin puffiness from disordered blood vessels among those already known manifestations of allergy following small intake of the drug. But its relation to asthma is their special interest and, among such patients, they cite estimates of from two to ten per cent as demonstrating this type of sensitivity.

In the September 8, 1951, issue of the *Journal of the American Medical Association*, two physicians from Cornell University Medical College report on the case of a 74-year-old man who experienced 8 years of continuous intestinal bleeding as the result of the prolonged use of aspirin. We know now that aspirin or other drugs containing salicylic acid block the action of vitamin K in our bodies. And vitamin K is chiefly concerned with the ability of our blood to clot properly. Now probably one aspirin will not cause an instantaneous and fatal hemorrhage. But we know people who take aspirin every day of their lives and especially when they have colds!

The *United States Armed Forces Medical Journal* for January, 1952, published an article describing 6 cases of salicylate poisoning of children, for two of whom the aspirin had been prescribed by physicians. In one case, a 5-month-old child, who was already taking (for a cold) several different kinds of medicine including penicillin, was given aspirin every 4 hours in addition by her parents, who did not even mention to the doctor that they were giving her aspirin! This child died of salicylate poisoning 4 days after she became violently ill.

We would say very positively that aspirin is not for you if you would be healthy. And we especially deplore the giving of aspirin to children. Aspirin especially for children has been getting a big play in the family magazines. It is temptingly flavored so that the child can chew it like candy. Here is another alarming hazard. Mother persuades Junior to take the aspirin "candy" to make him well. And what is to prevent Junior from seeking out the aspirin box and swallowing a lethal dose of the "candy" when mother isn't around? Why not go through your medicine chest today and just quietly throw away all the half-empty bottles of aspirin?

153. Shun the Antihistamines

For quite a long time, Americans took up the fad of antihistamines for colds. Medical journals were full of pros and cons. Experiments were conducted in hospitals and universities and among private patients. Reports came in of high percentages of "cures" for a while, then further investigation revealed that these were not cures at all. Symptoms had disappeared for a while, but nothing more. Then the reports of serious side effects began to come in. A death was finally scored up to the credit, or discredit of the antihistamines.

In the July 23, 1950, issue of the *Journal of the American Medical Association,* Hugh G. Rives, M.D., and associates report on the death of a 16-month-old girl in Dubuque, Iowa, who was poisoned "accidentally" one day in March, 1949, was rushed to the hospital and died the following morning. The poison which the unguarded child took *within the limits of the average adult dose* was one of the antihistamines, so-called because they reduce the efficiency of the action of "histamines," a vaguely understood substance formed in and released from body tissues during allergic reactions, such as those incidental to hay fever, colds and so forth.

The dictionary defines histamine as an amine (that is, a compound prepared from ammonia) containing 5 atoms of carbon to 9 of hydrogen and 3 of nitrogen. When produced in the body, it is a powerful stimulant to the female uterus and also lowers the blood pressure. Other reactions include those of the allergy group, for the treatment of which these "anti-histamine" drugs were originally created.

Dangers of the Antihistamines

Dr. Rives' article states that the incidence of unfavorable reactions following use of the antihistamines is estimated at ranging from 24 per cent to 46 per cent, even the average of which is surely sufficiently high to question the validity of calling them remedial, if not to justify their being banned. Other complaints against them are given in an article in the *Annals of Allergy* for May-June, 1950, by S. W. Jennes, M.D. He announces that two men patients were made sexually impotent as a result of treatment with two different types of antihistamine drugs. Though the impotence disappeared with discontinuance of the medicine, they might have been rendered permanently sterile if the dosage had been continued.

In addition, Dr. Jennes gives us an imposing list of other disastrous results including dizziness, heart palpitations, nervousness, nausea, diarrhea, dryness in the mouth, headaches and general weakness. A somewhat smaller number of patients were afflicted with rectal bleeding, abdominal pains and premature menstruation in women. More recently added to this list in other articles are fainting spells, severe prostration and mental conditions varying in gravity from simple confusion to serious mental illness. Concludes Dr. Rives: "That present indiscriminate use of these antihistaminic agents needs a critical review is evidenced in the medical literature. Although we have found no (other) report of a fatality, there have been serious reactions."

It appears clear to us that the discomfort of a common cold, while it may bother you for several days, is certainly not painful enough to warrant taking chances on any of the above-mentioned side effects. Perhaps you will not have any bad aftereffects at all. But considering the serious nature of some that have been reported, do you want to make it a practice to take any substance which, in other people, has such drastic results?

Finally, we have the report of Drs. Howard S. Triasman and L. Martin Hardy of the Children's Memorial Hospital in Chicago who, according to an Associated Press dispatch, tested 159 cold patients in their hospital with two treatments. One group was given Grandma's remedy—bed rest, fluids in abundance and (we must report it truthfully!) aspirin if needed. The other group received the same treatment plus sulfa drugs and antibiotics. All patients had the same symptoms. Of the group receiving Grandma's remedy, 56 per cent recovered in one week, 34 per cent in two weeks and the remaining 10 per cent took longer. Of the drug-treated group, only 39 per cent recovered in one week, 48 per cent in two weeks and 13 per cent took more than two weeks.

So why spend money for a drug that will not cure you any faster than no drug at all and may, in addition, start all kinds of unwholesome processes to work inside you?

[603]

154. How About a Shot
of Penicillin?

With every passing month, the medical magazines add one or two more pieces of evidence to the case against the antibiotics. We have come upon a great deal of information on harmful reactions to penicillin among hospital personnel who are not taking the antibiotic themselves, but have been so exposed to it while they were giving it to patients, that they are now extremely sensitive to it. Of course, the rest of us do not come in contact with the antibiotics every day. But what proof do we have that a dose of penicillin from time to time—for a cold, for a cut finger or for almost anything else—may not in time make us sensitive, too?

In addition, we have been warned over and over again by anxious medical men that we are now developing a much more powerful and stubborn kind of germ that can withstand the antibiotics. After a few more years of dosing with these medicines, we are likely to find that they are no longer effective against anything. What will we invent then to destroy these virulent germs? Another stronger poison? And what will happen when the germs become resistant to *that* poison, too? No, it seems to us that a far wiser course is to develop instead, bodies strong enough to withstand germs without any help from antibiotics. And certainly the most foolish course we can take is to rush for the penicillin at the slightest pretext, such as a common cold!

Allergic Reactions To Penicillin

Reporting in the *Armed Forces Medical Journal* for October, 1950, R. L. Gilman, M.D., calls attention to the fact that the severity of reactions to penicillin, currently being administered as a last-minute cure-all in the treatment of even non-infectious complaints, is greatly increasing. Whereas previous sensitizations produced by the wonder drug had resulted principally in skin eruptions, such as itching, wheals, nettle rash and hives, the list of newly observed post-injection effects now includes prostration, symptoms of arthritis, shock, chills and fever. All require protracted periods of readjustment for recovery, which may be marked by still further irritations. Dr. Gilman calls for a renewed and careful study of the use of the powerful antibiotic and states flatly that he considers its administration prior to any and every surgical operation to be unsound. He also demands that it not be employed in the case of maladies that have no infectious origin.

An army medical man warned the medical profession and the general public of the misuse of the antibiotic drugs, says the *New York Times* of November 2, 1951, reporting on a meeting of New York surgeons. Colonel

Edwin J. Pulaski of the Walter Reed Hospital disclosed that one hospital recently reported that 40 per cent of its pharmacy bill was for antibiotics!

Colonel Pulaski goes on to say that resistant strains of disease organisms are appearing which have acquired immunity to the antibiotic drugs, such as penicillin and aureomycin. Continued misuse of the drugs will increase the number of resistant strains. Actually, he tells us, all the wonder drugs do is halt the growth of germs which the body's natural defense mechanisms then destroy. The usefulness of the drugs depends therefore on the condition of the patient, his state of nutrition and his general stamina. "If the natural defense is at a low stage, the antibiotics are not apt to help much," he says. He also declares that antibiotics in powder or ointment form are probably of little benefit, and the combined use of several antibiotics together appears to be of little value.

155. How Harmless Is Menthol?

Any winter day in the bus or trolley car, among the coughers, sneezers and blowers, you will observe that practically everyone considers a box of mentholated cough drops as necessary as a handkerchief. Above the heads of the wheezing passengers, the cough drop ads and the mentholated cigarette ads plead with you to cool your throat and check your cough with so-and-so's mentholated remedy.

What is this menthol and how much do we know about it? Our medical dictionary tells us it is the crystalline substance derived from oil of peppermint and is used extensively in neuralgia, in skin diseases associated with itching and in colds. Menthol does indeed produce a cooling sensation for skin and throat irritations, but is this all it does?

An article in *Consumer Reports* for September, 1951, started us on our investigation. It reports the case of a young woman who went to a doctor complaining of small bleeding points that appeared on the skin of her arms, legs, face and chest. Laboratory studies indicated that some factor was interfering with blood coagulation, increasing the time necessary for clotting. Trying to reveal any possible factor that might be the source of her trouble, the young woman mentioned casually that she usually smoked a pack or two of mentholated cigarettes every day. On the doctor's advice, she discontinued the cigarettes and the eruption gradually and completely disappeared. She was then given test doses of pure menthol and the eruption reappeared; when the drug was stopped, the eruption vanished. She was then asked to smoke the mentholated cigarettes once more and again the symptoms of the blood ailment appeared. When she finally discontinued these cigarettes, all her symptoms vanished. This kind of an experience in today's America, where menthol is used in numerous products that can be bought at the corner drug store, set us to searching medical journals for further evidence.

Dangers of Menthol to Children

As early as 1909, we find that the Society of Pediatrics in Paris, France, debated the question of the possible dangers of menthol. The meeting was reported in their *Bulletin* for January 19, 1909. Dr. P. F. Armand-Delille described how he had treated a 3-month-old child with mentholated oil, two drops of which he placed in each nostril. The results were horrifying. The child had a violent convulsion and appeared about to die of asphyxiation. It took a quarter hour of warm baths to re-establish normal respiration. In the discussion following this story, several other French doctors related similar occurrences. It seemed that most of them had observed the ill effects of menthol on young children, and had tried various substitutes.

By 1935, menthol was, of course, being widely used in commercial preparations. The *Bulletin of the Academy of Medicine* of France for November 19, 1935, describes a "serious accident attributed to the ingestion of 6 milligrams of menthol in an infant aged four and a half." This little girl's mother gave her 3 cough drops containing two milligrams of menthol each. An hour later, the child asked to be put to bed, became pallid and cold, her respiration irregular and spasmodic, her pulse rapid, then irregular. Vomiting ensued. By the next morning, after an injection of camphorated oil, she was well again.

"Avoidance of the administration of menthol to all young children is a well-established opinion," says Dr. Chapeau, who made this report to the Academy of Medicine. He goes on to say that the irritating effect of menthol on the nose and throat membranes can "by way of reflex" bring about complete stoppage of heart and respiration. It is similar to the reflex of taking chloroform, he says, the dangers of which are well recognized. Accidents have apparently happened so often, especially with young children, that doctors should make it a rule to "abstain absolutely from the administration of mentholated preparations in the case of young children and particularly in that of nurslings."

On the basis of this report, the Medical Congress of Evreux in its general assembly of October 1, 1935, adopted a two-fold resolution: (1.) That on each package of products with a menthol base there be printed in large letters . . . "Medicament for adults. Usage dangerous for children," and that (2.) the Faculty of Medicine and of Pharmacy impress the dangers of the use of menthol by children.

Effect of Suppositories Containing Menthol

Our fourth medical experience relating to menthol appears in the *German Medical Weekly* for May 12, 1939. Dr. Wilhelm Gronemeyer describes the case of a woman patient, who had been apparently quite well all her life, developing suddenly a violent inflammation and itching in the anal region. She had been using suppositories for hemorrhoids and had discovered that the substances she had been using for some time, which had always helped her hemorrhoid condition, now apparently seemed to increase the intolerable itching and inflammation. After several tests which proved negative, Dr. Gronemeyer experimented with the patient and a number of test volunteers. In this way, the cause of the complaint was finally discovered.

All the suppositories the patient had used, except one, had a menthol content. Salves of menthol in concentrations of one per cent, two per cent and five per cent were placed for 24 hours on the skin of the patient and the volunteers. None of the volunteer experimenters showed any reaction to the menthol. The patient, however, showed positive reactions to all 3 concentrations: with the one and two per cent, obvious reddening of the skin; with the 5 per cent, inflamed redness with severe itching irritation. As soon as the patient stopped using suppositories containing menthol, her complaint ceased. Dr. Gronemeyer's conclusion was that he was "working with an eczema which originated from sensitization with menthol as a result of chronic use."

The Use of Inhalants

More recently, a series of tests of various inhalants is reported in the October, 1943, issue of the *Archives of Otolaryngology*. Testing 266 subjects, D. B. Butler, M.D., and A. C. Ivy, M.D., made some interesting discoveries. They found, for instance, that inhalers containing benzedrine showed no effect on pulse or blood pressure, but did show slight alterations in electrocardiograms. As a result, they warned that inhalation of benzedrine or compounds containing it may bring on anginal pain in patients with angina pectoris.

Other tests involved two substances called vasoconstrictors—that is, substances which constrict the blood vessels. In the case of commercial inhalants containing these substances, the doctors found that the pure drug was much more effective in relieving nasal obstruction than the commercial products, which included perfumed oils and other compounds. However, in the case of menthol, they found that inhaling pure menthol produced a rapid and striking increase in "nasal resistance." That is, instead of clearing the nasal passages, the menthol clogged them even more. Incidentally, the subjects being tested reported that the menthol made their noses *feel* cool and perfectly clear, even while the test was showing an increased amount of congestion.

The greatest congestion the experimenters encountered was when they administered an inhalant containing menthol along with several other substances: camphor, synthetic oil of wintergreen, oil of pine needles and oil of sassafras. While the subjects breathed in this inhalant, the nasal congestion rose as high as 212.9 per cent above basal level. And, once again, the subjects reported that their nasal passages "felt clear and cool."

So it would seem, say Dr. Butler and Dr. Ivy, that the undesirable

[607]

effects of menthol are strictly shown, not only in solutions, but in inhalers as well. They explain that menthol "feels good and cool" because the drug is an anesthetic which paralyzes many of the nerve endings and also stimulates the sensory nerve endings for cold—so that inhaled air feels cooler than it is and gives the subject the impression that a lot of fine cool air is circulating through his nostrils, when as a matter of fact, his nasal passages are more congested than before he inhaled the menthol.

Until much more extensive research has been done, then, we recommend the attitude taken by *Consumer Reports:* "Since menthol continues to be found in such common consumer products as cough drops, nose drops, inhalers, cough syrups, lotions and cigarettes, there is need for the establishment of some serious research projects to settle the question of whether the widespread use of menthol should be condemned or whether the drug should be exonerated." In addition, we counsel our readers to avoid mentholated products, from cough drops and inhalers to cigarettes and salves, until sufficient evidence of the human reaction to the drug will have established a fuller understanding of its potentialities. The cooling sensation produced by menthol is pleasant, but the aftereffects may prove to be serious. We want to caution readers especially against using any kind of mentholated product on very young children.

156. Smokers Have a Higher Percentage of Colds

The *Reader's Digest* for January, 1950, published an astounding article on smoking, in which the following aspects of the tobacco habit were reviewed: the effect of smoking on the throat membranes, on lungs, on stomach and digestion, on the skill of athletes, on the heart, on the blood pressure and the blood vessels, on Buerger's disease patients, on cancer incidence, on mortality figures, on colds. Author Roger William Riis came to the inevitable conclusion that smoking does nothing but harm. His own personal testimony is as follows: "When I began research for this article, I was smoking 40 cigarettes a day. As I got into the subject, I found that number dropping. As I finish the article, I am smoking 10 a day. I'd like to smoke more but my investigation of the subject has convinced me that smoking is dangerous, and worse—stupid."

Mr. Riis tells us that, if you smoke a pack of cigarettes a day, you take in 840 cubic centimeters of tobacco tar in a year. That means, he says, that you have exposed your throat and lung tissues to 27 fluid ounces or 15 full cocktail glasses of tobacco tar containing benzopyrene. The ugly, greasy tar that is left in your ash tray, on your fingers or in the filter of your cigarette holder is not nicotine. It is instead the "soot" that is left from the incomplete combustion of the tobacco—just as disagreeable and dangerous as the soot from your chimney. Many physicians agree that, as an irritant, it is more dangerous to heavy smokers than nicotine is.

He tells us that, of 100 smokers examined in one test, Dr. Frederick B. Flinn found 73 with congestion of the throat, 66 with coughs, 7 with irritation of the tongue. Dr. Emil Bogen reported on another 100 smokers, 30 of whom had mouth irritation and 30 of whom suffered from coughs. It appears that the way you smoke has something to do with how much injury you may encounter. The way you puff your cigarette, how long you hold the smoke when you inhale, how far down the butt you smoke your cigarette—all these have some bearing on how much irritation you are subjecting your throat tissues to. Rapid smoking, for instance, causes more irritation, because the smoke enters the mouth at a higher temperature.

Most of the nicotine escapes into the air when you smoke. About a third of it gets into your mouth where some of it is absorbed. Perhaps a fifth of what gets to the lungs is absorbed. Smoking one cigar gives the same effect as smoking about 4 or 5 cigarettes. The nicotine effect from a pipe is a little more than that from a cigar. The smoke coming into your mouth reaches temperatures up to 135 degrees Fahrenheit. The hotter your smoke, the more nicotine you absorb.

Says Mr. Riis, "In pure form, nicotine is a violent poison. One drop on a rabbit's skin throws the rabbit into instant shock. The nicotine content of a trifle more than two cigarettes, if injected into the blood stream, would kill a smoker swiftly. If you smoke a pack a day, you inhale 400 milligrams of nicotine a week, which in a single injection would kill you quick as a bullet."

Quoting *Risk Appraisal* published by the National Underwriters Company, Mr. Riis tells us that "Habitual smokers have 62 per cent higher incidence of gas on the stomach, 65 per cent higher incidence of colds, 76 per cent higher incidence of nervousness, 100 per cent higher incidence of heartburn, 140 per cent higher incidence of labored breathing after exertion, 167 per cent higher incidence of nose and throat irritation and 300 per cent higher incidence of cough." Insurance companies make it their business to do careful research; their business depends on it.

Colds and Smoker's Asthma

Surely this news should come as a surprise to no one. And we want to remind our readers, too, that "having a cold" is not the end of it. A cold, with its weakening effect on the body, may well predispose or lead directly to much more serious conditions.

An Associated Press news release of April 17, 1953, quotes a Detroit physician, Dr. George L. Waldbott, as saying that there is a very definite disease known to medical science as "smoker's asthma." He told of a group of 58 cases of smoker's asthma, 28 of whom recovered immediately as soon as they stopped smoking, 24 others who recovered by discontinuing tobacco and taking other treatment as well and the remainder of whom did not improve, even after they gave up smoking.

He described smoker's asthma as "chronic inflammation of the Adam's apple area of the throat; wheezing, shortness of breath, a tendency to respiratory infections, constriction of the chest above the heart and prolonged coughing in the morning, sometimes requiring several hours to clear the throat of mucus." He advised that other physicians should always make allowance for the possibility of "smoker's asthma" when they are diagnosing ailments.

Possible Effect of Tobacco Smoke on Others

Perhaps even more frightening is an article in the *Journal of the American Medical Association,* October 21, 1950, recounting the story of a one-year-old infant brought to the hospital with a history of watery eyes, nasal discharge and sneezing. At the age of 10 months, she had had an asthmatic attack. When the baby's allergy tests showed that she was allergic to tobacco, her parents were questioned, and it was found that her mother had been an incessant smoker for many years, smoking even while she fed, nursed and diapered the baby. All smoking was stopped in the house and, within a few days, the baby's symptoms disappeared completely.

A year and a half later, the baby developed a dry hacking cough, and it was found that the mother had started to smoke again. When she stopped, the baby's symptoms once again disappeared. Asthma is a very serious ailment, especially in the case of a baby. The extreme difficulty an asthmatic patient suffers in trying to breathe can result in death. Yet, from the story above, it seems quite possible that many of our asthmatic children today are the product of a household constantly blue with tobacco smoke. Perhaps much of the watery eyes, nasal discharge and sneezing that cause more absenteeism from school than any other reason, may be traced to a family which smokes and encourages visitors to smoke. Surely, even if parents will not make an effort to stop smoking for their own sakes, they should take into account the possible harm being done to children and other susceptible people who must breathe in the tobacco smoke they exhale.

Effect on T.B. Patients and Post-Operative Patients

A question to the Editor of the *Journal of the American Medical Association,* September 30, 1950, asks whether or not smoking should be permitted in a tuberculosis hospital. The Editor answers that tobacco smoke causes "hyperemia of the mucous membranes"—that is, excessive blood congesting the membrane. He states that some specialists in bronchial diseases can tell from the condition of the membranes whether the patient is a one, two or three packs-a-day smoker. In addition, he says, smoking causes coughing, which is, of course, much more harmful for a T.B. patient than for a healthy individual.

[610]

In the *Lancet*, 1:368, 1944 (a conservative British medical publication), H. J. V. Morton writes on the incidence of pulmonary complications in patients who have undergone operations. Patients were grouped into 3 categories: smokers, light smokers and non-smokers. The first category included anyone who smoked 10 or more cigarettes a day. The conclusions were that smoking definitely increases complications of many kinds in patients who are undergoing operations. There were 257 patients in the study, and results showed that the rate of complication for smokers was about 6 times greater than that of non-smokers. In addition, Dr. Morton says that smokers are more likely to develop complications associated with serious constitutional disturbance.

Undoubtedly, a thorough search of medical literature would reveal much more evidence of this same nature. Since the respiratory membranes —nose, throat, larynx and lungs—are more directly exposed and hence, more irritated by tobacco smoke than other parts of the body, it seems only reasonable to assume that all the most pesky nose and throat disorders (including colds) would be more common in smokers than in non-smokers. Once again, though, we must remember that families and friends are constantly exposed—though to a lesser extent—to the smoke of the tobacco user.

Authoritative Evidence Against Smoking

Smoking uses up vitamins that protect us against colds and other disorders—especially vitamin C and vitamin B. So the smoker, aside from irritating his nose and throat membranes, at the same time deprives them of food elements that might help to protect them against these poisons. Considering the fact that his respiratory membranes are pretty constantly in a state of irritation, is it any wonder that, when the cold bugs attack, they find good pickings in these depleted, sick membranes? The weapons that might defeat them have already been used up and the smoker becomes easy prey for the sniffles, the tears, the fevers, the chills, the coughs, the hoarseness and, perhaps, finally the pneumonia.

When you show this information to some friend who may be a chain smoker and who may have little regard for anything having to do with health, don't let him get away with sneering that we are cranks and crackpots. We didn't make up the figures on cold incidence among smokers just to frighten people. We don't have anything to sell in place of tobacco. The figures—65 per cent higher incidence of colds, 167 per cent higher incidence of nose and throat irritation and 300 per cent higher incidence of coughs—come from an insurance handbook put out by the National Underwriters Company.

Perhaps there really are people who are living wrapped up in a tight secure little cocoon of ignorance about what medical experimentation has shown in regard to the harmful effects of smoking. If you have a friend or relative like this, tell him to stop in at the local library and look through the *Readers' Guide To Periodical Literature*. All the magazine articles for

[611]

the past 50 years or so are listed there. Ask him to look up smoking or tobacco or nicotine, and marvel, as we have, at the number of articles on the harmfulness of smoking that have appeared—and this in a country where many millions of dollars are paid out by tobacco companies for advertising in current periodicals! *Index Medicus* is a listing of all the articles in medical journals all over the world. Any one page of any one year of *Index Medicus* will yield enough information on the harmfulness of tobacco to cause the most hardened smoker to think a long, long time before he lights that next cigarette.

157. Low-Carbohydrate Diets for Respiratory Disorders

Too much and the wrong kind of carbohydate in the diet is apparently closely related to colds and other troubles of the respiratory organs. In an earlier chapter, we have talked about an experiment in which colds of quite a large number of patients were reduced decidedly when the patients were put on a diet that included no foods high in carbohydrate. Now we find evidence that eating lots of starches may have a lot to do with getting tuberculosis and with suffering from sinus trouble.

The information on sinus trouble comes from Dr. E. Seaver, Jr., in an article in the *Transactions of the American Laryngology, Rhinology and Otolaryngy Society,* Vol. 44, 302-309, 1944. Dr. Seaver tells of his treatment of 30 office patients suffering from sinus trouble of varying degrees of severity. Every patient also had some involvement of the middle ear.

Prescribing diets for these patients, Dr. Seaver asked them to substitute natural carbohydrates for refined ones (potatoes instead of spaghetti for example). They were also told to eat plenty of meats of glandular origin like liver, green leafy vegetables, dairy and poultry products. In addition, he gave all of them a food supplement consisting of a finely powdered spinach concentrate which was especially helpful, he says, in cases of individuals who did not like and hence tended to avoid eating leafy greens.

The results of the investigation showed that there was no case that did not show some improvement, many showed a marked benefit and a few made a complete recovery—that is, a continuous freedom from the symptoms for which they had originally visited the doctor. Dr. Seaver tells us that the patient's frame of mind strongly influenced his progress. Fear inhibited good results. Faith made good results easier to attain. He found, too, that those patients who went back to their original way of eating invariably got their symptoms back again.

We think that Dr. Seaver has made an excellent analysis of why refined carbohydrates have a bad effect on throat, nasal and sinus passages. He tells us it is generally accepted by nutrition experts that a diet high in refined carbohydrates (white sugar and white flour products) is automatically low in minerals and vitamins, as well as the cellulose needed to assure the proper working of one's digestive tract.

In addition, if you eat a high-carbohydrate diet, your need for B vitamins is automatically increased.

Carbohydrates which have had their B vitamins removed (and this happens when foods are refined) must have B vitamins from some other source in order for the body to use them properly. So, if your diet is high in refined carbohydrates and you do not supplement it with enough B vitamins, you are bound to suffer from a shortage.

"Among other known factors that raise the vitamin B requirement above the normal amount are fatigue, chilling, infection, fear and fever. Probably the commonest form of fear is worry, which in reality is chronic fear, the basis of the anxiety neuroses so frequently associated with malnutrition . . . A diet adequate in B vitamin requirements may fail in assimilation under conditions of diarrhea or persistent use of laxatives and cathartics," says Dr. Seaver.

Low-Carbohydrate Diet for Tubercular Patients

An even more startling indictment of refined carbohydrates as the cause of respiratory diseases comes from an article hidden in the files of medical literature since September, 1942. It appeared in the *American Review of Tuberculosis* for that month. Its author is Benjamin P. Sandler. He is the author of two books: *Diet Prevents Polio* (available from Lee Foundation, 2023 West Wisconsin Avenue, Milwaukee 3, Wisconsin) and *How to Prevent Heart Attacks* (available from same publisher, Lee Foundation). In both of these books, he stresses the extremely harmful part played in the diet by refined carbohydrates and the great importance of a high protein diet.

In this article, he describes what happened to 10 patients with advanced pulmonary tuberculosis, so sick that they had to be hospitalized. All 10 of them responded by gain in strength, general improvement, healing of cavities in their lungs and clearing of infiltrations of the disease. They experienced what Dr. Sandler calls an "early and sustained relief from digestive, cardiac, respiratory, nervous and mental symptoms."

Dr. Sandler declares that rest plays a part in the treatment of tuberculosis because it makes available for the healing process the glucose and oxygen that might have been used up in physical activity. He tells us that a diet low in carbohydrates regulates the blood sugar level, thus providing an ample supply of glucose and oxygen, and hence, reduces susceptibility to colds.

He tells of a study of colds in an English boarding school. The

[613]

dormitory with the lowest sugar consumption had colds at the rate of 5.5 per head. The dormitory with the largest sugar consumption had a rate of 24.6 per head. Almost 5 times as many colds!

This is how the actual physical mechanism works, according to Dr. Sandler. The high-carbohydrate diet results in low blood sugar. This means that less glucose (blood sugar) can be used by body tissues. These tissues use oxygen in proportion to the amount of glucose they use, so low blood sugar results in tissues being asphyxiated for lack of oxygen. Then, too, people may suffer from the sometimes drastic symptoms of blood sugar levels falling too rapidly. Dizziness, faintness, nervousness, sweating, flushing, heart palpitation—all these may be simply indications that blood sugar is too low as a result of a diet high in carbohydrates.

Here are several case histories from Dr. Sandler's article. A 57-year-old patient, who had shown no improvement after 5 months of bed rest in the hospital, was put on a low-carbohydrate diet, and within two weeks, there was definite improvement. He felt stronger and his appetite was better. He had less belching. His breathing was much lighter. He had more pep and ambition. A year later he was discharged virtually cured of tuberculosis. A 49-year-old patient had become steadily worse with tubercular symptoms in both lungs. He also went home cured after a year on the low-carbohydrate diet.

Other case histories from Dr. Sandler's article show again and again that the high-carbohydrate diet his patients were on originally in the hospital brought no relief of symptoms. But when his low-carbohydrate diet was begun, improvement began almost at once and proceeded rapidly.

Here are some interesting comments by Dr. Sandler on the diet. He says that patients complained of being hungry after meals when they began the diet. They did not have that feeling of fullness that one experiences after a meal loaded with carbohydrates. So they were encouraged to take between-meal snacks—not carbohydrate ones, of course. After a few weeks, this feeling of hunger disappeared.

"Practically all the patients had to be encouraged at the beginning of the treatment. Sensing the experimental nature of the diet, they were reluctant to give up foods they always enjoyed eating. They were skeptical when told that bread and cereals were preventing their recovery. After a few weeks, however, when they began to feel stronger, appear healthier and when they began to lose some of their symptoms, they realized the value of the diet and were glad to continue on it," says Dr. Sandler.

Patients may show improvement within a very short time. There is usually a quick improvement in appetite and common digestive complaints such as fullness after meals, belching, heartburn, gas, cramps and a feeling of heaviness in the stomach. All of these symptoms disappeared soon. Patients were surprised to learn, says Dr. Sandler, that foods like cereals and baked potatoes, generally regarded as "light" and easily digested, were responsible for their distress after meals. They were also surprised to learn that meat and fish could be eaten often and in liberal quantities without digestive disturbances.

Low-Carbohydrate Diet Helps Frame of Mind

What about their state of mind? Here, too, great improvement was noticed. Patients became more hopeful and less depressed. They worried less about their illness, became more sociable and less irritable. Dr. Sandler believes that changes like this are a direct result of the regulation of the blood sugar level, which allows plenty of glucose and plenty of oxygen for the brain and nervous system.

This is the diet these tuberculosis patients were placed on. It comprised 101 to 129 grams of protein, 114 to 124 grams of carbohydrate, 161 to 212 grams of fat. These were the forbidden foods: bread, cereals, potatoes, sugar, corn, rice, tapioca, split peas, noodles, macaroni, spaghetti, cake, candy, ice cream, pancakes and all other white flour, white sugar products. Muffins made from soybean flour were sometimes allowed. (Soybeans are extremely high in protein.)

Breakfast consisted of a low-carbohydrate fruit, 2 eggs, butter, cheese and cup of a milk-cream mixture. Dinner was broth, meat, low-carbohydrate vegetables (cooked and raw), low-carbohydrate fruit and the milk-cream mixture. For supper the menu was the same except that fish was substituted for meat.

Patients were encouraged to eat nuts between meals. And they were allowed to have two "soda crackers" with each meal. We assume this was a concession to the feeling that one *has* to have some bread product at a meal. Of course, we believe this is not the best diet for healthy people to follow. We would skip the butter, cream and milk and, of course, the crackers.

158. What Is Constipation and What Causes It?

Our earliest record of constipation appears in a famous Egyptian medical document which is believed to have been written about 1553 B.C. At this time Egypt was at the height of her medical achievement. In those days a patient sent to a temple of health a description of his symptom and a doctor skilled in that particular disease was immediately dispatched to the sufferer's house. We are told by Donald T. Atkinson in *Magic, Myth and Medicine* (World Publishing Company) that the largest part of the manuscript is taken up with remedies for constipation. "For an overtaxed colon," says Dr. Atkinson, "the first prescription would be found superior in effectiveness to many of our modern remedies."

Here it is: "Take thou: fresh dates, one part; seasalt, one part; sebbet juice, one part. Mix in water, place in an earthen receptacle and put therein: crushed gengent beans, cook together, cool and let the patient drink warm. Thereafter let him drink sweet beer."

We don't know what sebbet juice is, or gengent beans. But we imagine these were common foods in those days, foods probably rich in minerals and cellulose.

Dr. Atkinson tells us that constipation was one of the common ailments of the early American colonists, too. Dr. Benjamin Rush, the famous eighteenth century physician of Philadelphia, believed that much of the colonists' difficulty lay in their eating of what he called "indigestible foods." Hot breads were supposedly the cause of much indigestion. The other foods disapproved of (and in this we heartily agree) were the salted pork, bacon, ham and "sowbelly" which were so salty that they had to be washed down with enormous quantities of fluid—milk, buttermilk and coffee. Of course, overeating was common and such things as fruits and vegetables were almost unknown except during the summer and fall.

Constipation in England

During early times in England, constipation was called "costiveness" and was quite prevalent. Drummond and Wilbraham, writing in *The Englishman's Food* (Jonathan Cape), tell us that the poorer people who lived chiefly on coarse, wholemeal bread scarcely knew what it was. In all probability, there was so much residue in their diets that two or three bowel movements a day were the rule.

[616]

However, they tell us, the wealthier classes ate large amounts of meat, which, leaving little residue, tends to result in sluggish bowels. Most primitive meat-eating races are constipated and sometimes resort to eating rancid fat which apparently acts as a laxative. Our authors tell us that "May butter" was used for this purpose in England. Purges were used in those olden times to rid the body of "vapors" or melancholy, so it is impossible to tell how much of the actual taking of physics was due to constipation and how much was due to "vapors" created by superstition. The purges used were laxatives such as rhubarb and senna. Others which were recommended were more in the nature of spring tonics and probably brought good results because they contained vitamin C—dandelion, scurvy grass and so forth. Drummond and Wilbraham tell us that they are inclined to think that the population of old England was a good deal less troubled by constipation than we are today.

Kinds of Constipation

Most authorities agree that there are two kinds of constipation: atonic and spastic. Atonic constipation usually affects the cecum, that is, the very beginning of the large intestine. Spastic constipation usually affects the transverse or descending colon or the rectum.

The name indicates the difficulty in atonic constipation—the intestine has no "tone." So, like any muscle without tone, it falls down on its job, which in this case is propelling food residues through the excretory tract. In spastic constipation the bowel is spastic—that is, it contracts in a spasm so that food residue does not pass along as it should.

Here is a partial list of causes of atonic constipation as given in *Lippincott's Quick Reference Book—Medicine and Surgery*: habitual neglect of the calls of nature; sedentary life; habitual use of laxatives or enemas; insufficient food; food deficient in residue; sometimes too much residue; not enough water-drinking; over-digestion and absorption of food; chronic stomach disease; chronic invalidism; debility or weakness; obesity; anemia; poor nutrition; senility; worry or grief; weakness of the diaphragm caused by chronic, unhealthy conditions of the chest; constricting corsets; enlarged abdominal organs (such as enlarged prostate, tumors, etc.); the taking of astringent foods or medications such as tea, red wine, or medicines containing alum, copper, iron, lead, bismuth, tannic acid preparations.

Here is a partial list of causes of spastic constipation, according to the same source: overuse of purgative drugs; irritating foods; too much acid in the stomach; mucous colitis; intestinal ulceration; mental strain from overwork and irritation; melancholy. In addition, of course, there are many diseases which are accompanied by constipation.

Some Causes of Constipation

Medical Treatment by Geoffrey Evans, M.D., a British publication, lists these as the causes of constipation: (1.) Habit. One of the factors assisting defecation is the passage of 24 hours of time, according to Dr.

Evans. This is one reason why establishing the habit of defecating at a certain time of day is so valuable. (2.) Posture is especially important. Since we walk upright we are inclined to have more trouble with posture than the animals which walk on 4 feet. And slumping results in crowded organs and pressure on the intestines. (3.) The gastro-colic reflex is the scientific name for the "call of nature." This reflex works when food is taken which causes the bowels to begin their work of peristalsis—that is, pushing the residual mass along. There is a time lag in the working of this reflex so there may be no urge to defecate for a half hour to an hour after food is taken. But it should normally occur. And if it is ignored, the reflex is weakened and gradually ceases to function as it should. (4.) Fatigue may be a cause of constipation. Dr. Evans says that some people live habitually over-tired. They do not waken naturally in the morning, but must be awakened. They feel too tired to get started at their daily activities until they have the stimulus of coffee, food, exercise or interest in the day's work. He goes on, "chronic constipation may be the first or only symptom of over-fatigue." (5.) Emotions may cause constipation. They may bring about loss of appetite, nausea, flatulence (gas), diarrhea or constipation. In cases like these, getting rid of the constipation hinges on getting the emotional problems solved. (6.) Drinking not enough fluids can cause constipation. Dr. Evans recommends 2½ to 3 pints daily. (7.) Rest and exercise are important. For those who suffer from atonic constipation, exercise is essential, particularly walking, horseback riding or some other form of rhythmic exercise. In cases of spastic constipation or mucous colitis, rest is important.

More Causes of Constipation

Jean Bogert in *Nutrition and Physical Fitness* (Saunders) lists these as the things which affect the tone of the intestinal muscles and hence the things which are involved in constipation: general condition of health; diet; posture; exercise; individual nervous sensitiveness; habit; psychic influence; amount of water; cellulose and gas present in intestines; lubrication of fecal mass (determined in part by the amount of water and also the undigested fat in the intestines); lack of the organic acids, especially in fruit and milk. If an individual is in "rundown" condition, the intestine may be flabby and in poor tone, so that contractions take place infrequently and with insufficient force. Such a condition is often the primary cause of constipation, Dr. Bogert tells us.

Differences in nervous sensibility may be responsible for the wide differences in individuals as to the frequency with which they must empty the bowel to feel comfortable. If we ignore the clear "call of nature," the desire and ability to defecate will pass. When this is repeated frequently, as it is in many people's experience, the sensitiveness to this stimulation becomes dulled and the individual no longer knows when his bowels need emptying. Thus, bad habit becomes one of the most important causes of constipation.

There are some experts who believe that psychic factors have as much to do with constipation as anything else. What do we mean by psychic factors? Hurry, nervousness, worry about one's ability to have a bowel movement and concern over the necessity of defecating every day. In toilet-training children, mothers often make such an unpleasant thing out of the daily session on the toilet that children become unnecessarily anxious about it. Eager to please, they try too hard and failure results. Such experiences can determine the habit of a lifetime. Neurotic adults are frequently constipated for psychic reasons.

The content of the colon in the normal unconstipated individual is semi-solid, non-irritating, free from undigested food remnants and of sufficient bulk that it secures good peristaltic movement and easy moving of the mass of feces along the course of the intestine. Of course, what you eat is largely responsible for the condition of the intestinal contents. Food which contains enough residue must be taken. This means fruits and vegetables, all of which contain some cellulose which is only partially digested, and whole grain cereals. That is, cereals from which the bran has not been removed, for bran is largely cellulose and hence contributes to the bulk of the intestinal mass.

159. Constipation Is Related to Other Diseases

Diabetes is nearly always accompanied by constipation. Individuals who have thyroid trouble suffer from constipation. It is common in obesity and almost as common among those who are reducing, if they have reduced so greatly the bulk of their meals that there is not enough to push the undigested residue through the elimination tract.

Fairfax T. Proudfit in *Nutrition and Diet Therapy* says, "The frequency with which constipation coexists with epilepsy and seems to predispose to an attack makes it seem very desirable to have good elimination."

It is pretty well established that gall bladder difficulties are caused by overeating. Persons who suffer from gall bladder distress are very commonly constipated.

In an article in *Gastroenterology* for December, 1950, A. Littman, M.D., and A. C. Ivy, Ph.D., M.D., tell us that the percentage of stomach ulcer patients who are constipated is very large. They quote other authorities from Europe who claim that as high as 60, 70 and 72 per cent of their ulcer patients also suffer from constipation.

Dr. Ivy and Dr. Littman came to the conclusion that much of the constipation among their own ulcer patients was caused by their treatment of this disease. They gave their ulcer patients a diet low in residue, the usual diet prescribed for ulcer patients. Then they gave them antacid drugs to reduce the acid in their stomachs. This caused more constipation. Seventy-nine per cent of their patients suffered from it while they were being treated for ulcer. And as usual, it did not occur to the physicians to try to prevent the constipation. Instead they gave laxatives. In other words, they continued to give the constipation diet and drugs, with 'the understanding that they would then have to give the laxative.

Clues to the Cause of Pruritus Ani

Finally, we have evidence that one of the most baffling and annoying conditions of all may be due to one aspect of constipation. Geoffrey Evans, writing in *Medical Treatment* (published by C. V. Mosby Company) says that after defecation, the rectum and that part of the colon which empties into the rectum should be completely emptied of food residues. Incomplete emptying of this part of the elimination tract is as much constipation as is a wholesale delay in the passage of food residues through the colon as a whole. He goes on, "Incomplete evacuation of the rectum, as much as complete failure of the rectum to empty its contents one day, is a cause of a variety of symptoms including a sensation of local fullness or discomfort, and perhaps *proctalgia fugax* (pain in the anus or rectum). It may be a cause of *proctitis* (inflammation), hemorrhoids and *pruritus ani.*"

Pruritus ani means an itching anus. For a long time we have been collecting information on the cause and cure of this most embarrassing and distressing symptom. We have uncovered evidence showing that it may be due to food allergies. Mentioned most often is allergy to citrus juice. Other foods sometimes spoken of in this respect are chocolate, alcohol and other fruit juices. The taking of antibiotics has also been indicated as a possible cause.

Now, however, it seems that we are on the trail of even more significant information. If you suffer from pruritus ani, and if you are constipated, the solution may be simply to correct the constipation. If by chance you have pruritus ani and are not constipated, your trouble may be this incomplete emptying of the lower bowel as Dr. Evans describes. Since this is, after all, a form of constipation, we are sure that these same suggestions will benefit you greatly.

Finally, it seems that the relationship between these various conditions and constipation cannot be just a casual one. Nor does it seem that the constipation is necessarily responsible for other conditions. It seems, rather, that the same things are causing both the constipation (an unhealthful state) and the diabetes, the ulcers, the epilepsy and so forth. If you re-arrange your life and your diet to eliminate constipation, it seems to us you have a very good chance of preventing the more serious disorder.

160. Exercise to Fight Constipation

The average time between the intake of food and the expulsion of its waste from the body is from 12 to 20 hours. This period of time is subject to the habits of the individual, for it has been established before that many perfectly normal persons do not empty their bowels for periods of several days at a time. Whatever one's regular routine for bowel movements, when the routine is upset the results can be headache, acne, discomfort in the abdominal area, distention of the abdomen and other unpleasant symptoms. We know this condition as constipation.

Muscular Action Is Necessary for Elimination

For persons who suffer from this problem often, there may be some relief through the use of exercises which are calculated to put tone into the muscles which assist in eliminating bodily waste. These muscles are especially apt to grow lazy when the individual leads a sedentary life, lacks regular exercise or is obese. Normally there is regular activity in the muscles of the stomach and intestines which push food and waste through the body at a proper rate. If the muscles lag in their job and are sluggish, constipation is often the result.

The book, *Massage and Remedial Exercise,* by N. M. Tidy, offers some suggested activities which are intended to strengthen the muscles needed for normal, regular elimination. Mr. Tidy urges "vigorous and energetic" application to these exercises, but we caution those of our readers who try them to start slowly, building endurance with each session. Overexertion is always far more dangerous than any lack of exercise can be.

For the first exercise perch on a surface high enough above the floor to allow the feet to dangle freely, let yourself go completely limp—head hanging on the chest, arms hanging loosely at the sides. Then straighten up—shoulders back, chest out, head far back and back arched, the arms extended to the sides. Hold this position a short time, then repeat the whole procedure about 10 times or until tired.

For leg-swinging exercise stand on one leg, swing the other far out and far back. Change legs every 5 or 10 times. Individual swinging of the arms is good exercise, too. Trunk-rolling is another exercise commonly employed to strengthen abdominal muscles. In this the patient stands with hands on hips and rotates his torso in a circular motion without bending the knees or moving the hips.

Difficult But Effective

A difficult, but very effective exercise suggested by Tidy is that in which the individual lies flat on his back, with his hands at his sides. Extending his hands in front of him, he raises himself to a sitting position and leans over to touch his toes, without bending his knees, or pushing himself up with the hands. We recommend the exercise in which one sits Indian fashion, with arms folded and legs crossed, then rises to a standing position while keeping the arms folded. It's tough, but very good exercise for the abdominals.

Nutrition and Diet Therapy by Proudfit suggests that a good exercise to relieve constipation consists in lying on the back, then raising the legs, extended as high as possible 10 or 20 times at each session. Proudfit says this should be done two times daily, morning and evening.

Aside from the setting-up exercises recommended here for relief of constipation, both books mentioned above advocate plenty of spontaneous activity and exercise—long walks, stooping, gardening, running, skipping, dancing and other activities that demand some physical exertion.

Exercise As Part of Your Daily Routine

Many of us think we don't have time to exercise. It's easier to take a laxative, we figure. But those of us who have found that we can easily work exercises into our daily routine have found increased benefits from doing so. Any time of day, no matter where you are, you can exercise your abdominal muscles. Simply straighten your back, tuck in your buttocks and pull in on those tummy muscles! You can do it sitting down as well as standing up. Press your back against the back of your chair, pushing hard against that hollow place where you probably curve in too far. If your muscles are lax and droopy, it will take some time to get them to respond. But once you do, you can be sure that you can easily keep them firm and tight from then on, which will mean a great improvement in posture and appearance, as well as in health.

More Exercises for You

Another good lying-down exercise is to bend your knees, bringing your thighs back against your chest, or as far as you can get them. Keep in mind about all exercising that it isn't really important whether or not you accomplish the final position of the exercise. You derive the benefit from *trying* to do it. While you're lying there so cozily in your bed, just before you go to sleep, you might try this one, too: lie flat, with hands behind your head, elbows out and flat against the bed. Now, not lifting your shoulders from the bed, bend your right knee and bring it over and touch the bed on the left side. Bring it back to position. Bend the left knee and touch the bed on the right side.

Just after you've had your bath is a good time for these next exercises. Hold both arms straight out at right angles to the body and walk on tiptoe back and forth. It is almost impossible to do this one comfortably without pulling in on your abdominal muscles. If you have a full length mirror you might study your posture while you do this exercise. The minute you pull those abdominal muscles in, you'll suddenly look as graceful as a ballet dancer preparing for a difficult step. Here's another exercise: keeping your abdominal muscles in tight, place your hands on your shoulders, elbows up, then bend forward from the waist, then back, then to the right and then to the left, slowly. Exercising rapidly only wears you out and gets you to puffing without actually flexing your muscles, which is the main purpose of exercise. Now stand tall. Then, holding your back straight, squat down on your haunches, slowly, then rise erect again.

Abdominal Massage

A technique that is often applied in cases of constipation is abdominal massage. It is believed that certain constant pressure on the abdomen sometimes activates the peristaltic reflex (the contractions of the intestines which move the waste matter to the rectum) and causes renewal of the desired habits of elimination. *Lippincott's Quick Reference Book—Medicine and Surgery* tells us that the massage may be practiced for 15 or 20 minutes twice daily, and preferably before rising in the morning, or after retiring. The massage is done with the hand, while the head is slightly raised, and the legs slightly flexed to relax the abdominal muscles. The massage should begin at the upper abdomen, and with a slowly kneading motion should progress downward to the pubic area. The Lippincott book even suggests that one might use a leather- or felt-covered two-to-ten pound bowling ball or cannon ball for this job, if the palm of the hand isn't up to it.

Tidy's recommendations are equally as strenuous, if not quite so inventive. He suggests that "vigorous kneading should be administered to the whole of the front and sides of the abdomen. Double-handed kneadings . . . are excellent, and also strong, deep 'picking-up' movements . . ." This is an old and much-practiced aid to elimination and is infinitely preferable to the use of laxatives and drugs.

In connection with the question of constipation, it should be noted that perfectly normal bowels will rebel in spite of exercise if proper foods are not included in the diet, or if the call for elimination is neglected or postponed. Eat well at regular times. Have a regular time at toilet and don't rush yourself. If you feel the need of a bowel movement, go and relieve yourself at once. These rubs, plus some daily exercise, will quickly lead you to untroubled regularity.

161. Try Natural Foods to Treat Constipation

If one doesn't take laxatives or enemas when constipation occurs, what can one do for relief? Certainly a good diet is an excellent preventive, but what can be done for people who don't always eat well, or for people who have just begun to eat naturally and are still plagued with constipation problems? The answer lies in a careful selection of natural foods which have the desired properties for moving waste through the intestines and into the rectum for elimination. It has been established that bulk is one property essential to stimulating the colonic muscles in the wave-like activity which pushes the undigested debris through the alimentary canal.

Why We Need Bulk

The needed bulk is usually contained in the necessary amounts in a good diet. If the meals you eat consist of natural foods in balanced proportions, and you cultivate regular habits and exercise, the problem of constipation should never plague you. If you've missed up somewhere and irregularity has taken hold, there is still much you can do to help yourself before resorting to laxatives. Many natural foods are high in cellulose content. This cellulose is an element in foods which cannot be used by the body and is eliminated once the nutrients contained with it have been absorbed. It might be compared to a honeycomb which is discarded once the honey has been drained from it. This cellulose is also capable of absorbing large amounts of water, and like a sponge increases in bulk, pushing at the walls of the intestine and stimulating the peristaltic action which pushes it through. With this, of course, comes any other waste that has been rejected by the body as useless.

Foods Rich in Cellulose

There are long lists of foods known to contain important amounts of cellulose. It is these foods that a constipated individual should concentrate on including in his diet. Some mentioned in *Nutrition and Diet Therapy* by Proudfit (Macmillan) are: figs, dates, dried peas, nuts, navy beans, seeds, grapes, plums, apricots, cantaloupe, raisins, lima beans and raw tomatoes. The list could be continued if space would permit, but it is apparent that bulky, juicy foods are important, such as tomatoes or cantaloupes, and foods with edible skin such as dried peas, beans and raisins. Tough foods such as nuts and seeds are also worthwhile.

It is easy to understand the effectiveness of these foods. The juicy, bulky ones with high cellulose take a lot of space and mechanically move the waste matter by their very presence. The unpeeled vegetables and rough

[624]

nuts, dates and raisins are more resistant to intestinal bacteria and make for a slightly abrasive surface that prods the intestinal wall into doing its muscular duty.

We are cautioned in *Dietary of Health and Disease* by Gertrude Thomas (Lea and Febiger) that too much cellulose in the diet can have an adverse effect, too. Taken in excessive amounts it may influence the absorption of other foods. Tests proved that loss of protein parts in digestion increased as the proportion of indigestible foodstuffs increased. Cellulose is classed as an indigestible part of food, since it is not actually assimilated by the body, but cast off as waste.

As in all things, eating to relieve constipation must be done with intelligence and a consciousness of overall health. Of course, increase your cellulose instake, but not to the exclusion of other important food elements. Cut it down at some meals, and eat the protein you need. When your elimination has righted itself, stop concentrating on cellulose foods.

The Question of Fluids

The question of fluids always arises in a discussion of constipation. Does one have to consume 8 glasses of water per day? Do juices and teas count?

It has been our opinion that compulsory drinking of certain amounts of fluids is no more natural, hence useful, than the idea of being forced to eat a certain amount of meat each day. As with any other animal, we know when we're thirsty. The healthy body, used to healthful foods, and not misled by processed foods which might dull its innate discretion, is naturally aware of what it needs in the way of food or drink. No preordained amounts need be set to avoid illness. The kind of food and drink is what really matters.

When the body is not well, as in the case of constipation, the natural appetite cannot always be depended upon to act as it should. In some cases of constipation, simple lubrication is what is lacking. The waste matter is so hard and dry that even the peristaltic action can't get it to move. In *Dietetics Simplified* by Jean Bogert, Ph.D. (Macmillan, New York, New York), we're told that water is the best lubricant. In such conditions we say forced liquids are worth trying.

The how and when of this water drinking evokes other great discussions. It is generally conceded that a glass or two upon rising is most effective. In *Medical Treatment,* Evans says that hot or cold fluids are more effective than tepid ones. Physiologists point out that just about any liquid at that time would act to make the bowels move, since it is the first activity of the day for the stomach, and reactivates the stomach's dormant muscles. The muscles that move the body's waste are activated, too. There is also evidence to support both views that say it should only be warm and it should only be cold. The "warm" opinion seems to have the edge.

Some people swear that only hot tea or coffee will activate their

[625]

bowels. Others put lemon juice in water, some use lime. Mary T. Quelch in her book, *Herbal Remedies* (Faber and Faber, London), recommends saving the water in which green vegetables have been cooked, and drinking it in the morning. Again the choice is yours (though we recommend a low limit on citrus juice because of its effect on the teeth among other reasons), for no matter how the fluid comes into the body, physiologically it should have some effect.

If lubrication is the problem, fluid—water in some form, preferably plain—should help. The general recommendation is for 8 glasses of water a day. Make an effort to remember to drink this much until the constipation clears up, after that in our opinion, you should drink water only when you're thirsty.

Fats as Lubricants

Another group of lubricants suggested to help in constipation is fats. *The Handbook of Digestive Diseases* (C. V. Mosby) tells us that fats act as lubricants in neutral states (when they go through the body in their original form) and as mild irritants in their split state (broken down by body processes). The unsaturated fats, such as olive oil, safflower oil, peanut oil, corn oil, etc. should be excellent for this purpose. A few tablespoons per day would give the body valuable unsaturated fatty acids whether the constipation condition were relieved or not. Salads are another excellent way to make use of these valuable oils for alleviating problems of this type. The fibrous greens as well as the oil act to promote evacuation.

Dietetics Simplified tells us that wheat germ and brewer's yeast may be taken to attempt an increase in muscular tone and bowel activity. We are reminded by this that one of the most beneficial properties of yogurt and whey is their ability to increase useful intestinal bacteria vital in processing foods through the stomach and intestines on their way to the alimentary canal.

Your regular diet, if it is free from processed foods and high in proteins and fresh fruits in proper balance and fortified with food supplements, will prevent a recurrence of constipation. Try these natural remedies and prove to yourself that laxatives are unnecessary.

162. Is Water Drinking Important for Preventing Constipation?

There are few subjects in the health field more controversial than "How much water shall I drink?"

One school of thought believes that the drinking of quite large amounts of water is not only beneficial but absolutely necessary for good health. Drink as much as 14 glasses a day, say some authorities. Don't drink any water at all, say others. You are loading your tissues with water, washing out vitamins and minerals and you get plenty of water in food.

Animals drink when they are thirsty. And the horse's aversion to drinking more water than he happens to be thirsty for has been immortalized in the proverb, "You can lead a horse to water, but you can't make him drink." Animals won't drink unless they are thirsty. Is it possible to use the same rule for human beings, or have our abitrary food habits so disrupted our thirst mechanism that we don't really know when we need water?

Certainly it is easy to know when one feels thirsty. It's also obvious that a juicy piece of fruit, a stalk of celery or a cup of herb tea will quench thirst as effectively as a glass of water will. It is also obvious that people who eat lots of salt will want more liquids than those who eat very little salt, for salt attracts and holds water. Refined sugar does the same, for this, too, is an almost pure chemical from which all fiber and other things that accompany it in food have been removed. Eating something overly sweet is almost bound to make you thirsty.

On the basis of this reasoning, it seems that people who eat healthful meals which contain no white sugar or salt, meals in which fresh, raw, juicy vegetables and fruits play a big part would need to drink far less water than the average American eating the average American diet, grossly oversalted, deficient in raw foods and sticky with sugar.

Fruits contain anywhere from 75 to 90 per cent water. Vegetables contain from 75 to 95 per cent water. Meat, eggs, nuts, cheese, cereals and concentrated fats like French dressing and butter contain far less water. Fresh whole milk is about 87 per cent water and most fruit and vegetable juices are about 87 per cent water.

So we might decide that the person who lives on a diet of highly concentrated foods—animal proteins, cereals, seeds, nuts, and fats—should drink far more water than someone whose diet is rich in the less concentrated foods. It seems reasonable to assume that drinking large amounts of water, whether or not you are thirsty, would do considerable harm in dissolving water soluble vitamins and perhaps even in washing away those minerals which are not easily absorbed.

In Bridges' *Dietetics for the Clinician* (Lea and Febiger) it is suggested that drinking generous amounts of water with meals may decrease bacterial activity in the digestive tract. This could be beneficial or harmful, we suppose, depending upon whether the helpful or the putrefactive bacteria were washed out!

Possible Harm of Too Much Water

Yet down through the years health literature has been preaching "You must drink more water" almost as if water were something very unpleasant that people had to be urged and forced to partake of. Perhaps one reason for this is the fact that undoubtedly plenty of water is necessary in the intestines if constipation is to be prevented. And, if you are not going to get enough water in fresh foods to supply this, then undoubtedly you will have to drink your water out of a glass.

Water forms the bulk of the body and its loss is continuous. In *Dietetics for the Clinician* it is stated that the normal requirement for water is about two quarts a day. By "forcing fluids" we mean taking a glass every hour. Three quarts a day should be the limit.

Says John P. Peters in the chapter on "Water Balance in Health and Disease" in the book, *Diseases of Metabolism* (Saunders), "Animals normally drink water after eating. This dilutes the food in the alimentary canal, rendering it more soluble and diminishing the quantity of fluid that would have to be secreted (by the body) for the same purpose, and provides water for the excretion of the indigestible residue and the end products of metabolism derived from the food. If all or most of the nutrient elements of the diet are given in solution, thirst becomes a limiting nutritive factor. In this case, water is taken in behalf of the sense of hunger, but only so long as the load of water in the body, the normal regulator of thirst, does not exceed tolerable limits."

In other words, if you drink large quantities of fruit and vegetable juices, your body is counting on these juices for their food value, rather than their water value, so the sense of hunger is involved rather than that of thirst. However, it does appear, according to Dr. Peters, that we do need considerable amounts of water to keep the food in the digestive tract well moistened, so that residue can be carried out of the body.

So it appears that getting not enough liquid in your diet may be a cause of constipation. An article in the July, 1950, issue of *College and University Business* described an experiment involving constipated patients of a proctologist (that is, a specialist in diseases of the rectum). Fifty-five per cent of his patients were constipated. It usually occurs, the article tells us, in persons whose dietary bulk is far less than it should be and whose fluid intake is inadequate for wetting the residue in the bowel.

The average fluid intake of the constipated patient was 2½ pints (about 5 cups). The non-constipated individuals had an average fluid intake of 3½ pints—about 7 cups. This physician recommended to his constipated patients that they drink a full 8 ounce glass of water every waking hour. In addition, he insisted upon fresh or stewed fruit for breakfast, fresh fruit and bulky salad for lunch and salad and two servings of high-residue vegetables for dinner. In addition, fresh raw fruits should be eaten during the evening.

163. The Relationship between Vitamins and Constipation

Bran relieves constipation, not only because of the large amount of cellulose it contains, but mostly because it is a rich source of B vitamins. Treating alcoholic neuritis with B vitamins has resulted in regularizing the intestines. Giving rice bran or rice polishings has relieved constipation— again mostly because of the B vitamins.

G. Spiegel, M.D.
La Clinique, Paris,
March, 1939.

*   *   *

In the majority of pellagra cases, the patient is constipated. Patients complain of abdominal pain, discomfort and distention especially after meals. Pellagra is a disease of vitamin deficiency—a lack of B vitamins. As an experiment, thiamin, one of the B vitamins, was withheld from a group of individuals. Loss of appetite, nausea and vomiting followed. Constipation was the rule. Young men subjected to hard physical work and living on a diet deficient in B vitamins, especially thiamin, were victims of easy fatigability, apathy, muscle and joint pains, lack of appetite and constipation.

Clinical Nutrition
Jolliffe, Tisdall and Cannon
(Hoeber)

*   *   *

Experiments with animals reported by Dr. Clive McCay of Cornell University, showed that powdered brewer's yeast (rich in B vitamins) and the pulp left from making tomato and citrus juices (vitamins C and P and a wealth of minerals!) might help many older persons suffering from habitual constipation.

Science News Letter
November 19, 1950

*   *   *

We have known for many years how important is the vitamin and mineral content of the diet in preventing constipation. There is a great disturbance of the movements of the intestinal tract in vitamin B deficiency, for instance. The stomach and intestines are relaxed and sluggish. The emptying time of the intestine is twice as long in vitamin-B-deficient animals. And such animals respond with a greatly improved activity of the intestine when vitamin B is added to their diet.

Robertson and Doyle (*Journal of Nutrition,* Vol. 9, p. 553, 1935) showed that animals fed on a diet low in minerals were noticeably constipated while other animals fed the same diet, but with added minerals, were not.

Vitamins A, C and B_1 and B_2 are all needed to keep the mucous lining of the digestive tract in a healthy condition. Constipation and many ill-defined digestive disorders frequently clear up when additional amounts of these vitamins are given.

> *Dietetics Simplified*
> L. Jean Bogert, Ph.D. and
> Mame T. Potter, M.A.
> (Macmillan Company)

*   *   *

The need for vitamins and minerals to prevent constipation is not generally appreciated. For instance, the lack of thiamin (one of the B vitamins) produces many and varied disorders of the stomach and intestines. For patients who cannot take the rougher vitamin-carrying foods (he means bran here, we suppose) brewer's yeast is a valuable food.

> *Nutrition and Diet in Health
> and Disease*
> James S. McLester (Saunders)

*   *   *

In an experiment on deficiency in thiamin (vitamin B_1) it was found that the persons in the experiment who were eating a diet from which all thiamin had been removed suffered, among other things, from the following: fatigue, lack of appetite and constipation. The other symptoms were loss of weight, nausea and vomiting, backache and sore muscles, numbness, burning feet, mental depression, headache, very little digestive juice in the stomach and so forth. The diet which produced these symptoms was: polished rice, tapioca, cornstarch, sugar, white bread, butter, cottage and American cream cheese, egg white, cocoa, tea and white raisins. We are told that, had the diet been unknown, their physician would probably have told these individuals that they were suffering from chronic nervous exhaustion.

"The high-vitamin diet has wide application in the treatment of disease." Among conditions for which a high-vitamin diet should be prescribed are chronic gastro-intestinal disorders—constipation, colitis, diarrhea, gastric atony, hypochlorhydria (lack of hydrochloric acid in the stomach), visceroptosis (fallen abdominal organs), ulcer, sprue, pellagra.

Laboratory work with animals shows that deficiency of thiamin (vitamin B_1) and/or pantothenic acid (another B vitamin) and probably other members of the B complex as well causes loss of intestinal tone and decreased movement of the intestines. It is not easy to confirm these findings in human beings because relief from constipation often occurs after the taking of very bulky food. And one does not know whether it was the bulk or the B vitamins that did the trick. However, we know that our American diet is deficient in B vitamins. Hence brewer's yeast should be included in the diet. Wheat germ is another good food to include.

Bridges' Dietetics for the Clinician
(Lea and Febiger)

*   *   *

Dr. Gustav Martin and co-workers at the Warner Institute of Therapeutic Research studied the effects of different B vitamins on the intestinal tract. Separate vitamins were given and the researchers studied the movements of the intestines as each was taken. Only inositol (a part of the vitamin B complex) caused a marked increase in the intestinal movements. Poor appetites became normal and constipation was relieved. Of course more and better absorption of food occurred, as intestinal movement increased. One of the richest sources of inositol is blackstrap molasses.

Patients taking synthetic vitamin preparations are likely to become constipated because the imbalances of B vitamins created by such preparations can produce shortages in the very vitamins needed to protect against constipation.

A partial deficiency of potassium in animals causes constipation and gas formation. (Potassium is plentiful in fresh fruits and vegetables.) Sodium—table salt—in the diet causes your body to lose potassium. Cooking fruits and vegetables brings about great losses in potassium.

If so much fat is eaten that it cannot be absorbed, both fat and calcium are lost, for they combine to form a soapy substance which is excreted. This often becomes hardened in the intestine causing constipation.

Lack of calcium can cause spastic constipation. Plenty of calcium in the diet prevents cramps and spasms. Spasms in the intestines called by physicians spastic colitis or spastic constipation, can be relieved by getting plenty of calcium in the diet.

Enough protein in the diet is necessary for healthy intestines. The walls of the stomach and intestines are muscles which contract and relax alternately. When there is not enough protein in the diet these muscles cannot function as they should and the flabbiness resulting may cause the entire intestinal structure to "fall," so that organs are displaced and constipation results. Food remains undigested when the flabby walls of the intestine cannot contract normally.

Let's Eat Right to Keep Fit
Adelle Davis (Harcourt, Brace and Company)

[631]

164. A Chance to Fight Cystic Fibrosis

The story of cystic fibrosis has been told often in the picture magazines and newspapers, so most persons have had an opportunity to find out about this killer. The symptoms, life expectancy figures, average incidence per capita, amount of money spent per year by parents whose children are afflicted—all of this has been made public with the hope of bringing this problem to national attention. The only thing that was never included in all that publicity was a potential cure, some hopeful sign for stopping the advance of this inevitable killer once its presence was known. For almost 20 years the cause of cystic fibrosis, or CF, eluded every attempt at detection. Perhaps the situation is changed now.

An Almost Perfect Fatality Record

For those who are not familiar with cystic fibrosis, we can fill in a few facts on the disease. Its most tragic aspect is that it attacks only small children, and its record for fatality seldom varies in its completeness. The lubricating mucus secreted inside the body to help carry on the digestive processes, as well as other important body functions, is the source of the problem. Instead of the normal watery consistency, the mucus in cystic fibrosis victims is as thick as molasses. It blocks ducts in the pancreas so that essential enzymes cannot be secreted, and, in the case of the lungs, oxygen cannot pass through as it should. The activities thus curtailed are so basic that life without them is exceedingly difficult to sustain, and, necessarily, short.

Where the lungs are affected the problems of pneumonia and lung infection are a constant threat, and CF victims are often kept on daily doses of antibiotics to defend against these complications. The children build natural immunities to these antibiotics, one after the other, and eventually parents are faced with the possibility of exhausting the potency of all known drugs.

Enzymes Shut Off and True Digestion Impossible

Most commonly cystic fibrosis attacks the pancreas. It is in this organ that the enzymes are made. These juices are secreted into the intestines and they break down the foods we eat into nutritional components the body needs for self repair and normal function. When these enzymes do not appear, the food passes through the body intact, without having had the least bit of nutrition extracted from it. This is the case when CF affects this organ. It becomes coated with a thick layer of mucus which prevents the enzymes from being excreted into the intestines where they are needed. Eventually the victim of such a situation is bound to die of starvation, no matter how much he eats, because his food does him no good whatsoever. Parents and doctors try to forestall this eventual consequence by feeding foods that are very rich in nutrition, hoping that some will remain behind, and by feeding large doses of vitamins to the patients. But neither of these can be effective for very long. The all too vivid proof of that conclusion lies in the fact that the oldest living victim of cystic fibrosis is 21 years of age.

While we know what cystic fibrosis is, little has been discovered up to now about how and why it occurs. We have seen that CF occurs in about one in 600 live births. For some unknown reason, Negroes rarely have it, and CF is unknown in Orientals. It is hereditary and often occurs more than once in a single family. There is no problem of contagion involved. The victim has symptoms similar to bronchitis and asthma, with chronic coughing and wheezing a common feature. He also shows a very strong appetite, though his heavy eating only results in poor weight gain. There are frequent bowel movements throughout the day, all of them bulky and foul.

Diagnosis Difficult Until Recent Years

Because of the symptoms presented by cystic fibrosis, it was often confused with other diseases and difficult to diagnose accurately. A great step forward came not long ago when a simple test was devised to ascertain the presence of CF. It was discovered that CF patients sweat profusely and that their perspiration contains an unusually high percentage of salt. An easy system was devised for obtaining and analyzing samples of perspiration taken from the hand of the suspected victim.

Now, at least parents know what lies beneath the frightening picture presented by a child suffering from this disease. The doctor can say it is cystic fibrosis, and explain just what is going on inside the young body. The parents will want to know *why* it is happening to their child. What have they done that caused this terrible thing; what can they do to stop its advance?

This Could Be the Great First Step

An answer might lie in a piece by 3 researchers, W. A. Blanc, J. D. Reid, and D. H. Anderson written on the subject in *Pediatrics*, Vol. 22, p. 494, 1958. They discovered that the presence of an excess of fat in the stools is a major clinical indication of cystic fibrosis. This means that fat is not being properly absorbed by the body. The authors believe the reason for this is involved with a deficiency of vitamin E. They were able to find signs of fatty degeneration in the muscles of CF victims which were similar

[633]

to those found in experimental animals whose diet was intentionally kept short of vitamin E. Deposits of an insoluble pigment usually found in livers afflicted with cirrhosis are also found in the organs of cystic fibrosis patients. This same deposit can be induced in laboratory animals by withholding vitamin E from their diets. The important aspect of this discovery is that the added formation of this deposit can be *prevented* in animals by administration of vitamin E, though that which is already present is not affected.

It remains, of course, to discover whether or not the vitamin will affect humans in the same way. The authors are definite, however, in saying that these deposits in both animals and humans are chemically identical. The relationship between cystic fibrosis and this ceroid pigment deposit is strongly established by the fact that one examination of 38 three-year-old cystic fibrosis patients showed 37 to have such deposits. Of 392 patients not having pancreatic deficiency, cirrhosis of the liver or closure of the bile ducts, not a single one had any sign of this accumulation. We wonder though why a simple control experiment isn't set up, using two groups of similarly affected cystic fibrosis victims, giving extra vitamin E to one group, withholding it from the other. If the deductions above are correct, there should be some difference between the two groups regarding the development of the disease.

We are indeed happy to print this hopeful development on cystic fibrosis. If vitamin E is the answer, there need be no further incidence of this disease which is estimated to kill more children annually than cancer, polio, cerebral palsy, tuberculosis, muscular dystrophy or rheumatic fever. Prospective parents who suspect that their genes might carry this killer can hopefully increase their vitamin E intake; children in whom it is discovered early can fight its advance with a diet high in vitamin E, extending their life expectancy indefinitely.

Hope to See the Research Continued

On the face of the research of these 3 men, the role of vitamin E in the cystic fibrosis picture certainly demands further investigation. Unfortunately, vitamin therapy is often considered too tame and researchers ignore its possibilities in favor of the dramatic drugs with numerous x's and y's in their long names. We hope this will not be the case here. The mothers and fathers who have seen the awful effects of this disease should make every effort, through their local organizations and alone, to promote further inquiry into this most promising development yet seen in the fight against cystic fibrosis.

Vitamin E Can't Work Alone

And if vitamin E should emerge from all the testing with its effectiveness proven, parents must be cautioned that a single vitamin can't work in the body without the help of other nutrients. A diet of candy, cake and vitamin E tablets washed down with soda, won't prevent a case of cystic fibrosis, nor halt a case that is already developing. The nutrients of other

[634]

foods are important in processing the vitamin E before it can do its work. The B vitamins, for instance, appear in many of the same foods as vitaman E—seeds, nuts and whole cereals. The unsaturated fatty acids are found in these same foods. A diet which does not include unrefined natural sources of these vitamins is bound to be short in all these elements. Most American diets are like this.

Let those who use vitamin E, or any vitamin which seems to be in short supply in their body, as a preventive or a cure, be certain that their body has a full supply of other nutrients if they expect results. When experimental animals are tested with specific nutrients, the balance of their diet is carefully gauged to give the experimental factor every chance to prove itself. If you wish to achieve the results they get, you can do no less for yourself. A good diet is the surest way to include all the necessary nutrients in an adequate, natural manner. When this is being done, then the use of special vitamins to prevent or cure specific problems can be effective.

It is our belief that everyone should be taking a vitamin E supplement, even if he takes wheat germ and eats nuts, seeds, vegetable oils and other sources of vitamin E.

165. The Nutritional Aspect of Cystic Fibrosis

While most researchers concentrate on new ways to treat cystic fibrosis patients with antibiotics to prevent infection, some, we are glad to say, are working on another angle—nutritional deficiency. As we reported in the preceding chapter, it is known that the muscles of cystic fibrosis patients show the same kind of fatty degeneration which is found in the muscles of animals deficient in vitamin E. A certain substance found in the livers of these deficient animals is also found in livers of CF patients. Additional formation of this substance can be prevented in animals by giving them plenty of vitamin E. Whether or not this will happen with human beings is not known.

Now we have additional information along these lines. An article in *Pediatrics* for January, 1960, tells us that "most patients with cystic fibrosis have low levels of vitamin E in the blood." Harry Schwachman, M.D., author of the article, goes on to say that adding vitamin supplements to the diet is extremely important for these patients. He gives, he says, twice the commonly recommended dose of vitamins. Vitamin K is important, especially for children who have been operated on.

There may be signs of vitamin A deficiency, according to Dr. Schwachman, although, since water soluble vitamin A has been available, this is less common. He strongly recommends that vitamin E be added to the diet. You may have noted that all of the vitamins so far mentioned are fat-soluble vitamins. It seems reasonable that cystic fibrosis patients would be deficient in these, since one symptom of the disease is a disorder in the way the body handles fat. In addition, Dr. Schwachman states that the B vitamins are extremely important, too, so that, although laboratory evidence is lacking concerning requirements for the B vitamins, he recommends always supplementing the diet with these vitamins.

Some Children Very Deficient in Vitamin E

As we were doing research on cystic fibrosis, we were very interested to discover an article in the *Canadian Medical Journal* (May 28, 1960) on the subject of the condition of infants and children where vitamin E is concerned. Richard B. Goldbloom, M.D., of Montreal, author of the article states that for reasons not yet clear, infants and children are much more susceptible to a lowering of the vitamin E in the blood by a deficiency in diet than are adults. So individuals of the younger age group offer far greater opportunity for the study of possible effects of deficiency in vitamin E.

Interestingly enough, Dr. Goldbloom discovered that the levels of vitamin E are especially low in infants and children who suffer from diseases which cause steatorrhea (one of the difficulties in cystic fibrosis) and also that the vitamin E levels are much higher in the case of infants which have been breast-fed. He asks at the end of his article whether we should not consider adding vitamin E to the formula of children who are bottle-fed. He says that this is even more important in the case of premature children who are fed on skimmed milk formulas. Since the fat has been removed from the milk, there is no chance of their getting any vitamin E from it, since the vitamin E is contained in the fat—and precious little of it there is in milk to begin with—a "trace."

Dr. Goldbloom goes on to say that there has been understandable hesitation in recommending that we supplement milk formulas with vitamin E. And it is not yet established what harm may befall an infant who goes through the first year of life with little vitamin E in his blood and tissues. He says that the symptoms shown in a cystic fibrosis patient which seem to indicate deficiency in vitamin E do not occur until after the child is two years old.

He says, too, that "it is of some interest" that the United States Food and Drug Administration has recently decided that vitamin E is essential in human nutrition. We want to point out that, since vitamin E seems to be involved one way or another in many other diseases, like muscular dystrophy, skin disorders and heart disease, might it not be true that lack of this vitamin during infancy may be one of the main reasons for the high incidence of these other diseases as well as cystic fibrosis?

And the final clue to the whole tragic picture may turn out to be the substitution of a formula for mother's milk. There are many reasons why breast-feeding is infinitely preferable to bottle-feeding and the one we have discussed above is additional evidence to bolster the case of breast-feeding. Doesn't it seem possible, too, that even breast-fed babies may not get as much vitamin E as they should if their mothers are living on diets short of vitamin E? The chief source of the vitamin is the germ of cereals which is carefully removed in the processing of such foods as white flour, white rice, degerminated corn meal and so forth.

Even though the Food and Drug Administration has declared that vitamin E is essential for good health in human beings, they have consistently maintained that everyone gets enough vitamin E in his daily diet, so there is no need to take vitamin E as a supplement. How they know this, we cannot conceive, unless they have personally followed every American throughout every day and observed what he eats.

But how can they continue to say this, when there is now ample proof that bottle-fed babies have far less vitamin E in their blood than breast-fed ones and lack of vitamin E seems to be related to a number of serious diseases of childhood? Children fed on milk formulas seem to be getting so much less vitamin E than they should have that a Canadian researcher proposes adding the vitamin to all formulas!

Does it take a great deal of imagination to suppose that supplementing everyone's diet with plenty of vitamin E just might result: (1.) in mothers who are able to breast-feed their children; (2.) children who can withstand diseases like cystic fibrosis, muscular dystrophy and so on, even though they have an inherited tendency toward them; and (3.) a considerable decline in the incidence of other diseases related to vitamin E deficiency—heart diseases, skin diseases, etc.?

One More Note on Cystic Fibrosis

Dr. Schwachman in his article in *Pediatrics* stresses the importance of a diet high in protein and low in fat. He says that the amount of fat allowed depends on the patient's reaction to it. Most patients can tolerate the amount of fat in homogenized milk, he says, but he may advise not giving them butter, ice cream, peanut butter, potato chips, fried potatoes and mayonnaise if these foods produce cramps, discomforts or bulky or frequent bowel movements. In some patients considerable reduction in fat intake is necessary, he says.

We would, of course, not advise any of the foods listed above except the peanut butter, if it is made from fresh peanuts and no hydrogenated oil is added.

Since Dr. Schwachman names highly processed items in his list of possibly forbidden foods, doesn't it seem possible, too, that it may be this quality of the food that is causing harm in these patients who obviously have difficulty with fatty foods to begin with? We doubt that completely

[637]

natural food like sunflower seed (also high in fats) would cause any trouble.

It seems to us that the answer to preventing cystic fibrosis is certainly near at hand, if our researchers will pursue the path they have started out on—diets for both mothers and children that are rich in all the vitamins—especially vitamin E—and every effort made by physicians to encourage breast feeding as the finest and most nutritious method of feeding infants.

SECTION 30: DIABETES

166. Diabetes in Modern Times

Diabetes afflicts close to a million Americans and it is believed by experts that another million may have the disease without knowing it. What causes it? We do not know. We do know that it is a disorder of the glands, chiefly the pancreas. Because of the complicated way glands work, the pituitary and the adrenals are also closely involved in what goes wrong inside the disturbed body processes of the diabetic. Mild diabetes is easily controlled by diet. More severe cases must take insulin and, furthermore, must look forward to taking insulin the rest of their lives. Insulin is the substance secreted by the pancreas. The diabetic is unable to produce enough insulin to keep his metabolic mechanism running efficiently, so insulin made from the glands of animals is injected to replace his own.

What is a typical "liberalized" diet for a diabetic? According to H. J. John in the December, 1951, issue of the *Annals of Internal Medicine,* the diabetic patient eliminates sugar, pastry and soft drinks; restricts bread to two slices per meal, and omits bread if he eats potatoes; uses fresh fruit (or fruit canned without sugar) or crackers and cheese for dessert. If he gains weight he cuts down a bit.

We ask you, wherein lies the hardship in eating like this every day? It is exactly the kind of diet we recommend except that we would never recommend eating so much bread. And certainly not crackers and cheese for dessert. So we cannot wail with the diabetic whose complaints are that his health forces him to eat such a diet as this. We think everybody should!

For years we have known that the body of the diabetic has difficulty in dealing with carbohydrates. We also know that the B vitamins are absolutely necessary for the proper use of carbohydrates by the body and we know that B vitamins have been removed from our food at just about the same rate that the incidence of diabetes has increased. Doesn't it seem possible that the lack of B vitamins may be one of the causes of diabetes?

Vitamin B Is Important for Diabetics

We find a number of authorities recommending that diabetics should get more B vitamins than normal folks get. *Diseases of Metabolism* (edited by Garfield G. Duncan, M.D., and published by W. B. Saunders Company) tells us that there is considerable evidence that diabetic patients require more of the vitamin B complex—especially thiamin, niacin, vitamin B_{12} and riboflavin—than do normal people. Many of the nondescript aches and pains of the diabetic are prevented to a large extent by taking brewer's yeast with every meal. He goes on to remind us that refined foods simply do not contain all the vitamins that the original food possessed. Calcium, too, it seems is lost by the diabetic to such an extent that decalcification of bones is common in elderly diabetics. A sure thing that bone meal should be added to food supplements.

Elmer Alpert, M.D., writing in the *New York State Journal of Medicine,* for November 15, 1953, tells us that diabetics whose intake of vitaman B is low will find that taking a food supplement rich in vitamin B may decrease the insulin requirement, and bring about considerable improvement in the diabetes.

He also reminds us that the diabetic's liver is likely to be functioning improperly. This will result in the patient not being able to get all of the possible vitamin A from vegetable foods like carrots that have a lot of it. In this case, of course, vitamin A should be taken in a supplement. We must remember that at the onset of diabetes great thirst is a symptom. Satisfying that thirst with large quantities of water can "wash out" the B vitamins and vitamin C, both of which are soluble in water. So it seems likely that the diabetic may be short on vitamins B and C.

We are told by Bicknell and Prescott (*Vitamins in Medicine*) that an injection of insulin lowers the level of vitamin C in the blood and seems to redistribute it to the other parts of the body. They include a picture of a diabetic patient suffering from a terrible skin eruption which was cured completely within a few days by massive doses of certain B vitamins and brewer's yeast.

In Bridges, *Dietetics for the Clinician,* a classic book for doctors on this subject, we find this comment on diabetes and refined foods: "Increasing evidence is accumulating to indicate that vitamin deficiencies are more common in average dietaries than formerly supposed. Present-day milling processes with the production of highly refined flours are robbing American foods of much of the greatly needed vitamin B complex. It has been estimated that only about 9 per cent of this substance derived from grain is now present, as compared to the flours of a hundred years ago . . .

"Since these facts obtain in the average unrestricted American dietary

[639]

of today, it is to be expected that it will be all the more true where special restrictions are imposed as in diabetes. Apparently the greatest danger of inadequacy is in the B complex. (We want to point out, however, that vitamin E is also removed from flour when it is refined.) . . . Deficiencies in the vitamin B group have been reported in diabetes even where the calorie needs were well supplied. It would appear that pellagra-like symptoms may be induced by the rapid metabolizing of carbohydrate stores. Glossitis, cheilitis, delirium and other pellagra-like symptoms seen in certain cases have been caused to subside by the administration of nicotinic acid (or niacin, one of the B vitamins). The so-called "protective foods" such as dairy products, eggs, green vegetables and fruits, though excellent sources of minerals and certain other vitamins cannot be taken in sufficient quantity to compensate for the low vitamin B concentration in highly refined flour. It would seem wise, therefore, especially in diabetic diets, to avoid highly milled products and in certain instances to add the vitamin B complex in the form of concentrates or food adjuncts." We, of course, advocate taking brewer's yeast, richer in all the B vitamins than any other food.

Vitamins for Diabetics

Here is a sample of the amounts of vitamins one physician (Dr. Alpert) believes necessary in case there is evidence of deficiency. He gives his diabetic patients a formula containing: 10 milligrams of thiamin, 10 milligrams of riboflavin, 100 milligrams of niacin, 300 milligrams of vitamin C, 5000 International Units of vitamin A and 400 units of vitamin D, in addition to other lesser members of the B complex of vitamins. Take a glance at the food supplements you and your family are taking at the present time. Do they give you anything like this amount of B vitamins? Of course, as you know, you should get the B vitamins from natural sources like yeast—not synthetics.

Vitamin E for diabetes? Some researchers say yes, others say no.

We know that disorders of the blood vessels are common among diabetics. Some time ago we received a letter from a diabetic M.D. suffering from advanced gangrene whose leg had to be amputated. In an effort to save his other leg, he took large doses of vitamin E. Not only did the other leg and foot return to normal, but his blood pressure and blood sugar did the same. He had no need for insulin from that time on.

Drs. Evan and Wilfrid Shute of the Shute Clinic, London, Ontario, Canada, who treated this physician use vitamin E regularly in the treatment of diabetes and report outstanding success with it.

Exercise Is Good for the Diabetic

We were gratified to find in several articles on diabetes the most emphatic recommendation of exercise for the diabetic. In *Diseases of Metabolism* we are told that exercise is "of inestimable value." It improves the patient's tolerance for carbohydrate foods and reduces the need for insulin.

Exercise lowers the blood sugar level. Then, too, the many diabetics who are overweight can take off pounds by exercising. Sugar in the urine tends to occur when the patient is physically inactive and subsides when he is active.

Of course, in the case of underweight diabetics whose bodies have begun to waste away, diet and insulin are necessary before the patient can begin a course of exercise.

Laurance K. Kinsell, M.D., writing in the journal, *Diabetes*, for July-August, 1955, tells of a diabetic friend, 47 years old, who plays strenuous tennis year in and year out. He believes the excellent condition of this man's arteries is the result of this exercise. And apparently the very fact that he exercises every day allows him far greater freedom in diet than he would have otherwise.

Dr. Kinsell also tells us that the average diabetic child who goes to camp in the summer finds that his insulin requirement has decreased by more than 40 per cent. "Factors other than exercise may play some part in this remarkable change, but it seems reasonable to assume that increased physical activity is the major factor which is responsible."

If you already have diabetes, you will undoubtedly find that exercise will benefit you. Does this mean you must enroll at a gym or take up tennis or golf? Not at all! The best things in life are free and one of the very best things in life, we believe, is walking. Every day, summer or winter, walk for a half hour, if that is all the time you can spare. An hour, or even two or 3 are better! Not only will you be busy manufacturing insulin while you walk, but you will be breathing in good fresh air which will carry oxygen to every cell of your body. You'll feel better, you'll sleep better, you'll be better!

167. Good News for Diabetics

Diabetes is a disorder of the body's mechanism for dealing with carbohydrates—starches and sugars. So we commonly think of it as a disease related only to the starch part of our diet. Yet diabetes specialists know fat metabolism is also disordered in the diabetic patient.

In fact, a diet too high in fat may be one of the most important causes of diabetes.

It is not surprising, therefore, to find that diseases of the heart and arteries are common among diabetics, for these conditions have been shown to be closely related to the amount and kind of fat eaten throughout one's lifetime.

We are told that arteriosclerosis or hardening of the arteries can be expected in practically all cases of diabetes, if they live long enough. Diabetics are particularly susceptible to coronary disease (disease of the coronary artery which leads into the heart). More than half of all living diabetics will die of some disease of the blood vessels or heart caused by "occlusion"—that is, blocking of an important artery, usually the heart artery.

In a study of 349 diabetics, compared with 3400 non-diabetics, it was found that 51 per cent of the diabetics had a significant amount of hardening of the arteries with narrowing of the heart arteries or blockage. This compared with only 18 per cent of non-diabetics.

So we see that the way the body uses fat has a great deal to do with the health of diabetics and their chance for a long and useful life. Accumulations of fatty materials (chiefly cholesterol) in the blood appear to be the cause of many heart and vascular disorders. So anything which contributes to lowering the blood level of fatty materials would seem to be beneficial for the diabetic.

We were especially pleased to find an article on this subject in the *Lancet* for January 9, 1960, in which certain food substances were tried to see what their effect would be on the level of fats in the blood of young diabetics. The results are most interesting and suggest that diabetics can do much to improve their condition and possibly to decrease the amount of insulin they must take, by including certain kinds of food in their daily meals.

Unsaturated Fatty Acids Important for All

The secret ingredient that made these hopeful words possible? The unsaturated fatty acids. These are certain fatty compounds that appear chiefly in fats of vegetable origin. We have written about them in relation to prostate gland disorders, skin conditions, heart and artery ailments and many more. Now we find that diabetics can profit greatly from the use of food products containing large amounts of these fats. In the experiments, it is well to note, these fats were *substituted* for fats of animal origin —they were not simply added to diets already heavy with fat.

The authors, Drs. Salt, Wolff, Nestadt and Lloyd of the Children's Hospital, Birmingham, England, tell us that complications involving the blood vessels may begin very early in young diabetics; the level of fats in the blood may be higher in those patients whose blood sugar is higher, and the high level of fat may be responsible for the vascular conditions.

Much as a diabetic may try to control the variations of his blood sugar through diet and insulin-taking, our authors say that "in practice one cannot expect that blood-sugar control will be maintained through the years strictly enough to keep the serum lipids (fats) always at a minimum." So they experimented with diets high in unsaturated fats—sunflower seed oil or corn oil. When they substituted these fats in exactly equal amounts (speaking in terms of calories) to match the animal fats that the children had been getting in their diets, they found that the blood fats were reduced to levels they could not achieve with insulin and these low levels of fat in the blood were maintained even when less insulin than usual was given.

Fourteen young, diabetic patients between 2 and 14 participated in the experiment. Some were given sunflower seed, some took corn oil. During part of the experiment, the usual fat in the diet was reduced and an emulsion of the vegetable oil in water "suitably flavored" was given 3 times a day. Altogether the patients took 50 grams of oil which contained about 30 grams of linoleic acid—the one fat supposedly most effective in lowering the blood cholesterol.

The patients taking sunflower seed oil took it for 28 days. The amount of cholesterol in the blood was reduced decidedly and remained so throughout all the trial period. When the oil was discontinued, the level of cholesterol returned to what it had been before the experiment.

The same results occurred with patients on corn oil. Two of these were taken off corn oil during the experiment and then returned to it. In both cases the level of cholesterol fell when the corn oil was returned to the diet.

Why do results like this occur? What is the relationship between sugar in the blood and fat in the blood? Our authors admit that the cause "remains obscure." However, they are quite sure that too-high levels of fat in the blood can be reduced by insulin, or, equally well, by giving unsaturated fats instead of saturated fats—note those words "instead of." The object is not to add fat to the diet, but rather to substitute one kind of fat for another.

Circulatory Diseases Threaten Diabetics

The authors of this article feel that their experiment has great significance for diabetics, especially young diabetics, because in the young people complications involving blood vessels may be prevented before they develop into something serious. They point out that if, by taking unsaturated fats, the diabetic can reduce his insulin dosage, this too is a great advantage, since taking insulin must be carefully regulated over a lifetime and, if a bit too much is taken, the patient runs the risk of insulin shock.

We would go on a bit further and suggest that the healthy person might see that his diet contains plenty of unsaturated fats as a possible help in regulating his blood sugar so that he will never risk getting diabetes. For diabetics, of course, it seems apparent that the wisest course is to get plenty of these healthful fats in every day's diet.

The patients in this experiment took 50 grams of oil daily. This would be roughly 3 tablespoonfuls of oil—surely not a large amount to include regularly in every day's meals, especially if you also delete most fats of animal origin and use nothing but vegetable fats. This means no butter, lard, chicken or pork fat of any kind. No milk or other dairy products such as cheese which are quite high in animal fats. It means using fatty foods like nuts, avocados, sunflower seeds and, finally, salad oils—seed, cereal and vegetable oils like corn oil, sunflower seed oil, olive oil, cotton-seed oil, peanut oil and so forth.

It might be best to start such a program by checking exactly how much fat from animal sources you are using at present, then begin to substitute vegetable fats, while at the same time you increase your intake of the foods listed above and cut down on fatty meats. Incidentally, fats from fish are good sources of unsaturated fats—the kind that reduce cholesterol—so do not cut down on these. And, of course, wheat germ oil and fish liver oil (two food supplements you should be taking) contain considerable quantities of the unsaturated fats. Be sure to include them with your daily supplements.

168. A New Diet

A new theory on diets for diabetics came our way recently from a Cuban medical journal, *Acta endocrinologica Cubana* Vol. 2, p. 79, September-October, 1954.

Described in the *International Medical Digest* as "a simplified new method for the management and instruction of diabetic patients which offers a new way of living for diabetics," the article presents the experience of Dr. Carlos P. Lamar with a group of his own diabetic patients.

Dr. Lamar tells us that diabetes is a disease involving the incorrect use of both fat and carbohydrates by the body. The ill effects of diabetes, he says, are produced by the incomplete combustion of fats, either from food or from the body store. This is the result of not enough sugar being "burned" either because of the lack of insulin (the gland secretion made by the pancreas) or because the diet is too restricted in sugars in proportion to the amount of fat eaten. This, he says, is how the usual diabetic diet is planned—far too much fat and too little sugar.

We have said above that, in order to "burn" sugar, that is, turn sugar into energy, the body must have an ample supply of the pancreas hormone known as insulin. The diabetic cannot supply enough of this from his own glands, so he must take it in the form of an injection.

But if we could find a sugar which the body can turn into energy without calling out any insulin, wouldn't this make the diabetic's life much simpler? Dr. Lamar says there is such a sugar and that by using this sugar wisely in prescribed diets he has revolutionized treatment for a group of his patients. The sugar which does not need insulin for its conversion into energy is fructose which occurs in fresh fruit.

"When sufficient fructose is provided in the diet, the body cells obtain most of their necessary fuel energy from this sugar and less insulin is then required," says Dr. Lamar. The fructose also makes the protein in the diabetic's diet go farther and thus helps from that angle, too.

However, fruits also contain glucose. And glucose is a sugar which does demand insulin for its proper use by the body. So, says Dr. Lamar, a certain amount of glucose remains in the body, unburned, and passes into the blood and the urine. But, he says, this does not cause the usual symptoms of diabetes "so long as enough of the fructose and of the glucose are properly utilized by the metabolic system." In other words, the diabetic who provides his digestive machinery with enough fructose can maintain a normal metabolism and health by by-passing the use of insulin entirely and thus avoid all the disturbances of fat digestion which, according to Dr. Lamar, are the real cause of the symptoms and signs of diabetes.

Patients Confirmed Dr. Lamar's Theory

He has kept some patients in conditions of very high blood sugar for months at a time, he says, and they have experienced no thirst, no increase in urine output and, most important at all, no "ketonurias," the term given to the presence of certain undesirable substances in the urine. Furthermore, much smaller amounts of insulin are required and there is less danger of *hypoglycemia* or so-called "insulin shock" because on Dr. Lamar's diet, the level of sugar in the blood is always kept high.

Providing large amounts of sugars high in fructose (that is, those which occur in fruit) seems to relieve the stress on the pancreas, he tells us. All of his patients have needed less and less insulin as time went on and some of them are taking no insulin at all, even though in some cases they had used it for more than 20 years previously.

"Every one of the patients . . . has experienced an impressive subjective improvement to an almost unbelievable degree . . . Nervousness, irritability, depressions . . . circulatory disorders, diabetic (nervous disorders), impotence and menstrual disorders have improved or disappeared and have been replaced by a state of euphoria with increasing energy and vigor."

Provisions of Dr. Lamar's Diet

We think that any reader who is diabetic or is threatened with diabetes should take this information to his doctor and ask him to send for the copy of *International Medical Digest* for October 1957, in which Dr. Lamar's article is reviewed in English. For there he will find, on page 220, the core of the basis for this new treatment. Dr. Lamar states that the chief purposes of his diet are to provide a maximum of fuel energy from sugars in which the proportion of fructose is as high as possible. So foods should be chosen in which there is more fructose than glucose, or at least as much. Such foods are fruits. In starchy foods, such as potatoes and cereals (and, of course, refined carbohydrates like white flour products), there is a large amount of glucose with little, if any, fructose. So such foods should be avoided. •

[645]

The second provision of Dr. Lamar's diet is to keep it low in animal fats which, he says, will keep the cholesterol content of the blood low and avoid difficulty with hardening of the arteries, high blood pressure, fatty liver, diabetic gangrene because of obstruction in the blood vessels, and so forth.

If the patient is underweight, he may wish to take enough insulin to use all the glucose he is getting in his diet. If he is overweight, then he can simply let this sugar "spill over" into his urine and be excreted. In this way it will not be turned into unwanted fat.

We do not think that any diabetic should try an experiment like this for himself. That is, we would be the last to recommend that anyone skip insulin shots just to see how his new diet is working. As long-time diabetics know well, you can get into serious or perhaps fatal trouble this way. But we do think you should talk over this idea with your doctor and ask him to work out a new diet for you along these lines in terms of your present insulin requirement.

And for those of us who have no diabetes but want to eat so that we never will have diabetes, doesn't it seem that the best part of wisdom is to get your sugars from fresh fruits? Keep your diet low in starchy foods (omitting entirely those made from refined starches) and cut down on foods high in animal fat.

169. Diabetes and the Weather

"Fair today. Cloudy and colder tomorrow." What does such a weather forecast mean to you in terms of health? Is it true that the weather makes a difference in the way you feel or do you just imagine it?

In his book, *Medical Climatology* (published by Charles C. Thomas in 1939) Clarence A. Mills, Ph.D., M.D., presents a theory that climate and weather play a very important part in man's health; then he traces the influence of these on a number of different diseases. In the section on diabetes, he explores all the information available on the severity and frequency of this disease in different climates.

Dr. Mills' discoveries about diabetes are astonishing. In the United States, for example, diabetes causes more than twice as many deaths in the colder northern section as in the gulf states. You would expect to find a great deal more diabetes in New England, says Dr. Mills, since it is a disease of middle and old age and the age level of the population is higher in New England than in other regions. But he found, instead, that Iowa and Nebraska are highest in the incidence and severity of diabetes and he ascribes it to the high climatic weather stimulation in that region—that is, the sudden changes in temperature and the bitter winter storms.

[646]

It appears from evidence he has gathered that the heat and energy produced by the body are directly dependent on climatic conditions and on the ease with which heat is lost from the body. Because all the energy created by combustion of food is not used by the body, there is a lot of waste heat to be disposed of, which makes a cooling system necessary, just like in a gasoline engine. This loss of heat can be accomplished much more easily in a cooler climate. However, in climates where there are great changes from season to season and where stormy periods of weather have a far-reaching effect on body mechanisms, the terrific stimulation of such a climate produces some unwelcome symptoms in the health of the individuals who live there.

Relationship Between Weather and Existence

Dr. Mills says that human development, resistance to infection and energy level of existence are closely linked to "the degree of climatic drive" under which the individual or population mass lives. In the damp heat of the tropics, for instance, existence may be depressed close to the purely vegetative level, because body heat loss is difficult. But in temperate regions —specifically the northern part of the United States and Europe—too severe stimulation by cold and storms and constantly changing weather may cause exhaustion and body breakdown to such an extent as to lower mass efficiency and "set limits to human advance."

Because heat and energy produced in the body seem directly dependent on climatic conditions and ease of heat loss, you would expect to find most disturbances in the organs and tissues chiefly involved in this combustion process. Diabetes is the functional breakdown on the body's combustion engine in handling and burning glucose. And the body normally depends on this combustion of glucose for about 85 per cent of its heat and energy.

So we find that diabetes develops with great frequency among people who move from the south to the north and it occurs most often within the first few years after they move. This Dr. Mills ascribes to the vigorous stimulation of the northern storm belt. In any world survey of diabetes, it is found that practically the only places where it is frequent and serious enough to cause alarm are the stormy, cooler regions of Europe and North America. It occurs so seldom and in such a mild form in the tropical countries that very little attention is paid to it there.

The Effect of Diet and Weather

We were interested to see that, in his studies of diabetes among the Chinese, Dr. Mills found that Chinese who "indulge in European food extensively are prone to have diabetes, while on their native diets they are very free from it." Furthermore, when they return to their usual diet their symptoms disappear. Among the Chinese, as among dwellers in the tropics, insulin must be administered to diabetics with great care, for the reaction to even a very small dose can cause death, whereas the amounts of insulin taken by northern European or American diabetics would surely prove fatal.

But, you may ask, why all this talk about climate? Isn't it true that diabetes is based on—or possibly caused by too heavy a consumption of sugar? Therefore those people who consume the most sugar should have the highest rate of diabetes. In Dr. Mills' chart showing sugar consumption in relation to diabetes incidence, we find that 11 countries highest in sugar consumption are among the 13 highest in diabetes. But on the other hand, Hawaii, Argentina and Cuba, with relatively high sugar consumption have relatively low diabetes rates.

Of course, adds Dr. Mills, the excessive stimulation of the weather in those regions where diabetes is high may cause an increased desire for sweets, for quick added energy. Also in the regions where diabetes prevails, standards of living are high, so that this desire may be satisfied to the full. In many of these regions, too, less hard physical work is done, and the sugar that is eaten becomes still more excessive in terms of the body's ability to consume it.

So Dr. Mills advises that whenever it is practical and can be arranged without too great disruption of family or economic arrangements, diabetes patients should consider moving to a warmer climate, in fact, the farther south they go, the more their symptoms are likely to abate. Going south for just the winter will also help, he says, provided they take some pains to accustom themselves to the stimulating northern weather when they return.

While Dr. Mills' theory is interesting, we cannot help but wonder whether, just on the basis of the Chinese experiment, diet has not a great deal more to do with symptoms of diabetes than climate or any other one factor. Or, taking it from another point of view, if the reaction of the climate on our internal combustion engines is so important (and it seems to us that it is), how much more important must be the fuel that we stoke into that combustion engine! If we feed it with devitalized fuel from which all the nourishment has been taken, can even the most favorable weather counteract the smoky, slow-burning flame we manage to coax into being?

So our advice would be—yes, go south in the winter, if you can, to avoid symptoms of diabetes. But, the year 'round, prevent the possibility of diabetic symptoms by watching closely the fuel you stoke into your metabolism furnace: avoid salt and sugar. If you possibly can, eat organically grown foods, stressing those whose vitamin content is richest; supplement this diet with brewer's yeast, bone meal and vitamin preparations from natural sources. Then, summer or winter, sunshine or storm, no fear of diabetes need distress you.

170. Carob Flour for Diarrhea

In the *South African Practitioner* for January, 1959, appears an article the subject of the effectiveness of carob flour as a treatment for diarrhea written by Thomas R. Plowright of Fresno, California.

Dr. Plowright was faced with treating cases of diarrhea among the children of migrant workers living under typically poor conditions during the harvest season. The children were all under 4 and most of them were under one year of age. While their parents were working in the fields, these youngsters had not had proper care, resulting in an average of 50 cases of diarrhea a month at the local hospital.

Tests for bacteria showed that the children were not suffering from some infectious disease. The cause of the diarrhea, according to Dr. Plowright, was probably a combination of these: poor eating habits, inadequate diet, excessive exposure to heat and poor sanitary conditions at the labor camps where the migrants lived. The children were brought to the hospital suffering from vomiting and diarrhea that resulted in as many as 15 to 20 stools a day. The doctors had tried all the usual anti-diarrhea medications without results.

Tried Carob Flour

Dr. Plowright decided to try a preparation of carob flour. Twenty of a group of 40 babies were placed on the usual hospital treatment—a period of not feeding at all, followed by a highly mineralized preparation given with diluted boiled milk. As the child began to improve, the strength of the milk was increased until the child was on the "going-home" formula.

The other 20 babies received exactly the same treatment except that they also got a 5 per cent solution of the carob flour preparation—as much as could be tolerated every 4 hours. As soon as a true-formed stool was passed, the carob preparation was diluted half-and-half with the infant's "going-home" formula.

The results were striking. The average number of hours needed to secure a formed stool in the babies who did not get the carob was 174.3. Those which did get the carob were on their way back to health *within 47.95 hours.* The total hospital stay of the first group was 14.15 days, whereas the children getting the carob could leave the hospital within a little more than 7 days. The average number of hours before complete cure in the first group was 339.6 while in the group given carob it was 120.05.

These figures leave little doubt as to the effectiveness of carob in controlling this condition which, of course, can be extremely serious, especially in very young children. It seems to us that exactly the same results can be obtained at home, since carob is a delicious and nutritious food which can be given in any quantity without a moment's hesitation.

What is carob flour and why are we so enthusiastic about it? It is the finely ground pods of the carob or honey locust tree. These pods are believed to be the "locusts and wild honey" that John the Baptist lived on in the wilderness. It is also thought that the "husks" in the story of the prodigal son may have been the pods of the carob tree.

Some Further Facts About the Carob Tree

Dr. Plowright goes on to tell us, "Cultivation of the tree began in historical times and was diffused by the Greeks in Italy and Greece and was carried by the Arabs as far west as Spain and Morocco. In these countries the fruit has been used for forage, as food by the poorer people, and for the manufacture of syrups and various fermented drinks. It was the main sustenance of Wellington's troops during the Peninsular campaign. It has been said that an acre of carob trees on arid soil yields much greater quantities of food matter than an equal area of alfalfa. These trees were introduced into the United States in 1954 from Spain.

"During the Spanish Civil War it was noticed by Ramos of Barcelona, Spain, that the children of the poorer classes in Barcelona who ate the fruit of the carob tree had fewer diarrheal disturbances, than did those of the wealthier classes. Using this as his criteria, he made a concoction using the dried pulp of the roasted carob mixed with starch for the treatment of diarrhea. The product was manufactured abroad under the name of Arobon. Since the time of this original study of the material, numerous reports have been published in the foreign literature."

We like to recommend carob flour as food rather than medicine. And it seems to us that using carob rather than sugar is a fine idea. It has a sweet taste, rather "chocolaty." You can use it in recipes that call for sugar, you can sprinkle it on fruit or use it to flavor fruit drinks. It is a very worthwhile food containing vitamins and minerals in ample quantity and, since its sugar content is as natural as that of fresh fruit, we approve of it highly.

Whether or not you make carob part of your menu-planning, do keep some on hand, especially during the summer months for use in case of sudden attacks of diarrhea. It is not easily available, so it is best to keep a supply.

171. Buttermilk or Bananas for Diarrhea and Dysentery

The advice of most experienced responsible pediatricians and obstetricians to the prospective mother is: "Nurse your child, if at all possible, for at least 6 months." That is the way nature meant the child to be nourished and that is the way he should be nourished to insure maximum growth and good health. It should be remembered that cow's milk and other types of infant feeding were improvisations when mother's milk was unavailable. They were, and are, a substitute, a poor second, intended for use when the real thing—human breast milk—is not sufficient to feed the child.

Over the years the use of this substitute milk has become more and more commonplace. Mothers often don't even make the attempt to nurse their babies. They say they haven't the time to nurse; they are afraid of losing their figures; they say nursing ties them down; they say nursing is painful; they worry about the pain they might have in drying their breasts when the nursing months are over. In short—they don't want to nurse their babies.

Baby Comes First

It may be an old-fashioned concept, but we feel that the baby's comfort and development should be the primary concern here, not the mother's. About the only valid argument listed above is that nursing does tie a mother down. She must be available when her baby is hungry. But, practically speaking, a new mother is usually there when her baby is hungry anyway. In the first few months after childbirth, mother usually wants to be close to home, to tend to her new baby, to be sure he is taken care of as only she can do it. What difference is it to her then if she nurse him at her breast or hold a bottle for him? The difference to the baby is great, however, for he gains much in the security of the sucking he does and the caressing his mother gives him. He gains much from the nutrition contained in the natural formula of his mother's milk. Scientists are agreed on this, and even the most modern doctors must admit that this is so. The baby who is bottle-fed is missing something.

Now there are cases in which for one reason or another breast-feeding is not possible, and the decision on whether or not to nurse is really out of the mother's hands. It is for such situations that bottle-feeding was intended. The aim, then, should be the closest possible approximation of human breast milk. Cow's milk does not really fill the bill. Ass' and mare's milks are actually better. Of course, availability dictates what is used, to a large extent. Cow's milk is easiest to get and, consequently, the cheapest. The baby's fed that unless he shows that he cannot tolerate it.

[651]

The Value of Buttermilk

Over the years, since the mid-nineteenth century, it has been common practice to modify cow's milk by dilution, the addition of certain carbohydrates, etc. This procedure can become extremely complicated and such complexities led to the popular canned formulae many doctors order. One simple answer to what to do with whole cow's milk to make it more digestible for more infants was discovered by the Dutch in 1865. They sold butter to Britain and Germany, and in looking for a use for the surplus buttermilk, they found that hogs and babies thrived on it. The usage for babies became so popular that almost the entire supply was given over to infant feeding. Soon a cultured whole buttermilk was introduced to meet the demand. That is, fresh or pasteurized whole milk—not merely the residue from butter-making—could be made into a smooth buttermilk merely by the addition of a "starter" that consisted of a souring bacteria. Eventually, further scientific evaluation of buttermilk and sweet milk showed that the main difference between the two is that buttermilk contains .75 per cent lactic acid. Adding this amount of lactic acid to sweet milk was found to be the easiest, most efficient way to make good buttermilk. Later, apple cider, vinegar and lemon juice were found to be fairly good substitutes for lactic acid in this procedure.

Why is buttermilk so much more desirable than sweet milk in formula? For one thing, it is a complete change in composition. After all, add sugar, dilute cow's milk, or whatever else you wish, and essentially you still have cow's milk. However, when milk is soured, some of the work digestion does to change the structure of whole milk (curdling it) has already been done. The body must release hydrochloric acid to transform sweet milk to the proper acidity. In buttermilk the lactic acid has already performed this job.

Doctors Testify

In their article on this subject in *Postgraduate Medicine* (July, 1956), Drs. Willis Blue and Wilburt Davidson of Duke University School of Medicine and Duke Hospital, Durham, North Carolina, asserted that digestion is not an advantage in acidified over sweet milk. Both, they say, are interchangeable as far as weight gain and digestion are concerned. But, "lactic acid milk will prevent intestinal infections and will remain sterile for 3 days at room temperature. The widespread use of lactic acid milk in North Carolina has undoubtedly been an important factor in the reduction in the incidence of dysentery and diarrhea in this locality. Furthermore, as far as could be learned, epidemics of infantile diarrhea in northern hospitals have occurred only in those institutions in which acid milk has not been used. Dysentery in infants and adult dysentery carriers are still hospital problems, and a bactericidal milk is advantageous."

Convincing evidence of the powers of acidified milk against intestinal infections appeared in the *Canadian Medical Association Journal* (November 5, 1960) in an article by Antoine La Rue, M.D. He wrote, "Modification of the contents of the intestinal tract by varying the chemical components of milk, as well as by acidification or alkalization of the infant's feeding, has long been recognized as an acceptable pediatric procedure. Before the discovery of antibiotics, this was the favored form of treatment. Since the advent of modern research, we have become inclined to forsake diet manipulation and have chosen to center our attention on intestinal antibiotic therapy, rather than on preventive feeding measures . . . Numerous failures have cast a shadow on this approach and compel us to find a type of feeding that will prevent epidemics of gastroenteritis in the newborn, from birth to 3 months."

A Prevention and a Cure

Dr. La Rue decided to make an actual test on the efficiency of acidified milk in preventing diarrhea and dysentery caused by *E. coli bacilli*. When usual forms of treatment failed to check an epidemic at a hospital in Quebec, Crèche St. Vincent de Paul, an attempt was made to combat the *E. coli* bacteria which caused it by preventive feeding measures. Three connecting dormitories were used with 12 newborns in each. The babies in the central dormitory were given acidified milk, while the dormitory occupants on either side of that one received ordinary pasteurized milk. Sixteen of the 24 fed pasteurized milk became infected. The 12 on acidified milk showed no signs of infection. Even when the babies were brought closer together, in alternate rows, the results were the same, except that now all of the babies on pasteurized milk were affected, while all of the others were still free of infection. This proved to Dr. La Rue that the preventive value of acidified milk must be admitted.

He was anxious to see what the acidified milk would do for a child who already suffered with the disease. Ten *E. coli* carriers were isolated. At the end of the first week on the acidified milk, all but those who were persistent carriers were shown to have normal stools—and the normalcy continued thereafter. Not one of these children received an antibiotic.

One would think that with such impressive results at hand, acidified milk would be used in every hospital and ordered by every doctor. But apparently this is not the case. As Drs. Blue and Davidson put it, "What our pediatric colleagues did not endorse was the advisability, let alone the necessity, of a bactericidal feeding. In the South and Middle West, lactic or citric acid often was added to infant feeding, but on the Eastern Seaboard, no credence was given to our belief that acid milk was superior to sweet mixtures."

The authors go on to list their reasons for favoring an acidified milk (in this case, evaporated and canned for easy keeping). (1.) It is as good, digestively speaking, as breast milk; (2.) contains sufficient protein and calcium for proper development; (3.) it is safer, especially for allergic infants, than pasteurized whole milk, and the lactic acid prevents the growth of organisms that cause dysentery and other organisms which can cause infection—lactic acid milk cannot be contaminated by mother's fingers as she attaches the nipple to the bottle; (4.) it is universally available, unlike other special formula ingredients or special animals' milk; (5.) it is inexpensive in its evaporated form—half the cost of dairy milk. Of course, most of these are equally applicable to whole cultured buttermilk in bottles or cartons.

We have long disputed the high place assigned to milk in the nutritional scheme of things. We have many reasons for this, but mainly we believe that milk offers no more to an infant or grownup than any other vitamin-protein-mineral-rich food, and the adverse effects are often disproportionate to the good a child gets from it. Many formulations—equally good and safer—are available. However, as with yogurt, buttermilk, or acidified milk, offers more than milk alone, enough to justify its use in the newborn. The allergenic possibilities of sweet milk are reduced, and the climate of the intestines for fighting infections is greatly improved. We believe that this is a natural means of fortifying one's child against serious illness and intestinal upset. We think it is worth a trial in treating diarrhea and dysentery before invoking antibiotics and other possibly dangerous medications. And if milk is to be used as an infant food, why not make it buttermilk? It comes well recommended.

Bananas and Diarrhea

For most mothers, the anti-diarrheal action of bananas is the most important and most reassuring of all of their powers. In the *Journal of Pediatrics* (37: 367, 1950) J. H. Fries attested to the fact that bananas have superceded apples and other raw fruits in anti-diarrheal action. This view is supported by E. W. Brubaker in the *Journal of the Michigan Medical Society* (36: 40, 1937) who tells of his experience with 56 cases of diarrhea in infants and children. It was found that those who were treated with bananas recovered faster than controls who were given other therapy.

International Medical Digest (32: 369, 1938) carried Drs. Bethea and Bethea's article which contained a description of the banana treatment for diarrhea in children. Babies are given ⅓ of a ripe banana as mashed pulp for each pound of body weight every 24 hours. (For example, if the baby weighs 6 pounds, he would receive two mashed bananas in a 24 hour period.) This pulp is, of course, given in small feedings of 2 or 3 ounces each, 8 or 10 times a day. The fruit may be given with water or incorporated in 1½ ounces of skim milk or buttermilk for each pound of body weight in the first 48 hours. (A 6 pound baby would drink his banana pulp in 9 ounces of liquid.) In the second 48 hour period, just about any accepted infant liquid is able to be used with the banana pulp. Diarrhea generally subsides after 4 days of treatment.

What is the reason for the effectiveness of bananas in conquering diarrhea? Dr. Fries, mentioned above, gives several properties of bananas which have this effect: (1.) the pectin contained in bananas swells and causes voluminous, soft, bland stools that clear out the intestines; (2.) the number and kind of intestinal organisms are changed favorably because bacteria are absorbed by this pectin, and the growth of beneficial bacteria species is promoted; (3.) from the outset of the illness, bananas help to maintain nourishment and weight.

The inclusion of bananas in the diet of small children and infants would appear to be one of the wisest things a mother can do. She has plenty of support from researchers and the more practical word of the New York Foundling Hospital, which regularly gives bananas as the first solid food for all infants who come there, and has done so since 1931. Aside from these points, consider the high nutritional content of bananas, and the flavor appeal they seem to have for all children. Finally, and most important from our point of view, if bananas can be effective in treating diarrhea, why not prevent the occurrence of this condition by including bananas in the child's diet regularly?

SECTION 32: DIGESTION

172. Some Digestive Tract Symptoms of Vitamin Deficiency

When you consider that every mouthful of food we eat must pass through our digestive system, you can see how important to our health is the well-being of that system. It is particularly important in cases of vitamin deficiency.

Louis A. Rosenblum, M.D., and Norman Jolliffe, M.D., in an article in the *Journal of the American Medical Association* for December 27, 1941, point out that patients suffering from gastric ulcers, colitis, gall bladder trouble or any disease of the liver are much more likely to develop vitamin deficiencies, both because of the diets they may be on and because their condition prevents the body from absorbing vitamins.

Various types of medication, too, are certain to result in vitamin losses. In the presence of alkalis, for instance, vitamin C, riboflavin and thiamin and perhaps even more of the vitamin B complex are destroyed in the body. (A good reason for avoiding bicarbonate of soda or the prolonged use of any medicine that alkalizes the body.) The use of several medications (magnesium trisilicate and aluminum hydroxide) for ulcers probably destroys the beneficial effects of vitamins B and C. Also the continual use of mineral oil will destroy vitamins A and D in the body.

Drs. Rosenblum and Jolliffe also point out that after an operation (especially a stomach operation) dextrose fluids are often given by injection so that the patient will not have to eat. These fluids, which are largely carbohydrates containing no vitamins at all, will deplete the body's vitamin B reserves within a few days.

Diarrhea and Vitamin Deficiency

Continued diarrhea will produce the same effect. This is partly because of the rapid passage of the food through the body, not leaving time for the vitamins to be absorbed and partly because the normal digestion of food may be prevented by the absence of digestive secretions. Then, too, in cases of diarrhea the processes of digestion that take place in the intestine are slowed down or eliminated entirely. Fever increases the body's metabolism and hence increases its demand for vitamins. Nausea and pain incline one not to eat and again vitamin supply becomes low—at a time when there is more need for the vitamins than in a perfectly healthy state. So the whole problem becomes one of a vicious cycle in any gastrointestinal disorder. Absorption of vitamins is prevented by the disorder. Vitamin deficiency interferes with absorption even more, and so on.

In addition to symptoms in the digestive tract, noticeable symptoms of vitamin deficiency occur in the mouth. Drs. Rosenblum and Jolliffe suggest that any such condition of the mouth should lead one immediately to suspect vitamin deficiency, whether or not there are any other symptoms. Vitamin C deficiency produces swollen and boggy gums that bleed easily and may go on to become ulcerated. Chewing is difficult and eventually the teeth may loosen and fall out.

Deficiency in niacin (one of the B vitamins) causes swelling and redness of the tip and sides of the tongue. As the deficiency grows worse, these portions become fiery red and ulcerations may appear on the tip and under-surface of the tongue, as well as on the mucous membrane of other parts of the mouth. The administration of the entire vitamin B complex will heal the mouth condition in 48 to 72 hours.

Riboflavin deficiency may produce sores of the mouth and also a scaly substance around the nose, mouth and ears. Again, the vitamin B complex must be administered before the mouth and tongue return to normal.

We have indicated here several symptoms of vitamin deficiency that should guide you in seeking a cure should any of these symptoms bother you. However, as usual, we suggest that you do not wait till such symptoms appear. Get your vitamins from a well-rounded, vitamin-rich diet. Eliminate sugar and cut down on salt. Eat plenty of protein, fruits and fresh vegetables. Finally, supplement your diet with brewer's yeast (for all the B vitamins), bone meal (for calcium, phosphorus, fluorine and other minerals) and fish-oil tablets for vitamins A and D. Say "good-by" to vitamin deficiency and "hello" to radiant good health!

173. Garlic

"Lack of time and space prevents me from going into more detail on the interesting history of this plant (garlic) as a medical and popular remedy. Its use is age-old. It was used by Hippocrates and Paracelsus and is frequently mentioned in the herbals of the middle ages as a remedy. Its range of uses was extremely varied. In recent times garlic has been highly recommended in France, particularly as a remedy in the case of lung diseases attended by copious and ill-smelling expectoration as well as a remedy against hypertension."

We are quoting Professor E. Roos of St. Joseph's Hospital, Freiburg, Germany. These words form the introduction to an article of his telling how he has used a garlic preparation in his own practice, treating patients who suffered from a variety of intestinal disorders, most of them involving diarrheal conditions. We found this article in an old (September 25, 1925) copy of *Münchener Medizinische Wochenschrift,* a medical magazine which is, of course, published in Germany.

Dr. Roos speaks mostly in this article of cases of intestinal complaint arising from the presence of disease-causing bacteria in the intestine. Generally speaking, the more serious forms of diarrheal diseases seem to result from the presence of some such bacteria. At any rate, large numbers of one or more of such bacteria are found in the stool of these sufferers. An overabundance of the harmful bacteria in the intestine can completely crowd out the helpful ones which normally live there, and unpleasant consequences may result. One of these may well be diarrhea—acute or chronic. And you may be sure that, if the helpful bacteria are not soon re-established, the diarrhea will continue.

How to Use Garlic

Dr. Roos tells us in the 1925 article that he had, at the time he wrote it, treated 96 patients with a garlic preparation which he made himself. He gave his patients garlic in dosages of one gram or more and one of his tablets which weighed a gram contained the same amount of raw garlic —one gram. He tells us that he feels garlic is effective against 3 different kinds of digestive or intestinal upsets which could conceivably occur all at the same time in the same patient. "There is in garlic," he says, "a special intestine-soothing and diarrhea-allaying effect which occurs in various colonic affections." There is an effect, also, that cleanses the intestinal flora (the bacteria that live in the intestines) of disease-causing bacteria or at least abnormal mixtures of bacteria. Then, too, there is an anti-dyspepsia effect in the taking of garlic. "Probably," he says, "the same healing influence on the intestinal mucous membrane lies at the basis of all 3."

The first effect which soothes the intestine is almost, he says, like the effect of a narcotic. So far as the diarrhea is concerned, it is frequently

[657]

stopped within a very short time and at the same time the pains, the stomach ache or other difficulties disappear, too. If you give narcotics for diarrhea (and this seems to have been the standard treatment at that time) constipation is likely to follow. It seldom does when garlic is taken.

"Quite to the contrary," he says, "we have even observed, following week-long use on the part of patients who do not have diarrhea, regular daily stool, though sometimes in these cases a mildly inhibitory influence makes itself noticeable. It makes little difference what kind of diarrhea you are dealing with or where it principally has its origin. A favorable result has been obtained in the great majority of cases treated, even in stubborn, chronic cases with recurrence." He reminds us that good results cannot be hoped for if the diarrhea is the symptom of some serious organic disorder—cancer or tuberculosis.

Then, almost as if to contradict the statement he has just made, Dr. Roos goes on to describe the case of a young woman who did have tuberculosis and was suffering from a severe diarrhea. In addition, she was subject to spells of vomiting, severe body swelling and pain on pressure. He prescribed his garlic preparation. "The patient took the remedy in the same dose for 6 weeks. Appetite quickly became very good, the general condition improved, the temperature after 6 weeks still showed only occasional light rises. After 4 weeks the stool was practically normal, for the most part once a day."

The lung inflammation subsided and the swelling disappeared. Says Dr. Roos, "Even if the probable tuberculosis was not cured by garlic, still one receives the distinct impression that the patient has been relatively quickly tided over the serious stage through the rapid improvements in the intestine and the appetite."

In other cases of serious organic trouble, the garlic preparation helped. Dr. Roos tells us of a 41-year-old farmer who had a case of dysentery for many years complicated by rectal polyps. This unfortunate man also suffered from what Dr. Roos describes as a "constant restlessness of body," abdominal rumblings and colic-like pains. For 3 months he took two grams of the garlic preparation 3 times a day, and finally two grams twice daily. For as long as he remained under the influence of the remedy, his trouble was much improved. His stools became for the most part much more solid and less frequent. He became happier and was able to work. He took a long trip each week to obtain the garlic remedy. Four months after completion of treatment, he told Dr. Roos that his condition was still more supportable and his body quieter than before, even though the diarrhea and slimy evacuations reappeared from time to time.

More Case Histories

A scholar who was troubled with abdominal pains, stomach trouble, hyperacidity and diarrhea found that he apparently had appendicitis and prepared for an operation. By chance the surgeon was not available and meantime the patient took some of the garlic preparations, two grams, twice daily. After a few days he declared that he was perfectly well and didn't want to hear any more about an operation. A couple of months later he wrote for more of the prescribed medicine and Dr. Roos suggested that he have the operation. He says, "I record this not for the purpose of recommending substitution of garlic medication for an indicated appendectomy, but in order to show its soothing influence even in organically conditioned troubles."

One final case history. This was a laboratory assistant who had by accident infected herself with a bacteria which causes dysentery. Her symptoms were alarming. Loss of appetite, vomiting and diarrhea were followed by bloody stools. The girl was pain-racked and weak. She was given the garlic preparation, two grams, 5 times daily for 6 days. The vomiting stopped almost at once, and she began to take food. It was not until the nineteenth day of illness that the illness began to subside, but quite some time before this, the patient was out of bed cheerful and feeling like herself.

"I could not maintain," says Dr. Roos, "that the length of time of actual illness was considerably shortened, only that convalescence transpired in a surprisingly rapid manner. To everyone experienced with cases of dysentery, the contrast must be extremely surprising between the obviously very severe form of the disease and the extremely light discomfort following introduction of treatment, along with only a mildly exhausted condition."

Other Conditions Also Cured

In the second part of his article, Dr. Roos goes on to give case histories of other patients, suffering from different conditions, who improved when they used garlic. Here are some of them.

1. A churchman, 33 years old, who suffered from chronic colitis which manifested itself in frequent diarrhea, along with pain and other unpleasant sensations. In the beginning, he took two grams of garlic twice daily for 14 days, then once daily. Within the first few days he felt better. Three weeks after treatment began he had two normal stools daily.

2. Acute enterocolitis. A 24-year-old woman who suddenly experienced terrific body pains, nausea, chills and fever combined with persistent diarrhea. She took two grams of garlic 3 times a day and by the fifth day her condition was perfectly normal.

3. Subacute colitis. A doctor of 35 years. Fell sick with diarrhea and colic pains. He took two grams of garlic 3 times a day and soon became normal.

4. Acute enterocolitis. A 28-year old doctor whose diarrhea occurred every time she took food. A dose of garlic—two grams 3 times a day for 3 days—brought her back to normal.

5. A case of nervous diarrhea. A patient who suffered from this complaint when he became excited. The diarrhea was improved from time

to time, by the use of garlic. Dr. Roos notes that the patient came for the remedy quite often.

The second group of patients discussed by Dr. Roos are those whose intestinal contents showed evidence of large numbers of harmful bacteria. For 17 years the first patient, a professor, had suffered from gas, dyspepsia and colitis. At times his diarrhea alternated with spells of constipation. Two grams of the garlic preparation taken 2 to 3 times daily were prescribed. In two and a half months this patient was fully satisfied that his troubles were over.

The second patient was an eccentric who had been starving himself. Examination of the stool showed copious infiltration of harmful bacteria. It took 4 weeks of treatment with garlic to bring this patient back to normal.

Another patient was a woman of 59 who had always been delicate and had formerly been constipated. She had suffered from diarrhea for about 9 months. When she began to take garlic, there was at first only a slight improvement, but by the end of 6 weeks, she was in good health and her stools were normal. Her appearance was better and she had gained weight. When she came for treatment, examination showed rather copious infiltration of harmful bacteria in her stools. After treatment these had disappeared.

Anti-Dyspeptic Effects

Patients who suffered from "dyspepsia" are next described by Dr. Roos. The first was a 23-year-old student who complained of excessive gas, restlessness, loss of weight, general feeling of ill health and diarrhea. After taking garlic, he returned to normal with only one brief relapse.

A master baker of 48 suffered from intense pressure pains in the upper abdomen. This pain had bothered him for more than a year and sometimes it was present for the entire day. He did not suffer from gas. Taking two tablets of garlic 3 times a day, he found that he experienced great improvement within a matter of days, and within 6 weeks he declared himself in perfect health.

An inspector of 31 suffered from diarrhea, poor appetite, gas. He had taken many drugs with no relief. By the end of the fourth week on garlic, he was satisfied that he was cured.

Two school teachers—one of 35 and the other 47, both suffered from diarrhea, gas, frequent bloating and belching, also headache and heart palpitations. Six weeks on garlic sufficed to do away with these symptoms.

Therefore, says Dr. Roos, we see that garlic preparations show special anti-dyspeptic effects, no matter whether they cause any great change in the consistency of the stools. "Often, after a very short time, the difficulties improve, the patients feel relieved and look better. One has the impression of a complete alteration in the intestine and of its complete transformation. So far as our patients could later tell, the effect also seems to last."

How does garlic achieve its effects? We do not know exactly, he says, but it appears to have a purifying effect on the bacteria of the intestine, brought about probably by some biological healing of the intestinal wall and its glands. But, he adds, in cases where there is no evidence of any unfavorable or abnormal concentration of harmful bacteria in the intestine —that is, for instance, in cases of "nervous" diarrhea—garlic is also helpful, apparently because of this same healing effect on the mucous membrane.

Naturally, he says, treatment with garlic, as with every other kind of treatment, has as well its unsatisfactory results, its failures and its limitations. He recommends as the best possible daily dose for intestinal complaints, two tablets 3 times daily. In severe cases one should take two tablets 5 times daily; in lighter ones two tablets once to twice daily. Most important of all, these tablets can be taken without any fear of disagreeable side effects.

174. Garlic Therapy in Diseases of the Digestive Tract

By E. E. MARCOVICI, M.D.

In recent years, the question of the therapeutic value of garlic and preparations derived from garlic has been the object of repeated discussions in medical and lay literature. The pros and cons have been more or less evenly divided, so that physicians, having no personal experience, encounter difficulties in forming an opinion as to the merits of garlic therapy.

My experiences with garlic medication originated in the year 1915 when, as an army physician on the eastern front, I had the opportunity of studying and treating innumerable cases of gastrointestinal infections (acute and chronic bacillary dysentery, cholerine, cholera and various kinds of postinfectious and non-infectious catarrhs). In an attempt to check the spread of these disabling conditions and to find new means for their treatment, investigations were carried out on the effect of various aromatic drugs, spices and etheric oils—that is, volatile oils given off from food substances. It so happened that my interest was directed towards the garlic plant. In spite of its widespread use as a vermifuge, mainly against pinworms, and its recommendation for all kinds of ailments in domestic medicine, nothing authentic was known at that time about the true medicinal properties of the drug.

The initial results of my experiments with gastrointestinal infections of various origins were so encouraging that they called for further investigations, including bacteriological studies. These findings, meanwhile confirmed and complemented by the work of other authors, and 25 years of personal experience, have led me to believe that there can be no doubt about the valuable therapeutic properties of *Allium sativum* (garlic). This conviction, moreover, induces me to urge physicians to make wider use of this harmless and excellent medicament even if, hitherto, crystalline active principles have not been isolated, and the exact mode of action has not been fully elucidated. (That is, garlic has not been completely analyzed in the laboratory and we do not know exactly how it works.)

Preliminary investigations were conducted with the fresh raw plant. One bulb per day was administered to patients suffering from acute and chronic dysentery. Rapid subjective and objective improvement occurred, the number of evacuations decreased, appetite returned and the general state of the patient was markedly improved. One drawback of this procedure, however, was the unpleasant taste and burning sensation resulting from the ingestion of the crude plant. Steps were therefore taken to overcome these difficulties and to bring the medicament into a better tolerated form. (Dr. Marcovici then describes the making of a tablet from garlic.)

This product represents the active principles of the fresh plant adsorbed to vegetable charcoal, and has the advantage of being devoid of the characteristic odor and taste. On account of the adsorptive properties of charcoal, the release of the active substances occurs gradually during the passage through the gastrointestinal tract. Any irritative effect is thus prevented. The unpleasant odor of the breath resulting from the passage of volatile oils into the respiratory system, occurs only with very large doses.

Garlic for Cases of Dysentery and Intestinal Catarrh

The original investigations were carried out in 91 cases of acute dysentery. The therapeutic results were good and in some cases recovery occurred in less than a week. A second series of experiments was conducted on 25 patients suffering from acute nonspecific intestinal catarrh with emesis (vomiting), fever, colicky pains and watery stools. These patients were frequently benefited within two to three days. Further gratifying results were obtained in the chronic postinfectious catarrhs following cholera and in the gastrogenous diarrheas (originating in the stomach). This procedure was later introduced as a routine treatment and prophylactic measure in hundreds of cases of digestive disorders.

Encouraged by the clinical results, it was decided to attack the problem from the experimental angle. Since experimental studies on humans brought no enlightenment regarding the mechanism of action of the drug, animal experiments were undertaken. The fact that garlic was widely used in all parts of the world as a prophylactic and food preservative suggested that garlic might possess specific bactericidal properties. A large series of rabbits were, therefore, fed dried garlic powder. This procedure was maintained as a prophylactic measure for several days, following which increasing amounts of dysentery toxin were administered intravenously. It was found that powdered dry garlic administered to rabbits in quantities of 2.5 grams daily protected the animals against a tenfold lethal dose of dysentery toxin. In the rabbit, protection is not limited to the intestinal tract but also includes the typical nervous manifestations of the dysentery toxin. Garlic not only exerts a preventive action, but also seems to have curative properties when administered with dysentery toxin. The poisoned animals became seriously ill, but if adequate quantities of garlic were administered, the series receiving the drug did not die, while the controls perished in all instances. The mucous membranes of the rabbits which had received 2¼ to 5 grams of the dried powder showed no pathological alterations—that is, no signs of harm from the powerful toxin.

How Garlic Works to Kill Bacteria

Frenkel and Lenitzkaja found that an addition of 3 per cent allium (garlic) to the food inhibited gastric putrefaction and the formation of gastrointestinal toxins. Kolle, Laubenheimer and Vollmar studied the bactericidal action of garlic on staphylococcus cultures (one of the most virulent of germs). They found that the volatile components evaporating from freshly cut garlic exerted a considerable inhibitory action on the growth of this bacterium. The phenomenon occurred even at a distance of 20 centimeters and reached its maximum within two hours. Sterile agar plates prepared with solutions of garlic remained free from growth after inoculation with staphylococcus.

Waugh conducted interesting experiments with the blood and serum of patients who had previously taken large quantities of garlic. He found that the blood of these individuals exerted an increased bactericidal action on staphylococcus cultures. The bactericidal properties were found to continue for about 10 hours of normal incubator temperature, after which time free growth commenced.

All these experiments, even if not fully convincing, are interesting in view of the fact that garlic is not only utilized for the treatment of gastrointestinal infections, but has been recommended for the treatment of various other infectious conditions. Thus Cooks and Gabriel obtained gratifying effects with diluted garlic juice in the treatment of purulent wounds. It is also widely recommended for the treatment of infections of the respiratory tract. Huss administered allisatin (garlic) to a large series of Swedish school children during an epidemic of infantile paralysis.

Bacteriological studies of the feces of humans suffering from diarrhea have revealed that garlic brings about a characteristic change in the bacterial growth. This product has also been found to be a valuable prophylactic in veterinary medicine. Nohlen recommends it for the treatment of the well known gastrointestinal catarrhs from which monkeys in captivity are known to suffer, and which are responsible for the loss of many a valuable animal in zoos and experimental laboratories.

Becher and Fussgaenger determined the excretion of indican (a waste product) in the urine which they considered an index for the degree of intestinal putrefaction. They observed that, in pathological cases, the excretion was distinctly diminished during periods of garlic medication.

How Garlic Combats Toxemia

In this connection, I should like to give expression to my belief that a large part of the beneficial results observed following the use of garlic in chronic hypertension of the aged are due to the control of intestinal putrefaction and consequent prevention of absorption of toxic substances from the digestive tract. These patients are known to suffer frequently from chronic constipation, cecal stasis (intestinal obstruction) or chronic appendicitis. As a result of these disorders, foodstuffs incompletely predigested in the stomach on account of subacidity or hyperacidity, reach the cecal region where they undergo pathological putrefaction. As a consequence, toxins are absorbed and carried into the blood stream. This toxemia is responsible for the varying symptoms from which these patients suffer: headache (migraine), dizziness, fatigue, capillary spasms, etc. I believe that the favorable effects attributed to garlic therapy in these conditions are not due to any direct vasodilatory effect of the drug, but to the mechanism described above.

General Improvement in Digestion with Garlic

Examination of the gastric juice by Bonem showed that a marked increase of secretion follows ingestion of allisatin (garlic). He maintains that a prolonged emptying time is the result of this stimulation of the secretory apparatus and leads to a more thorough sterilization of the chyme (the partly digested food). Varga performed gastric lavages and found an increase of free hydrochloric acid and total acidity. This effect was demonstrable even in previously completely antacid stomachs. The physiological stimulus, exerted on the secretory mechanism of the pancreas and bile by the increased production of hydrochloric acid, is enhanced by the action of etheric oils of garlic—that is, the oils released when the garlic is pounded or cut. Etheric oils have also been found to increase peristalsis— the movement of the intestines which carries the partly digested food along.

Roos, who has done extensive work with garlic, does not attribute its peculiar effect on the pathological intestinal flora to any direct bactericidal mechanism. He advances the theory that garlic brings about an alteration in the general reaction of the intestinal mucosa, as a result of which, the disturbed physiological symbiosis or relationship between the intestinal organisms is restored by means of a "crowding out" process. The return of normal gastrointestinal activity, brought about by these various factors, changes the environmental conditions for pathological organisms and deprives them of the medium favorable to their growth.

The question as to whether garlic has a direct effect on the liver has been studied by various authors. Kretschmer found that the excretion of bile was markedly increased. Schindel, experimenting on a patient with a biliary fistula (ulcer of the gall bladder), found that both the quantity and the constituents of gall were increased by the ingestion of garlic.

All these theories give no satisfactory explanation for cases of non-

[664]

infectious diarrhea. Beneficial effects obtained with garlic in "nervous" diarrhea, flatulence, distension, etc., are probably due to a mechanism related to the action of the simple stomachics and carminatives. The marked increase of appetite following the intake of garlic preparations obviously is due to the same mechanism.

Summary

It is thought that the antiputrefactive properties are responsible for the gratifying results with allium (garlic) therapy in gastrointestinal intoxication and the subjective complaints of the aged patient with chronic essential hypertension. A wider use of this harmless and effective drug available in the odorless and tasteless form of the new preparations is recommended.

175. A Natural Treatment for Intestinal Disorders

The revival of interest in the use of *Lactobacillus acidophilus* as a means of preventing, as well as curing, constipation and other intestinal disorders, is periodical. This bacterial organism, which is responsible for the formation of a preparation somewhat like buttermilk and yogurt from fresh, whole milk, was written up in two articles in *Drug and Cosmetic Industry* (October, 1958, and March, 1959). We soon acquired two more authoritative testimonials for the value of *L. acidophilus:* one from the *Lancet* (September 21, 1957) and another from *Certified Milk Magazine* (June, 1956). We think our readers will be interested in the findings shown in these papers. We think, too, that they will benefit, healthfully, from the inclusion of *L. acidophilus* in their diets.

The cultured milks are often confused in the minds of lay people, and understandably so. They are basically the same in their effect on the intestinal climate, though *L. acidophilus* seems to be more positive and surer in its effect. Buttermilk is simply acidified milk; that is, a small amount of lactic acid, vinegar or lemon juice will cause the desired change in skim, fresh milk. Yogurt requires a particular bacillus culture, which, when added to milk, produces a smooth, very thick almost solid food, which must be eaten with a spoon, rather than drunk.

If the yogurt is warmed slightly, a separation of the curds from the whey occurs. The separated curds are called pot cheese or cottage cheese. The whey is the yellowish liquid which remains. It is the "plasma" part of milk—whole milk modified by the lactic acid culture, the curds and butterfat removed. Whey is available in a dehydrated form. It comes without any of the disadvantages of and contains 20 times the mineral value of liquid milk, and 50 times as much lactose as yogurt or buttermilk. Lactose is the element in milk which acts to make desirable changes in intestinal bacteria. *L. acidophilus* is not to be confused with any of these other cultured milk preparations.

The Value of L. Acidophilus

The theory upon which the value of *L. acidophilus* is based is this: It is well known that great numbers of the countless bacteria, commonly found in the intestinal tract, contain or give off certain definite poisons. They can also produce products that have offensive odors as they stagnate in the intestines. Now these bacteria can be replaced by *L. acidophilus*, a type of bacteria which neither contains nor produces poisons, nor does it result in any bacteriological products which have offensive odors. Furthermore, this substitution is a safe and wise one because *L. acidophilus* is a natural inhabitant of the intestinal tract. It is found in appreciable numbers in the intestinal excretions of young, healthy children, and persists in varying degrees—but usually much smaller numbers—in the intestinal tracts of adults. It is reasonable to assume that larger numbers of these bacteria would remain, if the diet of the human host produced the proper conditions for their existence and development. In other words, if your *L. acidophilus* count is low, it's your fault. Increasing the amount of this valuable substance in the intestine can be done by the ingestion of foods which are rich in this particular friendly bacteria.

Common in Europe

Two similar foods, buttermilk and yogurt, are eaten frequently in Europe. People there have used them for years not only as a common table food, but also to fight disorders of the intestinal tract. They probably never knew the physiological theory that surrounds the value of cultured milk, but they have enjoyed the benefits of its use for many years. In Austria, Norway, Holland and Switzerland, yogurt appears regularly on the breakfast table. In Bulgaria, the healthy, long-living peasants have long added *L. acidophilus* and its twin, *L. bulgaricus,* to their milk. These people have good digestion and resistance to intestinal disease as the result of what they eat. We, on the contrary, suffer from these very diseases, at least partly because of what we eat.

The laboratory studies on what *L. acidophilus* will do show astounding conclusions. The article in *Certified Milk Magazine* was written by 4 researchers working in the Department of Bacteriology at Rutgers University. They wrote this: "That proper *L. acidophilus* therapy will bring relief to at least 75 per cent of individuals suffering from uncomplicated chronic constipation, constipation accompanied by biliary symptoms, mucous colitis and chronic ulcerative colitis is beyond question."

Arthur H. Bryan, Associate Professor of Biological Science, at Jacksonville University, Jacksonville, mentioned some other advantages in an article in *Drug and Cosmetic Industry* (October, 1958). He wrote that *L. acidophilus* is especially valuable in treating infant diarrhea. The difficult-to-deal-with "gas" that so many adults complain of will tend to be reduced or at least retarded by the ingestion of *L. acidophilus.* "Gas pains and excessive persistalsis (the intestinal motion which moves waste to the bowels), particularly in middle-aged groups, are far less frequent" when these bacteria are ingested.

Postoperative Gas Pains Preventable

It has been suggested that physicians might try giving their patients yogurt or buttermilk for some time prior to an operation, in an effort to build up *L. acidophilus* in the intestines, and thereby to prevent those terrible postoperative gas pains. (We believe this is an excellent idea for anyone facing abdominal surgery and, unless a physician specifically advises against it, we would recommend a special effort to include *L. acidophilus* milk, buttermilk or yogurt in the daily diet.)

Dr. Bryan states that one of the predisposing causes of gastric and duodenal ulcers, excess acid in the stomach, appears to be reduced by cultured milk therapy. It is also recommended for the management of existing ulcer conditions.

Even the skin appears to benefit from the ingestion of *L. acidophilus.* It is called a buttermilk complexion, as opposed to pimples, acne vulgaris and skin blemishes. The physiological and enzymatic action of the culture on the body's use of carbohydrates is thought to have some bearing on the skin's response.

In a later paper, which appeared in *Drug and Cosmetic Industry* (March, 1959), Arthur H. Bryan, in company with Charles A. Bryan, discussed the more technical biochemical aspects of *L. acidophilus.* One interesting point was made: Proteus colonies, those bacteria which cause the formation of foul-smelling hydrogen sulfide gas and indole, were held back by milk cultures of the *lactobacilli.* Carbon dioxide is formed in place of the more unpleasant gases.

A Guaranteed Safe Antibiotic

One of the most important assets of *L. acidophilus,* insofar as disease is concerned, is its antibiotic activity. It is so strongly associated with this activity, that the Byrons refer to it as "Nature's Gastrointestinal Antibiotic." They show slides of *L. acidophilus* in a field containing infectious organisms, such as Salmonella and Shigella. The action of the *L. acidophilus* is to build a wall around the infective organism and cut it off from further growth or expansion. It is said to be effective even where staphylococcus is concerned.

Other values which belong to acidophilus include its value in re-establishing a proper intestinal climate after the oral administration of antibiotics. These antibiotics cause their harm by destroying relatively harmless bacteria, which by their very presence in the intestine, normally pre-

[667]

vent the development of certain more aggressive, disease-causing bacteria. The researchers at Rutgers recommended the joint oral ingestion of *L. acidophilus* with any therapeutically administered antibiotics, to prevent undesirable, disease-carrying bacteria from getting a good start in the intestines, or to replace them if they have become established.

Sudden Spread of Dangerous Bacteria Possible

The investigation went on to suggest that a very real danger in the intestine's harboring of disease-causing bacteria lies in their sudden spread throughout the body, as a result of the shock of any injury. Shock reaction tends to make the walls of the intestine abnormally easy for bacteria to pass through. These bacteria, plus the other factors involved in the injury, tend to delay very strongly the possibility of recovery. This is another good reason for retaining, whenever possible, a climate in the intestines which will not release harmful bacteria in case of injury or other shock to the body.

A typical shock which can cause this superpermeability in the intestinal wall is radiation injury. If the bacteria which slips through the intestinal wall is dangerous, it can do great harm, because of the body's defense mechanisms having been weakened, and it is helpless against staphylococcus, Salmonella, Shigella, etc. It has been shown that such bacteria may play a significant role in the causation of death following exposure to ionizing rays. It is known that animals, whose intestines normally contain a large number of *L. acidophilus,* are comparatively resistant to radiation injury.

A summary of clinical reports on the value of *L. acidophilus* showed the following results: Of 10 researchers treating a total of 356 cases of chronic constipation with nothing but acidophilus-cultured milk, 305 showed "good" results, 51 had "poor" results; 5 separate reports on "Functional Diarrhea," which included 50 patients, 46 had "good" and 4 "poor" results. Thirty-nine cases of irritable colon and diverticulosis were treated with an acidophilus preparation: 32 showed "good" response, 7 "poor." Thirteen out of 13 cases of antibiotic colitis responded well to an acidophilus preparation. In each of the above cases, the report was made by a recognized scientist and appeared in a professional journal.

Low Cost and Easy Preparation

One of the most attractive aspects of the use of this milk product is the low cost. It doesn't take laboratory training for one to make one's own supply of this valuable food. *Drug and Cosmetic Industry,* in its first article (October, 1958) says acidophilus "can be easily cultivated in whole, homogenized, pasteurized, reconstituted or condensed milk. . . . Pure cultures of these organisms can be obtained initially from the Dairy Division of the United States Department of Agriculture, Washington, D. C., from the bacteriology or dairy division of local state universities, from pharmaceutical houses . . . or commercially from some dairy laboratories and the like."

Once one acquires the *Lactobacillus acidophilus* culture the rest is easy. Just mix it into the regular whole milk you can buy at any store. Even dry or condensed milk, reconstituted with previously boiled water to the equivalent of the total solids in whole milk, may be used. You use about a teaspoon of the pure *L. acidophilus* culture to a pint of the milk to be cultured. Let it stand at room temperature for about 24 hours. The milk solids will have begun to separate by then. Shake well and use as desired. Then, to keep yourself well-stocked, merely add more fresh whole milk to the cultured mixture you have already prepared and let stand another 24 hours and your next supply is ready. To stop the bacterial action after 24 hours, place the cultured milk in the refrigerator. The cold will hinder further development.

Not Really Milk

We view the product described in these pages as something other than milk. The milk products which we are opposed to—whole milk, butter, cheese, etc.—retain the very elements which make them objectionable to us, in spite of any appearance changes. Acidophilus-cultured milk, yogurt, buttermilk and the like, on the other hand, are free of the allergy-causing elements of milk; they are sometimes particularly recommended for reversing allergenic trends. Digestive problems caused by milk are taken care of nicely by the acid action of the *L. acidophilus,* which, so-to-speak, partially digests the milk in which it is placed. It offers friendly bacteria with which to populate the intestines, and this bacteria defends the body against any new growth of harmful bacteria by isolating what is already there, and by displacing any new bacteria which might grow. *L. acidophilus* milk contains all of the vitamins and minerals which are the real value of milk, but the disadvantages are largely eliminated.

It is for these reasons that we feel we can recommend the use of acidophilus without compromising our original, and still steadfast, position against milk. Acidophilus would be an excellent addition to one's diet, even when no physical problem exists. However, if any of the diseases mentioned earlier are present—constipation, colitis, ulcer, diarrhea, etc.— we would certainly recommend giving *L. acidophilus* milk a try in view of its therapeutic values. It is certainly to be preferred to the commercial laxatives and other drugs which, rather than add to good health, actually drain it from us. Acidophilus has a positive action. It relieves the symptoms of a disease by curing the cause. This is rare in the treatments we are subjected to today. Let acidophilus work for you.

176. A Low-Carbohydrate Diet

Can a diet low in carbohydrate cure ulcerative and mucous colitis? It seems much to simple, doesn't it? Yet the physician who made this discovery has a very special knowledge of this kind of diet and its effect upon health. He has used this diet as a weapon against polio and tuberculosis. He not only proves that a diet low in carbohydrate has a healing as well as a preventive power in colitis, he also explains his own theory as to why this may be so, on the basis of the amount of oxygen used by the body on this kind of diet.

Benjamin P. Sandler was living in New York when he wrote the article we are talking about, which appeared in the *Review of Gastroenterology* for March-April, 1941. At present, he is a resident physician at a veterans hospital in North Carolina. Dr. Sandler is well known for his book, *Diet Prevents Polio* (available from Lee Foundation, 2023 West Wisconsin Avenue, Milwaukee 3, Wisconsin) in which he shows how a diet low in carbohydrates stopped a polio epidemic in its tracks.

Listen to how Dr. Sandler begins his article on colitis. Peptic ulcer, he says, is due fundamentally to a disturbed carbohydrate metabolism which can be discovered by a test for blood sugar. He means by this, simply that the person with ulcer cannot properly use carbohydrates. He eats them and possibly he does not experience what we call "indigestion," but nevertheless, the many chemical changes that are supposed to take place involving these carbohydrates simply do not take place as they should, and everything goes wrong from that point on.

Dr. Sandler's Diet

Since ulcerative colitis patients seem to respond to the same low-carbohydrate diet, it appears that the two disorders have something in common. The diet which Dr. Sandler used for his colitis patients allowed no more than 35 grams of carbohydrate at every meal, and this carbohydrate is chiefly in the form of fruits and vegetables which are extremely low in starch. Some food is given between meals and at bedtime so that the patient eats frequently. The patient is instructed to have his meals regularly and never to miss a meal. Foods that contain a great deal of "roughage," like lettuce, asparagus, spinach, cole slaw are given at the start of the treatment, indicating, Dr. Sandler says, that such foods do not cause local irritation and aggravation of symptoms, because the patient begins to improve at once.

These are the forbidden foods on Dr. Sandler's low-starch diet: sugar, cereals, bread, corn, rice, potatoes, bananas, tapioca, beans, prunes, cake, candy, ice cream, spaghetti, noodles and anything else made from cereals or sugar. One "soda cracker" is allowed with each meal and with each between meal feeding. High protein gluten bread may be used later, as the diet proceeds—only one slice per meal.

The following symptoms disappeared or were greatly alleviated while the patient was following the diet: abdominal cramps, flatulence (gas), belching, straining at the time of evacuation, rectal discomfort, headache and dizziness. "There was a marked improvement in the general physical and mental status of the patients."

Improvement in patients with mucous and mild ulcerative colitis may be noted after one or two weeks, Dr. Sandler tells us. The amount of pus and mucus diminishes. Blood disappears. The number of stools falls steadily until there are one or two formed stools per day. In general, of course, the more recent the onslaught of the disorder, the quicker the improvement. A patient who had been suffering from colitis for 10 years improved more slowly than other patients. It is interesting to note that two patients with arthritis also showed improvement in joint symptoms as the colitis improved.

There were 3 patients whose case histories are so dramatic that we want to discuss them. Each of these had severe ulcerative colitis. They had had high temperatures for months; they were emaciated and had such further complications as osteomyelitis, rectal abscesses, arthritis and serious skin conditions. Previously, they had been given transfusions, sulfa drugs, liver extract, various medicated enemas and diets high in calories and in vitamins. Nothing helped.

"The response to the change to low-carbohydrate diet without other form of therapy was dramatic and sustained," says Dr. Sandler. The diarrhea with blood, pus and mucus stopped. The number of bowel movements soon became normal. Cramps and straining at stool disappeared.

More Case Histories

Here are some more case histories. (Dr. Sandler gives a total of 10 in the article.) A woman patient of 42 had had repeated attacks of loose bloody stools for 10 years. Examination at the hospital showed numerous bleeding ulcers in the colon. Nothing done for her in the hospital helped at all. She was given blood transfusions, put on a *high-calorie, high-carbohydrate, low-residue* diet and lost another 20 pounds. When Dr. Sandler first saw her, she could not raise her head from the bed or feed herself.

A blood sugar test revealed some very significant things to Dr. Sandler, who put her on a low-carbohydrate diet—like the one outlined at the beginning of this chapter. Within a week, she felt better and was able to raise her head and feed herself. After two weeks, stools were less frequent and contained less blood. After 3 weeks, the diarrhea had ceased, no blood or mucus was present. After 6 weeks, the stools were normal and other symptoms the patient had were greatly improved. At the end of 10 weeks, she had gained 20 pounds and an examination showed healing of all ulcers. After 8 months, she was free of symptoms—stools were normal.

[671]

A second case history is that of a young girl of 22 whose condition after admittance to the hospital became progressively worse. Attacks of nausea and vomiting alternated with bloody and frequent stools. There was painful swelling of the joints, much loss of weight and strength; the girl was irritable, depressed and had frequent crying spells. She also had been given a high-carbohydrate, high-vitamin diet, transfusions and liver injections. She was put on a low-carbohydrate diet without other therapy.

There was noticeable improvement after 3 days, says Dr. Sandler. After two weeks, her stools were practically normal, the joint symptoms began to subside, her appetite improved and she began to put on weight. She was later discharged, completely free of colitic symptoms and with only slight joint pain. An examination showed healing of the ulcers and improvement of the appearance of the lining of the colon.

A few months after she was discharged from the hospital, she broke her diet and had a recurrence of diarrhea which lasted for two weeks. A return to the low-carbohydrate diet once more brought her back to normal. The taking of a small amount of candy or sweetened prunes had resulted in an attack of diarrhea lasting two days.

A third case history is that of a child of 8. This little girl had had mumps, measles, whooping cough, frequent infections and colds. Examination revealed that she had osteomyelitis with abscesses on her legs. Examination showed that the colon was inflamed with bleeding ulcers. She failed rapidly after being admitted to the hospital, but once again the low-carbohydrate diet brought improvement. Nothing else was done in the way of therapy. Yet 8 months later, this child was perfectly well with absolutely normal stools and a steady gain of weight.

How can you explain such astonishing changes wrought in very very sick people by the installation of a simple diet?

Dr. Sandler's Theory on Low-Carbohydrate Diet

Dr. Sandler explains it on the basis of the way the body uses sugar (of course, starchy foods are changed to sugar as soon as they are eaten). It seems there are two kinds of sugar important for purposes of this explanation—that which occurs in food the patient eats and that which the liver makes and releases gradually for the body's use. Sugar in food is not used as readily by the body as is the sugar produced by the liver.

It seems that, when sugar is eaten, the sugar from the liver is suppressed and the body must get along on this food sugar, which is not used nearly so well. One evidence of the misuse is that less oxygen is consumed when the body is burning sugar from food. When it is burning sugar processed by the liver and released gradually for use, it uses more oxygen. Dr. Sandler states, "It is the opinion of the writer that any interruption in the discharge of glucose (sugar) from the liver is to be regarded as unphysiological (that is, unwise and not natural) in that it brings about a reduced glucose and oxygen consumption." When protein is eaten, there is apparently no such depression of the production of sugar by the liver. And there is a greater use of oxygen by the body.

Why should all of these various complicated processes involving the liver and eating sugars have anything to do with colitis, ulcerative or mucous? Dr. Sandler believes that when large amounts of sugar and starch are eaten rather than protein, the reduced amount of oxygen brought into use results in a poor flow of blood to various parts of the body. And this, of course, would include the colon and other parts of the digestive tract. Occasionally one sees patients who have both peptic ulcer and colitis, he says. In such people, both the upper and the lower parts of the digestive tract are suffering from lack of oxygen and lack of blood.

We don't think it matters much for our purposes what the reason is that a low-carbohydrate diet produces such splendid results. The main thing, we think, is that it does. Many people have written us about problems of this kind. Many of them have been placed on diets high in carbohydrate, low in fresh raw foods (because of the "roughage") and low in protein. They have told us they cannot follow the natural food diet because they must eat only "bland" foods which means, so far as we can discover, foods which have been refined, puréed and cooked to nothingness.

Doesn't the experience of Dr. Sandler show clearly that the important thing in the diet of the colitis patient, like that of anyone else, is natural food as little processed as possible?

177. Diet Care to Prevent Colitis

"There is no evidence to support, and in fact there is much evidence against, the assumption that man is better equipped to digest carbohydrate than protein and fat." Walter L. Voegtlin, M.D., of Seattle, Washington, made this statement in a speech before the Seattle Academy of Surgery in 1938. He was speaking about the use of a diet low in carbohydrates (starches and sugars) for the treatment of disorders of the colon.

Bland Diet Usual for Colitis Patients

It is almost a universal practice, he says, to give a colitis patient a bland diet. It is chosen, he goes on, probably because it satisfies our tactile sensibilities of smooth texture and our preconceived notions of easy digestibility. Is this what the colon needs? Apparently not.

"It has been known since the time of Moses," says our author, "that the fermentation of sugars and other carbohydrates by bacteria causes the liberation of gas and the production of alcohol and certain by-products." Bacteria exist in large numbers in the colon. These bacteria will ferment carbohydrates if such carbohydrates should arrive in the colon. "The products of this fermentation are definitely noxious to the large bowel and their continued presence in the colon leads, first, to a minor and later, a more severe irritation of the organ."

Undigested Carbohydrate Should Not Reach Colon

It seems that, under normal conditions of digestion, probably little or no undigested carbohydrate should reach the colon. The digestion of these substances should take place in that part of the digestive tract above the colon. However, in the colitis patient, the partially digested food is rapidly propelled through the upper or small intestine, which does not allow time for the complete absorption or digestion of food, so considerable amounts of fermentable carbohydrate may be deposited in the colon. The rate of passage of partially digested food in the colitis patient is two to three times that of normal individuals.

So, undigested carbohydrate is deposited in the colon, ferments there, gives off gas and, in the process, produces substances irritating to the lining of the colon.

Fermentation of starches and sugars in the small *upper* intestine is of less importance, because there is a difference between the lining of the two organs. Carbohydrates are just not absorbed in the colon or lower intestine, says Dr. Voegtlin. What happens to the protein and fat? Certainly the substances created when proteins are broken down in the intestine do not cause irritability in the colon, says Dr. Voegtlin.

Fats Important to Colitis Sufferer

Fat is digested very slowly and the substances liberated so slowly during its digestion do not occur in sufficient quantity to cause irritation of the colon. Then, too, fats are important in the diet of a colitis sufferer because they keep the stomach and intestine from being so active and nervous, so that the patient does not need "antispasmodic" drugs, if he has enough fat in his diet.

His idea, says our author, is that colitis should be treated by means of a low-carbohydrate and high-fat-protein diet, because, of the 3 food groups making up the human diet, carbohydrate is most apt to become irritating to the colon, either if fed in excess or if it is improperly digested. Improper absorption and digestion may occur if certain digestive enzymes are missing or if the whole digestive tract is working too fast, so that food is not processed at the point where it is supposed to be taken care of.

Dr. Voegtlin says that laxatives have a great deal to do with the problem. Nervous tension has the same effect as laxatives, he points out. Nervous strain, after a long period of time, results in a most unhealthful condition of the colon, and digestive tract in general. The combination of nervous instability, present or past taking of laxatives and colitis is so well established that physicians are surprised when all 3 conditions do not go together, and they look for something organically wrong with the bowel.

[674]

Fermentation Mechanism May Cause Irritation

"The usual diet prescription in colitis is predominantly carbohydrate and, while it may be entirely bland upon ingestion, it may become very irritating to the large bowel because of the fermentation mechanism described above," says Dr. Voegtlin.

The diet that he recommends for colitis patients results in rapid disappearance of symptoms and the appearance of formed stools in 7 to 10 days. He goes on to say that patients who have been taking laxatives for many years must be assured that a daily evacuation is not essential, or even normal, under certain circumstances of diet, and that laxatives are never necessary. In patients who have been "whipping" their systems with laxatives, a period of apparent constipation will follow their withdrawal. He recommends an oil retention enema if the bowel has not moved within 4 days after laxatives are stopped.

Low-Carbohydrate Diet for Colitis Patients

Here are Dr. Voegtlin's recommendations for a low-carbohydrate diet.

The following foods are to be avoided entirely:

CEREALS: starch, flour, macaroni, bran, spaghetti, breakfast cereal, bread (all kinds), crackers, rice, bakery products.

VEGETABLES: potato, cabbage, cauliflower, radishes, lettuce, celery, broccoli, cucumber, corn, rutabaga, turnip, onion. No raw vegetables are to be eaten.

FRUITS: pineapple, berries, citrus fruits. No raw fruits are to be eaten except bananas.

MISCELLANEOUS: candy, syrup, sugar, honey, milk, pastries, chocolate, condiments, French dressing, nuts, pickles, creamed gravies and sauces, carbonated or sweetened drinks, alcoholic beverages.

The following foods may be eaten freely:

SOUP: cream or purée made with cream and water instead of milk (the vegetables listed below should be used in a purée), clear soups, bouillon, consommé.

VEGETABLE (must be cooked and sieved): carrots, spinach, beets, asparagus, peas, prunes, tomato, string beans, rhubarb, squash (summer), beet greens, mushrooms.

FISH: all varieties cooked in any way except fried, shellfish.

MEAT: all varieties cooked any way except fried.

CHEESE: all varieties, cottage cheese is beneficial.

SALADS: made only with cottage cheese, gelatin, cooked fruit or avocado with mayonnaise.

FRUITS: all except those noted above. Fruits must be cooked and unsweetened (except bananas).

EGGS: cooked in any way except fried.

DRINKS: coffee, tea, postum, cream (no milk), buttermilk.

DESSERTS: gelatin with whipped cream, bananas, cooked fruit, sherbet.

MISCELLANEOUS: peanut butter, mayonnaise, olive oil, butter, salad oil, cod liver oil.

A Few Words of Dietary Advice

Health-conscious readers know which of the foods above we have a different opinion on—we would skip all dairy products, soups, coffee and tea. Aside from these, we think the diet should be the perfect answer for anyone suffering from colitis. Of course, you should not forget your food supplements—for some vitamins are bound to be deficient in a diet where practically everything is cooked. For that matter, if you have a blender, why not make your purées of *raw* vegetables and fruits—so much richer in vitamins and minerals than cooked ones!

178. Ulcerative Colitis

From time to time, in the consideration of correct eating, we run across theories about proper combinations of foods. It has never seemed wise to us to plan menus which group all proteins in one meal, carbohydrates in another, and so forth, even though such diets have been advocated frequently in the past. William Howard Hay, M.D., who enjoyed considerable popularity, based his diet menus on this principle.

However, we read a book on ulcerative colitis which appeared so reasonable, authoritative and sound that we are reviewing here its author's theories on food combinations. Some of our readers—especially those who are victims of ulcerative colitis—may wish to experiment with them. We can recommend wholeheartedly the sincerity and background of the author, N. Philip Norman, M.D. The entire title of the book is *Postulating a New Concept of the Etiology, Pathology and Treatment of Chronic, Idiopathic Ulcerative Colitis—Is It a Hemorrhage Disease Caused by Nutritional Imbalances?* It is published by the Lee Foundation for Nutritional Research at Milwaukee, Wisconsin.

The first part of Dr. Norman's book is, as its title would imply, a highly technical treatise on the disease itself, which he has studied for 30 years. In commenting on the treatment he prescribes for patients, Dr. Norman outlines his ideas on mixed meals and improper nutrition. "It should always be kept in mind," he says, "that proper nutrition goes back to the seed and the soil, plus what is done to food before it reaches the shelves of your local food distributor, and what you do to it before it is served on your table." He then describes how nature has balanced the chemical composition of all natural foods so that they may be easily digested and absorbed. When a grain of wheat is milled, it is separated into 5 parts, each of which is then used separately, without the others. Although there is a lot of talk these days about "enriching" foods, there is actually no such thing as ever putting back part of a natural product which we have destroyed.

Natural Foods and the Mixed Meal

So, says Dr. Norman, for all his ulcerative patients he insists on natural foods. He knows that they are difficult to obtain and may cost a little more. He knows that it is a lot of trouble for a housewife to shop for natural foods, to serve fruits and vegetables only at the height of their freshness and ripeness, to cook foods exactly right and to regulate all the other angles of a good natural diet, but he insists on it with his patients. Case histories of 12 cured patients, whose ailments received widely varied diagnoses and treatments before the sufferers came to Dr. Norman, show that, in most cases, those who followed his diet directions to the letter were cured. In all cases, those who did not follow directions continued to suffer.

In addition to the eating of natural foods, Dr. Norman says, "the ulcerative colitis patient should permanently renounce the mixed meal." He goes on to describe the experiments of Pavlov, the great Russian scientist, who proved that a meal consisting of fats, carbohydrates and proteins resulted in faulty digestion of the carbohydrates or the proteins. If the proteins were well digested, the carbohydrates were not, and the residue would bring about an unhealthy state of intestinal flora. If the carbohydrates were well digested, the proteins were not.

Pavlov found that the quantity of digestive juice poured out to digest meat was largest during the first or second hour after eating. To digest bread, the quantity of juice was greatest during the first hour; to digest milk, the quantity of digestive juice was greatest during the third hour after drinking the milk. Not only the quantity, but the digestive power of the juice is important. In digesting meat, the stomach uses the most active juice during the first hour; bread, the second and third hour; milk, the last hour of digestion, which may be the sixth hour after the milk has been taken. Pavlov also discovered that if a quantity of fat is taken into the stomach just before, during or after a meat meal, it will stop off the flow of digestive juice for a period of one to two hours. Then a rapid outpouring of the juice occurs at a time when the meat should normally be half-digested. This often brings about a condition of hyperacidity one or two hours after meals.

The mixed meal, when regarded in the light of the newer knowledge of nutrition, has no purpose and is totally unscientific, says Dr. Norman, and the fact that we continue to serve mixed meals makes our nutritional shortcomings even worse than they already are.

No one has ever disproved Pavlov's theories, he adds. Why, then, do

[677]

doctors and nutritionists continue to recommend the mixed meal? Just because they are as much creatures of habit as anyone else. The mixed meal is an established American custom. Would you have Thanksgiving turkey without bread stuffing, potatoes and pumpkin pie? Would you have Sunday dinner without a roast, browned potatoes and dessert? These are institutions that must not be tampered with. When the average American sits down to his meal, says Dr. Norman, it is not only a mixed meal, against all the known discoveries of science, but it is also a meal composed of foods that have been "refined, pasteurized, sterilized, homogenized, fortified, enriched, restored, chemicalized and otherwise sophisticated by food technologists, who seldom question or investigate the far-reaching effect of all forms of food processing upon public health."

Planning Menus for Ulcerative Colitis Patients

In planning meals, then, for the ulcerative colitis patient, the patient must be taught with great care all the shortcomings of processed foods, and also the necessity of including vitamins, minerals, enzymes and hormones as they are contained in natural foods. Then the patient must cooperate completely with the doctor's suggestions. The plan for meals which Dr. Norman has worked out for ulcerative colitis patients is: (1.) concentrated carbohydrates should not be combined with concentrated proteins; (2.) concentrated fats should not be combined with concentrated proteins; (3.) fruits, raw or cooked, should not be combined with concentrated carbohydrates. (The reason for this is that digestion of starch must take place in an alkaline or neutral medium. The acid in fruits delays the digestion of starch.)

Meals, then, fall into this pattern. Breakfast: only fresh, uncooked fruits, berries, melons, unsulfured dried fruits, milk or buttermilk and unsweetened coffee and tea, or substitutes; no bread or protein. Lunch, the starch meal: a vegetable soup without meat base, an unprocessed starch, a raw vegetable salad, cooked fresh vegetables, butter and a milk beverage. Dinner, the protein meal: a vegetable soup that may contain meat but no starch (that is no potatoes, etc.), a meat or meat substitute such as cheese, nuts or legumes, two or more properly cooked vegetables (one preferably of the leafy variety), a large green salad, fresh fruits, berries or melon and unsweetened coffee, tea or substitutes for them; no starch is allowed at this meal—that is, no bread, crackers or starchy vegetables; and, *never at any meal,* desserts such as pies, cakes, puddings, etc.

A typical day's menu on this diet would be:

Breakfast
2 slices pineapple
1 sliced pear
2 sliced peaches
½ cup dates or raisins
1 pint of milk

[678]

Lunch

Cream of asparagus soup
Whole corn muffins
Mixed vegetable salad
Butter
1 pint of milk

Dinner

Broiled chicken, broiled lamb chops or broiled lobster
(note: no fat is used in the preparation)
2 or more fresh vegetables such as spinach, cauliflower and cress
Salad of mixed greens
Sliced fresh pineapple without sugar

Dr. Norman recommends eating between meals for those who are underweight—fruit and milk at 10:30 in the morning, 4:30 in the afternoon and bedtime.

Editor's Note: We do not approve of dairy products, soups or coffee, tea and substitutes for them.

179. Ulcerative Colitis, Bread and Milk

Ulcerative colitis is defined in the *International Record of Medicine* for May, 1957, as involving: (1.) abdominal pain and griping; (2.) diarrhea which is often profuse, frequent and bloody; (3.) many bacteria in the stools; (4.) weight loss which may be severe; (5.) fever; (6.) general malaise or feeling of discomfort, associated with anemia and malnutrition.

It is understandable that anyone suffering from ulcerative colitis would be badly nourished, since whatever he eats may pass through his digestive tract so rapidly that he gains little nourishment from it. Jerome Weiss, M.D., of New York, in his article in the *Record*, tells us that the most important step in treating colitis is to stop the diarrhea. "Diarrhea in these patients results in incomplete digestion of food, excessive loss of nutrients, fluids, electrolytes and minerals. This obviously leads to a state of malnutrition if permitted to go on uncontrolled."

Dr. Weiss controls the diarrhea with drugs. It seems to us that a far better idea would be to prevent it before it occurs. And it seems to us that anyone who studies colitis must agree that it is a disease caused by improper diet. A great deal has been written on the personality traits of colitis sufferers, indicating apparently that people with certain emotional make-up are most susceptible to the disorder.

[679]

Says Dr. George L. Engel in *Gastroenterology,* Vol. 40/2II, 313-317, occasionally a family may show a striking susceptibility to ulcerative colitis or regional ileitis. He goes on to say that the disease usually becomes manifest when the patient feels hopeless or is attempting to defend himself against such feelings. Real, threatened or imagined loss of or separation from loved persons, goals, objectives, ideals or possessions are apt to precipitate onset. Other diseases may also be evoked by similar factors, but these factors are constant in the colitis patient.

Re-establishment of the threatened relationship is usually associated with relief of the helplessness and relief from the disease. Patients with chronic and relatively irreversible changes in the bowel, however, no longer show such fluctuations in symptoms. Only certain people are capable of developing ulcerative colitis, he goes on, and they must possess a certain "factor," which they inherit or develop early in life. A knowledge of these characteristics, he says, makes it possible to predict the circumstances in which an attack of colitis may develop.

It doesn't seem to us that this would help much if one couldn't do any thing to prevent or treat the attack. We are impressed by the fact that mistakes in diet can cause the very insecure personality and nervous temperament which Dr. Engel relates to colitis patients. So it seems reasonable to us that the very diet which brings on the nervousness, the helplessness, the insecurity, also may bring on the colitis.

Food Patterns Run in Families

Could such traits be inherited so that they would run in families? Certainly a tendency toward such personality might run in families, because of inherited patterns of metabolism and because of inherited diet patterns. This latter seems to us most important.

We know that we tend to eat as our families brought us up to eat. If, in your part of the country, pork and cornbread and fried chicken are staple foods every week, there is a good likelihood that you will like these foods and eat them throughout your life. If you live by the sea, fresh fish and shellfish may make up a large part of your menus, and it may surprise you to find that inland folks may not like these foods at all. If one of your grandmothers won prizes for her doughnuts or cakes or pies or jams, chances are that these foods have become an important part of your family tradition, featured at festive meals and Sunday dinners. If your children discover that you don't like broiled liver or fresh salad greens, it's quite likely that they will decide they don't like them either; in fact, they may not even have a chance to eat them until they grow up and their food patterns may, by then, be firmly established.

Bread and Cereals May Be a Contributing Cause

What foods in one's eating pattern might be responsible for causing ulcerative colitis? We presented the findings of W. L. Voegtlin of Seattle, Washington, who wrote in *Northwest Medicine* for July, 1939, that he is convinced the carbohydrate foods are largely responsible for colitis. This may sound strange, since diets high in refined carbohydrates are widely prescribed for colitis patients. ("Eat only white bread, shun all roughage in the form of raw fruits and vegetables," colitis patients are told by their doctors.)

Dr. Voegtlin believes that carbohydrates are the difficult-to-digest foods, not proteins or fats. The reason why bland, refined carbohydrate foods are recommended to colitis patients, he says, is that such foods seem to be smooth and non-irritating to the touch. But, once in the colon, they may ferment, producing irritating products of a chemical nature (that is, not rough, but dangerous, as many poisons are dangerous). Because food passes so rapidly through the digestive tract when one has colitis, carbohydrates may not be properly digested. The irritating substances this undigested starch forms in the colon may cause such a bad condition of the colon that food is passed even more rapidly and the situation becomes worse.

Dr. Voegtlin thinks that the taking of laxatives is very often responsible for the beginning of colitis. He says the patients have been "whipping" their bowels with cathartics. The diet he recommends is extremely low in starch, high in fats and protein. No refined carbohydrate food is permitted.

In addition he forbids the use of vegetables high in carbohydrate, such as potatoes, and others which are, he believes, difficult of digestion. He also forbids raw vegetables and fruits, except for bananas. No pineapple, berries or citrus fruits are to be eaten.

We think this last provision is interesting. Probably he objects to the seeds in the berries and the fibers of the pineapple. The citrus? Could it be the citric acid? Or the fact that citrus is taken almost universally as strained juice from which many valuable parts of the fruit have been removed? Dr. Voegtlin also forbids all sweets, including soft drinks and alcoholic beverages.

We are completely willing to agree with this author in his opinion of foods high in starch. We say, avoid them. And we point out especially that bread of any kind is mentioned by Dr. Voegtlin as being possibly responsible for colitis. We believe readers, to be healthy, should avoid bread and all cereal products.

Milk Is Investigated

Now we find that another medical researcher has incriminated milk as a possible contributor to colitis. Dr. S. C. Truelove of the Radcliff Infirmary, Oxford, England, has studied groups of colitis patients on different diets and has found that one group showed marked improvement when milk and certain milk products, such as cheese, were eliminated from the diet. In the case of several patients, milk was then brought back into the diet as an experiment. On every occasion when this was done, the patient suffered from another attack of the disease.

According to *Consumer Bulletin* for June, 1961, the number of patients studied was small—13 out of 200. But it shows, certainly, that milk can be an important contributing factor in this rather mysterious disease. Dr. Truelove believes that his studies may indicate that colitis is not a single disease, but a family of different diseases. Allergy to certain foods may be involved—in this case, an allergy to milk.

Health-minded readers know that we believe milk is not a food for adults. Man is the only animal who drinks milk after he grows up. It is Editor Rodale's opinion that milk is a food for babies and children only, and should not occupy too much of the diet of these, even. Present-day milk comes from cows which are little more than milk factories. To keep production figures high, milk cows produce far more milk than is natural to them. The way they are fed and the drugs given to them for various illnesses also affect the milk, of course.

Mixed Meals May Cause Colitis

One other suggestion on colitis. Dr. N. Philip Norman, M.D., of New York City, believes that this trouble is caused by eating modern processed and refined foods and eating them at mixed meals—that is, without any regard for the starch, protein or fat content of the foods. Dr. Norman puts his patients on diets completely free of refined and processed foods. He then recommends menus in which concentrated carbohydrates are not combined with concentrated proteins, concentrated fats are not combined with concentrated proteins, and fruits, raw or cooked, are not combined with concentrated carbohydrates.

We believe that Dr. Norman's patients get their results chiefly from omitting refined and processed foods and would get just as good results without bothering to arrange to separate foods at different meals, but we think readers who want to experiment with the non-mixed meal should go right ahead. Perhaps in your case it may be beneficial.

In any case, it seems to us the lesson to be learned is that refined foods, especially bread and other cereal products, can best be left out of the healthful diet—and should certainly be omitted, if you are suffering from ulcerative colitis. White bread, that mockery of good food, should never be eaten by anyone. It is Editor Rodale's firm belief that even good homemade bread is not a food for the health-conscious person following the natural foods program. We think, too, that milk is better left to those who are meant to drink it—infants and young children.

For ulcerative colitis patients who are afraid of the "roughage" of fresh fruits and vegetables, the cellulose strands and fibers which apparently irritate the sensitive or inflamed lining of the colon, we suggest buying a blender or a juicer and reducing fresh, raw fruits and vegetables to a purée or a juice which should give no trouble. Such a preparation should be eaten or drunk immediately after being made, for vitamins are lost rapidly with every minute such a food is stored.

[682]

180. Dizziness—A Mysterious Symptom

"Doctor, I sometimes feel so dizzy that I simply have to lie down or I'll fall down!" While such a condition is far from normal, doctors say that it is one of the most common complaints they hear from their older patients.

Everyone has, at one time or another, experienced dizziness, and it is easy to recall the unsettling giddiness, tinged with nausea, that characterizes this sensation. It might have been the result of a childhood game, a merry-go-round ride, a plane ride or a sudden rise in an elevator—whatever the cause, it is likely that you could link the cause and effect, and promise yourself to avoid such activity in the future. Comforting, isn't it, to know that you needn't experience such unpleasantness if you carefully stay away from the type of motion that caused it? It is easy, then, to understand the anguish and alarm experienced by persons who have long spells of dizziness or vertigo, as it is termed, and who can find no cause, no apparent reason, for feeling this disturbance. They are dizzy for minutes or hours at a time and can't imagine why.

Be Sure It's Actually Dizziness

When a doctor is confronted with a case in which the patient describes dizziness as one of the symptoms, he must first make certain that the patient isn't using the term to describe quite a different thing. For example, feelings of faintness, weakness, pressure on the head, etc.—these are not really dizziness. A sensation of turning motion is a true indication of vertigo. This motion may seem to be in objects or environment which surround the patient (objective vertigo); it may be a motion in which the patient feels himself moving in space around stationary objects of his environment (subjective vertigo); or the motion may seem to be confined inside the head of the patient. The physician tries to get a description of *exactly* what the patient is experiencing, for each type of dizziness can be a clue to its physiological cause.

Some Common Causes

By way of illustration let us catalogue some of the causes of vertigo, or dizziness, listed in the *Canadian Medical Association Journal* (June 15, 1957) in an article on the subject. Since the sense of balance rests primarily

[683]

in the inner ear, it is readily understood that trouble in the ear can result in the feeling of unsteadiness and turning of which we are speaking. A most obvious cause would be any blow to the head affecting the inner ear —a concussion or a skull fracture, for example. Such an injury might leave symptoms of dizziness long after external healing has been accomplished and the patient is engaged in normal pursuits.

Circulatory disturbances, common in many persons past middle age, can lead to vertigo of mild as well as alarming proportions. The *Journal of the American Medical Association* (March 13, 1958) tells of observations made of 476 elderly persons in Sheffield, England. The incidence of vertigo was found to be 47 per cent in the men, and 61 per cent in the women seen. In the majority of cases, the vertigo seemed to be associated with hardening of the labyrinthine arteries.

"Small stroke," so-called because of its relatively mild nature, is a slight blood-clot injury to the brain which usually occurs during the night when blood pressure is low. This injury often results in a sudden feeling of turning or unsteadiness. Both high and low blood pressure can affect symptoms of vertigo by altering the supply of blood to the brain, especially when the patient changes position too suddenly, as in springing from a chair to answer the telephone, or bouncing out of bed, to turn off the alarm clock. Bending to pick something from the floor will often make persons with poor circulation or abnormal blood pressure feel dizzy. Anemia can even cause dizzy symptoms, due to the fact that in anemic persons, the vital supply of oxygen to the brain is sometimes seriously curtailed.

Infections in any part of the inner ear sometimes lead to dizziness. The *Journal* article remarks that the administration of medications such as aspirin, quinine and streptomycin can result in toxic labyrinthitis, as can infections and diseases which are accompanied by high fever, especially "flu."

The labyrinth is the system of canals formed by bones in the inner ear, and labyrinthitis is an inflammation of this area. Usually, labyrinthitis comes on quite suddenly. The victim is seized with severe dizziness and vomiting, and complete bed rest is the only known means of relieving the uncomfortable symptoms. These slowly subside until, after approximately 3 weeks, the patient is well but for a slight residual dizziness. Sometimes there is a hearing loss on the affected side.

Meniere's Disease Is a Catchall

For many years, it has been the practice of some physicians to label all dizziness complaints as Meniere's disease. Thus many of those who complain of dizziness automatically assume that the terms are interchangeable. Actually, Meniere formulated, through observation, a group of symptoms in which dizziness played an important part, but which also consisted of other definite symptoms as well. These are loss of hearing, ringing in the ears, dizziness, distortion of sound and feeling of pressure in the ears. The

[684]

dizziness varies from simple unsteadiness to violent, whirling vertigo. A natural or induced sleep while the patient is suffering from an attack seems to take care of all unpleasant symptoms. The patient awakes feeling refreshed and healthy.

Although no one will say for certain, it is believed by some that Meniere's syndrome is due to a hemorrhage of the small, delicate parts of the inner ear known as the semicircular canals. Others suggest some imbalance of fluid and pressure in the inner ear. As can be imagined, theories on a cure are just as sketchy. One treatment consists in giving the patient 50 to 100 milligrams of niacin (a B vitamin) about 20 minutes before each meal. Low salt intake is another remedy used by medical men. Some doctors say that giving up smoking might help. We don't pretend to know how effective these efforts might be, but any of these 3 measures would certainly improve one's general health.

There are even psychological causes for dizziness. The same article in the *Canadian Medical Association Journal* says that, when no organic disorder or disease is found to explain dizziness, tension might be the answer. Tension sometimes gives rise to feelings of uncertainty or insecurity, and these might show themselves in the form of dizziness.

Tight Collars and Insect Sprays

Among the more bizarre causes of dizziness is a condition called the carotid sinus syndrome. It is a term used to describe cases in which victims simply get dizzy and black out, at times, from wearing a tight collar. The *Journal of Living* (August, 1954) describes this condition and suggests that soldiers who faint on parade might be victims of this circumstance, rather than simple fatigue or sunstroke. A sudden turn of the head sometimes has the same effect on these people.

Another unsuspected cause of dizziness lies in uneven dental bite, says *Science News Letter* (January 5, 1957). Research showed that 96 per cent of sufferers of vertigo examined by a physician-dentist team had teeth that did not properly support the upper or lower jaw. This improper support is said to affect the area of the ear and disturb the semicircular canals that control equilibrium. If this theory holds true, dizziness is sure to be more and more common as our children grow up, since the worthless foods they eat have already led to alarming numbers of deformed dental arches and extracted teeth.

Editor Rodale once recounted a curious experience with dizziness. He noticed persistent dizzy spells that seemed to have no explanation. As is his custom when he notices some irregularity in his health, Mr. Rodale began to review his diet, searching for some clue as to what could cause this unsettling symptom. It was quickly apparent to him that he was eating large amounts of those tasty black cherries that are so plentiful and popular in the summertime. While the cherries themselves are a natural, and therefore healthful, food, Mr. Rodale soon was reminded that most growers boast that the plump perfection of their crop is due to spraying and more spraying with insecticides. As in the case of grapes and berries, the dangers of sprayed cherries are multiplied because they are a fruit one doesn't bother to peel. As a result the consumer ingests all of the residual insecticide that a quick rinse under the tap won't eliminate. Mr. Rodale concluded that this was the seat of his dizziness problem. He quickly eliminated the cherries from his diet, and was pleased to see his vertigo disappear simultaneously. This was many years ago.

The *General Practitioner* (November, 1953) had the clearest explanation we've seen of just how dizziness works. We are told that each time the posture of the head is changed, the gelatinous substance in the semicircular canals of the inner ear begins to flow. This flow then stimulates nerve impulses which normally go to various parts of the body in equal intensity and degree. But should there be an imbalance and the impulses be unequal, vertigo results. The varying impulses reaching the cerebrum make the victim aware of disturbed equilibrium; some reach the emetic center of the body and cause vomiting. In certain cases, the nerves of the eyes are affected, and a jerky to and fro motion of the eyeballs results because of the uneven stimuli originating in the inner ear. This phenomenon is known by the medical term *nystagmus*.

The far-reaching effects of antibiotics were demonstrated in a test described in *Diseases of the Chest* (October, 1950 and September, 1951). It was found that prolonged or intensive antibiotic therapy can cause serious nausea, vomiting and dizziness. Of 28 patients treated with streptomycin, 18 per cent complained of dizziness after therapy. *Arizona Medicine* (September, 1949) also mentions the possibility of damage to the labyrinth, with the likelihood of resultant dizziness, due to the use of drugs.

An Answer to Labyrinthitis

Another disease involving dizziness is labyrinthitis. The results achieved by Theodore R. Miller, M.D., in treating labyrinthitis with bioflavonoids, as reported in the *Eye, Ear, Nose and Throat Monthly* (September, 1958) are very promising. Labyrinthitis is a disease of the inner ear, characterized by varying degrees of dizziness, loss of balance and nausea. A typical attack begins with a feeling of seasickness, which acts as a sort of warning in time for the patient to lie down. This is usually followed by a sensation of external rotating and a headache on the side of the ear that is affected. Any attempt to look at surrounding objects greatly aggravates the symptoms.

Dr. Miller based his experiments on the established theory that such cases are the result of something going wrong with the capillaries in the ear, a disturbance in balance of minerals in the body. Since it is generally recognized that bioflavonoids are beneficial in treating capillary injuries of all kinds, and since salt is often the cause of mineral imbalance, Dr. Miller simply treated his patients with citrus bioflavonoids and a restriction on their salt intake.

The report written by Dr. Miller was based on his treatment of 9 cases diagnosed as labyrinthitis. They were all given 4 to 6 capsules of bioflavonoids per day with a decrease in salt intake, and results were shown in 3 to 6 days. The author stresses that one of the great advantages of this treatment is the complete freedom from side effects in bioflavonoids. They are nontoxic and can be given freely in large doses.

Several case histories are included in the report. One tells of a man 62 year of age, who developed a severe attack of giddiness at work and had to be brought home. He found that he couldn't sit up without a return of the symptoms, and he vomited often the following day. His doctor prescribed dramamine, a motion sickness remedy, and achieved some relief, but the dizziness persisted. An examination revealed that the patient was not suffering from any organic disorder.

The dizziness was not relieved for 4 months, and the patient was finally referred to Dr. Miller. Labyrinthitis was the diagnosis. The patient was placed on a low-sodium diet and given 6 capsules of citrus bioflavonoids per day. "He had almost immediate relief, in 3 days, and was able to follow his regular routine."

He remained well until the following January when he again developed symptoms. The treatment was begun once again and relief followed swiftly. The patient was advised to stay on a low-salt diet for about 3 months and to continue with the capsules 3 times per day.

Bioflavonoids an Integral Part of the Treatment

In another case, it was shown that the bioflavonoids were an integral part of the treatment. The patient, a 42-year-old male, suffered a severe cold and it was followed by dizziness, with a sense of rotation to the right when he changed his position while lying down. Symptoms would worsen when the man bent forward. His doctor treated him with dramamine and restricted his salt intake, but dizziness and nausea persisted. Again there was no organic disease.

When he was referred to Dr. Miller, his salt restriction was maintained and the only change in treatment was the prescription of 6 bioflavonoid capsules per day. In 3 days the symptoms were completely gone and there was no recurrence.

Here is another exciting use for a natural food supplement in the treatment of disease. Doubtless there are other treatments with natural substances, which are just as effective and dramatic, waiting to be discovered by enterprising scientists and physicians who are aware of the powers of natural foods in restoring and maintaining good health. Until they are found, it is well to remember that prevention is still the most desirable way of remaining disease-free, and that a diet rich in the food elements we must have is the best way of avoiding any impairment of our body's functions. Add the bioflavonoids to your daily supplement list.

From what is printed in medical journals, we have come to conclude that vertigo is one of those phantom annoyances which seem to be caused by anything in general and nothing in particular. There is no one vitamin to take or a single bad habit to give up which will guarantee a recovery from dizziness. But if we were suffering with this problem, we would certainly do the following: review our diet. Too much salt? Enough sources of B vitamins? Enough unsaturated fatty acids to control cholesterol? Do we violate the other taboos of good health by using sugar, refined flour products, coffee, tea, smoking, drinking, etc.? Do we use plenty of vitamin C to give our bodies a chance to knock out infection and neutralize the large number of anonymous poisons our bodies take in every day, through food and atmosphere? Is a source of vitamin E included in our diet to help the blood keep up its oxygen supply? Do we bother to exercise—a walk, a few knee bends?

If we were suffering from vertigo those are the things we'd check first, and it is quite likely that a trip to the doctor, followed by a series of treatments, would never be necessary. Don't let vertigo scare you into inactivity. Do something about it! Make sure you're living as healthfully as you should, and that may be all you'll have to do to solve your problem.

~~~~~~

SECTION 34: EPILEPSY

~~~~~~

181. Epilepsy

From biblical times, individuals have been afflicted with "seizures"— mysterious fits during which they fell to the ground and foamed at the mouth. Perfectly normal, happy, intelligent people the rest of the time, they suddenly appeared to have been bewitched when a seizure overtook them. Seizures, being unpredictable, often occurred in public, to the horror and fear of onlookers. Thus, during past ages, a whole tradition of the supernatural grew up around epilepsy. Plainly these sufferers were possessed of demons. Why else would they froth at the mouth, twitch convulsively and be unaware of what had transpired after they awoke from the sleep that follows epileptic seizures?

As superstition waned and people ceased to believe overtly in witch-craft, some other notions grew up to explain the phenomenon of epilepsy. Perhaps, since this disease seemed to be hereditary, it was caused by sins of the parents. It led to insanity, people said, or it led to feeble-mindedness. It was caused by masturbation, they said. Epileptics became criminals, they said, they should not marry or have children. In fact, laws were passed in many states forbidding the marriage of epileptics.

Today, medical learning has wiped out once and for all every single

one of these misconceptions of epilepsy. However, much of the old superstition remains in those dark, unexplored corners of people's minds where
are hidden all the silly fallacies we hate so much to give up, because giving
up the fallacies means that we have to make an effort to think our way
through to the truth. So the families of epileptics still conceal the disorder
from their friends and neighbors. Epileptics themselves feel shame, as
though there were some terrible disgrace attached to epilepsy which does
not apply to diabetes, arthritis or tuberculosis, for example. Yes, incredible
as it seems, there are still individuals in our enlightened twentieth century
who whisper dark, shameful gossip about those unfortunates who suffer
from one of the most mysterious and dread disorders—epilepsy.

What Epilepsy Is Not

Lewis J. Pollock, M.D., writing in *Today's Health* for May, 1951, has
this to say about epilepsy: "What is epilepsy? It is not a disease; it is not
related to feeble-mindedness; it is not, nor does it lead to insanity; it is
not associated with, nor does it lead to delinquency, vice, crime or mental
deterioration. In most instances it should not interfere with good health,
education, technical or professional training, or commercial, manufacturing
or professional pursuits. It is compatible with courtship, marriage, bearing
and rearing children, the pursuit of happiness and normal social life and
good citizenship. It bears no shame. It deserves only that amount of com-
passion freely given to those who have some other illness."

Beyond the mouldy vestiges of superstition, why do we persist in
talking and thinking of epilepsy as something shameful, which should be
hidden from others? It may be because of the violence of the epileptic
convulsions. A teacher in a classroom may have an exaggerated fear of
the possible disruption caused by an epileptic student. Yet, diabetics in
coma or insulin shock exhibit frightening symptoms, too, and there is no
shame attached to diabetes. We heard of a splendid student who was asked
to leave one of the women's colleges after the college physician discovered
that she was epileptic. Surely such treatment is monstrously unfair and
can only be the result of ignorance. True, an epileptic may be injured
in a convulsion, and the question of responsibility arises in the mind of
his employer or school principal. But there are thousands of ways for
people to injure themselves and we do not refuse education or employment
to anyone else on the basis of possible injury on the premises. It seems that
a lot more educational work must be done before the epileptic will be
accepted as a person *who is sometimes ill,* just as most of us are.

Epilepsy Is Commoner Than You Think

Almost anyone to whom you mention epilepsy will tell you that it is
an uncommon disease. So it is surprising to find that there are as many
epileptics in this country as there are sufferers from diabetes, or from active
tuberculosis. One American out of every 300 or 400 people has epilepsy.
Measured in money—and not counting lost man hours—epilepsy accounts

for more than 60 million dollars annually. Yet 80 out of 100 epileptics can at present lead almost normal lives.

What is epilepsy? In our research, we studied about 5 learned medical articles debating the question. In many aspects of the problem of defining epilepsy, the authorities were not agreed. We have found out many things that epilepsy is *not*. But we still know little of what it *is*. We do know that it is not, in itself, a disease. It is rather a symptom of some kind of disorder in the body. Says Dennis Williams, M.D., D.Sc., F.R.C.P., Physician in charge of Neurology at St. George's Hospital, England, in the January 24, 1953, issue of the *British Medical Journal*: Every ordinary doctor sees many patients with symptoms of loss of memory or consciousness, muscle-twitching, feeling of faintness or unreality, disturbances of vision, and so forth. Since the patients are usually quite well when they come to see him, he can diagnose the illness only from their descriptions of their feelings. How many of these are epileptics and where does the physician draw the dividing line between epileptics and non-epileptics? "We know that epilepsy can occur without loss of consciousness, without amnesia, without involuntary movement and without any of the simple features which would enable us to make a certain diagnosis of epilepsy. None of the definitions will do, for they are all too narrow," says Dr. Williams.

We do have an instrument which will diagnose epilepsy—the electroencephalograph. "Encephalo" means "brain" and "graph" means "writing," so this jawbreaker of a name refers simply to an instrument which records the electrical workings of the brain in writing. The brain, like the heart, gives off electrical currents. In using the electroencephalograph, the patient merely sits while electrodes are attached to his head through which his brain's electrical currents are recorded. The brain of an epileptic records a different kind of pattern from that of a non-epileptic.

The Types of Epilepsy

There is pretty general agreement on the different kinds of epilepsy. *Petit mal* (meaning *little sickness* in French) is a form of disorder which is much more common in children than in adults. Seizures generally are quite frequent—in fact there may be hundreds in one day. They last only a few seconds and may be overlooked, because they may give no indication except for a slight hesitation or confusion. The child may drop whatever he is holding, or he may fall and immediately get up. There may be rhythmic twitching of the eyelids or eyebrows. *Petit mal* attacks are usually worse in the morning hours and they usually grow less frequent and serious as the sufferer grows older.

Grand mal (big sickness) is what most of us mean when we think of epilepsy. The patient becomes unconscious and falls. Saliva may appear on his lips, he may cry out (although he is not feeling any pain), his muscles tighten into a spasm or convulsion and he twitches violently for a minute or two. Actually the seizure does not last long, although it may

[690]

seem long to the helpless observer. During an attack of *Grand mal,* the patient may mimic normal movements. He may appear to be beckoning with his fingers, his eyes or head may turn to one side or another, as if he were actually looking to that side. He may get up after the attack and feel dull and drowsy for a time, or he may go into a deep sleep and sleep for hours.

Psychomotor epilepsy is the most difficult to diagnose because symptoms vary from patient to patient. This is the kind of disorder that may cause individuals to do things which they later do not remember, such as suddenly going to a strange city, unreasonably beginning to push the furniture around or throw things. Jacksonian epilepsy involves twitching of muscles on one side while the patient remains conscious. Many epileptics have a warning when they are going to have an attack. It is called an "aura" by physicians. It may be a strange feeling in the stomach, a dizzy feeling or it may involve an unpleasant odor that the patient believes he smells.

Not many, but some, cases of epilepsy are caused by damage to the brain either at birth or later in life. In the other cases, the disorder is called "functional" or "idiopathic," meaning that a physical examination reveals nothing wrong with any organ. However, it is possible that functional epilepsy may result eventually in injury to the brain or other parts of the body, if seizures are frequent.

The difference between an epileptic seizure and a "faint" is that the first is a disturbance in the brain, the second involves a sudden lowering of the blood pressure, which causes the patient to become unconscious. A faint generally has some outside immediate cause—the sight of blood, bad news, etc. But an epileptic convulsion comes without any such circumstances. Dr. Williams, concluding his definition of epilepsy, says, "It might be said in criticism of this didactic and rigid distinction between epilepsy and other states that the borderland between epilepsy and psychopathy is a narrow one, hardly explored and that the basis of neither state is understood."

At present, drugs are given which are effective in relieving epileptic convulsions. Dilantin and mesantoin for *Grand mal* and triodone for *Petit mal* have proved to be effective in many cases. However, as with all drugs, there are side effects and sometimes very serious ones, which necessitate the closest supervision by the physician and constant testing to make certain that these side effects are not fatal.

Can We Prevent Epilepsy?

What about prevention of epilepsy? We began our research on the subject with an article in the *Quarterly Review of Allergy and Applied Immunology,* June, 1952, by Hal. M. Davison, M.D., of Atlanta, Georgia. Dr. Davison presents and discusses evidence that allergies cause symptoms and disease conditions in the nervous system. Many of these symptoms are the same that are encountered in multiple sclerosis and epilepsy. Drawing from an enormous amount of reference material (192 articles and personal communications are listed in the bibliography), Dr. Davison describes many patients whose convulsions disappeared when the food to which they were allergic was removed from their diet. For instance, "in one patient with *Petit mal* and *Grand mal,* attacks were produced 5 times by the ingestion of cauliflower and were relieved by the omission of this food. . . . One child aged 4 with asthma, headache, mental and emotional symptoms, and convulsive attacks all relieved by injections of extracts of pollen to which the patient was sensitive. . . . Four patients were definitely proven to have epileptic attacks due to specific foods, one to eggs, one to milk, one to mushrooms and one to cereals. . . . Macready and Ray reported patients with convulsions beginning in infancy with the first real change in their diet. Some of these attacks persisted for years and were still present; some had been relieved by removing certain foods from their diet. . . . Eastlake reported one patient with epilepsy shown to be due to beef, in whom the subcutaneous injection of 4 drops of sterile beef broth produced an attack of such intensity that heroic treatment was necessary. The woman's eldest daughter also had epilepsy proven to be due to certain meats. . . . Eighteen allergists reported 33 patients with *Grand mal,* two with *Petit mal* and 3 with both *Grand* and *Petit mal,* all relieved by allergic treatment alone. . . ." We could go on and on giving most convincing case histories from this article.

Refusal of Allergy As a Cause

"The fact," says Dr. Davison, "that some of these patients with allergy and other symptoms involving the nervous system suffered from periods of unconsciousness without convulsions, some had convulsions, and some had twitchings and spasmodic contractions of muscles over various parts of the body without unconsciousness, led us to believe that epilepsy itself could be a manifestation of allergy." He goes on to tell of sending a letter to 1494 specialists in allergy, asking for their opinion of allergy as a possible cause of epilepsy. Of the 207 answers he received, typical ones were: "not suspected, never occurred to me, overlooked," and so forth. This, in spite of the fact that articles on allergy and epilepsy have appeared frequently in medical magazines throughout the past 30 years, as Dr. Davison's list of references testifies.

Dr. Davison tells us how epileptic attacks frequently begin with some manifestation of allergy—a 6-year-old boy who developed epileptic symptoms along with eczema, digestive disturbances, hives, hay fever, asthma and finally convulsions. A 32-year old woman who had digestive upsets, then hay fever, hives and migraine, followed some years later by convulsions. He also says that precipitating factors which often bring about convulsions are: fear, anxiety, fatigue, chilling, sexual excess, or overindulgence in alcohol or some unusual food.

[692]

In spite of the splendid array of evidence, Dr. Davison concludes, "No one believes that allergy is a causative factor in all cases of idiopathic epilepsy. It is evident and already proven that epilepsy is a symptom complex produced by many different causes. In some individuals, the epileptic attacks may have several causes cooperating to produce them." He pleads for a greater realization of the part that allergies may play in this tragic disorder and outlines the steps that doctors should take to check *first* on allergy as a possible cause.

Further Evidence of Allergy As a Cause

Dr. Foster Kennedy, writing in the *Archives of Neurology and Psychiatry* for June, 1938, adds some astounding evidence, including the case of a 21-year-old nurse who had an epileptic attack every time she ate chocolate. Dr. A. H. Rowe, in the *Journal of Nervous and Mental Diseases,* May, 1944, tells us of allergies to eggs, tomatoes, cereals, milk, veal, pepper, pollen and animal hair which brought on symptoms of dizziness, fatigue, headache, depression, confusion, spots before the eyes, tinnitus (ringing in the ears), tingling in hands and feet, and so forth, in addition to convulsions. In every case, the symptoms disappeared on Dr. Rowe's "elimination" diet by which various foods were omitted one at a time, until the villain was found.

In *Modern Medicine* for December 1, 1951, Susan C. Dees, M.D., and Hans Lowenbach, M.D., report on 37 children under the age of 14 with *Petit* and *Grand mal* who also had a wide range of allergic symptoms —asthma, eczema, colds, etc. In 24 of the children, all symptoms were controlled by finding the offending allergen and eliminating it from the diet. The brain patterns of these children improved steadily. However, as soon as the program was stopped and full freedom was allowed to eat anything they wished, all symptoms returned again.

Now, tracking down an allergy is a tedious and expensive business. It involves going back to the specialist week after week for tests which may go on for months or even years until the allergen is found. A friend of ours turned out to be allergic to everything! After weeks of frantic testing, his doctor finally gave up, then he made one last try in which he discovered that our friend was allergic to the serum in which the various tests were being administered. Then they started all over again and finally tracked down the villain.

An elimination diet would seem to be an easy enough solution for discovering whether you have any food allergies. We suppose any physician can make up such a diet. Of course, it must be adhered to without fail if you really want to uncover a food to which you are allergic. And possibly you might make up your own elimination diet by simply omitting one certain food every week and seeing whether the allergic symptoms may disappear. Of course, such things as alcohol and tobacco, coffee, tea and so forth should be suspect, too.

Now finally we come to our last suggestion which appears to us to be the most sensible of all. We have referred many times in these pages to a book by E. M. Abrahamson, M.D., *Body, Mind and Sugar,* published by Henry Holt and Company. Dr. Abrahamson writes in this book about low blood sugar, which he says, is far more prevalent in America than its opposite, which is diabetes. He tells almost unbelievable stories about curing allergies with a diet which keeps the blood sugar at its normal level and does not let it fall below. Asthma, hay fever, alcoholism, depression, neurosis (so-called), fatigue, dizziness, headache, migraine, weakness and many more common ailments take flight never to return, sometimes after only 3 weeks on the prescribed diet.

Allergies and Low Blood Sugar

Dr. Abrahamson believes that it is not necessary to have allergies at all. In fact, he claims that no one who adheres rigidly to the prescribed diet *can* have allergies. In speaking of epilepsy, he says, "at a meeting (Dr. Myerson) attended, some psychiatrist advanced the hypothesis that epileptics are men who hate their fathers. Myerson commented that he knew a lot of epileptic cats who had never met their fathers." He continues, "Among the signs and symptoms behind which hyperinsulinism (low blood sugar) masquerades, Seale Harris included those of *Petit mal.* It is significant that some women who suffered from epilepsy appeared to improve during pregnancy, as rheumatoid arthritis and peptic ulcer patients did— when the blood glucose (sugar) tends to be higher. Other pregnant epileptics, however, seemed to suffer more severely. A number of persons subject to epileptic seizures were given the glucose tolerance test which indicated low blood sugar curves. *It has also been found that the brain wave tracings of persons afflicted with Petit mal were similar to those of hyperinsulinism victims (that is, people who had low blood sugar).* (Italics ours.) While these facts are insufficient in themselves to indicate that epilepsy is a manifestation of hyperinsulinism, they provide enough evidence to warrant further investigation of the relationship between the two diseases."

We do not know how long it may take for the medical profession to get around to this "further investigation." Research is expensive and, we suppose, some people actually prefer drugs rather than adhering to a diet. However, those of us who believe in the effectiveness of diet in preventing disease can surely do ourselves a big favor by trying out Dr. Abrahamson's diet, which, incidentally, has a lot to recommend it whether or not you suffer from allergies, headaches, epilepsy or any other disorder. It is an extremely simple and inexpensive diet to follow and we can just about guarantee that anybody will feel better on it, no matter how good they felt to begin with. (See chapter 78 for Dr. Abrahamson's diet.)

Is Epilepsy Inherited?

There is a lively controversy in scientific circles over whether or not epilepsy is inherited. Incredible amounts of investigation have been done to prove one side or the other. In one article we read, 20,000 relatives of 4000 epileptics were interviewed, and the conclusion drawn was that "the genetic factor in epilepsy is probably no greater than it is in many other common diseases. Assets that are transmissible, such as sound vital organs, good intelligence, personality and social responsibility, may outweigh the liability of a tendency to seizures. Hence, advice regarding marriage and children must be individualized." Other researches show us that the inheritance factor in epilepsy is 1/10 of that in diabetes, and 1/25 of that in migraine. Surely no one would question the advisability of marriage for someone who suffers from migraine headaches, and is worried for fear he or she might transmit the disorder to children. Yet migraine headaches "run" in 25 times as many families as epilepsy does! And speaking of inheritance, we can't fail to come back to a favorite question of ours—how much is inherited and how much is due to food patterns?

Very early in life you are conditioned to the foods you like and those you don't like. It comes about largely through your family's ideas about food. If no one ever eats lamb in your family, chances are you won't eat it after you are grown. If your family has spaghetti once a week, you'll probably serve spaghetti often in your own home, while the family that lives next door may never have tasted spaghetti and so are convinced they wouldn't like it. If epilepsy is indeed related to allergies, and allergies are unquestionably related to food patterns, then, without studying the daily menus of everyone involved, how can we be sure that any predisposition to epilepsy is "inherited"? And what about those members of an epileptically inclined family who break away from the established food pattern and free themselves from prejudices where food is concerned? Might they not be the very ones who do not "inherit" the epilepsy?

One last statistic. It has been found that one person in every 10 has some irregularity in brain wave patterns when being tested by the electroencephalograph. Only one person in every 200 has epileptic seizures. How many of us then can say that we do not have a tendency toward epilepsy if we are the one person in 10? Robust health is our best safeguard against such a tendency. This means—whether you follow the Abrahamson diet or not—no foods that contain white sugar or white flour. No soft drinks. Only whole grain cereals. Plenty of fresh vegetables and fruits, as many raw as possible. And enough of the protective foods—meat, eggs and nuts. In addition, because all of our food has been robbed of vitamins and minerals before it reaches our tables, take natural food supplements: brewer's yeast or desiccated liver for vitamin B, fish liver oil for vitamins A and D, rose hips for vitamin C, wheat germ oil for vitamin E and bone meal for minerals.

182. Epilepsy and Other Mental Disorders

We see a great deal of medical information at our offices. We subscribe to medical journals from all over the world, written in many languages. We get weekly and monthly federal, state and city health reports, bulletins and abstracts. Add to this the dozens of books that come to us monthly for review, the many others we buy and those we get from libraries to help us in our research. Then our readers send countless clippings from newspapers and magazines from every corner of the world. We mention all of this merely to indicate that we are not naïve about medical reporting and not uninformed about what is being done in various branches of scientific research. We don't often see information that strikes us as revolutionary or world-shaking. However, of all the periodicals we see, none presents news as consistently dramatic as the *Summary* published by the Shute Foundation for Medical Research.

The Shute Foundation is devoted largely to bringing to the attention of the world experiments and observations on the therapeutic values of vitamin E. In each issue of the *Summary,* we see truly astounding news of the effectiveness of vitamin E in the treatment and cure of diseases often abandoned as incurable by orthodox medicine. Oftentimes vitamin E offers a simple answer to disease problems usually treated with strong-acting drugs which present dangerous side effects. Heart disease, diabetes, infertility, miscarriage and many other diseases have shown quick response to vitamin E.

An Important Letter

In the *Summary* (June, 1961) we saw what will probably be, for many, the most valuable and hopeful information yet. A letter from A. del Guidice, Chief of Child Psychology, National Institute of Public Health, Buenos Aires, Argentina, is quoted in full, and it tells of the success of vitamin E as a treatment for mental defects in children. Let us quote for you his initial remarks:

"Dear Sir:

"Our extensive experience with vitamin E therapy in children has taught us a good deal about the management of psychosomatic (physical disorders of mental origin) aspects of their problems.

"We use dosages of alpha tocopherol which vary with the age of the patient and the gravity of his disease, as well as the time permitted for treatment. However, the guiding principle has been massive dosage and continuous administration, never omitting a single day in our effort to achieve and maintain tissue saturation—one continuous course of treatment, until one sees the child's mental state improve.

[696]

"We have treated many complications in our infantile psychotics, such as the ophthalmological (visual disorders) where we have had brilliant results in myopia (nearsightedness), nystagmus (involuntary, rapid movement of the eyeball); strabismus (crossed eyes), cataract and other conditions, as will be noted in more detail below (case histories following the letter). No child remained unimproved when properly treated.

"Generally we have begun treatment with 200 to 300 milligrams of vitamin E daily, increasing over a period of as long as 6 months to doses approximating two grams daily—depending on the age of the child and his type of disease.

"Vitamin C was also given in doses of 500 to 1500 grams (most likely a misprint for milligrams) daily. It was added because of my belief that it reinforces vitamin E—it being clear, always, that the latter is the basic item. Vitamin C seems especially indicated in organic deficiencies and old cataracts."

Dr. del Guidice then presented a group of short case histories. We think his results with vitamin E are most gratifying and certainly deserve the attention of doctors in the United States. What doctor or parent would allow the opportunity of using a healthful nutrient therapeutically, to slip by, if he could hope for such results as Dr del Guidice describes?

Epilepsy Responds to Vitamin E

The first case concerns epilepsy, a not-too-rare problem in children. Its control is largely confined to rather powerful drugs which are given on an increasing scale, as required, until their side effects become so intolerable that some other form of therapy must be introduced.

Judge for yourself if the epilepsy cases treated by Dr. del Guidice could have merely disappeared in so short a time, or if vitamin E is the answer.

CASE I: Involved a little girl aged 3. She had experienced a severe fall at 9 months, and the epilepsy was attributed to that. She had her first seizure at the age of two. It lasted 4 minutes with unconsciousness, spasm and frothing at the mouth. Afterward, the child suffered with a violent headache and other slight disturbances for 6 hours. She was unable to speak for the first one and one-half hours of that period.

She fell frequently thereafter, wet the bed, was restless in sleep, nervous, had crying spells and did not get on well with other children. Tocopherol medication was begun as her sole treatment. In 3 months time, she had improved, was far more tranquil, played with other children, had no more convulsions.

After 10 months of treatment, she still had had no more convulsions, or seizures, had conquered her bed-wetting problem, had become quite friendly and calm, had gained weight, slept well, rarely cried and was a happy child.

CASE II: A 9-months-old boy who, after electroencephalograph tests,

[697]

(EGG) was diagnosed as an epileptic. He had convulsions several times daily during which his eyes pulled to one side, his neck retracted and became rigid and he lost consciousness. There was great instability in his movements and he was nervous while awake and restless in sleep.

His previous treatment had consisted of hormonal preparations and sedatives, but to no avail. Previous medication was halted by Dr. del Guidice, and the boy was given tocopherol only. After several months, he lost his convulsions, excitability and instability of motion. After 5 months' treatment, he had no more convulsions, slept peacefully and was much quieter.

Both of these cases of frank epilepsy responded to treatment with vitamin E when other treatments had failed. This is not an infrequent course of events. We do not know if such results could be achieved with adult epileptics. Dr. del Guidice does not discuss any patients but children, but we can see no reason for not trying vitamin E to treat adults as well.

Why Does Vitamin E Work?

The fact that vitamin E can prolong the retention of oxygen in the blood stream is probably the key to its effectiveness in treating mental disorders. The brain needs an optimum supply of oxygen if it is to function properly. Perhaps in some systems, the demands for oxygen elsewhere in the body exhaust the supply before the blood reaches the brain. This could be the result of an inadequate supply of oxygen in the first place, or because of an inability to retain it in the blood long enough to meet all necessities. Vitamin E could be very effective in preventing or reversing such a situation.

Dr. del Guidice gave 20 more case histories in his letter to the *Summary*. In each of them, mental disorder was effectively treated with vitamin E. It is not true that all of them were completely cured with vitamin E, but all were benefited sufficiently so that the change was clinically observable.

Here, briefly, are some of the other cases discussed by Dr. del Guidice. A 12 year old girl who was a congenital idiot exhibited aggressive impulses which called for restraint of her arms by her parents almost all the time. She shouted and cried for no reason and was extremely moody. The girl could not speak properly. She could not comprehend questions and was unable to manage her own toilet routine. For 6 years of medical treatment, there had been no improvement.

After 40 days of tocopherol therapy, she had made more progress than in all of the previous 6 years. At the end of a year, she was fairly subdued, sat correctly and watched her surroundings calmly. She lost her babbling, crying and aggressiveness, sat at table and ate by herself for the first time.

Case 12 was a female, aged 3, who stuttered and had a severe inferiority complex. Her mother was almost unaware of what the child's voice was like. She couldn't even play with her little brothers and sisters. On the third day of tocopherol therapy, she was improved. In 3 months of tocopherol treatment, she was completely free of stammering, could recite 3 verses of a poem with ease and fluency, and played happily with other children.

Psychosomatic Paralysis and Blindness Yield

Case 14 concerned a 5-year-old girl whose both legs were paralyzed, and her mind deficient. She had never talked, could not balance herself on her feet, did not walk, and had had no results from any of the considerable medical treatment taken since birth. After 7 months on tocopherol, she began to walk and talk, articulating some words clearly. Four months later she could walk well, even run, and her mentality was improved.

This is an obvious case of so-called psychosomatic illness, the type in which the mind is largely responsible for a physical disability. The child's legs were certainly able to function, had she willed them to do so.

A case much like this was number 15, a 23-year-old man who had physically normal eyes, but suffered from a mental deficiency and "blindness." Though he was equipped with normal visual apparatus, the man could not see. Eight years of treatment under his own physician had been futile.

In less than two months on vitamin E, he could vaguely count the fingers on a hand almost 7 feet away, and recognize people 10 feet away, with his left eye. With his right eye he saw a little less, but he could now dress and feed himself, travel alone on a train and walk through city traffic. He was mentally improved as well.

Cataracts Slowly Disappear

Of special interest to us were several cases, described by Dr. del Guidice, in which vitamin E proved an effective cataract treatment. In one instance, a 10 year-old-girl who had been born with cataracts on both eyes, was totally blind, even to the point at which she could not distinguish light, even after an operation on her right eye. She was depressed and extremely quiet. After 6 months on tocopherol, her personality had changed for the better, and she could detect light. The cataracts were less dense, and the corneas more brilliant. In the right eye the pupil was now visible.

Another child of 10, also born with cataracts of both eyes which had been operated on unsuccessfully, tried vitamin E. In 8 months, the child could see small objects at short distances.

A boy of the same age had congenital cataracts of the right eye and and other defects of both eyes. He was also mentally deficient. In 1955, vitamin E therapy was begun. His mental capacity increased, and the congenital cataract disappeared as the Opthalmological Institute, which had been watching him, testified. His vision improved in both eyes. (The slow disappearance of the cataract began as soon as the tocopherol treatment started.)

[699]

These cases are of more than passing interest. If the results obtained by Dr. del Guidice can be repeated by other doctors, surely vitamin E is at least a partial answer to one of our most vexing problems, mental illness. And if all cataracts will show a similar response to vitamin E, many inoperable cases can hope for relief.

It is to be hoped that more work will be done along the lines of Dr. del Guidice's. We hope other clinicians will be sufficiently impressed with the doctor's position and prestige to listen to him when he tells of his results of vitamin E, and use the treatment themselves. If there had been no Dr. del Guidice to use vitamin E on them, would those patients about whom he wrote have progressed as they did? No one really knows, but the record would indicate against it. Treatments of as much as 6 and 8 years along conventional lines had done no good. Several weeks or months with vitamin E had been rewarded with strong indications of improvement or complete recovery.

Will Our Children Have a Chance?

Will our children be given a similar opportunity for recovery? Will an American doctor who sees progressive epilepsy or some other mental involvement in a child, try vitamin E? Will he do so in the case of congenital cataracts? Will he try to *cure* nervousness instead of merely tranquilizing it?

Dr. del Guidice's experiences are truly monumental in the field of treatment for emotionally disturbed children, an increasingly common disorder in modern society. We can only guess why vitamin E is so effective in this area, but it apparently does work, so why not make the most of it? We are using drugs which merely dull symptoms and do not reach the causes of illness at all. Vitamin E is a nutrient, and if it is effective, it is effective because it fills a need which has not been met by diet. Meet this need and you have conquered the problem, not merely pacified or disguised it. Modern medicine seems satisfied to pacify disease instead of curing it. Aspirins don't cure headaches, they merely help to dull the pain; cortisone doesn't cure arthritis, it merely dulls the symptoms; phenobarbitol doesn't cure epilepsy, it merely quiets it. But this is the kind of treatment doctors prescribe. Why should we settle for temporary relief without trying for a possible permanent cure?

Talk to your doctor about vitamin E. Ask him to write for a copy of the *Summary* at the Shute Clinic, London, Ontario, Canada. How can he help but be interested in such a strong advancement in the treatment of so many physical and mental disorders?

[700]

183. The Asiatic Flu

The *Journal of the American Medical Association* for August 31, 1957, in speaking of influenza, announces that, "A properly constituted vaccine containing the new strain of type A virus represents the only preventive tool at our command." Earlier in the article, the author, LeRoy E. Burney, M.D., announced quite casually, "Influenza is one of several acute infectious diseases involving the upper respiratory tract that may occur in epidemic form. Such infections as adenovirus, exudative pharyngitis, the common cold and others cannot be differentiated from influenza without appropriate confirmatory laboratory tests. An outbreak of influenza may occur simultaneously with one of the other respiratory infections. However, influenza usually spreads more widely and more rapidly and its presence may be suspected when an epidemic shows this characteristic."

In other words, if more people get bad colds at the same time, then we'll call it Asiatic flu. Isn't that what the good doctor is saying? There seems to be no other way to decide whether it's a cold or the flu. Except, of course, that we have a vaccine for the flu.

Authorities Speak Out Against the Vaccine

Here are a few comments from our file on the Asiatic flu vaccine. The *Binghamton* (New York) *Press* for August 16, 1957, quotes Dr. Hobart A. Reimann, Director of Medical Services at the Binghamton Hospital, as saying, "There is no reason to believe that the infection (Asiatic flu) is any more serious than are ordinary epidemic colds such as we have every year." According to the *Press,* he also questioned the desirability of the vaccine. Said he, "A vaccine will be available, but I will not be vaccinated nor will my family. Vaccine may prevent or lessen the severity of influenza, but at times the reactions to vaccine are more uncomfortable than the influenza itself, and the duration of protection it gives probably does not last more than a few weeks."

Lest anyone fear that Dr. Reimann is one of us "health cranks," let us hasten to give you his qualifications to speak on the flu vaccine. For the past 20 years, Dr. Reimann has prepared an annual review on infectious diseases for the American Medical Association. He was a pioneer in describing virus pneumonia, has taught in several universities and is "an internationally-recognized authority on infectious diseases."

Our local county medical societies published much the same opinion. "Considerably exaggerated" said one county president. "Appears to be less severe than at first thought," said another. An M.D. wrote to the *Lancaster* (Pennsylvania) *Intelligencer-Journal* (in part), "Everyone with a touch of old-fashioned grippe, cold or even poor compatibility of food will be diagnosing himself as having the Asiatic flu, and when they go to the doctor, he will ask if they had shots for the flu. If they did, then they have the grippe or something else, but if they didn't have the shots—Mr. Public, you have the Asiatic flu."

Headlines in the *Washington* (D.C.) *Daily News* for September 11, 1957, ask "Is the Big Flu Scare Worse Than the Flu?" The article goes on to quote one doctor, "Catching the flu is the least of my worries right now. The whole thing has been blown way out of proportion. So far, the typical case has been comparable to a heavy cold." Another comment, "Although the public has almost ignored flu vaccines available since 1945 for other virus strains, the Asian flu has suddenly become 'fashionable.' "

A clipping came in, too, about a young girl who died from the vaccine. There has been considerable comment in much of the adverse publicity about the possible danger to folks who are allergic to eggs, since the vaccine is prepared from eggs and hence could do grave damage to such a person. One note tells us that among children, who are particularly susceptible to flu, as many as 20 per cent are allergic to eggs!

What is our advice if you would avoid the flu? We believe you can lick a cold, even after it has its clutches on you, if, at the very first symptom, you increase your intake of vitamin C to massive proportions. Take plenty of natural vitamin C at frequent intervals—every couple of hours. It is a natural antidote to poisons. It does its work in the white blood corpuscles which the body calls out to fight infections.

184. Using Vitamin E on Gangrene

An article on the use of vitamin E in the treatment of small areas of gangrene brings us much valuable information about vitamin E and why we should take it every day of our lives.

Did you know, for instance, that vitamin E can and does produce new blood vessels around the site of an obstruction in a vessel, so that the blood can continue to circulate there? In some cases, it has been found that the new artery is as large and sound as the old obstructed one. Did you know that vitamin E has the power of dilating the veins? That is, if they are narrowed by deposits so that the blood has trouble getting through, vitamin E widens them. Did you know, too, that vitamin E is an anti-thrombin? This means that it has the power of retarding or preventing the coagulation of blood—a good guarantee against a clot in the brain or heart artery. It does not, however, predispose one to hemorrhages, as many of the anti-coagulant drugs do. Finally, did you know that vitamin E makes the tiny capillaries stronger so that hemorrhaging is unlikely?

The authors of "Alpha Tocopherol in the Management of Small Areas of Gangrene" (*Canadian Medical Association Journal,* May 1, 1957) are Stephen Tolgyes, M.D., and Evan Shute, M.D. They go into the story of arteriosclerosis or hardening of the arteries with a most unusual theory. They quote a recent researcher, J. B. Duguid, as believing that the "hardening" that appears on the walls of arteries may be just an accumulation of old blood clots. It seems that a careful examination has shown that this troublesome substance does indeed contain fibers of blood protein. Is it the result of blood clots attaching themselves to the walls of the arteries? If this is indeed correct, then the role of vitamin E becomes even more important, for it may do much to prevent the formation of such clots.

Then, as perhaps its most important function in the body vitamin E "enjoys an unrivaled role among physiological agents in its ability to improve tissue utilization of oxygen," according to our authors. All of us know the importance of oxygen to good health. We learn about this in physiology classes in grade school. Conserving oxygen and helping tissues to utilize to best advantage what oxygen there is, becomes an increasingly important function of vitamin E when you contemplate the ever-lessening amounts of oxygen we must get along with in an atmosphere polluted day and night, in homes that are well-insulated and stuffy and often blue with tobacco smoke.

Treating Gangrene with Vitamin E

In treating gangrene with vitamin E, the authors treated patients with arteriosclerosis, diabetes and thrombo-angiitis obliterans or Buerger's disease. Of 48 patients, they saved from pending threatening amputation "a good percentage."

The first patient whose case history they give, aged 30, had gangrene patches on the fingers of the left hand. He was given 500 units of vitamin E by mouth and a vitamin E ointment was applied. No other treatment was given and, within a little more than two months, healing was complete.

The second case, a woman of 85, was an unsuspected diabetic. Gangrene of one of her toes had spread down the inside of her foot. Treatment with vitamin E and insulin, along with a low calorie diet, brought about complete healing within 4 months.

A third patient smoked heavily, we are told. She was urged to stop smoking, but did not. It is well known that smoking is at least one of the causes of Buerger's disease, if not the leading cause. The usual story in cases of Buerger's disease is that the disease can be halted so long as the patient does not smoke. In this case, the vitamin E treatment halted the progress of the gangrene, even though the patient did not adhere to the diet she was given and did continue to smoke heavily.

Most Successful in Diabetic Gangrene

In discussing these and other cases, the authors say that while vitamin E cannot cure every case of gangrene, it appears that it can "save many toes and feet that otherwise would be sacrificed." It is most successful in cases of diabetic gangrene. In 50 per cent of these cases, the insulin requirement was subsequently decreased. This often happened long before there was noticeable change in the gangrene, and in two cases, it happened within 3 days of beginning the vitamin E treatment.

Patients with Buerger's disease may find that treatment with vitamin E brings pain, as the blood returns to the area that has been gangrenous, in much the same way that a frozen toe or finger aches when feeling returns. The authors recommend that vitamin E be used on frostbite, and on feet or fingers suffering from long immersion in water.

Our readers will not, of course, be treating gangrene with vitamin E, we hope. We present the above information merely to show the power of this mild, fat-soluble vitamin which is almost nonexistent in our modern refined and processed foods. If vitamin E can work near-miracles like these with the horribly degenerated tissues of gangrene, where the only alternative may be amputation, what can it not do to strengthen healthy tissue? Now, while you are healthy, now, when there is no fear of gangrene or blood clots or any other affliction in your circulatory system—now is the time to take vitamin E in supplement form as well as getting plenty of it in everyday meals.

It is most plentiful in whole grains—real whole grains—vegetable and cereal oils, legumes, brown rice, eggs and salad greens.

~~~~~~

SECTION 37: GOITER

~~~~~~

185. The Riddle of Goiter

For an understanding of the condition we call goiter, we must first know something about the thyroid gland and its function in the human body. Located at the base of the neck, over the Adam's apple, the thyroid is a ductless gland. That means it is an organ of the body which secretes a fluid, but it has no "duct," or opening, through which this fluid passes to some other part of the body. So the fluid manufactured by the thyroid gland passes directly into the blood stream. This fluid, or hormone, thyroxine, is made by the thyroid gland out of iodine and the amino acid, tyrosine. (Amino acids are forms of protein.)

Importance of Thyroid Hard to Overestimate

The importance of the thyroid gland to health can hardly be overestimated. The thyroid, through the hormone thyroxine, determines growth, controls body temperature, regulates the metabolism or the burning of food in the body and influences, to a great extent, mental and emotional balance. Also, it is of special importance for a proper functioning of the reproductive system. The inter-relationship between reproductive functions and thyroid functions is very complex and not entirely understood, but it is known that various changes, especially in girls and women, are apt to cause changes in thyroid function. For instance, a slight enlargement of the thyroid gland is common at puberty, during pregnancy and the menopause.

When the thyroid gland is functioning properly, we are hardly aware of its existence. It stores practically all of the body's supply of iodine, releases thyroxine into the blood stream at intervals and regulates all the bodily functions we have mentioned above. Disorders of the thyroid gland are apparently caused by two conditions: (1.) lack of sufficient iodine in the diet, so that the thyroid cannot obtain enough to manufacture thyroxine; or (2.) some disorder of the body which creates a demand for far more thyroxine than the gland can manufacture and hence, more iodine than is available in the diet.

What Is Goiter?

Goiter, generally speaking, refers to any abnormal enlargement of the thyroid gland. *Simple* goiter, called also *endemic* goiter, is an enlargement of the thyroid caused, apparently, by increased need for the thyroid secretion. The gland becomes larger in an effort to produce more and more thyroxine. This condition is not accompanied by other symptoms, except possibly a feeling of fatigue. *Toxic* goiter, called also *exophthalmic* goiter, is marked by the suddenness of its appearance, and its accompanying symptoms of extreme nervousness, emaciation, irritability, sweating and rapid heart beat. We do not know what causes toxic goiter. *Myxedema* occurs in complete atrophy of the thyroid gland. That is, this gland does not function at all, and all the other body operations which it regulates are affected, with resulting headache, lassitude, obesity, depression, subnormal temperature and mental dullness. Children whose thyroid glands are atrophied at birth, because they have inherited this condition, are said to have "cretinism." Such children are mentally defective, lethargic and dull, with scanty hair and pasty, thick skins. Many do not survive to adulthood. Adult cretinism is the result of thyroid deficiency over many generations. It frequently results in heart trouble, deafness and deaf-mutism.

What Part Does Iodine Play?

J. F. McClendon, Professor of Physiological Chemistry at the University of Minnesota, is one of the leading authorities in the branch of thyroid study that has concentrated on iodine deficiency in the diet. His book, *Iodine and the Incidence of Goiter,* published by the University of Minnesota Press in 1939, includes a full discussion of the world distribution of the ailment, as compared with the distribution of iodine in food, water, soil and rocks. In 1910, Professor McClendon noted that a woman who had lived in a region where goiters were common was relieved of this illness when she began to eat quantities of sea food, which contains a lot of iodine. This observation convinced him that iodine is an essential food constituent and that lack of it may lead to a deficiency, just as lack of a vitamin may. The deficiency disease in the case of iodine would be goiter.

Though Dr. McClendon admits that many of the more complicated phases of thyroid function need much more investigation before they are adequately understood, he believes that enough is already known about goiter for us to relate it purely and simply to the iodine content of the diet.

Where Goiter Occurs Most Frequently

In the United States, the only complete goiter survey of one section of the population (in this case, men) was made by the draft board during World War I. Only goiters so large that military collars would not button around them were recorded.

The figures show that the following states ranked highest in goiter among the drafted men: Idaho, with 26.91 goiters per 100 men, Oregon with 26.31, Washington with 23.40, Montana with 21., Utah with 15.72, Wyoming with 15.37, Wisconsin with 14.02, Alaska with 13.14 and Michigan with 11.43. Goiter was least common in these: Maine, .66, Delaware, .59, Rhode Island, .55, New Jersey, .43, Massachusetts, .32 and Florida, .25.

From these figures, it was noted that goiter was most common in the Great Lakes region and the Pacific Northwest and least common along the Atlantic and Gulf coasts and in most southern states. In a Public Health survey published in *Public Health Report,* 1926 and 1929, Oelsen revealed that goiter is 10 to 50 times more prevalent in America than these statistics would indicate. His figures were based on a survey of school children in 43 states. He conducted actual medical examinations of these children, whereas the draft board had concerned itself only with observations and statistics of men whose goiters were already too large to be confined within military collars.

Iodine Supplements to the Diet

Those medical men who believed that addition of iodine to the diet was all that was necessary, searched for the best ways of administering it. In a number of places in the world, salt is a government monopoly, and in some of these countries, iodine in the form of potassium iodide was added to the table salt. In this country, Marine and Kimball, working on a grant from the American Medical Association, divided the school children of Akron, Ohio, into two groups, one of which was given two grams of sodium iodide in broken doses twice a year. The other group was used as a control group and was given no iodine. Among 2190 school girls who took this preventive treatment for 3 years, only 5 developed goiter. Of 3205 who did not take it, 495 developed goiter.

At the same time, various European countries were experimenting with iodized salt. By 1932, Switzerland (where goiter is very common) was using enormous quantities of iodized salt. After 1923, the Austrian government sold iodized salt exclusively for a 5-year period. In Vienna (Austria) in 1923, 43 per cent of the school children had goiter. In 1927, the incidence had fallen to 31 per cent. Since then, the health authorities of many other countries have recommended dietary supplements in the hope of reducing goiter rates.

In the United States, the taking of iodized salt has been up to the individual. But Professor McClendon recalls that in Detroit, the school cafeterias used nothing but iodized salt in meals for 50,000 students in 1931. The 1924 goiter rate of 46 per cent dropped to 12 per cent in 1931. This is in contrast to the rate in Cleveland where iodized salt was not used. In 1924, there was 34 per cent goiter among Cleveland school children; in 1931, 30 per cent. From a comparison of these figures it is apparent that the decline in Detroit's percentages cannot be attributed to pure chance, for in Cleveland (considered an equally goitrous region) where no iodized salt was used in the schools, there was no comparable reduction in the percentage of goiters.

Other researchers have favored the use of sea food to obtain ample iodine in the diet. Dr. McClendon points out that the Indians of the northwest coast of North America ate salmon and were relatively free from goiter. The same is true, he says, of the Pomo Indians of the California coast, "who ate octopus, barnacles, sea urchins, sea anemones, sea cucumbers, lobsters, crabs, mussels, abalone and fish." Curiously enough, in Japan, where iodine is scarce in water, soil and food, there is practically no goiter problem, whereas Formosa, also low in iodine, has a very high rate. The difference seems to be explained by the fact that the Japanese add to their body store of iodine by eating seaweed, carefully prepared into appetizing dishes.

Are Iodine Supplements the Answer?

A book called *Iodine Facts,* which is published by the Chilean nitrate and iodine producers, in order to make available to the general public the facts about iodine, brings out a great many more aspects of the whole riddle. This book tells us, for instance, that rheumatism, anemia and diseases of the ear, nose and throat are much more prevalent among people who have goiter. Abortions and stillbirths are more common among women whose thyroids are deficient. An average survey of mental defectiveness shows 5.8 per cent of defectiveness among goitrous children and only .7 per cent among non-goitrous children.

There is a general decalcification of bones in hyperthyroidism or goiter, which would seem to indicate that these patients are not getting enough calcium or that their bodies are not making proper use of it. It is known that the thyroid gland influences the metabolism of calcium—that is, the way the body uses it and the amount it uses. Some researchers believe that goiter indicates an overabundance of non-absorbable calcium in the diet— in "hard" water, for instance.

As you know, in many foods there are certain very small, or, as we call them, "trace" amounts of mineral elements which in large quantity would be poisonous. Some plant foods contain arsenic, for instance, or fluorine, or cyanide. Organic cyanide is present in "trace" amounts in cabbage, soybeans, peas, lentils, mustard seed, peanuts and other foods. Now, while these foods are good for you if you eat them in the amounts you normally would, they are not healthful if you eat them in large quantities to the exclusion of all other foods. For instance, during the first world war, there were people in isolated sections of Europe who could get no other food but cabbage and turnips. After they had lived for quite a while on these two foods, they all developed goiter. Scientists then tested these foods in laboratories and found, sure enough, that animals placed on diets which consisted almost exclusively of cabbage, for instance, developed goiters. This led them to believe that there is a connection between goiter and too much cyanide in food or water. We are quite sure that people who live in so-called goiter belts have lots of other things in their diets aside from cabbage and the other "trace-cyanide" foods. So how else might they be obtaining too much cyanide?

Water Pollution and Goiter

Sir Robert McCarrison, a famous British physician, devoted his life to the study of the causes of goiter. Starting off in his search with no preconceived ideas of what might or might not be the cause, he traveled widely, to obscure corners of the world, looking for clues.

He visited the country of Hunza described in Editor Rodale's book, *The Healthy Hunzas.* He found that, in nations in the territory surrounding the Hunzas, goiters were common. The terrain, the amount of iodine in soil and water, the climate of these nations were similar to that of Hunza. Yet, among the Hunza people, goiter is unknown. Sir Robert studied the water supply of Hunza and found that it was carefully guarded against pollution. Aside from the fact that the Hunzas themselves are meticulously clean in their way of life, they know that water for drinking must be pure. They keep their drinking water in roofed tanks or closed cisterns inaccessible to animals and well protected from any kind of contamination.

In 9 villages about 60 miles from Hunza, says Sir Robert, "the water comes from a single source and is conveyed to the different villages in open kuls or channels . . . it will be observed that there are two main channels on the banks of which the villages are situated, one below the other. Each village in this way receives the drainage of the village or villages above it, till at the last village, Kashrote, the drinking water has been polluted by the 6 villages above.

"The water in these open channels not only supplies the inhabitants with drinking water, but it irrigates their extensive crops, serves as an open sewer, is used for the cleansing of their bodies, household utensils and wearing apparel. The drainings from cultivated and manured fields flow into it. It can readily be imagined, therefore, that considerable organic impurities find their way down to the lower villages."

Sir Robert then gives the goiter statistics for each village and says, "From this table, it is seen that the percentage of infected houses, of infected individuals in these houses and of the total population suffering from goiter, goes on increasing from the highest to the lowest village on the water-channels."

Goiter and Cyanide

Ralph Scobey, M.D., has conducted many investigations which prove that there is a relationship between polio and goiter, and cyanides in food and water. Remember that cyanides in large enough amounts are poisonous. They will produce both goiter and polio in experimental animals. How they do this is complex. Dr. Scobey figures it out as follows. When cyanides are present in the blood stream in sufficient quantity, they prevent one of the most important functions of vitamin C, which is its part in the process of the oxidation of cells. The less vitamin C present, the greater the danger of this function being cut off. Vitamin C is important for the utilization of calcium by the body, too. There are symptoms of calcium deficiency in goiter, says Dr. Scobey, which may be the result of this chain of events: cyanides enter the blood stream, forming hydrocyanic acid, vitamin C is used up in fighting the poisonous action of the acid, calcium is not assimilated, and the body requires more iodine to counteract the effect of the cyanides. If iodine is not supplied in sufficient quantity, the thyroid gland may react by enlarging.

Goiter and Polio Result of Imbalance in Nature

So, says Dr. Scobey, diseases such as polio and goiter result from a lack of balance in nature and, later on, in the diet, between vitamin C, iodine and the cyanides. Vitamin C and iodine act as protectors against cyanide. When there is not enough of either or both of them to counteract the amount of cyanide in the system, our bodies succumb to the poison.

Now how might this cyanide come about in food and drink? Barbiturates produce hydrocyanic acid in the body and the increasing use of these drugs undoubtedly influences the present-day goiter statistics. Goiter, like polio, is more prevalent in rural districts. The government estimates that about three-fourths of the wells in rural areas in this country contain water that is polluted. During periods of floods, which are the result of deforestation and lack of conservation measures, the streams, rivers and other waterways fill up with organic matter. If a drought follows the flood, which happens frequently, this matter becomes concentrated as the amount of water decreases. Cyanides are produced in water by this organic matter. During floods around large cities, the water supply is bound to become contaminated with sewage. This also results in cyanides in the drinking water supply. Goiter epidemics have been observed after rainy seasons and during droughts, when polluted water is concentrated.

Fish Can No Longer Live In Polluted Waters

Dr. Scobey reminds us how rapidly our inland fish are dying. Fish can live in water that is not fit for drinking. So what must be the condition of our water when the fish are dying in it? During polio epidemics, there is a noticeable rise in the destruction of the fish, apparently because the pollution in the water has increased to a lethal point for the fish. Now think of all the clams, oysters, mussels, scallops, fresh and saltwater crabs and fish that must be taken from polluted water and undoubtedly contribute to the sum total of cyanide released into the digestive tracts of the individuals living in a given area. No wonder goiter appears sometimes as an epidemic! No wonder it often afflicts people of one locality and not people of another! Why should it not afflict *all* of the people in the region? Perhaps some of these who escape regularly eat more foods that contain vitamin C, so this one part of their defense mechanism is strong.

On the other hand, if you want to imagine the most extreme case of a person surely destined to get goiter, wouldn't it go something like this? Have him move to a farm located in the "goiter belt." There's a shallow well on the farm that has been used for years and has never been tested. It's fairly close to the cesspool. Then instruct this poor victim to avoid any fresh fruits and vegetables that might contain vitamin C and live on cooked turnips and cabbage.

What We Conclude

To sum up our conclusions on goiter:

1. It appears that iodine is necessary in the diet for the prevention of goiter, but this is not the whole story.

2. It also appears that polluted drinking water contains cyanides which, in the absence of sufficient iodine and vitamin C in the diet can result in goiter. While it is important for individual families to check on their private water supply to make certain it is pure, it is also the concern of everyone to safeguard the purity of our national water supply. The constant and ever-increasing use of commercial fertilizers, the ruthless cutting down of forests, the dumping of sewage into waterways and the waste of organic materials which should be returned to the soil are responsible for the floods which regularly cost millions of dollars worth of damage in property alone. As we have seen, pollution of water is to be expected following floods. So one of the best preventives of goiter, from the national standpoint, is for each of us to preach the principles of organic gardening and organic farming to our friends, neighbors, doctors, the people we buy our produce from and, most important of all, our senators and congressmen.

3. One last comment on behalf of the wisdom of Old Mother Nature and the way she has planned and provided for our welfare. The foods which are most likely to be contaminated from cyanides in the water supply—fish—also contain iodine, which helps the body to defend itself against cyanide. Cabbage and many of the other foods that contain trace amounts of cyanide contain also large amounts of vitamin C—the other warrior against cyanides. So a well-rounded, fully adequate diet, with all of its natural goodness preserved in its preparation for eating, and a pure water supply are probably the two best guarantees against goiter in the long run. Kelp, prepared seaweed, is an excellent source of iodine and other trace minerals.

186. Some Environmental Causes of Goiter

"In articles, and even in books, on the possible influence of the soil (and the water that springs from it) on man, it is generally stated that the only known example of such an influence is that exerted by iodine on the thyroid." These words are from a startling and valuable book, *Soil, Grass and Cancer*, by André Voisin (published by the Philosophical Press, New York). Dr. Voisin points out that iodine has been used to treat goiter for about 140 years. In some parts of the world, such treatment is successful. In other parts, iodine is plentiful in food and water and yet, goiter is extremely common among the people.

Dr. Voisin tells us that goiter is a disturbance of the entire system of glands of the body, not just the thyroid gland. Of a representative group of patients suffering from goiter, 79 per cent also have disturbances of the pituitary gland, 68 per cent of the adrenal glands, 60 per cent of the hypothalamus and 52 per cent disorders of the liver. So, deciding that goiter is caused simply by lack of iodine in food or water, gives us no answer as to what lack is causing the disorders of the other glands and how they are related to the goitrous condition.

Goiter is a reaction on the part of the thyroid to a disturbance in the metabolism of iodine—that is, the way the body uses iodine, says Dr. Voisin. One extremely important clue to the way the body uses iodine is the amount of vitamin A present in the diet. For the last 20 years, we have known that lack of vitamin A is one cause of goiter. A thyroid gland already goitrous contains about 1/10 of the normal amount of vitamin A. If the epithelial cells present in the thyroid are deficient in vitamin A, then enough thyroxine will not be made, for it is apparently in these cells of the thyroid gland that the hormone is manufactured.

It is true, too, that a lack of vitamin A disorders the function of the pituitary gland. The pituitary gland secretes a substance which regulates the thyroid. Lacking vitamin A, this entire process goes awry. Night blindness is one of the first symptoms of vitamin A deficiency. It has been observed that people who suffer from night blindness also suffer from goiter, another indication that lack of vitamin A is involved. Dr. Voisin quotes a Dr. Rhein of Strasbourg, who believes that an original lack of vitamin A probably is responsible for setting in motion both these two disorders. He thinks perhaps the vitamin lack may sensitize the thyroid to some goiter-causing element in the environment.

Increase in Goiters Result of Changed Environment

Dr. Voisin goes on to tell us that after World War II, there was a wave of goiters throughout Germany and Austria. In Saxony, one locality where the disease was practically unknown before this time, ¾ of the native and 4/5 of the refugee child population developed goiters. In sections of the continent where goiters due to *too little thyroid* activity had been common before, the wave of new goiters were of the kind caused by *too much thyroid* activity. So, apparently, something was bringing about a complete change in the environmental causes of the disease.

It could not be lack of iodine, because goiter, at that time, affected 40 per cent of the children of one city right on the seacoast where, of course, iodine is plentiful in food and water. Children of American Army personnel did not suffer incidentally.

It was believed at first that plain lack of food might be causing the rising incidence of goiter. But it was found that some populations, among whom the disorder was rising, still had plenty of food and were not even rationing it. Then it became apparent that the quality, not the quantity of the food was at fault. Among these mountain peasants, who lived chiefly on bread and milk, the chief source of vitamin A was butter from their cow's milk. The vitamin A content of the butter had been reduced. A researcher was able to show that the frequency of goiter among the children in this locality—the Bavarian Alps—increased in direct proportion as the amount of vitamin A in the butter decreased. In one neighborhood where the percentage of children affected by goiter was 85, the vitamin A content of the butter supply was 486 micrograms per 100 grams. Where 79 per cent were affected, the vitamin A content was 489. Where only 32 per cent had goiter, the vitamin A content of the butter was 618 micrograms and where only 13 per cent were affected, the vitamin A content of the butter was shown to be 1015 micrograms!

Why did the butter suddenly decline in vitamin A content? It has been shown, Dr. Voisin tells us, that the vitamin A content of milk fat is the direct result of the vitamin A content of the grass eaten by the cows. A lack of mineral fertilizers in their pastures was partly responsible for reducing the vitamin content so severely that, along with a restricted use of butter because of war conditions, the end result was a disorder so serious and so widespread in the young population of those mountainside communities.

Here is some further evidence on the causes of goiter, collected by Dr. Voisin. In two neighboring towns, hardly a mile apart, it was found that a 32 per cent incidence of goiter went with a low vitamin A content in the butter supply, while in the other village a 13 per cent incidence of goiter occurred where the butter contained 65 per cent more vitamin A. What could have caused such a difference in vitamin A content of butter from cows on two neighboring pastures? The difference seems to result only from the geographical location of the two villages. The one which has the low incidence of goiter is located high on a mountain, facing the south and the sunshine. The other is located in the valley, beside a lake, with a cold, foggy climate. It is estimated that the upper village gets anywhere from

3 to 6 weeks more sunshine than the lower one. Analyzing the grass, it was found that the grass higher up the mountain contained 60 per cent more vitamin A than that of the lower village.

Weather and Goiter Are Related

In 1800, 3 books were published by a French doctor, Francois Emmanuel Fodéré, in which he pointed out that goiter and the mental deficiency that accompanies it in many regions of the country may be the result of weather and geography. He pointed out in his books that goiter is relatively more frequent: (1.) on damp northern slopes than on southern slopes of the same hill; (2.) in deep, narrow valleys suffering from frequent fog than in wide valleys where the sun can penetrate; (3.) in misty areas along the sides of lakes and by the mouths of rivers. Dr. Fodéré's work was greeted with gibes and jeers, according to Dr. Voisin. One commentator remarked sarcastically that, on the average, there are no more idiots among the inhabitants of London than among those of Rome.

However, Fodéré was right. He did not, of course, know at that time the connection between weather, hours of sunshine, vitamin A content of grass and goiter. But he did know, by observation alone, that *something* about the misty, sunless terrain produced more goiter than there was higher up where the sunshine came for many more hours a day.

One last bit of evidence on the extreme complexity of the relationship of environment to incidence of goiter. Dr. Voisin tells us that a certain strain of white clover will produce goiter in animals fed on it. The reason is that a substance contained in the clover makes it impossible for the animal's thyroid to take up iodine and use iodine from the blood.

Analyzing the plants, as is done in laboratories to determine the mineral and vitamin content, it was found that these particular clovers were especially rich in iodine, containing about 14 times more than ordinary white clover. So, according to all our ideas about thyroid glands and the necessity for iodine to keep them healthy, one would naturally think that such clover might be deficient in other things, but certainly, so far as the thyroid gland was concerned, this clover would be the best for that important gland. But, says Dr. Voisin, chemical analysis is not enough, because the analysis did not reveal that the poisonous substance, also present in white clover, would completely negate the beneficial effects of the high iodine content, since it prevented the thyroid glands of the animals from making any use of the iodine. When the clover was finally fed to animals, the truth came out.

Dr. Voisin is making the point here that in modern agriculture, we are ignoring the needs of the animal and concentrating on fodder that is important for some other agriculture reason. "These new varieties of grass," he says, "have been and are being selected from experiments on tiny squares which are cut with the shears. There is hardly any concern for the methods of practical management in which these new varieties will have

[714]

to 'live.' But the most serious matter which has not been—and is not being —considered is the influence of these varieties on the production and health of the animal."

Complications of This Kind of Research

Dr. Voisin's book contains many ideas on goiter and the possible causes of it. He has done much fascinating research on the problem. We think it is important, chiefly because it illustrates so well the complexity of our biochemical life and the overwhelming importance to our welfare of almost any detail of our existence. Nothing is unimportant, nothing must be overlooked as we search for the reasons for disease.

Dr. Voisin, who is concerned chiefly with the effects of various kinds of fertilizers on soils and hence on the health of people who eat food grown on those soils, tells us that the problem becomes more complicated all the time because of our modern way of life. "Modern civilization has multiplied means of transport," he says, "with the result that our diet today includes wheat from Canada, oil from Senegal, oranges from Spain, etc. Our cells therefore contain mineral elements originally existing in the soils of all these various countries. The time for people living in small rural communities and making do with the produce of their own fields and the water from their own springs for their sustenance is past. In these days, it was easy enough to track down the deficient local 'dust' giving rise to malfunctioning of the human cells and causing goiter, for example. It is much more difficult today to determine the influence of the soils of England, Senegal, Spain, etc., in causing disorders in the functioning of the cells of one man or group of men."

187. Hemorrhoids

Our research has shown us that the most important thing to remember about hemorrhoids is this: avoid them! The measures one should take are simple and sensible. Since hemorrhoids are generally caused by straining the abdominal muscles in difficult bowel movements, heavy lifting, etc., avoiding such strain is your best defense against the problem.

What Hemorrhoids Are

Hemorrhoids (or piles) are veins that have become distended and stretched thin due to strain. These veins may be situated just inside or outside the rectum. They do not lie buried deep in the flesh, but they are close to the surface where they can be irritated easily. These veins serve as an auxiliary pathway for the blood and are not meant for hard use. If there is heavy pressure on the abdominal cavity, the blood takes the unimpaired alternate route. This puts a heavy load of blood on the hemorrhoidal veins, and these were not meant to do heavy work. If the strain lasts any length of time, or if it is often repeated, the walls of these veins gradually expand until the strain is past. Soon the elasticity is gone from them and they no longer regain their original shape. They then expand to the point at which they can be seen and felt. These veins are then extremely sensitive, and can cause true misery, as well as bleeding, with even the slightest strain on the abdominal muscles.

Some Causes

Perhaps it would be well to mention at this time that there are several other possible causes of hemorrhoids. They can often be an indication of a much more serious disorder. Cancer often leaves hemorrhoids as its calling card, and cirrhosis of the liver will often announce itself with a suddenly acquired case of hemorrhoids. Pregnancy is also a quite common cause.

In most cases, though, hemorrhoids can be best avoided by avoiding strain of the abdominals. First of all, learn to lift heavy objects properly. Do not bend over at the waist to lift something heavy, since the strain is transmitted directly to the stomach and back muscles in such lifting. Rather, bend the knees and crouch to a level as close to the object as possible. Now, when you are raising the object, you have some of its weight distributed to your legs, and the strain on the abdominal muscles is minimized. This is one way to keep the hemorrhoid problem out of your life.

The Most Common Cause

It is extremely likely that the majority of hemorrhoid cases are the result of constipation and straining to cleanse the bowels. An article in *Today's Health,* August, 1956, touches on this subject. The author emphasizes that careful control of the bowels is most important. It is wise to be aware of some definite pattern in one's elimination processes. For many people, a bowel movement each day is the normal order of things; however, it is quite common for many apparently healthy persons to pass several days between bowel movements. It is important, therefore, that each individual should know what is, for him, a normal interval and not try to force his bowels into frequent action when they are not geared for it. A person is constipated only when a normal, easy movement does not occur even after the normal interval has passed. But don't take a laxative just because you've missed a bowel movement one day. Give yourself a chance to get back to normal without artificial means.

How to Defeat Constipation

In view of the role constipation plays in acquiring hemorrhoids, it might be wise to review a few points regarding prevention of that disorder.

Most medical authorities agree that one cause of constipation is that we ignore nature's call too often. There should be a regular time for this function, a time which is most convenient, and easiest to adhere to. You should be relaxed and unhurried. Give yourself ample time for this duty as you do for other necessities such as grooming and meals. Make this interval as easy and pleasant for yourself as you can: if it seems to help if you read, then by all means read; if a hot drink beforehand seems to help, then do have one—in short, use any means that seems to ease the effort involved in defacating.

The proper amount of exercise can make a great deal of difference in one's regularity. If yours is a sedentary job that allows for little moving about, then manage to do some walking every day. If it is feasible, walk to and from work each day, or get off the bus a good way from home and walk the rest of the way. Use any form of exercise but make sure you put as many muscles into play as possible—and make a habit of it.

Food and Constipation

Of course, what you eat has a lot to do with your ease of elimination. The abdominal muscles are set up to deal with all types of fibrous and bulky materials. The modern processing methods have eliminated these characteristics from many of our foods, and as a result, these muscles have less and less to do. They soon lose tone and become too lazy to do a job when they get one. The result is, of course, poorly digested food which gives rise to elimination difficulties. The poor digestion plus the lack of enough of the bulky and fibrous foods, which help to push the waste through its proper channels, are keys to the problem of constipation.

Raw fruits and vegetables contain more bulk and fewer calories than any other food, so they serve as an excellent food for those who wish to maintain healthy elimination. In an article in *College and University Business* (July, 1950), a group of experts suggested the following to be included in a diet to prevent constipation: fresh or stewed fruit for breakfast (rather than juice); lunch should include a fresh fruit or a bulky salad; dinner should 'include a large salad and generous servings of two such vegetables as cabbage, sprouts, green beans, peas, asparagus, corn, spinach, okra or baked squash. Raw carrots, celery, lettuce, water cress and tomatoes should be used freely, too. Fresh fruits should be taken daily, especially as an evening snack, and one should drink a full 8 ounce glass of water every waking hour.

If you are eating plenty of this kind of food, it's obvious that you simply won't have room for sweet, gooey desserts, lots of bread and refined carbohydrates, noodles, spaghetti—things like that. So your elimination system will benefit two ways—more fresh foods with bulk and also with necessary vitamins, and fewer refined foods from which both 'the bulk and the vitamins have been removed.

Vitamins Play A Role

Only healthy intestines are capable of doing a proper job of working the food we eat thoroughly and at a proper rate. To keep the intestines healthy, one must eat all of the necessary food elements. Vitamins are necessary in the body's proper use of proteins, carbohydrates and fats.

Experiments have shown that inositol and niacin, two of the B vitamins, prevent constipation in animals. Laboratory volunteers on diets short in thiamin, another B vitamin, become constipated. If one does not get enough B vitamins, the body simply cannot handle the carbohydrates and fats one eats!

Vitamin K is another food element that is necessary in the prevention of constipation; calcium, phosphorus and other minerals must be included in the diet, too.

It will be noticed that most of the recommendations given for avoiding constipation are the general ones for maintaining good health. If you wish to be certain that any one part of your body is healthy, you must make every effort to see that all parts of the body are well-nourished. Stay with a simple diet of unprocessed fresh foods, avoid white flour products and sugar and salt. On a diet such as this you'll never know what constipation is.

If you can keep yourself free of constipation and you will take care to avoid bad habits in heavy lifting, you will certainly have done the most important things towards keeping yourself free of hemorrhoids. And if you're eating as you should, you need fear none of the other diseases that plague those who are careless of their diet and their health.

[718]

188. Hernia Is Easily Avoided

Most persons who have never actually experienced a hernia, or rupture, as it is commonly called, are not very clear on just what it is. Technically, hernia is the escape or protrusion of an organ, or part of an organ, from its natural cavity. By this definition we can see that hernia can occur almost anywhere in the body—the brain, the lungs, the iris of the eye, etc. Any of these is an organ that is contained in a specific area of the body, and if some part of one of them should spill over the bounds set by nature for its containment, or should push through the skin walls that holds it in place, a hernia of that organ has occurred.

More commonly a hernia refers to the escape of some part of the intestine from the abdominal cavity, through an opening in the abdominal wall. It then pushes along the natural paths of the body, often to a point just below the surface of the skin. When it reaches this point, a hernia is usually visible. At first it is about the size and shape of a marble, and grows larger as more and more intestine escapes. The victim often notices a "dragging" feeling in the abdomen, coupled with severe constipation and tenderness.

How Hernia Is Discovered—Three Common Sites

Sometimes the hernia is not visible and can only be discovered by a physician examining the common sites of hernia. He places his hand over the suspected area and asks the patient to cough. The sudden increase of abdominal pressure caused by the cough, creates a "pulse" that can be felt if a hernia is present.

There are 3 areas in which the occurrence of intestinal hernia is most likely: the groin or the base of the abdomen, the point at which the legs and torso meet (inguinal hernia); the upper part of the thigh (femoral hernia); the region of the navel (umbilical hernia). In each of these cases, some loop of the intestine will have broken through the abdominal wall and followed the easiest path to one of these points.

The inguinal hernia occurs most frequently in men. The inguinal canal is a passage, from the abdominal wall to the groin, through which the unborn male's testes descend to the scrotum, and certain ligaments in the female descend to the genital area. Normally this canal closes once its purpose has been accomplished. However, if the closure is not complete, it can be seen that the passage would offer an excellent avenue for the descent of an escaping intestinal loop. In the male, this loop can descend into the scrotum, and remain undetected, but for discomfort, until the patient undergoes a physical examination.

There is also a type of hernia more peculiar to females. Most female hernias are of the femoral type. The femoral canal leads from the pelvis into the thigh, and serves as a sort of tunnel for the main vein, returning blood from the leg to the heart. Normally this vein and a few small lymph glands are the sole occupants of the canal. When a hernia develops here, a sac composed of a weak spot of the inner abdominal tissue, and some small portion of the intestine, pushes into the canal, causing a visible and painful bulge on the upper inside part of the thigh.

The umbilical hernia is the result of a giving way of the abdominal wall tissues near the site of the navel, a weak area in many babies. The protrusion is usually quite visible, and sometimes easiest to treat.

The Varying Causes

The causes of hernia vary, but most of the immediate causes relate in some way to sudden or unusual pressure on the abdominal wall. The most widely recognized cause is heavy lifting, and putting the weight of the object on the stomach muscles instead of the stronger arms, shoulders and legs. Another frequent cause of hernia is constipation, and the resultant straining at stool. This puts a tremendous strain on the abdominal wall, and is a dangerous practice which should be carefully avoided. Excessive coughing can result in hernia, and vomiting is another physiological activity which puts great pressure on the tissue that keeps the intestines in place.

The accumulation of fat in the intestinal area causes a downward pull against the abdominal wall which can result in hernia. Persons who are heavy about the middle should make every effort to reduce, lest hernia be added to the other problems of overweight. Pregnancy can effect a similar strain on the abdominal wall; however, if proper nutritional procedures are followed, the body can compensate for this natural condition with ease.

High jumps to a solid surface are to be avoided. The intestines' weight is augmented by a high jump and sudden stop. Again the abdominal wall must, so to speak, "catch" the intestines when one lands. If the tissue is weak, this type of activity can easily lead to hernia.

The intestines are rather like a long hose coiled carefully within the abdomen. If a hernia should occur, and a part of the intestinal hose should escape, it is like a hanging loop. If caught soon enough, it can be pushed back through the hole and into its normal position quite easily in surgery. If the hernia is let go, it can grow and become twisted, just as garden hose can become twisted, so that no blood can pass through it. The result can be infection and gangrene. It is therefore extremely dangerous to ignore a hernia, for, unless it is repaired, it can easily become serious enough to cause death.

Using a Truss

Where does the truss fit into the hernia picture? The truss is a pad

RULES FOR HEAVY WEIGHT LIFTING

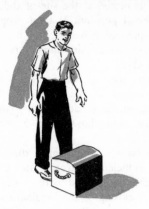

FIGURE 20: Face heavy weights, keeping the feet 18 inches apart and close to object.

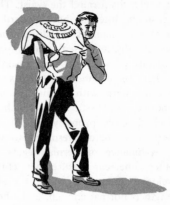

FIGURE 23: Carry loads on the shoulders wherever possible. Don't carry on hips.

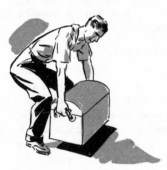

FIGURE 21: Lift from the floor with bent knees.

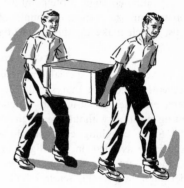

FIGURE 24: Get someone to help if you need it.

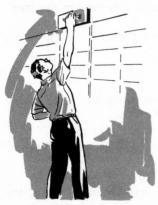

FIGURE 22: Don't reach too high for big parcels.

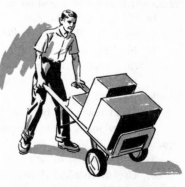

FIGURE 25: Use mechanical devices where you can.

of some kind (wood, hard rubber, plastic, etc.), usually fastened to a belt which fits around the waist. The pad is placed at the site of the hernia to push the intestine back toward its normal position. If used properly it can relieve much of the discomfort and pain of a hernia, but it is not a cure. Usually it is used as a temporary measure in case surgery might not be readily possible, for one reason or another.

In a small child, the truss is sometimes used to better effect. Children are often born with hernias around the navel. If the hernia is properly supported, the tissue from which it escaped, may, due to the youth of the child, grow properly over it. Doctors often allow up to 3 years for this to occur before resorting to surgery.

Avoidance of hernia begins in the womb. The proper diet of the mother-to-be can assure her child of sufficiently strong and properly developed abdominal walls. Protein is the main need here. Such tissue strength is normal enough, as is the proper closing of the inguinal canal. If the materials are available, the developing baby will make use of them, it is certain.

Continued high protein intake will keep the abdominal wall in good repair, and the proper amounts of vitamin C will help in keeping the cells, which make up this tissue, tightly knit.

Exercise and Avoid Colds

Exercise, with special emphasis on the abdominal muscles, is another preventive measure that should be taken by all health-conscious persons. Such exercises as sit-ups, in which one rises from a supine position to a sitting position without use of the hands, are especially useful in this.

Since coughing can contribute to intestinal strain, colds are to be especially avoided in the light of what we know of hernia. Vitamins A and C are two excellent preventives. To keep clear of constipation, a diet high in protein, natural bulk and unprocessed foods, especially raw fruit and fresh vegetables, will help. Also, try for foods rich in the B vitamins, for they aid in maintaining friendly organisms in the intestinal tract, which helps in digestion of foods.

In lifting, follow the rules offered in the United States Public Health Service pamphlet, *Workers Health Series* #3:

1. In lifting heavy weight, face the object, keep the feet close to it and space them about 18 inches apart. (Figure 20.)

2. Lift from the floor with knees bent, using leg rather than back muscles. (Figure 21.)

3. Don't reach too high for heavy packages. (Figure 22.)

4. Carry loads on the shoulders where possible, rather than on the hips. (Figure 23.)

5. Get someone to help you if you need it. (Figure 24.)

6. Use mechanical devices where you can—hoists, elevators, trucks, etc. (Figure 25.)

189. Avoiding Indigestion

Possibly every individual has a different definition of indigestion. The symptoms may vary from person to person and from one attack to another. But, in general, these are the conditions we associate with indigestion: pain in the stomach or the chest, "heartburn," gas, distention of the abdomen, regurgitation of acid, acrid liquid into the mouth, belching, coated tongue, unpleasant taste in the mouth, nausea or vomiting, "nervous indigestion," "acid indigestion."

We are told by John Tebbel, M.D., in *Your Body* (Harper and Brothers), that 50 million working days are lost annually by the American people due to indigestion. The cost to industry is more than 250 million dollars a year. Only respiratory illnesses take a greater toll in day to day absences from work.

Indigestion or dyspepsia arising from organic disorders need not concern us here. It is obvious that, in conditions in which the digestive tract is badly disordered, digestion will suffer accordingly. Gall bladder disorders, stomach ulcers, anemia (preventing proper blood supply to the digestive tract), diabetes and other glandular disorders, cancer of the stomach—all these and many more will result in indigestion. In fact, indigestion is one of the first symptoms of stomach cancer. Generally, someone suffering from such ailments expects his digestion to be upset.

However, there are plenty of us who suffer from functional indigestion, acute or chronic. There is apparently nothing organically wrong with us. This is the indigestion that plagues millions of us and results in drug-store shelves crammed with "remedies," many of which are simply baking soda preparations, others being sedatives or aspirin concoctions. There is no evidence anywhere that such remedies can improve the situation; they will probably make it worse.

What can you do, then, to prevent functional indigestion? There are a few simple rules to follow. If you are certain your discomfort does not arise from an organic defect or disease (better check pretty carefully on this, first), you can correct indigestion and you can make certain that you will never suffer from it again.

Consider first the structure of your digestive tract—a very long tube (relatively speaking) containing certain pouches and storage spots. From the walls of this tube pour out the digestive juices, chiefly enzymes of one kind or another. These combine chemically with the food, making other compounds, until the food is gradually broken down into substances that can be transported through the walls of the intestine into the blood stream. The digestive tract contains many bacteria which change according to the kind of food eaten. Undigested food is broken down by these bacteria with the formation of gas. Food which is properly digested proceeds on its way with no such difficulty. The contractions of the intestines move the food mass along at the proper rate of speed, elimination of waste material is normal and all is well.

The Role of the Enzymes

Enzymes are perhaps the most important element in the process. These are made chiefly of protein substances, underscoring the great importance of protein in our diets. Enzymes cannot be formed in the digestive tract unless plenty of protein is available to manufacture them. Lack of enzymes means food will remain undigested. Another important function of protein is to keep the walls of the digestive tract strong and healthy. The muscles in the intestinal walls have the job of contracting almost continually, to break up the food mass and to push it along to the next step in the digestive process.

The sufferer from indigestion may blame his condition on protein foods. ("It's the meat I ate last night," or "Eggs don't agree with me.") So he cuts down still further on good protein and his condition becomes worse. How many of us reach for a cracker or a piece of toast when we feel twinges of indigestion? A boiled egg or a piece of meat or some fresh fruit is a far better idea.

Digestion and the B Vitamins

Two B vitamins are universally mentioned by all the experts in relation to digestion—niacin and thiamin. One of the symptoms of pellagra is indigestion. Pellagra is the disease of vitamin B deficiency, involving chiefly niacin. Thiamin is needed every moment in the digestive tract whenever we eat carbohydrates of any kind. It is an essential part of the enzyme system, necessary for breaking down carbohydrates into easily digestible substances. If the carbohydrates you are eating are beans, potatoes, bananas, nuts, peas and other perfectly natural foods, then you are getting plenty of these two B vitamins to assure your good digestion of the starches. If, however, you are eating refined cereals, bakery products, candy, soft drinks or other starchy or sweet foods made of refined products, then you are certainly heading for indigestion, or perhaps it has already overtaken you, for you will lack niacin and thiamin—it has been removed from these carbohydrates when they are refined.

Lack of niacin over a long period may result in a decrease of hydrochloric acid in the stomach, which will lead to further indigestion, since this is an important digestive juice. A lack of thiamin changes the entire digestive tract. There is a loss of appetite, the stomach and intestines cannot contract normally and food is not well mixed with digestive enzymes. Hydrochloric acid decreases as well the flow of digestive juices from the pancreas and the gall bladder. The thin person, hoping to gain weight by eating lots of starchy foods, is fighting a losing battle, for the undigested food is wasted. Adding plenty of B vitamins to the diet will make the job of gaining weight easier and prevent indigestion.

What kind of diet should you eat, then, to guard against indigestion? First of all, abandon your ideas of foods that "disagree" with you, unless you have a proven allergy to them. For instance, eggs are among the most easily digested foods in the healthy digestive tract. Meat is digested almost as easily as breathing. Fatty meat takes longer to digest because fat is handled more slowly by our digestive apparatus. But this does not mean that it is indigestible. On the basis of what we have said above, the smooth, tasty starches and sweets are the hardest of all to digest.

Other Aids to Good Digestion

In addition to diet, other aspects of living are important if you would avoid indigestion. It is important not to hurry through meals. Chewing is part of the mechanism that calls forth digestive juices. It is much more important that carbohydrate foods be chewed, because of the purely mechanical breaking down of food particles in the mouth. This leaves a greater surface available to the digestive juices and enzymes when the food reaches the stomach and intestine. In addition, part of the digestion of starch is begun in the mouth. Bolting your food in a few minutes because you have not allowed time for a relaxed meal, is not giving your digestion a fair chance to save you from harm. Don't grab a sandwich, a cup of coffee and a piece of pie at a lunch counter. Eat lunch, as well as breakfast and dinner, in as quiet and relaxed and unhurried a state of mind as you can possibly manage. Protein food is digested largely in the stomach and intestines, so this need not be chewed.

In *Nutrition and Physical Fitness* (Saunders), Jean Bogert has this to say about the importance of your frame of mind to good digestion: "Fear or worry, anger or irritation, nervous fatigue or strain, emotion or excitement—all exert a strongly unfavorable influence upon digestion (especially in the stomach), both by suppressing the flow of digestive fluids and by inhibiting the muscular activity of the digestive tract . . . Such conditions as introspection or concern about one's self, monotony or boredom, mental preoccupation or overstimulation have similar unfavorable effects and are often associated with lack of appetite, which in itself constitutes an unfavorable factor . . . Peace and quiet, cheerful but not overstimulating companionship, appetizing food with attractive surroundings and table service—all are factors that favor good digestion." Perhaps excitement and overstimulation are important factors in the so-frequent heart attacks and strokes after big banquets. Of course, the starchy food and rich, sweet desserts are certainly to blame, too.

However, it is obvious that a quiet and serene outlook especially at mealtime is important. The clear association of "nerves" and digestion is apparent in the naming of one kind of ailment—"nervous indigestion."

Exercise and Posture Are Important

Perhaps more important than anyone knows in the prevention of indigestion, is the matter of posture and exercise, pointed out by Dr. Bogert. Poor posture may result in the stomach and intestines being badly out of position, crowded, lying on one another so that they cannot possibly function as they should. "A stomach which is so badly out of position that it cannot empty properly will not only give immediate distress signals, but the continual irritation that results may eventually cause gastric ulcers or even cancer of the stomach," says Dr. Bogert. "The poor blood supply to the intestines which results when they are crowded down into disadvantageous positions in the abdomen, causes the muscular walls of the intestines to become flabby and is one of the contributory factors in constipation."

Good posture is partly the product of good eating (plenty of protein and minerals to provide strong muscles) and partly the result of habit and exercise. Don't allow your stomach muscles to become flabby, so that you exhibit a "paunch" in front. It may indicate that your stomach and other digestive organs are out of place, since they do not have the support they need from these exterior muscles. You need to develop these muscles. It can be done easily over a period of time. All you need is determination. Wherever you are and whatever you are doing, practice pulling the muscles of your stomach in, in, in, until you can control them at will.

Walking is the best exercise you can engage in. Aside from providing a perfect time and place to practice good posture, walking will improve your circulation, it will improve your appetite so that you will want to eat a hearty meal rich in proteins, vitamins and minerals, it will help to abolish constipation, if that bothers you, and it will relieve boredom, nervousness, worry, irritation and hence, improve digestion.

Don't Overeat

One last caution about indigestion. There is no doubt that overeating plays a big part in our national indigestion. Pushing back from a table at the end of a too-big meal with grunts, groans and belches is not to be advised. It is interesting to note that, if you are eating a diet of natural foods, you are not so likely to overeat. Dr. H. L. Cleave of the British Royal Navy said, in an article in the *Journal of the Royal Naval Service,* spring, 1956, "Nearly all the harmful consequences that arise from this (overeating) are due to the concentration, leading to a definitely excessive consumption of the carbohydrates. Their taste (in concentrated form) is too highly geared for the tongue to be able to know when to stop." A bar of chocolate, for example, contains as much sugar as a dozen average apples. The tongue would know when to stop eating the apples, but not the chocolate bar.

We are not likely to overeat on apples or bananas or any other completely natural foods. The fibers they contain are bulky and filling. We are not likely to overeat on meat or eggs. Normal amounts of them satisfy our appetites. But when starches and sugars are changed completely from their natural forms by refining, they have a deceptive quality which leads us to eat too much of them. Our natural appetite control has no automatic gauge for determining how much of such foods we should eat. So there is no check on us and we overeat time and again on such foods.

To summarize, here are some basic rules if you would avoid functional indigestion: (1.) Get plenty of B vitamins and proteins. This means eating foods in which they are plentiful and taking food supplements like brewer's yeast and/or desiccated liver. (2.) Check on your posture and, if it is bad, do something about it. (3.) Exercise—especially walking—is essential, especially if you lead a sedentary life. (4.) A happy frame of mind, freedom from noise, worry and hurry, and a relaxed and pleasant atmosphere are conducive to good digestion. If these seem impossible of attainment, resolve to attain them no matter what the cost. If it means changing the habits of a lifetime or making completely different arrangements for taking your meals, make the changes. It's *your* digestion, and no one else but you is going to be concerned with it. Finally, avoid overeating. The best way to accomplish this is to eliminate from your meals all foods that are not completely natural ones. It's doubtful that you will overeat if your diet contains nothing but meat, fish, eggs, nuts, fruits and vegetables.

190. Garlic Triumphs
Over Indigestion

One of the most common annoyances for modern man is still old-fashioned indigestion. The symptoms may vary, but it is a condition which many recognize as a constant visitor, and some view with serious alarm because of the frequently accompanying sensation of heart palpitations and severe headache.

At the first sign of this condition, the regular sufferer reaches for one of dozens of stomach-settlers in the form of minty tablets or fizzing seltzers which are on the market. They all do about the same thing; neutralize the hydrochloric acid in the stomach. It is essential that the climate of the intestine maintain a balance of acid and alkali, it is true, but this balance should be brought about by natural diet; that is, the consumption of foods which are acid, such as meat, and alkaline foods, which include fruits and vegetables. To eliminate entirely the acid of the stomach by the frequent use of these bicarbonate of soda compounds is a very dangerous practice. The stomach acids are essential in breaking down foods so that their component parts may be used to nourish the body. Without these acids, calcium, for example, cannot be fully digested. It either passes through the intestines and is eliminated, as though it had not been eaten at all, or it is inefficiently used, not properly absorbed and can result in the formation of calcium deposits (stones) in the kidney or bladder.

Nature's Relief

As any reader who is interested in the study of nutrition should know, Nature has a way of taking care of the hyperacidity problem without any danger of overalkalizing. The natural device which performs this service is our old acquaintance, garlic. The value of garlic in this connection has often been hinted at, and people from ancient times to this have used the herb to relieve gastric distress brought on by the accumulation of gas. It remained for Frederic Damrau, M.D., and Edgar Ferguson, chemist, writing in the *Review of Gastroenterology* (May, 1949), to arrive at some concrete, scientific basis for this usage.

In their paper, these researchers class garlic as a carminative; that is, "aromatic or pungent drugs, used in flatulence and colic, to expel gas from stomach and intestines, and to diminish the griping pains." The theory on how a carminative can do such things follows along this line: the oils of carminatives, upon reaching the mucous membrane, cause a decrease in the movements and tone of the stomach wall. This weakening action probably extends to the sphincters (muscles) and their relaxation may explain the feeling of relief from distention and gas in the stomach after the administration of these oils.

Observation by X-Ray

Damrau and Ferguson decided to observe, from a truly scientific point of view, just what action garlic would have in the stomach. They proposed to accomplish this by means of X-ray. They would give the subject barium sulfate (the usual tool for a study of the intestines by X-ray) with and without garlic, and study the speed at which the barium was processed by the stomach in each case. Slower processing would indicate that the needed relaxation of the stomach had been accomplished. Twenty-five patients were included in the study, 12 males and 13 females. The average duration of the complaints, which included abdominal pain, abdominal discomfort, belching and nausea, was one year. In each case, X-ray comparison was made with and without garlic, after a 10-day period. The so-called medication consisted of 6 garlic tablets, each containing 4¾ grains of dehydrated garlic. Two tablets were given with the barium, two 2 hours later, and two after 4 hours. With the use of garlic, the size of the barium residue in the stomach after 6 hours was definitely larger than without it. This meant, of course, that, with the garlic, the stomach operated at a more relaxed, more comfortable pace. The researchers were impressed with the patients' reports of relief of all symptoms.

In another series of studies, which included 29 patients complaining from heaviness after eating, belching, flatulence, gas colic and nausea, two garlic tablets were given twice daily, after lunch and dinner, for a period of two weeks. Again the garlic dosage was 4¾ grains per tablet.

Remarkable Results

The results were gratifying. Heaviness after eating, present in 25 cases, was completely relieved by the treatment in 15 cases, partially relieved in 6, and 4 cases had no relief. Belching was present in 25 cases, and was completely relieved in 13 cases, partially in 9, and not at all in 3 cases. Flatulence was present in 25 cases, and 20 cases were completely relieved, one partially, and 4 not at all. Gas colic, present in 24 cases, was completely relieved in 13 cases, partially in 8, and no relief in 3 cases. Nausea, present in 8 cases, was completely relieved in 6, with no relief in two cases.

As can be seen, the garlic did not bring only temporary relief, but permanent freedom from these gastric disorders. It is to be presumed that garlic was included in the diets of these patients in some kind of maintenance dose, but since it is a natural food, there need be no fear of dangerous accumulation in the intestines of a harmful substance. There is no fear either of a dangerous habit-forming drug. Quite to the contrary, garlic is really an excellent food in its own right, with many valuable nutrients contained in it, and its use might beneficially affect other parts of the body.

191. Dyspepsia from Starch Eating

Fullness in the abdomen, especially just after eating, usually more common at the right side. Painful gas in the intestine with immediate relief when the gas is expelled. Constipation, sometimes alternating with diarrhea.

These are symptoms of a disorder which seems to plague many people —a nameless discomfort which does not seem to have a beginning or an end, for it may go on for years. A British M.D., Sir Arthur Hurst of Guy's Hospital, London, calls it "carbohydrate intestinal dyspepsia." Describing the disorder in the *British Encyclopedia of Medical Practice,* Vol. 4, Sir Arthur tells us that this kind of dyspepsia comes from not being able to digest starch properly.

"The only possible explanation of the condition," he says, "appears to be hypermotility of the small intestine, which allows sufficient time for the digestion of meat and fat, but not for the starch contained within its cellulose envelope." Hypermotility means that food is passing too rapidly through the intestine so that digestion is not complete.

Cooking swells and softens but does not break the cellulose envelopes containing starch. Under normal conditions, the enzymes responsible for breaking down starch penetrate the softened cellulose and digest the starch, which is then gradually changed into glucose which is rapidly absorbed from the intestine. No fermentation of the starch takes place because there are no bacteria in the upper part of the small intestine.

But in individuals with starch dyspepsia, the undigested starch reaches the colon, where the sugar is attacked by the many bacteria which are present. The whole mass of food ferments, producing carbon dioxide gas. Pain may precede defecation, says Sir Arthur. Immediate relief follows the evacuation of the gas. "Attacks are most likely to follow overindulgence in starch-containing vegetables, new potatoes and young carrots being the most indigestible."

Carbohydrate dyspepsia may remain for years without getting any better or worse and without affecting the general health. In fact, we suppose one might get so used to living in this condition that he might believe it to be normal. However, in early stages, complete recovery follows proper treatment. In long-standing cases, the deficiency may be permanent and the individual may have to live on a sharply restricted diet for the rest of his life.

Sir Arthur's Treatment

The treatment prescribed by Sir Arthur is, as you might suppose, to cut down sharply on starchy foods. He says, "All foods containing more than a very small quantity of starch in its original cellulose envelope must be excluded from the diet."

He forbids his patients to eat the following: potatoes, onions, carrots, beets, artichokes, parsnips, green peas, lentils and rice. He suggests avoiding cereal products altogether, except for possibly one slice of bread for breakfast. These restrictions are often all that is required, he says. If constipation is present, fruit should be eaten with each meal. There are many non-starchy vegetables, too, which add bulk to the diet and thus help prevent constipation. We would certainly recommend that these vegetables be served in quantity. They are such things as greens of all kinds, tomatoes, asparagus, avocados, cabbage, cauliflower, celery, broccoli, cucumbers, peppers, squash and so forth.

After a time, one after another of the forbidden foods may be brought back into the diet. If no discomfort or gas occur, they may remain and several others can be tested. If there is no return of symptoms when all these high-starch foods have been returned to the dinner table, then apparently the intestinal glands have recovered and no more difficulty will be experienced with digesting starch. In more serious cases, however, some or all of the restrictions may have to be continued indefinitely.

We are inclined to lay most of the blame for difficulty with carbohydrates on cereal products rather than on vegetables. Part of the reason for this is that today's cereals are generally so processed by the time they reach us that nothing much but starch is left, with none of the vitamins or minerals that went along with it in the original cereal to aid in its digestion.

Vitamin Loss and Vegetables

In the case of vegetables, of course, one's method of cooking can result in almost the same condition. We know people who never cook a vegetable without soaking it first in cold water. Most of the vitamins and minerals leech out into the water and disappear down the drain when the water is thrown away.

Then, if the same vegetable is cooked in a large quantity of water, more of these precious substances are lost. The B vitamins (vitally concerned with starch digestion) disappear in escaping steam. Vitamin C, so perishable, dissolves into the water. Calcium and potassium have already been discarded, if the vegetables are peeled, for minerals lurk close under the skin. Whatever remaining minerals might still be in the vegetables are probably thrown away with the cooking water.

Vegetables should never be peeled before cooking them. Whether or not you eat the skins depends on the quantity of insecticides you think may be on them. If they are store-bought, you can depend on it—there are plenty. Cook vegetables in as little water as possible for as short a time as possible—just until tender. And, of course, *never soak any fresh food.* You soak dried foods only to restore to them the liquid that they lost when they were dried.

It seems to us that if you are bothered by the symptoms of starch dyspepsia described by Sir Arthur, it should not be too difficult to get back your good health. Omit everything starchy for a while—and, of course, when we include cereal products in this, we mean everything made from grains—not just bread and breakfast cereal. The starchy, incorrectly named "meat-extenders" are the worst offenders—macaroni, spaghetti, noodles, along with all floury desserts. When it comes time to try putting back some of the starchy foods, just forget about the cereals and all the cereal products. Potatoes, carrots, onions and all the other vegetables are good foods—natural, unprocessed and full of vitamins and minerals if you prepare them properly.

Beware of Cereal Products

An interesting comment on Sir Arthur's article appears in a letter to the editor of the *British Medical Journal* for February 1, 1958. J. Pepys writes that the unpleasant digestive tract symptoms that sometimes follow treatment with antibiotics may be caused partly by the eating of products made of wheat. He goes on, "I have now observed 5 cases in whom the eating of bread excited severe cramp and diarrhea, associated with a sometimes remarkable degree of intestinal flatus (gas). In all cases, *pruritus ani* (itching anus) was also present, but appeared to be unrelated to the eating of bread."

[731]

It seems that the effects of eating products made of wheat were related to the amount eaten, and each patient was able to find for himself the amount which could be tolerated. One may be able to give the patient complete relief by simply restricting the amount of bread eaten, says Dr. Pepys.

We want to add only one comment: bread is not the only wheat product most of us eat every day—remember, wheat flour is used in all the starchy foods we mentioned above, in desserts, in gravies and sauces. And breakfast cereals—the cold, processed kind—are perhaps the worst foods, nutritionally speaking, to which we are exposed today, whether they contain wheat or some other grain.

~~~~~~

SECTION 41: INSOMNIA

~~~~~~

192. Insomnia Is a Frustrating Problem

For persons who sleep well, insomnia is hard to understand. The good sleeper lies down, closes his eyes and off he goes. Once he hits the pillow, he couldn't stay awake if he wanted to!

The insomniac's experience is decidedly different. He lies down, closes his eyes, only to begin a nightly struggle to get enough sleep to keep going through the next day. He will plump-up his pillow a dozen times, rearrange the covers, change his position at least that often and be exhausted, but wide awake, as the living room clock strikes three.

The person who has trouble sleeping seeks outside help soon enough. He begins by asking his friends how they manage to fall asleep so easily. He is deluged with theories. One will tell him to take a hot bath before retiring, another will recommend a short walk, another, warm milk. Our insomniac tries them all and is likely to conclude that these tricks work for everyone but him.

Desperate for Sleep

Desperation for a decent night's sleep drives the insomniac to the doctor. "You've got to help me get some rest, Doc. I can't get through the day anymore!"

Now, the doctor could give this fellow a complete physical examination, with all of the laboratory tests, to see if the sleeplessness is a symptom of a more serious disease. The doctor could also take an involved case history to see if some facet of the patient's surroundings or some particular occurrence in his recent past might be the cause of the insomnia. These things are often at the root of a sleeping problem. But it is more than likely that the doctor will skip these preliminaries and give the patient instant relief—an envelope of sleeping pills.

The threat to good health that is bound up in a sleep-inducing drug is apparently not considered by the physician. He sees his job as done if the patient sleeps at night.

Should the patient be satisfied? Of course not! The sleeping pill is not a cure, just a postponement; it may have a toxic reaction that is immediate, or side effects that sneak up with no warning. Soon the patient is sleeping only fairly well with one tablet, so the dose is upped to two; eventually, 3 or 4 might be needed to knock him out for a peaceful night. And the idea of even attempting to sleep without the nightly quota gives our man the squirms. Meanwhile, instead of a wide-awake day, the drugged insomniac is bleary-eyed and exhausted at work. Pep? Drive? He never expects to experience them again. His emotional reactions have even changed. He's cranky, disinterested, unenthusiastic; his wife gets on his nerves and he can't stand the children. Before he was unhappy for maybe two or four of the hours he should have been sleeping, now he's miserable for the 16 hours he's awake, then he slams himself into senselessness with his sleeping tablets. Some improvement!

Is There a Better Way?

There must be a better way to conquer insomnia, you say. Of course there is, and the weapon lies within you. You can *learn* to go to sleep, just as you can *learn* to play ball or to dance. It takes practice for some, and others can do it naturally. There are many theories on how one can go about this learning, but the central idea, no matter what technique you use, is the relaxation of tension.

In his book, *How to Sleep Well* (Vantage Press, New York, $2.95), Dr. Samuel W. Gutwirth maintains that the ideal invitation to sleep is to simply do nothing. Apparently for an insomniac, this directive is not easily accomplished. Dr. Gutwirth says that, unless the nerves or muscles are diseased, one possesses the ability "not to do." Tossing, for example, is doing something; so is counting sheep or changing position. This doesn't mean that one can't move around in bed, for holding a set position when you are yearning to turn is just as likely to cause tension. You've got to learn to let yourself go when you lie down at bedtime. Cease doing anything about sleep or anything else—cease all activity.

Practice Sessions for Relaxation

Dr. Gutwirth believes that this is what the good sleeper does automatically. He is convinced that anyone can learn to do the same thing, no matter how wide-eyed an insomniac he is. The method is called scientific relaxation. It calls for regular practice sessions aside from bedtime, of about 45 minutes each day, until you become proficient. These periods take place in a quiet room, with the student lying on his back, outstretched. He then begins to tense each group of body muscles for several minutes (the arms, legs, trunk, facial muscles, eye muscles), then relax them, consciously allowing them to grow more and more limp. Dr. Gutwirth theorizes that such a procedure teaches the subject the contrast between tension and relaxation. Once the sensation of complete relaxation is firmly embedded in the subject's mind, he need only point his consciousness in that direction and sleep will follow with ease. Though the book offers much more detailed directions for achievement of this, the above outline gives the essentials of the method.

Dr. Gutwirth offers the thought that an insomniac can help himself to sleep by arranging for as many of the following as possible: a dark room, no undue noise, a hot bath before retiring (with a gentle massage if possible), a regular hour for retiring, a large bed with a good mattress, potsponement of worries or fears until tomorrow, avoidance of excitement before bedtime, mild fatigue, proper ventilation and satisfaction of any hunger pangs.

Coffee, Tea and Aggressions

In a paper on the subject of sleeplessness, published in the *Medical Journal of Australia* (May 2, 1959), Dr. Barry Mulvany makes several interesting observations which might be of some help to the insomniac. First of all, tea and coffee should be taken out of the patient's diet. While these beverages do not interfere with the sleep of every person who drinks them, sensitivity to the caffeine they both contain is extremely common among insomniacs.

Dr. Mulvany also suggests that one needs a means of releasing aggressions that pile up during the course of a day. This sounds terribly psychiatric, but it simply means that one needs a challenge that one can meet effectively. Some people find such a challenge in their jobs, and find release for aggressive impulses in doing their jobs well. Others find that a hobby affords the feeling of accomplishment they need; sports are another outlet. The insomniac might not have discovered the valve he needs to let off steam, and this psychological steam can boil in him, keeping him awake with nervous energy.

Another point made in this same article is that many tense and anxious people can relax better on a hard surface. Such an unyielding support induces a sense of security and firmness, which is translated into relaxation of the muscles. This psychological reason is not the only one for using a hard surface for sleeping. Many physiologists show evidence proving that the alignment, and eventually the health of the body, is bound to be impaired by sleeping on a soft, yielding surface.

The Harder the Mattress, the Better the Rest

Editor Rodale determined to test this theory some years ago, and found that the harder the mattress, the better his rest. He eventually tried a bed board under his mattress and relished the support it gave. He then began to wonder about an even more rigid surface, since the mattress with the board under it still had some "give." In discussing the problem with a friend of his who is a mattress manufacturer, Mr. Rodale asked if it would be possible to cover a bed board with about ¾ of an inch of padding, so that it could be put on top of the mattress. Indeed it could. The result was a product with a wooden frame which fit nicely over the sides of the bed where the mattress would ordinarily have been. The padded board was so successful, that it became a commercial item offered by the Bethlehem Furniture Company of Allentown, Pennsylvania.

Returning to the problem of insomnia, Mr. Rodale found in his experience a basis for a theory on insomnia which holds that the problem is often an imaginary one. He had considered himself an insomniac for many years, until he began to notice that he was often oblivious to storms and street excitement which had occurred just outside his house during the night. He thought he had spent a sleepless night, yet he must have slept through these noisy incidents.

Sleep Will Return

Mr. Rodale concluded that he must be sleeping much of the night but was aware only of the awake periods, for he could naturally have no memory of the time he was actually sleeping. This discovery changed his whole attitude toward sleep. When he awoke, during the night, he relaxed, and simply let sleep overtake him once more, rather than his worrying about not being able to sleep again or counting sheep. Such activity builds up the tenseness that fights sleep. These periods of wakefulness and sleep vary with the individual. For some, the waking lasts barely long enough for a shift in position; for others, it can last for a minute or 10 minutes, but sleep will come again if the subject calmly expects it and waits relaxed.

Still Awake?

Why not face it? Some of us do not sleep as well as others. Accept this and you can enjoy what sleep you do get. Try the remedies for insomnia; they might help, but to be calm and unexcited about the condition is the first requirement. You will notice that lack of tension is the basis of all insomnia remedies. Do what you can to teach yourself relaxation, be certain that your bed is comfortable, firm and that all possible steps have been taken to make your surroundings conducive to sleep. Relax when you lie down, enjoy just lying there and resting. Try to let sleep overtake you, but don't be aggressive about chasing after sleep. If you've learned your lesson well, it should come to *you*.

If, after lying in bed for a while, you find that you're not enjoying the rest and relaxation you should and you're beginning to thrash around, get up for a while. Read a chapter of a favorite book, glance over the evening paper and read the things you didn't have time for earlier. After about a half an hour try again. This time, you've relaxed a little more, you have some new and pleasant thoughts, you're ready to let sleep capture you.

~~~~~~

SECTION 42: LEUKEMIA

~~~~~~

193. Leukemia in Infants and Young Children

By W. J. McCORMICK, M.D., Toronto, Canada

In recent years, mostly within the last decade, there has been an alarming increase in the incidence of leukemia in infants and young children, the cause of which has led to much investigative research and conjecture. In the United States, more children 5 to 14 years of age are victims of this disease than of any other, and it is invariably fatal.[1] In a recently published report from the Sainte Justine Children's Hospital in Montreal, the admissions for leukemia in infants and young children for the 5-year period ending with 1958 were almost twice the total of the previous 10 years.[2] (Leukemia is cancer of the blood. There is an increase in the white blood corpuscles, and enlargement of the spleen, the lymphatic glands and the bone marrow.)

Regarding the cause of this disease, Pierce[3], of the University of Chicago, states that the pathogenesis (origin) of congenital leukemia (that is, leukemia present at birth) is as obscure as it is in the childhood form, but that existence of this disease in utero (that is, in the unborn child) suggests that maternal and genetic (hereditary) factors are etiologically (etiological means pertaining to the cause of the disease) significant in both forms. Forty-five cases in the literature are reviewed (by Pierce). Most of these with signs of leukemia at birth had severe systemic involvement and died within a few years. Hemorrhagic manifestations occurred in all cases, ranging from scattered petechiae (small rounded spots of bleeding under the skin) to confluent ecchymoses (large patch-like bleedings under the skin) and bleeding from the umbilical stump, the gastrointestinal (digestive) and genitourinary (elimination) tracts.

Concurrent Leukemia in Mother and Child

Cramblatt and his associates,[4] in an article in the *New England Medical Journal,* make the first report of the concurrent incidence of leukemia in a mother and her infant. Near the end of the seventh month of pregnancy, petechiae and ecchymoses developed spontaneously on the abdomen and lower extremities. Three weeks before delivery, gingival (gum) bleeding also developed. Eight days after spontaneous labor and birth of an apparently healthy boy, the mother developed symptoms, of acute leukemia with white-cell count of 25,000 and died about two months later. Her son, at 9 months of age, also developed the same disease with white-blood-cell count of 40,000 and the usual hemorrhagic manifestations—easy bruising, bleeding from the gums, petechiae, ecchymoses and purpuric areas (purple patches of bleeding under the skin) were scattered over the trunk, the extremities and skull. The correlated incidence of these two cases is strongly suggestive of the likelihood of unsuspected and unrecognized maternal transmissions of this disease in many such cases (Dr. McCormick believes).

The most generally accepted culpable etiological factor (that is, the circumstance we should blame) has been the exposure of the pregnant mother to diagnostic or therapeutic X-ray, thus exposing the unborn child to unintentional radiation. However, from a careful analysis of this factor, Swartz and Upton[5] (in the magazine *Blood*) conclude that prenatal irradiation can account for only a small part of the increasing incidence in infantile subjects.

There is, we think, another major factor in the possible solution of this problem which has been apparently overlooked or ignored, and that is the tobacco smoking of mothers during pregnancy. Tobacco smoking by our female population began on this continent about 40 years ago, following the first great war, and it must be admitted that the female addiction in this respect is rapidly overtaking that of the male. It must also be recognized that, by this time, a rapidly increasing number of our female population have become heavily addicted (30 to 50 or more cigarettes daily), while at the same time qualifying as contributors to our exploding population.

About 26 years ago, a scientific study of the effect of cigarette smoking by prospective mothers on the heart function of their unborn babies was conducted at Antioch College, Yellow Springs, Ohio, by Doctors Sontag and Wallace[6] as part of a study on the effect of prenatal environment. They made over 80 tests on several prospective mothers who were habitual smokers. To begin with, during the interval between smoking, their babies' heartbeats averaged 144 per minute, which was 14 beats faster than normal average, 130, as reported by obstetricians at the turn of the century, before women began smoking.

Then, when they resumed smoking for the tests, their babies' heartbeats, within 10 minutes, were speeded to an average of 149 to the minute, thus making a total of 19 beats per minute above the normal average.

It should be pointed out that, when these tests were made, very little was known about the carcinogenic (cancer-causing) tars and other toxic elements in tobacco smoke. When one considers that many millions of our unborn progeny are continually receiving these and other toxic food preservatives through the medium of their mothers' blood, it is little wonder that, at the present rate of increase, it has been estimated that one-third of our present population may expect to die of cancer. Incidentally, lung cancer and blood cancer (leukemia) are the two most rapidly increasing forms of this disease today.

In confirmation of our hypothesis, we cite the observations of Lawrence and Donlan[7] in *Cancer Research* as follows: "It seems clear that several types of embryonic tissue have a high degree of sensitivity to carcinogenic (cancer-causing) agents. The acute leukemias are an example of diseases that may have such an origin. Leukemia seems to be increasing in recent years, especially in young children under 5 years, suggestively due to carcinogenic stimulation in prenatal life."

In further support of our hypothesis, we cite the work of Ehrhart, Stich and Benoit reported in the German publication *Blut*,[8] in which they gave a toxic chemical ("indole") to a strain of mice with a normally low incidence of leukemia. To one group, they gave 50 milligrams of this chemical in divided doses, resulting in an incidence of leukemia in 55 per cent of the animals. To another group of the same strain of mice they gave a smaller dose of the chemical—30 milligrams in divided doses—which led to an incidence of only 16 per cent of leukemia. These observations give definite support to our concept that tobacco carcinogens, transmitted maternally in prenatal life, may be the culpable agent in the recent upsurge in incidence of infantile leukemia.

A striking feature in all the leukemic cases referred to in this treatise is the uniformity in the incidence of hemorrhagic manifestations—easy bruising, petechiae, ecchymoses, gingival bleeding, bleeding from the mucous membranes of the gastrointestinal and genitourinary tracts and so forth—all of which are suggestive of a scorbutic background. (That is, a background involving scurvy, the disease of vitamin C deficiency.) It is also quite possible that many of the scurvy victims of centuries ago had leukemic complications which were not recognized in the absence of microscopic hematology (the study of blood conditions with a microscope). As a matter of fact, the great plague, "The Black Death," which ravaged Europe and Asia in the fourteenth century got its name from the prevalence of "black and blue" patches on the skin, the result of subcutaneous bleeding—in reality a manifestation of scurvy.

It is also worthy of note that an ulcerative and hemorrhagic prelude is usually associated with cancer, which Martini[9] (who wrote in the seventeenth century) thus relates to scurvy and the plague, all of which is indicative of an unrecognized etiological situation warranting investigation—suggestively vitamin C deficiency. The recent increase in the incidence of

[738]

infantile scurvy in our children's hospitals lends support to this concept. However, infants and young children are not unique in this respect. By chemical test, we find that fully 90 per cent of our adult population is definitely deficient in vitamin C. The increasing use of tea, coffee and alcohol, with their phenomenal advertising propaganda are the major contributing factors to this debacle. We regard tobacco as the major offender in this respect, since the toxic fumes are known to have a neutralizing effect on vitamin C and this may be a preconditioning factor in the pathogenesis of leukemia, and cancer in general.

Summary

The author reports a marked increase in the incidence of leukemia in infants and young children, which he attributes to prenatal transmission of carcinogens (cancer-causing substances) from smoking mothers. Several citations are made in support of this concept and correlation of vitamin C deficiency (subclinical scurvy) is postulated as the basic etiological factor in the development of the hemorrhagic manifestations of leukemia, and cancer in general.

REFERENCES

1. METROPOLITAN LIFE INSURANCE CO., *Statistical Bulletin*, Dec., 1958.
2. SUPERINTENDENT OF THE MONTREAL CHILDREN'S HOSPITAL, report, "Les Cancers Infantiles a Sainte Justine," *L'Union Medicale du Canada*, Tome 87: 905, 1958.
3. PIERCE, MILA. I., "Leukemia in the new-born infant," *Journal of Pediatrics*, 54: 691, 1959.
4. CRAMBLATT, HENRY G., et al, "Leukemia in an infant born of mother with leukemia," *New England Medical Journal*, 259: 727, 1958.
5. SWARTZ, E. E., and UPTON, A. C., (Oak Ridge National Lab.), *Blood*, 13: 845, 1958.
6. SONTAG, L. W., and WALLACE, R. F., (Antioch College, Yellow Springs, Ohio) as part of a study on effect of prenatal environment, *Associated Press* dispatch, Feb. 7, 1935.
7. LAWRENCE, E. A., and DONLAN, E., "Neoplastic diseases in infants and young children," *Cancer Research*, 12: 900-904, Dec., 1952.
8. EHRHART, H., STITCH, W., and BENOIT, W. S., *Blut*, 6/1: 11-17, 1960.
9. MARTINI (1609), cited by LIND, JAMES, *Treatise on the Scurvy*, Edinburgh, 1753.

194. The Appearance of Lupus Erythematosus and Aplastic Anemia

A blood disease, lupus erythematosus, characterized by disk-like patches on the skin with raised, reddish edges and depressed centers and covered with scales and crusts, is growing increasingly common among us. The disease can be fatal. Sometimes this disease is present in the blood stream, without skin blotches showing at all. A blood test, developed by Dr. Malcolm M. Hargraves of the Mayo Clinic, Rochester, Minnesota, has made detection possible even when the skin eruptions are not present. In any case, this disease has emerged from the status of a medical rarity to a relatively common disorder. The *Roche Report* (February 6, 1961) printed an interview with Dr. Hargraves on the subject of this systemic disease, and we believe his answers are important and interesting.

When asked what reason he would assign to the increase in the number of lupus cases, Dr. Hargraves first insisted that the increase of the disease was an actual fact, not due just to increased detection of already existing cases. Then, "This absolute increase, I think, is associated with our more extensive exposure to antigenic agents (vaccines) which stimulate and activate our reticuloendothelial system (that which aids in the formation of antibodies). A few such agents are polio and flu vaccines, various antibiotic agents and drugs, to say nothing of the tremendous influx of new chemical products in our environment. . . ."

Detection Routine But Cause Unknown

The difficulty presented with erythematosus is that, while detection has become fairly routine, there is no specific treatment for the disease. Exactly how it enters the body or just how it is produced are mysteries which have yet to be solved. There are many symptoms that might be an indication of the presence of lupus erythematosus—dysfunction of the lungs, the blood, the spleen, high fever, etc.—so it can be seen that even a physician who knows of Dr. Hargraves' blood test might not suspect lupus when he examines a patient, and hence might neglect the test.

We wondered, in the light of Dr. Hargraves' statement about the lack of a specific cure for lupus, just what advantage there would be to discovering the fact that the disease were present. The answer from Dr. Hargraves was this: ". . . the diagnosis will spare him (the patient) the injudicious use of drugs, vaccines, unnecessary surgical treatment or other therapeutic procedures which might only aggravate the underlying disease." Dr. Hargraves was then asked just what steps he would take when confronted with a case of lupus erythematosus, considering the fact that no specific therapy is known.

Difficulties Brought on by Environmental Agents

"Since I believe that the difficulties of most of these persons are precipitated by environmental agents, I attempt to take as careful a history as possible, particularly relating to exposure to noxious agents. Experience has taught me to suspect vaccine, bacterial infections, medications, actinic rays (X-rays) and cosmetics (such as hair dyes and permanent waves), together with household and industrial materials which contain the various aromatic, aliphatic (oily) and chlorinated hydrocarbons . . ." Dr. Hargraves then tries to protect the patient from the agent he deems responsible, and he recommends total rest in bed for a period of months.

Dr. Hargraves appears to be one of the few physicians we read about who is willing to say he is aware of and frightened by the danger of the poisons in our environment. He wrote some time ago of the many serious, even fatal, effects of insecticides upon those who breathed them, or somehow came into physical contact with them. He mentioned Hodgkin's disease, leukemia and aplastic anemia as being possible results of insecticide poisoning. He spoke specifically of farm sprays and of the aerosol bombs many people use to rid their homes of insect pests.

Drugs and Sprays Blamed

Dr. Hargraves received some support in the views of Dr. M. M. Wintrobe of the University of Utah (reported in an Associated Press dispatch date lined Salt Lake City—no date). Dr. Wintrobe, chairman of the American Medical Association's subcommittee on blood abnormalities, blamed the increased frequency of blood disorders on drug misuses, crop sprays and radiation.

One of the most worrisome of the blood diseases is aplastic anemia. In this disease, there is an upset in the bone marrow where red blood cells are made, resulting in a red cell shortage. Other disorders strike the white blood cells or the clotting factor in the blood. Any of these can be fatal, yet early diagnosis is not always possible. Victims become weak and anemic. Breathing is difficult and heart flutter is apparent to the physician. These are the symptoms of a hundred diseases, so an observant and intuitive doctor who is willing to run all necessary tests is the one most likely to uncover such disease.

Said Dr. Wintrobe, "The Food and Drug Administration has suggested in studies that there is an increase in aplastic anemia, and we have known for a long time that certain chemical agents can produce aplastic anemia and aplasia in bone marrow. . . . In recent years, we have begun to recognize that, in an occasional person, sensitivity to a certain drug, which does no harm to anyone else, might cause aplastic anemia."

Coal Tars, Sulfa Drugs among Causative Agents

Dr. Wintrobe, named as causative agents: benzol, coal tars, sulfa drugs, excessive radiation and some crop sprays. What an odd situation; the Food and Drug Administration and at least two very respected researchers in the medical field assert the danger of drugs, certain chemical food additives, sprays and X-rays, and seem to be completely ignored. When we point out these drawbacks, we are branded faddists and the public is told to ignore us. Why are these dangers such an obscure truth? Why are dangerous drugs available so easily and used with such abandon? Why does the government actually urge spraying with deadly pesticides and, through the Department of Agriculture, carry on spraying programs over wide areas of our country? Why are aerosol bombs containing the same dangerous preparations available for home use? Can you think of many processed foods which have not been treated with coal tar derivatives, the very hydrocarbons mentioned by Dr. Hargraves?

Even someone who is ready to accept the fact that the problem is serious, cannot—positively cannot—avoid every type of environmental hazard that might do him physical harm. Imagine what happens to those who don't give the problem a thought. They eat oranges dyed with coal tar, they drink sodas colored in the same way. They spray clouds of DDT and parathion on every bug in every room. They get X-ray treatments for acne, for psoriasis, for bursitis. They beg for penicillin shots when sniffles appear, and take sulfa drugs in spite of a bad liver or poor kidneys.

Doctors Coöperate

Even more amazing is the fact that doctors coöperate in much of this. In the *Medical Journal of Australia* (April 8, 1961), a correspondent, S. C. S. Cooke, hit on this very thing when he expressed concern over the possible long range dangers in drugs such as the antihistamines and the phenazones. Dr. Cooke was worried about the fact that "thousands of psychiatric patients are being sent home with instructions to take phenazones for the rest of their lives. Are we sure that the increase of leukemia, aplastic anemia and even cancer (in the widest sense of that word) is not due as much to the regular and sustained use of phenyl-group drugs as to the excessive use of X-rays for diagnosis?"

It is important to know that Dr. Cooke's question, along with others asked by conscientious medical men, has yet to be answered. Unfortunately, orthodox medicine would have us all live as though the answer were already ours, as though we knew that no harm could come of this.

Gradually the true facts are emerging and cannot be ignored. Los Angeles General Hospital has severely clamped down on the use of the drug, chloromycetin, strongly suspected as a cause of aplastic anemia. A test showed that newborn babies given chloromycetin (formerly a regular routine at Los Angeles General) to prevent any infant infection, had a death rate 300 per cent higher than babies given no antibiotic whatsoever. Now an order is in effect stating that only in extreme emergencies can this drug be administered at this hospital.

What About Other Drugs?

The danger in the use of chloromycetin has been common knowledge for several years, yet most doctors use it more than ever. We wonder how many other hospitals will order its strict control, if not discontinuance? Why just this one drug? The cortico-steroids, the sulfas, the antihistamines are all used with utter recklessness. They, too, carry a great potential for harm, yet they are avidly advertised in medical journals throughout the United States and samples of each appear as if by magic in the mailboxes of doctors, lest they forget about using them.

The problem we face is in educating our doctors to the long view demonstrated by Drs. Cooke, Hargraves and Wintrobe. They are looking beyond the slogans and the single treatments with drugs that may show a quick effect on symptoms, but don't really alleviate, and sometimes actually aggravate, the true physical problem. They are interested in what will happen as the result of a year of injections or 5 years of pills. They know that the continued breathing of polluted air and non-stop ingestion of additives and the continued use of drugs, must have some unwanted effect on bodies whose organs are not equipped to handle such things.

We Must Awaken the Country

We must do what we can to awaken the rest of the country to the dangers we all face. Protest to food manufacturers about the additives they use. Write to newspapers, asking that they review the books by William Longgood (*The Poisons in Your Food*) and Franklin and Bicknell (*Chemicals in Your Food*) which deal with the problems presented by our treated food and poisoned environment. Review the books yourself for your club and, of course, avoid these dangers yourself by shopping carefully, by reading labels to discover which foods are least contaminated by additives, by eating as much fresh fruit and vegetables as possible, by drinking bottled spring water when the municipal supply is fluoridated, chlorinated or otherwise questionable. Taking food supplements is a positive action one can take as a defense against the unavoidable poisons one must cope with today. Vitamin C and the B vitamins are the nutrients most urgently needed to protect the body.

195. Mental Illness

The slick picture weeklies and ladies' magazines periodically investigate and expose our mental hospitals. The subject is sensational and of concern to everyone, and the facts are so shocking in themselves, that there is no need to color them to make an interesting story. The authors usually wring their hands over the lack of facilities we have to take care of our mentally ill and end with a plea for more funds to be used for new buildings and larger staffs.

But all this is merely a delaying action. More and more of our people are the victims of mental illness each year—the current estimate in *Scope Weekly* (February 11, 1959) is that some 17,500,000 persons in the United States have nervous or mental disorders serious enough to warrant treatment. What of next year, and 5 years after that? What hope is there for these people? We are told of tranquilizers and shock treatments, and of the mysteries being uncovered by psychiatry, but the yearly increase in the numbers of our mentally ill testifies to the fact that these measures are inadequate to the problem. If tranquilizers are all they're supposed to be, we should be emptying our mental hospitals instead of building more. We are convinced that there is a better, cheaper, less dangerous and more efficient means of helping these unfortunate people, and preventing new disasters, than the standard methods now being employed. The logical answer lies in bolstered nutrition.

A Theory Shows Promising Results

For many years it had been suspected that mental illness has its origin in nutritional deficiencies. While the theory was widely known, little was done to test it. Many authorities scoffed at it, as they often do when nutrition is mentioned as a treatment for disease. It's too simple. The problem of proving the value of nutrition was complicated greatly by the fact that measuring changes in mental illness, as a result of this or that treatment, is extremely difficult. Each case is so highly individual that comparisons with other patients, not receiving the experimental treatment (controls), actually cannot give the type of scientific evidence that stands up as undeniable proof.

Dr. George Watson reported on an experiment in the *Journal of Psychology* (1957, 43: 47-63) in which these problems seem to have been solved. The article proves quite conclusively the effectiveness of nutritional supplements in treating mental disorders. Dr. Watson states that psycho-neuroses and psychoses can be induced experimentally by dietary restrictions. It is presumed then that such conditions which already exist have been caused by the lack of certain dietary requirements. A formula was worked out which included large amounts of all the vitamins and minerals known or believed to be important in human nutrition. This was to be the experimental substance used in treating a test group of patients.

A group of 19 emotionally disturbed patients was to make the test. It was planned that these same 19 would act as their own control group. Each of these patients was maintained at first on a capsule which contained no active ingredients whatsoever (a placebo) for a period of from 1 to 2½ months, to see if they would react to the mere psychology of a pill. They were then transferred to the experimental capsule of nutrients for an average period of 2.9 months, though some were treated for as long as 6 months.

The evaluations of the treatment were based upon subjective and objective factors. Changes in attitude (loss of resentments, interest in job hunting, feeling of well-being), as well as improved scores in a psychological test, were considered the criteria of improvement.

Each of the group of 19 patients was given a month's supply of capsule-shaped tablets to be taken orally and daily, 3 at each meal. At the end of the month, the patients reported for a fresh supply of capsules and an interview to assess their progress. Of the 19, 16 improved significantly, one got worse and two showed no change. Certainly there is no other treatment currently being given to alleviate mental disorders which can boast of a better percentage of good results.

A Young Man with Dermatitis

What type of cases were these that responded so well to a nutritional supplement? The answer to that question is best illustrated by describing several of the case histories.

There is the case of a young man of 19 years who had developed a psychosis due to a facial dermatitis. He would not leave his room, nor talk with his family. He was depressed and afraid to meet anyone. The young man was enrolled in the experiment. During the period in which he was given the placebo capsule, the boy got worse. However, after only one month of treatment with the vitamin capsule, he was more at ease. He began to join the family in the living room to watch TV. Also, he began to have long, confidential talks with his father, whom he had especially ignored before. His mother was so amazed at the change in her son that she reported "His recovery, frankly, is more than we had hoped for." His score in the psychological test, given at the end of treatment, was normal.

Another of the patients was a woman of 42 years. In her initial interview, she reported feeling depressed, frustrated and generally inadequate;

she had not been able to seek employment or do anything for several years. To the interviewer, she appeared to be mentally confused and spoke with a slow, childlike voice pattern.

The placebo trial of one month saw no change in her condition. After a month on the vitamin treatment, she reported that she had re-enrolled in school; her voice pattern was normal once more and she appeared to be more alert. At the end of the third month of treatment, she had secured a job. She appeared calm and relaxed for the first time since the experiment began. The lady's score in the psychological test also improved.

Attempted to Run Away

Another lady, aged 53, reported extreme fatigue, flights of anger and excessive hostility. Her family said she had delusions and had attempted to run away. In her first interview, she was hostile and excitable. She told of being hungry all the time and eating constantly. Her family doctor had been treating her with reserpine (a tranquilizer) for 6 months.

The placebo period saw a change for the better, but then a quick return to her former pattern. The vitamin capsule was begun, and after one month of treatment, her voice pattern became normal; she was no longer irritable or impatient. In two months, her family reported that she had lost her aggressiveness, and her appetite was normal. After 4 months, she appeared clinically normal and obtained a job as saleslady in a department store.

Tried to Smash TV Set

Finally, let us look at the case of a 26-year-old man who was so easily frustrated to anger, that he tried to smash a TV set when his father told him to change a station. He was hostile and slightly depressed.

He showed some unsustained improvement on the placebos, but once he began the vitamin treatment, his father said the son's condition was vastly better. He was more at ease and more alert. He wanted to find a job, where before he was uninterested in anything.

Because he was also receiving medication for epilepsy, which was considered not to be involved with his mental condition, it was decided to stop the vitamin capsule to see if the other medication was the cause of the pleasant change in the patient. After 3 weeks without the nutritional support, the mother called to say her son had regressed. He was irritable, his attacks increased and he was inactive and sleeping all the time. He had lost interest, was increasingly tired, forgetful, confused. Upon resuming treatment with the vitamins, he improved to the point of obtaining a job without aid.

These are typical of the cases treated, and they prove that nutrition is a major factor in mental health. The victory over this problem lies, then, not in building new hospitals or paying psychiatrists for the time they give to public institutions, but in educating the public to proper nutrition. More emphasis must be laid on the value of careful diet in preserving health. If some of our public dollars were spent to publicize Dr. Watson's findings, perhaps some of our potential inmates could be detoured from serving time in a mental institution.

Whatever happens, you are fortunate enough to have read of Dr. Watson's work. You know that, if a full quota of vitamins can bring one out of a mental problem, the same can help one avoid such an illness in the first place. Protect yourself and your family by giving them, as Dr. Watson did his patients, "large quantities of all the vitamins known or believed important in human nutrition." Fresh, unprocessed foods and natural food supplements can guarantee this.

196. The Nutritional Approach to Nervous Disorders

We can't help but wonder how many of the country's doctors and psychiatrists are familiar with the work of Norman Jolliffe, M.D. He wrote a paper on the subject of "Treatment of Neuropsychiatric Disorders with Vitamins," and it was printed in the November 1, 1941, issue of the *Journal of the American Medical Association.* Dr. Jolliffe was then on the staff of the Psychiatric Division of Bellevue Hospital in New York and on the staff of New York University College of Medicine. Clearly, Dr. Jolliffe had the approval and respect of his colleagues, yet his findings have gone into a limbo which would make one think they were utterly worthless. Almost no one even tries vitamins for mental illness. Still, it is not as though mental disease were being effectively dealt with through other means. The cases mount and the hospitals overflow. Tranquilizers, shock treatments, sedatives and other commonly used measures are patently ineffective in curing most cases of mental illness, but they are still used with hopeless desperation. Strangely, few doctors are desperate enough to resort to the one treatment proven by Dr. Jolliffe to be useful in improving many mental conditions; that is, the use of nutritional supplements. Said he, in his article, "Almost every vitamin has also been credited with playing a role in the maintenance of a normal nervous system. The more important of the vitamins thus accredited are thiamin hydrochloride, nicotinic acid, riboflavin, pyridoxine and alpha tocopherol. . . ."

Pellagra Symptoms Equal to Mental Illness

Dr. Jolliffe equated the mental symptoms which occur in pellagra (a classical manifestation of thiamin deficiency) with those of most psychoses. They include memory defects, disorientation and confusion. Periods of excitement, depression, mania, delirium and paranoia occur frequently.

Often these mental symptoms appear before other signs of pellagra are evident. Without these other signs, an observer would certainly not differentiate between this mental response and that shown by any other patient with similar psychiatric attitudes. Thiamin lack causes such symptoms; who is to argue that the frankly mental patient, whose symptoms are the same, could not be helped by increased thiamin in the diet, or by injections of this vitamin alone or in liver extract? Dr. Jolliffe pointed out that, in treating such symptoms, the physician should be certain that other dietary factors necessary to brain metabolism are also present, in order to obtain a maximal therapeutic response.

Nicotinic Acid Therapy Greatly Reduced Mortality

Another series of symptoms which shows a mental nutritional connection is known as nicotinic acid deficiency, encephalopathy. This illness is characterized by exaggerated sucking and grasping reflexes, alternating rigidity of the body and progressive clouding of consciousness. Dr. Jolliffe says that this syndrome is seen most frequently in cases of chronic alcoholism, endemic pellagra, senility and cirrhosis of the liver. "In our study of 150 cases, mortality was reduced from 90 per cent to 15 per cent by nicotinic acid therapy."

In discussing chronic alcoholism, the author also mentions delirium tremens, the terrible mental aftereffects of too much alcohol in the system. "In delirium tremens, the decided increase in total metabolism raises the vitamin requirements to such an extent, that an acute deficiency may be precipitated, from which the patient may die unless attention is given to insuring adequate nutrition."

Shaking Palsy Relieved

Paralysis agitans, a condition characterized by continual shaking of one or more extremities which become less facile in execution of everyday exercises, was another disease which Dr. Jolliffe submitted to vitamin therapy. He first chose 15 patients who were completely incapacitated and administered to each, 50 or 100 milligrams of pyridoxine either daily or every other day for at least 4 weeks. Of the 15, 4 showed definite improvement, one of whom later regressed.

Another group of 46 ambulatory patients was treated with pyridoxine. Fourteen of these, all of whom showed no improvement, abandoned the treatment in less than 3 weeks. The 32 who continued were considered by Jolliffe to have shown "worthwhile results."

Nutritious, Natural Diets Plus Vitamin Supplements

Dr. Jolliffe outlined in his report the procedure he believed necessary in preparing and treating psychiatric patients to whom specific therapy is to be administered:

1. A full, nutritious diet of natural, refined foods. No sugar, candy, jellies, white flour products, refined cereals, polished rice or alcoholic drinks.

The patient gets each day, citrus juices or tomato juice, milk, meat (including liver and pork muscle), eggs, butter, salad of raw vegetables and/or fruit, salad oil and potatoes. The balance of the diet is selected from vegetables, fruits and whole grain bread.

2. Vitamins by mouth include fish liver oil containing 10,000 units of vitamin A, and a source of the entire B complex (brewer's yeast, vegex, liver extract, wheat germ)—all "preferred to synthetic products in capsule form from which some factors as yet impossible to encapsulate are likely to be missing."

3. Injections of vitamin B complex in liver extract, or as thiamin hydrochloride—10 milligrams, riboflavin—1 milligram and nicotinic acid —100 milligrams.

Safer to Give too Much

"Specific treatments . . . are based on the principle that, when biochemical or reversible anatomic lesions (injuries) are present, it is safer to err on the side of wasting the vitamin, than to give too little for too short a time. . . . If the patient has liver disease or diarrhea, or is an alcohol addict, the larger dose should be given. Clinical evidence, as well as experimental evidence, indicates that, in these conditions, much larger doses of vitamins are required to produce maximal response than when absorption is unimpaired and the liver normal.

"In view of recent expressions concerning toxic effects of vitamins, I believe it pertinent to state that, in treating more than 3,000 patients with clinically manifest deficiency disease, I have not observed any toxic effects when the vitamins were administered as a crystalline vitamin dissolved in saline solution without added preservative, in the doses described, and while the patient was maintained with a good diet and the entire vitamin B complex (except, of course, the vasomotor phenomena of nicotinic acid)." Dr. Jolliffe refers here to the expanding and contracting action of blood vessels that can be caused by synthetic niacin.

Field of Nutritional Therapy Should Be Expanded

That was the feeling and experience of an eminent man in the field of treatment for mental illness in 1941. From time to time, we still see expressions of Dr. Jolliffe's faith in nutrients for mental as well as other illnesses, but the field is notably unexplored in proportion to the enormity of the problem. Many types of mental illness are known to withstand all of the commonly used medications and treatments, and the doctors do no more. They do not try nutritional therapy, in spite of the scientific foundation it boasts of. They merely throw in the towel and announce that there is nothing to be done. The doctors have no experience with nutrients, they don't know whether they would work or not. They simply refuse to try them.

197. Retarded Mentality Means Nutritional Need

The sad plight of a family whose child is mentally retarded is becoming less and less unusual. This impression is borne out by the judgment of Dr. I. Newton Kugelmass, who is quoted in the *New York Times* (October 10, 1954) as saying, "Since the turn of the century, there has been a progressive increase in the number of mentally defective children, and a progressive decline in the intelligence of the population as a whole." Why is this happening now? Why within the last 50 years?

We believe that the answer lies in the type of diet we eat. Fifty years ago, processed foods were largely unknown, candy was a sometime treat, ice cream an event and soda had barely been invented. Nowadays, the child or adult who goes through a day without all of these is considered underprivileged. In all of these foods, if they may be called that, are elements which are destructive to good health. When they are included in the diet, the body cannot hope to run at its peak efficiency. They contribute almost nothing in the way of nutrients, and what is worse, they squelch the normal appetite for healthful foods, and destroy many of the nutrients which might happen to be present in the body. Directly, or indirectly, these nutrients are involved with the development of our intelligence.

Diet of the Mother-To-Be

A recognized source of the problem of mental deficiency in children's health is the poor diet of the mother-to-be. Experiments cited by Dr. Albert G. Hogan, Professor Emeritus of Animal Nutrition at the University of Missouri, indicated that rats receiving inadequate rations tend to produce unusually large numbers of defective offspring. So predictable is the response to a diet deficiency among these animals, that it is known that, if their diet is lacking in vitamin B_{12}, 20 per cent of the rats born of such parents will be mentally abnormal.

Another experiment, reported by the Missouri Agricultural Experiment Station, *Journal Series, Number 1254,* showed that rats born of dams fed a ration low in folic acid and reared to near maturity on the same ration, showed inferior ability in learning their way through a maze, as compared with control rats. Supplementation of the diet of the pregnant rats with folic acid resulted in offspring which learned as readily as the control animals. This was the first study which suggested such a functional deterioration of the central nervous system. Of course, folic acid is another of the B vitamins. These are the vitamins in which the average American diet is so sadly lacking. We eat few foods rich in the B vitamins, and are fond of foods which, when eaten, destroy as much of the B vitamin supply of the body as they possibly can.

Obvious Parallel

Now, if we put the results of these two experiments together with Dr. Kugelmass' statement that more and more mental deficiency is showing up in our society, the parallel becomes obvious. True, we do not test our children's intelligence by putting them in mazes, but we do put them in school and challenge them to be graduated. Many of them don't make it, and the drop-out rate is going up, according to authorities. Would a supplementation of the expectant mothers' diets have helped to correct this problem, as it did in the case of the rats?

A 7-year test (*Time*, March 28, 1955) illustrated that question. In it, 2,400 women were observed. They were of low income families and ate poorly balanced diets. Controls were given pills containing nothing at all and the rest given nutritional supplements during pregnancy. Without a doubt, the children of the women who had received supplementation were found to be of higher intelligence than those who had gotten the placebo and maintained their regular diet.

In 1943, in a Louisiana parish (county) called Ascension, the problem of poor efficiency in classwork was becoming acute. The scholastic rating of the parish's schools was embarrassingly below the national average. A whole new approach to the problem was taken here when it was found that the dietary habits of the children who attended school were also appallingly bad. A survey disclosed that one per cent of the 2,500 school children concerned ate what would be called a "good diet." Over 33 per cent ate what had to be called an actually "poor diet." Then a change took place. The school superintendent inaugurated a program aimed at making everyone—children and parents—diet-conscious. Perseverance made the program a success, and proper eating habits of the pupils became usual. With the improved nutrition, came a miraculous increase in scholastic accomplishment. By 1950, the parish was well above the national average in the rating of its students' learning ability. (The *Sign*, February, 1952.)

Here was a definite indication, on a large scale, of what diet can do. No other changes were effected which could have accounted for the improvement. It was simply a matter of nourishing the children's brains, if you will. Does this not raise wonderful thoughts of what could be if all of our schools would adopt a similar program? If we could replace the penny candy and cookies of the grade schooler, and the potato chip, candy bar and coke of our high school pupils, our whole national scholastic average would surely rise.

Early Start Essential

In *Bio-Dynamics* (winter, 1957), this conclusion was further bolstered. An article there asserted that a definite relationship exists between nutritional status of children and their I.Q.'s. The younger they are when good nutrition is introduced, the greater the chance for improvement in retarded children. This study supported the value of a planned nutritional program for preschool children of two to four years.

Does this hold true in the more serious forms of mental retardation? In the *Journal of the American Medical Association* (June 27, 1953), an article by Levingson and Goldenberg told of 4 cases of mental retardation definitely due to nutritional deficiency. As soon as steps were taken to improve their nutritional picture, one of the children was made completely normal, and the other 3 showed definite improvement.

When Is Abnormality Apparent?

Apparently, one of the most important factors in improving the intelligence of retarded youngsters is to begin early. The problem here is how to tell if a child is normally "slow" about doing things, or if he actually has not got the mentality to develop skills. Arguments rage among pediatricians on how soon one can tell this. In the *British Medical Journal* (July 2, 1955), an article was printed which typified the opposing views. The author quoted one authority, Kirman, who had written, "It is only very seldom that a child of less than two can safely be diagnosed as definitely mentally defective." On the other hand, Gesell is quoted as saying, "Practically every case of mental deficiency can be diagnosed in the first year of life, excluding cases due to secondary causes later in life." An interesting clue to suspected mental deficiency was offered in this article by R. S. Illingworth, M.D., the author. He noted that the mentally retarded child is late in learning the basic function, chewing. Such a child is likely to vomit all solid foods given to him at an age when most children are able to handle them. A history of repeated unsuccessful attempts to introduce solid foods is usual in the development of mentally retarded children.

We are not sure which opinion on the recognition of mental deficiency is correct. Though there are undoubtedly signs of low mentality which an expert can interpret in even a very young child, we lean to the more conservative view that a definite diagnosis can hardly be foolproof before the child is two or so. Other factors, such as environment and personality, could inhibit a normally intelligent child, and keep him from exhibiting the expected signs of normalcy, even though he had the ability to do so.

The lesson, however, is obvious. Good nutrition is important from the moment the mother becomes pregnant, on through the birth and growth of the child. A good diet for the mother does not guarantee that the baby she carries will be born a genius, but it does offer the assurance that the baby will be born with its full share of native intelligence, and normal mental and physical capacity. Once the child has arrived, plenty of love, mother's milk, plenty of B complex-rich foods, bone meal for calcium and fresh fruits and vegetables rich in vitamin C, should be the heart of his diet. All white sugar, white flour products should be absolutely forbidden. A foundation like this will give the brain and body a chance to develop normally. No need to wonder about the mentality of a child with this kind of nutritional history. Is your child as safe from the danger of mental deficiency as you would like him to be? Will you be certain that your next child is safe?

[752]

198. Mental Illness and Vitamin B$_{12}$ Deficiency

The whole question of mental disease, its causes and treatment, is taking on a new look. The psychiatrist's couch is being displaced by the laboratory. The chemical make-up of the blood has been proven to have a very definite effect on the health and operation of the brain, and it is in this field that the greatest advances against mental illness have been made. Strangely enough, the doctors who deal with mental disorders seem reluctant to take advantage of these new developments, in spite of the fact that the more commonly used treatments are obviously ineffective in most cases, can be dangerous and often lead to recurrence. We have seen startling evidence of the effect an unbalanced blood sugar level can have on the mind; the lack of a proper amount of thyroxin in the blood has been seen to cause mental disorders; treatment with nothing more than a potent vitamin-mineral supplement has brought about amazing results in returning the mentally ill to normalcy. Each of these measures has been written up in respected professional medical journals, and has elicited favorable comment from authorities in the field. In spite of this, attempts by patients or their families to have such treatments instituted are almost invariably fruitless. To hope that the doctor himself would be familiar with the procedure and suggest it on his own is to be unrealistic.

Nothing Could Be Safer Than Course of Treatment

If the new findings called for the use of dangerous drugs or delicate surgery, one could understand the reticence of the doctors in using them (though the dangerous and harmful tranquilizing drugs seem to have found immediate acceptance). However, the measures we have outlined in the following pages, as advocated by Drs. Abrahamson, Roberts and Masor, call for nothing more than careful diet, food supplementation, and, in the case of Dr. Masor, the use of a hormone (thyroxin) whose shortage can be shown by a simple test. Giving such treatment to patients who are shown by tests to be deficient, certainly entails no risk; however, refusal to administer such vital therapy might have serious consequences. The diet, the vitamins, the thyroxin are essential if good health is ever to return. Psychoanalysis, shock treatments, tranquilizers and confinement in a mental hospital are not going to help a bit if the need is nutritional, as is often the case.

The findings of Drs. James Wiener and Justin Hope, as printed in the *Journal of the American Medical Association* (June 27, 1959), are another example of the relationship between mental health and nutritional deficiency. This time, research has shown that mental illness and pernicious anemia (which is largely the result of a vitamin B$_{12}$ shortage) often go hand in

[753]

hand. This connection was first suggested in 1902. In 1915, Pfeiffer recorded an unquestionable case. By 1927, McAlpine was able to write, "Mental changes occur not uncommonly in pernicious anemia. They range from states of depression accompanied by loss of mental energy, to definite psychosis. They, like the nervous symptoms, may precede the characteristic changes in the blood by many months." In other words, the patient might become ill mentally long before his doctor could discover, from tests, that he had anemia.

Little Consideration in Standard Textbooks

The *Journal of the American Medical Association*'s article calmly states that the cerebral (mental) manifestations of a vitamin B_{12} deficiency have received little consideration in standard textbooks. In other words, a doctor would probably never hear of this possibility in medical school. After graduation, he probably would have missed it, unless he came upon the 1927 reference of McAlpine, until June, 1959. Imagine the number of patients who have consulted doctors on mental trouble, who might have needed vitamin B_{12} and nothing more, yet were pronounced hopeless.

The effectiveness of the vitamin B_{12} therapy depends largely on the duration of the deficiency before beginning the therapy. The importance of early diagnosis is apparent in the report by Holmes quoted in the article. Holmes treated 14 patients for a vitamin B_{12} deficiency, all of whom had well-marked mental symptoms. In all but two, the mental symptoms disappeared, or were greatly relieved after intensive treatment. The two patients who did not respond had been psychotic patients at a mental hospital for several months before treatment. Psychosis, in these cases, had developed and progressed over a period of 7 or 8 years.

Diagnosis Difficult

The diagnosis of mental problems due to pernicious anemia is often difficult, because they may occur without the changes in the blood usually expected when anemia is present. However, the article describes two tests for vitamin B_{12} levels in the blood which are helpful in such cases. It is also worth noting that tests show consistently low values of oxygen consumption in the brain in patients with mental disturbance due to pernicious anemia, as compared with normal people and those with anemia due to blood loss.

When mental symptoms occur along with the classic symptoms of pernicious anemia—weakness, sore tongue, an increase in the size of red corpuscles, absence of digestive juices in the stomach, etc.—diagnosis is easy. However, these are often absent, and the mental symptoms are not consistently characteristic. They range from mild moodiness, with difficulty in concentrating and remembering, to violent maniacal behavior, severe agitation, stuporous depression and hallucinations.

The common nervous symptoms of a vitamin B_{12} deficiency are different, and not connected with the mind at all. They include "pins-and-needles" sensations, numbness, stiffness, feelings of heat and cold, local feelings of deadness, tightness and shooting pains. If any of these are present with the mental symptoms, the diagnosis is again made somewhat easier.

The Treatment Is Simple

In the actual treatment of mental illness resulting from a deficiency of vitamin B_{12}, much larger doses are needed than in the treatment of simple blood count conditions of anemia. The treatment outlined by Wiener and Hope in their article is extremely simple: intramuscular injection of 1,000 micrograms of vitamin B_{12} for the first treatment, followed by 500 micrograms twice weekly for one month, then 100 micrograms of vitamin B_{12} once a week for 6 months. The authors tell us that results can be expected in 3 to 6 months.

Now this is certainly a worthwhile avenue of investigation for the doctor confronted with a puzzling case of mental illness. Determining a vitamin B_{12} deficiency is not an involved procedure. Each patient can be tested for this possibility. Such testing for all nutrients should be a matter of course when any physical problem presents itself. This is especially true when a precedent has been set through responsible treatment, given by a respected physician, with good results. The tragedy of mental illness requires us to use any means we have to combat its appearance and development, and we see no reason why proven nutritional therapy should not be given a chance to show its effectiveness.

Note that injection is used. The reason is simply that, by the time such conditions have appeared, the stomach does not contain any, or possibly enough, of a certain substance which must be present to absorb vitamin B_{12}. So vitamin B_{12} taken by mouth would be wasted. Injecting the vitamin into the patient's blood or muscle assures its absorption, since it does not pass through the digestive tract at all. Of course, injection of a vitamin must be done by a physician. Meanwhile, to insure oneself against the ever-increasing threat of mental illness, include some food and food supplements rich in B vitamins (including vitamin B_{12}), such as beef liver and other organ meats, brewer's yeast and desiccated liver in your regular diet. Remember, if vitamin B_{12} can be used to cure mental disorders, it should also be an excellent preventive.

[755]

199. The Thyroid

Probably the most frustrating illness of all for both the victim and the doctor, is mental illness. No one can actually watch the mind function, except as these workings are translated into actions or attitudes or emotions. When we see that the results of the mind's workings are somehow off-center, that they do not conform to accepted standards for living with our fellow men or they show a violent reaction to the normal stresses of life, we suspect that there is a mental problem. There is no way to X-ray the brain to find the quirk of memory or emotion that has been disrupted. There is no swelling or discoloration to be seen as a clue to the site of the problem. Just what is affected, we do not know.

Compounding this basic difficulty of mental illness is the relative lack of past experience in treating mental disorders. For centuries, the insane were shackled, tortured or left alone to die because their affliction was thought to be a mark of demoniac possession. No one even considered therapy before the nineteenth century. Freud and his colleagues made the first important contribution to the rehabilitation of the mentally ill, largely by recognizing that such illness can be treated, and that there is a cause and effect in it, just as in other breakdowns of the body's functions.

Several Eras of Mental Treatment

The discovery of psychiatry, the science which seeks to explain mental abnormalities by uncovering unconsciously suppressed experiences or motives, generated more and more interest in the treatment of mental illness. It soon became apparent, however, that psychiatry is not the whole answer. A large number of cases would not respond to this probing type of therapy. Experiments with shock treatment followed, in the hope that an electric charge directed to the brain might, largely by chance, rearrange the molecules in the disturbed part and restore complete sanity. The danger that such a charge might, also by chance, disorganize perfectly normal parts of the brain is ever present, and the use of shock treatment has been ebbing, except for specific cases in which reasonable assurance of its total effect can be ascertained.

Tranquilizers Did Not Bring a Cure

Then came the era of the tranquilizer. It was found that certain drugs have a depressing and calming effect on the brain. The subject, it is hoped, becomes passive upon taking these drugs, and loses all sense of rebelliousness and concern. The condition usually holds only until the medication is discontinued, whereupon the entire mental problem seems to erupt with renewed vigor, as after a long sleep. Tranquilizers are not a cure. At best, they calm a serious mental case while other treatment is prepared. At worst, they are dispensed to suppress any helpful symptoms in mental patients who might be effectively treated. They are also given to persons who are mentally normal, but for the nervousness bred by stressful situations we all face, and seek to forget their troubles with this easily-acquired narcotic. The habit, once created, is hard to stop; the possible injury to the body's organisms by the chemical components of these drugs may be irreparable.

The Biochemical Approach

In more recent years, organic causes of mental illness have been emphasized by forward-looking researchers. Even with the relatively small amount of work that has been done, the tremendous possibilities of curing mental illness by correcting systemic disorders in the body are obvious. We have come across a book, *The New Psychiatry,* by Nathan Masor, M.D. (Philosophical Press, New York), in which the strong effect of the thyroid gland upon the proper operation of the brain is discussed.

Dr. Masor broached his theory on the biochemical approach to mental disease at the Second International Congress for Psychiatry, Zurich, Switzerland, in September, 1957. He introduced his remarks with this statement, which must have crumbled the complacency of many a doctor listening: "The many deleterious side effects of tranquilizing and other drugs used in suppressing psychiatric symptoms dramatizes the present great need for a therapy which would not destroy the stability of the individual."

In his speech, Dr. Masor went on to cite many successful experiments in which the chemical make-up of the blood showed its influence on the mind. In an experiment at the University of Southern California, spiders fed blood serum from schizophrenic patients became listless and indifferent, spinning patternless webs without system or purpose. At Tulane University, studies showed that, by injecting protein from the blood of schizophrenic patients, doctors could induce psychotic behavior in normal subjects.

A Meeting Ground

In this context, the findings of Dr. Nathan Masor are especially impressive. He has explored the effect of an underactive thyroid gland in relation to mental disease. Using, in his experiments, patients who had undergone some previous psychiatric treatment without success, and who were still acutely disturbed, Dr. Masor had phenomenal success in restoring their sanity by administering a compound of thyroxin and certain B vitamins. It is Dr. Masor's view that too much emphasis is placed upon the use of psychoanalysis in treating mental disease, with the result that the biochemical possibilities for treatment are neglected. He feels that "there is a meeting ground between the biochemical approach and a more rounded type of psychiatry. Each complements the other, doing what the other cannot do. The biochemical approach brings about the metabolic changes that are required in order to make proper psychological functioning."

Thyroid's Influence Long Known

Dr. Masor's use of the thyroid-produced hormone, thyroxin, is not based upon any new discovery of thyroxin's activity. It has been known for many years that a shortage of this iodine-carrying hormone in the body can result in a slow down of both physical and mental processes. That more advantage has not been taken of this fact in treating mental patients, is truly indefensible. How often does one hear of thyroid treatment, or even a test for thyroid disorder, given to a mental patient? Almost never. Shock treatment and psychoanalysis are the common tools most psychiatrists use. Yet, this amazing statement made by a Dr. Lahey appeared in *Postgraduate Medicine* (9:400) in 1951: "We have always known that hypothyroidism is related to emotional states." What Dr. Lahey means by "always" we do not know, but 25 years ago, doctor-novelist A. J. Cronin, in his book, *Between Two Worlds*, described a classic case of hypothyroidism in a patient whose physician had recommended his admittance to a mental institution, without even having thought that a thyroid disorder could be the cause. Cronin repeated the description again in one of his most famous novels, *The Citadel*. He describes the symptoms of hypothyroidism as including defective memory, slow mentation and attacks of irritability culminating in an outburst of homicidal violence. Reading that makes one wonder how many of the beds in our mental hospitals are taken by patients who need nothing more than additional thyroxin in their diet to become as mentally normal as any of us.

Literature Aplenty

There is plenty of scientific literature available on the subject of thyroid and mentality. Aside from those already given, the *British Medical Journal* of May 26, 1951, told of testing 541 psychoneurotic and psychotic patients for thyroid activity. Over 50 per cent of the males showed a tendency toward below normal thyroid function. In the female schizophrenics, the thyroid output ranged from normal to subnormal in the chronic forms of the disease.

In the *Canadian Medical Association Journal* (December 15, 1956), Drs. Ferguson and Rayport noted that the thyroid is shown to have a direct connection with the central nervous system of the body, in a network which also involves the hypothalamus and the pituitary gland.

In the Allentown (Pennsylvania) *Morning Call* (January 2, 1958), in a regular column on medical topics, the author calmly stated that an emotionally distraught person may go to a psychiatrist, thinking he has mental trouble, when his real problem is an underactive thyroid gland. He did not say whether or not every patient who goes to a psychiatrist is tested for thyroid irregularity—or if even 5 per cent are so tested.

A Near Tragedy Due to Thyroid Lack

A book published in 1957 entitled *Kathy* (E. P. Dutton Company) by Katherine Homer Fryer, offered an almost tragic illustration of what can happen when a hypothyroid condition is not properly diagnosed. The story, a true one, is of a young girl who changed, with alarming rapidity, from a normal healthy child, to a shadow of herself. Her weight steadily dropped;

her good spirits and energy simply disappeared and she suffered from a frustrating inability to keep warm. One doctor after the other was consulted, and each was forced to admit that he could find nothing wrong with Kathy. As a last resort, the child was taken to a psychiatrist who declared that she was suffering from a psychosis and should be sent to a mental hospital. Almost by accident, shortly thereafter, she happened to be in the office of an M.D., who decided to test her thyroid gland's operation. He found it dangerously deficient, and gave Kathy a thyroxin preparation to supplement the short supply in her system. In a matter of hours, her condition was noticeably improved. In a few weeks, the terrible ordeal was over and she was back at school, a perfectly normal girl. Without the alertness of the doctor who suggested the thyroid test, Kathy might have been condemned to years of confinement in a mental institution and, eventually, a premature death.

Thyroid Shortage Sometimes Unnoticed

In a *Reader's Digest* article (February, 1959), science writer Albert Maisel writes of a survey which shows that 8½ million Americans are victims of hypothyroidism. We presume that very few of these are aware of it. A slowing thyroid may not be suspected, even when its function is 15 to 20 per cent below normal. At this stage, the victim has vague and chronic symptoms such as tiredness, muscle weakness, headaches, constipation, nasal congestion, menstrual disturbance or just general below par feeling.

Until recent years, there was some justification for misdiagnosis of thyroid abnormalities. The decision was usually based upon the basal metabolism rate (BMR) test. Metabolism is the name given to the process by which the body converts food into energy. Now this test seeks to determine just what this metabolism rate is when the patient is completely at rest. Even the act of digestion can make this reading shoot up, so it is easily seen how the result could be inaccurate if the patient is emotionally disturbed or exhausted. For example, anxiety over some problem may so elevate the reading that it might falsely indicate normal thyroid function.

A Reliable Thyroid Test

Recently, a new test was developed for measuring thyroid activity, and it is much more reliable. Called the protein-bound iodine (PBI) test, it requires nothing more from the patient than that he allow a small sample of his blood to be taken. The sample is analyzed for iodine content, which must be sent from the thyroid, and if the amount of iodine exceeds or falls below an established norm, there is trouble suspected in the gland's working. The PBI test is easily available to your doctor, who has only to send a sample of blood to one of 250 medical centers and laboratories throughout the country which are equipped to make the test. The fee is no more than the fee for the BMR test, and this test is a lot more accurate.

It would seem important that the thyroid has a sufficient supply of iodine through the diet, so that it can be released in thyroxin when needed. Sea kelp is an excellent natural source of iodine, as are all sea foods.

Mr. Maisel makes two other points of special interest to us: (1.) thyroid deficiency can cause habitual abortion; (2.) of 4,500 industrial workers, supposedly in good health, PBI tests showed that 5 per cent were hypothyroid victims.

We Know What Affects the Thyroid

What causes all of this thyroid trouble? Well, a lot of the problem is in the way we eat. Many of us include salt in our diet, for example. In *Endocrinology* (56:387, 1955), mice tested for goiter-activating foods showed an enlargement of the thyroid could be caused by salt. With omission of salt, goiters decreased in size. As we know, it is the amount of iodine released by the thyroid gland, in thyroxin, which determines whether or not one is faced with goiter problems. A healthy thyroid will release the proper amount of iodine if it has been made available through foods. The *Journal of Endocrinology* (November, 1953) tells us that aspirin, a "must" for many of us, has an immediate antithyroid action, and hypothyroidism is often the result of its use.

In the *Journal of the American Medical Association* (November 23, 1957), Arnold S. Jackson wrote that "the most important single factor responsible (for symptoms of thyroid disturbance in 228 patients he observed) was the overindulgence in the use of stimulants—coffee, tea and nicotine." Many of these patients smoked two or three packs of cigarettes a day, and some drank from 5 to 30 cups of coffee each day.

Are You a Potential Victim?

Do you use salt, aspirin, coffee, cigarettes, etc.? Perhaps your habits are not as excessive as those outlined above, but then perhaps your symptoms are milder. Could you be one of the 5 per cent of supposedly "well" industrial workers who were found to be victims of an underproductive thyroid? Could your thyroid be only 10 or 15 per cent below par, so that your symptoms are more or less indefinable, such as tiredness, weakness, headaches, constipation, etc.? Try a month or so without the stimulants—no liquor, cigarettes, coffee; no barbiturates, salt or aspirin—and watch the change. Perhaps iodine-rich foods are missing from your diet. Try kelp.

There is hope for the slightly affected and hope for those who appear to be seriously mentally ill, if the thyroid is considered when diagnosis is made. The biochemical phase of treatment for mental illness is coming into its own, and when its importance is fully appreciated, we believe we will see, for the first time, a reversal of the upward trend in the number of cases of mental illness.

200. Blood Sugar and Mental Health

In a book written by an eye, ear, nose and throat specialist you would hardly expect to read much about mental and nervous disorders. Yet, here is a paragraph from such a book:

"All age-groups are subject to metabolic dysfunctions, even the allergic-asthmatic child . . . The symptoms are mostly bizarre and simulate a neurosis, at times even a psychosis . . . It may also be the precursor (forerunner) for many pathologic conditions which are today of unknown etiology (cause) . . . It is the enigma that prompts most patients to report to physicians, or to clinics, for a complete check-up because of 'utter exhaustion.' "

This paragraph is quoted from a book on *Ear, Nose and Throat Dysfunctions Due to Deficiencies and Imbalances,* by Sam E. Roberts, M.D., Associate Professor of Otolaryngology at the University of Kansas School of Medicine. The publisher is Charles C. Thomas, Springfield, Illinois.

Treated in chapters of this remarkable book are such subjects as migraine headaches, deafness, multiple sclerosis, allergy, sinus disorders, Menière's disease, headaches and many other conditions of ill health. All these can be improved with diet and diet supplements, according to Dr. Roberts, plus hormone substances when there is evidence that glands are badly out of balance. The thread that runs all through the book is that the importance of cell nutrition and metabolism far outweighs the virulence and toxicity of germs.

Dr. Roberts believes that many patients who go from doctor to doctor seeking cures for nervousness, anxiety and exhaustion are suffering from low blood sugar. Instead of being told they are neurotics, they should be given a diet to overcome the low blood sugar conditions. He says that rapid fluctuations in blood sugar, common in this kind of condition, often give rise to many bizarre symptoms that suggest mental disorders. "Before the final diagnosis of any nervous or mental disease is made, the patient should be given the therapeutic test for at least 3 months. As previously stated, I am certain that the population of our institutions for patients with nervous and mental disturbances would be greatly reduced if this regimen were followed."

The test he refers to is simply a test of the amount of sugar in the patient's blood at given intervals after he takes a dose of sugar. This is called the "glucose tolerance test."

If the test indicates low blood sugar, the patient can be cured permanently by a simple diet, no medication or other treatment being necessary.

Some Symptoms of Low Blood Sugar

His own patients, who are described in this book, suffered from symptoms like these: fatigue, exhaustion, a feeling the patient called "rubber legs" (as if the legs would not support one), tightness in the chest and pain in various parts of the body, Menière's disease, migraine, deafness, nasal allergy, nervous habits such as fingernail biting, bed wetting, pain in the shoulders and hips, constant hunger, eye ache, mental depression, sleeplessness, swollen feet. Many of the patients were chain-smokers and/or drank numerous cups of coffee all day long.

In some of the cases, the patient had been to a family doctor who discovered the low blood sugar condition and prescribed a diet high in sugar. This made the situation progressively and rapidly worse. In every case, the correct diet brought about complete improvement, and in a re- markably short time. In addition to diet, Dr. Roberts treated his patients with food supplements containing vitamins and minerals. He also gave hormone substances to adjust the function of glands when this seemed necessary.

In his discussion of low blood sugar, Dr. Roberts points out the relation of the adrenal glands to the regulation of blood sugar, and the importance of vitamin C to the health of the adrenal glands. Diets which produce low blood sugar seem to be low in vitamin C, a deficiency which undoubtedly helps to bring about the conditions he found in his patients.

He speculates on the reason for the widespread occurrence of low blood sugar and reminds us that 25 billion, 51 million bottles of soft drinks were consumed in this country in 1951. This is in addition to all the soft drinks dispensed at fountains. Of course, this figure increases every year. On a per capita basis, in 1940, an average consumption of all sweetened beverages was 88.6 bottles and in 1952, it had increased to 163 per capita. Estimates indicate that over 100 pounds of sugar are consumed by each person each year.

Why Low Blood Sugar Is So Common

This does not mean that each person in the United States sits down at the sugar bowl and eats by the spoonful 100 pounds of sugar a year. It does mean that all the many foods that contain "hidden sugar" add up to this terrible total every year. And, when you take into account the number of diabetics and people on special diets who never eat sugar, of course the amount consumed by each of the rest of us must be far above 100 pounds a year.

Says Dr. Roberts, "When one considers that each 6-ounce bottle of a sweetened, carbonated beverage contains from 3½ to 5 teaspoonfuls of sugar, one can easily compute the large quantity of sugar consumed each day in this manner.

"Assuming that each person had one or two sweetened desserts each day, such as the American favorite, apple pie, this would add another

[762]

7 teaspoonfuls of sugar for each serving. To metabolize this intake, the sugar carburetory of the body must be thrown wide open and the Islands of Langerhans (a gland) must secrete at an abnormally high speed to produce an *overabundance*, causing a hypoglycemic (low blood sugar) state with all its disagreeable, and at times, dangerous sequelae. What makes the situation worse is that the persons who are prodigious consumers of sweets seldom consume fruits, fruit juices or vitamin C-rich foods which are extremely essential in the control of nearly all bodily ills."

He also tells us that a calcium deficiency usually goes along with a low blood sugar condition.

How often have you heard the statement, "Unless I have my breakfast on time, I'm sure to have a headache." Such a statement is an almost certain indication of low blood sugar. How many people do you know who are hungry, weak, cranky or fatigued by 11 in the morning and 4 in the afternoon? Significant symptoms of low blood sugar. Observe those people you know who are habitually nervous, irritable, hard to get along with, tired, complaining. Aren't they the same ones who cram themselves with soft drinks and sweets and coffee and, if they smoke at all, chain-smoke? Although Dr. Roberts does not go into this, it is believed by some authorities that alcoholism, too, is a disorder of low blood sugar.

How to Avoid Low Blood Sugar

What a terrible waste of people's happiness and lives to allow them to spend most of their time in unhappiness and despair going from one doctor to another when a simple, easy diet can mean good health! The tricky thing about the low blood sugar diet that you must keep in mind, is that *low* blood sugar is caused by *too much* sugar in the diet. So the cure, and the preventive, is to cut out sugar and with it, those starchy foods which are rapidly changed to sugar in the body.

Cigarettes, coffee and alcohol must go, too, for these react almost instantaneously on the blood sugar level, raising it first, then plunging it way below normal and adding to the sufferer's symptoms in the long run, although they appear to alleviate them for the moment.

The secret of the diet that prevents low blood sugar is to eat often and to eat wisely. All sugars and starches are forbidden. The only foods allowed are proteins (meat, eggs, fish, nuts, soybeans), fruits and vegetables. Bread must be whole grain and should consist of no more than two very thin slices daily. We recommend eliminating cereals and bread.

Eat a piece of fruit, like banana, first thing in the morning when you get up; eat a hearty high-protein breakfast (fruit, eggs and meat or both, no starches); have another snack a few hours after breakfast—this should be fruit or a protein food like nuts or sunflower seeds. For lunch, we like Dr. Roberts' suggestion of a glass of tomato juice which contains a teaspoonful of brewer's yeast, and a teaspoonful of wheat germ. He adds lemon juice and rind. We would suggest rose hip powder. Lunch and dinner consist of meat, eggs or fish with salad, cooked vegetable or both and nothing but fruit for dessert. You must eat again 3 hours after lunch. Dr. Roberts suggests a glass of milk. We suggest another protein snack. Eat something an hour before dinner and again two to three hours after dinner. Grape and prune juices are not recommended because they are rich in sugar. Grapes and dried fruits are sugary, too. Sauces and gravies made with flour are taboo. No sugar may be added to anything.

"The object of this nutritional regime is to prevent blood sugar starvation by keeping a trickle of usable sugars constantly going into the blood stream," says Dr. Roberts. This prevents the sudden rush of an overabundance of sugar, which is what causes the trouble by stimulating the secretion of too much insulin, resulting in an almost immediate need for more sugar.

Food supplements are extremely important, too. Calcium from bone meal, lots of natural vitamin C from rose hips, minerals from kelp, B vitamins from brewer's yeast—these will help make your dieting easier and your recovery quicker.

201. Low Blood Sugar, Crime and Mental Illness

How many times have you said to yourself, reading crime headlines in the newspaper, "Surely, something can be done to prevent people from becoming criminals! Why doesn't somebody find out what causes people to commit horrible crimes?"

Perhaps somebody has found out, but the investigation produced facts that might insult or irritate a very large industry, and certainly would eventually decrease this industry's profits.

We are speaking of the people who produce and sell sugar and products made from sugar. And we say what we have said above because there is already a large body of evidence indicating clearly that wrong diet —chiefly a diet too high in sugar—has a great deal to do with criminality and with mental illness—both top problems in our society.

Joseph Wilder, M.D., of New York City, observed as long ago as 1943 that a chronic state of low blood sugar produces mental symptoms in individuals which are not only characteristic of persons committing crimes, but are also quite common among people we generally think of as "neurotic" or "unbalanced" or even just "difficult."

Here are some of the symptoms Dr. Wilder has found in patients suffering from low blood sugar: slowing of mental processes, dullness, difficulty in making even minor decisions, depression, anxiety, irritability, tendency to be negative, also physical symptoms like double vision, dizziness, changes in voice texture and so forth.

The qualities of mind most easily and earliest affected are spontaneity and initiative. Difficulty in thinking may progress to a temporary arrest of thought, and abstract thought may be almost impossible. There are disorders of orientation and consciousness, there is mental and physical fatigue, apathy and indifference, irritability and aggression.

Many of Dr. Wilder's observations were made on volunteers whose blood sugar level was normal, but who deliberately experimented with greatly reduced levels of blood sugar in order to report on their own feelings. "Very interesting observations and self-observations on fine changes in moral feelings have been made," says Dr. Wilder in an article in the *Nervous Child* for April, 1943-44.

Low Blood Sugar in Children

Where children are concerned, it seems that low blood sugar may be far more serious than for adults. For, says Dr. Wilder, "The importance of nutrition for mental (and physical) functioning is much greater in children than in adults. In adults, faulty or insufficient nutrition may alter or impair specific or general mental functions and eventually cause reparable or even irreparable structural damage of the central nervous system. In children, we face a grave additional factor. The development of the brain may be retarded, stopped, altered, and thus the mental functions may become impaired in an indirect and not less serious way." He also says that repeated attacks of low blood sugar may give rise later to true epilepsy.

Here are some of the symptoms of low blood sugar in children: the child overeats or does not want to eat at all. Impairment of memory in the form of amnesia is one of the most common happenings in more severe cases of low blood sugar. When the child states that he did not do or say a certain thing, he may actually not remember. The child may not sleep well. Nightmares, sleep-walking or even bed wetting may be symptoms. The child does not learn. Cases have been reported in which the child failed in one subject only. He may be absent-minded or michievous or cannot remember anything. Such things occur generally during morning classes, around 10 or 11 o'clock. This is the time at which the child's blood sugar is probably lowest. "Laziness may be caused by hypoglycemia (low blood sugar)," says Dr. Wilder, "with mental fatigue, dullness, indifference, lack of initiative and above all, severe inability to make decisions." Dawdling is a symptom of low blood sugar.

The child may be neurotic, psychopathic or have criminal tendencies, says Dr. Wilder, anxiety, running away, aggressiveness, a blind urge to activity, destructiveness with impairment of moral sensibilities like shame. "In its simplest form," he says, "it is the tendency to deny everything, contradict everything, refuse everything at any price . . . It is no wonder that a considerable number of criminal and semicriminal acts have been observed in children in hypoglycemic states, ranging from destructiveness or violation of traffic regulations, all the way to bestiality, arson and homicide."

Proof of Dr. Wilder's Statements

Strong statements indeed, to be based on the observations of one person only! But Dr. Wilder's beliefs were tested in Argentina by researchers N. Rojas and A. F. Sanchi, who wrote an article on "Hypoglycemia and Delinquents" which appeared in the *Archives of Legal Medicine*, Vol. 11, p. 29, 1941. In this article, they told of doing blood sugar tests on a group of apprehended delinquents. There was a striking percentage with low, sometimes even very low, blood sugar.

Of the 129 delinquents examined, most were juveniles and the offenses were in 32 cases against persons, 65 against property, 10 sex offenses and so forth. In 48 cases, the blood sugar was less than 75 milligrams per cent, in one even as low as 38 milligrams per cent and in 64 cases between 75-90 milligrams per cent. Only in 13 cases was the blood sugar strictly within the normal limits of 90-100 milligrams per cent.

Furthermore, in an investigation in New York, A. S. Church found and reported in the *New York State Journal of Medicine*, 1954, Vol. 45, p. 74, that there were evidences of malnutrition or undernutrition in not less than 80 per cent of 750 boys admitted to an institution for juvenile delinquents.

"Criminal acts have been committed time and again in abnormal psychological conditions impairing judgment or self-control. Alcohol and other poisons, fever delirium, psychoses, epileptic equivalents and so forth, are among the best known causes of mental conditions conducive to abnormal or criminal behavior. Since hypoglycemia (low blood sugar) is capable of producing more or less severe mental changes, followed mostly by amnesia, there is no reason why such acts should not occur in hypoglycemic states," says Dr. Wilder in another article which appeared in the *Handbook of Correctional Psychology*, published in 1947.

He goes on to say, "the well-known-problem of the relation of poverty to crime calls for an investigation from the angle of hypoglycemia. In such an investigation, we must also keep in mind the possible irreparable anatomical damage and arrest of development in young brains caused by malnutrition in childhood, even if the patient or criminal does not present any metabolic abnormalities at the time of investigation."

In this article in the *Handbook of Correctional Psychology*, Dr. Wilder proceeds to discuss many well-documented cases of criminal acts performed by individuals suffering from low blood sugar. Tests indicated without a shadow of a doubt that each individual was in a state of low blood sugar at the time the crime was committed. The crimes range all the way from homicide to sadism, arson, serious traffic violations, mutilation, violent aggressiveness, etc. In fact, the article sounds as if you might be reading today's and yesterday's newspaper.

[766]

And recurrent throughout are paragraphs like this: "After the patient's arrest, his family physician notified the defense that two years prior to the crime a sugar tolerance curve (blood sugar test) had shown a tendency to hypoglycemia."

Causes of Low Blood Sugar

Low blood sugar may be caused by a number of disorders: tumors of the pancreas causing an overproduction of insulin, diseases of the liver interfering with the storage and release of sugar, diseases of the adrenal glands and of certain centers of the brain. By way of damage of the organs mentioned, many poisons may produce the same effects. Liver diseases are important, since most poisons causing low blood sugar act by way of the liver.

At the time Dr. Wilder wrote these words, thousands of chemical poisons to which we are today exposed had not been discovered. Chlorinated hydrocarbon insecticides like DDT were unknown. Today, they are everywhere. They are liver poisons. They are cumulative poisons—they accumulate in the fatty tissues of the body so that small doses over a lifetime are perhaps more poisonous than one big one.

The brain differs from most other organs of the body in that it cannot make use of its own stores of sugar and convert them into the glucose which is needed for brain functioning. It must get its sugar from the blood stream. The study of electrical brain waves (electroencephalography) shows graphically the changes in the brain function when changes in blood sugar level take place. In chronic states of low blood sugar, the level is permanently low and returns to normal or nearly normal only for short periods following meals or sugar injections. Symptoms of chronic low blood sugar are, according to Dr. Wilder, apathy, dullness, indifference, laziness, lack of initiative and possibly paranoia and other psychotic conditions as well.

"For the problem of delinquency," he goes on, "it is important to know that children, as a rule, not only show a more marked tendency to low blood sugar but seem to get symptoms much quicker."

The Real Cure for Low Blood Sugar

During the time that Wilder was making his astonishing revelations about the relationship of crime and mental illness to low blood sugar, it was generally assumed that conditions of this kind were caused either by the various disorders we mentioned above or by getting insufficient amounts of sugar in the diet. In fact, Wilder recommends giving sugar to bring patients out of the low blood sugar state.

However, even then he realized that more was involved, for he reminds us that, if you are going to add sugar to a diet, you must be certain to balance the rest of the diet accordingly—especially, you must be sure to add plenty of vitamin B_1, thiamin, for this is essential if the body is going to use sugar properly.

[767]

But he also says, "Apparently, too copious feeding of sugar may, in the long run, cause an overfunction of the islet cells of the pancreas and increase the tendency to hypoglycemia; on the other hand, there are cases in which a diet extremely poor in carbohydrates and sugars may improve or even cure the condition."

Later investigators have shown that this is indeed the right way to improve or cure low blood sugar, especially where no disorder of liver or pancreas is involved. In other words, most Americans today are eating far, far too much sugar. The low blood sugar condition which is frighteningly widespread (far more common than diabetes according to authorities) is not caused by any obscure disorder of the glands which necessitates drugs or operations. It is caused simply by our enormous consumption of sugar (over 100 pounds per year per person) in soft drinks, candy, pastries, chewing gum and all the other foods and drinks whose content is largely some form of sugar.

It seems obvious that such an overconsumption of sugar is going to result in damage to the apparatus that has the job of dealing with sugar in the body—the pancreas. Overworking constantly in an effort to deal with this problem, the pancreas secretes too much insulin. The individual whose blood sugar is chronically at a low level is suffering from too much insulin, just as the diabetic is suffering from too little insulin. The regulatory apparatus no longer regulates. After a dose of sugar, the blood sugar level shoots up far above normal, so that a very brief period of well-being is experienced. But almost at once, the blood sugar level begins to decrease rapidly, and feelings of hunger, weakness, irritability, nervousness ensue until more sugar is taken.

Dietary Cure for Low Blood Sugar

The only permanent relief from this chronic condition we now know is a diet in which there is as little sugar as possible, in which there are frequent meals high in protein and fat (because fat stays long in the stomach and tides one over to the next meal without hunger). The entire story of low blood sugar and its relation to a number of diseases (epilepsy, alcoholism, allergies, asthma, neuroses) is related in a book entitled *Body, Mind and Sugar* by E. M. Abrahamson, M.D., and A. W. Pezet, to which we have previously referred. Dr. Abrahamson devotes many pages to outlining the diet that should be followed by patients with low blood sugar. (The diet appears at the end of chapter 78.)

In many case histories, Dr. Abrahamson shows complete relief from all low blood sugar symptoms when the diet is followed to the letter. Get the book, read it, give it to your friends, especially those who may be suffering from the disorders discussed.

Then see if you don't agree with us—that the crime is not the illegal or violent act performed by an individual whose glands and mentality have been crippled by sugar. The crime is that such a person should be considered a criminal, rather than a poor victim of a food industry which does nothing to control our national intake of sugar products, but instead spends millions to persuade our people to use increased amounts of sugar and millions more to suppress or discredit irrefutable facts such as Dr. Wilder, Dr. Abrahamson and many other reputable medical men have presented.

~~~~~~~~~~~~~~~~~~~~~~~~~~~~~~~~~~

SECTION 45: MISCARRIAGE

~~~~~~~~~~~~~~~~~~~~~~~~~~~~~~~~~~

202. Preventing Miscarriage

In the *Canadian Medical Association Journal* (January 9, 1960), Dr. Evan Shute presents an interesting discussion of a question of concern to all who are capable of becoming parents. What should be done in the case of spontaneous abortion or miscarriage, that is the spontaneous interruption of pregnancy up to the twenty-eighth week? Can it be prevented? Should it be prevented?

Spontaneous abortions are generally estimated to occur in about 10 per cent of pregnancies, but some doctors believe this figure to be unrealistic, citing the large number of abortions not reported, and those which occur before a physician has been consulted, as well as those induced by criminal means and which remain statistically silent. Rock and Hertig believe that about 34 per cent of embryos are lost before pregnancy is even recognized as such.

What About the Threat of Abnormal Birth?

It is the view of many physicians that spontaneous abortion is nature's way of rejecting a fetus which has been poorly formed, or had an unhealthy start. They say, if spontaneous abortion or miscarriage begins, it is best to let it run its course, rather than to try saving a fetus which will be born abnormal to full term.

Dr. Shute is not of this opinion, and quotes figures to show that this is far from the rule. He refers to E. S. Burge who, in the *American Journal of Obstetrics and Gynecology* (44: 973, 1942), remarks that of the threatened abortions in 12,000 cases, no more than 1.5 per cent ended in the birth of major defectives. On that percentage, Dr. Shute suggests that, of 100 mothers threatening to abort, 98.5 should produce babies free of any major defect. Such odds offer every reason for attempting to avert threatened abortion, says Dr. Shute. It is not at all a rule that congenital defects are bound to appear in infants whose spontaneous abortion was reversed.

Dr. Shute then goes on to tell of his 25 years experience, in which he has administered vitamin E routinely to every private obstetrical patient registered with him, from the beginning to the end of the pregnancy. He has administered alpha tocopherol to every patient with threatened abortion (except two special cases in which estrogen was used). The doses have ranged from two drams of wheat germ oil 25 years ago to 50-450 milligrams of alpha tocopherol (vitamin E) per day at present.

Half the General Average of Abortions

Of 4,141 private, consecutive, unselected cases, all given alpha tocopherol, there have been 134 recognized abortions and miscarriages, an incidence of 3.2 per cent. Dr. Shute suggests that this percentage be raised to 5.2 per cent to account for abortions reported over the phone before there has actually been time for an office visit, and for incidents casually mentioned at a later office visit. The 5.2 per cent figure is still only about half of that reported in literature generally. Surely, this fact lends support to the idea that alpha tocopherol is helpful in preventing abortion in a large number of cases treated both preventively and therapeutically.

Of Dr. Shute's 4,141 patients, there were 139 threatened abortions and 98 threatened miscarriages (the term differs only to designate the first 3 or second 3 months of pregnancy), and the abortion or miscarriage was reversed in 76 per cent and 96 per cent, respectively. Therefore, 182 normal children were born, in a ratio to 13 abnormal children, 6 of whom died at birth.

Dr. Shute further holds that the administration of alpha tocopherol just before or just after conception is helpful in the prevention of congenital defect, and this theory has been borne out in literature concerning animals made vitamin E-deficient by special diets. The placenta is the foundation of good circulation for the fetus. Presumably, if there is a good foundation, a good infant will develop and the mother remains normal. On the other hand, a defective placenta may alter the whole pregnancy and its product for the worse.

The placenta provides the embryo with nutrients of all types, but especially oxygen. Alpha tocopherol has been shown time and again to be an oxygen-conserving agent. This alone would make it a valuable agent in pregnancy.

The placenta can also be regarded as a great sponge, a net of capillaries. Their being kept intact is vital to the life of the fetus. Alpha tocopherol has unique properties for preserving normal capillary strength and in maintaining their proper width.

We believe that the evidence Dr. Shute presents on behalf of the use of vitamin E in pregnancy is indeed convincing. It is obvious that vitamin E is effective in maintaining the health of the fetus, as well as in providing the fetus with the best possible atmosphere for normal development. Of course, the question of whether or not to attempt to reverse a spontaneous abortion is a question to be decided by the attending doctor and his patient. However, scientific warning on the possible malformation of a child which threatened to be aborted does not seem to scare most people. Doctors and patients usually do all they can to see that such a pregnancy continues to term. It would seem, from Dr. Shute's figures, that such an attempt is justified, since the tragedy of serious malformation follows in only a very small percentage of these cases. It is of great interest to see that the use of vitamin E as a means of preserving the fetus, is effective in threatened miscarriage—76 per cent in the first 3 months, and 96 per cent in the second 3. But even more important is the low incidence of this problem in Dr. Shute's practice, for which he credits vitamin E. We believe that everyone should be taking a vitamin E supplement daily, but this is especially so for a pregnant woman.

Aside from vitamin E, the B vitamins, notably vitamin B_1 and niacin, and vitamin C, have shown themselves to be of value in maintaining a normal, comfortable pregnancy. A diet which is rich in foods containing these nutrients, as well as supplementary dosage, is the best guarantee a woman can have for a successful pregnancy.

SECTION 46: MONGOLISM

203. Hope Seen for Mongoloid Children

The relative novelty of vitamin E therapy has led to constant surprises when used in new fields. So often, it has shown effectiveness in treating diseases long considered hopeless. It is unfortunate that skepticism and suspicion on the part of many doctors and researchers have led to a reluctance to try vitamin E in such cases, even though there is no other resource, and no danger from side effects.

An experiment that we hope will achieve wide publicity and attention from the medical world is that reported by Dr. Anna Szasz of Budapest, Hungary. She has had results in her observations which indicate that there is a strong connection between a lack of vitamin E and other nutrients in the diet of a pregnant woman, and the subsequent birth of a Mongolian

[771]

idiot child. Also, vitamin E therapy for such children seems to bring about definite improvement in their condition.

What Mongolism Means

As most readers probably know, Mongolism is one of the most tragic of birth defects. Such a child has a short life expectancy—usually about 10 or 12 years is maximal. Both bodily and mental development are drastically arrested. These children have neither the concept nor capacity for self care. They seldom speak and their comprehension is seldom advanced beyond that of a 3- or 5-year-old child. The skull is markedly flattened, and the eyes have a decidedly oriental appearance, hence the term Mongolian idiot. Another characteristic is an abnormally short thumb and little finger.

Dr. Szasz remarks first that the number of Mongoloids born during times of war and siege is higher than at any other time. She speculates that, aside from known contributing elements in Mongolism (greater age of the mother, numerous previous births, hormonal dysfunction of the mother, nutritional deficiencies, etc.), overwork, stress and nervous excitement may also cause physical consequences which cannot be ignored.

However, in cases of Mongoloid infants and older children, vitamin E is Dr. Szasz's chosen treatment. This vitamin, she says, somehow favorably influences the tissues whose development is most backward in a Mongoloid child. Dr. Szasz, drawing from previous experimental evidence, knew that vitamin E acts upon the glandular system, the proper development of the fetus, the blood vessels, the neuromuscular system, the locomotor and supporting systems. Vitamin E also influences metabolism and, by its antioxidant and catalytic properties, protects the liver and mucous membranes of the stomach. It alleviates tiredness, increases working capacity and enhances mental efficiency. Dr. Szasz's conclusions were borne out, in part, when she was able to observe in *Monatschrift für Kinderhulkunde* (1949, p. 89, 5-6), a German journal, that, during pregnancy and nursing, women suffering from a vitamin E shortage are anemic, tired, somnolent, feel giddy and are hardly able to accomplish mental and manual work.

The First Success Story

Dr. Szasz describes a remarkable case history of a Mongoloid child born to a middle-aged couple, both of whom worked. The town in which they lived was besieged during the woman's pregnancy, and she was in a state of nervous exhaustion, as well as being nutritionally deficient. The child was born a grave Mongolian idiot.

Immediately following his birth, and practically without interruption for 13 years, this boy was given from 10 to 30 units of vitamin E daily, depending upon its availability. Occasionally this was supplemented with .1 gram of thyroid extract daily for a week. Given longer than that, the thyroid extract caused marked restlessness. For his first 3 years, the boy's bodily and mental development were arrested. After 3, however, he began to develop more rapidly. He began to walk, utter syllables and observe his surroundings. By the age of 5, he spoke fluently, and understood everything. At 7 he went to a normal school, and although he was a mediocre pupil, he showed a good grasp of geography and drew well. He now (13 years old) shows interest in everything, concentrates well and even speaks a little German.

Amazingly Near to Normal

Physiologically, he has developed remarkably. He is of normal height and weight for his age. His bone and muscle development has been satisfactory, but for defective teeth. His hair shows good growth and thickness. He swims well and shows a pleasant disposition. He is fairly resistant to infections.

When the boy reached the age of 11, an attempt was made to stop giving him thyroid extract and vitamin E; however, it was soon seen that a noticeable retardation of learning power was developing and the vitamin E treatment was resumed.

Since she began treating the above case, Dr. Szasz has treated 10 similar cases in a similar manner. Where the treatment was begun early and continued on a regular basis, parallel, slow, but very satisfactory results were obtained.

How many parents of Mongoloid children would thrill to such progress in their own! It hardly seems fair that the hopelessness which surrounds the birth of such a child should be endured in the light of Dr. Szasz's findings. What harm could there be in the administration of daily doses of vitamin E in the small quantities described here? At worst, it would be a nutrient, probably needed anyway, which, though it did not have the desired effect, should aid the child's physical well-being. At best, it could open the door to a reasonably normal existence for a child, whose hope for life as we know it would be nil without the treatment.

Vitamin E a Preventive

A further finding of Dr. Szasz relates to the parent of a Mongoloid. She tells of a middle-aged couple—the husband an epileptic, the mother anemic and tired, with low basal metabolism. Within 5 years, 4 daughters were born to the couple. The first 3 were all Mongoloid, with each one more serious than the last. At the fourth pregnancy, Dr. Szasz tried to improve the mother's health by giving her glanduantin, small doses of thyroid extract, liver, iron and all of the vitamins, including a plentiful dosage of vitamin E. The mother was sent to a mountain resort, rested a great deal, ate a high-protein diet plus plenty of liver and vegetables. The baby was born at the proper time—completely normal and healthy.

While it is true that normal children are frequently born to a mother who has given birth to a Mongoloid baby, with such an unpromising precedent as 3 Mongoloid children in a row, the chances are very good

[773]

that, without the special treatment of Dr. Szasz, still another unfortunate birth might have occurred. Why should any mother take a chance? It is true enough that few mothers can take a few months in the mountains, and probably few need thyroid extract and other glandular stimulation, but no mother-to-be should chance a pregnancy that has not been insured with supplementary food elements.

In the following chapter it will be shown that drinking of fluoridated water by pregnant women results in an increase in the frequency among them of Mongoloid births. Especially, therefore, should Dr. Szasz's findings be considered of grave importance. Women who live in communities whose water is fluoridated should give extra care to proper nutrition, with the accent on vitamin E. For those who have borne Mongoloid children, vitamin E offers some hope and certainly deserves a try.

204. Mongolism and Fluoridated Drinking Water

A University of Wisconsin researcher has discovered a frightening relationship between the incidence of Mongolism and fluoridated drinking water.

Ionel Rapaport of the Psychiatric Institute of the University of Wisconsin has written some very interesting articles on the relationship of the incidence of Mongolism to fluorine in the water supply. The first article appeared in the *Bulletin of the National Academy of Medicine* in France, Vol. 140, 1956, pp. 529-531.

Dr. Rapaport became interested in the subject of fluorides in water when he noticed, in studying the problem of Mongolism, that such children have little tooth decay compared to normal children, who eat the same diet. He also discovered from the work of other researchers that oxygen consumption in the brain of Mongoloid children is lowered, resulting in their characteristic brain deficiency. This indicates, he tells us, an incomplete development of the enzymatic equipment of the brain. We know that fluorine has a definite effect on certain enzymes. It is an "inhibitor"—that is, it stops their activity. And some enzymes present in brain tissue are fluoride-sensitive.

Fluoride Passes from the Mother to the Child

It is true, too, that fluoride in the blood of the pregnant woman passes into the blood of the unborn child. The fluorine content of the placenta (through which nourishment passes from the mother to the unborn child) increases with the amount of fluorine in the drinking water. The amount of fluorine in the baby's blood in turn increases along with the amount in the mother's blood. In this way, fluorine reaches and affects the developing brain of the unborn child.

Dr. Rapaport studied the incidence of Mongoloid births in 4 states— Wisconsin, Illinois, North and South Dakota—and found that *there is a definite relationship between the concentration of fluorine in the drinking water and the frequency of Mongolism.* It is particularly in areas where mottled teeth indicate a too-high concentration of fluorides in water, that there is the highest prevalence of Mongolism. Enamel mottling, it should be remembered, is one of the earliest signs of fluorine poisoning.

More Incriminating Evidence

In another article, which appeared in the same journal, Vol. 143, numbers 15 and 16, 1959, pp. 529-531, Dr. Rapaport gives further figures for Illinois towns with water containing different concentrations of fluorine (Table 6).

Table 6: Frequency of Mongolism in Illinois Towns of 10,000 to 100,000
(January 1, 1950 to December 31, 1956)

Total Number Births	Fluorine in Water mg/liter	Cases of Mongolism	Number per 100,000
196,186	0.0 - 0.2	67	34.15
70,111	0.3 - 0.7	33	47.07
67,053	1.0 - 2.6	48	71.59

In other words, in towns where the fluoride content is 0.0 to 0.2 milligrams per liter of water, there are 34.15 cases of Mongolism per 100,000 population, whereas in towns where there are 0.3 to 0.7 milligrams of fluorine per liter of water, there are 47.07 cases of Mongolism per 100,000, and, finally, where there are 1.0 to 2.6 milligrams of fluorine per liter of water, there are as many as 71.59 cases of Mongolism per 100,000 population!

There seems to be no possible doubt that the increased incidence of Mongoloid births is directly related to the increased fluoride content of the water supply.

Does Artificial Fluoridation Increase Mongolism Cases?

The important question is this: does the artificial fluoridation of a water supply increase the incidence of Mongolism? In other words, is fluoridation actually causing Mongolism? Dr. Rapaport's statistics show that artificial fluoridation does indeed increase the number of cases of Mongolism, but he concludes that this increase is not "statistically significant." He is assuming, however, that *all* pregnant women consume the *same amount* of water *each day,* that the fluorine content of a city's water supply is controllable and can be *maintained at a constant concentration,* and that *all* pregnant women excrete fluorine *equally efficiently.*

Let us review some facts about fluoridation. Let us also see if his assumptions are scientifically justified. If they are not, then his conclusion about the harmlessness of fluoridation may be wrong.

We know that fluoride is deposited in bones. The older one is, the more fluoride one would have accumulated, other things being equal. Fluoride exists in the body in combination chiefly with the calcium phosphate in our bones. During pregnancy, calcium is mobilized, as the physiologists say, from the mother's system for use in forming the baby's skeleton. As the calcium is solubilized and transported from the mother's body to that of the baby, the fluorine also becomes soluble and goes along with it, since these two elements occur together in the same compound known as calcium fluorophosphate.

Mongolism Commoner in Children of Older Women

The older the expectant mother is, other things being equal, the more fluoride might be transferred along with calcium into the body of the child. Mongolism is commoner among children of older women, remember.

Now let us look a little further into the question of whether or not the fluorides in water might be responsible for Mongoloid children.

1. Is the fluoride content of all fluoridated water in any given city always constant?

2. Does every resident of a fluoridated city or town drink the same amount of water?

3. Does everyone excrete fluoride at the same rate or do some people accumulate more of it than others?

The answer to the first question is that many tests of the drinking water in fluoridated cities conclusively prove that the amount of fluoride released through water faucets in one and the same city varies widely from time to time and from place to place. It is absolutely *impossible* to control fluoridation so that every faucet delivers water with the same concentration of fluoride!

The answer to the second question is that, of course, all the residents of a city do not drink the same amount of water. Even you yourself do not drink the same amount of water every day. A survey showed that some children drink 7 times as much water as others. Amos Light in an article in the *Archives of Biochemistry and Biophysics,* Vol. 47, p. 477, 1953, reports that 6 pregnant women from Newburgh, New York, (artificially fluoridated) drank widely varying amounts of water.

As regards the third question, Gedalia and associates, writing in the *Journal of Dental Research* (May-June, 1959) tell us of an investigation of fluoride excretion by pregnant women. There were wide differences in the amounts of fluoride excreted in the urine of pregnant women who drank the same water.

Now let us consider a representative pregnant woman, say an older woman whose body normally contains more fluoride than a younger

[776]

woman's body contains. Suppose she drinks a lot of water. Suppose she is also one of those people who do not easily or efficiently excrete fluoride so that it tends to accumulate in larger amounts in her body than in that of some other woman. Under ordinary circumstances, that is, with a pure water supply, she would not give birth to a Mongoloid child, because the amount of fluoride needed to affect the brain of her developing baby is just below the critical threshold level.

Pregnant Women Might Be Vulnerable to Fluorine

But suppose she lives in a fluoridated city! Let's say, too, that she lives where the concentration of fluoride coming from her faucet is generally higher—perhaps in an area closer to the water works. Suppose such fluoride, which now accumulates in her body as a result of all these conditions, exceeds the limit necessary to produce a Mongoloid condition in her unborn child. *Under these circumstances, is not the fluoride in the drinking water directly responsible for the Mongoloid child which she may bear? Can fluoridation not tip the biological scale so as to be a direct cause of Mongolism?*

Are we talking about just one woman in whose life such a set of circumstances might happen? *Does it matter if there is only one such woman —if that one woman happens to be you or a member of your family?* Of course, all or part of these circumstances might conceivably happen to thousands of women. And, it would seem, from the statistics collected by Dr. Rapaport, that just such a situation might have brought about just such results for many women in the state of Illinois and elsewhere.

There are almost twice as many Mongoloid births in Illinois cities with high fluoride content as in cities with low fluoride content. Can it possibly be just coincidence?

It doesn't seem to us that it could be anything but direct cause and effect. However, even if it were coincidence, shouldn't such a coincidence have been investigated carefully by the Public Health Service *before* this agency spent so much of its time and our money trying to ram fluoride down our unwilling and resistant throats?

If there is a chance that 10 or 5 or even one pregnant woman is going to bear a Mongoloid child as a result of fluoridation of our drinking water, shouldn't the Public Health Service be doing everything in its power to persuade municipalities to remove fluorides from the drinking water? Is this not its function, its legal and moral obligation?

Public Health Service Advocates Fluoridated Water

Instead, the Public Health Service is the blindest and strongest advocate of compulsory fluoridated drinking water in this country. Incidentally, the Chief of the Department of Epidemiology and Biometry at the National Institute of Dental Research conferred with and advised Dr. Rapaport on his survey. The Department of Public Health of the state of

Illinois cooperated by sending him the chemical analyses of the drinking water of all towns with 10,000 to 100,000 inhabitants. So we see that the very people who are responsible for fluoridation are well aware of the possibility that their efforts to fluoridate may also cause Mongolism!

Those who have had the temerity to oppose or even question (without actually opposing) fluoridation have been branded by its proponents as uninformed, misinformed, anti-intellectual or even crazy and in need of psychotherapy. Some have even lost their jobs because they doubted the wisdom of fluoridation. Now, however, the shoe may be on the other foot.

If fluoride causes Mongolism, as now seems likely, then fluoridation may turn out to be the major medical blunder and the outstanding legal and moral injustice throughout all history. And the monument to those who so stubbornly and blindly fought to fluoridate their fellow men may well be the statue of an idiot!

205. A Treatment for Favorable Change in Mongolism

There seems to be a new interest and activity in scientific circles concerning Mongolism. This most serious birth defect of the mind and body had long been considered unpreventable and incurable. The first 3 months after conception are the most critical ones. If the mother's health and nutrition can be maintained at a high level at this time and throughout pregnancy, chances of her bearing a healthy, normal baby are greatly increased. Mongoloidal characteristics have been found in the fetus as early as the 8th week of gestation. It was, thus, assumed that the Mongoloid developed soon after conception and many factors such as diet, nervous stress, strains, etc. in the mother were considered to have been the cause. However, recently, it was found that Mongoloids have 47 chromosomes in their cellular make-up instead of the 46 which are found in normal individuals. No cause for this inborn abnormality has as yet been discovered. There are cases on record where fraternal twins were born of which one child was normal and the other a Mongoloid. It is now assumed that the abnormal chromosome may be in only one of the many eggs (ova) and as such, very little can be done medically to prevent the development of a Mongoloid. To explain the formation of a Mongoloid simply, we might say a Mongoloid is something like a 4-leaf clover among many 3-leaf clovers (normal) originating on the same plant. But as yet, no one has found the explanation for the "why" of the development.

In the field of improvement, progress has been most uncertain in

Mongolism. More accurately, any attempts at progress in improving Mongolism have been almost nonexistent, except for the work of a European doctor, Anna Szasz, whose gratifying results in treating Mongolism with vitamin E were discussed in chapter 203.

Learning and Social Activity

Now, in a paper by Henry Turkel, M.D., 8000 West Seven Mile Road, Detroit 21, Michigan, we read of an entirely new method of treatment for Mongolism. As Dr. Turkel defines it, treatment of Mongolism "is to prepare the Mongoloid patient for the process of learning, for social activity of which he was hitherto not capable, and for adaptation to newly perceived environmental stimuli." In other words, the goal of such treatment is to allow the Mongoloid to lead a life of near normalcy. This is a tall order when dealing with a condition which most physicians say is hopeless and cannot be helped.

Dr. Turkel, according to his paper, which he presented at the American Association for the Advancement of Science convention in Chicago in December, 1959, and at the Pan American Medical Congress in Mexico City in April, 1960, specifically points out that the medical treatment gradually alters the Mongoloid abnormalities and changes the various abnormal organs until each approaches near normalcy. Therefore, in time, these near-normalized glands and organs will produce more normal secretions which the body requires. As soon as this happens, the medicines may be reduced gradually and finally eliminated. Obviously, as the various structures and organs reach near normalcy, their functions, too, become more nearly normal. Just as the heart, lungs, etc. improve and become nearly normal, so, too, the brain improves structurally and assumes a near-normal function. Then, the Mongoloid becomes educable and requires teaching, just as does any normal child.

Since at the present time, one cannot halt the formation of a Mongoloid, at least the medical treatment can be started as soon as diagnosis is established. One of Dr. Turkel's patients, a 4½-year-old boy who was treated from the age of 7 months, is now able to read a children's book having 40 different words. Another patient, a 22-year-old female Mongoloid, after treatment, married, and is now the mother of a 6-month-old normal baby boy. She takes care of her home, cooks, shops, handles money and takes care of her baby entirely by herself.

Ideally, the treatment could be used on a Mongoloid before birth. To do so, it would be necessary for the expectant mother to take the medicines and, if a Mongoloid were being formed, it would already be treated in the womb.

Dr. Turkel emphasizes that any treatment of Mongolism must be based on the individual case. The type of Mongolism must be diagnosed, the specific kinds of abnormality present and the degree of their severity, as well as the age and response to treatment over a period of time, must all be considered. Since no two Mongoloids are exactly alike, medical treatment for them cannot be standardized. Skill and judgment of the attending physician are vital. There is a series of 11 compounds formulated by Dr. Turkel, all of which are to be taken daily by the patient. Each of them is intended to affect a separate function of the body, but, unless they are taken in combination, the desired effect cannot be expected. As the doctor notes, Mongolism is not a single type of disease with definite responsive treatment, as with glaucoma or a bone fracture. It involves widespread abnormalities in the formation of the body organs and tissues. Medication must take into account that the whole body of the Mongoloid has been adversely affected.

The "U" Series of Drugs

Dr. Turkel has designated his medications as the "U" series of drugs. There are 5 of them, each aimed at relieving a specific part of the general condition presented by Mongolism.

1. Unoid—a cerebral nutrient to stimulate and improve mental alertness.

2. Upeptoid—a supplement to aid digestion and to reduce cholesterol content in the blood.

3. Umorphoid—a supplement to normalize the shape of cells.

4. Upneoid—to relieve allergic manifestations, especially respiratory congestion.

5. Utrophoid—a supplement to normalize tissue nutrition and physiological functions.

The formula for each of these drugs is given in the paper by Dr. Turkel, and in all but one, vitamins, minerals, amino acids or enzymes do make up a substantial and important part. A timetable for the use of each capsule and a suggested beginning dosage according to age is also offered. From this point on, it is the job of the attending physician to decide on an increase or decrease of dosage. Indications are also offered for supplementation of the regular dosage with one or the other of the drugs to concentrate on specific aspects of the case. For example, for cases exhibiting severe mental retardation, Dr. Turkel suggests two Unoid capsules with each meal instead of one, plus an increase in glutamic acid and nicotinic acid.

Dr. Turkel is frank to point out side effects resulting from the treatment. Unoid may cause flushing of the face or the entire body, with a sense of accompanying itching and feeling of warmth. This is temporary. Umorphoid may cause insomnia. Compared with what one can expect from using just about any other medication, we feel that these side effects are minimal.

Dr. Turkel points out that the medicines are not the final word, but we feel, at least, he has shown that the hopeless condition can be markedly altered and further medical research may improve the treatment. Previously physicians and parents alike accepted the fatalistic view that nothing could be done. Now we can recognize that this condition is not hopeless. There are many other diseases which have abnormal chromosomes or genes, such as diabetes. And we all know that the diabetic can live a normal life even if he must depend for support on insulin or allied medication. Thus, too, the Mongoloid can hope for a future such as the diabetic.

Proper Diet Necessary

Dr. Turkel specifies that proper diet will make the medication most effective. He forbids white bread and bakery products made of bleached flour; no peanuts or peanut products, no pork products, no sodas. He recommends lean meats, fish, dark bread, cereals, margarine, especially that made from soybeans, and milk.

Probably the most interesting and convincing part of the paper, for a layman, is the series of pictures taken at measured intervals to show the progress of those Mongoloids under Dr. Turkel's treatment. Their results appear to be miraculous, and, when the treatment is stopped for an interval, the regression is readily apparent in the appearance of the patient.

Dr. Turkel closes his paper with an analysis of 60 Mongoloids and 3 severely retarded individuals not diagnosed as Mongoloids. The periods of treatment range from 3-6 months to 63-66 months. In only 14 patients was there any noticeable regression, and this was explainable by occurrences such as brain injury, infectious disease and interrupted medication. In most, the progress is impressive in everything from a favorable change in appearance to reduction in size of enlarged heart and a bettering of poor muscle coördination. Dr. Turkel feels that much is accomplished if the Mongoloid individual can reduce the unfortunate physical characteristics of the disease. If he can feel acceptable and be accepted socially by others, he will learn faster and develop the independence he needs and wants.

While Dr. Turkel's treatment is no cure-all and is not claimed as such by him, it is indeed a chance for the Mongoloid, and chances are rare where this disease is concerned.

206. Fighting Mononucleosis

By J. I. RODALE

Here is a disease regarding which very little was known until one investigator discovered what was causing it. That is why I am going to talk about it, because I love to seek out the causes of things. But first, what is mononucleosis? Mononucleosis is an acute infectious disease, which comes upon a person suddenly, with fever and inflammatory swelling of the lymph nodes, especially those of the neck region. *The Complete Medical Guide,* by B. F. Miller, M.D., says about it: "A communicable disease of unknown origin."

In reading the *Southern Medical Journal* for December, 1955, however, I came across a remarkable article that clears up the mystery surrounding this disease. It is an editorial, and I will quote parts of it: "Infectious mononucleosis is a disease seen, in an overwhelming majority of instances, between the ages of 17 and 25, and rarely over 40 years of age. Surely it is not a contagious disease to be ranked with the childhood diseases in ease of transmission, otherwise it would not appear in such high incidence in young adult life. Furthermore, this disease, so common in the experience of student health services of universities and colleges and of the medical officers of the armed services, has been noted to occur practically never among roommates or other close contacts, thus virtually ruling out droplet infection.

"Because of these facts and his epidemiologic investigations, Hoagland at the United States Military Academy, (Reference: *American Journal of Medical Science,* 229:262, 1955, 'The Transmission of Infectious Mononucleosis'), offers his theory as to the transmission of infectious mononucleosis. First, he casts doubt upon many of the 'epidemics' which have been reported in the past.

"Having considered the validity of these 'epidemics,' Hoagland goes on to develop his theory of the transmission of infectious mononucleosis. He first points to the report of 3 cases which developed on a destroyer, where the crew lives in crowded quarters for weeks on end, 5 weeks after a shore liberty. No other instances of the disease appeared. In his 6 years of study of infectious mononucleosis at the United States Military Academy, Hoagland has gone carefully into the epidemiology in 73 cases. Most of his cases appeared in February and August. His first case was in a cadet who became ill in February, 1951, and who had spent some hours on the train before Christmas in company with a female medical

[782]

student whom he had never seen before. They engaged in intimate kissing, permitting the mixing of saliva. In later correspondence, it appeared that she developed the disease 3 days before her contact with the cadet. They both were also exposed to a bottle which was passed around among a group of train acquaintances. This cadet contact thus had an incubation period of 47 days.

"In his 73 cases, Hoagland found that all except two had engaged in such intimate oral contacts 32 to 49 days before illness. Three had had only one such contact 42 to 45 days previously. Of the two without a history of kissing, one frequently drank from bottles passed to him by friends. He explains the February and August incidence in his cases by the fact that the semiannual vacations fall some weeks before this time, which, because of the restricted life at the Academy, offers practically the only possibility of the necessary exposure. This fits the pattern of the 3 cases on the destroyer.

"Hoagland points out that his hypothesis explains a number of facts. It explains the high incidence in the 17- to 26-year-old group. (He has never seen a patient under 14 and rarely one over 30 years of age in over 200 cases.) It explains why the disease does not appear in roommates or spread in a dormitory. Though infectious mononucleosis is frequent among nurses, medical students and internes, there are no cross-infections among patients in the hospitals. It explains why the disease is rare among married persons, there being less promiscuous kissing.

"No doubt this hypothesis of the epidemiology and transmission of infectious mononucleosis will be put to the test in student health services. With new thoughts of an extended incubation period and the probability of a virus, nonviable outside the body, further studies in experimental transmission will be needed, especially to establish the possibility of a carrier state, a probability suggested by some of Hoagland's cases.

"It will be interesting to await further observations by others."

The editor is waiting for observations by others. May I make a few? In the first place, shall young people stop kissing? It is not for me to say. This is a controversial point, and I have enough controversial points to deal with in my own sphere of work. But you know and I know that there is going to be a goodly amount of kissing. In fact, when I meet a certain old aunt of mine she insists on kissing me right on the mouth, but I am not afraid of getting mononucleosis because of my vitamin C intake, vitamin C acting as an antibiotic.

So—what do I suggest? That all young folks who expect to indulge in kissing go into training for it—that is, take plenty of vitamin C, and a few other vitamins for good measure, and cut down on the artificial sweets —the colas, ice creams, candies, etc., and other refined foods—make their bodies strong and healthy through good nutrition and exercise, build up a resistance to germs, and then they won't have to fear kissing their old aunts.

207. Multiple Sclerosis, the Crippler

We have seen the progression of the nerve disease, multiple sclerosis, hopelessly characterized in these words: "From canes to crutches to wheelchair to bed." Nothing to do, nothing to try. Imagine being faced with such a prognosis!

The picture of MS, as it is sometimes called, is not as bad as it would appear. Work done by several researchers throughout the world has shown that the disease can be successfully treated. We will present these findings in some detail, but first let us review the symptoms and possible causes of multiple sclerosis.

A Case History Tells All

Perhaps the case history of a typical MS victim will best illustrate how the disease attacks and what its symptoms are. This case was detailed in an article for the *New York Times* (April 20, 1947) by Howard A. Rusk, M.D. The patient, apparently well, first felt peculiar pricking sensations in his left foot and leg (pins and needles). Three months later, he complained of a weakness in the knees and blurring vision of the right eye. Soon his balance became poor and he had a tendency to stagger when walking. He felt dizzy upon closing his eyes. In the sixth month, he noticed a continual and severe itching of the face, and, with his worsening unsteadiness, it became apparent that he must give up his job. In the ninth month, the patient began to have lapses of memory, for recent as well as remote experiences. Finally, he experienced speech difficulties; the fingers of the left hand became numb, and the ordinary motions required for buttoning, tying shoes, etc., became chores that were impossible. The man's vision got worse, but even with glasses he was unable to correct the blurring. He was soon a complete invalid.

What Is MS?

The disease, which for some reason strikes mainly among young adults, causes the destruction of the protective sheath which covers the nerves of the brain and the spinal cord, acting as an insulation. When this covering is damaged or destroyed and the nerves exposed, the impulses from the brain center cannot pass through them properly, with the result that the muscles which normally do one's bidding are out of control. A progressive weakness ensues. The victim tries to move his leg, but he can't; he tries to focus his eyes, but they remain unfocused; he wills his knees not to buckle, but they do.

That is the path of multiple sclerosis. It is not always so fast in disabling its victim as in our case history, but such a case is not a rarity. One of the odd aspects of the disease is its property of complete or partial remission for periods of as long as 20 years. Sometimes an MS patient seems to become suddenly well, and remains so for quite some length of time, without even a sign that he has been attacked by multiple sclerosis. It is thought that, if doctors could discover the reason for these spontaneous periods of freedom from the effects of the disease, they could prolong them indefinitely, but the clue eludes them.

The Cause Is Still Unknown

The very reason for the occurrence of multiple sclerosis is not known. There have been some suggestions that a hereditary influence operates to bring on multiple sclerosis, but the evidence is not very strong. In the *British Medical Journal* (March 2, 1957), Dr. Douglas McAlpine expresses the opinion that, when any genetic influence is present, it is extremely weak and must be reinforced by environmental and constitutional factors. But then, MS also occurs in persons who have absolutely no history of the disease in the family. From this, it is reasonable to assume that environmental and constitutional factors are the main, and possibly the only, cause of the disease.

For some reason, it is known that multiple sclerosis appears most frequently in the colder climates. In the countries of northern Europe, the incidence is many times that of those in the south; in the United States, the incidence of MS in the northern states far outweighs the number of cases in the southern states. Just why cold weather seems to have such an effect no one seems to know. One theory advanced by several well-known researchers, including R. L. Swank (*American Journal of Medical Sciences,* Vol. 220, October, 1950), is that people in northern climates eat larger amounts of animal fats to maintain body warmth, and that these fats are in some way responsible for the deterioration of the myelin sheath. The factor of climate remains quite definite, but the theory that animal fats in the diet are contributory has been largely discounted in more recent years. In *Neurology* (2:369-460, September-October, 1952), it was reported that, in testing 65 MS patients, 24 per cent were shown to have a lack of fat in their system, rather than an overabundance.

Allergies Present in Many Cases

The main purpose of the article in *Neurology* is to show a relationship between allergies and multiple sclerosis. The researchers tested 65 MS patients for allergies to food, trees, grass, pollen, etc. They found a high percentage of allergic reactions to rye and wheat in the group. It is noted by the author that there is a high incidence of MS in countries where rye bread is one of the important food factors; also, there is a low incidence in those countries in which rice is a staple food.

A diet free of all suspected allergens was given to the patients and favorable therapeutic results were brought about in 31 per cent of the cases. In 12 of the cases, temporary reintroduction of the allergens brought about a recurrence of the symptoms.

Aside from the lack of fat shown in the systems of 24 per cent of the 65 patients, 50 per cent were also found to be short of calcium and iron, and 31 per cent were seen to lack the proper amount of protein.

Drs. Adams and Gordon of the University of California were reported, in the *Kansas City Star* (January 4, 1954), to have found a kink in the body's metabolism to be the cause. Normally, when food is broken down, ammonia is deposited in the nerve cells. This ammonia is quickly removed by other body processes, thus eliminating any chance for poisoning of the nerve cells. In many multiple sclerosis cases, the process for removing the ammonia from the nerve cells failed. It was discovered that a chemical normally present in the body, succinate, when injected into the vein, made possible the removal of ammonia from nerve tissue. This discovery seems to be pertinent, but we have seen no further material on it in subsequent issues of the medical journals.

What Science Knows about Treating MS

An indication of how much progress is being made in the treatment and cure of multiple sclerosis comes to light with a look at the *Publication of the Association for Research in Nervous and Mental Disease* (1948). Of 600 pages devoted to the subject of multiple sclerosis, only 30 pages have to do with treatment of the disease.

Of all of the efforts made at treating multiple sclerosis with a variety of modern drugs and techniques, the use of nutrients and the careful observation of diet have shown the most promising results. One might even say that such measures have shown the only results. The reason is apparent upon reading the words of T. J. Putnam, M.D., of the Neurological Institute of New York, as quoted from the *Journal of the American Medical Association* (August 5, 1950). Dr. Putnam says: "It is well known that recovery from traumatic lesions of the (spinal) cord are dependent on a good general state of nutrition and absence of infection. This is also true of other lesions of the nervous system."

The B Vitamins Bring Some Results

One attempt to use nutrients in treating multiple sclerosis is mentioned in the same article. Dr. George Schumacher tells of the use of thiamin hydrochloride, given intraspinally to two MS patients, with improvement noted to the extent that the patients "felt, ate, walked and talked better." Improvement was also noted when a group of 5 MS patients were treated with niacin (another B vitamin). The improvement was not seen to be permanent. Similar results were obtained through the use of vitamin B_6 and hydrocortisone (*Journal of the American Medical Association,* September 12, 1958), when 8 MS patients were given this mixture intraspinally. All of the patients reported a feeling of well-being. Two of them who were unable to walk were walking within two months after the treatments. In 5 patients, dizziness disappeared and spasticity diminished. One patient got no relief. The hydrocortisone was used to take advantage of its anti-allergenic and anti-infectious properties (both, incidentally, prominent properties of vitamin C), and the vitamin B_6 was used for its power to regulate the metabolism of the nervous system.

Blood Sugar Level Should Be Corrected

The famous Dr. E. M. Abrahamson wrote an article giving his views and experiences with multiple sclerosis in the *New York State Medical Journal* (June 1, 1954). Dr. Abrahamson saw 126 MS patients in 18 months and found high or low blood sugar in every case (as well as a lack of calcium). Because the central nervous system is restricted to the use of glucose for fuel, the level of sugar in the blood is of vital importance, and has direct bearing on the course of any disease in which the spinal cord and the brain are concerned. With a diet correcting the sugar level and injections of calcium, Dr. Abrahamson has had amazing results.

The level of sugar in the blood should be relatively constant—approximately 140 to 150 milligrams per 100 cubic centimeters of blood. Normally, the level drops slightly before meals, creating a hunger that tells you it's time to eat. The meal raises it for a short while, then the blood sugar subsides once more to its proper level.

When one is having trouble with low blood sugar, one notices hunger, fatigue and headache a few hours after eating; and these symptoms disappear immediately after eating. Many persons bring up the blood sugar level with a piece of candy or cake, or a bottle of soda at odd times during the day. But this habit only creates a deeper abyss into which the blood sugar falls when the stimulation of the added sugar wears off. A basis of good nutrition at meal times is what one needs to sustain a steady healthy level of blood sugar.

Dr. Abrahamson prescribes the Seale-Harris Diet in his book *Body, Mind and Sugar,* for low blood sugar patients. This diet appears in chapter 78.

Use of Chemical Fertilizers Linked with MS

Another approach to the problem came from James A. Shields, M.D., (*Southern Medical Journal,* January, 1947). It is his opinion that the use of inorganic chemicals in farm soils disturbs the mineral balance and natural bacteria of the soil. He noted that people whose food comes from soils fertilized with these inorganic fertilizers, appear to have more vascular and degenerative diseases than those who use natural organic elements. Of course, the connection is obvious: multiple sclerosis is a degenerative disease with vascular involvements.

Hewing close to Dr. Shields' attitude is that expressed by Dr. Evers in the German publication *Neue Medizinische Welt* (June 10, 1950). Dr. Evers has treated over 400 MS patients and 42 per cent showed improvement. His treatment is based largely on a diet he conceived. The ruination of our foodstuffs by processing, bleaching, refining, etc., says Dr. Evers, is one reason for the disease. He offers this diet as a treatment: raw fruits, nuts, raw roots, raw milk, raw eggs, bees' honey, uncooked coarse rolled oats, sprouted rye, wheat grains and whole meal bread.

Dr. Evers says this, too: "I do not give at all, leafy vegetables, stem vegetables or green vegetables, since in their raw state, they cannot be sufficiently broken up by the human intestine."

While we do not understand all of Dr. Evers reasons for the foods he permits and excludes from his diet, except that they are all natural foods, we cannot deny the fact that his results are impressive—more impressive than any others we've seen in medical literature.

Good Nutrition Is Always Worth Trying

As we can see from the above report, there are some things a multiple sclerosis victim can try before giving up his cause as hopeless. Why let such a disease take its toll just because no drug company has come up with an antibiotic or a hormone that they claim will arrest the progress of MS? Why not give nature a chance to effect a cure? The treatments with the B vitamins have shown some promise. Why shouldn't a person suffering from multiple sclerosis greatly increase his intake of natural B vitamins, just on the chance that a lack of these could be the root of his trouble? The nerves require the B vitamins for proper function, and multiple sclerosis is a nerve disease.

The blood sugar experiments of Dr. Abrahamson offer exciting possibilities. Correct level of blood sugar is a healthy condition that everyone should strive for, why not a victim of MS?

And Dr. Evers' treatment, is it not worth adopting his suggestions in diet since they have shown such remarkable results in the patients under his care? The treatment is not expensive—it is free. The diet is natural, and couldn't be safer. There is nothing to buy in the way of medication or gadgets. What could a multiple sclerosis victim lose by trying the treatment?

As Dr. Putnam said, good nutrition is of major importance in treating disorders of the nervous system. But good nutrition is important in treating any disease; it is important in simply maintaining good health. Until a multiple sclerosis patient has organized his diet and supplement intake, so that he can feel certain that his body is getting large amounts of all the nutrients it can use, he has not tried everything. He has not tried what is likely to be the most important thing of all!

[788]

208. Significant Facts about Multiple Sclerosis

A free translation of an article that appeared in the book, *The Waerland Therapies,* by Ebba Waerland, copyright 1955, Nords Förlag. Translation by Roland S. Moller.

It is hard to say which of our diseases of civilization, cancer or multiple sclerosis, is the most awful. Cancer is at present more widespread and takes away every fifth person here in the North in indescribable suffering. But the organic nerve disease, multiple sclerosis, has, during recent years, become so widespread that it probably soon will become as general as cancer. A horrible thing about this organic nerve disease is that it attacks young people, often even in their teens. It is an insidious and treacherous disease and orthodox physicians stand powerless before it. The person who is once attacked by it is, according to orthodox medicine, without hope of recovery.

Since the disease attacks the whole nervous system, it is not, like some other diseases, localized in a certain organ. The central nervous system regulates all of the body's functions and, consequently, if it is disorganized, the whole cell-state (the whole body) with all its organs is affected. When the disease has reached a certain stage, the mind becomes affected, and severe, paralyzing depressions, crying spells, apathy and complete hopelessness arise. It is heart-rending to see young people wither away from this dreadful disease.

Multiple sclerosis progresses inexorably onward, slower or faster, leading commonly to invalidism. It is a nerve disease which owes its occurrence to injuries in the white substance in the brain and marrow of the spine. The symptoms—paralysis, disturbance in balance, dizziness, difficulty of speech, poor vision—are connected not only with the diffusion of the disease, but also with its localization.

It begins often apparently innocently, with a certain weakness in the legs and a disturbance of the sense of balance. The leg muscles wither slowly and the walk becomes more unsteady until the patient staggers around as if he were drunk. It becomes more and more difficult for him to stand. The vision becomes poorer and poorer and the eyes become apathetic and expressionless. Gradually, symptoms of the withering and paralysis of muscles appear in the arms. The face loses its healthy color and becomes pale and sallow. As the disease progresses, the paralysis spreads and the end usually comes when the lung muscles become affected.

He who has seen at close range how young people, in the flower of their youth, are broken down by this implacable scourge and who, at the same time, knows and has proof that all this suffering is unnecessary, has no more peace in his soul. It becomes his duty to show as many sick people as possible a way out of this inferno before the disease has reached the stage where there is no return to health.

In Germany, there is a physician, a Dr. Evers (of whom we spoke earlier), who has become aware of the extraordinary importance of diet in this disease. He is the first who has succeeded in stopping this disease in its development and who has, in many cases, slowly built up new health. He rules out all processed foods from the diet and prescribes raw food. But in his dietary system are certain weaknesses or flaws which explain why improvement in his patients progresses so slowly and why he fails in some cases where the Waerland diet attains quick results. It would be desirable to have these two diet systems tested in some government hospital under strict control, so that later, the diet which has shown itself the most effective could be used as the basis of treatment.

In certain cases, Dr. Evers gives the patient raw meat and raw egg yolks. On the other hand, he forbids potatoes and green leaves. Since both potatoes and green leaves are very important constituents of a complete health-building diet, and since raw meat and egg yolks introduce putrefactive bacteria into the body, we have here, surely, the explanation why the otherwise fine diet used by Dr. Evers is not as effective as it might be.

The disease arises through a disorganization of the nervous system which is caused by an unnatural, unbalanced diet which poisons the body and is lacking in important nutritional elements. That so many young people become afflicted by this disease, must be caused partly by a tendency inherited from the parents, whose bodies are so deficient in body-building substances that the children are predestined to have this most dreadful of diseases. That all other nerve diseases have become so widespread among civilized peoples, is due to the same cause.

The only effective remedy against multiple sclerosis is a detoxification of the body and the supplying of substances which will build the health. But besides this, it is very important to stimulate the blood circulation and digestion by medical gymnastics, baths and massage. The sick person can do a very great deal to aid in his recovery. He must fight his way forward step by step and, with never-failing energy, exercise his benumbed muscles. An unheard-of endurance and endless patience are needed, and quickly bought victories are rare.

Some Case Histories

I. G., a young girl I met the first time up in Elmau in the spring of 1951. Dr. E. Rohling, a German physician who had studied our methods at first hand, had opened a sanatorium up in the Bavarian Alps. I. G. suffered from multiple sclerosis in an already far-advanced stage and was in a pitiful condition. She was completely helpless, broken in body and soul and absolutely without hope. When one tried to instill a little hope, she burst into tears. Dr. Rohling cared for her through the summer and, when I took over the large sanatorium in Elmau, I took over her care also. She was already on the way to recovery and continued to make rapid progress. It was the first of October that I came to Elmau. By the end of November, Miss I. went alone on a mountain climb in ice and snow. She began at dawn and did not return until late at night, after an achievement which many healthy people would envy.

A young Swiss lady, who had suffered from multiple sclerosis for several years, came to one of our sanatoriums in Switzerland. Thanks to the Waerland diet, she became so well that all the pleasures and possibilities of life opened again to her. She married a Swede and the young couple settled down in Sweden.

Another patient at this same sanatorium, Miss A. B. (in her forties), improved enormously in only 3 weeks. The improvement was able to progress so rapidly because she had had the disease only one year.

(There followed here 5½ pages telling of other cases of multiple sclerosis and similar diseases which were cured or greatly benefited by the Waerland therapy.)

Diet for Multiple Sclerosis

After a short fast, which can be repeated after a time, the patient receives, for a period of at least two weeks, a completely alkaline diet; that is, two raw food meals with the addition of sprouted wheat every day.

Then one may give the ordinary Waerland diet with the addition of sprouted wheat, for two weeks.

Bread consumption is reduced to one or two slices daily. Only bread made with sour dough is permitted. Butter is replaced preferably with cold-pressed oil. No cheese, except whey cheese in small quantities and cottage cheese, is allowed. Sugar consumption must be as low as possible.

If unpasteurized milk is not available, it is better to keep to two raw food meals.

The Ordinary Waerland Diet

Upon arising: One pint of liquid, preferably water in which vegetables have been cooked (potatoes, carrots, celery, parsley, onions, etc.); two level tablespoonfuls of wheat bran and two of flaxseed are put into this. vegetable water the preceding evening and allowed to soak overnight.

Breakfast: Sour milk (e.g., yogurt) with fruit, preferably raw, but even dried fruit may be used, pulverized rose hips or nettles, and milk sugar.

Lunch: A cereal (a 4- or 5-grain cereal, or even a one-grain cereal), very slightly sweetened compote such as apple sauce or cooked dried fruit. Sweet milk.

Dinner: A large raw vegetable salad, plenty of potatoes cooked in their skins and the skins eaten, sour milk, cold-pressed oil, a slice of bread, cottage cheese, possibly soybeans. DO NOT OVER-DO THE BREAD at this meal since it is the main alkaline meal. This is what the Swedes call the "rakost" (raw food) meal.

Between meals: Herb teas or raw fruit. You should get enough juices and liquids at these times to make it unnecessary to drink with meals.

Options: You may alternate the cereal meal with potato porridge. You may eat the vegetable meal at noon and the cereal meal in the evening, if you prefer it that way.

Mrs. Waerland points out that the cereals are cooked only about 5 minutes over direct heat and are then put into a preheated thermos jug and allowed to remain there until they reach the condition in which one desires to eat them. The minimum time is a half hour, but it may be 5 or 6 hours or even longer. The cereal should be hot when removed from the thermos jug. Mrs. Waerland also says that cereals may be eaten without any real cooking at all if one has a good stomach. In this case, one merely pours hot water over the cereal and allows it to stand for some hours.

A word of caution: People not used to salads, coarse bread and cereal, and raw fruits, should use great caution in adopting the Waerland diet; that is, go slowly. This applies to older people especially.

It is of very great importance to eat organically or biodynamically grown foods free from poison dusts, sprays, weed killers and other harmful substances. Also, raw milk, if a good quality, is greatly to be preferred to pasteurized milk.

SECTION 49: MUSCULAR DYSTROPHY

209. Muscular Dystrophy— A Multiple Deficiency?

In rabbits and other laboratory animals, muscular dystrophy (which means literally "faulty nutrition of muscles") results from a diet in which there is no vitamin E. One might believe that the same thing is true for human beings, except for two things: first, most human beings get *some* vitamin E, no matter how poor a diet they eat; second, most human beings do not get enough of the other vitamins necessary for good nutrition. Laboratory animals which live on carefully planned diets get plenty of all these. So perhaps the answer lies in combinations of vitamins.

[792]

A good diet should be rich in all the vitamins and minerals. Here is an article strengthening this point of view. E. L. Hove and D. H. Copeland, of the Alabama Polytechnic Institute, wrote, in the July, 1954, *Journal of Nutrition,* on progressive muscular dystrophy in rabbits as a result of chronic choline deficiency. Choline is a B vitamin. These authors tell us that one of the functions of vitamin E in the body is to bring about the synthesis of a substance called acetylcholine from choline and acetate. This tells us that vitamin E is bound closely with this particular B vitamin, choline, in at least one important body function. Another B vitamin, pantothenic acid, is also involved to a certain extent.

Therefore, say these authors, a deficiency in choline should produce muscular dystrophy as well as a deficiency in vitamin E. To see if it does, they designed a diet in which there was little or no choline, and placed a group of laboratory rabbits on this diet. Other groups of rabbits, eating the same diet, were given choline so they would not have this deficiency.

All of the rabbits whose diet was deficient in choline developed muscular dystrophy between the seventieth and hundredth day on the diet. The symptoms of muscular dystrophy were identical in all respects to those of the dystrophy of rabbits deficient in vitamin E. When choline was added to the diet, all signs of muscle weakness disappeared in 4 days. When the rabbits were examined at post-mortem, it was found that the degeneration of muscle which had taken place was similar to that found in vitamin E-deficient rabbits.

Then the investigators tried something else. They knew that a deficiency in choline produces damage to the liver. Damage to the liver interferes with the body's assimilation of vitamin E. Perhaps, reasoned the researchers, the muscular dystrophy produced by lack of choline was really the same thing they had seen before. Maybe the lack of choline simply resulted in a lack of vitamin E—and what they were actually seeing was the same thing they saw in rabbits who got no vitamin E in their diet. They would have to devise some way to test the choline-deficient diet only.

So they began to give their rabbits vitamin E in large quantities— about 10 times the amount they know is needed. Interestingly enough, they knew, from former experiments, that animals who develop liver disorders as a result of choline deficiency have a greatly increased need for vitamin E! So, at the same time their liver disorder is preventing them from making use of whatever vitamin E is in their diet, this same disorder is causing them to need more vitamin E than they normally would!

By giving large doses of vitamin E, the authors of this article managed to see to it that the animals were not deficient in vitamin E. They could tell this by testing the vitamin E content of their blood. In this way, they knew for certain that the disease was not produced by a vitamin E deficiency, but by a deficiency in choline. In some respects, they tell us, the kind of disorder produced by choline deficiency is more like that seen in human beings. The significance of the present findings, they say, is that dystrophy may result from dietary deficiencies other than a vitamin E deficiency. However, in human muscular dystrophy, there is not usually evidence of severe liver damage.

We have here another chain in the link showing the complexity of nutritional relationships and the harmfulness of tampering with food. Vitamin E (a fat-soluble vitamin) is closely related in its function to one of the minor B vitamins. Perhaps a deficiency in both of them might be partly responsible for human dystrophy. How are we to know what other vitamins will be found in future experiments to be related to these same functions?

We Are Deficient in Vitamins B and E

Would it be possible for a modern human being to be deficient in both vitamin E and choline, one of the B vitamins? It is not only possible, but almost completely certain that anyone who eats refined foods is bound to be short in both these vitamins. They are most plentiful in the germs of cereals—those living parts of our grains which we remove and discard when we make white flour, white rice, when we produce cold breakfast cereals, pearled barley, refined corn meal, cornstarch and all the many products made from these devitalized foods. "Use enriched flour," say the articles in the women's magazines. Cereal products are enriched by replacing synthetically a few of the vitamins and minerals that have been removed when the germ is removed. Iron and a few of the B vitamins are added. *Vitamin E is not replaced. Choline and all the other minor members of the B complex of vitamins are not replaced.* Since cereals are our richest, practical, everyday source of both these food elements, do you see what damage may have been done by food refining—especially to those people who may have abnormally large requirements for one or both of these vitamins?

In addition, remember that both vitamins are destroyed by a number of chemicals to which most of us are exposed frequently. Chlorine destroys vitamin E. Does chlorinated water? We don't know, but it seems likely. Most of us are eating many foods that have been bleached with chlorine compounds. Rancid fats destroy vitamin E. Foods fried in fats used over and over again are bound to contain rancid fats. How many Americans eat fried foods almost every day?

Proof of Vitamin Therapy

As proof of the importance of all the elements of good diet for prevention of muscular dystrophy, we present the following facts: Dr. Walter Eddy, writing in *Vitaminology* (Williams and Wilkins), states that definite improvement was noted in muscular dystrophy patients treated with wheat germ oil. He said, too, that adding the vitamin B complex to the vitamin E-rich wheat germ oil "appeared to increase the value of the vitamin E."

S. Stone, writing in *Archives of Pediatrics,* Vol. 49, 1949, tells us of 25 muscular dystrophy children treated with fresh wheat germ oil, vitamin

B and vitamin C every day, all of whom improved and one of whom recovered completely.

Finally, there is the muscular dystrophy case completely cured by Dr. W. Coda Martin, as described in *International Record of Medicine and General Practice Clinics* for February, 1954. Dr. Martin cured this 17-month-old girl with a diet and diet supplements, after she had been discharged as hopeless by physicians at Babies Hospital. His article stresses the fact that diet therapy, to be successful, must be *complete, intensive* and *persistent*. No laxness which permits you to "break rules" one or two days a week. No relaxing on rules for holidays or trips. Diet therapy must be *complete, intensive* and *persistent*.

A Diet for Muscular Dystrophy Patients

We are going to print here the exact diet on which this little girl returned to perfect health after a diagnosis of "hopeless."

1. *Low-cholesterol, low-fat diet,* free of refined sugars and carbohydrates. (The first provision is not to be recommended for normal children whose bodies can handle fat successfully, but the "free of refined sugars and carbohydrates" is surely an excellent recommendation for all.)

2. *Only whole grain bread and cereal.* (No bakery bread; no ready-to-eat cereal, in spite of all the inducements of the prizes every boxtop will bring.)

3. *Certified raw milk* (rather than pasteurized or evaporated milk).

4. *Fresh raw fruits and vegetables daily*—extra supplements of vegetable and fruit juices. (We suspect that most mothers these days try their best to get their children to eat lots of raw fruits and vegetables, but, we might as well face it, a child who has filled up on candy, ice cream and pop simply cannot be interested in a raw vegetable. And note that this child ate *not only fresh fruits and vegetables every day, but fruit and vegetable juices, in addition, every day*.)

5. *Raw fresh calves' liver* (juice or rare broiled liver) daily. (It seems logical to expect that eating liver, especially raw liver, would work wonders for someone with a liver disorder. Liver is a wonderfully healthful food for all of us, and how many children are brought up without ever having tasted it! Serve it at least once a week.)

6. *Lean meat, fish or fowl.* (To supply protein. If your children get enough first-class protein they will not be so hungry for the forbidden sweets.)

7. *Nutritional supplements.* Vitamin E (natural tocopherols). Desiccated liver. (What, in addition to liver every day at meals? Yes, indeed.)

Multiple vitamins. (This we suppose would include the B vitamins, vitamins C, A and D.)

Lipotropic substances. Crude liver and vitamin B_{12} intramuscularly daily. Thyroid.

210. A Cure for Muscular Dystrophy?

Dr. VanMeter, in the October, 1953, issue of *California Medicine,* announced that he had used amino acids and selected vitamins in 10 muscular dystrophy patients over a period ranging from two months to a year, with noticeable improvement in the patients. No drugs are involved—no expensive treatments. Dr. VanMeter's reasoning went like this: he figured that there might be, in dystrophy patients, a failure of the digestive system to split protein foods into amino acids. Normally, proteins (which are composed of amino acids) are broken down into these various amino acids by the digestive system. Then they are recombined by the various body enzymes, into new body-building tissues, like muscle tissue. If anything goes wrong in this process, the proteins cannot be utilized to build tissue.

Dr. VanMeter prepares amino acids by having them predigested so that the body does not have this job to perform. Certain doses of vitamins are also given in conjunction with the treatment, since vitamins form a part of the chemical structure in which enzymes can work in the body. The results obtained in patients included increase in size of wasted muscles, restoration of normal respiratory action and relief of depression. Says *Science News Letter,* reporting on the article, one woman, a complete invalid, was able to resume all her household chores, after treatment.

We do not know what causes muscular dystrophy, but all research has pointed to the fact that it is nutritional in origin. In 1861, it was first described as a disease separate from other forms of paralysis. Boys are affected more often than girls. The disease quite often afflicts members of the same family. Then, too, it has been found that the mother often gives a record of very poor diet before the birth of the child who later develops muscular dystrophy. The child may be born after several recurrent abortions, for instance, which appear to indicate serious lack in the diet of many important factors, including vitamin E.

In general, the disease may come on in the form of great muscular weakness in the legs and back, so that the patient has trouble walking. Gradually, the paralysis spreads until he is unable to move at all. Respiratory muscles may be affected to such an extent that the patient is unable to cough, so if he contracts even a slight cold, he may suffocate since he cannot cough to remove mucus from his throat or chest. Weakness of legs, lateness in beginning to walk, slowness in running, frequent falls, lordosis (sway back) and prominent stomach—these are easily recognized symptoms of muscular dystrophy in children. In some cases, the disease attacks the arm, shoulder and face muscles before the legs, resulting in a strange expression on the face and possibly inability to close the eyes.

Dr. VanMeter believes the answer lies in the body not being able to use proteins correctly. Earlier researchers have believed the cause of the disease to be the inability to use vitamin E properly. Perhaps the two are related. Perhaps diseases that result in destruction of vitamin E (such as sprue, celiac disease and other diseases involving diarrhea) may also bring about inability to use proteins properly. Perhaps vitamin E is necessary for proper usage of protein by the body. At any rate, whether or not both these factors turn out to be involved in producing this tragic disease, we can be sure that medical science is at last on the right track in ferreting out the cause of muscular dystrophy.

~~~~~~

SECTION 50: OVERWEIGHT

~~~~~~

211. Overweight Is a Mistake You Can Correct

A clever man once summed up the reason for overweight thusly: "There are only two real causes of being overweight—chewing and swallowing." We would add, ". . . the wrong foods." The important thing about this statement, however, is that it gets to the heart of the weight problem: eating. Of course, there can be other factors involved in overweight, but careful selection of foods is really the source of healthy body weight, and all the pills and gadgets in the world won't help a bit if one's diet is ignored.

There Is No "Easy" Way

Millions of dollars are made every year by investors who plan a campaign to take advantage of the heavy person's desire to reduce the easy way. Though the customer is well aware that reducing by simply taking a pill or spending an hour with a masseur is impossible, he is still hopeful enough of some miracle to risk a dollar or a hundred dollars on a "painless" reducing plan. The "pain" involved is the rejection of sweets, the elimination from the diet of pastries, salt, fried foods and second helpings.

Is it possible, somehow, to lose weight healthfully without giving up these things? Any responsible doctor or layman who knows even the most elementary facts about human physiology will tell you it is not. These foods contain the very stuff overweight is made of, so that eating them and hoping to reduce permanently and healthfully, is as foolish as heaping wood on a fire hoping at the same time that it will go out!

The Metropolitan Life Insurance Company issues a booklet entitled *Overweight and Underweight* which says this about the so-called miracle reducing preparations that are supposed to be a short cut to a normal weight. "Any drug which can increase the body's rate of burning calories enough to affect weight reduction without dieting is dangerous. One drug, released in the early 1930's without medical sanction, 'worked,' but it also caused deafness, blindness and paralysis before it was withdrawn from the market. Even if drugs are prescribed by a physician, they will be used in addition to—not in place of—a diet."

The Reason Dieting Works

The theory behind dieting is quite simple. It is based upon the fact that food is the fuel that keeps the body working. One's body can use only so much fuel per day to perform its job, just as a furnace can burn only so much coal to perform its job of keeping a house warm. In the case of the furnace, any extra coal piled into it will simply lie there, waiting to be used. In the body, extra food that the body can't use will lie there, too— in the form of fat.

To avoid having any leftover fuel that will pile up uselessly and unhealthfully, one can introduce either of two effective dietary systems into his eating. He may either weigh his food exactly to the body's needs by counting calories, or he may use fuel that will not be stored at all, by eating high-protein foods which will either be used by the body as they are eaten, or be thrown off as waste, should the body be so well nourished that it has no need for them. While either of these methods is worthwhile and sensible, the calorie-counting has its drawbacks. Many calorie-counters are of the opinion that they will lose weight and stay healthy on a 1200-calories-a-day diet even if the 1200 calories consist of two 600-calorie pieces of pie. This reasoning, of course, can only lead to a physical breakdown much more serious than overweight. The 1200 calories must be carefully calculated to give your body the nutrients it needs to operate efficiently. The foods must be packed with protein and vitamins. Worthless foods on a low-calorie diet are, for all practical purposes, suicidal.

Another objection offered against calorie-counting is the counting itself. The constant referring to a table of numbers, and the temptation to give oneself the benefit of the doubt in borderline cases, or in foods not mentioned in the list, can lead to discouragement and eventual impatience with the whole routine.

We believe the best plan for reducing is simply to rid your diet forever of any foods which the body might not be able to use or throw off. Use only completely natural foods, unprocessed and untreated and prepared in the simplest way—minus salt. This leaves out all white flour and white flour products, all refined sugars and processed fats. On such a diet

[798]

one can let his appetite rule him as it did early man, who ate what he wanted and could be sure his instincts would tell him when he'd had enough. There was no danger of getting fat, because one simply didn't want to eat enough of anything to do so.

With this scheme, there is no need to weigh foods or consult lists. You have only to limit your choice to natural foods—any kind—and you will soon revert to your proper, healthful weight.

The Official Opinion on Patent Weight Reducers

If you're tempted to use an "easy way" to proper weight, and hope thereby to lose weight without dieting, remember this slogan from *Overweight and Underweight*—"No easy way is safe; no safe way is easy." Though this type of statement has received wide publicity, patent reducing preparations are still being bought everywhere. In August, 1957, a Congressional Committee under Representative John A. Blatnik (Democrat of Minnesota) heard doctors and federal officials blast product claims of weight-reducing-pill promoters. Their conclusion, according to *Chemical Week* of August 17, 1957, was this: ". . . the pills just don't do the job and overweight consumers are wasting the money they spend on them." Under existing laws, all that the Federal Trade Commission can do is to order an end to extravagant claims. And what claims they must be! According to an article on these same hearings printed in the *New York Times* (August 8, 1957), a spot check on Washington, D. C. showed that over one million dollars a year is spent on reducing pills, candies and gums in that area alone!

Dr. Peter Farago, Deputy Medical Director for the Food and Drug Administration testified (according to the *New York Times* for August 9, 1957) that one drug, phenyl propanolamine, probably would have a mild effect on cutting the appetite if the dosage were doubled. But this might subject users to heart palpitations, high blood pressure and insomnia. In other words, the drug is useless except in dangerous doses.

Several years ago, the thyroid was often blamed for overweight problems. Thyroid injections and pills have since been discontinued as utterly useless in reducing. One thyroid-containing patent medicine has even been banned by federal court order, according to the Allentown (Pennsylvania) *Morning Call,* March 14, 1955.

What About Exercise and Steam Baths?

We know that reducing preparations are not the only means we hear of for losing weight. Many persons have definite programs of exercise which they are convinced will keep their weight down. Well, the principle of exercising to burn up excess calories is a sound one, but it takes a tremendous amount of exercise to make a dent in an armor of fat that's been built up over the years through ruinous eating. Many pound-foolish people consume 3,500 calories at a single meal, yet, according to the *Hand-*

book of *Physiology and Chemistry* (McDowall), it would take a day of active outdoor life to burn that number of calories in a man. How many eating that kind of food could label their day as one of "outdoor activity"? Even a 6-day bicycle rider only uses 10,000 calories per day, and his is a grind of continual physical exertion over long, long periods of time. There are few of us indeed who have the stamina for the kind of exercise that will take weight off a person who won't combine regular and careful exercise with better dietary habits.

Another of the "easy ways" that doesn't do much good, and can cost a lot of money, is the steam bath. After the prescribed period of "steaming," the patient rushes immediately to a scale and discovers, to his intense joy, that there is a weight loss! But he forgets to weigh himself again after he's thirstily drunk several glasses of water to relieve the dryness caused by the loss of water he sweated out, and which accounted for his temporary weight loss. It's all back on him before he's had time to pay his bill and get his clothes on.

Emotions and Overweight

As in many physiological problems, the blame can be traced, in some degree, to psychological sources. Overweight is such a problem (*Newsweek*, November 11, 1952). The article made the point that excess pounds are a sign that the personality is out of kilter. This opinion was the result of psychological tests on 130 overweight women volunteers. Their personalities were not nearly so well adjusted as those of normal weight who were tested. The main problems of these women were these: they were more tense, anxious and depressed than others; they were too preoccupied with themselves; they had a strong fear of failure; they did not seek out new friends; they did not enjoy social relationships. Any doctor will tell you that all of these things can lead to compulsive eating—a craving for food that is every bit as passionate and frenzied as the alcoholic's need for liquor—and just as dangerous.

Women Look Fatter, But Can Lose More Easily

Unfortunately, because their appearance means so much to them, it is sad to report that women look fatter than men, even when their weights are exactly the same. *Science News Letter* reported this in its June 15, 1957, edition, where it carried an article on the work of Dr. Stanley M. Garns, anthropologist of the Fels Institute, Antioch College, Yellow Springs, Ohio. Dr. Garns concluded that women carry more weight on the outside of their frames (where it shows) than men do. He made measurements on 107 healthy women and 81 healthy men by picking up and measuring rolls of fat, such as the "inner tube" around the waist, the upper arms, etc. Out of 9 places measured, the women's rolls of fat were larger in all but two. At the same time, the total body weight was not materially different for the two sexes.

If it is of any comfort to the women, the Oklahoma City *Times* of

November 29, 1954, carried an article quoting the United Nations Food and Agriculture Organization which says a woman can diet and lose weight faster than a man can. A woman only needs 2300 calories per day to keep going, while a man needs 3200. Women also do not radiate heat from their bodies as men do, so they can get along on fewer calories. The average woman should eat 900 calories less than her husband, says the piece.

The question of just how much one should weigh is too individual a one for exact designations, but *Parade* magazine for November 3, 1957, carried a guidepost that makes sense. One should weigh 14 per cent less at age 50 than at age 35. Dr. Charles F. Wilkerson, Jr., of New York University Postgraduate Medical School, formulated this norm. He explains it in this way: From age 35, body muscle is likely to decrease due to lowered physical activity, and as it does, it is replaced by fat. Thus, while the total body weight might stay the same, the percentage of fat is rising steadily. Nature accounts for these changes, says Dr. Wilkerson, by the fact that your body needs less food to operate smoothly after 35, and, as a result, you should want less to eat.

There are hundreds of facts, experiments and theories on overweight and diet which we cannot go into here, but they all have one thing in common: they all agree that weighing too much is seriously dangerous. The *Practitioner* for July, 1955, gives a few of the reasons. The article warns that the mortality rate of fat persons is high compared with the standard or expected mortality rate. The causes of death in overweight people are mostly degenerative diseases of the heart, arteries and kidneys. The latter rate is one and one-half times the expected one. Diabetes causes death in 4 times more obese people than in the average. Cirrhosis of the liver and gall bladder problems occur one and one-half times as often, and child-birth is always open to complications when the mother is appreciably overweight.

Excess poundage is a danger and a disadvantage in every way. Insurance is harder to get and chances for a job lessened as well when the applicant is beyond his best weight by many pounds. So do yourself a favor. Watch your weight carefully. Eat foods that will be used, not stored unnecessarily. Pay attention to sensible portions of food, and don't eat more than you're actually hungry for. Get enough exercise to help your body use its food effectively. Walking is the best possible exercise. Also, when dieting, or anytime, be sure that your body's needs are being met by taking plenty of supplemental foods, especially vitamins B and C.

If you're eating properly, weight won't be a problem for you. If you are not eating properly, it's a problem you can't avoid!

212. Overweight and High Blood Pressure

Everyone knows, in general, that overweight is unhealthful. It has been called, by many physicians, America's number one health problem. Statistics are constantly being quoted by insurance companies to show that overweight individuals are more susceptible to the degenerative diseases of middle and old age. Or should we say that the tendency to overweight seems to accompany a predisposition to the various degenerative diseases? Or do we mean simply that people who overeat are digging their graves with their teeth?

We know that overweight individuals are much more likely to die of cancer or heart trouble. What about high blood pressure? Is it, too, a condition which overweight makes worse?

Risk Appraisal, a book published by the National Underwriter Company, is a study of "the factors that determine length of life and the fullness thereof," according to its author, Harry Dingman. In the pages of *Risk Appraisal,* we find that blood pressure is, in general, higher when weight is higher. In an analysis which was done of 9,926 unselected life insurance policy holders, it was found that all of them showed an increase in blood pressure with increasing age and weight.

Generally, increasing weight goes along with increasing age. It doesn't have to, of course. In the table accompanying this information (Table 7), we find that, from the age of 10 to 60, higher blood pressure went along with overweight.

TABLE 7:
BLOOD PRESSURE VARIATION WITH AGE AND WEIGHT

Age	10	20	30	40	50	60
Weight			Blood Pressure			
Underweight	116	120	120	122	128	135
Normal weight	117	122	123	125	133	145
Overweight	120	125	125	128	137	152

Mr. Dingman asks "if 1000 heavyweight persons average higher blood pressure than 1000 lesser weight persons, will 1000 persons show step-up of blood pressure when they become heavier? And, conversely, will there be decrease of blood pressure with decrease in weight? Answer is yes."

He goes on to tell us that decreases in blood pressure reading with loss of weight are less than increases with gain of weight. In other words, if you are overweight and should decide to lose weight partly to reduce your blood pressure, it won't be nearly so easy as it would have been to keep your weight normal or below normal—and your blood pressure, too.

He tells us that Emerson and Irving, writing in the *Journal of the American Medical Association,* Vol. 11, p. 1174, 1938, describe an experimental study of 100 persons whose blood pressure was above 142. Fifty of these folks were overweight—an average of about 44 pounds. They reduced an average of 8 pounds each and their blood pressure dropped an average of 19 points!

In an article on obesity and hardening of the arteries in the *Canadian Medical Journal* for March, 1954, we read of a study of post-mortems that was done at Bellevue Hospital. S. L. Wilens studied 1,250 cases to determine whether the weight had anything to do with the progress of this disease. He found that, between the age of 45 and 54, 20 per cent of obese individuals had advanced changes in the walls of their arteries. Only 6.7 per cent of those who were lean showed such changes. Between the ages of 65 and 74, the proportions were 45.4 per cent for the overweight patients and 20.2 per cent for the underweight ones.

How Fat Causes Ill Health

Another article, mentioned in *Nutrition Reviews* for October, 1953, describes results of a survey among more than 3,000 employees of the Metropolitan Life Insurance Company, extending over 12 years. Between the ages of 35 and 44, high blood pressure was almost 3 times as common among the "fatties." Over the age of 45, it was twice as common. The article lists these 3 diseases as the leading causes of high mortality among the obese: diabetes, hypertension (high blood pressure) and atherosclerosis (hardening of the arteries).

How do you suppose added fat can be responsible for the much greater incidence and severity of these diseases of the blood vessels? For one thing, we must assume that obesity is an illness—the fat body is an unhealthy one. So perhaps the same things that produce fat also produce disorders of the circulation. Eating too much of the wrong kind of food is responsible for overweight. Could this also be the cause of high blood pressure? Perhaps those thin individuals who suffer from high blood pressure simply eat the wrong kind of food without eating enough of it to get fat.

Dr. D. D. Feller of the University of Washington School of Medicine is doing some research to determine, if he can, why and how fatty tissue shortens the lives of the overweight. According to *Newsweek* for April 12, 1954, Dr. Feller explains that the heart pumps blood through the vital organs about 10 times as fast as it does through the muscles and fatty tissues. As the ratio of fat in the body increases, there is an even greater decrease in the rate at which the blood moves through the body.

By means of an elaborate machine, Dr. Feller is able to measure the actual volume of blood in his volunteer subjects. He has found that the amount of blood per unit of body weight is related to the sex of the individual and also to his degree of obesity. Women have less red-blood-cell volume in proportion to their weight than men. And the fatter you get, the less blood you have circulating around, in proportion to your body weight. Lean people contain about one and a half times as much blood per pound as obese people. Dr. Feller believes that the lesser amount of blood circulating in the stout people creates extra demands on the heart and probably is at least partly responsible for the tendency to heart and blood vessel disorders associated with excess weight. It's easy to see that the less blood it has to work with, in proportion to body weight, the harder time the heart would have getting it to circulate properly to all parts of the body.

We found an account of another experiment which seems to indicate, better than anything else could, just how much reduction in weight may have to do with decreased blood pressure. A. P. Fletcher writing in the *Quarterly Journal of Medicine,* for July, 1954, describes an ambitious undertaking at the outpatient department of the London hospital in England. Overweight women were the subjects, because at this particular clinic they far outnumbered the men. Women were classified as "obese" when their weight was 20 per cent over the maximum ideal weight for their age and height. They were called "hypertensive" if their blood pressure was above 150/100.

A diet providing 600 calories a day was given to all the women, and the doctors "tried to persuade the patients to keep to it." Toward the end of the dieting period, the calorie count was raised to 1000. The doctors suspected that, even in the case of the women who managed to reduce their weight considerably, the diet probably was closer to 1000 calories throughout rather than 600. But, no matter whether they ate 600 or 1000 calories a day, the women did lose weight. And as they lost weight, their blood pressure went down. The blood pressure of those who did not diet and did not lose weight did not go down. So there seems to be no doubt, according to Dr. Fletcher, that the overweight was at least partly responsible for the high blood pressure and that reducing the weight also reduced the pressure.

Reducing Weight and Blood Pressure

It seems to us that this fact is of paramount importance for all of us who are overweight and hypertensive. Regardless of what the doctor may be giving us to lower blood pressure, regardless of what we are doing in the way of rest, relaxation, special diets and so forth, there is one ever-so-valuable thing we can do on our own—reduce. We all know the general principles of how to lose weight. A diet high in protein, low in carbohydrates and fats will take off the pounds. There are many physicians who allow you to eat all you want on a reducing diet, provided only that you stick to certain foods and eliminate others completely.

Dr. H. L. Marriott, writing in the *British Medical Journal* for July 2, 1949, believes that a simplified diet, where there is little or nothing to remember and no calories to count, will be more successful than a complicated one. He also believes you should never go hungry on a diet. On Dr. Marriott's diet, you may eat as much as you like of any of the following: lean meat, poultry, game, liver, kidney, heart, sweetbreads (cooked in any way but without the addition of bread crumbs, sauces or gravy); fish (not canned, boiled, steamed, broiled or baked only; no fats or sauces); eggs (boiled or poached only); potatoes (boiled, steamed, baked in skins but not fried, roasted, sautéed or chips); vegetables (any you wish, except that no fat or butter shall be used in their preparation); salads (any and all, without mayonnaise or oil); fruits (any kind, fresh or frozen, including bananas, but not dried fruits or fruits canned or frozen with sugar); clear soup, broth or bouillon, tea or coffee, up to a half a pint of milk daily (no cream); no salt; three very small slices of bread a day. *You may have absolutely nothing else whatsoever.*

Now surely such a variety of foods, of which you may eat all you wish could not impose any hardship on a dieter. In fact, we would suggest omitting the bread, soup, tea or coffee and milk entirely. And, of course, taking all your food supplements as usual—fish liver oils for vitamins A and D, brewer's yeast or desiccated liver for the B vitamins, rose hips for natural vitamin C, wheat germ oil for vitamin E and bone meal. With such a diet you cannot possibly become deficient in any vitamin or mineral. Everything you eat will nourish you and you will not be cluttering up your digestive tract with refined, processed foods.

It seems to us that, if you are overweight and have high blood pressure, a diet such as this is bound to take off pounds and reduce blood pressure. If you have high blood pressure and are not overweight, try the diet anyway. We'll even go so far as to recommend the diet for folks suffering from low blood pressure as well. If disordered blood pressure is actually caused by bad eating habits, then it seems only reasonable that any disorder of blood pressure might be prevented by eating properly and healthfully.

SECTION 51: PARKINSON'S DISEASE

213. Parkinson's Disease

Parkinson's disease, *paralysis agitans,* or shaking palsy is a chronic nervous disorder which usually occurs after middle life and is more frequent in men than in women. Its symptoms are muscular weakness, rigidity and tremors, or shaking. The muscular weakness results in an unusual way of walking, of holding the hands and the head. The part of the brain affected is that known as the *corpus striatum.*

For many years we have searched medical literature hoping to find somewhere a hint of something helpful for sufferers from this violent and most distressing disorder. The only information we could come up with, until recently, concerned itself with nothing but drugs and operations which, you know, we do not recommend to our readers. Any physician can recommend those. They practically never give any permanent relief and often they create a condition worse than the one they were supposed to alleviate.

Curing by Injury!

Science News Letter for June 7, 1958, carried an article about a method of using an injection into the brain which "causes a chemical lesion or wound, which relieves both tremor and rigidity." In other words, alcohol or some other substance is injected into a certain part of the brain in order to deliberately injure that part of the brain. According to the article some improvement was shown by Parkinson patients who had the injection.

The same day we read this article and marveled once again at a medical philosophy which believes that injuring one part of the body (especially the brain) is going to cure another part, we had in the mail an unpublished article by the Professor of Pharmacology at the University of Pretoria in South Africa, Dr. Douw G. Steyn. Dr. Steyn submitted to the *South African Medical Journal* his suggested treatment for Parkinson's disease along with a recommended diet. The *Journal* did not publish it, so he had it mimeographed and distributed it to other journals in the hope that someone might publish it.

He says, "To my knowledge, there have, from time to time, been reports (in medical literature) on the treatment of this malady with pyridoxine (a B vitamin). To my knowledge, one case of Parkinsonism of very long standing (approximately 25 years) responded to treatment with pyridoxine alone within two months."

He goes on to suggest that since Parkinson's disease is a nerve disease it would be wise to give, with the B vitamin pyridoxine, the other food elements known to be essential for the health of the nerves—vitamin C, glutamic acid and the other B vitamins. "I have very good reasons," he says, "for believing that the treatment suggested by me will yield much better results than if only pyridoxine were used. Further, pure drug treatment is only palliative and not curative." And a professor of pharmacology, dealing only in drugs, should know!

We believe firmly that one reason vitamins, minerals and other food elements used in massive doses as drugs frequently fail in treating diseases is simply because parts of food belong with other parts of food. Taking ever so much of a single vitamin and continuing to eat a completely non-nutritive diet, short in all the other vitamins, could hardly result in a cure. But adding the vitamin to a well-planned diet which includes ample amounts of the other food elements which naturally accompany it in food, how different the story can be!

Here is a statement from *Vitamins in Medicine* by Bicknell and Prescott (Grune and Stratton) on the subject of pyridoxine used for Parkinson's disease. They say: "Spies has used vitamin B_6 (pyridoxine) in 11 selected cases of Parkinsonism of at least 4 years' duration, 8 of the cases being arteriosclerotic and 3 postencephalitic. In the latter, considerable improvement was reported within a few minutes; rigidity was significantly decreased and the patients walked without their usual stiffness. Two of the arteriosclerotic patients showed definite improvement, 5 were unchanged and one was considerably worse. From a study of 46 cases Jolliffe concluded that no improvement occurred in postencephalitic cases and little or no improvement in patients hospitalized for over 3 years, but that a dramatic improvement resulted in approximately 20 per cent of cases of non-postencephalitic Parkinsonism that had been helpless for less than a year. All patients received 50 to 100 milligrams of vitamin B_6 intravenously. Jolliffe subsequently extended the series to 90 cases and reported permanent improvement in 9—that is, 10 per cent. Baker has also observed improvement in 8 cases out of 19 and Meller in 9 cases out of 10 receiving a similar dosage. . . . The introduction of such efficient drugs as the antihistamines, artane and kemadrin has now made these observations of historical interest only."

This is a typical attitude. No attention was paid to diet, no supplements other than this one isolated B vitamin were given and the conclusion drawn was that drugs were better.

We are happy to know that Professor Steyn, a Professor of Pharmacology, disagrees with this philosophy, for, in addition to the vitamins and the one amino acid (form of protein) which he recommends, he also outlines a complete diet to be followed by the patient.

Here are the food supplements he suggests:

1. Daily doses of 50 to 100 milligrams of pyridoxine, to be injected intravenously very slowly. This, of course, would have to be done by a doctor.

2. A vitamin B tablet with a very high content of niacin.

3. Vitamin C—four 100-milligram tablets daily, divided in 4 equal doses—that is, a total of 400 milligrams daily.

4. Glutamic acid—an amino acid, or form of protein. Eight tablets of one-half gram each to be taken in 4 equally divided doses, preferably not immediately before or immediately after meals.

It is advisable, says Dr. Steyn, to begin treatment with small doses of each of the above to make certain the patient is not allergic or otherwise hypersensitive to any of the preparations.

Here is the diet which Dr. Steyn recommends for the Parkinsonism patient:

1. Early morning—a glass of *fresh* orange juice with two tablespoonfuls of lime water added. Lime water contains calcium. No coffee or tea. (We would substitute bone meal and a natural vitamin C supplement and would recommend eating the orange rather than juicing it.)

2. Breakfast—fruit, lots of it, along with a breakfast cereal made

[807]

with crushed wheat or oats with one tablespoonful of brewer's yeast. If possible, says Dr. Steyn, use only whole wheat bread, groundnut butter (peanut butter) and a little honey. Limit the intake of sugar, jam, etc., as much as possible. Of course, we say omit them entirely. And we would certainly advise a breakfast higher in protein than the one outlined here. Eggs or meat are a "must" for a healthful breakfast. But, in any case, don't forget the brewer's yeast—important for its vitamin B content.

3. Eleven in the morning—the same as the before-breakfast snack.

4. Lunch—a piece of tender meat, preferably liver (we would add fish or poultry) with vegetables but not potatoes or rice, or, of course, any other starchy food. Do not mix heavy protein and heavy starch food, says Dr. Steyn, eat preferably salads prepared from fresh lettuce, fresh cabbage, tomatoes and grated carrot. For dessert—fruit salad. (This means fresh fruits—nothing canned or sugared.)

5. Afternoon—eat two pieces of fruit.

6. Supper—A soft boiled egg with salad, cheese, whole grain bread and peanut butter. (We suggest omitting the cheese and eating peanuts rather than peanut butter, since peanut butter is mixed with hydrogenated oils.)

Some other diet suggestions: Fatty foods, especially starchy foods baked or fried in fat must be totally avoided. Do not cook foods in vinegar or bicarbonate of soda. Limit your intake of starchy food. All food must be chewed very well. Patients can partake of any kind of fruit and fresh raw vegetables. *They are of very great value in our battle against allergic diseases, rheumatism, obesity, etc.*

Smoking must be stopped.

Undernourishment, overeating and malnutrition are to a very large extent responsible for allergic manifestations (migraine, hay fever, asthma, skin afflictions, etc.), colds, sinusitis, tonsillitis and liver, kidney, nerve and gastrointestinal troubles. All these afflictions, as well as the ever-worsening problem of obesity, can be very successfully combated by a properly regulated diet. The words are Dr. Steyn's. We agree wholeheartedly.

Now, how is a Parkinsonian patient going to follow all of Dr. Steyn's instructions to the letter? First, he must find an M.D. who will cooperate to the extent of giving the pyridoxine injections. We would suggest asking your doctor to write to Dr. Steyn for further information about this part of the program, if he is unconvinced. You can address him at the University of Pretoria, Union of South Africa.

Since our chief aim is prevention of disease, we once again remind all our readers that the best way of doing things is to see to it that you and the members of your family are never afflicted with Parkinson's disease. Every day, every month, every year, get in your diet and your food supplements enough of the vitamins, minerals and other things so important for the health of nerves and brain—the B vitamins chiefly, and vitamin C, protein and calcium.

214. Pernicious Anemia

The word "anemia" brings to mind someone who is pale, listless, weak and devoid of spirit and energy. Actually, the word comes from the Greek and means literally "not-blood" or "lacking in blood."

There are so many different kinds of anemia that even the experts get them confused sometimes, so it is not surprising that we laymen find ourselves baffled, if we try to thread our way through the maze of terminology—aplastic, cytogenic, idiopathic, lymphatic, myelogenous, macrocytic, hypochromic. These are only some of the terms used to describe various kinds of anemia. The one we are concerned with here is pernicious anemia, one of the macrocytic anemias.

Meaning and Symptoms of Anemia

Anemia is a deficiency of blood or a deficiency in the number of red blood corpuscles or a deficiency in the hemoglobin (red) content of the corpuscles. In macrocytic anemias, the body, trying desperately to provide enough red blood, produces abnormally large corpuscles. Hence the term *macrocytic,* which means "large cell." The laboratory technician, looking at a sample of blood in a microscope, can diagnose the pernicious anemia victim, for the corpuscles are few and very large.

Symptoms of pernicious anemia are: lack of hydrochloric acid in the stomach, an inflamed tongue and frequently, changes in the nervous system, all the way from painful neuritis to actual degeneration and destruction of parts of the spinal cord. The pernicious anemia patient lacks coordination of muscles, sways visibly when he stands with eyes closed, loses his sense of position, may become spastic, or have spasms. In addition, he suffers from upset stomach, extreme paleness, shortness of breath and indescribable fatigue.

Not a pleasant picture, is it, especially when you recall that before 1926 practically all cases of pernicious anemia had a fatal ending? No one knew what to give so that the red blood corpuscles would regenerate themselves and return to normal size. No medicine could relieve the painful symptoms; no amount of rest could relieve the terrible fatigue.

In 1926, researchers Whipple, Minot and Murphy were successful in using liver for pernicious anemia. In some ways this was an unwieldy method of treatment. Patients rebelled against eating the enormous amounts of liver that were necessary; liver extract sometimes caused allergies. There must be something in liver that could be isolated, scientists thought, and used by itself. Years of patient effort brought to light the magic "something"—vitamin B_{12}, which was first tried on a pernicious anemia patient in 1948.

Some Facts about Vitamin B_{12}

So powerful a substance is the pure, crystalline vitamin B_{12} that, we are told, one heaping tablespoonful of it has the blood-regenerating power of 28,000 tons of raw liver. It is 10,000 times as strong as the most potent liver extract—the most effective medicine per unit of weight ever discovered. Is pernicious anemia, then, caused by the patient not getting enough vitaman B_{12} in his food? Partly. But it also appears to be more complicated than that. Even if there is enough vitamin B_{12} in his food, pernicious anemia will occur if there is something lacking in the tissues or secretions of his stomach. What is this "something"? We don't know. So it has no name. It is called "the intrinsic factor," meaning something that occurs only in the stomach itself which cannot come from anything "extrinsic" or outside the stomach.

Normal stomachs secrete enough of this factor to get the vitamin B_{12} out of the foods in which it occurs—animal foods, mainly, such as meat, organ meats, eggs, milk. Pernicious anemia patients cannot make use of the vitamin B_{12} because they lack this mysterious "factor." There seems to be considerable evidence, however, that wrong diet may bring about this lack, just as there is evidence that lack of B vitamins can bring about a lack of digestive juices in the stomach. And that, of course, is one of the symptoms of pernicious anemia.

No Need for Pernicious Anemia Today

The main point we want to make about pernicious anemia is simply this—there is no need for anyone to suffer from this disease these days. And every week we receive letters from readers who are seriously ill from it and whose doctors do not know how to treat it. It seems impossible, after so many years, that anyone connected with the medical profession should not know how to treat pernicious anemia, yet this seems to be the case, judging from letters we receive.

Very often, vitamin B_{12} is injected by the physician because by injecting it he can be sure that it is going to be used by the patient's body. Giving it by mouth may not be successful until, by trial and error, he discovers whether there is any intrinsic factor in the patient's stomach or whether the vitamin B_{12} is excreted unchanged rather than being used. More often than not, the doctor gives the intrinsic factor by mouth, along with the vitamin. This preparation is made from material taken from an animal's stomach.

Sometimes people who apparently have pernicious anemia do not respond to treatment with vitamin B_{12} with or without the intrinsic factor. In cases like this it seems that another B vitamin, folic acid, will bring results, for this may not actually be pernicious anemia. And there are other kinds of anemia which respond only to folic acid. However, the fact remains that by using any or all of these substances, liver, liver extract, vitamin B_{12} and the intrinsic factor, and folic acid if it is necessary, these so-called macrocytic anemias can be overcome, rapidly, inexpensively and without any danger at all to the patient, for, of course, liver and the B vitamins are not drugs which may be dangerous in large amounts. They are food. And certainly anemia is a disease of malnutrition.

An article in the *South African Medical Journal* for November 2, 1957, tells us that a fair proportion of elderly patients who lack that important digestive juice, hydrochloric acid, in their stomachs, but show no signs of pernicious anemia, absorb vitamin B_{12} poorly. (In addition, we believe that elderly people in general tend to get much less food rich in vitamin B_{12} in their diets.) The editorial says that mild vitamin B_{12} deficiency is seldom diagnosed properly because there may be other kinds of anemia, like iron deficiency anemia, which mask it. The doctor may be giving his elderly patient iron in medicine to correct an anemia but may not notice that the symptoms of vitamin B_{12} deficiency persist—such things as a sore tongue, weakness, psychological disturbances, fatigue. "There would be some justification," the editorial goes on, "in occasional cases, for the insistence by practitioners that injection of vitamin B_{12} has a 'tonic' effect, particularly in elderly patients."

How do you get vitamin B_{12} in food and how can you be sure that you will absorb it properly so that you will not become anemic? The answer is easy. Include liver in your menu at least once a week and oftener if possible. Take desiccated liver daily. Include in your menu plenty of foods rich in the B vitamins, especially foods of animal origin like eggs and meat, for these, too, contain vitamin B_{12}. Be certain that your food supplements contain vitamin B_{12}.

~~~~~~

SECTION 53: POLIO

~~~~~~

215. Treatment of Polio Victims

Like it or not, the polio figures have been rising and, of course, with the incidence of the disease, comes the need for treatment and rehabilitation of the victims. In the earlier days, polio victims had their affected limbs splintered and bandaged into complete immobility until, even if there were a return of muscle power, the function had been partially or completely lost by atrophy of the limb. With the treatment devised by the gallant and forceful Australian nurse, Sister Kenny, a new attitude toward polio-paralyzed limbs was adopted. She proved that action, not immobility, was the key to bringing affected arms and legs back to usefulness. Massage and whirlpool baths, etc., all aimed at the patient's earliest possible attempts to use the affected part, became standard procedure in the treatment of paralytic polio. As a result, the National Foundation reports that, of every 100 new cases: 50 recover completely, 30 are left with some muscle weakness, but not enough to interfere with normal life; 14 have more or less severe paralytic involvement; and 6 die.

Dr. George Boines, whose article on the subject appeared in the *Virginia Medical Monthly* (June, 1956), told of how he improved on the recovery rates given above by using a unique course of treatment which includes: (1.) early ambulation, (2.) muscular relaxation, (3.) controlled and prolonged medical observation to attain maximum recovery and function of neuromuscular power still retained, (4.) special nutritional program. As can be imagined, we were especially concerned with the final part of the program—*special nutritional program.*

Polio Presents Added Nutritional Needs

Dr. Boines believes that the problem raised in the body by polio is a disturbed nutritional absorption by the muscles and a loss of protein. He feels that both of these conditions can be remedied by improved diet and supplementary feedings. Dr. Boines even suggests that susceptibility to polio may be the result of the shortage of protein. As he sees it, the fundamental defenses of the body depend upon the presence of antibodies in the tissues and body fluids. The antibodies are protein, so if the protein, intake goes down, the number of fighting antibodies is lessened and the chances for infection increase.

If the disease should strike, the protein situation becomes even worse. A negative nitrogen balance occurs with the usual high fever, and this results in a waste of the body's protein—the worse the infection, the greater the protein destruction. Now, with essential protein low to begin with, and further lowered by the fever, it must be replenished as quickly and generously as possible, if recovery is to take place. This will not occur on a regular diet. A special effort must be made to insure sufficient protein intake.

General Diet Inadequate

Dr. Boines believes it is necessary to institute a nutritional program as soon as the patient is admitted to the hospital. Even if he is too weak to eat, the protein and glucose are poured into him intravenously. At this stage, the shortages are most acute and the body is in its most desperate need of continuing nourishment to arrest weight loss and to restore the size and strength of muscles. It is alarming to note that Dr. Boines is of the opinion that the general diets in hospitals are often inadequate in protein for *any* patient. They definitely do not furnish enough protein to supply a polio patient's needs, so supplementary protein must be furnished.

If we cannot depend upon an adequate diet in a hospital, where can we expect to find such a diet? "Adequate" protein is not enough when one is so ill as to be hospitalized, for then the body needs super amounts of all nutrients just to "keep up." And what of the polio patients whose doctors are not conscious of the need for extra nutrition? If they must subsist on the general hospital fare, how much is their recovery hampered? How much do they lose in the process due to insufficient nutrition supply?

The Importance of Capillaries

Added to Dr. Boine's special interest in a sufficient supply of protein for the polio patient is his concern for the proper condition of the patient's capillaries. This he insures by prescribing a daily dosage of 600 milligrams of vitamin C and 600 milligrams of hesperidin, a bioflavonoid, for each patient. The importance of capillary health is best realized by an enumeration of the functions of these tiny tubes that transport blood between the main blood vessels of the body: (1.) They are part of the structure that supports the nerve tissue. (2.) They hold the mechanism for maintaining a balance between blood plasma and cerebrospinal fluid. (3.) They provide channels for the supply of nutrition and oxygen. (4.) They regulate the mechanism for control of the intestinal functions. (5.) They are a protective mechanism against disease. (6.) They are avenues for the evacuation of dead materials from centers of soreness or infection. (7.) They are sources of material for body repair. It is not surprising to find that one researcher has said that an "intact capillary system means a solvent body."

When polio strikes, as with any strong infection, the strength of the capillary walls is found to be diminished. The infection which is more safely contained in them tends to "leak" through the walls, attacking the more susceptible nerve cells. Vitamin C and the bioflavonoids have long been known to increase the strength of the capillaries so their use here is strongly indicated.

Other Polio Theories

In the light of the importance of firm capillary strength in preventing and controlling infection, the theories of several distinguished scientists concerning vitamin C and polio make more sense than ever. C. W. Jungblat in the *1939 Proceedings of the Third International Congress on Microbiology* in New York said, ". . . a study of the natural history of poliomyelitis suggests a vitamin C deficiency as one of the chief predisposing agencies. The tissues of the susceptible do not seem able to destroy the virus when it enters as they should." Dr. Jungblat, at another time, remarked that extremely small doses of ascorbic acid (vitamin C) are capable of inactivating many times the fatal dose of polio virus—two or three milligrams of vitamin C are enough to inactivate 10 to 20 thousand fatal doses of polio virus. Dr. W. J. McCormick has said (*Archives of Pediatrics, 69*: 151), "There is an unusually broad spectrum of antibiotic action in this therapy (ascorbic acid), including all bacterial and viral infections." H.

[813]

Scarborough (*Edinburgh Medical Journal*, 50: 85) says that ascorbic acid helps the vitamin P activity of hesperidin to increase the capillary resistance of man when given by mouth.

Doesn't it all add up to make one wonder if a careful support of vitamin C intake for everyone wouldn't cut down the polio rate without any vaccine? If there is such a thing as sectional areas of polio epidemic in our cities and states, can't it be that these poorer areas suffer, not from a lack of Salk vaccine, but a lack of vitamin C-rich foods and C supplements?

Dr. Boines' Record

Dr. Boines has used all this information to good advantage in treating his polio patients. He does not claim that the actual paralysis or permanent stiffness of limbs is decreased by his treatment. However, his methods do improve considerably over what the national statistics would lead one to expect. He has ⅓ fewer deaths among his patients than the expected average and 90 per cent less severely disabled. Only 17 of 474 patients in 8 years have had to use braces or crutches.

Food supplements are given and a check-up on the tray as it leaves the patient's room reveals whether or not they have eaten. If not, they turn up on a special fourth-meal tray. It is considered normal for the polio patient to have a weight loss of 10 to 40 pounds in the first 3 to 6 weeks. Many of Dr. Boines' patients maintain a normal weight, or even gain weight. The added protein and natural vitamin C and hesperidin are continued throughout the hospital stay and into the home life. The family is instructed on how best to prepare high protein foods and warned to withhold sweet drinks and candy from the patient.

It appears that Dr. Boines has a lot of good reference work and logic —not to mention results—to back up his choice of treatment. We can't imagine an excuse for a doctor's following any other. We think that the preventive measures for polio could well be based on Dr. Boines' theories. We hope that the authorities will seriously consider adopting them. You don't have to wait for a national movement, however. You can begin protecting your children right now. See that they get plenty of the protein that forms antibiodies to fight infections such as polio. Stuff them with vitamin C-bioflavonoid-rich fresh fruits and vegetables and C supplements. Skip the sweets and sodas. You won't need to depend upon vaccines to protect them. Good health fortified with good nutrition will do the job.

Remember, too, the Sandler diet for preventing polio, which is a diet high in protein in which starches, especially refined starches, are completely eliminated, and even natural foods that are high in starch are restricted.

[814]

216. Polio in Primitive Countries

Wrote an Associated Press reporter on September 11, 1954, "Polio was pictured Friday as the great leveler, attacking the highest and sparing the lowest of the world's civilizations. Its incidence rises with the standard of living. It seems to thrive where other diseases fail. Where infant mortality is highest, it is lowest. It probably will continue to advance along with civilization, until some dramatic new vaccine brings it to a halt.

"This phase of one of the world's problem diseases was presented Friday to the final session of the Third International Poliomyelitis Congress."

At the same congress, Dr. Rivers, Director of the Rockefeller Institute for Medical Research in New York, said, it is now well known among medical researchers that in primitive countries and in communities where the economic and social levels are low, antibodies against polio appear sooner than they do among the "privileged" children of the higher civilizations and communities. Said Dr. A. M. M. Payne of the World Health Organization, "Until the infant mortality rate falls to about 100 per 1000 live births, the incidence of poliomyelitis is generally below 2 per 100,000. As the infant mortality rate falls from about 50 to 20, there appears to be a tendency for the incidence of polio to increase alarmingly."

In our file on polio, we have some of the most astounding theories you can imagine—for instance, an observation that the paralytic aspects of polio may be much worse after the child has been transported in an ambulance to the hospital. We have theories on whether polio is hereditary, whether it attacks only certain racial groups and other equally nonsensical observations. And now we have the theory that, so long as children are living under the worst possible conditions of bad sanitation and squalor, they will somehow manufacture antibodies to combat polio when they are quite young, and so, will never get the disease when they are exposed to it later on. If there is indeed anything to this theory, then we see even less need for the programs of spraying with DDT which are carried out regularly in many parts of our country as a precaution against polio. We have never heard of any polio epidemic being stopped by spraying with DDT and we have heard of localities where the polio incidence rose after the DDT spraying.

But, to return to Dr. Rivers and Dr. Payne. You see where this line of thinking leads us—if we're just dirty enough and disregard even the basic laws of sanitation, our children will be safe from any threat of polio. Isn't that exactly what they imply in statements such as they made?

Polio Is a "Civilized" Disease

Disregarding the theory about antibodies being formed in the blood only of children who live in filth, let's consider for a moment the well-known facts (for they are well known by now) that children and adults in primitive countries simply don't get polio. And the more civilization they have, the more polio they have. The lower their infant mortality, as a result of wonder drugs and all the marvels of civilized medicine, the higher their rate of polio.

For instance, a letter from a Turkish correspondent in the *Journal of the American Medical Association* for August 6, 1950, assures us that polio is practically unknown in Turkey. Monthly reports submitted to the Ministry of Health and Social Assistance indicate that there are two or three cases of polio a year in the whole country. There is no evidence that an epidemic has ever occurred there. Medical students never observe the disease in its acute stage and seldom see a patient with recent paralysis. We are told that, in the summer of 1947, the child of a prominent physician, returning from a summer resort in Istanbul was the first patient admitted to the Ankara General Hospital with polio. Remember those conditions—the boy had been away to a summer resort on a vacation.

In *Science News Letter* for October 4, 1947, we read of a group of university scientists visiting the orient to take blood specimens in an effort to discover why American troops in Japan, India and North Africa suffered from an increased incidence of polio, while the native populations had no polio at all.

Dr. A. B. Sabin, writing in the *Journal of the American Medical Association* for June 28, 1947, discusses the same puzzling aspect of polio. Why, asks Dr. Sabin, in the same year, when polio epidemics are raging in cities like New York, Chicago, Los Angeles and Denver, do Chinese cities occupying the same latitude report only rare, rare cases of the disease?

Dr. Sabin tells how polio occurred among American troops in China, Japan and in the Philippines, in spite of the fact that there were no outbreaks of polio at the time among the native children and adults. In 1954, there were 246 cases of polio with 52 deaths among American troops in the Philippines. There have never been any outbreaks of polio among the native Philippines. For many years, medical magazines have been commenting and marveling on the scarcity of reports of polio among the races living in North China.

What Civilization Contributes to Polio

Isn't it discouraging how our experts will examine every aspect of the problem except the obvious one that is staring them in the face? They study the climate of Chicago compared to the climate of Shanghai. They study the blood of the children of China and compare it with that of American children. They note with care the number of flies in homes in Shanghai and on the South Side of Chicago. These and countless other angles have been investigated. Why have they never studied the food eaten by the people of these countries and compared it with the food eaten by Americans and Europeans, whether they are at home or abroad?

It's pretty obvious that American troops in all the fighting theatres of the last war ate, in general, the same foods they eat at home—including white bread, refined cereals, white sugar, soft drinks, ice cream, candy, canned vegetables and all the degerminated, devitalized, refined foods that "civilized" people eat. And the American troops went right ahead consuming their annual 100 pounds of sugar per person. Consumption of sugar in China is 3.2 pounds per person, annually. Why is it that no writers except the "faddists" have pointed out this fact?

What kind of food did the Turkish physician's son have at the summer resort that was different from the food he ate at home? Does it seem far-fetched to believe that, because he was a physician's son, his family could afford to buy him refined and processed food such as the other Turkish children could not afford to eat? What would a survey reveal about the food habits of this boy and those of the other Turkish children who apparently are not susceptible to polio?

We do not believe that the per capita consumption of 100 pounds of sugar annually is solely responsible for the high incidence of polio among Americans abroad and the low incidence of polio among the native peoples in the same countries. But when the Third International Poliomyelitis Congress announces to the world that the higher the scale of civilization, the higher the rate of polio, we believe that the time has come to investigate the part played in such a circumstance by "civilized" food as opposed to the more or less natural foods eaten by people who have not as yet attained our level of civilization.

We suggest that one of the best guarantees against polio is to keep yourself and your family as nearly as possible on a diet which is not "civilized"—that is, avoid the foods that have been put through the mill of civilized processing. Avoid foods made from white sugar and white flour, canned foods, prepared "mixes," ice cream, bakery products, cold cereals or any cereals that are not completely whole grain. Stick to the natural foods—fresh fruits and vegetables, as many raw as possible, for cooking is actually a form of processing, remember. Eat fresh meats, nuts, eggs, fresh or frozen fish. Even though you live in a civilized country, you do not have to suffer the penalities for that, if you will take just a little trouble to avoid the foods that civilization has turned into health menaces.

217. Vitamin A vs. Polio

A very strong case for the addition of vitamin A to the list of elements of health known to be necessary to build up resistance to polio, is presented by Dr. José Guadalupe Reyes of New York City in his article in the *New York State Journal of Medicine* for August 1, 1945. Of 84 children suffering from polio who were admitted to St. Francis Hospital during the epidemic of that year, 98 per cent showed skin symptoms of vitamin

A deficiency; and of these, all but two recovered under the proper care and with a well-balanced diet amply provisioned with vitamin A.

Dr. Reyes was especially interested in the skin manifestations of polio, because physicians can very often determine what is taking place inside the body as evidenced by skin changes. A science of the various skin conditions would open the way to easier recognition of diseased conditions of internal organs. Addison's disease, for example, in which one or both of the glands located above the kidney is destroyed, produces brown pigmentation on the skin, especially near mucous membrane areas and over the bony prominences. A disease called hemochromatosis, in which metabolism is disordered, produces a bronze shade of pigmentation of the skin occurring at the same time as an enlargement of the liver and changes in the pancreas, a gland producing digestive juices and insulin.

In the cases of polio described in Dr. Reyes' article, the skin disorders were symmetrically located below both kneecaps, over the ankle bones, the arches and on the soles of the feet. These areas were typically horny and appeared as patches of warty elevations or scattered pimples with roughness and dryness on the skin of the legs. They varied in size from a dime to a half dollar and sometimes were covered with fine scales. Children's skin may often show irritation at places where friction is present—where tight clothes or shoes rub the skin, for instance. But these horny and scaly patches resulting from vitamin A deficiency were not to be mistaken for friction skin diseases, even though they occurred in some areas where friction might be present.

Some children even had a horny hardening of lymph sacs under the skin in certain areas such as below the kneecap, on the tops of the toes, especially the big toes, and on the fronts of the hips and the backs of the forearms. These were not of an inflammatory or acne-form type.

Since mucous membranes are also readily affected by vitamin A deficiency, Dr. Reyes expected to find evidences of equal injuries to the internal organs. He was not surprised, therefore, to observe gastrointestinal symptoms such as nausea, vomiting, diarrhea and abdominal pain in 60 per cent of the cases. Moreover, 5 children had musical rales (a sound in the lung) all over the chest, with a cough similar to whooping cough without the whoop.

Investigations of vitamin A deficiency have revealed the course of the resultant changes in the body beginning with general disturbances and followed by structural changes affecting, primarily, the skin. There is a hardening and shrinkage of the outer layers with excessive multiplying of the basal cells. This occurs in the skin as well as in mucous membranes, such as the under surfaces of the eyelids, the tongue, mouth, nose and throat, the passages of the lungs, the urogenital system and "possibly the whole gastrointestinal tract." The hardening may also take place in the ducts of the mucus or the skin glands, with the formation of cysts or abscesses produced by the blocking of the duct passages. A description

[818]

of the effects of vitamin A deficiency on the spinal cord and nervous system is given in Sollman's *Manual of Pharmacology*, indicating that degeneration of the myelin sheaths (or coverings) of surface nerves, especially the sciatic nerve and of scattered areas in the spinal cord, begins several days before other signs of deficiency appear in rats, and increases until the animals die, with muscular weakness, lack of coordination and final paralysis of the hind legs. The progress of this degeneration can be stopped by supplying the deficiency (of vitamin A). In its effect on the rest of the body, this deficiency makes it easy for bacteria to enter into the deeper layers of the skin and nerves, and hence lowers the body's resistance to infection, since vitamin A is essential for the normal cellular metabolism of the body.

Dr. Reyes suggested that "It may be possible that this modified skin or mucous membrane may be one of the portals of entrance for the poliomyelitis virus, since the vitamin A deficiency has diminished or impaired the normal resistance of these structures. It is now known that this virus is highly neurotropic (nerve-loving) and that it travels mainly in the nerves through the myelin sheath. . . . Vitamin A deficiency also produces changes in the myelin sheath of the nerves, probably facilitating in this way the destruction wrought by the virus. . . . The final changes in the nerves, however, may be due to the combination of both factors."

Although vitamin A deficiency may be a factor in many diseases, it seems to have a special connection with polio. Children admitted to St. Francis Hospital for other diseases showed the skin manifestations described above once for every eight polio cases in which they occurred.

Many vegetables and fruits, such as carrots, yellow squash, broccoli leaves, beet greens, escarole, apricots, etc., contain carotene, which is converted into vitamin A by the body. Fish liver oils contain large quantities, in addition to vitamin D. Since the vitamin concentration of the blood depends on the amount eaten, it is good to eat plenty of carotene-bearing vegetables in summer when they are fresh. Vitamin A is fat-soluble, hence oils and fats favor its absorption, so put plenty of dressing on your salads. Beware, however, of mineral oil, which prevents absorption of vitaman A as well as of calcium.

As Dr. Reyes recommends: "Routinely, a diet rich in vitamin A should be administered to all children, especially during the periods of epidemics, and this diet should be supplemented by cod liver oil." Rose hips are rich in vitamin A as well as vitamin C—they contain about 25 times as much vitamin A as oranges contain. So keep rose hip powder, syrup or puree on hand.

218. Infantile Paralysis and Vitamin B Deficiency

By W. J. McCORMICK, M.D.

Early History of Infantile Paralysis and Sleeping Sickness

During the last century, two modern diseases, poliomyelitis (infantile paralysis) and encephalitis (sleeping sickness), have made their appearance in epidemic form in civilized countries.

Epidemic poliomyelitis was first reported by Heine, a German orthopedic surgeon, in 1840. Epidemic encephalitis was first reported in 1917, during the food deprivation of the Great War, at which time a serious outbreak of the disease occurred in Austria. In the United States, at the present time (1951), poliomyelitis and encephalitis take an average annual toll of 800 and 2500 lives, respectively, besides leaving a much larger number of physical and mental cripples in their trail.

Microscopic examination of the nervous system in these two diseases reveals a very close relationship in the disease processes. In poliomyelitis, the motor nerves of the spinal column are attacked, whereas in encephalitis, the nerve structures of the brain suffer most. The disintegration of the nerve cells and fibers and the inflammatory reactions are almost identical, the variation in symptoms being due to the different function of the nerve tissue involved in each case.

In the earlier history of these diseases, only the pronounced cases, exhibiting gross injury to the nervous system with resultant paralysis or pronounced mental symptoms, were recognized. However, with accruing knowledge from repeated epidemics, it has become apparent that a much larger number of mild forms of these diseases accompany the more frank cases. In poliomyelitis, it is now generally conceded that there are at least 100 mild cases to one paralytic case. It is thus evident that some basic constitutional defect, hereditary or acquired, provides the cause for the selective incidence of paralytic effects in these mysterious diseases.

Vitamin B Deficiency

A correlated study of the various forms of paralytic disease which have been treated successfully by vitamin B, first suggested to the writer the possibility of a deficiency of this nerve-protective element in poliomyelitis as the cause of the paralysis.

Beriberi was the first paralytic disease found to be definitely attributable to vitamin B deficiency. In 1897, Eijkman found that paralysis could be produced in birds by an exclusive diet of polished rice. In 1911, Funk showed that beriberi could be cured and prevented by feeding extracts of rice polishings. After much research work, the nerve-protective element,

[820]

designated vitamin B, was isolated. More recently, it has been produced synthetically, and is now available in chemically pure form for medical use.

Recent reports of the successful treatment of many diseases of the nervous system by vitamin B give support to the theory of a deficiency of this food element in poliomyelitis and encephalitis. Favorable results have attended the use of vitamin B in the treatment of alcoholic and arsenical neuritis, diphtheritic and typhoid paralysis, diabetic and anemic paralysis, and the paralysis associated with cases of pernicious vomiting in pregnancy (based on the assumption that the growing embryo increases the maternal demand for the vitamin, while persistent vomiting decreases the intake).

Similarity of Diseases

In a comparative study of poliomyelitis and beriberi, many features common to both diseases provide a striking similarity. The former attacks mostly young children and adolescents, with a marked preference for males, while the latter has its greatest incidence in infancy and young adult males. Poliomyelitis has its peak of incidence in the hot weather— July, August and September in northern temperate climates, and the corresponding summer months in the southern hemisphere—while beriberi prevails in tropical climates where the weather is warm almost constantly. Both diseases are characterized by flaccid paralysis, the leg muscles being mostly affected. Alimentary disturbances and muscle tenderness are common symptoms, while nerve disintegration with inflammatory exudates and edema are present in both. Physical overexertion is a well recognized predisposing factor in both diseases.

There are a number of determining factors in relation to the vitamin B requirements of the body which have a direct bearing on the question of the possible deficiency of this vitamin in poliomyelitis and encephalitis. In the first place, it has been shown that the storage of vitamin B in the body is very limited. It has also been shown that the vitamin B requirement bears a direct relation to the metabolic rate (rate of food utilization), which has its highest peak at the period of most rapid growth and activity, childhood and adolescence. The metabolic rate is also noticeably higher in the male. Furthermore, with fever or increased physical exertion, there is an increased bodily demand for vitamin B. It is perhaps, therefore, not without significance that the age and sex requirement for vitamin B bears an almost parallel relationship to the age and sex incidence of beriberi, poliomyelitis and encephalitis. Since digestive disturbances are usually associated with these diseases, the depletion of the nerve-protective vitamin is not only hastened thereby, but the intake of new supplies is impeded. Under the combined action of all these factors, it would seem reasonable to assume the possibility of the precipitation of a severe vitamin B deficiency. This in turn might so condition the nervous system that it would be more vulnerable to attack.

[821]

It has been shown that the central nervous system provides the greatest means for storage of vitamin B in the body, the storage of the vitamin in all other parts of the body being more rapidly exhausted on a diet void of vitamin B. On the assumption that the nerve cells of the brain and spinal cord provide the vitamin storage in much the same way as a battery stores electricity, and that mental and physical activity discharge the storage while sleep and rest effect recharge, it would seem reasonable to conclude that mental exertion depletes the storage in the brain while physical exertion reduces the reserves in the spinal motor nerves. It may thus be possible to account for the seasonal incidence of these two diseases, poliomyelitis being more prevalent in the summer when physical activity predominates, and encephalitis occurring more often in the winter when mental activity is generally greater. Professor W. T. Porter, of Harvard University, found, as the result of the observation of 3000 school children, that the period of greatest growth and weight increase was during the summer and early fall. Undoubtedly, the summer vacation is the period of greatest physical activity of children and young people generally; whereas the winter months are devoted more to mental activity in school and college life. The greater incidence of leg paralysis may be accounted for in the same way, by the predominant use of the leg muscles in sport and general activity with proportionate depletion of the vitamin reserves in the lumbar spinal nerves. A further observation which supports this theory is that, in animal experiments, it has been found that physical exhaustion produces certain changes in the nerve cells almost identical with those observed in poliomyelitis.

Quarantine Ineffectual

By the assumption of vitamin B deficiency in poliomyelitis and encephalitis, not only are the peculiar features of age and sex incidence of these diseases accounted for physiologically, but the conspicuous lack of contagious relationship between the cases and the recognized ineffectual control by quarantine are explained. In a recently published paper on poliomyelitis in the *American Journal of Diseases of Children,* Davison says: "Isolation for 3 weeks of patients and contacts is required by most boards of health since 1916, but the evidence then and now does not indicate that anything is accomplished by this procedure. The disease rarely attacks more than one member of a family, and cases developed by contact are conspicuously rare. Of 2,070 persons definitely exposed, only 14 contracted the disease. Patients with the nonparalytic type of the disease must be so common that nearly the whole population should be isolated."

Diet Supplement

In recent years, considerable prominence has been given, in both the medical and commercial world, to the importance of the vitamins, particularly the A, C and D vitamins, as reflected in the increased use of fish liver oils, the irradiation of food products, the more liberal use of citrus fruits and leafy vegetables, and exposure of the body to ultra-violet-ray lamps and sunshine. Vitamin B, however, seems to have been left in the background. The infant and young child of today are amply supplied with vitamins A, C and D in the form of cod liver oil, orange and tomato juice; but no routine measures are employed to contravene vitamin B deficiency in the diet of young children at a time when rapid growth and intensive physical activity make increased demands for this essential food element. McCollum, in his *Newer Knowledge of Nutrition,* points out that there is very clear evidence that nutritive disorders have a far-reaching influence in controlling the health of children, bringing about many borderline cases of malnutrition. He emphasizes the danger to health in adherence to a diet in which milled cereal products, particularly white bread and sugar, syrup, tubers and meat of the muscle type predominate—all deficient in vitamin B.

Average Diet Faulty

According to a recent editorial in the *British Medical Journal,* the British soldier's ration in 1670 contained 1000 international units of vitamin B daily, based on the flour portion being of the whole-wheat variety. In 1782, the diet of the "parish poor" contained 660 to 850 units and in 1832, the poor-law diet (London) contained 1,230 units. A very different condition prevails in England today. The daily vitamin B intake now ranges from 200 units in the lower income levels to 500 units in the high income levels. Thus, the best-fed today, while getting twice as much vitamin B as people on low income, yet consume less of this essential food element than the "parish poor" of the eighteenth and early nineteenth centuries.

The situation in America, in respect to vitamin B consumption, is no better. The average diet, in which meat, potatoes, root vegetables, white bread, white sugar, corn syrup, jam, coffee and pastry products predominate, is sadly lacking in vitamin B. The consumption of milk, eggs, leafy vegetables, whole-grain products and fresh fruits is still considerably insufficient in this country. A recent survey shows that the consumption of white bread is still 5 times that of all varieties of brown combined, aside from the fact that very little of the latter contains the wheat germ. Polished rice is still also a staple commodity.

In view of these facts, it may not be merely coincidental that the adoption of the modern steel-roller system of milling white flour, from which the vitamin-carrying elements of the wheat (the bran and the germ) are excluded, very closely preceded the historical appearance of infantile paralysis and sleeping sickness in epidemic form. This new method of flour milling was adopted in central Europe in 1839. The first epidemic of paralysis was reported in Germany in 1840. Steel-roller milling was not generally adopted in western Europe and America until near the end of the century. In 1890, the Swedish epidemics of poliomyelitis were reported, and following this, perennial outbreaks have been recorded in England, France and America.

[823]

If the basis of the theory herein advanced is found to be physiologically sound, it would appear that a fair trial should be given to this natural nerve-protective agency, vitamin B, which has proved to be so effective in the treatment of other paralytic diseases of undoubted similarity. At least the use of preventive dietetic measures would not be fraught with any of the dangers that have attended the use of serum and chemical agents.

Suggestions

The following suggestions are offered to parents by the author of the above in the hope of protecting children from poliomyelitis:

1. Make sure your children are supplied with a liberal vitamin-balanced diet, giving special attention to the extra need for the nerve-protective vitamin B. Vitamin B is found in wheat germ, whole-grain products, yeast extract, egg yolk, spinach, asparagus, green beans, soybeans, red kidney beans, nuts, rolled oats and tomatoes. Vitamin A is found in fish liver oils, milk, cream, butter, cream cheese, eggs, carrots, bananas, sweet potatoes and green leafy vegetables. Vitamin C is found in grapefruit, lemons, oranges, apples, peaches, raspberries, strawberries and blueberries. Vitamin D is found in fish liver oils, irradiated milk, egg yolk, and by exposure of the body to sunshine.

2. Provide for plenty of sleep in well ventilated and screened sleeping quarters.

3. Guard against overexertion in work or play.

4. Live outdoors as much as possible and wear light clothing.

5. Make liberal use of water, internally and externally.

6. Banish fear. Cultivate optimism. "A merry heart doeth good like a medicine."

Note: Since this treatise was submitted for publication, the author, through the coöperation of physicians throughout the country, has had opportunity to make practical application of the theory advanced. A number of acute cases of both infantile paralysis and sleeping sickness have been successfully treated by the medicinal use of synthetic vitamin B. The recovery was so rapid in some cases that the attending physicians were inclined to question their diagnoses. A number of last summer's convalescent "polio" cases have also shown a marked response to the new vitamin treatment.

As a further check on the validity of the theory, the writer has made a survey of the dietary habits of a considerable number of poliomyelitis victims, and has found that, almost invariably, they have been exclusive white-bread eaters prior to their illness.

Reprinted from GOOD HEALTH, *Oshawa, Canada, July, 1938.*

219. Vitamin E for Post-Polio
Disorders

With polio still showing every sign of shattering previous marks for incidence, the problem of caring for recovering victims of the disease becomes more important than ever. A letter, appearing in the *Canadian Medical Association Journal* (July 15, 1959), written by W. H. Jaques, M.D., Medical Director at Riverdale Isolation Hospital, Toronto, Ontario, Canada, suggests a very interesting therapeutic measure for chronic polio patients—vitamin E.

Dr. Jaques writes that polio victims with extensive residual paralysis often suffer from painful muscle cramps, tingling sensations and a feeling of coldness or numbing in the affected limbs. Because of previous success with the use of vitamin E for treating aged persons suffering with nocturnal muscle cramps, Dr. Jaques decided to try the vitamin on polio patients suffering from the above symptoms.

The results were most gratifying, as can be seen from the case histories Dr. Jaques includes in his letter. For example, a 28-year-old man who had been paralyzed completely in his extremities for 4 years, complained of painful cramps and ankle swelling. A month's treatment with vitamin E (1600 International Units per day) resulted in complete disappearance of cramps and a definite decrease in the swelling.

Pain Disappearance Complete

A 19-year-old female, with extensive paralysis and wasting of the left leg, suffered from cramps and a feeling of coldness in the left leg. Eight hundred units of vitamin E per day, for 4 weeks, were prescribed and complete recovery from cold and cramps followed.

An attack of polio resulted in complete paralysis of the right leg and part of the left in a 42-year-old female patient being treated by Dr. Jaques. She, too, was troubled by crampy pains, tingling and numbness in the right leg. Conventional therapy was attempted, but to no avail. Three weeks of vitamin E therapy, consisting of 800 International Units per day, did the trick. Interestingly, it was found that, when the vitamin E treatment was discontinued, the patient experienced a return of her symptoms within 10 days. A maintenance dose of 400 International Units of vitamin E per day was prescribed indefinitely.

Polio and Menstruation Difficulties

In some cases of polio involving women, the infection has the effect of disrupting the regular menstrual flow. The usual treatment consists of hormone injections. Dr. Jaques tells of two female patients who developed menstrual irregularity: one did not menstruate for 14 months, the other for 9 months. Hormone drugs proved useless. Vitamin E was tried, and after only one month of receiving a dosage of 400 International Units per day, complete regularity returned. The patients experienced no further difficulty even after the vitamin was discontinued. Three other women with irregularity after polio attacks, though not so pronounced, are mentioned as having equally good success with vitamin E.

Further Investigation Is Needed

We hope that the experience of Dr. Jaques will influence others who work with chronic polio patients, causing them to experiment with vitamin E therapy for the relief of the symptoms described. What is more important, we hope to see increased use of vitamin E among doctors treating similar disorders in patients who have not suffered them as an after-effect of polio. The numbness, tingling and cramps in the extremities are common ailments of victims of poor circulation. If vitamin E will work in relieving such complaints among those whose limbs have been impaired by polio, why not with persons who are able to move about freely and do not have the phantom, and real, pains often associated with paralysis?

The usefulness of vitamin E in treating menstrual disorders has been established before, but the classic medical treatment for such conditions is still hormones, dangerous as they are. Again, if vitamin E can help in polio cases, where some physiological damage is likely to have caused interrupted menstruation, why not in cases where the extra hurdle of polio does not have to be met? Why not try vitamin E for hot flashes, painful or irregular menstruation, etc., before using drugs that are known to have severe side effects? The work of such men as Evan Shute, M.D., and Dr. Jaques offers excellent evidence upon which to base further investigation of vitamin E's powers in relieving such disorders.

220. The Sandler Diet for Preventing Polio

Beneath all the hullabaloo over the Salk polio vaccine runs a consistent thread of hesitation and doubt expressed by responsible medical men throughout the world. There are doubts as to its safety; doubts as to whether this is the best way to make the vaccine; doubts as to whether, even if the vaccine does conquer the present-day forms of polio virus, we will not then be confronted with a host of viruses just a little different, each of which will also have to have its own vaccine.

Reports from other nations indicate that events in this country during the spring of 1955 understandably did much to discourage these people from going ahead with their own vaccination programs. A press release from the World Health Organization indicates that, in France, vaccination was used on only a very small group of children, each of whom was carefully followed up. No ill effects were observed and no cases of polio were reported among these children. Even so, France had not at the time of this report decided whether or not to go ahead with polio vaccination.

In Great Britain, Salk vaccine was made, but was never issued for use because American experience in May, 1955, raised questions as to its safety. Sweden decided in April, 1955, to discontinue the use of the Salk vaccine they had made until "better proofs could be obtained of its safety."

Why not look elsewhere for a way of preventing polio? Dr. Benjamin P. Sandler of North Carolina stopped a polio epidemic in its tracks by going on the air and into the news columns with a diet for preventing low blood sugar. He stopped the epidemic, and he caused such a drop in the profits of ice cream and soft drink manufacturers that the diet was very soon buried from sight, even though Dr. Sandler's experiments had been published in the highly respected *American Journal of Pathology* for January, 1941.

Dr. Sandler came to his conclusions by studying rabbits—animals generally highly resistant to polio. Rabbits normally do not ever have low blood sugar. On the other hand, monkeys, who frequently have low blood sugar, are highly susceptible to polio. In his experiments at Morisania Hospital in New York, Dr. Sandler lowered the blood sugar of rabbits by injecting them with insulin. Those inoculated with polio during the time their blood sugar was low got the disease, some dying of infection within 14 hours.

Chronic *hypoglycemia* (low blood sugar) is a common disorder, especially among children and adolescents, being readily induced, according to Dr. Sandler, by overexertion and wrong diet. This would explain the high incidence of polio in the summer when the children are racing around playing and consuming unbelievable amounts of soft drinks, ice cream, candy and so forth.

Dr. Sandler was at the Oteen Veterans Hospital near Asheville, North Carolina, in 1948 when a polio epidemic struck the state. He claimed that he could establish complete immunity to the disease within a 24-hour period. On Thursday, August 5 of that year, the United Press carried the story through North Carolina and several neighboring states who were also suffering severely. The polio epidemic stopped in its tracks after the diet had been highly publicized in the local papers and radio.

What Is the Diet?

The diet Dr. Sandler recommends is not one that the average American will look on with great enthusiasm, for it eliminates some of his favorite dishes. Your neighbor will laugh at you when you say that too many sweet foods may be the chief cause of polio. Yet, your neighbor knows that sweet

[827]

things are not good for him; deep in his heart he knows it. And the evidence against modern, refined sweets is so overwhelming that they seem to be implicated in almost every disease of our century.

In a book called *Body, Mind and Sugar* by E. M. Abrahamson, M.D., and A. W. Pezet, we read of low blood sugar being the cause of a variety of disorders, as epilepsy, asthma, hay fever, allergies, rheumatic fever, ulcers, neuroses, alcoholism, fatigue, migraine and so forth. How does Dr. Abrahamson know that these were caused by low blood sugar? He cured the patients with a diet designed to raise their blood sugar to normal levels. If you doubt us, read the book and get a new outlook on life!

A Diet to Reduce Low Blood Sugar

Now about the diet that will bring blood sugar levels back to normal. It is not at all difficult to follow and it is certainly the most healthful diet anyone could eat, low blood sugar or not. Can you go on the diet for a day or so, then go back to your former ways of eating and expect to be immune from polio for the rest of your life? No, you cannot. But it has been our experience that, if you stay on the diet for a month or so, you will have no wish to go back to your old ways of eating. This holds good whether you are 9 or 90.

Actually, the diet boils down to a few very simple rules. Eat lots of protein; go easy on the starches and sweets. Eliminate entirely products made from refined sugar—that means desserts of all kinds. Don't forget that prepared dessert mixes, as well as most mixes of any kind (muffins, pancake, etc.), contain white sugar and white flour.

Now is this really such a difficult diet to follow? Will this cause you any real hardship in preparing meals? What will you serve for dessert? Fruit, of course, fresh and raw—as delicious and satisfying a dessert as anyone could want. How can you do without spaghetti and macaroni, noodles, pancakes, pie, doughnuts, pastries? Just forget that they exist; cross them permanently off your grocery list. And in addition, forget about bread. Dr. Sandler forbids bread entirely on his diet.

Here is the diet, and we heartily recommend it as a year-round diet, except for a few slight changes of which health conscious readers are well aware. We believe that fruits are not damaging to the blood sugar level and we would say go on eating bananas, apples, etc., in any quantity. We would advise going easy on milk products, skipping bacon and ham because of their high salt content and taking not more than several oranges or grapefruit a week.

Make selections from foods listed below. Take special note of foods to be avoided:

Foods allowed in unlimited quantities: All dairy products—milk, buttermilk, cream, cheeses, eggs, butter. All meats, fish, poultry—prepared any style; no breaded cutlets or breaded chops; no gravies thickened with flour; no stews with potatoes or rice. Nuts—all kinds allowed except peanuts, cashews, chestnuts. Try to have meals on time. Take some milk, tomato juice, cheese or nuts, between meals or at bedtime. Avoid sweet drinks.

Avoid completely: Sugar, potatoes, corn, rice, barley, lentils, hominy, split peas, bananas, tapioca, macaroni, pancakes, noodles, spaghetti, cake, candy, pastries, malted milks, prunes, raisins, canned fruit juices, cereals, bread, rolls, toast, ice cream.

Vegetables allowed: asparagus, string beans, wax beans, Brussels sprouts, cabbage, celery, spinach, cauliflower, kale, tomatoes, lettuce, olives, fresh peas, eggplant, endive, water cress, broccoli, green pepper, radishes, pumpkin, carrots, onions (cooked), squash, turnips, beets.

Fruits: oranges, grapefruit, lemons, limes, honeydew, cantaloupe, watermelon, apples (peeled), pears (peeled), peaches (peeled), pineapples, strawberries, blueberries, blackberries, raspberries, grapes, cherries, fresh plums (peeled).

Take only one portion of fruit at a meal; i.e., don't eat more than one orange or apple at a time. Apple sauce prepared without sugar is all right; apples may be baked without sugar. Don't use dried fruits.

Suggested Meals:

Breakfast

1 small orange or ½ grapefruit
2 eggs (any style) with or without bacon or ham, or fish if desired
cheese
butter
glass milk; light coffee without sugar.

Lunch

1.	2.
tomato juice or clear broth	tomato juice, fruit, broth
meat, fish, poultry	combination salad (egg,
cooked vegetables	sardine, salmon, cold cuts,
salad	etc.; no potato salad)
fruit	cheese
milk	milk, light coffee, no sugar
	nuts

Dinner

soup (clear broth, or vegetable soup cooked with permitted vegetables)
entree (fruit, oysters, tomato juice, etc.)
meat, fish, poultry
vegetables
salad
butter
fruit, cheese, nuts
milk
coffee—cut down as much as possible—take light coffee.

Note: Don't sleep late and miss breakfast. If necessary, get up and eat and return to bed. Have something between meals at 10 A. M., 4 P. M.

Tobacco—cut down as much as possible; don't smoke before mealtime.

For more details about Dr. Sandler's diet and the historic events at Oteen, North Carolina, when diet prevented polio, read Dr. Sandler's book on the subject, *Diet Prevents Polio*, published by the Lee Foundation for Nutritional Research, 2023 West Wisconsin Avenue, Milwaukee, Wisconsin.

221. Garlic Tablets and Polio

Attempting to cure a disease after it has reached epidemic proportions is the usual formula. Trying to prevent a disease before it has reached the proportions of an epidemic is the hard, but worthwhile, way of doing things that we admire so much.

When he was appointed borough medical officer of the town of Malmo, Sweden in 1935, Dr. Ragnar Huss decided that he would make some practical experiments with preventive treatment of polio as soon as signs of an impending epidemic would warrant it. In an article in the Swedish medical magazine, *Svenska läkartidningen,* Vol. 35, p. 216, he describes such an experiment.

Dr. Huss tells us he has long been impressed with the fact that an unimpaired mucous lining of the intestine might give protection from polio. Much laboratory work has shown that animals in whom the intestinal tract is damaged, irritated or inflamed are far more susceptible to infection by polio. He quotes Dr. Mayerhofer, a German biologist, as saying that an initial digestive "catarrh" is necessary before one can contract polio. Catarrh is a term used generally to signify inflammation from whatever cause.

Mayerhofer tried to prevent polio by protecting children from intestinal catarrh. He kept no records of these trials so we do not know how successful he was. However, says Dr. Huss, "Mayerhofer found in garlic a suitable means for the prevention of intestinal catarrh. This vegetable has a property—well-known from European folk medicine and tropical experience—of preventing intestinal catarrhs as well as therapeutically influencing an already existing ailment of that kind."

Another researcher, Nohlen, in Düsseldorf, used garlic preparations to keep 45 monkeys in the city's zoological gardens free from disease during the fall, when inflammations of the intestinal tract are most common.

Dr. Huss Begins His Experiment

In September, 1937, then, signs were apparent in Malmo that a polio epidemic might be on the way, Dr. Huss tells us. In July, the first case appeared. In August, there were 8 more cases and a new one when school began in September. By the time the epidemic ceased in the middle of November, it had caused 67 cases of polio, almost half of them without paralysis.

Dr. Huss arranged to have the children in 3 schools take a garlic preparation at school under supervision of the teachers. They were asked to bring a signed letter from their parents granting permission for the experiment. Only 2.3 per cent of the parents declined to participate. Each day the teacher laid out the garlic tablets on her desk, the children filed past and each took two tablets which he carried back to his desk. Then, at a signal from the teacher, everyone in the room downed his garlic tablets. Altogether, 1,204 children were given the preventive tablets. There were, altogether, 13,829 children in the Malmo school district. No case of polio occurred among the children given the garlic pills.

Dr. Huss concludes that no cases among the treated children compared to 67 among those who were not treated, is a significant percentage which was probably the result of the treatment rather than mere chance.

Interesting as this experiment is as a polio prevention measure, it assumes an added significance when you consider all the other disorders that are undoubtedly preconditioned by an unhealthful state of the intestinal tract. Might one not assume that taking garlic would tend to prevent these disorders, too?

What We Recommend

Our advice, then, is to do everything possible to prevent polio the year round—not just at the polio season. A diet high in trashy foods cannot possibly contain enough of the good foods. You must make good foods paramount in your diet and even then, you will not be getting enough vitamins and minerals unless you take food supplements. Considering the value of garlic for keeping the intestinal tract in a healthy state, don't you think you should add garlic to your supplements, too, making it part of your everyday meal planning?

Garlic is especially useful in cooking when you have cut down on salt or eliminated it entirely, for the zesty garlic flavor is delicious in almost all meat dishes and vegetable salads. Garlic perles contain the essential valuable oils of garlic in a preparation that will never taint your breath, for the perle does not dissolve until it is well beyond the point in your digestive tract where its fumes might reach your breath.

One more point on the subject of polio which we are sure will interest you. A Portugese researcher, writing in the *Arquivos mineiros de Leprologia,* Vol. 17, p. 110, April, 1957, announces that injections of vitamin E have been found to be powerful against muscle-wasting in lepers. Injections of 30 to 300 milligrams, given at intervals varying between one and three weeks, showed satisfactory results in all patients. It is unusual for an experiment of this kind to react favorably in all cases. We might expect that at least several of the subjects would react less favorably. But

[831]

we are told that, in every one of the lepers, the volume of the muscles increased, the muscle tone and muscular movements of hands improved. Partial or total functional recovery was obtained.

Furthermore, the results were permanent. Patients did not relapse to their former condition when the injections were stopped.

Why not try such injections for polio patients, asks Dr. H. C. deSouza Araujo, author of the article? And indeed, this strikes us as a most sensible suggestion. We know that vitamin E is the muscle vitamin. We know that vitamin E, and plenty of it, is essential for muscle health. Why not shoot this wonder-working vitamin directly into the wasting muscles of polio victims? The Portugese article was reported in the *Journal of the American Medical Association* for February 1, 1958. We hope sincerely that many American researchers and physicians will experiment with vitamin E for polio patients.

222. Iodine Against Polio

By J. I. RODALE

I was amazed some time ago, in reading the September 1, 1955, issue of the *Canadian Medical Association Journal,* to come across a letter written by a physician to the editor, in which he shows some astounding facts about iodine and polio. It is surprising during all the talk and hullabaloo about the Salk vaccine, that not a word was mentioned about iodine as a factor in polio, in view of what this doctor proved. And the *American Medical Association Journal,* which abstracts so carefully from the medical literature of the world, did not deem this item fit for comment.

First let me reproduce the letter. I am giving the letter in full even though parts of it are very technical. When Dr. Edwards refers to iodine as a "virucide," he means that it destroys viruses. Here is the letter:

"To the Editor:

"The highlight of my attendance at the recent meetings of the British and Canadian Medical Associations in Toronto certainly was not the panel discussion on poliomyelitis. Though it was very well organized, one came away feeling that the profession is permanently sold on the idea 'there is no treatment for poliomyelitis.' Therefore, we must suffer its horrors until Salk vaccine or its counterpart is perfected and made 100 per cent effective. And our British colleagues are content to wait and see.

"Fortunately for many, but not nearly enough, a few of us have been successful in therapy in the acute case of poliomyelitis. I refer to the work of Drs. Ortiz and Calcada of Mexico City; Dr. R. R. Scobey of Syracuse, New York; and myself. Working independently and unknown to each other we have found that iodine therapy will control acute poliomyelitis.

"Quoting from Drs. Ortiz and Calcada, 'Colloidal iodine solution was the only medication used. Symptomatic relief was prompt and remarkable in all cases. Headache, spinal rigidity, pain in the neck, fever, tremor, irritability and positive Kernig sign all disappeared within 12 to 24 hours of the first injection. Recovery was complete, with no sequelae of infantile paralysis.'

"Dr. Scobey and I concur in this finding and recommend its use, or some modification thereof, to any practitioner faced with a poliomyelitis problem. The response to this therapy is most rewarding.

"I have also learned that a German doctor is linking poliomyelitis with hypothyroidism. I have, I am sorry to say, failed in obtaining his reports.

"My personal findings, during the epidemic years of 1952 and 1953 and with endemic cases in 1954 and 1955, link poliomyelitis control and immunity very closely with iodine metabolism. Dr. Louis Gershenfeld of Philadelphia has confirmed my opinion that iodine is a virucide, proving its virucidal quality in solutions of a few parts in a million in 5 to 10 minutes' contact with poliomyelitis virus Type I. But in the human subject, the virucidal reaction is not always 100 per cent, as two of my 1954 cases made a complete recovery on iodine therapy while expelling poliomyelitis virus Type I in the stool. This would imply that a secondary reaction shortly comes into play, a reaction I have observed since 1952. This appears to be an activation of antibody reaction.

"Another rather unexpected reaction noted in 1954 was that, in two of my patients, antibody titres after recovery were so low that they are, I would say, lacking in immunity against the type they have already had. Could these be representative of the group who fail to immunize with Salk vaccine?

"As a prophylactic medium, iodine appears to be of value for approximately 60 days, after which the iodine level falls below par and must be renewed.

"The success of this therapy rests in early diagnosis and early treatment. It would be of tremendous help to clinical diagnosis if we had a rapid confirmatory test for poliomyelitis.

"My present therapy is 7½ grains sodium iodide, intravenously every third day in bulbar polio, and Iodaminal, one tablet 3 times a day for 10 days in spinal cord poliomyelitis.

"May I again urge the use of this simple, harmless therapy by any treating acute poliomyelitis.

J. F. EDWARDS, M. D.
Winnipeg, Manitoba"

The amazing thing is that iodine is not only effective as a cure, but may be depended upon as a preventive for this dread disease.

The fact that some iodine is lost in perspiration could be one of the reasons why polio generally strikes in the summer, and after undue exertion, when one would tend to perspire freely. During the summer, also, the secretions in the thyroid gland are lowest, thus resulting in less iodine available to the body. These two items—less iodine in summer due to underactivity of the thyroid, and loss of iodine due to perspiration—could very well be the main reasons why polio strikes during hot weather.

In Dr. Edwards' report on his therapy written up in the *Manitoba Medical Review* for June, 1954, he puts himself in a group of "we farmers." Farmers usually are much more concerned about the health of their animals than of their own families. Thus, a long time ago, Dr. Edwards learned about iodine deficiencies in animals. If you will go to an animal feed store, you will find on each sack of feed a list analysis of the food elements contained in it. This you will never see on foods intended for human consumption.

And talking about farming, I wonder whether present-day farming methods, with the use of chemical fertilizers, are not partly responsible for the great increase in polio? We once made a test of wheat that we grew by the organic method (that is, with the use of decomposed organic matter, such as manure, weeds, leaves, etc.) compared with the same variety of wheat grown by a neighboring farmer with chemical fertilizers. Some iodine was present in our wheat, and not in the other. Organically grown foods are generally richer in minerals and in vitamins.

We believe we have unearthed something in medical literature which is extremely significant. It should be given wide publicity. It should be brought especially to the attention of Parent-Teacher Associations and given full discussion there.

223. The Slow Death of the Salk Vaccine

For the most part, people who dread the grim possibility of polio's striking in their family rest easy once the children have had their third Salk shot, and easier yet if they've had their fourth. How soothing to know that the children are safe. How reassuring to read the words of Basil O'Connor, President of the National Foundation, spoken in March of 1959: "Because of it (Salk vaccine), no child in this country or anywhere else in the world need ever suffer the paralysis of one disease—polio." How calming, the words of Dr. A. D. Langmuir of the United States Department of Health, Education and Welfare, which he wrote in the *Journal of the American Medical Association* (171: 271, 1959) ". . . the marked downward trend of poliomyelitis in the past 4 years is due in large part to the immunization program . . ." How wonderful to know that, according to a publication of the Health Information Foundation (March, 1959), "Until recently, polio was a widespread and increasing danger, and little could be done to control it. But medical progress, culminating in the Salk vaccine, has reduced this disease to its lowest levels in many years. The evidence is now overwhelming that the full series of 3 or more Salk inoculations provides a high level of protection from paralytic polio." How deceiving! In 1959, more than 5,000 paralytic polio cases occurred—50 per cent more than in 1958, and 100 per cent more than in 1957. This trend has developed in spite of 300,000,000 doses of Salk vaccine administered in the nation by the end of 1959.

The True Situation

Dr. E. Russell Alexander of the United States Public Health Service Communicable Disease Center in Atlanta, Georgia, faces the issue a bit more honestly as he is quoted in the *New York Times* (April 21, 1960). Commenting on the growing incidence of polio in the United States, he said "it has been a sobering experience for those enthusiastic epidemiologists who had anticipated a progressive disappearance of this disease with increasing use of Salk vaccine." In the October 16, 1959, Public Health Service report on polio, we find that, of 3,389 paralytic cases, whose vaccination records are known, 595 cases of paralytic polio were recorded among persons who had received three or more shots of Salk vaccine, another 302 had had two shots. Dr. Harold Faber predicted in the *Journal of the American Medical Association* (April 9, 1960), that, of a probable 6,000 paralytic cases expected by the end of 1960, 1,000 were likely to have had the 3 shots.

Scope Magazine (June 29, 1960) reported on an outbreak of polio in British Columbia, Canada. Of 17 cases of paralytic polio from January, 1960, to March 25, 1960, 6 were fully vaccinated and 4 were partially vaccinated with Salk polio vaccine. One of the paralyzed children had had two complete series—a total of 6 injections! In the *New York Times* (April 24, 1960), we see this statement: "About ⅔ of the polio cases are among unvaccinated persons." This means that ⅓ *of the persons who contract polio are among the vaccinated!*

The point of all this is that the expected, the promised immunity from paralytic polio, which is implied or guaranteed for those who have had the Salk vaccine, simply does not exist. One can hardly label as deliberate and unashamed lies, the assertions that the polio rate is going down steadily spoken by such persons as Basil O'Connor and Dr. A. D. Langmuir —who have much better reason to be aware of the published figures on rising polio rates than we do. Yet, these respected personages, and others in similar positions, persist in creating the impression that the child who has been vaccinated with the Salk vaccine is guaranteed safe from paralytic polio. The actual fact is that there is no absolute proof that the vaccine works in humans at all, and no scientific assurance whatsoever that your child with 3 or 4 or 5 shots of Salk vaccine is any safer after receiving them than he was before.

What About the Decrease in 1956?

When the people who are pro-vaccine are forced to defend their position, they point to the impressive decrease in polio from 1955 to 1956, the first year of the vaccine. The drop was 37 per cent, reported the United States Public Health Service pridefully, and there was no doubt that Salk vaccine had been responsible. Interestingly enough, in the same period infectious hepatitis decreased 38½ per cent—no vaccine, no inoculations, no explanation by the United States Public Health Service. The record of polio shows it to be one of the diseases which runs in cycles, up one year, down another. Polio naturally decreases after a high incidence year. In 1953, it showed a drop of 42 per cent over 1952's high incidence. In 1916 to 1917, the drop was equally impressive, but there was no vaccine which could receive the credit for the improved state of things. It had just spontaneously happened.

Unfortunately, the Salk vaccine is not willing to take the rap when the polio rate rises, in the same way it is willing to take the bows when it falls. When polio goes up, the authorities say it's because not enough people have availed themselves of the shots. Yet, in 1956, when the rates went down, the polio experts assured us that the decrease occurred only because so many people had had their vaccine shots. Now if enough people had been vaccinated after the vaccine was in use only one year, how, after 5 years of vaccination, can we be expected to believe that polio rates are rising because not enough people have availed themselves of the vaccine?

The Facts Don't Match the Hopes

The claims are one thing—the ideal of how everyone wishes the Salk vaccine had worked out—the facts are something else. It began with the field trials of the vaccine prior to its national release in 1955. After these trials, the public was told that the vaccine was 90 per cent effective in preventing polio. These same field trials get this evaluation from K. A. Brownlee in the *Journal of the American Statistical Association* (50: 1005, 1955): ". . . 59 per cent of the trial was worthless because of a lack of adequate controls. The remaining 41 per cent may be all right, but contains internal evidence of bias in favor of the vaccinated. . . . The reviewer (Mr. Brownlee) would point out that gamma globulin was triumphantly proclaimed effective by the National Foundation after a similar trial. . . ." (Gamma globulin has since been shown to be valueless in preventing polio.) Doesn't it seem to be a grave omission that this opinion by a top statistician, appearing in a technical magazine devoted to statistics, was never referred to in the *Journal of the American Medical Association?* If one is searching for the truth about the effectiveness of the Salk vaccine, the results of the field trials are obviously not the place to look. The truth is that no one knows where to look. Officials of the Public Health Service are preconditioned to expect nothing but success from the Salk vaccine, no matter what the situation seems to be. When persons who had one or two shots get polio, we are told that they were not "fully protected," although the National Foundation's pamphlet for physicians says that paralytic attacks should be 75 to 80 per cent lower among persons with one or two inoculations than among the unvaccinated. That's just a little less than the 90 per cent we're led to expect from the full series of shots. However, in the same pamphlet, we read that the frequency of paralytic polio is 59 per cent in the unvaccinated, 47 per cent among those who have had one shot, and 32 per cent among those with two shots. When one considers the vast number of unvaccinated over vaccinated, the percentage does not seem to mean much as an advantage.

Some Statistical Principles Violated

According to Dr. Ernest Ziesler, Clinical Associate Professor of Medicine at the Chicago Medical School and Ph.D. in mathematics, in the *Minority of One* (June, 1960), the position that polio among the vaccinated is less frequent than among nonvaccinated is not quite proven. First, he notes that a primary statistical principle is that no reliable conclusions can be drawn from samples that are not random. No sample, consisting of volunteers for some procedure, such as vaccination, is random. The people who volunteer have to be different from those who do not volunteer to an extent that may affect the experiment. Mothers who bring their babies in to a doctor for vaccination may be more informed of the current medical thinking, they may be more concerned about their children's health, they may be able to spend more money on their children, they may be free to bring them to a doctor when other mothers have to work, they may have only one child or only a small family, they may feed their children more carefully, supervise their rest more consistently. These and many other factors might make one mother volunteer to have her child vaccinated while another does not.

Any one of these might also have had a bearing on whether or not the child contracts polio, regardless of his having been vaccinated. It is as though a parent were to have his child inoculated against snake bite, then forbid the child to go anywhere snakes might be found. If the child does not then ever suffer from snake bite, one cannot claim that the inoculation was any more responsible than the fact that other precautions were taken to avoid the possibility of snake bite. Yet this is precisely the assumption of the promoters of the Salk vaccine. They simply refuse to recognize the possibility that any of the above factors could influence the occurrence of polio, or lack of it, in the vaccinated. Without good evidence of equality, comparisons between volunteers and nonvolunteers should not be made.

No Attempt to Eliminate Personal Bias

Also, there has been no attempt to eliminate personal bias in diagnosing polio. There are a dozen illnesses due to viruses other than poliomyelitis which are difficult to distinguish from paralytic polio, except by special

[837]

virus tests—tests which, incidentally, are not readily done by the average practicing physician. When a doctor sees a patient with one of these paralytic illnesses, he asks if the patient has had the Salk injections. If the answer is yes, he will begin serious testing for one of the other illnesses, and, if a doubt arises, he is likely to say it is not polio. How could it be? The patient has had the shots that the physician believes effectively protect him from polio!

If the patient admits that he has not had the injections, the physician is likely to be less careful in his diagnosis. He is likely to assume even without exhaustive tests, that the disease that looks like polio is polio, especially since the patient has not had protection from the vaccine. All of this may be done in the best faith and with complete honesty on the part of the physician, but chances for complete objectivity are slim, and such diagnoses provide a poor basis for the scientific tabulations being made by the United States Public Health Service.

Where Outbreaks Occur

Much has been made of the stand taken by the National Foundation and the Public Health Service which intimates that polio outbreaks occur in the slums or in areas in which the people are not interested in protecting their children. Each time there is an epidemic, each time the polio rate goes up, that is the excuse—polio has been concentrated among those who did not receive their inoculations. In *California's Health* (May 15, 1960), the publication of the State Department of Public Health, we are told that, except for a higher incidence in the preschool group (the group, incidentally, which is very highly immunized, since most babies are receiving the injections as part of their pediatric schedule), there are no concentrated cases in any particular segment of the population. California is a state with wide variations in its population and geography. It goes from the plush beach houses of Malibu to the squalor of skid row in Los Angeles, from the Mexican quarter of Los Angeles to Chinatown in San Francisco, from the heat of Bakersfield in the desert to the snows of Squaw Valley in the Sierra Nevada mountains. Los Angeles is one of the largest and most thickly populated cities in the world, while some of California's desert towns are made up of only a dozen families. If the theory of sectionalism were valid in the case of polio incidence, it would certainly show up in California. Incidentally, 16 per cent of the cases of paralytic polio in California in 1959 occurred in persons who had 3 or more Salk injections.

The Public Health Service cites Negroes living in the slum areas, Indians on reservations, certain religious groups who keep to themselves and residents of housing developments for military personnel as being higher than the national average in polio incidence. In each case, there are many obvious extraneous factors which would have bearing on the occurrence of any disease, whether the victims had been vaccinated or not.

[838]

None of these situations is average or ordinary. Chances are very good that their incidence rate of any disease would be higher than average.

The experience in Massachusetts in 1959 provides an added illustration. In that state's epidemic, the 157 cases (137 paralytic) were scattered throughout the state and through all economic levels, and a remarkably high percentage of the victims had received 3 or more Salk shots.

Does It Work or Not?

How good is the Salk polio vaccine? The *New York Times* (April 24, 1960) will tell you that the results ". . . of the Salk vaccine have shown that it is even more effective than had been predicted from 1954-1955 field trials. . . ." Four days previous to that statement, which means that the vaccine was more than 90 per cent effective against all 3 types of polio virus, the same paper carried a news story on a purified and concentrated Salk vaccine giving an even higher rate of immunity. Yet, before the announcement, vaccinated persons were already made by many public health figures to feel 100 per cent safe from polio.

In the *Saturday Evening Post* (July 25, 1960), we read, in connection with trials on the new live-virus vaccine, that there ". . . is recent evidence that Salk vaccine has not been as effective as it was hoped it would be . . . (the) report evaluating the 1954-55 field trials rated the vaccine 80 to 90 per cent effective. Many people subconsciously thought of this as almost 100 per cent protection and hailed the end of polio." Not the least of these "hailers" was the National Foundation, which turned its attention to other things, having finally caused the end of polio. Even Dr. Salk was looking for new research fields to conquer. Now everyone is rolling up his sleeves again, promoting the new oral vaccines, and Dr. Salk is trying to salvage his doomed vaccine by making superconcentrated batches that are better than the old kind.

The oral vaccine discovered by Dr. Albert Sabin consists of live polio viruses that have been so weakened that they no longer cause the active disease, but do cause the body to manufacture a resistance against any stronger polio virus which might attack. Dr. Sabin says, in *Archives of Internal Medicine* (July, 1960), that the vaccine has proven itself.

Will the Oral Vaccine Take Over?

The United States Public Health Service demanded to know the answers to several questions before approving the new vaccine. You will note that (where they apply) the questions have yet to be answered about the Salk vaccine:

1. How much immunity is conferred by the vaccine, and for how long?

2. Should the mono- and trivalent vaccines be given early in life?

3. Is it significant that attenuated strains can and do revert to forms virulent to monkeys?

[839]

We don't know yet how much Salk vaccine is good for how long, yet we're urged to take it. We don't know about the safety of the injections of Salk polio vaccine for tiny babies; we just do it, taking a chance that it will be all right. As to the question of the safety of a vaccine whose virus becomes strong enough to kill monkeys, the consideration of the possibility is admirable, but what of the danger in the Salk vaccine mentioned in *Medical News* (June 22, 1960): There is a dangerous virus sometimes present in the kidney cells of monkeys used to make the polio vaccines for humans. "Virus-infected culture fluids used to prepare killed poliomyelitis or adeno virus vaccines are commonly contaminated with simian agents. . . ." This statement was made at the Second International Conference on Live Polio Vaccines.

The Sabin vaccine has been extensively used overseas, and the reported results are heartening. The *British Medical Journal* (June 4, 1960) tells of two countries (Estonia and Lithuania) who used the Sabin vaccine on all between two months and 20 years of age. Estonia's polio figures for the years 1955 to 1959 read like this: 1955—180; 1956—213; 1957—102; 1958—963; 1959—8. Lithuania: 1955—411; 1956—247; 1957—124; 1958—264; 1959—17. The results are said to be similar in the Soviet Union. The figures certainly qualify for the "startling if true department." We have no reason to doubt their authenticity, but can we be certain that the vaccine and nothing else was responsible? More time is needed.

It is interesting to see that Dr. David E. Price of the United States Public Health Service agrees. He is quoted in the *Saturday Evening Post* (July 25, 1960) as saying: ". . . there are serious objections to drawing conclusions about its (the Sabin vaccine) effectiveness after such short observation periods." He said he would like more evidence that the drops in polio incidence are not simply due to fluctuations in the polio pattern. This is an extremely sensible viewpoint, one with which we wholeheartedly agree. But where was this watch and wait attitude with the Salk vaccine? The trials weren't nearly so extensive when the results were published, yet the United States Public Health Service was pushing the vaccine as a great advance on the day it was released to the public. In the next year, the same conservative Health Service was pointing with pride to the toppling polio-incidence figures. The Health Service never mentioned that there are natural fluctuations in the polio pattern until it questioned the Sabin vaccine. Could it be that a postponement of the okay on the Sabin vaccine was dictated by powerful drug firms who would be left high and dry with millions of unsalable Salk doses if the Sabin vaccine were approved at once?

We do not know how effective or safe the Sabin polio vaccine is. No one does. It would appear from available data that it is safer and more effective than the Salk vaccine was shown to be when it was approved. It is our guess that the Sabin vaccine will take over the leadership, and the Salk vaccine will be allowed to fade peacefully into the background as "a great advance," a "real pioneer," "the almost-perfect vaccine." Its short-

[840]

comings will never be truly explored. The story of the money thrown away on it, the people fooled by it, the faith wasted on it, will never be told. Let us hope that the next polio vaccine, whatever it is, will be safe and effective —if there can ever be such a thing. We prefer to rely on the common sense of good health, carefully fortified with good diet and food supplements, to fight the body's battles against all infections. Vaccines can never take the place of sanitation and the natural immunity of a healthy body in counteracting disease.

224. Scientific Experts Reveal
the Salk Vaccine Hoax

In a series of two articles, the respected *Illinois Medical Journal* (August, 1960 and September, 1960) has had the courage to expose the Salk vaccine as a frank and ineptly disguised fraud. And don't think it didn't take courage to publish a direct contradiction to the releases and pronouncements of the AMA, the United States Public Health Service and just about every other organization and agency that has anything to do with health and medicine in the United States. It took courage, and it took a solid foundation of proof furnished by qualified, reputable experts whose opinions and statements could not be discredited. The opportunity to present such evidence came through a panel discussion moderated by none other than Herbert Ratner, M.D., Director of Public Health, Oak Park, Illinois, and Associate Professor of Preventive Medicine and Public Health, at Stritch School of Medicine in Chicago. The panelists were Herald R. Cox, Sc.D., a leading authority on live virus vaccines, as well as killed vaccines, and at that time, president-elect of the Society of American Bacteriologists; Herman Kleinman, M.D., an epidemiologist from the Minnesota Department of Health, and co-author in 1957 of a paper entitled "The Efficacy of Poliomyelitis Vaccines with Special Reference to its Use in Minnesota, 1955-56," wherein it was concluded that "analysis has revealed (that) the use of two doses of Salk poliomyelitis vaccine . . . (was) 83% protective against paralytic poliomyelitis"; Paul Meier, Ph.D., a biostatistician from the University of Chicago, who is known in the field of polio for this analysis, "Safety Testing of Poliomyelitis Vaccine," which suggested, futilely, that a searching study of the entire Salk vaccine program by an appropriate body be conducted; and Bernard G. Greenberg, Ph.D., of the Department of Biostatistics of the University of North Carolina, School of Public Health, and former chairman of the committee on Evaluation and Standards of the

American Public Health Association. This distinguished panel presented its views before the Section on Preventive Medicine and Public Health at the 120th Annual Meeting of the Illinois State Medical Society (May 26, 1960). There can be no question of the qualifications of these men, and their conclusions have yet to be answered or disproved.

The chairman, Dr. Ratner, began the session with a review of the increasing rise in the polio rate in the United States, quoting Dr. Langmuir (in charge of polio surveillance for the United States Public Health Service) when he said that the polio trend ". . . has been a sobering experience for overenthusiastic health officers and epidemiologists alike." Dr. Langmuir made a prediction in the fall of 1955, that, by 1957, there would be less than 100 cases of paralytic polio in the United States. This has proven to be grossly optimistic. The 1959 figure for paralytic polio was 6,000 cases, 1,000 of which occurred in persons who had received 3, 4 or more doses of Salk vaccine.

Data Handled in a Misleading Way

Statistician Dr. Bernard Greenberg, spoke first: ". . . my primary concern, my only concern (as a statistician) is the very misleading way that most of this data (on the Salk vaccine results) has been handled from a statistical point of view." He goes on to tell of the rise in polio incidence in 1958, 1959, and the resultant alarm sounded by officials of the Public Health Service and "one large voluntary health organization" over every mass communications media, to persuade more Americans to become vaccinated. ". . . the misinformation and unjustified conclusions about the cause of this rise in incidence gave concern to those interested in a sound program based on logic and fact rather than personal opinion and prejudice," says Dr. Greenberg. "One of the most obvious pieces of misinformation," he goes on, ". . . is that the 50 per cent rise in paralytic poliomyelitis in 1958 and the real accelerated increase in 1959 have been caused by persons failing to be vaccinated. This represents a certain amount of 'double talk' and an unwillingness to face facts and to evaluate the true effectiveness of the Salk vaccine. . . . If the Salk vaccine is to take credit for the decline from 1955 to 1957, how can those individuals who were vaccinated several years ago contribute to the increase in 1958 and 1959? Are not these persons still vaccinated?" Dr. Greenberg refers to an Associated Press release warning of the threat of increased polio and giving as the main reason that "millions of children and adults have never been vaccinated." If all of these millions never were vaccinated, undoubtedly the number given as vaccinated during 1955, 1956 and 1957 was exaggerated, for then the same officials were claiming that the polio reduction was due to the vaccine and all those who had taken advantage of it.

Effectiveness Is "Unknown and Greatly Overrated"

Dr. Greenberg states flatly that, "A scientific examination of the data, and the manner in which the data were manipulated, will reveal that the true effectiveness of the present Salk vaccine is unknown and greatly overrated."

The Francis report of the field trials of 1954 actually says no more than that the vaccine *used then* was 72 per cent effective in preventing paralytic polio *for one season*. For 1955, changes in the manufacture and testing of the vaccine were introduced. Methiolate was removed. Live viruses were found in several lots and the foundation of Salk's theory of inactivation was questioned. Great variations in the potencies of different lots from different manufacturers became alarming, especially since the product was to be administered on a mass basis. To insure "absolute safety," an extra filtration step was introduced in November, 1955. The effects of all of these changes, and any other since then, upon the present vaccine are unknown.

Reported Rate Had to Decrease

If the vaccine was indeed less effective, one might wonder why the tremendous reduction occurred in the years 1955, 1956 and 1957. Dr. Greenberg offers this explanation: prior to 1954, any physician reporting paralytic polio did his patient a favor by qualifying him for subsidized care, and he was doing his community a favor by reporting a communicable disease. All that was required was an examination on admittance and another 24 hours later; if the classic polio symptoms were discernible, the patient was considered to have polio. No lab test, no residual paralysis were required to establish a paralytic polio case definitely.

Criteria of Diagnosis Were Changed in 1954

In 1954, the criteria were changed—unless there is residual paralysis 60 days after onset, polio is not now considered paralytic. This is actually a new disease, namely paralytic poliomyelitis, with a longer lasting paralysis. So the minute this new rule of diagnosis for paralytic polio was introduced, with the simultaneous introduction of the Salk vaccine, the number of cases of paralytic polio was bound to decrease. All the cases in which paralysis lasted more than 24 hours and less than 60 days would no longer be listed as paralytic polio. Many of the cases that doctors had always considered to be paralytic polio simply were not reportable as that any longer. Fewer cases reported meant less incidence shown on the Public Health records. When one considers the possibilities in such sure-fire insurance against failure of the vaccine's early reports, it is surprising that the authorities weren't able to report an even greater drop in the incidence of paralytic polio than they did! Even if there hadn't been a bit of vaccine used, the reported incidence rate had to drop.

New Forms of Diagnosis

Another reason for the reported decrease of paralytic polio, when the Salk vaccine came out in 1955 and through 1957, was the new forms of diagnosis. Publicity had us convinced that paralytic polio in a vaccinated child was practically impossible. When such a rare event did occur, every

[843]

known test was made to be sure of the diagnosis. When an unvaccinated child showed signs of paralytic polio, there was less skepticism. It is as though a 60-year-old woman were to announce that she is pregnant. The testing to make certain would be much more extensive than if a 22-year-old woman were to make the same announcement. Physicians have been conditioned to consider the first circumstance extermely unlikely, and they would use every opportunity to prove their preconceived notion to be correct. The second case would get a casual examination, really just to confirm what was already accepted as true. One cannot term such examinations as unbiased and objective. The attitude was, and is, exactly the same in examining suspected victims of polio, depending upon whether or not they have had the shots. These, among other more technical things, were the highlights of Dr. Greenberg's opening speech.

"I Am Getting Nervous"

Dr. Kleinman, who had actually been a forceful promoter of the Salk vaccine in his home state of Minnesota, was next to make a statement: ". . . Let me tell you why I am getting nervous about the Salk vaccine. My first reason is the definite increase in paralytic polio. In Minnesota, we have found that 20 per cent of our 1959 paralytic experience has occurred in triple and quadruple vaccinees. . . .

". . . Laboratory findings are another reason why I am getting nervous. If polio antibodies mean anything in respect to protection, then I am forced to conclude that much of the Salk vaccine we have been using is useless. . . .

"I should like to emphasize Dr. Greenberg's remarks on the changing concepts of polio. It is now extremely difficult to get a Minnesota physician to make a preliminary diagnosis and report of paralytic polio. . . . As a result, the only polio that is being reported today are cases with frank paralysis."

"Absolutely Silly"

"I would also like to agree with Dr. Greenberg that the insistence upon a 60 day duration of paralysis for paralytic polio is absolutely silly. There isn't a doctor in this room who hasn't seen a case of frank paralytic polio which has not recovered within 60 days. . . .

"I would like, then, to have my position understood . . . as that of an agnostic so far as the Salk vaccine is concerned. I am not against it. I think it is the only medium we have which has some degree of reliability; but I think there are better methods, and I think we should take advantage of these methods if it seems at all reasonable."

Disappointment of Former Salk Vaccine Proponent

These are the words of one of the foremost promoters of the Salk vaccine in Minnesota. His disappointment is evident and his characterization of the vaccine as "the only medium we have which has some

[844]

reliability" is a far cry from the high estimates of 92 per cent immunity which we've been told we can expect from the Salk vaccine. And even the "some degree of reliability" Dr. Kleinman mentions is hard to accept on the face of the other statements made by this panel.

Dr. Cox spoke next: "First let me say that I am convinced that living virus vaccine is going to be the final answer. I base this statement on my experience in the virus field since 1928. I am not against killed virus vaccines. I was the first person to prove they could be made. . . .

". . . The reason our company refused to make the killed Salk vaccine was because we knew it was impossible to produce enough virus by known tissue culture methods to make a good killed polio virus vaccine."

Manufacturing Methods Deficient

Dr. Cox went on to say that a worthwhile killed virus vaccine must have at least 100 million particles per dose. In mass production the Salk vaccine manufacturers don't often get more than 10 to 30 million. This means that the vaccine would have to be concentrated 5 to 10 times to get a proper end product. This means that the 39 cents a cubic centimeter it costs to make the killed vaccine would have to be multiplied 5 or 10 times, plus labor costs, to make a proper vaccine. Dr. Cox's company didn't think it worthwhile to risk such large sums, when other companies were not above making and selling the cheaper product. "No one manufactured the vaccine that would properly have 100 million particles per cubic centimeter. Actually no one ever got the proper vaccine."

Dr. Cox continued, ". . . the killed (virus) does a fairly good job . . . against Type II polio virus. But Type II represents only about 3 per cent of paralytic cases throughout the world. The killed vaccine does a poor job against Type I, however, which causes 85 per cent of paralytic cases, and Type III, which causes about 12 per cent. In other words, the killed vaccine is doing its best job against the least important type . . . it was proven in Israel in 1958, when it had its big Type I epidemic. They did not see any difference in protection between the vaccinated and the unvaccinated."

Potency Varies Astronomically

Dr. Cox was asked if he knew of any variations in the potency of the Salk vaccine that is on the market. He replied that it varies considerably. Dr. Ratner added to this in detail: "New York State Health Department investigations reported in September, 1956, that there was a six hundredfold variation in the potency of commercial Salk vaccine on the market. . . . Today many inoculations of Salk vaccine are needed to accomplish the same results that were claimed in 1955 with one inoculation. In the history of drug therapy there are few drugs, if any, which become progressively inferior with increasing years."

A little later, Dr. Ratner made one of the most amazing declarations of a very amazing panel discussion: "To close the discussion on potency,

[845]

back in May, 1957, the largest producer of Salk vaccine in the United States had several million dollars worth of vaccine on hand which did not pass the minimum potency requirements of the United States Public Health Service. Subsequently, the Division of Biological Standards reinterpreted the minimum requirements to make possible the commercial utilization of this vaccine."

Salk Issue Confused?

Dr. Meier of the University of Chicago then commented upon the little one has heard of any doubts concerning the Salk vaccine. He said, "How is it that today you hear from members of this panel that the Salk vaccine situation is confused; yet what everybody knows from reading the newspapers, and has known since the vaccine was introduced, is that the situation, as far as the Salk vaccine is concerned, was and is marvelous? The reason for this discrepancy lies, I think, in a new attitude of many public health and publicity men. It is hard to convince the public that something is good. Consequently, the best way to push forward a new program is to decide on what you think the best decision is and not to question it thereafter, and further, not to raise questions before the public or expose the public to open discussion of the issues."

(Does that not sound like the entire fluoridation scheme?)

Dr. Cox and Dr. Ratner then spoke of the testing procedures for insuring safety of the Salk vaccine. Each offered evidence to show that, in mass production, testing procedures were pared to a minimum, and only one test, not the recommended 3 was done to determine the vaccine's safety. Figures submitted show that the vaccine used in 1955 was inadequately tested, and the cases of vaccine-induced polio which followed were not wholly a surprise to the scientists.

Live Viruses Found

Even with the recommended procedures, the vaccine's safety was doubted by some. Dr. Ratner tells us that, "In 1953, experienced investigators at the Michael Reese Hospital in Chicago failed to produce a safe vaccine by the Salk formula. Their findings were dismissed by the backers of Salk.

"In the spring of 1955, one of the manufacturers using safety tests more rigid than those required by United States Public Health Service found live virus in its own vaccine, in another manufacturer's vaccine on the open market, and in one of Dr. Salk's vaccine preparations, used as a standard for commercial vaccines. . . . Some of the released vaccine of this manufacturer, however, had already been used in Massachusetts, which experienced an epidemic. . . .

Safety Testing Inadequate

"It should be stressed that safety testing was inadequate when Dr. Salk developed his vaccine and when the vaccine was commercially prepared for the field trials of 1954, and for licensing and use in 1955. The claim of long duration of effectiveness, then, . . . really applies to a vaccine that did not exclude the presence of a live virus. *It does not apply to current vaccine in which potency has been sacrificed for safety.* (Italics ours). . . . At present, epidemiological methods employed by the United States Public Health Service to assure safety of the vaccine are inadequate."

A question was asked of the panel as to whether any state health department at present advised against the use of the Salk vaccine. Dr. Ratner said he knew of none, but presumed it to be unlikely that such a department could oppose the mass propaganda and its effect on public opinion, by doing so.

The discussion concluded with a long and rather technical talk by Dr. Cox concerning the theory and development, as well as the safety and effectiveness of the live-virus vaccines. There seemed to be little disagreement among the panelists that, if a vaccine is to be effective against polio, it will have to be a live-virus vaccine.

Public Owes Gratitude to Panelists and Journal

We believe that we owe a great debt of gratitude to the men who had the courage to participate in this panel discussion. There is no question that they have laid themselves open to professional and private reprisals. They have accused organized medicine and the government's medical authorities of conspiracy to deceive the public about the effectiveness and safety of the Salk vaccine. You can be sure this will not be taken lightly by these groups. This is especially true because of the stature of the panel members in their profession. These men can't be brushed off as cranks or know-nothings. Each of them has been especially honored by his profession for his expertness in his chosen field. These men speak with undeniable authority.

A bow should go, too, to the *Illinois Medical Journal* for printing the transcript of the discussion. We wonder how it went with the editor when his intention was made known. We wonder if he is still editor.

Complete Investigation of Campaign Is Necessary

Of course, it is impossible to carry the entire discussion in these pages, but its essence is here. Show this material to those who have been depending on the Salk vaccine to keep them and their children polio-free, in spite of bad diet and careless exposure to crowds during the season. Urge them to write to their congressmen demanding a complete public investigation of the campaign that has led Americans to believe that a Salk-vaccinated child is safe from polio. The grim fallacy of this impression is all too evident in the statistics, yet the papers, radio and TV blare out the lie again and again. The Salk vaccine is a fiasco, and the public must not be deluded any longer into believing it is anything else.

225. Confusion Reigns over the Salk Vaccine

There must have been a gasp from coast to coast on the day the *Journal of the American Medical Association* for February 25, 1961, hit the mail boxes of America's M.D.'s. The doctors who turned to the Questions and Answers pages of the *Journal* found a startling answer to a question from a Wisconsin physician concerning the effectiveness of the Salk polio vaccine. The answer, highly critical of the vaccine in general, most particularly noted the variations in the manufacturing procedure which result in "an unstandardized product of an unstandardized process." The author of this opinion is Herbert Ratner, M.D., Health Commissioner of Oak Park, Illinois. He went on to state that 335 million of the polio shots given until now were a waste because they were too weak to be effective. He went on to imply that the Salk shots are undependable, and that, unless one were to be inoculated with a complete series of an improved vaccine, one's chances against polio, regardless of the previous number of shots, were no more dependable than those of someone who had not been inoculated at all.

It was not too many hours before accusations and denials as to just what the American Medical Association meant to convey by carrying such a statement in its official publication began to fly. Dr. Ratner was identified by *Journal* spokesmen as a "competent authority" and a "qualified health officer" whose opinion "must carry weight."

"A Little Inclined to Agree with Him"

John Troan, who wrote the story for the Scripps-Howard Newspapers (*New York Herald Tribune*, March 1, 1961), quoted two of the *Journal's* staff from conversations he had with them over the phone. Dr. Wayne C. Brandstadt, an editorial assistant who chose Dr. Ratner to answer the questions, said, according to Troan, that he was "a little inclined to agree with him (Dr. Ratner)." Dr. Brandstadt held his opinion in the face of Dr. Jonas Salk's blaming the failure to use the vaccine, not the vaccine itself, for the continued occurrence of polio; and in the face of the assertion of Public Health Service epidemic expert, Dr. Alexander Langmuir, that 3 Salk doses reduce, by at least 80 per cent, a person's chances of being crippled by polio, and 4 doses cut the risk by at least 90 per cent. Said Dr. Brandstadt, "The interpretation of statistics is open to some question." He charged that the United States Public Health Service got into "an embarrassing position" by "jumping the gun a little on the Salk vaccine," and has been compelled to continue backing it "to save face."

Dr. Ratner's statement in the *Journal of the American Medical Association* was at variance with the American Medical Association's House of Delegates proclamation that the vaccine "has proved to be effective" and its urging "widest possible use" of it, pending the availability of the new live virus preparation. In an immediate effort to extricate itself from an embarrassing situation, the *Journal* announced that Dr. Ratner's answer was his own and did not represent the official view of the *Journal of the American Medical Association,* nor of the Association itself. Any signed material in a publication is legally the responsibility of the signee, not the publication. Therefore, the *Journal* was on firm ground in disavowing Dr. Ratner's opinion, at least technically.

A New Editorial Policy?

Practically speaking, the insistence on this editorial practice leaves one to wonder about the sponsorship of the rest of the answers in the Questions and Answers section of the *Journal.* Will we see more answers that are not strictly in agreement with AMA pronouncements? We would be gratified, for instance, to see an answer from Dr. Fred Exner, famous anti-fluoridationist, to the next question on the value and safety of water fluoridation. We would like to see Dr. W. C. Hueper, famous cancer expert, comment on the danger of food additives and Dr. Shute of Canada write on the value of vitamin E for heart and vascular disorders. Perhaps the *Journal* has introduced a new policy by publishing the contradictory view of Dr. Ratner on the Salk vaccine. If so, one can only applaud its forthrightness. However, in the interests of preventing a repeated misunderstanding such as that caused by Dr. Ratner's remarks, it seems to us it would be well to make this policy known more fully, perhaps in an editorial. Currently, we are convinced, most M.D.'s who read the Questions and Answers section in the *Journal of the American Medical Association,* believe that the answers reflect the current thinking of the *Journal* and of the American Medical Association. According to a regular, but inconspicuous statement on the editorial page, this is not true.

Actually, the American Medical Association has not, of itself, made a full investigation of the Salk vaccine. The Association's approval of the Salk vaccine has been based not upon its own evaluation of the vaccine, but on that of the National Foundation and the United States Public Health Service. When these two organizations decided that the Salk vaccine was effective, the officers of the American Medical Association got together to make a *policy* decision—not a scientific or medical decision, but a *political* one. They agreed that it would be to the interest of the AMA, as an organization, to go along with the National Foundation and the government health service in the approval of the Salk vaccine. Nothing more than that.

A Business Matter

The American Medical Association has a great deal of influence in the field of medicine, but it should be understood that this is a business group.

It is the job of the Association to look out for the business or professional interests of its members. It has no responsibility to us to check on the value of a medication, to warn us of its danger or its lack of effectiveness. One has as much right to demand that the United States Chamber of Commerce rule with exactness on something like the entertainment appeal of Philadelphia. The main function of the Chamber of Commerce is to look out for the business of its members. It will take the word of the mayor of Philadelphia and, perhaps, the governor of Pennsylvania, that Philadelphia is a wonderful place to play. It will tell ànyone who asks that Philadelphia is a hot bed of entertainment: (1.) because it likes to say something positive about a member city; (2.) because it trusts the opinion of the mayor and governor; (3.) because the United States Chamber of Commerce has never sent anyone to check Philadelphia's entertainment firsthand. and doesn't know differently.

One tends then to put more stock in the word of such a group than is actually intended or desired. If the Chamber of Commerce says that entertainment in Philadelphia is tops, that is a policy decision to promote the charms of Philadelphia, because the Chamber of Commerce thinks it good business to do so. If the House of Delegates of the American Medical Association decides to support the Salk vaccine, it is because the House also thinks it is good business and good policy to do so.

This is not to say that the American Medical Association ignores doing any scientific investigation on its own. To the contrary, when a question of science reaches grave proportions of controversy, as has the value of the Salk vaccine, then the AMA appoints what is termed an Ad Hoc Committee (an objective scientific group) to investigate in full detail the claims of the Salk vaccine.

Official Responsibility

Who is responsible officially for the popular opinion that the Salk vaccine is 96 per cent effective? The United States Public Health Service and the National Foundation. The National Foundation (formerly the Polio Foundation) is, again, a private organization. We have no control over its conclusions and promotions. It poured plenty of money into the Salk vaccine at a time when it needed a winner in the polio fight. The Salk vaccine was ordained to be that winner on the day Dr. Salk thought he had found the answer in his dead monkey virus. Even if it had caused polio instead of preventing it, as indeed it did in the horrible Cutter Laboratories incident, the National Foundation would probably have pumped advertising money into its sinking ship to keep it afloat. The Salk vaccine *had* to pay, or the National Foundation might have been dealt a blow from which it could never recover.

The United States Public Health Service promotion of the Salk vaccine is not so easily explained. This is a government agency, not a private one. It is an agency whose specific job it is to protect us from any dangerous or fraudulent health measures, and to investigate, scientifically, before it

[850]

approves or disapproves of anything in the health field. You pay this agency through your taxes to do only this. It is answerable to you if a mistake is made, answerable to you if its conclusions are open to question. It is, in short, answerable to you concerning Dr. Ratner's statement that 335 million Salk shots were useless due to inferior potency. Dr. Ratner gave a reputable reference for the proof of the potency variations. You have a right to insist that the United States Public Health Service disprove this finding, or modify its stand which gives the impression that the Salk vaccine has no limitations or drawbacks.

The statistics compiled and released by this government agency to prove the Salk vaccine's value have been seriously questioned by statistical experts. The very criteria for diagnosing a polio case have been changed, with the approval of this agency, in favor of the Salk vaccine, since its approval of the vaccine in 1955. The other ingredients (aside from the actual vaccine) in a standard polio shot have been blamed for causing other serious diseases.

The statements as to the number of shots needed to ward off polio have been changed so often by the United States Public Health Service that no one seems sure—even our doctors—of just how many shots are required to confer maximum immunity. (We have these current recommendations: 3, 4, 5 and 8 shots. Some say a shot a year, no matter how many the individual has had!) Yet each recommendation is made with the assurance and positiveness of the Ten Commandments. The Public Health Service's epidemic experts fluctuate in their public statements about the vaccine between its being "a disappointment" and its being "96 per cent effective." Can they actually be talking about the same vaccine? In early statements, the United States Public Health Service was jubilant about their estimate of the Salk vaccine's 85 per cent effectiveness. Can they be disappointed now when they can say that it is 96 per cent effective?

Plenty of Personnel and Money

The editorial assistant at the *Journal of the American Medical Association* suggested that the Public Health Service had "jumped the gun" on its approval of the Salk vaccine. Why should it have done such a thing? It has the personnel, the money and the duty to investigate thoroughly, and as long as necessary, any question which affects our health. The announced Sabin live-virus vaccine was under study for years before it was given an okay by this agency. It was used on millions all over the world before it was approved. The Salk vaccine was in the hands of the doctors even before the official Francis Report of its effectiveness was made known, and this was permitted without an official, independent investigation by the United States Public Health Service. This government agency took the word of the Francis Report as the basis for its approval of the vaccine for the use of United States citizens. The Francis Report was commissioned by the National Foundation, the group which sponsored the Salk vaccine. The United States Public Health Service's acting on that recommendation alone was as though one were to write to an aspirin manufacturer and ask him if his aspirin is effective, and order it on the strength of his saying yes. The answer was bound to be yes.

Hard to Turn Back

Once committed to the positive value of the Salk vaccine, the Public Health Service could hardly change its mind publicly, without looking silly and losing public confidence. So, instead, it has ordered changes in manufacturing procedure; it has changed the potency requirements up and down, and it has increased the required number of shots.

We defy the United States Public Health Service to state that the bottle of vaccine your doctor is using in his office today is even approximately the same vaccine approved by this organization in 1955. It is not, of course. The vaccine of the Francis Report is no longer being made. The vaccine we are now using has been modified for safety. This is less potent, and therefore should be, by all the laws of logic, less effective. The United States Public Health Service has increased by 10 per cent the original estimate of its effectiveness. What basis is there for so much controversy over the Salk vaccine? It is a question that must be answered. The answer should come through an open Congressional investigation of the Salk vaccine and the part played by the United States Public Health Service in promoting it. Let all of the evidence, pro and con, be gathered together so that it can be discussed and evaluated. We pay the Public Health Service to be as anxious as we are to know the truth about the Salk vaccine. They should be demanding an investigation so that they can justify their position in all of this confusion. Perhaps Senator Kefauver is the man to initiate such an investigation. Perhaps he is only waiting for the suggestion from us that he do so.

SECTION 54: PRURITUS ANI

226. Pruritus Ani

The number of articles appearing in medical journals on the subject of pruritus ani (itching or burning rectum) would seem to indicate that the disease is an extremely common one. Assuming this to be the case, we are pleased to carry a report on a very informative article by Louis H. Brooks, M.D., on his experience with a different method for relieving pruritus ani, which appeared in *Diseases of the Colon and Rectum* (September-October, 1958). In this article, Dr. Brooks tells of past findings which indicate that patients whose bowel discharges are markedly alkaline are most likely to suffer with pruritus ani. He reasoned, then, that if the rectal discharges could be somehow changed from an alkaline to an acidic character, the irritation might cease.

Attempts to transform the contents of the colon to acidic reacting substances were made. Buttermilk was somewhat successful, but malt soup extract was found to be much more effective in turning the fecal matter toward an acid reaction. This malt soup is an extract of barley which has been neutralized with potassium carbonate and concentrated into heavy syrup. Though newly applied to the problem of pruritus ani, malt soup extract has long been used in infant feeding to prevent constipation.

Malt Soup Extract Creates an Acid Climate

The malt soup extract creates, in the colon, a field in which acid bacteria are able to exist healthfully. When these bacteria predominate, the growth of putrefactive bacteria is lessened, as is the growth of certain yeast-like fungi. The putrefactive bacteria and yeast-like fungi have been shown to produce substances which are irritating to the anal canal and perianal tissues, and which are probably responsible for the itching in that region. Get rid of the undesirable bacteria and fungi, says Dr. Brooks, and the condition should correct itself in a matter of days.

Dr. Brooks tested his theory on 12 patients who suffered from the symptoms of pruritus ani. He treated each of them with malt soup extract, and in all cases, they experienced relief within 10 days of the start of treatments.

Good Results for 80 Per Cent

Careful records were kept of another group of 46 patients suffering from the same rectal problem. They ranged in age from 25 to 68 years of age, and some had suffered from pruritus ani for as long as 10 years. The administration of malt soup extract produced "good" results in 37 cases. This means that they experienced complete relief from the characteristic itching and burning, and there was a marked improvement in the tissue involved. Four cases reported "fair" results, which indicated that they had experienced relief, but that symptoms had recurred in a few weeks or months. Of the 5 in the "poor" group, who experienced inadequate relief, 3 were found to require surgery in the perianal region, and one admitted that he hadn't bothered to cooperate.

We think that such results are indeed promising and make malt soup extract worth trying when pruritus ani is the cause of discomfort. Dr. Brooks' course of treatment is quite simple. He instructs his patients, first of all, to keep the anal and perianal area scrupulously clean. To avoid any unnecessary irritation, he suggests the use of wet cotton in place of cleansing tissue, and the application of talcum powder to help in keeping the area dry. In the way of diet, Dr. Brooks forbids eating between meals, and strongly limits the intake of foods rich in sugars. In stubborn cases, reduction of meat and eggs is advised, to lessen the growth of putrefactive organisms in the colon. Alcoholic beverages are strictly forbidden. Dr. Brooks favors a liberal milk intake since it favors the growth of bacteria that thrive in an acidic medium. Yogurt and whey do exactly the same thing, and we feel that these are more desirable foods than plain milk. Mineral oil or any preparation containing it is absolutely prohibited.

The Doctor's Suggested Dosage

The author's suggested dosage for malt soup extract in pruritus ani cases is quite simple to follow: two tablespoonfuls twice a day, to be continued for several days after the symptoms have been relieved. He directs that the dosage then be reduced—we would guess to one table-spoonful two times a day, then one tablespoonful once a day—and finally discontinued. Should the symptoms return, original dosage is to be resumed. Diabetics who use malt soup extract are presumed to take account of its carbohydrate content with relation to the diet they are following.

Most doctors will tell you that there is little to be done for pruritus ani aside from surgical removal of hemorrhoids which sometimes cause similar symptoms. Malt soup extract might be the effective means of reliev-ing certain cases. However, we object to the internal use of potassium carbonate. We do not know if the malt soup extract would be effective without it. Furthermore, we know of no commercial means of obtaining the extract Dr. Brooks uses. However, if his theory is sound, any food which induces an acid-supporting environment in the colon should be effective. Again we must mention that yogurt and whey should fill this requirement very well, and they are easily obtained.

~~~~~~

SECTION 55: RABIES

~~~~~~

227. Rabies—Fact or Fancy?

Rabies, according to medical terminology, "is a virus-produced disease which causes swift destruction of the nerve cells in the hindbrain." Although it is usually carried to man by dogs, other animals also spread the infection. After a person is bitten and infected, the disease usually requires from 4 to 8 weeks to develop, but it may lie dormant for as long as a year.

Medication prescribed is to wash the wound thoroughly with soap and water, or more likely the wound is cauterized or burned with some strong acid. The animal that did the biting is then watched carefully for at least 12 days for any symptoms of rabies. If any develop, vaccination of the patient starts at once. Pasteur is given credit for developing the first vaccination for rabies when he inoculated a boy, Joseph Meister, who had been bitten by a "mad" dog.

There has been much-to-do about rabies through the years, especially since Pasteur brought rabies into the limelight with his anti-rabies vaccine. Medicine heard much of the startling cure of Joseph Meister by Pasteur, but little mention is made of the fact that 3 relatives of the Meister boy were bitten by the same dog and, without benefit of the Pasteur treatment, recovered completely.

Effectiveness of the Pasteur Treatment

Many are now beginning to question whether there is such a disease as rabies. Dr. William Brady, a popular medical syndicated writer wrote in the Berkeley *Gazette* for September 1, 1954, "I have never seen a case of rabies in man and I have never met a doctor who has seen a case, yet we know that preventative inoculation of Pasteur virus sometimes causes death. This disease is so rare in man that if it ever does occur, health authorities may well cease and desist from frightening people about 'Mad Dogs'." Dr. Brady also states, "The Pasteur treatment for rabies is a blind treatment and no one knows whether Pasteur treatment confers any protection against rabies. I'd never willingly receive Pasteur treatment or give it to anyone under any conceivable circumstances, because I fear the material so injected has a disastrous effect in some instances. It is not always successful and occasionally paralysis follows its use."

To quote an article on rabies treatment, appearing in the *San Francisco News*, July 16, 1954, "Injections with rabies vaccine themselves are hazardous. About one out of every 600 persons who undergoes the Pasteur treatment will be permanently paralyzed by the treatment itself. The doctors call these 'neuroparalytic accidents,' and the disturbing possibilities of such a fate (which some might think worse than death itself) arise every time the Pasteur treatment is begun."

The article goes on to say: "There is a popular idea that, if you are bitten by a rabid animal, you are sure to get rabies unless you undertake the Pasteur treatment; and another that, if you do undertake the Pasteur treatment, you will surely be saved from death. Both these ideas are false. It has been estimated that only one person in 10 who is bitten by a rabid animal will get rabies. And in a place like California . . . the prospects of being bitten by a rabid dog are very small. In fact though 68,000 persons are bitten in California every year (mostly by dogs), human rabies is exceedingly rare. The last case was in 1951." And even for those who are not paralyzed, the Pasteur treatment is prolonged, painful and deeply disturbing. It takes two to three weeks, depending on what course of treatment is offered. The site of the repeated injections becomes swollen, painful and feverish. And even after all this, the treatment may fail.

[855]

Some Classic Stories about Rabies

It seems the cure is more deadly than the disease. In the book, *Bèchamp or Pasteur,* by E. D. Hume (published by the C. W. Daniel Company, Ltd.), a case is recorded which is pertinent to this point. A young postman and another man were attacked by a dog supposed to be mad. The postman actually wasn't bitten, for the dog's teeth did not penetrate his clothing, but his companion received severe bites. The latter refused to go to the Pasteur Institute for inoculations and remained in perfect health. The postman was forced by the postal authorities to undergo the treatment. Several symptoms set in with pain at the point of inoculation. A few days later he died of paralytic "hydrophobia," the new disease brought into the world by Pasteur.

Another interesting recorded case is that of a young lady, who, returning from swimming, stated that she had been bitten by a dog. The anxious parents rushed her for Pasteur treatments, she became violently ill and death followed. On the way home from the funeral, the girl's companions who were swimming with her told the parents of the dead girl that she was not bitten by a dog, but by her young man friend.

An article in the *Archives of Neurology and Psychiatry* for January, 1951, gives an account of two patients who became paralyzed after they had been treated by the Pasteur vaccine. Both these young men had had anti-rabies injections in their childhood. Both developed acute paralysis after the later injection, and one of them died.

In speaking of the incidence of fatalities, the article reports that incidence "ranges from one in 280 treated patients to one in 8,287." No explanation is given to show why two statisticians should arrive at two such different sets of figures. World-wide incidence of death from rabies vaccine is said to be one in every 6000 or so.

Medical Authorities against Pasteur Treatment

A report in the *Journal of the American Medical Association* for January 14, 1956, relates the happenings at a meeting of the Academy of Medicine in France, where a Dr. Hasegawa and his co-workers spoke sharply against the use of the Pasteur vaccination for rabies. They pointed out that it may be followed as long as 20 years later by a disorder called Korsakoff's psychosis, which is a state of delirium. Twenty years after the injection! They also said that, in a study of 460 patients treated with the Pasteur injection after being bitten by a rabid animal, 20 died.

They had prepared a different kind of vaccine which they claimed gave complete protection without fatalities. We have no way of knowing what may happen to *their* treated patients 20 years from now, though, do we?

The *Indiana State Medical Journal* for December, 1950, reported the case of a man of 25 bitten by a rabid dog in 1948, who received the Pasteur treatment at once. At the end of the full course of treatment he became paralyzed from the waist down and died shortly thereafter. The authors say that no one knows what causes these paralytic reactions! However, it has been definitely established, they say, *that they are not caused by the rabies virus.* In other words, vaccination, not rabies, is the danger here. The authors go on to quote Sellers, another authority, who believes that "not hydrophobia, but rather rabiphobia is the most troublesome problem." Fear of rabies, then, is what we have to fear most.

Time magazine in their November 19, 1951, issue gave some advice on what *not* to do if you get a dog bite. It seems there is conclusive evidence that a dog bite, like any flesh wound, should not be cauterized or burned with a strong acid. "It was proved 8 years ago that rabies virus can be removed from a wound more thoroughly by soap and water than by nitric acid or any other cauterizing agents." A doctor using these agents converts the wounds into acid burns which will leave permanent, disfiguring scars.

Meaning of the "Rabies Scare"

Most occurrences of rabies turn out to be nothing but "rabies scare." A dog may die from the heat or from some other cause, due to poor treatment, and right away the "rabies scare" gets out. All dog owners are then urged to take their dogs to get inoculated against rabies, and in some localities it is compulsory.

A famous ex-dancer of the World War I era, Irene Castle, spent the last 3 decades fighting for a better life for dogs and other animals. Miss Castle, fighting measures taken by Chicago Public Health authorities to combat rabies, once challenged the Board of Health to let a rabid dog bite her. She was willing to bet 5,000 dollars that she would not die, but the head of the board refused to accept the bet.

The "rabies scare" seems to be another outgrowth of Pasteur's false assumptions, which have been accepted by medicine blindly without proper investigation. The best preventive measure of course is to keep animals in such a healthy well-nourished state that they cannot possibly develop any disease. And keep yourself and your family in that same blissful state, too. If by chance—and the chance these days is very slim indeed—someone should be bitten by a rabid animal, we would suggest washing the wound with water, letting it bleed so that any foreign matter will be washed away, and then taking massive doses of vitamin C, which fights and destroys all kinds of poisons, including so-called "viruses."

One last story which indicates clearly that probably thousands of deaths from Pasteur treatment go unreported. An acquaintance of Editor Rodale died recently, from a heart attack supposedly. His family told us that he had been bitten by a dog and rushed to the doctor for the Pasteur treatment. There was no waiting to see whether or not the dog was rabid. No tests were given to the patient. He was a diabetic. Should this not have made some difference in the treatment he received? Is it not possible that any number of disease conditions might make for many and serious complica-

[857]

tions in the presence of vaccinations as potent and devastating as the Pasteur rabies treatment?

The patient died, but the family is convinced he did not die of a heart attack. They say he died as a result of the Pasteur treatment. How many other cases like this happen regularly all over the country?

And what about the undisputed medical fact that morbid complications can occur as long as 20 years after the Pasteur treatment is given? Might not the same be true of the Salk vaccine? Is it possible that we will not know for 20 years the full effects of all the "needles" our children get these days? And by that time who is going to trace the cause and the effect? Who is going to be able to?

~~~~~~

SECTION 56: SCURVY

~~~~~~

228. Scurvy Yesterday and Today

In 1753 appeared a medical manuscript that revolutionized thinking about medicine and disease. Dr. James Lind's *A Treatise of the Scurvy* was printed. Dr. Lind believed that scurvy (a plague responsible for many deaths) had something to do with food. So he performed the first well-controlled experiment in human nutrition of which we have any record. He used 12 sailors who had scurvy. He fed all of them a diet typical of the food eaten on sailing ships at that time—mutton, hardtack, sugar, rice, barley. Two of the sailors got nothing but this diet, the rest got the following additions: two got one quart of cider a day, two got 25 drops of sulfuric acid in water, two got vinegar, two, sea water, two, oranges and lemons. The two men who got the oranges and lemons began to improve immediately. All of the rest became worse, except for the two who got the cider. They improved, too, but very, very slowly. So Dr. Lind showed by this experiment, not just that scurvy is caused by the lack of a certain kind of food, but he also showed what kind of food that is. It was not until 50 years later, however, that the British Navy made use of this knowledge by requiring all of its sailors to take lemon juice daily. Twenty years after that, the American Navy followed suit.

It is hard for us to understand—at our period of history—what a frightful thing was scurvy and what a tremendous influence it had on the course of history. The Crusaders suffered from scurvy. It was a plague that devastated country after country. Listen to this description taken from an account written by Don Sebastian Vizcaino who came to the California coast in 1603: "We did not enter (the harbor) because the state of our health was so bad and the sick were clamoring, although there was neither assistance nor medicines nor food to give them except rotten jerked beef, gruel, biscuits and beans and chick peas spoiled by weevils.

"The mouths of all were sore, and their gums were swollen larger than their teeth, so that they could hardly drink water, and the ship seemed more like a hospital than a ship of an armada. Affairs were in such a condition that anyone who had ever in his life been at the helm steered, climbed to the main topsail, and did the other tasks, and all who could walk assisted at the hearth, making gruel and porridge for the sick."

Scurvy Was Sometimes Cured

When they finally landed they found a small fruit (possibly a cactus) which they ate raw. Within six days, there was not a sore mouth among the sailors. Vizcaino lays this healing power to the "strength" of the fruit, claiming that it caused the ulcers to slough off and bleed profusely.

Soldiers, sailors, explorers of olden times were fit victims for scurvy, for the food carried on the ships or military expeditions was similar to that described above by Don Vizcaino. But, in addition, scurvy was frequently an epidemic disease among civilian populations until quite recent times. Before the days of refrigeration and modern transportation, northern countries were completely without fresh fruits and vegetables for months at a time. There were 30,000 cases of scurvy among the soldiers in our own Civil War. During the first World War, there were more than 11,000 cases of scurvy and 7,500 fatalities from it among Allied soldiers fighting in the Near East. More sailors have died of scurvy than have been killed in all the naval battles ever fought.

Captain Cook, the famous sailor who took his ship on a 3-year voyage around the world, carried a supply of barley on board which was sprouted and made into a drink. The Captain decreed at first that only officers were privileged to have this drink. The sailors got the idea that it must be something very special, so they insisted on having a daily drink as well. Although Captain Cook could not possibly have known it, sprouted grain is rich in vitamin C. None of his men got scurvy during those 3 years.

In the early days of colonization of this country, a group of sailors desperately ill from scurvy was put ashore on the New England coast to die. Indians who found them gave them a tea made from evergreen needles which cured their scurvy almost overnight and they rejoined their ship. From incidents like this, sprang the notion that scurvy had something to do with the sea and that "the circumambient Air and the Fruits of the Ground will prove the best Remedies," as one eighteenth century authority puts it.

[859]

What Is Scurvy?

Eddy and Dahldorf, in their book, *The Avitaminoses* (Williams and Wilkins), define scurvy as a disease in which defective materials are formed in the cement between the body cells. When vitamin C is completely lacking in the diet, certain skeletal tissues form a fluid material rather than their natural products, dentine and bone. If vitamin C is given, this material rapidly jells or solidifies.

One group of scientists believes that lack of vitamin C causes the skeletal tissue cells to atrophy or become useless. This results in less oxygen consumption by the cells, reduced digestive juices in the stomach, reduced content of hormones in the adrenal glands, retarded hematopoiesis (the formation of blood) and a decrease in the ability of the individual to fight infection.

It is interesting to note that another researcher, Glasunow, defines scurvy as the "loss of the ability of differentiation" by the mesenchyme. The mesenchyme is that part of the body which produces all the connective tissues—the blood vessels, the blood, etc. We have been told by cancer researchers that cancer is nothing more or less than the body's loss of the power to differentiate between two kinds of cells—the normal cells and cancerous cells. Do the two statements above seem to you to indicate that one's dietary supply of vitamin C may be closely related to one's susceptibility to cancer?

Guinea pigs develop scurvy and die very rapidly on a diet completely deficient in vitamin C. Their blood vessels become fragile, their teeth develop disorders, they waste away and generally die at the end of the third week of a diet containing absolutely no vitamin C at all. If they are given diets just partly deficient in vitamin C, they develop a condition much like scurvy in man. Researchers have discovered many interesting things about scurvy in guinea pigs in relation to man's need for vitamin C. For instance, the condition of the bones and joints of guinea pigs with scurvy resembles very much the condition of the bones and joints of human beings with arthritis and rheumatism. Eddy and Dahldorf tell us that many researchers believe these diseases, especially when they occur in the winter and spring, are due to partial vitamin C starvation.

They go on to say, "Boyle has described the effects of scurvy on the alveolar bone (the tooth socket) and states that vitamin C deficiency is the only nutritional disease, in his experience, which produces the characteristic features of systemic pyorrhea." Guinea pigs with scurvy often have premature litters. The young may be born dead or may grow slowly. Animals with scurvy suffer from anemia which can be cured by giving vitamin C. Their joints are tender and swollen. There may be disease of the thyroid gland. The nerves degenerate.

In human scurvy, there may be hemorrhages in any part of the body. The bones become deformed. The teeth become diseased. The gums swell and bleed easily. The skin is subject to bruises. The person with scurvy is pale and anemic. His heart may be enlarged. His stomach may be congested and there may be small ulcers.

Say Eddy and Dahldorf, "Mild, atypical cases of scurvy are much more frequent than clinically definite ones. They masquerade as rheumatism, gingivitis (gum inflammation), purpura (hemorrhages), hemophilia (bleeder's disease) and osteomyelitis . . . But there are still more individuals who lack even these symptoms of scurvy and yet who prove to be depleted of the vitamin." Doctors use the term "subclinical scurvy" to describe such a condition. The most common symptoms are lassitude, lack of appetite, fatigue and rheumatic pains. Does that describe anyone you know?

How Many of Us Are Deficient in Vitamin C?

Today, we believe scurvy is perhaps even more a menace than it was in the days when it carried off thousands of people in epidemics. Today, we suffer from subclinical scurvy. Colds, infections, sinus trouble, bleeding gums, pyorrhea, mineral deficiency, rheumatism, cancer, loose teeth, cataract—the list of ailments is almost endless—how many of these can be related to a daily diet in which we get enough vitamin C to keep us from going to bed ill with scurvy, but not enough vitamin C to keep us healthy?

An article in the *American Practitioner and Digest of Treatment* for August, 1954, reviews the findings of a physician, G. E. Morris, who declares that 5.45 per cent of the new patients seen by him were suffering from "frank or latent scurvy." Laboratory tests revealed that they were short on vitamin C, although, of course, many of them had come to the doctor for other complaints.

These patients were from all walks of life and all believed that they were eating good nutritious diets. Eight of them had scurvy symptoms and the rest showed low vitamin C levels in their blood. Four of the patients were students in a theological seminary and eating the diet served there. All of them got well as soon as plenty of vitamin C was added to their diet.

The *British Medical Journal* for November 13, 1954, reports 6 cases of infantile scurvy—and the article begins with a quotation from a prominent physician who says, "Today, in its grossest manifestations, (scurvy) may be said to have ceased to exist." Yet the 6 infants, living chiefly on boiled milk, had scurvy just as surely as the sailors who were too sick to get their vessel to shore in California in 1603. One of the children, incidentally, was diagnosed as a case of "multiple arthritis" until the diagnosis of scurvy was proved when vitamin C worked a complete cure. In the January 1, 1955, issue of the same medical journal a further case of infantile scurvy is reported. In this case, the diet since birth had been boiled milk with cereals and some orange juice *diluted with boiling water!*

The *New York State Medical Journal* for June, 1953, reported a case of scurvy in a breast-fed child. In this instance, the mother herself was so deficient in vitamin C that her milk could not supply enough of the vitamin

[861]

to keep the child healthy. A report in the *Bulletin of the Johns Hopkins Hospital* for December, 1950, describes the prevalence of scurvy at autopsy during the first two years of age. The bones of 1303 children were examined. Sixty-nine cases of scurvy were found. It is interesting that only 6 of these had been diagnosed as scurvy when the child was brought to the hospital. Two-thirds of the infants with scurvy had had acute diseases, most of them infectious. It was clear that the scurvy ante-dated the infectious diseases. In the *Journal of the Medical Society of New Jersey,* for February, 1951, 3 cases of scurvy in infants are described. The *Canadian Medical Journal* for December, 1950, relates the story of 37 cases of scurvy seen at the Children's Hospital in Halifax. Undoubtedly, a thorough search through medical literature would reveal much more information along these lines.

But, you may say, these isolated cases simply indicate that some mothers have not been well enough educated to the importance of vitamin C. This is true and we believe that American infants in general are far less likely to be deficient in vitamin C than their older brothers and sisters. The *Journal of Tropical Medicine and Hygiene* for August, 1950, describes an appalling deficiency in vitamin C among residents of a tropical town. Ninety per cent of all those examined had blood levels of vitamin C below normal. Sixty per cent were far below normal and 30 per cent showed levels suggestive of scurvy. The *Journal of the American Dietetic Association* for August, 1952, carried an article about a survey among Louisiana children. Say the authors, Margaret H. Dallyn and Dorothy S. Moschette of Louisiana State University, "The serum ascorbic acid values of Louisiana school children were found, on the whole, to be low. A serum concentration of 0.6 milligrams or more per 100 milliliters has been used by many workers as a standard . . . Only 48.6 per cent of the 463 children studied had serum levels of at least 0.6 milligrams per 100 milliliters." Only about 61 per cent of the 8 and 9 year olds and 44 per cent of the 10 and 11 year olds were receiving the daily allowance of ascorbic acid recommended by the National Research Council. When the children were examined, it was found that there was a "significant association" between vitamin C intake and blood content and the changes in the gums that mean "too little vitamin C."

Subclinical Scurvy Is Today's Disease

W. J. McCormick, M.D., of Toronto, tells us, in an article in the *Archives of Pediatrics* for January, 1954, that he has examined more than 5,000 patients and has found *that less than 10 per cent of them had the optimum amount of vitamin C in their blood at any given time.* The *Journal of Periodontology,* Vol. 23, p. 228, 1952, describes patients suffering from one form or another of gum diseases, in which 44 per cent showed signs of vitamin C deficiency. *California Medicine,* Vol. 74, p. 105, 1951 tells us that, of institutional inmates over the age of 50, 87 per cent are deficient in vitamin C. The *New York Times* for July 11, 1954, gave the results of a two-year study by Rutgers University scientists who interviewed 600 men in industrial plants. Nearly one-third were low in vitamin C.

Who says scurvy has disappeared from the scene? Of all the individuals mentioned in the statistics above, probably not one was put to bed with "purple spots two fingers high" and so forth, as scurvy was described in the old accounts. But aren't all these folks suffering from scurvy—to a greater or less extent? Our official research council has decided upon a given amount of vitamin C as the least anyone can take every day and avoid scurvy. Yet, vast numbers of people, as the statistics above show, are not getting even that minimum amount in their food. And the rest of us are apparently getting only enough vitamin C to prevent us from being actually sick.

229. Don't Wait for a Scurvy Diagnosis

No one knows, yet, the full impact of vitamin C in the diet. Since this vitamin is the very thing which holds our cells together, and since every bit of the body—the eyes, the liver, the heart, the hair, the fingernails, the skin, everything—is made up of cells, the value of vitamin C cannot be overestimated. When the cement of the cells is missing, tissues tend to give way. Skin breaks develop, capillaries and veins rupture under the stress of their normal job; stomach linings become weak enough to be attacked by gastric juices, and the result is ulcers. So it is true that, as we become more and more deficient in vitamin C, we quite literally fall apart.

How is this "falling apart" recognizable? Dr. Ian A. Kellock, M.D., described the condition in the *Medical Press* (July 12, 1961). He also told how a vitamin C deficiency can occur to the point of scurvy, even in a country where fresh foods are available. Social scurvy (scurvy is the technical name for extreme vitamin C deficiency) occurs chiefly in older males (usually widowers) who live alone in a place where sleeping quarters alone are provided. They have to fend for themselves for the first time in old age, and they tend toward an amazing uniformity of diet which is usually inadequate. They might eat corn flakes at every meal, or a steady diet of bread and jam. Sometimes it's because these men don't know how to cook anything else, or they don't want to learn; sometimes they can't afford much else and sometimes they are perfectly content to eat only these simple and nutritionally barren foods. These conditions may last for months, even years.

Iatrogenic Scurvy

There is another group subject to what the author calls "iatrogenic or therapeutic scurvy." These people take special diets—often on medical advice—and stay with them religiously. These diets often consist of milk drinks, cereals, custards, soups, mashed potatoes, etc., and are almost completely lacking in vitamin C.

One should mention here that self-imposed diets are often not well-rounded, and might be distressingly short of vitamin C or some other vitamins. Any diet should have ample amounts of all the vitamins and minerals, plus enough protein, to keep the body functioning well.

The bare minimum of vitamin C is 30 milligrams per day. That amount, it is thought, will keep one from being confined to bed due to a vitamin C shortage. We feel that this figure is grossly inadequate to the needs of anyone who must live in the day-to-day civilization we know. With every breath and with every bite of food, we acquire noxious poisons which require vitamin C for their safe neutralization.

Perhaps it is because of the many unrecognized thieves of vitamin C today, that the frank scurvy that was once considered to be a clinical curiosity now occurs with fair frequency. Dr. Kellock tells of 11 cases seen in the wards of two London hospitals within a period of 6 years. Another doctor described 75 cases of scurvy seen over a period of 15 years. As one expert put it, ". . . to describe the condition as a rarity or a clinical curiosity in this country (England) is surely an overstatement." We are certain that the same statement applies in the United States as well.

The Way Scurvy Acts

What is scurvy like? Dr. Kellock lays out the symptoms for us. It is painful, and the pain is characterized as a "rheumatic" feeling, usually an aching in the legs or in the back. Sometimes there is a stiffness of the legs. The patient often believes himself to be a lumbago victim. Aside from the pain, the scurvy patient feels weak and tired; his appetite is almost nonexistent. He may have a dry cough, get dizzy spells on the least exertion. His gums may be sore and may bleed. He might even spit blood.

That is the way the patient feels scurvy. The signs the doctor must look for are these: bruising—spontaneous bruising is one of the most common signs of scurvy in adults. Touching the skin lightly is often enough to cause this phenomenon in such persons, because the capillary walls which contain the blood are so very weak, due to a lack of vitamin C. Hemorrhages of the mucous membranes—around the nose and mouth and the eyes may also occur. Bronchitis is a fairly frequent manifestation of subclinical scurvy.

The outward manifestations are practically endless, as can be imagined when one reflects upon the place of vitamin C in maintaining our physiology. There can be eruptions of the skin around hair follicles or an inflammation in the area, fever, jaundice, grey skin color, aggravation of acne conditions, low blood pressure and stoppage of circulation announced by the blue color of the skin. Anemia is often present.

A Case of Scurvy

An interesting example of the way improper diet can lead to scurvy is presented by Dr. Kellock. A widower, aged 64, was admitted to the hospital. Ten years prior to his admission, he had been told he had a duodenal ulcer for which he was given a diet sheet. The sheet actually made provision for the addition of vegetables after the third week, but the patient hadn't noticed this, so for 10 years he firmly held to a diet consisting mainly of fish and eggs, with occasional porridge (much like our cream of wheat), bread, butter and jam. He ate no vegetables at all.

Two weeks before admission to the hospital, he noticed purple bruises on his legs. He also complained of pain in his ankle.

The examining physician reported his general appearance to be pale and sallow. He had no teeth, but his gums were healthy, in spite of "blood spots" on the roof and floor of the mouth, and large red and purple swellings at the knee and ankle. X-rays showed generalized conditions compatible with bronchitis and shortness of breath.

The treatment consisted of nothing but vitamin C—1,000 milligrams each morning. The response was gratifying and all outward abnormalities soon disappeared. His legs were almost completely normal in less than 3 weeks and his blood count had greatly improved to well above the minimum. He was discharged with a maintenance dose of 150 milligrams of vitamin C plus added ferrous sulfate.

Interestingly enough, after 10 years on what he thought was a proper ulcer diet, X-rays showed that the patient's ulcer was still present. Of course, we know that with a diet that is short of vitamin C, it would be useless to hope for the healing of a break in the tissue, which is what an ulcer actually is. Several researchers have shown that high dosages of vitamin C serve as an excellent therapeutic measure in cases of ulcer.

One is amazed to imagine how the patient managed so long on the low vitamin C intake he was getting. Imagine his plight if a serious infection had attacked him. The need for vitamin C in such a case cannot be overemphasized. Dr. Kellock recommends, especially for the elderly, self-imposed or deliberate diets planned to contain adequate amounts of vitamin C.

We believe that everyone should keep a close eye on his diet to assure proper vitamin C intake. While special situations faced by older people do present a hazard as to sufficient vitamin C foods in their diets, it must be admitted that most of us face the same possibility. Children whose parents allow them to indulge in sweets, in sodas, in pretzels and potato chips, at the expense of their appetites when nutritional foods are presented to them, have cause to be concerned over possible vitamin C deficiency. Mothers who rush through the busy day on a few cups of coffee and a bun or two, and fathers who snack on a soda and a hot dog for lunch, or maybe a candy bar in between, are excellent candidates for vitamin C shortage.

No Sense in Waiting for Scurvy

There is no sense to waiting for bruises, bleeding gums or swellings to appear before taking stock of one's vitamin C intake. We say take no chances on missing out on sufficient vitamin C. You can never be sure you have enough, unless you actually run daily tests. Each day's needs are different. If your nerves are taut because the children have been particularly trying, if nothing has worked smoothly that day, if you are seething because of a disagreement, if the boss has been demanding too much of you, you are using extra vitamin C. If you are exposed to weather that is unusually hot, or unusually cold, if you've slept poorly, burned yourself on the stove, smoked even one cigarette, you are using extra vitamin C. If you've eaten foods with chemical additives, drunk liquor, been in a poorly ventilated room, breathed exhaust from a car or smelled cleaning fluid, you've needed extra vitamin C. If infection is in the air, vitamin C is needed to combat it. If you're having an operation—or a baby—you'll need more vitamin C to help your body to function properly.

You see, the day's need for vitamin C is utterly unpredictable and the body does not store this vitamin. How can the same amount that gets one through a peaceful day of vacation be enough on a day of crisis? How can a person who suffers from arthritis get along on the same amount as a high school pupil? He cannot, of course. So we say everybody should eat plenty of fresh fruits and vegetables which have a high vitamin C content, and a daily natural supplement of vitamin C as well. If there should be an excess, the body will quickly eliminate it, and no harm done. The important thing is to have what is needed when it is needed. Proper supplementation is the only way to do that.

Scurvy is not so rare as we thought and we are sure that cases of "almost-scurvy" are really quite common. Don't let it happen to you.

230. Modern Infants' Diets Can Lead to Scurvy

It was not until about 100 years ago that scurvy became known in small children. Doctors didn't believe it. They diagnosed all around it, but could hardly bring themselves to call it scurvy. "Acute rickets" was a favorite designation. Finally, the disease was defined as infantile scurvy, and treated as such.

The strange thing about all of this is that scurvy in small children has persisted even until today. In an article discussing this phenomenon, in the *Medical Journal of Australia* (August 22, 1959), the authors, Turner, Pitt and Thomson, tell us this shocking fact: "All over the Western World, where the general standard of nutrition is good, infantile scurvy appears to be on the increase. An increase has been recorded in certain states of the U.S.A., in Canada and in Glasgow . . ." They go on to say that Australia is worst of all, however, and note that 5 children's hospitals there recorded 256 cases from 1954 to August, 1958.

What Is Responsible?

It is interesting to note here that the first cases of infantile scurvy occurred only after the introduction of artificial feeding for babies. It is understandable when one discovers that human milk contains about 4 times as much vitamin C as cow's milk. Also, the infants' shortage of adequate vitamin C is explained by the fact that, if a pregnant woman is possessed of an adequate vitamin C diet, she can pass enough on to her child before he is born to last for his first 5 months after birth. This is the much talked-of immunity to disease babies are said to be born with. Of course, with the diet followed by many modern mothers-to-be, the baby they carry is quite likely to miss even enough vitamin C to hold him for a single day after birth. And then, if he is not nursed by the mother and drinks only cow's milk, with what little vitamin C it had boiled out of it, scurvy is not far behind.

A Survey Shows Similarities

In order to understand more thoroughly just what can cause scurvy so frequently in these times, a survey was made of cases by the State Department of Health in Victoria, a province of Australia. The patients all ranged between 7 and 10 months of age. Symptoms were similar: the child, at first, lost his appetite and was unduly irritable. Following this, some kind of infection set in—tonsilitis, earache or a fever. Then the actual signs peculiar to scurvy would begin to show. The child resented any movement, and screamed at even being touched. It would not crawl or walk, but lay quite still. Tenderness and weakness were present in the lower limbs of all patients, and some had tender swellings along the shafts of the long bones. Because of the pain and immobility, physicians sometimes diagnosed the illness as polio. However, the telltale swollen gums and skin hemorrhages were present in many of the cases and helped with the diagnosis.

Little Mother's Milk and Plenty of Canned Food

It was determined that none of these children had been breast fed for more than 3 months, and almost half had been weaned in less than two weeks after birth. Solid foods had been given in most cases, but usually canned foods. In most cases, no vitamin C had been given in any form, be it tablets, drops, juices or fresh fruits. Some mothers said they had

[867]

administered multi-vitamin preparations. Still, when therapy was begun, their children responded as immediately as the rest.

All of the scurvy cases were the youngest of several children in the family, usually about fourth. The mother had become careless about supplementary nutrition by this time. Many of the youngsters were of poor families living in slums, and some were families who did not understand the English language and did not know the value of fresh fruits, juices and supplementary vitamins.

The response to treatment with ascorbic acid, 50 to 100 milligrams two to three times a day, was so dramatic (freedom from symptoms in the following 3 to 4 days), that the parents were not at all impressed with the importance of the disease. How could it be serious if it were cured so easily? Yet it must be considered that the suffering experienced by the babies is not to be invited again by feeling parents.

A Lesson for Americans

The attending physicians noted one cause of scurvy in infants which should hit home among Americans. Parents tend to abandon older food customs and discontinue breast feeding, although they readily cooperate with sterilizing milk formulae and other foods. They do not realize that, by sterilizing, they automatically cut down the infants' ascorbic acid intake. Say the authors: "There is a general tendency to abandon the use of home-cooked infant foods and rely more and more on sterilized, tinned, pasteurized, autoclaved and denatured foodstuffs, *without a corresponding adequate realization of the importance of supplementary practices.*" (Italics ours.)

We hope that the work of these Australian doctors will serve to answer the question of the American mother who hesitates to give her child food supplements, lest he have some difficulty in digesting or absorbing them. A child cannot afford to be without them! Vitamin C in the form of a rose hip or acerola tablet should be crushed and added to every day's cereal or batch of formula, along with a teaspoonful of B complex-rich brewer's yeast for good digestion and calmness.

Think over the causes of modern infantile scurvy and consider the ease with which it could occur in babies you know, perhaps even in your own child. Take steps to prevent this most preventable of all diseases. Make sure the mother-to-be and the child, once it is born, have a certain supply of vitamin C through natural foods and natural food supplements.

231. The Sinus

The sinus can be most easily defined as a hole in the head—except for the fact that we have not just one hole in the head, but many. Sinuses, that is. Their purpose is surely not just to cause us trouble, yet sometimes it seems as though they had been created specifically for that.

Actually, the sinuses in one's head are holes in the bones of the skull. They help to lighten the bony structure which would otherwise be quite a burden to carry around. In addition, they act as sound boxes for the voice. The vocal chords might be compared to the strings of a violin. The sinuses, then, are like the space enclosed in the violin proper in which the sound waves reverberate. It is not by accident that many of our greatest singers have come from the sunny countries of the south, such as Italy, where vitamin D is plentiful and hence bony structure is good. The nasal passages, sinuses and throat of a Caruso have a great deal to do with the magnificence of his voice.

Names of the Various Sinuses

Here are the words of a famous sinus expert, describing the different sinuses and their location. Says Dr. Lucius Bush, in his book, *The Secret of Sinusitis and Headaches* (Liveright Publications), "Let us see how these sinuses are arranged. I mentioned previously the sphenoid sinuses, a pair of sinuses high up and toward the back of the nasal passages. The openings from these sinuses point almost directly forward. In front of them and slightly below are the posterior ethnoid sinuses which drain inwardly toward the nasal septum, the partition which separates one nasal passage from the other. There may be a half a dozen or more of these posterior ethnoid sinuses. In front of them, lie the anterior ethnoid sinuses which drain mostly in an outward and downward direction. Both anterior and posterior ethnoid sinuses lie in the ethnoid bone about the middle turbinate (another bone). Near the anterior ethnoid openings are the openings of the frontal sinuses and antra. The frontal sinuses lie in the forehead above and between the eyebrows and their openings point downward, while the antra lie in the face under the eyes and drain upward into the nasal passages. In all, we find an average of fifteen or twenty nasal sinuses in the normal head. Some open outward, some inward, some up and some down."

There is no reason to remember all the names of the various sinuses, unless your doctor uses them in diagnosing your case and you want to have some idea of what he is talking about. What it boils down to is that all these various holes are grouped about your nose, and drain, one way or the other, into your nasal passages. Sinusitis and sinus trouble of any kind are involved chiefly with the drainage problem. As you can see from Dr. Bush's statement, the sinuses open up or down or out or in.

You see, the openings from most of these sinuses into the nasal passages are no bigger than the thickness of the lead in a pencil. The secretions that accumulate when one has a cold are thick and gummy. They can't get through! Dr. Bush explains the peculiar position in which the sinuses open by saying that we were meant to clear the sinuses of mucus by blowing our noses. Air can be blown forcibly through the nasal passage, says he, and it is blown over the 15 or 20 individual sinus openings, if the nasal passage is normal. The passage of air creates suction which draws the liquid up so that it can be expelled by the air. So in the normal nose, it is easy to empty all of the sinuses simply by blowing the nose. Hence many people never have any trouble at all with their sinuses and don't know what it means to suffer the excruciating pain of sinusitis.

The sinusitis sufferer, on the other hand, has obstructed nasal passages for one reason or another and so fluid secretions collect in his head. The pressure of the fluid is what makes the pain. Someone whose nasal passages are narrow may be able to keep them well drained most of the time. But when a cold comes along and the mucous membrane inside his nasal passages swells, fluid may accumulate and sinusitis may be upon him.

232. How's Your Sinusitis?

If you have a healthy and well-formed nose, you probably won't have sinus trouble. If you were born with nasal passages that are too narrow to perform their function, or if you have suffered from a blow on the nose, chances are that you have or may develop sinusitis.

The sinuses (cavities in the bones of the skull) open into the nasal passages. In some cases, this small opening is at the bottom of the sinus; in some cases, it is at the top or the side. Normally, blowing one's nose clears all secretions from the sinuses, for, as the air passes over the sinus openings, the suction created draws the fluid out into the nose. However, if the passages of the nose are too small to accommodate the air, or if some injury to the nose has closed up those passages, the mechanism will not work and secretions begin to accumulate in the sinuses. Then, too, when you get a cold, the mucous membrane of the nose swells and may shut off the nasal passages. Most cases of severe sinusitis start from a bad cold.

Lucius M. Bush, M.D., (in his book, *The Secret of Sinusitis and Headache*) tells us that man has a long history of sinusitis. Ancient skulls show the effects of surgery which was performed apparently to ease the pain of sinusitis. In fact, Dr. Bush goes so far as to say that more than half of the human beings who ever lived have had acute or chronic inflammation of the nasal sinuses. He also believes that at least two-thirds of the world's headaches are related to sinus disorder.

He tells us that the nasal membrane is extremely sensitive to all kinds of influences. A little loss of sleep, cold or wet feet or a draft at the neck may be all that is necessary to cause the membrane to swell and become congested. Many people even have some nasal congestion after a heavy meal. In head colds, the inflammation spreads along the mucous membrane into the sinus. It cannot get out, since the membrane has swollen, so it causes more mucus, which produces pressure inside the sinus. The accumulated fluid becomes coagulated, thick and gummy. When there is enough of this fluid to overflow, it is forced out into the nasal passage, but the sinus is by no means drained. If the nasal passages are too narrow, or swollen with congestion from the cold, the rest of the mucilagenous matter remains in the sinus and causes more and more irritation.

Operations for sinus conditions are not notably successful. When surgeons make new openings into the sinus cavities, the bones and cartilage tend to grow back together, so the project fails and the sinus fills up with fluid once more.

Dr. Bush's Treatment

Dr. Bush has developed a unique method of treatment which resulted from a cold that he himself contracted. Using his finger, he pushed against the side wall of the nasal passage, which relieved the congestion in his nose. When it became stuffed again, he repeated the massage and found that gradually his nose cleared and he was able to breathe once again. Trying the treatment on his patients, he found that he could obtain a marked clearing of their noses and eventually complete relief from their symptoms of congestion.

One patient of his had breathed through one side of his nose for years. The nasal passage on the other side was almost completely blocked. After a number of treatments, the passage opened and his breathing became normal once again. Polyps in the nose also seemed to disappear when the proper ventilation was provided in these passageways. Dr. Bush also found that many patients suffering from asthma had narrowed nasal passages which he could manipulate to relieve the stuffiness in their heads.

Diet Can Prevent Sinus Difficulties

It is well to keep in mind how important diet is in the formation and maintenance of well-formed mouth and nasal passages. Prospective mothers can assure their children of good bone formation by eating diets in which refined foods are reduced to a minimum and vitamins A and D are plentifully supplied, as well as calcium and the other important minerals. Of course, what the child eats while he is growing is important, too. Dr. Weston Price, in his book, *Nutrition and Physical Degeneration,* available from the

Lee Foundation for Nutritional Research, 2023 West Wisconsin Avenue, Milwaukee, Wisconsin, presents priceless evidence that primitive peoples who have never known our "civilized" food show, without exception, broad, well-constructed mouth and nose formation. Just as soon as they begin to eat our diets, including white flour and white sugar products, the bone structure begins to change within one generation. Their teeth become crowded, the dental arch is small and narrow and their noses take on a narrow pinched look.

The best book we know on the subject of sinus and diet is that by Egon V. Ullmann, M.D., entitled *Diet in Sinus Infections and Colds*, published by Macmillan Company, 60 Fifth Avenue, New York, New York. Dr. Ullmann believes firmly that modern diet is largely responsible for sinusitis. We have come to think of colds and sinusitis chiefly in terms of infections, says Dr. Ullmann, and our concept of infection has led us to believe that the infection—present through some mysterious means—is responsible for the cold and also for the feelings of ill health that go with it.

Instead today, he says, "the trend is to look for constitutional changes which render our organism more susceptible to colds and their consequences. For want of a clearer definition we shall call the combination of constitutional weaknesses, which so often leads to a series of colds, *lowered resistance* or a *run-down condition*." The one symptom that is present in all patients with colds and sinus infections is acidosis, he continues. In other words, these patients have not been getting enough of the alkaline-forming foods in their diets.

Going further in his discussion of foods, Dr. Ullmann tells us that one of the early symptoms of vitamin A deficiency is lowered resistance to colds. Vitamin A is necessary to maintain the tissues in the skin of the body and the linings of body openings, such as the throat and nose. The mucous membrane in these linings is known to dry up considerably during the early stages of a cold. Exactly the same condition can be produced in laboratory animals by depriving them of vitamin A. Dr. Ullmann recommends natural vitamin A as it occurs in fish liver oil—not the synthetic vitamin. Vitamin A appears in most yellow and green foods, such as butter, carrots, salad greens and so forth, but there is a question as to how much of it is absorbed from these foods in a person who has any difficulty with his liver. So the wise thing to do is to take fish liver oil the year round, but especially during the fall and winter months when the cold danger is ever-present.

Proteins are important to a good diet, says Dr. Ullmann, and it is very difficult to get enough good, first-class protein without the animal foods—meat, fish and poultry. However, it is well to remember that these foods are acid-forming in the body and must be balanced with foods that have an alkaline reaction. These are, in general, the fruits and vegetables.

However, there is one other group of foods that form acid in the body—the cereals. Dr. Ullmann gives in his book, an excellent description of what happens to a grain of wheat in processing it to make bread. "If we consider the efforts other nations have to make in order to obtain the necessary amount of grain for their daily bread, it is a sorry sight indeed that the people of the United States who dispose of such wealth of grain do not make better use of it. But in the United States, a singular civilization, with all its habits and styles, is responsible for the restriction to bread made almost entirely of refined, white, wheat flour which is eaten either as toast or as any of the marketed products such as crackers, biscuits, rolls, buns, doughnuts, cakes, pies, puddings, waffles, wafers, etc. The consequences are lack of calcium and valuable minerals, a tendency toward acidosis, poor teeth, gas, constipation and sluggishness," says Dr. Ullmann.

He tells us that sufferers from colds and sinusitis should keep to rye bread, graham bread and pumpernickel whenever possible. All of the cereals used should be unrefined. Sugar is another evil, says he, which should be omitted entirely from the diet if you would avoid colds and sinusitis.

Salt May Be Responsible for Sinusitis

Dr. Ullmann's chapter on table salt is the most interesting in the book. He tells us that almost all of us eat far too much salt. The amount of salt necessary to produce hydrochloric acid in the stomach is amply supplied in the food we eat, without any additional salt at all. Too much salt, therefore, can result in too much acid in the stomach, which is believed to be a reason for stomach ulcer. Taking salt is merely a habit, says Dr. Ullmann. Experts tell us that more than 8 grams of salt per day is injurious to the full utilization of the proteins we eat, yet many of us eat as much as 20 to 25 grams a day. Our kidneys cannot keep up with the job of eliminating this amount of salt, so it accumulates in our tissues.

However, from the point of view of sinus trouble, the reason for not eating salt springs from its relation to calcium in body metabolism. "If large amounts of sodium chloride are taken, a good deal of it will be stored in the skin, mucous membrane and other tissues, and calcium will be liberated. Therefore, each sodium molecule retained in the tissues will diminish the calcium effect. And this is important in preventing colds and other inflammations of the nasal passages." To prevent colds and sinus trouble, the diet should be what Dr. Ullmann calls "salt-poor"—not more than 5 grams of salt per day.

We are in 100 per cent agreement with Dr. Ullmann's diet recommendations, particularly as they apply to salt, bread and sugar. In fact, we would go so far as to recommend no salt, no sugar and no bread at all for the individual who would avoid sinus infections. There are two excellent reasons for avoiding cereal products, especially in the case of children whose diet is likely to consist largely of cereals. First, they are acid forming. And secondly, they are so filling, that they simply do not leave room for the fresh fruits and vegetables that are so necessary, both because they form alkaline residue in the body and because they are rich in vitamins. Study the average cereal eater. You will find that he gets not nearly enough fruits and vegetables—that he has little interest in eating them at all.

How can one go about using the information we have given here to prevent or cure a sinus condition? First of all, the diet we have outlined seems to us an excellent one, whether you fear sinus trouble or not. By all means, begin now to cut down on salt until gradually you are doing without it entirely in cooking and at the table. Of course, this means no salty foods like potato chips, olives and so forth. Then, if you are eating much cereal food, cut down on that, too. Of course, the part of your meals that used to consist of bread should now consist of fresh raw fruits and vegetables.

If you are suffering from sinus trouble, we think you should tell your doctor about Dr. Bush's discovery. He will want to get the book or write to Dr. Bush and find out more about it. In other words, we don't think you should try to give yourself this treatment, for the nose is a delicate piece of machinery and should be manipulated only by an expert.

~~~~~~

SECTION 58: STAPH INFECTIONS

~~~~~~

233. Staph Infections Create New Problems

"Hospital acquired staphylococcal disease is now recognizable as a formidable contemporary cause of illness and death." So said Dr. Reimert T. Ravenholt, noted Seattle authority on causes of epidemic diseases. He was quoted in *MD* for May, 1958.

Dr. Ravenholt was speaking of a disease which is an anachronism. Formerly thought of only in connection with filth, poverty and lack of proper medical and nursing care, staphylococcal infection (staph) now invades modern hospitals where complete antiseptic cleanliness has been taken for granted for years; it races into maternity wards where all the latest medical genius is brought into play for the benefit of the mothers and the new babies, where childbirth is so antiseptic, controlled and managed that one hardly recognizes it as a natural function. Staph infects the hospital nurseries where the new born infants, surrounded by gleaming plastic, glass, nylon, sterilized formulas, masked nurses and so forth, go down like wilting flowers before the powerful germ. Wards full of old people and desperately sick people, fresh from the operating table, are infected. Nurses and doctors break out with boils and abscesses and the terrible word is whispered through hospital corridors like the sound of a death knell—"Staph."

What is the explanation of this seeming contradiction? Why, in modern times when supposedly most of our troubles with infection have been conquered, should such a bug (for bug it is) take such a toll? Why don't they stamp it out with antibiotics?

That is a key question, for it seems that antibiotics are probably the main cause for the epidemics. There are two reasons for this. First, antibiotics (good old reliable bug-killers that they are) have made hospitals and doctors careless about the necessity for such a high degree of cleanliness that no bug can survive. Blankets laden with germs are shaken out, dirty laundry is stuffed carelessly into chutes, rooms are cleaned only casually before new patients are brought in, dressings from infected wounds are not disposed of properly and so forth.

Presence of Staph Reveals Bad Practices

The bad housekeeping at hospitals that has come to light since staph became a major problem is understandable because of the dependence on antibiotics which has characterized these past 10 or 15 years. The slackening in antiseptic procedures is due to an unconscious, or perhaps conscious, reliance on antibiotics. They can get rid of germs easily, why bother with so much tiresome and dull cleansing and sterilizing procedure?

Every article we read on staph in medical literature stressed this aspect of the problem, especially articles from nursing journals, for, of course, nurses are vitally concerned in hospital housekeeping. By the same token, they are the most sensitive to criticism of hospital cleanliness. But, like most of the rest of us, they have come to depend on drugs to take care of infections—there's no longer any need to scour and scrub and disinfect. If one antibiotic won't get the germ, another will, or perhaps a combination of several.

Antibiotics Are Largely Responsible

However—and this is where the second area of blame must be laid on antibiotics—staph germs have become resistant to antibiotics. We are told that staph germs, studied in a laboratory, *become resistant to one kind of antibiotic within 7 days.* How? No one is sure just how. But the fact remains that one generation of *staphylococcus aureus,* which is the bug we are discussing, produces another generation every hour. Somewhere along the line, within a very short time, the resistant bug arrives on the scene. The antibiotic ceases to be effective from that time on, no matter what dosage is given.

Another antibiotic is then tried, and for a while, seems to work. But once again, the resistant member of the family eventually develops, and another antibiotic must be discarded, where this particular infection is concerned.

So we have a situation where the very hospitals which use the most antibiotics have the most staph. "Researchers have discovered that the pool of resistant strains in a hospital, for instance, will increase in direct proportion to the number of patients receiving an antibiotic." Ironically, these staph germs eventually feed upon the very drugs that are intended to kill them, says a report on *Staphylococcus, The Problem, Its History and Significance,* published by Dial Research Laboratories.

Overcrowding in nurseries is regarded as certainly a contributing cause for the spread of staph among infants and mothers. Time and again epidemics have been halted or reduced in severity by moving infants to other, less crowded locations. There is no doubt in anyone's mind that babies, packed in nurseries end to end, like peas in a pod, are much more likely to "catch" any germ that is present in even one of them or in the nurse who tends all of them.

Home Delivery of Infants Is Impractical Solution

An article in the *Ladies' Home Journal* for February, 1959, says, "There have been suggestions of a return to home deliveries for child-births which are expected to be normal, at least until the hospital staph is brought under control. Doctors have computed that, in about 10 per cent of childbirths, conditions are present which indicate possible diffi-culties, for either mother or infant. These are usually indicated in ad-vance. Where this is the case, it is conceded, the mother should have the benefit of hospital facilities. But permitting home deliveries for normal, healthy women who prefer to have their babies at home would, it is felt by many, not only prevent infection of these mothers and infants by hos-pital staph, it would also lower the possibility of infection for babies who need hospital care."

Here is a revolution indeed! Doctors advising home delivery of infants! And this suggestion, of course, runs headlong into the present acute short-age of doctors. Who is going to deliver and care for these babies, when it entails house calls for doctors already so busy they hardly have time to care for patients who are all neatly arranged under one roof in a hospital? This is a problem for which the American Medical Association, with its deliberate program of limiting the number of doctors, must provide the answer.

Take a Long Look at the Killer

What are some of the symptoms of staph infections and who is most likely to get them? These bugs have been around a long, long time, we are told; they are nothing new. Boils, carbuncles, abscesses are staph in-fections. Impetigo, conjunctivitis, infected wounds and burns, hard-to-cure infections of the digestive, urinary and respiratory tracts, food and blood poisoning, and staphylococcus pneumonia, which is often fatal, are all staph infections. Osteomyelitis is a staph infection of the bone. If the germ penetrates into the inner heart chambers, it can cause heart failure and death.

The hospital-caused epidemics, which are causing today's concern, may show up as boils and abscesses on infants. Breast feeding new babies who are infected may bring on breast abscesses in the mothers. Surgical patients may develop suppurating wounds that cannot be healed.

Carriers who do not become ill themselves may infect hospital patients. It is estimated that more than half the people in the world carry staph in their nose passages or on their skin. It can survive and maintain virulence for great lengths of time, especially in fine dust which has extraordinary powers of movement and penetration. Newborn babies and their mothers, leaving the hospital, apparently well, may carry staph with them when they go home, infecting fathers and other children. The *Ladies' Home Journal* told of a survey in Ohio which showed that three-fourths of the mothers and one-third of the fathers and other children in families with newborn babies developed staph infections from 3 to 6 months after the return home of the hospital-infected baby. In one family, 3 of the 5 members were still carrying the epidemic strain two and one-half years after the baby's birth.

Who Is Susceptible to Staph Infection?

Who gets staph infections? People whose resistance is low, we are told. Newborn babies, especially in our chemicalized age, have little resistance to disease. Sick people, old people, patients recovering from operations— these are logical candidates. Are you surprised to learn also that people taking cortisone, X-ray treatments or insulin are especially susceptible? We did not find this information in any of the articles we read, but we believe probably those most susceptible to staph infections would be people whose body supply of vitamin C is dangerously low. Deficiency in other vitamins may share the responsibility, but lack of vitamin C leaves tissues weakened and flabby so that they fall easy prey to germs.

You hear little about staph—why is it considered so dangerous a problem? Here is the story of one hospital epidemic reported in the *New England Journal of Medicine* for May 12, 1960. Ninety-four families had children born in a California hospital during a staph outbreak there. A survey conducted 16 months later showed that the germ had become disseminated among 65 per cent of the families, although only 12 of the children had actually contracted the disease while they were in the hospital. Boils, abscesses, skin disease, pneumonia, mastitis had developed among the mothers, fathers, brothers and sisters of 65 per cent of the families.

Staph Epidemic Is Almost Uncontrollable

Another frightening story, reported in the *Journal of the American Medical Association* for October 24, 1959, tells of a hospital where 750 children are born every year. A two-day-old baby developed an abscess.

Within 7 days, 11 other infants developed abscesses, too. The nursery was closed and every effort was made to stamp out the sources of infection. Improvement was only temporary and the epidemic broke out again when 29 out of 48 newly born infants were found to be infected with staph. In this instance, the only way the disease was controlled was compulsory "rooming in" of the infant with the mother. That is, each baby stayed in the room with its mother—there was no central nursery.

In one hospital 35 per cent of the babies born developed infections, 10 per cent had infant mastitis, 19 per cent of the mothers had infected breasts. Staph infection on a country-wide basis accounts for 12 per cent of infant mortality! These figures came to light in a survey conducted by Dr. Ravenholt whom we quoted at the beginning of this discussion. Dr. Ravenholt's survey revealed, too, that more than 100 of the 7,837 deaths that occurred in one county in Oregon in 1956, could be attributed to staph.

Staph did not choose to reside only in American hospitals. It appeared simultaneously in countries all over the world, where antibiotics are in regular use. A letter to the editor of the *Lancet* states, "There is little doubt that most hospitals are now infested with resistant staphylococci."

What Can Be Done About Staph?

The medical profession is understandably a bit reluctant to talk very much publicly about staph. But when an epidemic starts in a hospital (and many of these have occurred in the past 5 years or so), some explanation must be given, some cause found and, most of all, some end put to this devastating plague which, once started, can run like wildfire through a hospital ward or nursery. And no drugs will help stamp it out.

The answer most of the medical articles give is revision of ideas and practices of cleanliness in hospitals. This means the most scrupulous attention to every detail—making hands antiseptic before tending patients; placing infected dressings, bedding, clothing etc., into receptacles immediately upon removing them; introducing more effective methods of laundering and cleaning, which may mean changing the kinds of equipment used. Floors must be wet-mopped with disinfectants.

Great Antiseptic Care Is Given Staph Patients

An article from the *Journal of the Albert Einstein Medical Center* for April, 1960, gives recommendations on such matters as how to change sheets and pillow cases on the beds of staph patients. They must be carefully folded inward to avoid air contamination, placed immediately in a special "contaminated laundry" bag which is closed with a drawstring. The plastic covers of mattresses and pillows must be washed every day with disinfectant. Floors, walls, furniture and especially flat surfaces where dust collects, like windowsills, must be scrubbed with disinfectant. It was discovered, in a survey reported in *Hospitals* for June 16, 1959, that the

[878]

"extra" blanket which is brought in every night and distributed indiscriminately to any and all patients may carry as high as 5,000 staph germs per blanket. Not only is the recommendation made that this kind of distribution be discontinued, but the question of disinfecting blankets, especially woolen blankets that cannot be boiled at high temperatures, becomes a hard one to solve. The *Journal* advises, too, thorough cleaning of everything in the hospital room with water "containing soap or detergent. Staphylococci may develop resistance to antibiotics, but not to 'elbow grease.'"

Imagine a modern medical journal coming out in favor of "elbow grease" as the best deterrent to infection!

There is a lesson—a serious and eternal lesson—to be learned from the saga of staph. The *Dial Report* tells us that "although staph's exact role in nature's scheme of things is not known, microbiological experience indicates staph is a part of the bacterial balance in nature. It plays—or did play—some part in the balance of bacteria within and surrounding the human population." It may play a helpful role in performing a metabolic or waste function or it may—listen carefully—"hold other disease-carrying bacteria in check. If staph were banished—a seeming impossibility—other bacteria that cause disease might well sweep the world."

We Are Producing Resistant Staph Strains

Did you ever read anything like this before—in regard to another aspect of today's living? Just as we are producing resistant strains of bacteria like staph, so we are producing resistant insects with our new insecticides. Just as, when we take antibiotics, we kill off helpful bacteria in the intestinal tract, along with harmful ones, so we destroy with insecticides, the helpful living things that keep the insects in check and preserve the balance of nature. As germs (or insects) become resistant to one after another of our drugs or insecticides, it becomes necessary to attack them with ever stronger and more poisonous substances. This, in turn, results in even more powerful, more resistant germs (or insects) in future generations. Using our present weapons, we are fighting a losing battle and the germs (and insects) are bound to win.

The answer to staph infections is the same as the answer to insect infestation. Leave the balance of nature alone. For millions of years she has kept harmful pests controlled by other organisms which prey on them. Just as there are birds, insects and animals that destroy other insects, so there are germs that destroy harmful germs. By trying to kill all germs or all insects, we succeed only in destroying this balance and making our enemies more powerful.

Prevention Best Defense against Staph Infection

How, then, do you prevent staph infections? The medical magazines themselves have shown the way. All the experts say, in essence, there is no way we can destroy the staph germ once it has caused illness. The only answer is good housekeeping, cleanliness, much stricter observance of rules for antisepsis. The other part of the answer is to develop bodies so strong, so healthy that they can and will resist all diseases—staph included. People whose resistance is poor get staph infections. Prevention is the only answer left for us—not cure.

What is the alternative to a program of prevention rather than cure? Dr. Mary E. Godfrey and Ian MacLean Smith of the State University of Iowa, writing in the *Journal of the American Medical Association,* somberly predict that, when or if staph is brought under control, some equally virulent organism may arise to take its place. Experience of many years' standing indicates, they say, that this possibility does indeed exist, so long as the overcrowded central nursery remains in existence.

SECTION 59: TOBACCO AMBLYOPIA

234. Tobacco Amblyopia

By H. S. HEDGES, M.D., Charlottesville, Virginia

Amid all the heated controversy as to the relation between lung cancer and cigarettes, I find practically nothing about the damage to eyesight; but, frankly, if the findings in my small-town practice are any indication of the possible results to our smokers all over the country, there must be thousands of men (and women, too) who are on the way to industrial blindness if they keep on long enough.

Of course, we all know that thousands and thousands of people smoke all their lives with no apparent trouble except the formation of a vicious drug addiction, which is *very* hard to overcome. Not long ago, a big strong man came into my office with the story that "when driving, often everything goes black before me." His eyes showed typical, early tobacco trouble, and I begged him to stop smoking. He came in again a few days ago telling me "It was the hardest thing I ever had to do, but I haven't had a blackout since."

In these tobacco eyes, the first symptom is usually premature presbyopia (the condition most middle-aged people develop, in which you must hold reading matter rather far from the eyes to be able to focus on it). A strong man of 38, with perfect distant vision, came complaining of headache on close work and utter inability to read at all. He could read with a glass for a person 10 years older than he was. He stopped his cigarettes short, and in less than 3 weeks, all of his headaches were gone and he reads as well as anyone without a glass.

We see this condition so often among our women. They have not been smoking long enough to have developed the late nerve changes, but the premature presbyopia is my concern. Nearly all of them also complain of cold finger tips in the morning, after the first cigarette. In many of these women, if you get them quite early in the morning, place a delicate thermometer between the finger tips, let them smoke one cigarette and you can measure a definite fall of temperature. Among many, the flow of blood in the arterioles will fall 30 per cent; in men, about 10 per cent. And please tell me, if the arterioles of the fingers are so affected, why cannot the little vessels of the heart show the same trouble? I am told that they are controlled by a different nerve supply.

The next commonest symptom is a central loss of red and green. (Dr. Hedges is speaking of color blindness.) The test is easily made. Fix a deep red circle about ¼ inch in diameter on the end of a small rod. Sit facing your patient about 4 feet away, close one of his eyes, and with the other, let him look straight into one of yours. Now, move the little circle slowly before his eye as he fixes yours. If the color fades in the very center of the field but remains clear in the periphery (around the edges), you may be sure that trouble is starting; and later on, all central red and green will be lost. By the time this has come about, the central distant vision is failing fast; and in some, it will be down to 20/200 (industrial blindness). Very marked changes will have developed in the nerve head, the whole of this area carrying the papillomacular bundle becoming a dirty gray. Fortunately, however, if these patients will really stop all use of tobacco, most of them will make an excellent recovery.

This spring, a cigarette smoker came in, the picture of despair, a man about 50 who had been a truck driver. "Doctor, my eyes have failed so that I have lost my job; I can't see well enough to do any work, I have a family to care for and I have nothing."

Vision 20/200, unimproved with glasses (industrial blindness). To make a long story short, he had typical tobacco eyes. I begged him to stop his cigarettes and he said he would. He came in again a few weeks ago— the happiest looking man I have seen in a long time. "Doctor, my sight has all come back," (it tested normal) "and I have the best job I ever had."

We could give you dozens of case reports, but the best description of tobacco amblyopia that I know is found in Dr. DeSchweinitz' *Toxic Amblyopia*, published by Lea Brothers, in 1896. The earliest I can find is by Beer, 1792, and the next by the great Scotch MacKenzie in 1832. So, you see, the trouble has been known for a long time, but many still know nothing about it. One of the scientists on the Tobacco Investigating Committee wrote me he "had never heard of such a thing."

As to the much publicized filters, while some of them doubtless remove some of the tar, they have very little effect on the unburned nicotine in the smoke. Nicotine, however, is very soluble in water, so one brand carries a damp sponge. The water in this will absorb most of the nicotine. I had a patient who needed to stop smoking, but would not; so I bought him a pack of the above type. Result: "I might as well not smoke at all." It is the nicotine that the old addict craves, and only a cigarette carrying the full percentage of the drug will or can "satisfy."

Reprinted by permission from the MEDICAL TIMES, *October, 1957.*

SECTION 60: TRICHINOSIS

235. Trichinosis Is a Threat to You

What do you suppose is meant by "U.S. Government Inspected," when you see it stamped on the meat you buy? If you believe, as we did, that it means the government has certified the meat as free from infectious disease, you are dead wrong. There is no such guarantee. There is every possibility that you can be infected with a fatal disease, trichinosis, as readily with government inspected meat as with meat that never got within a hundred miles of an inspector.

We were awakened to this unpleasant fact by a letter in the *Journal of the American Medical Association* (December 31, 1960). The letter, signed by two professors at the University of Missouri, John H. Walters, M.D., of the School of Medicine, and George C. Shelton, D.V.M., of the School of Veterinary Medicine, deplored the fact that most people in the United States think that animals are inspected for trichina and condemned if necessary. On the contrary, say the authors, no effort is even made to detect the presence of trichina. Almost 50 years ago, the Department of Agriculture decided to abandon all efforts at detection on the ground that no detection technique was sufficiently accurate. Instead of inspection, then, the housewife was instructed to cook all pork products before they are eaten.

This country, advancing in every scientific way, shooting satellites into space, inventing nuclear weapons and color television has yet to find a way to uncover trichina in meat. Somehow, one gets the impression that our scientists are not expending much effort on this project, especially since many other nations have been able to work out some criterion for con-

[882]

demning meat infected with this parasite. As a result of our lack of effort, we, in the United States, suffer from 3 times as much trichinosis as the rest of the world put together. The number comes to one out of every 5 persons, and of these, one out of 20 dies.

Named for the Worm

The disease is named for the parasitic worm that causes it, *Trichina spiralis*. In its larval stage, it embeds itself in the muscles of animals, mainly pigs. Human beings then acquire the disease by eating uncooked or undercooked meat that is infected. Once in the human body, the digestive processes liberate the larvae from the meat, and they attach themselves to the lining of the lower intestine. As they mature they are carried to the lymph nodes, the heart, lungs, brain and everywhere else in the body.

At each stage in their progress, they produce some symptom of invasion. It might be nausea, diarrhea, abdominal pain and/or fever, when it is in the intestine. In the lungs, the symptoms might suggest pneumonia; at the heart, the larvae may coil themselves around that organ and interfere with the function of it; at the brain, they produce inflammation. Eventually they seek out their natural haven, the skeletal muscles. There they coil up and work a cyst around themselves which causes stiffness, pain and swelling of the muscles, and fever, sweating and insomnia in the patient. Many victims carry encysted trichina larvae in their muscles throughout life, with symptoms so vague as to go unsuspected.

The letter in the *Journal* goes on to say that the clinical symptoms of trichinosis often resemble a viral infection, and it is believed that many acute trichinosis cases are diagnosed as "flu" or "a virus."

An illustration of the prevalence of trichinosis is offered by a news story in the Allentown, Pennsylvania, *Morning Call* (February 1, 1961) in which it is reported that in Bethlehem, Pennsylvania, a number of trichinosis cases (6) occurred within a week. The county health officer reported that there were other cases of which he was informed by family physicians. He noted, too, that diagnosis of the disease is not easy, and absolute cure is impossible to predict. The symptoms usually arise 7 to 10 days after eating the infected meat, and may be so severe that hospitalization is required.

When hospitalization is necessary, it is the symptoms, not the disease, which are treated. When the symptoms have subsided—this may be from two to three weeks—the patient may never have any further difficulty with the disease, or the condition could cause muscle aches and pains for the rest of his life.

You Are on Your Own

The individual is on his own in protecting himself from trichinosis, and the best way to do that is to cook meat, especially pork and pork products, thoroughly. This means it must be cooked at a temperature which will kill any larvae which might be present—350°F. for pork roasts, for

35 minutes per pound. The temperature of the meat itself, taken by meat thermometer, should be at least 185°F. For fresh pork, a good rule is to cook the meat until it is gray in color, or at least white. Never eat pink pork. A special warning about frankfurters: they are usually a pork product, and should never be eaten raw.

Doctors Walters and Shelton warned that, in view of the high incidence of trichinosis being found in our population, a new effort should be made to perfect detection techniques, and the public should certainly be informed that the government inspection stamp does not mean that the consumer is safe from trichinosis. In closing they say, ". . . ultimate relief can come only with proper Congressional action and may well merit equal legislature time with such Congressional pastimes as investigation of disc jockeys and of quiz shows."

We think this is a worthwhile project for all health-minded people, and for anyone else who cares to avoid a serious illness. Our government is expending thousands of man-hours on fluoridation promotion and on keeping measles and whooping cough records. These projects may never yield any truly significant information or aid to the health of Americans.

In a system for detecting trichinosis, a concrete and valuable service would be done automatically. A known disease could be stopped in its tracks. Think how many cases occur in New York, Los Angeles and Chicago, if a town such as Bethlehem, Pennsylvania, can have 6 in one week, not counting others suspected but not officially reported. Trichinosis must be a very prevalent disease throughout the country, on that basis. Remind your congressman of this situation. Ask him to investigate the reason that no work has been done on such an urgent problem in the past 50 years. He may be as surprised as you were to know of the danger to which he is exposed.

236. Tuberculosis and Malnutrition

In our thinking, tuberculosis has long been associated with malnutrition and bad living conditions in general. We know it is frequent after wars and famines; we expect to find it in slums. But researchers have found it difficult to decide in all cases whether it was the actual lack of proper food, or whether perhaps overcrowding, inadequate housing, exposure to weather and so forth might have more to do with causing tuberculosis.

Some time ago it was discovered that tuberculosis patients had a deficiency of vitamins A and C in their blood—a discovery which led to the use of the "McConkey Cocktail"—cod liver oil in tomato juice, the oil for vitamin A and the tomato juice for vitamin C. However, it seemed that even very large doses of these two vitamins could not raise the blood level of the two vitamins when active tuberculosis was present.

Now further investigation has shown that a lack of these two vitamins in the diet may predispose to tuberculosis and, what is extremely important to prevention, that an ample supply of these two vitamins may be the finest protection anyone can have against the disease.

Research on Vitamins A and C

Horace R. Getz, Esmond R. Long and Howard J. Henderson, writing in the *American Review of Tuberculosis,* Vol. 64, 1951, describe the results of a survey among 1100 men, just for the purpose of establishing if possible, the relation of nutrition to tuberculosis susceptibility. All of the men were shown by X-ray to be free from tuberculosis at first examination. They were followed up and studied for a period ranging from one month to 5 years. Periodic X-rays were made, as well as nutritional studies, which included the following measurements of the content of their blood: the hemoglobin (red substance in blood which carries oxygen) the vitamin A and vitamin C content, the amount of protein, albumin and globulin, calcium, phosphorus and phosphatase (a substance necessary for proper use of phosphorus by the body).

During the years of the survey, 28 of the men developed tuberculosis, 4 of them dying from the disease. The charts of these 28 men showed approximately the same blood values for all of the items listed above, except for vitamin A and vitamin C. All cases of the active disease occurred in persons whose blood level of vitamins A and C was considerably lower than average, before the appearance of the disease.

We know that the need for vitamin A increases greatly in fevers, which is believed to be the reason why TB patients suffer from lack of vitamin A, which is evidenced by night blindness and other symptoms. We are told that an enormous amount of vitamin A (100,000 units) daily is necessary to keep the level of the vitamin in TB patients up to that of normal people. In addition, countless surveys have shown that vitamin A is deficient in American diets—not deficient enough to put people to bed from vitamin A deficiency, but enough to bring on a state called "sub-clinical" deficiency, just enough to lower their resistance to diseases, for example.

We have also known for many years that vitamin C is deficient in TB patients. *Nutrition Reviews* for April, 1947, tells us that as much as 1000 milligrams of vitamin C must be given to TB patients every day to keep their body supply of the vitamin at a normal level. Investigations of laboratory animals have shown that, in cases of re-infection with TB germs, the cells and tubes of the lungs are filled with an accumulation of vitamin C, which explains why the vitamin is so lacking in the blood of victims. Now they tell us that we cannot assume from this that quantities of vitamin C will cure or prevent TB. But why can't we? Isn't it obvious that the body, trying to protect itself against the germs, concentrates its strongest fighting force in the lungs, where the disease is concentrated? If this force is vitamin C, why is it not possible to prevent and cure TB with massive doses of vitamin C? We know from animal experiments that a vitamin C deficiency predisposes to the disease. Massive doses of the vitamin increase the weight of tuberculous animals and decrease the severity of their TB symptoms. Why then do we not publicize *these* facts about preventing TB rather than the always discouraging news about new wonder drugs!

Jolliffe, Tisdall and Cannon in their classical book, *Clinical Nutrition,* published by Paul B. Hueber, Incorporated, tell us that it has long been assumed that malnutrition predisposes to TB. Tuberculous animals are afflicted with scurvy unless they are given large amounts of vitamin C. Protein and vitamins A and C are the food elements missing, whose lack in a diet predisposes to tuberculosis, say these experts on the subject of nutrition. In the *American Journal of the Diseases of Children,* April, 1951, we find an account of premature children born to tuberculous mothers. The authors tell us that premature births are common among these patients —*not because of the tuberculosis, but because of the impoverished nutritional status of the mothers.*

Protein vs. Tuberculosis

Speaking of the necessity of protein in preventing TB, we have an article from *Diseases of the Chest* for April, 1950, by Benjamin P. Sandler, M.D., in which he discusses treating 38 patients with a high-protein, low-carbohydrate diet. Results were significant; improvement in cough, strength, weight, appetite and so forth. Dr. Sandler attributes this success to the fact that the diet adjusted the patients' carbohydrate metabolism so that their blood sugar level was more nearly normal. We stress all the time the importance of high-grade protein in the diet and the fact that most Americans eat far, far too many carbohydrates, especially in the way of white sugar and white flour products. Says Dr. Sandler, "A normal carbohydrate metabolism, with concomitant normal liver glycogen stores, is an essential and fundamental mechanism on which other defense mechanisms rest." How often, in TB prevention literature, do you see any mention of a high-protein diet as an essential?

Why Not Test for Vitamins, too?

Today, chest X-rays are the fashion. Local tuberculosis associations, with lots of publicity gather whole communities together in a drive for chest X-rays as a free service. Why not make it a practice hereafter whenever a chest X-ray is given, to also take a sample of blood and test it for vitamin A and vitamin C content? In this way, those individuals whose X-rays show no tuberculosis could be warned that they should watch out for vitamin A and vitamin C deficiencies in their diet, so that they would not become susceptible to tuberculosis in the future. Although, of course, there are possibly other things involved in contracting tuberculosis, at least the possibility of this one deficiency could thus be guarded against. Perhaps the cost would be too much for the local tuberculosis association to handle. But we are sure most people would be willing to pay for this part of the service, if the whole significance of nutrition and tuberculosis were explained to them in a very thorough way. Why not suggest such a project to your local tuberculosis association?

And meanwhile, of course, pay special attention to the amount of vitamins A and C and protein in your family's diet, especially for the youngsters. Vitamin A appears chiefly in foods whose color is yellow— sweet potatoes, squash, carrots and so forth, as well as many green leafy vegetables. Vitamin C is that one vitamin of which it is most difficult to obtain enough in daily diet. It is contained in some fresh fruits and vegetables, citrus fruit and tomatoes being the best source, as well as parsley, water cress, cantaloup. Protein is found in such foods as meat, nuts and sea food.

These elements are so necessary to health and we are so likely not to get enough of them in daily fare that it seems almost a positive necessity to use food supplements for these three—fish liver oil perles for vitamin A, rose hips for vitamin C and desiccated liver for protein.

[887]

237. Failure of B. C. G., the Anti-Tuberculosis Vaccine

The struggle with tuberculosis has been a relatively mild one in the United States since the 1920's. Most experts agree that the disease need no longer be a cause of major concern for the Public Health Service. Still we hear murmurings, now and then, from the National Tuberculosis Association about mass vaccination against tuberculosis with a vaccine that has been around for a good many years. It's name is B.C.G. (Bacillus Calmette Guerin), named for its discoverers. It is a live virus taken from cows which actually gives the patient a slight case of tuberculosis. Nothing unusual about that, as that is the premise upon which all vaccines are founded.

As sometimes happens with a new vaccine, for one reason or another, B.C.G. really caught on—especially overseas, where tuberculosis is a truly serious problem for many nations. On the recommendations of many health officials, great programs of mass vaccination were instituted. Strangely, the United States was not included in these—for we are a vaccine-happy nation if ever there was one—but we were certainly cheering along the sidelines. The World Health Organization was hip-deep in the project, giving aid to many countries so that they might buy the vaccine. In some cases, notably India, they practically insisted that the country accept this bounty.

How the Mortality Rates Tumbled!

As the years passed, the tuberculosis rate tumbled in these countries. It was disconcertingly clear, however, that the same thing was happening in places that had nothing whatever to do with the vaccine. In the United States, the rate of regression was similar to that of mass-inoculated Sweden. The same was true in the Netherlands, again without the use of the B.C.G. vaccine or any other. When these obvious facts began to filter through to the scientists who make a study of contagious disease and its prevention, it became all too apparent to them that B.C.G. was not causing any miracles.

But long before these realizations came to pass, the voices of scientists all over the world had been raised in protest against the use of the vaccine. From the time in 1921, when the bacillus was discovered, its career was rocky. The general line of objections was expressed again by Dr. J. Arthur Myers, Professor of Medicine at the Medical School of the University of Minnesota, in the *New York Herald-Tribune* (June 3, 1951). He said that the value of the vaccine was as yet unproven, and its safety open to serious question. It is a mixed, not a pure, culture and no two batches can ever be the same. They might be either too weak to produce immunity, or

[888]

so strong that they actually produce the disease instead of protecting against it!

The First Step to Tuberculosis

The safety of the vaccine raises several interesting points. Most important is this: the first infection with the tubercle bacillus seldom results in a case of active tuberculosis. (In fact, a recent estimate put the number of such "primarily infected" persons in the United States at 50,000,000. Of these, about 5 per cent can expect to see active signs of the disease in their lifetime.) However, it is a necessary first step. When one acquires this mild infection, the ground is prepared for the serious "post-primary" infection. The body's natural immunity is stronger against this first infection than any vaccine yet discovered. In tuberculosis, permanent immunity does not result from the patient's having once had the disease, as it does with smallpox, polio, scarlet fever, etc. (*Journal of the American Medical Association*, November 7, 1959). Each new exposure can result in re-infection. With all of this in mind, the very idea of the use of B.C.G. seems to be homicidal! The subject is given a vaccination which cannot prevent the disease, but actually makes it more likely that the disease will appear in a more virulent form.

Deficiencies Invite Infection

Dr. Myers, mentioned above, remarked that, in experiments with B.C.G., animals suffering from dietary deficiency frequently died when they were inoculated with the vaccine. Now the idea of nutrition introduces a whole new problem into the discussion. It is well established that poor nutrition is one of the primary causes of tuberculosis. If these people are inoculated with B.C.G., their chances of contracting tuberculosis are even greater. Yet these are the poor people of Latin America and Asia at whom the program for mass immunization with B.C.G. is aimed. For that matter, who, in this modern world is not nutritionally deficient? If such a program were begun in the United States, how many fully nourished subjects would there be?

Patients' Resistance Low When Vaccinated

A more concrete instance of this serious difficulty appeared in the *Journal of the American Medical Association* for January 14, 1956, as it was reported in a Swedish medical magazine. When an 8-month-old boy, who had been vaccinated with B.C.G. a few days after birth, died, an autopsy was performed. It showed the cause of death to be widespread tuberculosis. Three other fatalities, directly attributable to B.C.G. vaccination, were reported in the same article. In each case, it was supposed that the patient was in a state of low resistance to infection at the time of the vaccination. Of course, the physical inability to cope with even a slight infection is not always noticeable at the time of vaccination, and this fact is a strong argument against smallpox, scarlet fever and polio vaccination.

Why Do They Keep Trying?

Despite the obvious dangers, the National Tuberculosis Association keeps trying for mass immunization with B.C.G. in the United States. Listen to their appeal given in this headline in the *New York Times* (May 28, 1959): "B.C.G. Vaccine Found to Give Immunity When Inhaled— Convenience Stressed." The article described the Association's finding that B.C.G. could be released as a spray in theaters and auditoriums, thus vaccinating the patrons without their even being aware of it. (Shades of Fluoridation!) How incredible that all the evidence of B.C.G.'s danger should be ignored, and the lack of effectiveness of B.C.G. should be dismissed by an organization whose main job it is to keep abreast of any new developments in the field! How surprising that they were not aware of this statement by the man who introduced the principles for B.C.G. vaccination and sponsored mass vaccination in Scandinavia, Professor Arvid Wellgren: "The knowledge that such progressive B.C.G. diseases (referring to the 4 fatalities mentioned above) can occur in man must shake our faith in the harmlessness of the B.C.G. bacillus and perhaps induce us to reconsider the continuance of mass vaccination. We have hitherto encouraged, by publicity, as many as possible to have themselves B.C.G. vaccinated, even if there were no obvious risk of exposure. We can no longer accept the non-dangerousness of our propaganda." (*Nordisk Medicin,* January 5, 1956.) If they were aware of this statement, how shocking that they should make their ridiculous proposal for "mass gassing" with B.C.G. in the movies!

Or where was the Association's attention when this statement appeared in the *British Medical Journal* (April 30, 1955): "Progressive tuberculosis can certainly occur in previously tuberculin-negative persons who have been recently vaccinated with B.C.G. . . . No one believes that B.C.G. vaccine gives complete protection . . . Almost all forms of tuberculosis appear after B.C.G. vaccination." This means, of course, that even persons who have had no previous tuberculosis infection can get one after B.C.G. inoculation, and that the vaccine is utterly unreliable in preventing the disease it is intended to prevent.

Notice the Resemblance?

The whole story of B.C.G. bears a close resemblance to fluoridation in principle. Fluoridation, too, has been under attack for many of the same reasons B.C.G. is suspect, ever since its introduction. It has yet to be proven safe; its reaction varies with the individual and there is no sure way to control the exact composition of each dose. The effectiveness of fluoridation is open to serious question, and any results which are claimed to have been achieved by its introduction could be achieved more simply, safely and efficiently by other means. Even the fact that communities have tried mass fluoridation and have seen fit to discontinue it, resembles the situation in Sweden, where, after many years of mass immunization with

B.C.G., the very persons who introduced it are advocating that it be dispensed with.

The parallel holds up for the Salk vaccine, too. Nobody knows how safe it is and serious questions remain unanswered in that regard. It is unreliable both as to composition and effectiveness. Several nations which were advocating mass vaccination have dropped that policy. There are other safer, simpler, more effective means of protecting against polio which are available.

The story of B.C.G. offers a lot of good lessons, if we are willing to learn. We must not let ourselves be stampeded into a program that has not been sufficiently researched or proven safe beyond all question. It is for this reason that we must make our objections to fluoridation and compulsory Salk shots known, and inform our fellow citizens of the danger to which they are being exposed. The B.C.G. fiasco could have happened in the United States—it still might!

SECTION 62: ULCERS

238. Could You Get an Ulcer?

When the pain centers in the pit of your stomach, just below the breastbone, and recurs often, especially within ½ to 3 or 4 hours after a meal, with a gnawing or aching sensation, likely as not you have an ulcer. And if you do, you're a member of a club that's growing less exclusive every day. The current count of ulcer patients seems to be about 3 people in every thousand.

What Is an Ulcer?

If you want to know how an ulcer develops, most physiologists subscribe to the following theory: As you know, your digestive system produces strong acids and juices, that are designed to help break down the food one eats so that its components can be used to nourish the body. The lining of the healthy stomach is marvelously resistant to these juices and is not affected by their caustic nature. In ulcer patients, this defense of the stomach's lining against stomach acids has broken down somehow, so that, even when the ulcer patient's stomach is empty of food, the digestive juices pour forth and work away at his stomach lining as though it were food. The continued irritation of this now-delicate area soon produces a sore, which we know by the name of ulcer.

The several names one hears in connection with ulcers often confuse the layman. First of all, it helps to know that peptic ulcers and ulcers are the same thing. Duodenal ulcers are those ulcers which occur in the first 11 inches of the intestine, which is known as the duodenum. Gastric ulcers are those which occur in the stomach proper. Most ulcers are of the duodenal type.

Theories on What Causes an Ulcer

The theories on why ulcers occur are varied. Though some physicians and many psychologists are still of the opinion that tenseness and the hectic pace of modern living is the main cause, observations such as the following one, carried in *MD* magazine (September, 1957), would seem to cast doubt on that theory. A comparative study was made on the incidence of ulcers in various countries, and it was found that they are just as common in countries that are relatively free of industrial stress as they are in highly industrialized areas.

For example, in India, China and Malaya, ulcers are quite an ordinary occurrence. In Japan, the death rate for gastric ulcers among men alone actually exceeds the United States figure for all ulcer deaths by 5 to 1. The Japanese rate is by far the highest in the world. Chile is next to Japan in gastric ulcer deaths among men, with 7.1 per 100,000. The United States death rate for all types of ulcer, gastric and duodenal, in both men and women, is only 6.3 per 100,000 population, according to *Statistical Abstracts of the United States,* 1956. If stress and strain were the only factor in ulcer formation, certainly the United States, a country known for its hectic pace, should be far out in front of such industrially backward countries as China, Malaya and Chile. It is well to keep in mind that the incidence of ulcers is just about the same among pigs as among human beings. It's hard to imagine that pigs concern themselves over social and industrial problems.

At the same meeting of pathologists at which the above information came to light, the opinion that ulcers spring from an inborn characteristic of the tissues received strong support. Seeming to coincide with this theory is the information in *Northwest Medicine* (March, 1956) to the effect that people with blood type O have a 35 per cent better chance of developing an ulcer than anyone else. Also included in this report was the fact that persons whose relatives have an ulcer are likely to develop the same type (gastric or duodenal) as the relative has.

Dr. A. C. Ivy and a colleague, in *Good Health* (October, 1950), remark that they are impressed with the large incidence of ulcers in people who smoke and drink coffee. Both caffeine and nicotine are known to be enemies of vitamin C, and it is this vitamin which is necessary for maintaining healthy tissue, including that which makes up the stomach lining.

A psychological study of 25 female ulcer patients, mentioned in *Good Housekeeping* for May, 1952, showed a profound personality disturbance in each case. All had either lost their mother early in life, been rejected by her or had some other intense conflict with their mother. They then turned to a father or husband for emotional security. When the woman was, in turn, rejected by the male, the ulcer signs began to show themselves.

Drugs and Ulcers

An article in the *Journal of the American Medical Association* (January 19, 1957) points to certain drugs as a possible cause of ulcers. In an experiment with 9 groups of guinea pigs, all were fed or injected with 9 different drugs. In all other respects, their diet and environment were kept identical. After 30 days, all of the drugs given except two were found to have caused ulcers in some percentage (10 per cent to 40 per cent) of the group of guinea pigs to which they were administered.

A lack of a B vitamin—pantothenic acid—is a responsible factor in duodenal ulcer cases, says *Drug Trade News* (March 11, 1957). In rats whose diet omitted this B vitamin, hormone activity was shown to cause ulcers in 11 to 14 weeks. The same hormonal activity in rats who had been fed pantothenic acid did not produce any ulcers.

Ulcers Related to Nutrition

The United States Department of Health, Education and Welfare puts out a pamphlet on ulcers in which they describe the cause of ulcers as a disturbance to the nerves which control the blood supply to the stomach lining. If the blood does not flow freely, thus interrupting the supply of nourishment which the cells of the stomach lining depend upon for their health, these cells are in a weakened condition and open to attack. This logical interpretation of the cause of ulcers points, as do several other theories, to the need for proper nutrition throughout the body if ulcers are to be avoided.

Dr. D. T. Quigley, writing in the *Nebraska State Medical Journal* (April, 1945), best expressed our point of view in the matter of ulcers and nutrition. He speaks of the high incidence of recurring ulcer (about half recur within 5 years), and bemoans the custom of putting a patient on a bland diet for a few months while the ulcer heals, and then withdrawing supervision and allowing a relapse to the diet that brought on the ulcer in the first place. Says Dr. Quigley: "Peptic ulcer is a deficiency disease reflecting a relatively high intake of refined carbohydrates and inadequate amount of all vitamins and food minerals. . . .

"The so-called enriched flour is still lacking in many vital elements, and so it is a menace to these patients since it engenders a false sense of security. It should be forbidden the ulcer patient for life.

". . . All foods containing sugar or white flour are permanently forbidden. . . . Other forbidden foods are canned and packaged foods. These have been robbed of their value by high heat and long storage. They are stale and worthless. They crowd out good foods. . . . To sum up: the idea is to reject non-vitamin, non-mineral foods and to use natural high-vitamin, high-mineral foods and to keep this up for life."

In general, most doctors leave it to a careful diet to heal an ulcer. Usually, the foods are soupy or custard-like, if they aren't completely liquid. Any roughage that might call on the gastric juices for concentrated aid in digestion is to be avoided in the first stages. Though milk and derivatives of milk are highly respected in this regard, it should be noted that caution is to be exercised when such a prescription is made. Milk cannot be tolerated by everyone, as is evidenced by a case related in the *Southern Medical Journal* (February, 1955), in which an ulcer patient began a milk diet until it was discovered that he had developed a case of hypercalcemia; that is, his body was unable to utilize the large amounts of calcium that were being taken in, and calcium deposits were beginning to form in undesirable locations. He stopped the milk and the condition disappeared.

Two Natural Cures

As a substitute for milk, Dr. L. J. J. Nye suggests potatoes. Potatoes are higher in vitamin C than milk, and they also have an alkaline effect on the stomach, thereby helping to reduce any overabundant stomach acidity.

Another natural food—fresh raw cabbage juice—has been shown to be most effective in curing ulcers. *California Medicine* (January, 1956) tells of an experiment using cabbage juice on prisoners at San Quentin for management of peptic ulcers. The patients were given either concentrated cabbage juice or a facsimile which contained no cabbage juice. X-rays after 3 weeks showed the cabbage juice treatment to have been beneficial.

Patients being treated for diseases such as arthritis, with ACTH or cortisone are warned to be on the lookout for ulcers, even if their stomachs are normal. The *Journal of the American Medical Association* (December 15, 1951) tells of Boston doctors who gave ACTH injections daily for 3 to 4 weeks to arthritis patients whose stomachs were normal. In each case, acid secretions of the stomach rose to the level found in cases of active ulcer. Cortisone brought on similar results. The article goes on to tell of a young man who was given ACTH as a treatment for arthritis for 6 months. He developed an ulcer as a result. The ulcer hemorrhaged and he died in shock.

The *New York State Medical Journal* (September 15, 1956) tells a similar story of an arthritis patient being treated with a daily dose of prednisone. On the 32nd day, he developed perforation of a duodenal ulcer and blood poisoning.

A calm announcement in *Chemical Week* (July 18, 1953) should be kept in mind, too. The Upjohn Company introduced a new drug called Pamine for the treatment of ulcers. It is aimed at paralyzing the vagus nerve, the nerve which initiates the secretion of the acid juices in the stomach. It is described as "somewhat toxic in overdosages." How anyone would ever digest any food with his vagus nerve paralyzed is quite beyond us.

[894]

It is interesting to find that men show a greater susceptibility to ulcers than women do. In a survey of 6,047 people, as reported in the *British Medical Journal* (March 30, 1957) it was found that approximately 80 per cent of the ulcer patients were men. The largest incidence of ulcers in men was found to occur between 45 and 54 years of age. Also, duodenal ulcers are more likely to occur in laboring classes than in professional people.

Women who are of childbearing age seem almost to have an immunity to ulcers. The age at which ulcers are especially prevalent in women is 55, and even then the figure of incidence is well below that of men. Dr. Joseph Shaiken, of Marquette University Medical School, confirms this view. He told the American College of Gastroenterology that ulcers in women are more likely to occur during the change of life, or menopause. However, he says, pregnancy invariably has a beneficial effect on ulcer patients at an earlier age.

It is shocking to note the rise in the incidence of ulcers in children. The *British Medical Journal* (June 29, 1957) says that in 1925, in a survey of 8,260 cases of peptic ulcer, only two were children. In 1953, 45 children between the ages of one and eleven seen at a Children's Hospital in one year, were found to have peptic ulcers. The article further states that, in a group of 1,000 adult patients with duodenal ulcers, 26 dated the onset of symptoms to childhood—some as early as 4 and 5 years of age!

There you have the facts on ulcers, their cause, treatment and occurrence. We think the best treatment of all is to avoid getting them in the first place. We think this can best be done by exercising care with one's diet, following those suggestions for healthful eating as outlined by Dr. Quigley, quoted above. If you have recovered from an ulcer, start using a sensible diet free of processed foods, sweets and white flour products, and stick to it! You ate yourself into an ulcer, careful eating can keep you from another.

239. Views Are Changing on Ulcer Cause and Its Treatment

Doctors have been playing a sort of guessing game where ulcers are concerned. They usually have to wait until an ulcer actually appears before they can do anything about it. Even then, they're not agreed on the procedure for healing an ulcer. The traditional treatment has been to have the patient eating often, so that the stomach is never completely empty, and eating only the blandest of foods, liberally laced with milk and cream.

Doctors Disagree on the Need for a Bland Diet

The suggested diet usually contains mostly, foods designed to inhibit the functioning of the gastric juices or to neutralize them. Doctors usually rely on milk and cream to accomplish the latter. On the forbidden list, at the direction of many physicians, are raw fruits and vegetables, condiments, very hot or very cold substances. There is no proof that these foods actually do aggravate ulcers. Dr. J. W. Todd (*Lancet,* January, 1952) said he knew of no reason to avoid the roughage and condiment type of food usually forbidden an ulcer patient, unless the individual found that it caused immediate distress. A. M. Gill, in the same magazine (March 8, 1947), told of 20 consecutive ulcer patients he treated with nothing at all but a harmless and useless daily injection of one cubic centimeter of distilled water. They all healed in 4 to 8 weeks. He attributed the cure to the confidence he had imparted to the patients. They assumed he would make them well and he did. There are other similar testimonies in the medical literature, including one in which 3 doctors observed 121 patients and concluded that dieting with bland foods does not increase the rate of healing with peptic ulcer (*Lancet,* January 7, 1956). S. Wolf experimented by deliberately feeding forbidden foods, such as garlic, parsnips, radishes, onions, turnips, mustard, pickles, etc., to ulcer patients without producing any evidence of irritation.

Coffee, Alcohol and Smoking Dangerous

One thing that most ulcer experts do agree upon is the danger of coffee and alcohol when an ulcer is present. Coffee is known to cause increased flow of the digestive juices, which are responsible for continued irritation in the ulcerated stomach. The caffeine in coffee is also known to destroy vitamin C. This vitamin is the one necessary for maintaining healthy tissue in every part of the body. This includes, of course, the tissue which makes up the lining of the stomach. It is easily inferred from this that coffee drinkers who do not have an ulcer, as yet, are more likely to acquire one than the persons who avoid this beverage. In the case of alcohol, it is the loss of B vitamins, due to drinking, which is presumed to cause or aggravate ulcer.

Because of the value of vitamin C in maintaining the tissue of the stomach lining, another thief of this vitamin, nicotine, is to be avoided by an ulcer patient. We think that alcohol, caffeine and nicotine should be avoided, whether one has an ulcer or not. The loss of B vitamins and vitamin C is never to be taken lightly, for, aside from depriving the rest of the organs of these essential nutrients, one must realize that a lack of them makes one a likely candidate for ulcers.

Fried Foods Offer Clue To Ulcer Cause

The search goes on to find new causes of ulcer. Many phases of modern living are suspect. Fried foods have always been considered questionable, and an article in *Food Field Reporter* (June 22, 1959) confirms the danger. Dr. Robert S. Goodhart, Director of the National Vitamin Research Foundation, Incorporated, told the interesting story of the connection between heated fats and ulcer. In the mid-1950's, Dr. Max Horwitt began a study on vitamin E deficiency in human beings. Though it had been demonstrated in animals, no one knew what to look for as a sign of human vitamin E shortage. Dr. Horwitt set out to produce a vitamin E deficiency in man by means of a special diet.

It is known that unsaturated fats are rich in vitamin E, but that high heat destroys the vitamin E in them. Dr. Horwitt fed his subjects diets with heated unsaturated fats. It took some time for the signs to appear, but, eventually, the vitamin E level in the blood was seen to decline and the red blood corpuscles became fragile. This activity was taken to prove that vitamin E is a dietary essential for humans.

An unintended result of this experiment showed up about a year later; one-third of the subjects used in the vitamin E experiment were found to have duodenal ulcers. The percentage was considered extraordinary, and quite improbable as a mere coincidence. The ulcers cleared quickly when the subjects were taken off the special diet and given regular therapy.

Play Safe with Good Diet

The cause of the ulcers in these subjects is still being debated. It is known that the heating of the fats produced certain chemical formations not found in nature and not readily processed by the body. Whether it was the introduction of these so-called fat "polymers" to the stomach, or the lack of vitamin E, or some unknown factor, that caused the appearance of the ulcers, no one seems prepared to say. Everyone is agreed that it could have been any of these factors.

We have always deplored the use of heated fats, not only in this connection, but as suspected causes of cancer as well. We say, don't fry foods; roast or broil meats, and bake or boil potatoes. Serve other vegetables raw or steamed if possible. Use unsaturated fats in salads and supplement the vitamin E in them with fish foods and wheat germ. Get plenty of vitamin C in fresh vegetables and rose hips. Brewer's yeast and whole or desiccated liver are both excellent sources of all the B vitamins. Eating properly is your best defense against ulcer.

240. Low Blood Sugar as a Cause of Ulcers

A surprising discovery about stomach ulcer patients bulwarks our contention that stomach ulcers are mostly the result of eating refined foods. At a meeting of the American College of Gastroenterology, reported in *Newsweek* for October 29, 1956, Dr. Maxwell Berry disclosed the fact that 75 per cent of stomach ulcer patients also have hypoglycemia, or low blood sugar.

He said, too, that there is a significantly larger number of cells secreting acid in the stomachs of ulcer patients and there is a very large production of acid in the stomach of patients with low blood sugar levels. Putting these two facts together, he predicted that a big percentage of patients with low blood sugar will eventually develop stomach ulcers.

Then, as you might expect, he proceeded to show that the conventional treatment for ulcer (a bland diet and drugs) checks the excessive flow of stomach acid, the low blood sugar symptoms are relieved and the patients improve. Doesn't it seem too bad that he could not have taken hold of the matter the other way around and speculated on the (to us) perfectly obvious conclusion that the same circumstances which are responsible for the low blood sugar also cause the ulcer? Of course, medical men, in general, are not especially interested in causes or prevention so long as they have a drug they can use for temporary relief of symptoms.

What is low blood sugar and how could its cause be the same as the cause of stomach ulcers? It is the opposite of high blood sugar, which prevails in the diabetic person, and, we are told, it is much more common than diabetes. It comes about like this: eating a diet high in carbohydrates (especially refined carbohydrates) causes the level of sugar in the blood to spiral upward rapidly, so that an extremely high rate is reached immediately after eating. Then the level falls so fast that the individual begins to feel uneasy, nervous, hungry, tired. If he can, he eats something more, or he takes a cigarette, for smoking, too, will raise the blood sugar level temporarily.

If you are very well nourished, you can fast for several days and your blood sugar will stay at about the same level, for the liver keeps releasing sugar into the blood gradually so that the level is stabilized just where it should be. But badly nourished folks feel the need to eat every hour or so, because their blood sugar level zooms up and down so fast that they are uncomfortable, nervous and hungry soon after they have eaten.

Specialists in the field of low blood sugar find that it is easy to tell exactly what will happen to the blood sugar depending upon what you eat at any given meal. A breakfast of pancakes, syrup and coffee (all carbohydrates) shoots the blood sugar level up within a matter of minutes, and it falls sharply within an hour or so. A breakfast of meat and eggs causes a slight but steady rise in blood sugar level, which does not fall below normal again until time for the next meal.

Doesn't this explain a lot about present-day eating habits, especially the ever-present chewing gum, cokes, candy bars, doughnuts and coffee, most of us have to munch on practically all day in order to feel comfortable? If we were eating a proper diet, high in protein and low in the starches that cause the sudden abrupt falls in blood sugar, we would not feel the need to nibble at something pretty regularly between meals.

Since wrong eating brings about hypoglycemia, or low blood sugar, to begin with, doesn't it seem reasonable that wrong eating may be responsible for many other disorders, too? And if low blood sugar (caused by wrong diet) is prevalent among ulcer patients, doesn't it seem likely that the same wrong eating caused the ulcer just as it caused the low blood sugar? This is only one of the many pieces of evidence we have gathered over the years implicating present-day refined carbohydrate foods as the main cause of ulcers.

So what do we advise, if you would prevent ulcers? First, avoid refined foods as if they were poison. By this, we mean any and all foods that contain refined sugar or refined grain products—cakes, pies, candy—in fact, anything sweet except for fruits and vegetables. And, of course, any and all products made from white flour—bread, noodles, spaghetti, crackers, pretzels, and so on, and so on.

If your own feelings tell you you have low blood sugar (and you'll know it if you usually find it necessary to eat between meals), take protein snacks rather than starchy ones. Eat a slice of meat, an egg, a handful of nuts, rather than something starchy or sweet. And for meals, cut out the forbidden foods and eat lots of protein. You'll soon have your blood sugar level properly adjusted and you'll be able to feel certain, too, that you are safe from the threat of stomach ulcers.

241. Gastric Ulcers Can Be Prevented

"Life is so hectic these days that even the small fry get ulcers," says an International News Service dispatch from Kansas City. "Dr. W. E. Hendrickson of Poplar Bluff, Missouri, estimated today that 50,000 children from one to six years of age are suffering from gastric ulcers. The physician said even peptic ulcers no longer are rare among children. Hendrickson placed the blame on increased family tensions."

So now the kids are worrying themselves into ulcers! One of these days, some statistician will publish the figures on heart disease among children, along with a learned conjecture that "it's the pace" of present-day kindergarten and grade school that leaves our children cardiac cripples.

Fifty years ago, most kids grew up on the farm. They got out of bed long before dawn to do the chores. They walked miles to school where, as like as not, their teacher licked them soundly just for the exercise. They walked home again, did the chores again and fell into bed too tired even to get into mischief. Who is to say what "family tensions" existed then? But in those days, did anyone ever hear of a child below the age of 6 with a stomach ulcer?

Editor Rodale has covered the question thoroughly in his book, *This Pace is Not Killing Us* (Rodale Books, Incorporated, $1.00), showing that our lives are easier today than ever before and that actually, the emotional and nervous strains of times past were just as great as ours today. The only difference is that, in those days, folks were able to cope with their stresses and strains without developing ulcers, or heart trouble or nervous breakdowns. How? We believe the food they ate was largely responsible.

Here, for instance, is a quote from the Los Angeles *Examiner* for April 4, 1952: "Britain's health officers believe that the treatment of the nation's food with chemicals is having a serious effect on the people's health. After a national inquiry, they blame the increase in stomach ulcers and similar illnesses on greater use of chemicals to sweeten or preserve foods, color them and extend the fat content." Many people, in this country as well as in England, never have the opportunity of eating anything at all that is free from chemicals. Every mouthful of food they take has been refined, processed, degerminated, pasteurized and chemicalized until it resembles food only in the name and perhaps in the number of calories it contains.

Back in 1950, there was a great commotion over a new method of healing ulcers—the cabbage juice treatment. In the September, 1950, issue of the *Journal of the American Dietetic Association* appeared the article that started the hullabaloo. Garnett Cheney, M.D., of the Department of Medicine of Stanford University wrote of treating 65 patients with raw cabbage juice. No medicine was given. The average amount of cabbage juice given per day was one quart. Many of the patients took one quart of fresh cabbage juice for as long as 6 to 12 weeks without any discomfort. Several of the patients had a little difficulty with gas and bloating. But the large majority downed their quart of cabbage juice every day with no trouble at all. The juice was made in a juicer. But, Dr. Cheney says, it can be prepared (with a little more trouble) in an osterizer or even in a plain hand meat grinder. The pulp that results must then be squeezed through a cloth to obtain juice. The juice was taken in conjunction with meals, and also in midmorning, midafternoon and before retiring.

Cabbage Must Be Raw and Fresh

Dr. Cheney stresses over and over again that the juice must be freshly made, and must not be heated. His theory is that the "factor" which cures the ulcer (called "vitamin U" during this experimental period) is very sensitive to heat. Whatever juice is not taken at one time should be refrigerated immediately until it is used. Other vegetable juices or fruit juices may be added to it to increase its palatability. But the main ingredient should, of course, be the cabbage juice. Fresh celery, tomato, pineapple or citrus juice added in small quantities will improve the taste. Incidentally, all but 3 of the 55 patients who used the cabbage juice treatment consistently, were free from symptoms in from 2 to 5 days.

Dr. Cheney believes that "there is an anti-peptic ulcer dietary factor which is readily destroyed by heat. Cabbage in the form of the head, leaf or juice is only one source of this factor." He also reminds us that the whole subject is in the experimental stage and should be carried out only under a physician's direction. We wonder what has happened in the years since this article was published in 1950. Have any more experiments been done? We have seen no reports on any.

Possibly there is something to the theory that some magical anti-ulcer substance exists in cabbage juice. Certainly we doubt whether all the health-minded folks who regularly juice some cabbage or other raw vegetable and drink it ever get stomach ulcers. But we are inclined to believe that it is not the cabbage itself that creates the magic—but the fact that it is, *that it must be,* raw. Probably, for many people who suffer from ulcer, this quart of raw cabbage juice may be the first morsel of uncooked food they have had to eat for years and years. Consider for a moment the children below the age of 6 about whom we spoke earlier. How many of them live on a diet like this: breakfast—cereal, white toast, pasteurized milk (everything here has been cooked); lunch—sandwich, soup and pudding, or stewed fruit (everything here has been cooked); dinner—meat, potatoes, cooked vegetables and pastry or cake (everything here has been cooked). Between meals they have soft drinks and cookies or crackers and jelly.

Dr. Cheney's Convalescent Diet

It is interesting to note that, after Dr. Cheney has relieved the symptoms of his patients, he puts them on a convalescent diet which includes raw fruit or vegetables at every meal, and considerable raw fresh vegetable juice. We are sorry to see that he also allows bread products made from white flour and desserts made with white sugar. We are sure his patients would have a much more successful and rapid convalescence if just these two items were omitted.

242. Potatoes for Ulcer Patients

A potato diet for a peptic ulcer patient! Whoever heard of such a thing! Dr. L. J. J. Nye of Australia has been using it for years, according to an article by him in the *Medical Journal of Australia* for January 2, 1943.

Dr. Nye tells us that his interest in a potato-ulcer diet was first aroused when he visited Ireland and found that peptic ulcer was almost unknown there. Of course, the Irish diet was mainly potatoes. With the exception of the, we believe, relatively few people who are allergic to potatoes, it is an ideal food for ulcer patients. It is rich in minerals and vitamins. The fact that pasteurized milk contains very little vitamin C is another reason why potatoes which do contain considerable vitamin C seem to be best for ulcer patients rather than a milk diet. They need vitamin C, undoubtedly— all they can get, for vitamin C helps immeasurably in wound healing. Then, too, potatoes have an alkaline reaction in the body, thus helping to neutralize overabundant stomach acidity.

Dr. Nye says that he has found potatoes an admirable substitute for, or addition to, milk in the ulcer diet. He advises the patient to take two or more potato meals a day, and for the patient's permanent diet, he recommends that potatoes should be substituted, as much as possible, for bread, which has an acid ash, the potatoes being alkaline.

A Case History

He recounts the story of one ulcer patient, an engineer, and how he fared on a potato diet. His ulcer was a deep one. He agreed to an experiment of living almost entirely on potatoes for several weeks. Treatment was begun on July 23. A two-hourly regime of potatoes supplemented with milk and milk foods was instituted, but the bulk of the diet was made up of potatoes mashed with milk. His intake of potatoes averaged 3 to 3½ pounds a day—8 or 9 large potatoes. Does that sound monotonous? More monotonous than just milk?

Within a few days, the engineer was relieved of pain and returned to work. On August 9, an X-ray revealed a great improvement in the ulcer and on September 26, the radiologist could find no evidence of its presence after careful screening. The patient felt extraordinarily well and had gained 15 pounds during this 5 weeks. He was dismissed with the recommendation that he stick to a routine "bland" diet with frequent feedings and take at least two good helpings of potatoes per day. In the following two years, he had no recurrence of the ulcer, even though he was putting in many overtime hours of anxious work.

Dr. Nye tells us that many patients who could not take milk have been successfully treated with a diet consisting mainly of potatoes. Ulcer patients are frequently surprised when they are told to eat potatoes, for they are under the impression that they are indigestible. In this country, we frequently hear people say they are on a good diet because they don't eat bread or potatoes! Modern American bread is probably the worst so-called food available. But potatoes are excellent food for everyone, even folks who are reducing!

We believe ulcers can easily be prevented, even if you have had them at one time, by following a diet from which refined foods are completely restricted—that is, no cereals and no desserts—nothing at all that has been made from refined cereals or white flour or sugar. A diet high in protein and fresh raw fruits and vegetables will not leave any room for the degenerate foods that are, we are convinced, the main reason for ulcers. Meanwhile, if you are on a monotonous ulcer diet, why not vary it with potatoes, a delicious and very nourishing food!

Do we need to add that the potatoes should not be fried? Or fixed in any other way that involves cutting, dicing, slicing or mashing them. Baking or boiling in the skins results in loss of least vitamins.

243. Vitamin C Injections for Ulcers

In a work published in the *Medical World* for February 10, 1950, Dr. B. A. Meyer of London and his associate, J. I. Orgel, write on the subject of treating peptic ulcer with vitamin C complexes.

They tell us, in this article, that no one knows exactly what causes peptic ulcer, but we do know that a delay in healing an ulcer has been shown to be due to a vitamin C deficiency. We know that this important vitamin is necessary for the sound and rapid healing of wounds, since it is necessary for the formation of intercellular material. Its deficiency has been shown to cause a marked decrease in the tensile strength of wounds. When there is inadequate formation of the intercellular material, or collagen, the cells remain immature and blood vessels do not easily penetrate the poorly developed granulation tissue.

There is, Dr. Meyer believes, considerable vitamin C deficiency among ulcer patients. He gives us references to 4 articles describing studies of ulcer patients where extremely low levels of vitamin C were found. "Subclinical scurvy" is the name given to such deficiencies. In other words, these people have scurvy—not enough to put them to bed or bring fatal consequences—but enough to cause some of the symptoms of scurvy.

Why Ulcer Patients Are Vitamin C Deficient

There are 3 reasons for the condition of vitamin C deficiency in ulcer patients, Dr. Meyer believes. First, the diet for ulcer patients usually

[903]

consists of milk, fish, eggs, chicken and so forth, with little or no fresh fruits or vegetables. The original bland ulcer diet—the "Sippy diet"—contained only 5 milligrams of vitamin C per day for the first week and 15 milligrams per day in the fourth week, when other foods were gradually introduced. A satisfactory intake should be around 70 milligrams a day, says Dr. Meyer. We would add that far more than that would be even better, since we are surrounded every day by so many substances that use up the little vitamin C most of us get in our foods.

We want to point out, too, that individuals on other kinds of diets can suffer from this same difficulty. Ulcerative colitis patients are usually placed on "bland" diets because of their difficulty with tough, fibrous foods. Such diets are bound to be short on vitamin C. Since this vitamin is essential for the process of healing, it becomes apparent why ulcers in the colon are slow to heal.

A blender is the answer for the person who wants fresh raw foods without irritating fibers. Even the toughest vegetables can be blended into a soft mass or (with the addition of a little water) a fine drink which could never be irritating.

The second reason for a condition of near-scurvy in ulcer patients is that there is defective absorption of the vitamin by the intestines, so that even the little vitamin C available does not get into the blood. Vitamin C is not well absorbed in other ailments involving abnormal bowel conditions—ulcerative colitis, constipation which is relieved by daily cathartics.

The third reason for ulcer patients being short on vitamin C is, according to Dr. Meyer, a derangement of vitamin C metabolism. Then he says a very interesting thing—patients who got no better using the "usual" treatment showed improvement when given *vitamin C complexes.* We interpret this to mean that plain, synthetic vitamin C as such would not do the trick, for, apparently, you must have, along with the vitamin C, those additional things that accompany it in food—mainly, the bioflavonoids. Another argument for natural vitamins as opposed to synthetic ones. The synthetic ones contain only the vitamin—nothing more. But the natural preparation contains the other valuable substances that accompany the vitamin in foods.

It seems, then, that the typical ulcer patient is short on vitamin C, cannot absorb it properly through his digestive tract and has trouble using it after it is absorbed, unless it is accompanied by the bioflavonoids. Injections of vitamin C directly into the blood stream should solve the problem, it would seem. Apparently there is no risk of any unpleasant aftereffects from vitamin C injections. They are harmless even in quite large doses.

Patients Report Good Results

Dr. Meyer tells us that ulcer patients he treated with injections of vitamin C had these good results: (1.) Prompt relief of symptoms; (2.) No necessity for rest in bed or absence from work; (3.) No dietary restrictions;

[904]

(4.) No toxic effects; (5.) A general tonic effect which was apparent in most cases.

Here are some of the patients' stories. The first, a 69-year-old man, had a typical history of duodenal ulcer for many years. Dr. Meyer gave him 6 intravenous injections of vitamin C. Within a few weeks after treatment began, he suffered from no pain or discomfort, was eating normal meals, taking no medication, and even drinking beer.

Another patient, 69 years old, had not been able to eat any solids for some time. Within 4 days, he was eating solids and, inside of 10 days, ate a liberal diet with no discomfort. A 70-year-old patient reported improvement within two days and made a completely uneventful recovery from an ulcer of long standing. Other case histories are similar.

We do not advise injections. We believe in preventing diseases before they start. However, in instances of this kind, where the damage has already been done and the body is apparently unable to use some natural substance like a vitamin, then there seems to be no reason for not injecting the vitamin, since it is completely harmless and can have only beneficial results. So we would advise readers who are suffering from ulcers to try large amounts of vitamin C for the possible relief it may bring. If the vitamin C is not assimilated, possibly your doctor would be interested in knowing about Dr. Meyer's work so that he, too, could try injections of vitamin C.

The rest of us, who don't have ulcers, can learn a valuable lesson from Dr. Meyer's work. Vitamin C is essential for body activity every day for good health. And it is particularly important for healing wounds of any kind.

244. Bioflavonoids for Ulcers

The bioflavonoids, also known as vitamin P, are the source of some very encouraging news for ulcer victims, and for those suffering from that peculiar dizziness known as labyrinthitis. New research on both of these diseases has shown bioflavonoids to have a very beneficial effect in curing them.

Capillary Weakness Is the Key

In both diseases, weakness of the capillaries has been found to be a major causative factor. In the case of ulcers, it has been known for some time that inflammation of the intestinal area always precedes the appearance of an ulcer. This inflammation occurs when the capillaries, the tiny avenues which carry the blood to the surface of the skin, are weakened or damaged in some way so that they cannot do their job efficiently. The lack of nourishment to the skin surface results in soreness and, finally, eruption of an ulcer.

[905]

The capillaries are damaged easily if they are not properly nourished. (Almost any type of virus, and all bacterial infections, can cause capillary weakness.) And this damage, when it occurs in the duodenum, is the first step toward developing an ulcer. Even the type of bleeding common to a duodenal ulcer—a slow oozing of blood—is typical of damaged capillaries.

Relationship of Weak Capillaries and Ulcer Is Logical

When the bioflavonoids were discovered by Albert Szent-Gyorgi from citric solids and paprika (they also exist in other foods rich in vitamin C), they were known to be biologically active, and of therapeutic value. Tests and observation soon showed that they could be used effectively in treating abnormal capillary fragility and capillary bleeding. It was logical enough that the relationship between capillary fragility and ulcers would eventually lead to the employment of bioflavonoids in the treatment of ulcer cases. The imagination to see the entire relationship was the only thing lacking.

In the July, 1958, issue of the *American Journal of Gastroenterology*, it became apparent that the secret had been discovered. A paper was published in those pages in which Drs. Samuel Weiss, Jerome Weiss and Bernard Weiss told of their success in using the bioflavonoids in the treatment of 36 cases of bleeding duodenal ulcer.

Nothing But Diet and Bioflavonoids Used

The doctors used no other medication but the bioflavonoids compound, in capsule form, administered orally, at the rate of 3 to 9 capsules per day. Aside from this, only a change in diet was prescribed. The diet was of a type common to ulcer patients, and consisted of an orange juice-milk-gelatine mixture, given in doses of 4 to 6 ounces every two hours, with the bioflavonoid capsules, until bleeding was arrested, usually on the fourth day. After that, the patient was placed on a bland diet which was made up of oatmeal gruel, butter, lactose, pea soup, bouillon and eggs. These foods were given in small amounts 6 times a day. Vitamin supplements were added to the diet and bioflavonoid rations, when the need was indicated.

All of the 36 ulcer cases treated in this way responded with a return of the mucous membrane and duodenal contour to a normal state. This healing usually took place in a period of from 12 to 22 days, and was ascertained by means of X-ray examinations.

Of even greater importance to the relieved patients was the fact that the cure lasted. Twenty-three of the 36 patients had no recurrence of bleeding in two years or more. Twelve cases remained ulcer-free for one year or more, and the remaining case had been successfully treated and ulcer-free for 4 months, at the time this report was written.

No Generally Accepted Ulcer Treatment

There is still a mighty controversy raging as to which treatment is best in ulcer cases. As one authority put it, "We are still treating peptic ulcer blindly, and consequently, with embarrassingly poor results." About half of those whose opinions count still favor surgery in cases of bleeding ulcer, in spite of the results achieved with diet and the use of specific nutrients. The mortality insurance rates point in the opposite direction, however, They show that patients operated on for duodenal ulcer have a lower survival rate than those who are treated by other means. We think the odds make it well worthwhile to try the two to three week treatment described by the Doctors Weiss. If it should fail, surgery is always available as a last recourse. Better yet, keep ulcers out of your life by eating wholesome foods, fortified with food supplements, including bioflavonoids.

~~~~~~

SECTION 63: UNDERWEIGHT

~~~~~~

245. The Problem of Underweight

Being too fat is distressing, from the point of view of both health and happiness. But being too thin is almost as great a problem, as those of us who grew up to the derisive catcall of "Hey, skinny!" know.

Excessive thinness is not attractive. And it may produce unusual fatigue, nervousness and a predisposition to many ills. It is considered quite healthy to be slightly underweight. Deaths from most of the degenerative diseases—heart and blood vessel disorders, diabetes, cancer and so forth—are much fewer in that group of people who consistently maintain their weight at a little below "normal." But some diseases, such as tuberculosis, claim most of their victims from among those who are very thin.

We put the word "normal" in quotes above, for we have the idea that many of us tend to measure our degree of over- or underweight by the tables that are put out by the insurance companies according to age and height. But what is underweight for one person may be normal for another, so it is not wise to go entirely by the standard tables when you are figuring out just where you stand. These tables are compiled, not from any ideal weight, but from averages over the country as a whole. So, if you happen to be 35 years old and 5 feet six inches tall, the table does not mean that 142 is the ideal weight for you. It means simply that this is the average or "normal" weight for others of your age and height all over the country.

Two Types of Thin Persons

So don't spend too much time worrying if you show up quite a bit underweight according to the tables. It seems that it is perfectly natural and healthy for many people to be thin. Doctors call these people "sthenic." They have good muscles and the average amount of endurance and stamina. They have good resistance to disease, they are poised and emotionally stable. They have a well balanced nervous system, but their bodies somehow just don't deposit fat. If you are this kind of person, don't worry about your underweight. You will probably live to a healthy old age untroubled by the high blood pressure and diabetes that make your stout neighbors' lives unendurable.

The other kind of thin person is called "asthenic." Such a person lacks endurance, is easy prey to fatigue and diseases, is nervous and physically weak. He is not able to meet the demands made on him by society either from a physical or personality standpoint. Usually such an individual has a narrow, shallow chest, poor posture, flabby muscles and a weak digestion. Subconsciously he fights the idea of taking more food, for he is convinced that food does not agree with him. So he continues to grow thinner. If you are an "asthenic" type of thin person, you would do well to increase your weight if you can, for obviously your body is badly nourished and the outcome may not be a happy one.

Medical literature and the books on library shelves are full of suggestions on losing weight. Almost every month, a new book on reducing is published; a new reducing diet appears at regular intervals in monthly magazines; radio programs advertise countless diets and reducing medicines that line the shelves of drug stores. In fact, it seems that the plight of the overweight person gets much more attention than that of the thin one. One good reason for this is the large number of Americans who are overweight. Underweight is not nearly so general a problem. But there is another reason, too. It is pretty generally agreed that the overweight person can reduce by simply eating less. But it does not follow, apparently, that the thin person can gain weight by eating more. Throughout all the research we did in medical journals, we found very, very little material on the subject of gaining weight. And what articles we found specified that there is no one formula for success. Serious underweight is a hard problem to lick.

How Is Your Appetite?

There is general agreement on the fact that there are two kinds of underweight—exogenous and endogenous. That is, some people are thin simply because they don't eat enough of foods which will put on weight. This is exogenous underweight—coming from circumstances *outside* the body. But others are thin, apparently, from some reason that has nothing to do with how much food they eat, for they may have good appetites and (without gaining a single pound) may eat as much as others in their family who are overweight. This is the endogenous underweight—arising from something *inside* the body.

In the case of the first group, the answer is simply to eat more food. Yet perhaps we had better not say "simply," for sometimes there are complex reasons why people do not eat enough, just as there are complex reasons why others eat too much. Faulty habits of eating are perhaps as responsible as anything else for inadequate intake of food. An example is the child who gets up too late to eat breakfast, wolfs down a few bites for lunch because he is eager to get back to playing, and hastens through dinner with one eye cocked toward the television set. In the case of children, of course, the parents must play the biggest part in correcting bad eating habits, for the child cannot possibly foresee what difficulties may result later from these habits. But how can he be taught good food habits by a father who habitually gulps a cup of coffee for breakfast, skips lunch or eats a sandwich while he stands up at a drug store counter and then finds himself too exhausted to do justice to dinner? Or a mother who also skips breakfast and can't be bothered to make lunch because no one else is home at lunchtime?

Children and adults alike should be taught the importance of food and of mealtimes. Three times a day at least, all other activities should be dropped completely for meals. Meals should be eaten in a quiet, unhurried and unworried atmosphere, regardless of what television programs are at hand or what other activities are pending. Mealtime should, above all things, be a pleasant time—no scolding, no worrying, no arguing, no recitals of bad news should ever be permitted within 10 feet of a dinner table. Meals should be served at regular hours. If dinner is delayed an hour beyond the regular time, children and adults alike will be so hungry, that they are bound to be grumpy and cranky. If they have taken the edge off their appetites with crackers or candy, the worthwhile food served at the meal may go uneaten.

Psychological Deterrents to Appetite

Persistent worry, psychological upsets and a feeling of being unwanted or unloved can result in lack of appetite. In fact, the whole phenomenon of psychological disorders getting in the way of appetite has become so common, that it has been given a medical name—*anorexia nervosa*—nervous lack of appetite. As the appetite dwindles, and the individual eats less, his stomach shrinks accordingly, he has a desire for less and less food. As his body loses nourishment, he may develop an extremely serious condition that can result in death—death from starvation actually, although there is plenty of food around him.

In the case of children, one nutritionist, Jean Bogert, has put the matter quite directly in her book, *Nutrition and Physical Fitness* (Saunders, 1949)—we do not let our children decide on what clothes to buy, whether or not they wish to go to school or what time they go to bed, so why in the world should we leave it up to the children to decide what they will or will not eat? Obviously this is a matter needing mature judgment. And the child who is allowed to have as much candy, soft drinks, chewing gum and ice cream as he wants between meals, will not have any appetite for the meats, vegetables and fruits which he should be eating at his meals.

Bringing back appetite to adults is a little harder to accomplish. And sometimes it necessitates a firm hand and as much will power as the overweight person needs to refuse food. One element that should be kept constantly in mind is that a lack of vitamins—B vitamins particularly—results in loss of appetite. We have yet to see or hear of the thin person without appetite who can hold out against a whopping big dose of brewer's yeast or desiccated liver daily. He has no choice. Regardless of "nerves," stubbornness or a deep psychological hatred of food, 3 or 4 weeks of brewer's yeast or desiccated liver therapy *will* give him an appetite—it's bound to—unless there are conditions of ill health present that prevent him from absorbing the B vitamins.

Of course, we should not have to remind you that food should be attractively served to tempt the appetite of a thin person. A rest (yes, we mean lying down) from 5 minutes to a half hour before and after meals will bring enough relaxation that food may appear attractive again. If appetite has been poor for some time, it will take a while to establish normal eating habits again. The stomach must be stretched so that no feeling of disagreeable fullness results. Snacks in midmorning and midafternoon, as well as something to eat before going to bed, may be the answer, for it is hard to eat enough at only 3 meals, if you have been accustomed to nibbling.

Now, throughout all this discussion of how to get thin persons to eat more, we have not touched on *what* they should eat. Not so many years ago, the theory was that, since sweet and starchy food make a fat person fatter, a thin person should eat lots of them to gain weight. In fact, one medical article that we found, written only about 15 years ago, advised all kinds of starchy foods—spaghetti, macaroni, bread and butter—for gaining weight. But more recently the thinking has been that, just as high-protein diets regulate metabolism so that the fat person loses weight, so high-protein diets are valuable for gaining weight. True, the thin person need not watch calories on foods like potatoes, beans, butter and so forth. But he should certainly not try to put on weight by eating lots of refined cereals, foods like noodles, spaghetti, cake, pie or foods that are high in refined sugars, such as candy, ice cream and so forth. A diet high in protein and starchy vegetables (prepared to retain all their vitamin and mineral content) with a minimum of sweets and plenty of fruits and vegetable oils should certainly result in weight gaining.

Some Deterrents to Food Absorption

The second kind of thin person who wants to gain weight presents a much harder problem to solve. This is the individual who has a good appetite and eats as much as the average person, but who still remains scrawny and bony, in spite of everything he can do. In the book, *Diseases of Metabolism*, edited by Garfield G. Duncan, M.D. (W. B. Saunders Company, 1952), there is a full page list of factors which can produce undernutrition. Skipping those which have to do with lack of appetite, and purely mechanical causes such as bad teeth, diseases of the mouth and diseases such as peptic ulcers and so forth, we find quite an extended list of conditions that prevent absorption of food, which might be what is wrong with our thin person who cannot gain weight no matter how much he eats.

Here are some of them: 1. Those which increase destruction of food before the body has assimilated it—lack of hydrochloric acid in the stomach, or the taking of alkaline medicines such as bicarbonate of soda.

2. Those which interfere with absorption of food—absence of normal digestive secretions, dysentery, colitis and other diarrheal diseases; sprue; vitamin deficiencies; drugs which prevent absorption, such as mineral oil, cathartics and so forth.

3. Those which interfere with utilization or storage—impaired liver function, alcoholism, hypothyroidism, therapy with one or another of the sulfa drugs, or X-ray therapy.

Now, how does such information apply to those of us who are underweight? Well, have you had an illness during the past 10 years or so for which your doctor prescribed sulfa drugs? If so, it is quite possible that these drugs affected a very important part of your digestive tract—the intestinal flora—those friendly bacteria that dwell inside you and help in the digestion of food and the synthesis of some vitamins. This might be an excellent reason why you are short on B vitamins and why you are not assimilating your food as you should. Do you take mineral oil? If so, you're bound to be suffering from a shortage of all the fat-soluble vitamins —A, D, E and K—for these are dissolved and carried away in the presence of mineral oil. Do you suffer chronically from any condition involving diarrhea? If so, perhaps a great deal of your food is excreted without being assimilated, so that no matter how much you eat, your food is doing you little good.

Or perhaps you have not been eating correctly and so you have a real deficiency of many vitamins. This will prevent you from making proper use of your food. People who are underweight should try as much as possible to eat concentrated foods.

Food supplements are a much more highly concentrated food. For instance, let's say you are underweight and have been taking mineral oil and so are short on vitamin A. Don't try to get all that vitamin A from carrots. Although carrots are good for many reasons, you must eat more than one cup of diced carrots to get the amount of vitamin A that is contained in a few perles of commercial vitamin A product. Carrots are quite low in calories, so they will not help much in your weight building program.

Most advice on gaining weight will tell you to avoid bulky foods that are low in calories, such as salad greens. Under no circumstances would we advise cutting out raw green, leafy vegetables—you must have them. But you can cut down to, say, one salad a day, provided you get plenty of vitamins C, A and B in food supplements. That would mean taking rose hips, fish liver oil and brewer's yeast or desiccated liver—highly concentrated sources of these 3 vitamins.

Do You Know How to Save Energy?

Finally, authorities are agreed that the most common reason for underweight among people whose appetites are good is a waste of nervous and muscular energy. If they are children, they are striving to be the best student in the class or the captain of the team. If they are adults, they are perfectionists in everything they do—driving themselves all day long, never relaxing, and too busy to waste much time sleeping. If this is your difficulty, the only way to solve it is to begin to take it easy. Don't rush. Do everything with the least possible expenditure of energy. Don't walk if you can ride. Don't stand if you can sit. Don't sit if you can lie down. The more energy you use up in everyday activities, the more fat you are burning. And you need your fat. You need it to pad your bones. You need it to provide support for your abdominal organs so that they will not become displaced. And you need it against some possible future day when an illness may use up even more fat and energy than you expend when you are healthy.

In general then, this would be our advice for those of you who are worried about being underweight.

1. Watch your diet. Don't try to gain weight by stuffing yourself on desserts and candy. A diet high in protein—meat, fish, poultry, nuts and eggs—is best for you, along with plenty of vegetables and fruits, fresh and dried.

2. Relax and stop burning up so many calories in your daily activity. Take naps. Rest before and after meals if possible. Be sure that you eat 3 good big meals a day and have wholesome snacks between meals and at bedtime (if this does not spoil your appetite).

3. Eat concentrated natural foods high in calories. Remember, though, that refined foods—white breads, bakery goods and refined cereals—will do you no good and may do you considerable harm. Make certain you are getting enough vitamins and minerals by taking food supplements—the most highly concentrated foods there are. Take fish liver oil for vitamin A, brewer's yeast or desiccated liver for vitamin B and rose hips for vitamin C.

246. Too Fat—or Too Thin?

Remember the picture of Jack and his wife in the old Mother Goose book? Jack so lean and hungry, with his clothes hanging baggily on him, Mrs. Sprat round and ruddy, reaching for more and more food!

Doctors and psychiatrists studying obesity have now decided there is a "fat personality"—that is, a certain combination of personality traits that goes along with fat in a person's character. The study was made at the New England Medical Center by Dr. Benjamin Kotkov, a clinical psychologist, Dr. Stanley S. Kanter, psychiatrist, and Dr. Joseph Rosenthal, an internist. For several years, these scientists studied a selected group of 131 fat women and a control group of about 80 normal-weight women.

Standard psychological tests given to both groups revealed some very interesting things about the overweight women. They were more repressed, more given to daydreaming and less able to use their natural talents creatively than the normal-weight women. They were also more tense and anxious. This surprised us, for we have always thought of thin people as being nervous and tense. The obese women also had a tendency to turn their anger and frustration on themselves, rather than giving vent to it in a healthy outburst of wrath or remonstrance.

The overweight women did not seek out new friends, and it was agreed that sensitivity about their extra poundage was partly responsible for this. But they were also wrapped up in themselves and their own problems, with little interest in the joys or griefs of those around them. They did not enjoy social functions or other "worldly" pleasures as much as the normal women did. They did not feel happy or at ease in their clothes and so took little pleasure in their appearance. Furthermore, these personality traits were indicated by the tests in those who were only 15 per cent overweight as well as in those who were 50 per cent overweight. The 3 specialists conducting the tests were at a loss for any constructive help to be given these women, except for treatment by psychotherapy. "Unless the basic personality problem is solved," they declare, "the weight problem cannot be licked."

In the light of this discouraging conclusion, we were interested in a letter from Theodore Maday, M.D., a physician who is a longtime friend of Editor Rodale. Dr. Maday sent us some stimulating thoughts on the subject of underweight and undernourished individuals and what can be done about them. From his observations over the years, Dr. Maday believes that there is a "thin personality"—the kind of person who will never attain normal weight unless some of his habits are drastically changed.

The Reason Why Some People Are Thin

An undernourished person, he says, does not have fully developed taste buds, with the result that he simply does not enjoy his food. "From babyhood and childhood he has been a problem feeder," says Dr. Maday, "nervous and active and often harrassed, who boasts that he would rather be doing something else than eating. His face is usually long and thin-nosed (like Jack Sprat's we guess) and, whether he is nervous or phleg-matic, he can and does conceal his nervousness. . . . If we do taste tests, we discover mostly a meager development of sour, acid, salt and sweet taste buds. This individual obviously is undernourished for the simple reason that he has insufficient taste to make any food attractive. His taste buds have been undeveloped since childhood. His hunger will be from the stomach and he will eat only enough to satisfy that. . . . His taste buds must be developed by a common-sense explanation of just what is de-ficient. He should be asked to hold an apple or an orange or a bunch of grapes and smell them at frequent intervals until he develops a desire to eat that fruit. The sense of smell stimulates the taste buds. This will take time, but if you appeal to his reason, and if he expects improvement, he will cooperate. He should be encouraged to be with people of good appe-tites, and to try to taste foods in preparation or, if he is a man, perhaps even study cooking or become proficient in preparing barbecue meals for his friends."

Another kind of thin person, according to Dr. Maday, is the hollow-cheeked individual who concentrates on work and study. Desire for food is incidental. Keen hunger is lacking, even when food is needed. When this individual is eating, he reads or thinks of other things rather than enjoy-ing his food. The result is that he takes away energy from his stomach and digestive processes with resulting discomfort after meals. In his case, the taste buds are only dormant, and can be stimulated in the company of jovial, sociable people, at picnics, informal parties and, perhaps the best place of all, in the kitchen, preparing or helping to prepare delicious food.

Now surely in the light of what Dr. Maday says about thin, under-nourished people, you would not think of them as being especially well-adjusted and perfectly free from any personality problems. Why then do they not react as the overweight people do and take out their frustration and woe in eating? We have compared notes with friends and neighbors, and we find we know a number of overweight people who admit that they try to solve, or perhaps we should say avoid, their daily problems and frustrations by eating. If these people get really angry or sad or lonely, they want to eat, almost as if they were saying to themselves, "I'll get even with whoever it was that made me feel like this. I'll just eat a whopping big meal with an enormous dessert and top it off with a box of chocolates. I'll get even!" On the other hand, we know several thin and undernour-ished people who react in just the opposite way. As soon as they are upset or angry or sad, they stop eating entirely, almost as if they were saying, "I'll get even. I'll just stop eating and I'll waste away to a shadow, and then everybody will be sorry they treated me so badly."

Therapy for Those Not Interested in Food

We do agree with Dr. Maday that many thin, undernourished people simply do not enjoy eating at all, and many overweight people enjoy it too much. The thin people, especially as they grow older, tend to avoid variety in food and confine themselves to the same few dishes day after day. We are amazed when we read in medical journals case after case of older people who actually live on tea and toast, a little soup and crackers, or cereal and coffee. Sometimes they have the excuse of missing teeth or uncomfortable dentures. These can be remedied.

Then, as Dr. Maday says, these folks must simply be taught to enjoy food. We would suggest that the first step in this direction is to give them an abundance of all the B vitamins in the form of desiccated liver. Hundreds of laboratory experiments have proved that plenty of vitamin B is necessary for a good appetite. And we know that, once these "picky" undernourished folks begin to get enough vitamin B, their hunger is bound to increase, even though they may still like to pretend that their appetites are as bird-like as ever.

Once they begin to experience normal, wholesome hunger, this is the time to bring out your tastiest dishes and by this, needless to say, we do not mean chocolate pie and caramel cup-cakes. We mean meat—their favorite meat at first—cooked in some delectable way, seasoned just right, served attractively. We mean salads—huge salads of tender crisp greens, with a carefully made salad dressing, garlic and herbs. We mean eggs—cooked appetizingly with some tasty sauce, mushrooms or a sharp, spicy dressing. We mean vegetables—tender, raw and crisp, or cooked just a little. We mean fruits. Just as Dr. Maday says, you must teach these folks to enjoy the smell of the fruit first, then urge them to try more, and different kinds.

One other suggestion about that member of your family who won't eat enough to bring his weight up to normal. Perhaps through his disinterest in food, he eats very slowly. By the time everyone else is finished, he may have eaten only a few mouthfuls. If you rush through the meal and clear the table, he will never get a full meal. So try to make mealtimes more relaxed and unhurried. The children get impatient and must be off to play, so excuse them from the table, but keep the grownups occupied with fruit, nuts and cheese until the last slow eater is finished. Never rush him or complain that he holds things up by eating slowly. Encourage him to have a second helping of meat and vegetables, even though everyone else has long since finished dessert. And stay with him and talk to him while he eats.

247. A New Treatment for Brucellosis

The disease we know today as undulant fever, or brucellosis, may have been known as long ago as 400 B. C. We are told that Hippocrates described an intermittent fever which may have been this. Undulant fever existed along the shores of the Mediterranean for 5 or 6 hundred years. In the eighteenth century, it was studied by the medical profession. It was then called "Malta Fever."

Brucellosis is caused, supposedly, by a germ called the *Micrococcus melitensis*. It is found in the liver, kidneys, spleen, lymphatic glands and salivary glands, in the blood, bile, urine and in milk. The disease is very widespread around the world, apparently. It seems certain that the disease is transmitted from food animals to human beings. Apparently milk from infected cows, if it has not been treated to kill the bacteria, may cause the disease in susceptible persons.

Its symptoms are rather varied. Edwin C. Mick, M.D., of East Orange, New Jersey, writing in *Archives of Pediatrics* for April, 1955, tells us symptoms of a number of his patients who were suffering from brucellosis. Extreme fatigue, abdominal pains, and pains in other parts of the body, especially joints, loss of sleep, night sweats, loss of appetite and weight, digestive disturbances were the symptoms. In every case, recurrent fever was a symptom. Some of the patients had had brucellosis since childhood. In others, it was of more recent origin.

Dr. Mick describes 12 cases of his own. Then he tells us that, from reading articles by Dr. W. J. McCormick, he decided to use vitamin C as therapy for these patients. Dr. McCormick of Canada has successfully used large doses of vitamin C on many kinds of infectious diseases. Dr. Mick gave his patients as much as 3,000 to 6,000 milligrams of vitamin C a day, after all other medication had failed to show any results.

These are his reports on patients after they had taken the vitamin C:

1. Fatigue all gone. Abdominal pain gone. Occasional pains in joints. All other symptoms have disappeared.

2. Except for a slight skin eruption, he is symptom-free.

3. No further symptoms.

4. Free from all symptoms. Tremors gone. Numbness, pain, mental depression gone. Normal appetite. Working full time.

[916]

5. This patient had brucellosis since childhood. Dr. Mick is certain that, because of her acute intestinal disturbances, she did not absorb the vitamin C, for she showed no response.

6. This patient, too, had the fever from childhood and apparently did not absorb the vitamin.

7. Pain in legs eliminated. Headaches absent. No pain in eyes. Fatigue much diminished. New outlook on life.

8. Definitely improved. Almost free from pain. Appetite improved.

9. Sleeping normally. Nausea gone. Fatigue reduced. Temperature normal.

10. All pains gone. Fatigue almost gone. Temperature normal. Nausea gone.

11. Fatigue rapidly disappearing. No further swelling of ankles or dizziness.

12. Less fatigue. Pains gone. Symptom-free.

Dr. Mick quotes Dr. McCormick as saying that he had found ascorbic acid (vitamin C) better than any or all of the antibiotics for infectious diseases, bacterial or viral.

In New Jersey, alone, says Dr. Mick, there are estimated to be 30,000 new cases of brucellosis yearly. Some authorities believe that as much as 10 per cent of the entire rural population of this country is infected. In a booklet entitled *Crippler in Disguise,* published by the National Society for Crippled Children, Dr. Alice C. Evans states that the number of sufferers from brucellosis in this country must be around 8 million. Since milk is pasteurized in this country, says Dr. Mick, the number of cases in countries where raw milk is drunk must be staggering.

Another Way to Get Brucellosis

Another very interesting aspect of the cause of the widespread incidence of brucellosis comes to us in an article from Brazil, *Revista da Associacao medica brasileira* for July, 1955. This article says that brucellosis is one of the diseases that may be transmitted by a blood transfusion. Trying to determine the frequency of brucellosis in donors that come to the blood bank at the Hospital of the University of Sao Paulo, the writers of this article performed tests on the blood of a number of healthy persons. They found 9 positive reactions among 839 donors. That does not seem very high, but the number of donors who might have contributed brucellosis infection to the blood bank does not indicate of course what might happen to those who have blood transfusions from that particular blood bank. How much infection is needed to cause brucellosis in persons who are already ill who receive blood transfusions?

The Brazilian magazine goes on to say that, although the transmission of brucellosis by the transfusion of blood has been demonstrated in rare cases, the problem is of little practical interest because the disease is not common there. (In Brazil, that is.) Even so, those who slaughter hogs,

workers in refrigerators, butchers and veterinarians, and all those with suspected brucellosis, should be rejected as donors, or should be tested before
being allowed to donate blood.

Could our present mania for blood transfusions at the slightest excuse
have anything to do with the fact that brucellosis is apparently widespread?
At any rate, we have proof once again of the marvelous effectiveness of
vitamin C against bacteria, even in cases of long-standing infection.

SECTION 65: VARICOSE VEINS

248. Varicose Veins

"Alpha tocopherol (vitamin E) has been used successfully in the treatment of acute phlebitis. It seems to have very obvious advantages over
other agents used in treating this condition."

The quote is from an address made before the Second World Congress
of Obstetrics and Gynecology, Montreal, Canada, June 6, 1958. The speaker
was Dr. Evan V. Shute of the Shute Institute, London, Ontario, Canada.

He went on to say, "For example, it (vitamin E) decreases embolism
(blood clots) to the merest minimum. It not only prevents extension of
existing clots, as do the classical anticoagulants, but it quickly resolves what
clot is present. It acts very rapidly, especially in relieving associated pain
and tenderness. It has none of the side effects which dog the anticoagulants,
since it never produces hemorrhage, for example. Moreover, it does not
require frequent blood examinations, can be self-administered far from any
hospital or even medical care, and is as useful for clots in the vital organs
as for clots in the peripheral vessels. It has an extraordinary ability to increase collateral circulation . . ."

In simple language, Dr. Shute is saying that, for the greatest possible
improvement in the health of the circulatory system, vitamin E is the
thing. In diseases involving blood clots (of which phlebitis is one), it has
been customary to give certain drugs which keep the blood from coagu-
lating. This seems like a good idea except for one thing—when you are
destroying those substances in the blood that make it clot, how are you
going to know when to stop? Carrying the treatment too far will bring
about a condition where the thickening power of the blood is seriously
disturbed, and then hemorrhages are likely to follow.

A blood clot is indeed a serious thing, especially if it occurs in a
blood vessel leading to the brain or the heart. Permanent damage or death

may result. But a hemorrhage into either of these organs can be just as serious. When you begin to tamper with the blood's ability to clot, you can see that you can get into serious trouble. Vitamin E does not work this way. It is a natural constituent of the body—not a drug. So, instead, it regulates those substances in the blood that cause clotting or hemorrhaging.

Dr. Shute says further that vitamin E "has an extraordinary ability to increase collateral circulation." What does this mean? When some part of the circulatory system is injured, an effort is made by the body to repair it. Let's say a blood vessel is clogged with a clot. Naturally that part of the body to which this blood vessel carries blood is going to suffer from loss of blood. So another blood vessel is brought into activity to detour around the obstruction. Vitamin E, says Dr. Shute, has the ability to get this extra blood vessel into working order so that normal operations can proceed.

Patients Treated with Vitamin E Improve

Then Dr. Shute relates what happened to a group of 300 patients who were treated with vitamin E at the Shute Clinic. The first group consisted of 166 patients, all of whom had chronic phlebitis. This is an inflammation of the veins which usually occurs in the legs and feet. It is more common among women and occurs frequently as an aftermath of child- birth. Dr. Shute gives the following as the causes of the disorder in 74 of his patients: Pregnancy, 30; abdominal operations, 17; trauma, including fractures, 15; general or local infections, 5; intravenous injections, 2; other operations, 2; penicillin, 1; hospital bed rest, 1; food poisoning, 1. (It is interesting to note that a total of 23 of these cases of phlebitis resulted from some kind of medical treatment.)

Most patients had suffered from one to five years. Some of them had had phlebitis for longer than 6 years. The main symptoms were swelling and "ache." In addition to the phlebitis, many of the patients had varicose veins, arteriosclerosis and ulcers on the legs. They were given, at the clinic, no other treatment but vitamins. Results were as follows: 35 cases had slight relief; 20 cases had moderate relief; 79 cases had good relief and 32 patients had excellent results, or complete relief.

Some Histories of Phlebitis Patients

Here are some individual case histories. A man of 47 had suffered for 6 years. He was given 300 milligrams, and later 400 milligrams, of vitamin E daily. The trouble in one of his legs cleared 4 days after the dosage was raised to 400 milligrams. At his last visit, he could walk half a mile each day and there was no tenderness in his leg. His feet swelled very slightly and ached slightly on rare occasions.

A woman of 51 had had aching legs for 4 years. She had high blood pressure (160/104) and hence, the beginning dose of vitamin E was smaller—150 milligrams. (Dr. Shute has found that large doses of vitamin E may raise blood pressure in patients whose pressure is already too high.) Raising the dose gradually (225 milligrams within two months), he found great improvement including a lowered blood pressure—130/100. Nine months later, she was entirely well except for rare swelling and slight tenderness and her blood pressure was 130/80.

A 39-year-old patient complained of soreness and swelling in her right ankle for 3 years. She also suffered from cramps at night. She was greatly overweight. She was given 600 units of vitamin E daily, along with calcium and thyroid extract. She was also put on a reducing diet. Four months later, she had lost 21 pounds, the swelling had disappeared and she was feeling well.

Here is how Dr. Shute explains phlebitis and the varicose veins that practically always accompany it. He says that deep phlebitis should be looked for whenever there are varicose veins, "however mild or early." He says, "We are surprised nowadays to find a patient who has varicosities and still no evidence of chronic phlebitis in the deep veins." By this he means the veins deep in the muscles of the legs rather than on the outside where they can be easily seen.

The veins deep inside the leg muscles are designed to carry about 80 per cent to 90 per cent of the return flow of blood from the feet. If something goes wrong, so that one of these veins is plugged, the veins on the outside of the leg near the skin surface must take over. In the effort to cope with this additional work, these veins dilate, twist and do their best to empty the blood from feet and legs. They enlarge and the valves which control the blood flow cease to function properly. The veins which join the deep set of vessels to the exterior ones become filled with blood and big varicose veins spray out over the ankles.

If a doctor injects or cuts or strips away these ugly veins on the outside of the leg, he is removing the only possible channel for the blood to flow through, since the deeper veins are already plugged. So the patient may end up far worse off than before the operation.

The Way Vitamin E Acts to Increase Circulation

What does vitamin E do, if it is used instead of an operation? It "produces collateral circulation about the obstructed deep veins by calling into play the great unused networks of veins lying in wait for emergency utilization. We have such venous reserves just as we have reserves of brain, lung and liver. Alpha tocopherol mobilizes them. It does more. It has the unique power of enabling tissues to utilize oxygen better and hence, the devitalized and congested leg tissues of the chronic phlebitic who is given alpha tocopherol are receiving the equivalent of more oxygen," says Dr. Shute. It should be remembered, too, he adds, that taking vitamin E before you experience any of these painful symptoms is the best possible way of guarding against them.

The Condition of Collagenosis

A condition which frequently follows chronic phlebitis is called, by Dr. Shute, collagenosis, also cellulitis, or inflammation of cell structure. Of the 134 patients he treated for this condition, most of them had all but given up any search for treatment, since nothing that had been done for them seemed to help at all. Eighteen per cent of them had evidently come to this condition as a result of abdominal operations!

Sixty-five of the patients had varicose veins, 16 had arteriosclerosis and 74 had chronic ulcers on their legs. These were very severe cases, Dr. Shute says, which had been receiving drastic treatment before coming to him.

Here are some case histories. A man of 59 had had ulcers on his legs for 13 years. He was given 400 units of vitamin E daily, along with 100,000 units of vitamin A. Seven months later, he "felt like a young man" and had no further complaints. From that time on, he was completely well, but continued on the vitamin E and vitamin A. Incidentally, this is an extremely large dose of vitamin A, which we would not recommend as a permanent thing. Vitamin A accumulates in the body and can be dangerous if too much is taken.

A 46-year-old woman had had aching legs, cramps in her legs and varicose veins for several years. She was given 600 units of vitamin E, as well as calcium and vitamin D, for the cramps. "She returned a month later," says Dr. Shute, "unable to believe that she could be helped so much. She had been working day and night and yet her legs were not painful." Of course, she continued to take vitamin E.

The final history we want to give is that of an 84-year-old woman who had had enlarged veins in her legs for most of her adult life. She also suffered from arthritis. Two months of treatment with 375 units of vitamin E left her completely well.

Forty-eight of the second group of patients could be said to have gotten fairly good results, we are told. Dr. Shute concluded his talk by recommending that physicians look for deep phlebitis in every case of varicose veins they see. He believes that phlebitis is usually the cause of varicose veins. High dosage of vitamin E is the secret to successful treatment of phlebitis, he says. He has used as high as 1000 units per day.

Always, in speaking of high doses of vitamin E, Dr. Shute cautions against their use in patients with high blood pressure. An initial high dosage can raise the pressure sharply, causing serious trouble. So, if you have high blood pressure, it is best to begin taking vitamin E with small doses and increase them gradually.

We have used the terms milligrams and International Units interchangeably throughout this chapter, as they mean the same thing in the case of this vitamin.

Exercise Important, Too

We have one other suggestion for the prevention of phlebitis and varicose veins, apart from taking vitamin E and, of course, making certain that your diet is well chosen. Doesn't it seem likely that some of our present-day difficulty with the blood vessels of our feet and legs comes from the fact that we just don't use them enough? We were made to be active all day long—and by active we don't mean driving a car or punching a TV tuning button.

We need to exercise, all of us, every day. Walking is one of the best and cheapest forms of exercise. Walk in the country, if you can; walk barefoot, if you can; walk before breakfast and before lunch and before dinner, if you can. But regardless of how much you can walk, do plan your day's activities, no matter how much trouble it takes, to include at least one good long walk every day. You'll be amazed at how thoroughly the exercise will get the blood to flowing through in your feet and legs.

When you rest, put your feet up on something—a footstool if you're sitting, a pile of cushions or the arm of a chair if you're lying down.

249. A New Theory on Varicose Veins

We are always delighted when we can bring to readers a helpful idea from the medical profession—especially when it concerns something simple, practical and easy to understand. Such a theory was presented in the August 15, 1959, issue of the British medical journal, the *Lancet*—one of the most progressive medical journals.

The article was written by a surgeon-captain in the British Navy—T. L. Cleave. It shows the same thoughtful, searching point of view and the same everyday, common-sense-approach that distinguishes Dr. Cleave's other writings.

Dr. Cleave asks in the *Lancet* article, are varicose veins nature's error or man's? He tells us that medical opinion favors the idea that man is the only animal subject to varicose veins because he is the only one that walks upright, and his troubles with the veins in his legs began when he assumed his upright position. But, says Dr. Cleave, we know that animals (and man) adapt themselves to changes in their environment or perish. How does it happen, then, that nature could have made such a grievous error in the anatomy of man, by allowing him to assume an upright position many, many years ago and not in some way adapting him to this position so that he should no longer suffer from it?

Dr. Cleave says, "It is not as though varicose veins were rare, or confined to people above the reproductive age whose physical efficiency may be reckoned unimportant to the survival of the race. DeTakats and Quint found that 10 per cent of 1,000 otherwise healthy young workers suffered from varicose veins of some degree, and in older people, they are, of course, far more prevalent; for example, Foote considers that, in Great Britain, the number affected is in the region of 5 million, and it is now the commonest surgical ailment in this country. Such a tremendous incidence is evolutionarily quite incompatible with the view that the veins are a structural weak link—a failure in man's evolution. The struggle for existence has never been so kind as to permit a state of affairs like this."

People Are Not Born with Varicose Veins

Is it a congenital state of affairs, then? That is, are people born with varicose veins, or born with a tendency to have them? Obviously not, says Dr. Cleave, for congenital malformations in general affect not more than .5 per cent of the population, whereas varicose veins afflict 20 times this many people. Besides, malformations with which one is born are caused by an error in the fusion or joining together of certain parts in the unborn child; they are not errors in mechanical conception, as varicose veins are.

Varicocele, which is a dilation of the veins of the spermatic cord of the testicle, is much commoner on the left side. Ordinary varicose veins of the leg are about 10 per cent commoner on the left side. Severe varicosities, which have usually been preceded by a blood clot in the veins of the thigh, are commoner by 50 per cent on the left side. (These patients have generally been confined to bed for considerable lengths of time.)

A Common Condition May Be the Cause

Dr. Cleave believes that the cause of varicose veins is constipation, and he shows clearly that the greater incidence of these on the left side of the body helps to strengthen his theory.

The vein leading out of the left side of the testicle opens into the renal vein at right angles without a valve, while the right vein opens into the main vein obliquely, with a valve. The way the left vein leads into the main abdominal vein results in a greater pressure on that side. On the left side of the abdomen, is the part of the colon which descends to the rectum. It crosses directly over the left spermatic vein. On the right side, is the ascending colon which does not cross over the right ascending spermatic vein. This is the circumstance which, Dr. Cleave believes, holds the secret of varicose veins. Civilized life has created, suddenly, a new set of conditions which make this anatomical difference in the two sides important.

He goes on, "Thus, the removal today of so much of the fibre from foodstuffs often leads to delay in the passage of the colonic contents and hence, to increase in their weight. Since a relatively low pressure can arrest the blood-flow in even the largest veins, a loaded iliac colon (the left side) can easily obstruct the left spermatic vein, and ultimately induce a varicocele."

What about varicose veins in the legs? "How can we suppose," asks Dr. Cleave, "that the evolutionary forces which, during countless ages,

[923]

have adapted man's feet, hands, legs and arms, and countless other structures, to the erect posture, have failed to make the necessary adaptations also in his leg veins?"

Weight of Body Fluids Could Be Big Factor

In the standing or sitting position, the entire weight of the contents of the ascending colon, which are fluid, is transmitted down to the cecum (the place where the small intestine opens into the colon). If the colon is overloaded, says Dr. Cleave, this pressure will be considerable—more, perhaps, than the pressure exerted on the other side by the contents of the descending colon. This may explain why plain, everyday varicose veins are not much more common on the left side than on the right—a little more common, but not much.

How does such a consideration affect very serious varicose veins— the kind that confine one to bed? These are many times more common on the left side. Lying down in bed results in far less pressure by that part of the colon on the right side of the body, but there is still plenty of pressure on the left side where the colon, overloaded, lies over the large vein that goes to the legs.

Dr. Cleave goes into more detail in regard to the pressure involved when one arises from a lying down position to a standing or walking position. We do not think it is necessary to go into these rather complicated explanations, for we think he has made his point and made it well.

Individual Anatomy Makes a Difference

Now, how does the theory stand up in view of some of the things we know about varicose veins? First of all, granted that most people in the civilized world eat about the same kind of refined foods, why do some have varicose veins and others do not? Dr. Cleave says that is probably because they differ in the robustness and valvular arrangement of their leg veins and the arrangement of their colons. It is not hard to see what a difference would be made by even a small variation in the position or the fortitude of one or another of these abdominal organs. But in the absence of the primary cause—that is, constipation—these structural differences would not produce any disease at all.

What about heredity? If there are structural differences, they are likely to be inherited, and when members of one family with these structural weaknesses are exposed to constipation, they will probably have a greater frequency of varicose veins than another family without the predisposing weaknesses. But without the constipation, the weaknesses in structure would not bring on any symptoms at all!

"With perhaps 5 million sufferers in these islands alone, there is obviously little scope for any special incidence as far as occupation is concerned," Dr. Cleave goes on, "and it is hardly surprising to find that at least one English authority does not regard varices as more common in athletes, in people who stand a lot, or in the obese. Nearly all writers, however, agree that about three-quarters of the sufferers are women—who are known to suffer much more often than men from colonic stasis (constipation)."

What about primitive people who do not eat refined foods that Dr. Cleave has accused as the villain of the piece? They don't suffer from varicose veins. In Uganda, East Africa, for instance, a survey has shown that "varicose veins and varicocele had never been noted in any of these tribal areas by any of the 7 observers who have studied these peoples, and must be considered exceedingly uncommon." But this cannot be because of racial differences, for Negroes in America are just as subject to varicose veins as whites.

Compare Tooth Decay with Varicose Veins

Dr. Cleave then takes up the question of tooth decay and compares it with varicose veins. Tooth decay is, even in modern times, practically absent from primitive people who still live on primitive diets without refined foods. We know this from many studies that have been done on this subject. Yet we know that tooth decay, like varicose veins, appears rather early in recorded history. White flour was being produced in Greece as early as 500 B. C. Just as tooth decay came into being roughly at about this time, so it seems that varicose veins appeared about that time.

History Shows the Relation of Disease to Food

In England about the time of the Roman conquest, millers were beginning to sift flour to produce white flour, Dr. Cleave tells us. He goes on to say, "The increase in the consumption of refined sugar, derived from the sugar cane and sugar beet, is much more recent. Reaching England in the twelfth century, refined sugar remained a food of the rich for a very long time. Since 1915, however, consumption has risen from 15 pounds per head per annum to over 100 pounds today.

"If one disease produced by the refinement of carbohydrates—dental caries—can be seen already to have become noticeable in the earliest civilizations, there is no reason why another, such as varicose veins, if due to the same cause, should not have become noticeable, too; and the description of this disease by Hippocrates, therefore, presents no obstacle to the view advanced here—though, needless to say, in those days, the disease must have been very much rarer."

He concludes, "The evidence reviewed here suggests that the environmental change responsible for varices (varicose veins) is the adoption of a diet largely freed from vegetable fibre. In many people, the effect of such a diet is to slow the passage of food residues through the colon. Such slowing is compatible with regular action of the bowel, but it causes overloading of the colon. This process affects the venous return from the lower parts of the body" and results in that disfiguring, painful and usually chronic condition known as varicose veins.

How do you know whether you are constipated in the sense in which

Dr. Cleave uses the term? He says that many people suffering from varicose veins or varicocele would not admit that they are constipated. Many people suppose, he says, that their bowels are acting normally so long as they pass a stool each day, whereas the true criteria of normality are the diameter of the stool and its hardness, which increase steadily with delay. A person who thinks he is not constipated because his bowels move every day may actually have a 24-hour delay or more. Dr. Cleave is talking about delayed passage of the colonic contents—not necessarily constipation as we think of it.

There Can Be Only One Acceptable Answer

There is only one answer, according to Dr. Cleave's theory—and we see no reason for not accepting it. The only safe foods, if one would avoid constipation and possible susceptibility to varicose veins, are wholly natural foods from which none of the fibre has been removed. We mean by this fresh fruits and vegetables, as many raw as possible. There is no doubt that cooking, and especially overcooking, softens the fibre to such an extent, that it cannot function in the colon to prevent constipation. Raw fruits and vegetables, also so rich in vitamins and minerals, are the best sources of natural fibre.

By the same token, refined foods lack it completely. Sugar is refined from sugar cane—a tough, fibrous plant. The sugar we eat contains no fibre. It is as crystalline "pure" as a drug; it dissolves into syrup with the addition of liquid. Refined cereals are just as bad. White flour, used in making practically all the baked goods we eat, is as free from fibre as laundry starch, or face powder. These are the foods to be avoided. The less you eat of sugary and starchy foods, the more you will want of the nutritious, natural, unrefined foods which are best from every angle.

BOOK THREE

GENERAL DISCUSSIONS
OF DISEASES

250. Bananas and Disease

Bananas have been taking a quiet but effective place in the treatment of disease in the last half century. Doctors with access to the latest drugs and surgical techniques still find that including bananas in the diet sometimes works more effectively than other more complex therapies. The medical journals have yielded a great store of information on stubborn ailments which have responded to banana eating when other more conventional efforts have failed. Perhaps you will come across a problem that has been bothering you, and find evidence that bananas might be the answer. One could certainly not find a cheaper or more appetizing form of medication than a golden banana.

Bananas are best known as normalizers of colonic functions. They are instrumental in controlling constipation through their bulk-producing properties, as well as through their ability, beneficially, to change bacterial flora in the intestines. The bulk is produced by the water-absorbent pectin contained in bananas and their nonirritating fibre.

Constipation Relieved

In so-called spastic constipation, all irritants must be eliminated from the diet, for they can cause soreness and great pain in the intestinal lining if they are not completely smooth. The problem, then, is to select a food which will provide bulk enough for normal movements, without causing irritation. In the *Medical Times and Long Island Medical Journal* (62:313, 1934), Dr. E. E. Cornwall emphasizes this need, plus the requirement that animal protein be kept low to discourage (intestinal) putrefaction. He restricts starches moderately and feels that any resulting caloric deficiencies should be made up with fruits. Many clinicians believe that bananas deserve first place among the fruits in such a diet.

Dr. L. Weinstein, in *Archives of Intestinal Medicine* (6:21, 1939), remarks that he noted relief from constipation was often associated with the number of acidophilus bacteria in the intestinal tract. He instituted an experiment in which he observed 9 adults and 15 children, all of whom had suffered from constipation for over 4 weeks, with no relief from any other treatment. They began eating a diet which included 3 or 4 ripe bananas each day. Within one to two weeks, it was demonstrated that the bananas had produced normal movement in all subjects. The acidophilus in the intestinal tract rose to a count of 60-95 per cent by the end of the second week.

Soothing and Healing of Colitis and Ulcers

A related problem, ulcerative colitis, seems to cry out for the special properties offered by bananas. Once more, the difficulty is irritation, whether it be mechanical or chemical, which causes further soreness of the inflamed or ulcerated lining of the colon. Patients are plagued by nausea, lack of appetite and frequent bowel movements. The need is for adequate intake and absorption of foods. Bland bananas, ripe and mashed, are recommended and, if used early enough, can lead to complete remission of the disease, whereas most raw fruits are poorly tolerated.

The special texture and flavoring of the banana make it ideal as a food for the ulcer patient. It buffers or neutralizes the hydrochloric acid in the stomach, the acid which causes much of the ulcer patient's woe. Bananas are believed to coat the lining of the stomach in such a way as to lessen the irritation the ulcer is exposed to, as well as to promote healing and prevent recurrence. The banana feedings, small and frequent, are well tolerated, easily digestible and palatable. When they are mashed and added to a protein preparation, such as soybean milk, the buffer action is even more complete, and certainly the nutritional values are even higher.

Nonallergenic Properties of Bananas

Bananas are known to contain only benign protein constituents, and therefore, they are often used in cases of food allergies which manifest themselves in skin rashes, digestive ailments or asthma. L. W. Hill (*Journal of Pediatrics,* 47:648, 1955) remarks that he routinely includes bananas in a basic diet for allergic eczema. It is usually one or the other of the amino acids to which the body has a basic intolerance that causes one of these distressing allergy symptoms, which are actually manifestations of the body's defense mechanisms. Bananas can serve as an excellent background food, rich in needed nutrients, while food elimination tests are carried out, and, later, should a basic food be found to be the culprit, bananas can be retained in the diet to offset any deficiency.

Anemia is another condition which can be helped by adding bananas to the diet. The *American Journal of Public Health* (23:129, 1933) carried the opinion of W. H. Eddy, which held that iron in bananas is present in sufficient amounts to cause some regeneration of hemoglobin in anemic rats. In the book, *Chemical Composition of Foods,* by McCance and Widdowson (New York Publishing Company, 1940), this conclusion is supported with the added opinion that all of the iron in bananas is in a form that can be used for forming hemoglobin.

Pellagra is a disease due primarily to a shortage of niacin, and secondarily, to other factors of the B complex which are missing. The body simply does not make use of the B vitamins it takes in, due to an unfavorable climate in the intestines. Bananas help to make these conditions more suitable, so that the dietary intake of patients is used more profitably.

Kidney Diseases

In cases of uremia (presence of toxic urinary constituents in the blood) bananas are suggested by J. Raiboff, in the *Urological and Cutaneous Review* (40:850, 1936), as a help in avoiding an overloading of the kidney. His prescription is 9 bananas per day for 3 or 4 days.

In the *Journal of the American Medical Association* (69:440, 1917), the value of bananas in treating nephritis (inflammation of the kidney) was already being recognized by A. F. Chase and A. R. Rose, who suggested bananas with every meal for the patient with this kidney disease. Because gastrointestinal upsets so often accompany this disease, the bland, non-irritating, mildly laxative action of bananas is favored.

More Instances of Banana Versatility

Aside from those above, bananas are considered valuable in the treatment of other diseases, such as gout (since they have no purine and are adaptable to the soft diets often prescribed), heart disease (they are very low in salt and fat content and have no cholesterol content), typhoid fever (diarrhea is often a complicating factor and bananas have been shown to bring prompt relief and change the pH of stools from acid to alkaline, as well as to eliminate blood and mucus from the stools).

Hardly any diet for a diabetic can be found which would not recommend the use of bananas, both for slow absorption rate, high satiety value, taste appeal and easy digestibility. In the Mayo Clinic diet manual, bananas are recommended on standard and special diabetic diet menus.

Pre- and post-operative patients were known to benefit from the use of bananas in the diet. One of the main reasons for this is probably the high vitamin C content, which both protects from shock and aids greatly in the healing of wounds.

Bananas are obviously a valuable tool for maintaining good health, as well as for regaining it when it has been lost. The year-round availability of this fruit leaves little excuse for not including it regularly in your diet. It is inexpensive, easy to handle and prepare and even comes in a natural wrapper that surely protects the edible portion of the fruit from insecticides and sprays better than any other natural food.

251. Lung Cancer Isn't All A Smoker Has to Worry About

Cigarette manufacturers are desperately busy these days trying to create the impression that the tobacco-lung cancer connection is a form of persecution completely unfounded in fact. It is hard to believe that anyone could be influenced by these protests when the evidence being presented by leading scientists to prove this relationship is so conclusive and so clinical.

But just for the sake of argument, suppose that what the industry claims were true. Suppose that tobacco smoking and lung cancer had no more relation than cigarette advertising and honesty, could the average steady smoker rest easy? Would the consequences of puffing a pack or two a day stop with stained fingers if lung cancer were out of the way? One might as well ask if, aside from a corroded stomach, there is any other consequence of drinking a cup of nitric acid than the stain it might leave on the lips. In the consumption of any poison, we know that the entire body suffers even though the direct cause of death might be assigned to a specific organ.

Nicotine's Personal Reputation

The thing that makes tobacco what it is, is nicotine. Without this element, smoking a cigarette would be about as stimulating as smoking a shredded banana peel. It's the nicotine that swells the blood sugar reading, thereby giving one the "lift" a cigarette seems to promise.

Nicotine is classed, pharmacologically speaking, as one of the deadliest poisons known to man. The pure nicotine contained in a week's smoking at a pack per day, would kill as suddenly as a bullet to the heart, if the body were to get it in one concentrated dose. Further, to attest to the lethal qualities of nicotine, it is estimated that, if the nicotine contained in a year's consumption of cigarettes were to be doled out with precision, it would be enough to kill 1,000 times the population of the United States. These facts are contained in an article on the subject in *Reader's Digest* for January, 1950.

You are wondering, quite logically, "Then why are there so many smokers still on their feet? The streets should be littered with dead smokers!" The answer lies in the fortunate fact that the smoker does not get all the nicotine a cigarette contains. Only about a third of it enters the mouth, and this amount is further dissipated when the smoke is inhaled. Some of what remains is sidetracked on its trip through the body, until only about 1/10 of what nicotine the average puff contains is actually carried to the blood stream. Also, the body has a short time to recover between puffs, and the body elimination system gets rid of nicotine fast enough to keep a lethal dose from piling up in the system. Finally, the body of a smoker builds up a tolerance to expected quantities of nicotine, just as it can be forced to do with other poisons. These reasons are not advanced to accent the safe side of smoking, for there is none, but rather to explain why regularly consuming a poison as deadly as nicotine, doesn't kill the average smoker on the spot.

Acute Nicotine Poisoning

The tolerance factor is not to be lightly dismissed. It is probably more responsible than any other reason for the strong hold the cigarette habit can get on a person. How many smokers do you think there would be if each cigarette brought on the effects of acute nicotine poisoning that are experienced by the novice smoker? The *Ohio State Medical Journal* (December, 1950) describes these symptoms as nausea, vomiting, cramps, diarrhea, blurred vision and clammy perspiration. So characteristic of nicotine is this reaction, that drugs with similar results are said to exert a "nicotine action." With increased use of tobacco, this reaction is toned down, as the body adjusts to expecting this poisonous jolt. Still, there are many regular smokers who experience one or more of these symptoms with the morning cigarette or after particularly heavy smoking. If any other poison were involved (with the possible exception of alcohol), such a reaction would be enough to warn the consumer against its further use. As it is, smokers smoke and drinkers drink no matter how sick it makes them feel.

Official Medical Opinion on Smoking and the Heart

Cigarette companies spent much of their advertising budget, until recent years, trying to show that smoking is as healthful as eating an apple by picturing a "doctor" puffing a cigarette. The suggestion was, of course, that, if a doctor smokes (and he's an expert on health), why shouldn't you? The answer to that question comes in dozens of articles printed in medical journals and secular magazines which show smoking tobacco to be a possible factor in the breakdown of almost every physiological function.

Doctors have warned heart patients for years against the effects of smoking. In March of 1955, the *Journal of the American Medical Association* ran an editorial which erased all doubts as to the official position of doctors on smoking and heart disease. "There seems now to be definite evidence that smoking, even though it may not directly affect the coronary arteries, can have a damaging effect on the myocardium (muscular wall of the heart). . . . No patient with coronary disease should incur the added risk to his heart imposed by smoking . . ."

Science News Letter (February 26, 1955) says, "Smoking affects your heart whether you are a normal person or one with heart disease." There is even a series of symptoms—chest pains, irregular beating, breathlessness and dizziness—brought on by what is known as "tobacco heart."

Science has long ago established a relationship between the number of fat molecules in the blood stream and difficulties with the heart. A report in the *New York Times* (April 6, 1955) gave proof that smoking had definitely been found to increase the number of these dangerous fat molecules.

The *Journal of the American Medical Association* editorial quoted above also lists the results of a test of 37 patients with heart disease (including 6 nonsmokers). Of the 37, 30 showed an increased heart rate after smoking and 4 showed a decrease; 34 showed increased blood pressure. Add to these stresses the extra work the heart must do to force the blood through vessels which are narrowed with every puff of a cigarette, and you know that smoking is no better for the heart than a day at the races is for the rent money. Probably worse—at least at the races you have a chance to win.

A Circulatory Disease Closely Related to Smoking

Another in the category of circulatory diseases is Buerger's disease. Simply, this disease results from an impairment of circulation to the extremities. (Tobacco smoking constricts the blood vessels—the smaller the vessels, the tighter the constriction. Fingernail blood vessels close entirely.) The hands and feet tingle and feel numb as though "asleep." In time, the affected areas show splotches of dead tissue that soon result in gangrene and eventually, amputation must be resorted to. This disease is discussed in detail in chapter 106 of this book.

How Smoking Affects the Respiratory System

The respiratory system takes an awful knocking around from prolonged use of tobacco. In this case, it is not the nicotine so much as the accompanying tars which irritate these zones. It has been said by Dr. Mervin C. Meyerson, a laryngologist of Beverly Hills, California, that *all* smokers have postnasal drip. Dr. Meyerson maintains that "the mucus secretion of the nasal pharynx is affected by a single puff of the average cigarette. The larynx (of a regular smoker) shows anything from a mild infection to tumor formations."

The smoker's hack, well known to anyone who is often near a heavy smoker, is due to the irritation of the tars mentioned above. The *Practitioner* (March, 1952) says that smoking may irritate and cause inflammation of the mucous membranes of the entire respiratory system. Smokers have more colds that last longer, and sinusitis is more frequent and persistent in smokers.

Of course, one of the greatest of respiratory diseases, tuberculosis, is aggravated beyond measure by the smoking habit. The *Journal of the American Medical Association* has a number of reasons listed in the September 30, 1950, issue which are intended to illustrate disastrous reactions of smoking on tubercular patients. Smoking is irritating to the lungs

[934]

(whose texture tends to absorb any tars), causing inflammation. The smoker's cough (due to the strain it puts on the lungs) is another dangerous companion of the tubercular smoker. Appetite is known to suffer when one smokes, and, for a tubercular patient, there are few things of greater importance than a steady intake of healthful foods.

In view of these obvious dangers, for tubercular patients, contained in cigarettes, we were confounded by a squib in the *New York State Medical Journal* (January 26, 1954) which remarked that, out of 50 tuberculosis sanatoria canvassed, only 16 per cent had rules rigidly forbidding smoking —about 8 institutions have bothered to take so elementary a precaution on behalf of their patients!

How Cigarettes and Ulcers Are Related

Will a cigarette help bring on an ulcer? Consulting the *Practitioner* (March, 1952), we find that the general medical opinion is that tobacco smoking is harmful to the inflamed or ulcerated stomach and intestines, and should therefore be prohibited in such cases. New York University research has shown that patients who continued to smoke during ulcer treatment had more relapses than those who did not or had not smoked before. Ochsner Clinic in New Orleans, which specializes in treating ulcer cases, refuses even to undertake the treatment of any ulcer patient who will not stop smoking.

An article in the *West Virginia Medical Journal* (September, 1951) is the most definite of all. The authors insist that, in cases of peptic ulcer, a definite attempt should be made to break the patient of the tobacco habit. The article lists the following reasons: (1.) nicotine depresses the sympathetic nerve endings, allowing the vagus nerve to have greater effect, which results in increased gastric secretion and activity; (2.) tars dissolved in sputum act as irritants when swallowed; (3.) appetite is decreased.

Surgery

The smoker's troubles won't end with his ulcer. If he needs an operation, as ulcer patients often do, tobacco again multiplies his woes. The *Lancet* for January, 1944, tells of a study of 257 cases with all types of abdominal operations which showed that the morbidity rate for smokers taking more than 10 cigarettes per day is about 6 times that of non-smoking operative patients. Many anesthesiologists believe that smokers are more difficult to anesthetize than nonsmokers, says a piece in the *British Medical Journal*. (November 6, 1954). Then, too, these patients are likely to develop laryngeal spasms during the administration of such anesthetics as ether. Such constriction could easily lead to death, as in the case reported in the article of a healthy, young, adult male smoker who was about to undergo a simple appendectomy. He developed a laryngeal spasm and died when it could not be relieved. The writers advise that any person contemplating surgery should stop smoking a long time in advance of the

[935]

operation, and that a smoker should be sure to inform his surgeon of any observed effect he has noticed in himself as a result of smoking.

So you say none of these things bother you—you have no ulcers, no tuberculosis, no surgery impending? You're willing to take your chances if that's all smoking can do. Well, my friend, a poison so insidious as nicotine and its tars will not let you off so easily.

The Problem of Sterility

Perhaps the thousands of childless couples, one or both of whom are smokers, can trace a parallel to their cases in the one reported in the *Hawaii Medical Journal* (May-June, 1943). A young couple, wife 27, husband 33, had been married 5 years. The wife had been unable to conceive, although examination showed her to be healthy in every way, with no history of disease and a diet considered adequate by her physician. The husband showed up equally well in his report; however, it was noted that he smoked 20 to 30 cigarettes per day. A sample of the husband's semen was analyzed and showed a large number of well-formed sperm— but they were all dead. It was suggested that the husband stop smoking. He did so on November 1, and on December 1, an analysis of his semen showed a large number of sperm, well developed and perfectly alive! Sometime in January, the wife conceived and a healthy male child was born to them in October.

As a follow-up to this remarkable case, it is noted that the husband took up smoking once more, and on examination, the semen again showed sperm in large numbers, but again all dead. Once more he left off smoking and, sure enough, a semen analysis a month later showed healthy, live sperm in more than adequate numbers. These observations were considered as proof that smoking and reproductive function were definitely connected in this case.

The *Practitioner* (March, 1952) mentions, in this connection, an experiment carried on with rats to test any relationship between nicotine and reproductive processes. Dosing rats with nicotine resulted in an increased number of nonfertile pairs and fewer litters. Descendants of chronically poisoned pairs also proved less fertile than control pairs. Translated into human terms, this, of course, could mean that parents who smoke stand less of a chance of becoming grandparents than those who do not.

The *Reader's Digest* for December, 1953, says that many doctors agree that tobacco causes toxic changes in the blood which impede the formation of sexual hormones. The article tells of a German study of 5000 women which indicates that there may be a greater incidence of frigidity, sterility, menstrual disturbance and miscarriage among smokers than nonsmokers.

What of women who smoke during pregnancy? How much nicotine does the fetus get from a smoking mother? This question is almost

[936]

impossible to answer directly. However, the *Journal of the American Medical Association* offers a few indications in its January 9, 1954, number. We are told of experiments which show an actual rise in fetal heartbeat noted during maternal smoking. This change was taken to show that toxic products of smoke do pass through the placenta and enter fetal circulation. Animals exposed to cigarette smoke equivalent to 20 cigarettes a day showed a stillbirth rate 10 times as great as those not exposed.

Smoking can make things tough for a baby in his first few months of life, too—not his smoking but his parents'. In the *American Medical Association Journal* for October 21, 1950, an interesting case is catalogued in which a baby was brought to a doctor, at the age of one year. The child was having an attack of asthma and had been having similar attacks from the age of 6 months. The cause was found to be in the mother who admitted to being a constant smoker for many years. She even smoked when nursing the baby, as well as when feeding and diapering him. At the doctor's direction, all smoking in the house was eliminated and within a few days all of the baby's symptoms cleared completely. For 18 months, the baby was fine, so the mother commenced smoking once more. A dry cough developed in the child almost at once. The cough stopped as soon as the mother's smoking did.

Smoking Disturbs Function of Kidney and Pancreas

The deleterious effects of smoking, where the genito-urinary tract is concerned, do not stop with the reproductive problems just discussed. An enlightening experiment, recorded in the *British Medical Journal* (March 24, 1945), shows quite definitely that the kidney function is also impaired. After setting up a schedule of the average voiding times and the volume of urine excreted by a group of 9 healthy persons, these subjects were required to smoke at intervals to see what effect, if any, smoking would have on their regular voiding habits. In 7 of the subjects, voiding was delayed from 1¾ hours to 3½ hours, while two experienced no change. The *Journal* concluded from this that "It would seem that those with impaired kidney function should not be allowed to smoke." A conservative conclusion, to be sure. ·

Pancreas disturbances are often traced to smoking when a thorough investigation is made. Both of the most common pancreatic diseases, hypoglycemia (a condition in which too much insulin is manufactured by the pancreas, thus cutting down on the body's sugar to below optimum amounts) and hyperglycemia, or diabetes (a disease in which not enough insulin is manufactured by the pancreas, leaving the blood stream awash with vast amounts of sugar that it can't use), have been successfully controlled with an injunction against smoking. The *Journal of the American Medical Association* (May 10, 1946) found a "significantly higher incidence of thrombosed peripheral arteries" (the first step toward gangrene and amputation in diabetics) in the smokers among 301 male diabetics

[937]

than in those who did not smoke, regardless of other illness factors.

The symptoms of hypoglycemia (low blood sugar) are certainly frightening to experience. The victim gets the feeling that consciousness is about to be lost, and this is accompanied by blind staggers and dizziness. But look at the easy therapy: The *Practitioner* for February, 1954, tells of 38 patients suffering from this disease, of whom 36 were heavy smokers. Within one month after giving up tobacco, the 36 smokers were completely free from the symptoms. Those who returned to smoking found that a recurrence of the symptoms was lurking in their first package of cigarettes. The *International Medical Digest* (March, 1954) relates the history of a hypoglycemia victim who had ingrained in himself the habit of consuming ½ to ¾ pounds of sugar each day to maintain the level of sugar in his blood, for he was so victimized by symptoms that even in crossing a street he could not be sure he would retain consciousness until he reached the other side. He admitted that he had, for 40 years, smoked 2 to 3 packs of cigarettes each day. Even in this extreme case, as soon as the man stopped smoking, all symptoms disappeared within a month!

How About a Smoke for the Nerves?

Well, one thing, says the smoker, there's nothing like a cigarette when your nerves are jumpy. This fallacy is the product of advertising that has pictures of people engaged in nerve-wracking endeavors reaching greedily for a cigarette before or just after they make their champion effort. The 500-mile racer needs one, the man going over Niagara in a barrel wouldn't make the trip without first calming himself with a cigarette, a ballerina about to do a hundred consecutive turns lets it be known that she wouldn't even attempt First Position without the aid of a cigarette to make her steady. Referring again to the *Practitioner,* we are told that the nervous system suffers seriously from heavy smoking. "Chronic tabagism may lead to profound depression, stupor, melancholia and psychoneurotic states." One might find these attributes helpful for the trip over Niagara, but hardly for some of the other feats for which one is supposed to need a smoke.

A more visual illustration of the cigarette's effect on the nerves was an experiment written up in *Time* (June, 1948). Dr. Austin Edwards of the University of Georgia wanted to prove the thesis that smoking has a harmful effect on the nerves and he wanted to measure the results of smoking by noting changes in the steadiness of the fingers. Dr. Edwards invented a measuring device for the tests and called it a "tronometer." The finger tremors were measured before and after smoking. The tremor of regular smokers increased 39 per cent on one cigarette. In nonsmokers who did not inhale, there was no change. In nonsmokers who did inhale, the finger tremor increased 82 per cent.

As for endurance, factors were not considered controllable enough to obtain exact results, but Kapovich and Hale, whose effort is included in the *Journal of Applied Psychology*, felt impelled to conclude that "there are tobacco-sensitive people whose performance is impaired by smoking" and that the usual no-smoking rule for training athletes is a wise one. One of the greatest of all coaches, Knute Rockne, was quoted on the subject in these words, "Tobacco slows the reflexes and any advertising that says it helps an athlete is a falsehood and a fraud."

Etiquette has stepped in to frown on smoking at the table, perhaps because the satisfaction of fine cookery is sure to be dissipated by a cloud of smoke blown from across the table into one's face. And surely no true gourmet would consider numbing his taste buds with the harsh flavor of tobacco. More dangerously, smokers are prone to the ulcerative problems of lips and tongue that are associated with incipient skin cancer.

While we're in the area, what about the teeth and gums? Can smoking possibly have an adverse effect here? You bet! The *Journal of Dental Research* (June, 1947) tells of observation studies on 1,433 Danish Marines which showed that, while 1.5 per cent of these men who were nonsmokers had ulcermembraneous gingivitis, the count among regular smokers was 10 times that.

Smoking and the Senses

If you enjoy the smell of a roast or a whiff of your favorite perfume, the fleeting pleasure of a cigarette might permanently rob you of these delights. The *Journal of the American Medical Association* for May 19, 1951, states unequivocally that a loss of the sense of smell (anosmia) may result from excessive smoking.

The precious asset of good eyesight is in jeopardy when one is a smoker. The *Virginia Medical Monthly* carries a piece in its December, 1955, issue which tells us that tobacco poisoning will cause a dimness of vision. After one or two cigarettes, opthalmoscope examination shows that the whole area of the optic nerve which carries the fibres of accurate vision shows a dull, grayish outline and that gradually, the entire disk comes to appear paralyzed.

Dr. Charles Sheard of the Mayo Clinic asserts that smoking cigarettes definitely interferes with best night vision possible. Dr. L. Tuendenhall, in *Tobacco* (Harvard University Press), agrees and adds that optic neuritis plus dilated pupils and inability to focus are smoking consequences.

The effect of smoking on eyesight probably explains the statement of Dr. Robert Koons, Assistant Commissioner of the New York State Health Department, carried in the *New York Times* (March 26, 1957), in which he said that cigarette smokers seem to have more auto accidents than non-smokers. The Assistant Commissioner referred to studies that indicate a rise in an individual's auto accident rate as smoking increases.

As a parting barrage, let us quote the figures in Harry Dingman's book, *Risk Appraisal,* published by the National Underwriters Company. Note the added percentage of physical problems invited by the smoker. Habitual smokers have 62 per cent higher incidence of gas on the stom-

[939]

ach. Habitual smokers have 76 per cent higher incidence of nervousness. They have 100 per cent higher incidence of heartburn. The percentage of those who breathe in a labored way after exertion is 140 per cent greater in smokers than nonsmokers. Habitual smokers have 167 per cent higher incidence of nose and throat irritation and, finally, a 300 per cent higher incidence of cough.

Althouh cigarette smoking is the commonest form of tobacco use, these disorders can arise from any type of smoking, so that pipes and cigars are equally dangerous.

Somewhere a doctor we read about gave his patients this advice: "If you're feeling under par in any way, and you are a smoker, give it up for a month's trial. Chances are that you will be a new person as a result, without a single other treatment."

We think it is excellent advice and we are sure that the increase in vigor and the feeling of well-being a month free of smoking can bring will convince all but the most determined smoker against resuming the habit.

252. Vitamin Deficiency Plus Smoking Equals Trouble

A condition known as *tobacco amblyopia* has been known for many years. It is a dimness of vision or a loss of vision due to poisoning by tobacco. There are, incidentally, similar conditions caused by alcohol and other poisons. The one caused by smoking is seen only in people who smoke quite a lot.

An article in the British *Lancet* for August 9, 1958, relates the story of 3 physicians from the University of Bristol who found evidence of a deficiency in vitamin B_{12} in patients suffering from the tobacco-caused disease.

They tell us that, in their experience, people who smoke strong pipe tobacco are more likely to have the disease than are those who smoke cigarettes. Excessive drinking helps to increase the severity and incidence of the disease. One investigator found in 1954 that injections of vitamin B_{12} improved the condition whether or not the patient stopped smoking.

So our 3 investigators decided to find out by doing some research among their own patients. They laid out a set of rules to go by: the patient must be a smoker, he must display certain definite symptoms of amblyopia in the form of color blindness and blind spots in his eye. Of the 14 patients they studied, all of them who were given vitamin B_{12} recovered, whether or not they stopped smoking.

Some Typical Cases

One patient, aged 62, was advised to stop smoking and was given thiamin (a B vitamin) by mouth. In spite of this, his vision slowly deteriorated. When he came in at a later time, he was also complaining of a sore tongue, slurred speech and numbness in his legs. The level of vitamin B_{12} in his blood was low. He was given vitamin B_{12} by injection, and within 6 months, his eyes were normal.

Another patient, aged 75, who had been smoking for only a little over a year, was given vitamin B_{12} in injections and was allowed to continue smoking. Here again, improvement was rapid.

A third patient, aged 81, had visible known symptoms of vitamin B_{12} deficiency. His tongue was red, smooth and sore. He had numbness and tingling in his hands and feet and weakness in his legs. He did not stop smoking, but he was given vitamin B_{12} and his poor sight and other symptons disappeared within two months.

Of the 9 patients who were given vitamin B_{12}, all recovered more rapidly than would have been expected had they just stopped smoking. Three of them continued to smoke throughout. Our authors point out that a lack of hydrochloric acid in the stomach usually goes along with the anemia that is caused by lack of vitamin B_{12}. It is thought that this lack keeps the patient from absorbing the vitamin, even though he is getting it in his daily food. A considerable number of the patients treated had this hydrochloric acid deficiency.

A lack of hydrochloric acid in the stomach's digestive juices is quite common among older people and is one of the reasons they so often lack vitamins and minerals. If this important digestive juice is absent from the stomach, they simply cannot absorb vitamins and minerals.

Our authors say that vitamin B_{12} deficiency has been reported among "vegans," vegetarians who do not eat anything of animal origin. Diabetics, too, have a tendency to vitamin B_{12} deficiency so, as might be expected, there is an increased incidence to tobacco amblyopia among diabetics. "A dietary deficiency of vitamin B_{12} may be present in some elderly men, particularly if they live alone," say our authors. We assume this is probably because of careless or improper preparation of balanced meals. This deficiency might be expected to predispose towards the development of tobacco amblyopia long before producing anemia and symptoms like numbness and tingling in arms and legs. The increased severity of amblyopia among prisoners of war could be explained in this way.

What can we learn from these comments in the *Lancet?* The first lesson is, of course, to stop smoking, if you smoke. If you are over middle age, it seems that smoking may be even more harmful. Whether or not you continue to smoke, make certain you are getting enough vitamin B_{12} in your diet. Liver is the best and most economical source. If you know that you lack hydrochloric acid in your stomach (doctors can test you for this), then you would do well to get injections of vitamin B_{12} from your doctor from time to time, for this is a mighty important vitamin that you cannot do without.

If you have symptoms of tobacco amblyopia, ask your doctor to give you injections of vitamin B_{12}, for, chances are, you are deficient in this vitamin. You can refer your doctor to the *Lancet* article which he can see at the nearest hospital library. It was written by Drs. J. M. Heaton, A. J. A. McCormick and A. G. Freeman.

253. Researcher Cites Smoking as a Cause of Disease

"Cigarettes cause cancer.

"In 1954, I began the previous version of this book with that statement. The passing years have substantiated the statement with terrifying clarity. Indeed, in view of research by the American Cancer Society, the National Cancer Institute, the National Institutes of Health and scores of independent scientists throughout the world, it is appalling that anyone could doubt the shocking link between smoking and a dozen major health problems."

With these emphatic and terrible words, Dr. Alton Ochsner of Tulane University, one of the world's greatest lung surgeons, takes off after the confirmed user of tobacco, letting him know for 103 frightening and irrefutable pages that his addiction to nicotine is harming him in innumerable, and perhaps fatal, ways. We doubt that anyone who smokes can read this book and not decide that he should stop. The name of the book is *Smoking and Health* and it is published by Julian Messner, Incorporated, New York.

Dr. Ochsner is no crank or faddist. The list of professional honors and societies which appears in his biography marks him as one of our leading surgeons, and his specialty is lung surgery. Who would know better than Dr. Ochsner the ravages of cigarette smoke on the human lung? But he does not confine himself to lung damage in this sensational book. He writes of damage to nerves, to digestion, to circulation, to sex life.

Every page is peppered with fiery words and straight-from-the-shoulder statistics. Dr. Ochsner spares no one—not the part-time smoker, the chain-smoker, the tobacco industry, the advertising industry, nor the scientists who pooh-pooh experiments linking smoking and cancer. There is no doubt of the harm done by nicotine and tars, says Dr. Ochsner, "THE FEAR OF SMOKING CAN SAVE MORE LIVES THAN THE FEAR OF THE DISEASES IT CAUSES." These words appear as capitals in the book.

Listen to this one set of statistics on stomach ulcer: "—of 64 patients who continued to smoke, only 47 per cent gained satisfactory relief.

"—Of 26 who stopped smoking, all obtained satisfactory relief.

"—Of 40 patients who never smoked, 85 per cent responded to treatment.

"—Of those who continued smoking, 53 per cent suffered recurrence of their ulcers, while recurrence occured to only 11.5 per cent of those who stopped smoking and 17.5 per cent of those who never smoked.

"—Of 13 patients who stopped smoking, improved, then resumed smoking, 11 suffered immediate exacerbation of their ulcers."

How Can You Stop?

Chapter 6 is titled "You Can Quit—You Must Quit." And Dr. Ochsner outlines a 10-point program for quitting, which, he has found, works with patients he has been recommending it to for years. We have only one fault to find with the program—it does not mention the importance of good nutrition to bulwark your campaign to stop smoking. We have found that the well-nourished person can do without drugs of all kinds much more easily than the badly nourished person. The poorly nourished person is the one who has the "jitters," the "nerves," which make him believe he cannot give up smoking. The effect of smoking just on the blood sugar level is much more devastating on the individual whose diet has already disturbed his blood sugar level to such a point that he is always hungry, craves sweets, swigs coffee continually.

A diet high in protein from which the refined starches (all sweets and cereal products) are completely lacking will help immeasurably to gear the addict's bodily processes so that he will find it easier to give up smoking. A breakfast of eggs and fruit (no coffee) starts the day right. A mid-morning snack of fruit, nuts or sunflower seeds (no coffee) keeps the blood sugar level where it should be. A lunch which avoids dessert and concentrates on meat, fruit and salads, will keep the blood sugar steady until dinnertime. Dinner should be free of all cereal products and sweets —no macaroni, no noodles, no pies, no desserts, no crackers. A rigid adherence to this diet will prepare one amazingly well for the day when he stumps out his last cigarette and, as Dr. Ochsner recommends, "stops smoking abruptly, completely and permanently."

Food supplements help, too. The B vitamins in brewer's yeast and the calcium in bone meal are essential for calm nerves. Nuts, sunflower or pumpkin seeds are ideal snacks—high in protein and the healthful kind of fat. Snacks like these at hand will satisfy the new nonsmoker when he reaches automatically for a smoke.

What Cigarettes Do

Here is a partial list of the bodily conditions caused by smoking, as Dr. Ochsner states in his book, along with a few that we have uncovered in our research. Can any thinking person read this list and not realize what he is doing to his body when he smokes?

[943]

1. Increase the heartbeat—causing exertion for the heart.

2. Increase the blood pressure—as high as 75 millimeters.

3. Cause skin temperatures on toes and fingers to drop 6 degrees.

4. Cause some blood vessels to collapse entirely.

5. Slow down the flow of blood through the heart—so the heart has to pound to overcome the deficiency.

6. Cause coronary artery disease—victims of this die 4 years sooner if they smoke.

7. One pack of cigarettes in a day (inhaled) gives you enough nicotine to kill you if you got it all in one dose.

8. Cause a disease called *tobaccoangina*—pain in chest, arms, etc.

9. Constrict blood vessels.

10. Cause Buerger's disease—almost nonexistent in nonsmokers—results in gangrene and probable amputation of limbs.

11. Cause numbness in hands and arms.

12. In a lab, nicotine eats into animal tissue like lye—apparently does this in the stomach, too.

13. Cause outpouring of stomach acid, inviting ulcers.

14. Two cigarettes result in marked rise in stomach acidity lasting for more than one hour.

15. Harm taste buds—tobacco smoke is hotter than hot food, so it deadens taste buds even worse than hot food does.

16. Have cancer-causing (irritation) effects on mouth lining, lips, tongue, cheeks and throat, and, of course, lungs.

17. Cause dizziness, blind staggers, feeling of uncertainty, due to lowering of blood sugar.

18. One or two cigarettes cause pituitary gland to pour out a stream of hormones into blood stream sufficient to constrict the heart of a dog and possibly a man, too.

19. One or two cigarettes inhibit the flow of urine.

20. Cause heartburn, belching, flatulence, nausea and loss of appetite.

21. Acetaldehyde in tobacco smoke combines with protein the minute the smoke enters the lung—stiffens connective tissue in bones, skin, blood vessels, lungs, etc.

22. Cause *obstructive emphysema* (barrel chest disease); chest swells, air sacs in lungs are affected. More new cases of emphysema than of TB are turning up these days.

23. Cause chronic bronchitis.

24. Cause allergies. Can cause palms of hands to redden, postnasal drip to begin, eyes to itch, skin to itch, in those who have these allergies.

25. Destroy the body's supply of vitamin C, so important for good health.

26. Cause sterility, frigidity, impotence, possible abortions and miscarriages. The toxic changes tobacco produces in the blood hinder the formation of essential sex hormones.

254. Do Any Diseases Just Happen?

Leprosy is probably one of the rarest diseases we know of today. This fact makes it easy to forget what a scourge it has been in the past. Its hold on France during the Middle Ages made cancer and heart disease in our time seem very tame. In that country alone, 2,000 hospitals were continuously maintained to house and treat the leprosy victims of that era. And the France of medieval days was much less populous than the country we know today.

Of course, the people of that day were handicapped by ignorance, and with today's knowledge of leprosy, incomplete as it is, they might have stemmed the advance of this awful disease. They didn't know what caused leprosy, nor how to treat it. Diagnosis was often late—too late to prevent the infection from being passed on.

The strange thing about all of this is that leprosy suddenly retreated into relative inactivity. No one knew much more about preventing the disease in the fifteenth century than was known in the eleventh, yet it abated until its appearance in France became almost as rare as it is anywhere else. It is an instance of what Jacques M. May, M.D., in his book, *The Ecology of Human Disease,* calls a spontaneous change in the geographical pattern of disease.

How Disease Disappears

Dr. May writes that diseases disappear either because the environment in which they flourish is corrected, a medical treatment which cures them is discovered or the aforementioned spontaneous disappearance takes place. An example of a change in environment which affects the progress of disease can be seen in cholera, controlled by proper sanitation and quarantine, and yellow fever, greatly alleviated by elimination of swamps which acted as a breeding place for the disease-carrying mosquitos. As an example of treatment's doing away with a disease, Dr. May offers the response of syphilis and amoebic dysentery to antibiotics. He predicts a complete disappearance of such spirochetal diseases, controlled by penicillin, in the foreseeable future. While this might be true, Dr. May is quick to point out the undeniable fact that the intensive use of antibiotics might eventually and significantly change the intestinal bacteria of large groups of people. This will probably reduce the incidence of some intestinal diseases, such as dysentery, but might also open the door to so many biological changes that the results are as likely to be disastrous as they are to be beneficial.

It's hard to put one's finger on a single cause of a disease whose rate is particularly high. It depends upon so many factors that are seldom apparent until the disease is with us, and commands our attention by affecting large parts of the population. Probably the best illustration of this theory is the leukemia that has been advancing as a result of the radioactivity to which we are all being exposed. Now it is not too obvious, at first, as to how an explosion off a remote South Pacific island can cause a disease problem for us here in America, but science has given us enough hints to allow us to work out the rest.

Nobody Without Strontium 90

The splitting of the atom introduced a new element into our atmosphere called strontium 90. Each nuclear explosion releases new quantities of the stuff into our world, and the winds that blow in the substratosphere push clouds of it to every continent, where it rains down on the soil, and eventually comes into our systems. It has been stated that there is no person in the world whose bones do not have a quantity of strontium 90 in them.

How much we get of strontium 90 is largely a matter of chance. Dr. May tells us that, if the strontium 90 falls on ground that is high in calcium, the vegetation growing there will take the calcium from the ground rather than the strontium. If the ground is calcium-poor, whatever is raised there will be strontium 90-rich. If a cow grazes on strontium-rich grass, her milk and her meat will contain high amounts of this element. If you drink this cow's milk or eat her meat, you will contain higher amounts of strontium 90 than you did before. Since strontium 90 is known to be cancer-causing, you will be more likely to get cancer than you were before you drank the milk or ate the beef. Eventually, if the testing continues—and even if it doesn't—there's bound to be an increase in cancer cases in the world. Yet, chances are good that historians looking back at our time will scratch their heads at the increase in cancer during our century and chalk it up to a spontaneous occurrence.

Insecticides—A Present-Day Evil

As another example, we can consider the use of insecticides and what they have done to our bird life. Daily, we see reports of this or that bird's nearing extinction, or of the fact that it no longer returns from winter migration. Historians will cluck their tongues and speculate about sudden cold air masses that must have discouraged or killed a good many birds in the twentieth century, never even thinking of the deadly dusting of the crops that we carry on each year.

We wonder, too, what brilliant historian will have the imagination to figure that whatever is killing the birds so fast, has a hand in killing the people, too? Will he figure that the spray on fruit trees that killed the birds stayed on the fruit until we ate it, thereby ingesting another cancer-causer?

If statistics in the next 50 to 100 years should show our generation to have been plagued with kidney disease, how many scientists do you suppose there will be to point out that we used plenty of aluminum and that our society endorsed fluoridation, both showing evidence of danger to the kidney? Hardly likely that anyone will think of it. The whole problem of kidney disease will find its way into the record books of a few centuries from now as a spontaneous outbreak.

Our civilization holds history in its hand. We can still change our destiny as an era of cancer, heart disease and kidney ailments by doing our utmost to draw attention to the dangers to which we are exposing ourselves and our future generations. If we stop the nuclear testing now, if we outlaw insecticides used to spray our food, if we call a halt to fluoridation while we still have a chance to avoid serious physical consequences in everyone, we might change our era's label from "sick" to "sane."

Now, perhaps you are wondering, as we are, what went on in medieval France that spread the blanket of leprosy under which that country struggled for 400 years. It becomes less easy to label it "spontaneous," doesn't it? Nothing happens without a cause and leprosy didn't just happen either. Nor do cancer, heart disease and kidney disease.

255. Conquering the Infectious Diseases

How can we explain the seeming decrease in some of the infectious diseases that used to plague us many years ago? For instance, how can we explain that in 1900, pneumonia was responsible for 202.2 deaths per hundred thousand of our population, whereas in 1944, only 48.6 per hundred thousand persons died of this disease? Tuberculosis, which at one time was responsible for one-fifth of all the deaths in western Europe, has now decreased in incidence to a point where it seems to have become no plague at all.

There are several theories advanced as to this state of affairs. One of these is that our present-day sanitation and mode of living have greatly decreased the chances of infectious diseases being spread. However, a physician from Melbourne, Australia, has quite a different idea.

H. McLorinan, Medical Superintendent of the Fairfield Hospital in Melbourne, writes in the October 2, 1954, issue of the *Medical Journal of Australia* that extravagant statements have been made indicating that infectious diseases have now almost disappeared and are now no longer a social problem. He disagrees sharply. He tells us that beds in "fever" hospitals are almost as busy as they formerly were, and that the infections we have to deal with now appear to be more severe than they used to be.

True, he says, scarlet fever and diphtheria have almost disappeared. Twenty years ago, these two diseases alone kept four-fifths of the beds in fever hospitals occupied. But what of infectious hepatitis, he asks, which was practically unknown then and is becoming commoner by the year! Streptococcus infections are relatively mild and respond well to the antibiotics. But can anyone prove that the so-called "respiratory infections" are decreasing in incidence? Dr. McLorinan thinks not. There are fewer cases of infections of the skin, such as erysipelas, but there are many more cases of drug sensitivity and allergy.

Then he describes a set of symptoms that will sound familiar to all of you—headache, fever, vomiting and stiff neck. What disease is this, he wants to know. Sometimes we call it encephalitis, sometimes virus meningitis and so forth. Is it the same thing as polio—only in a slightly different form? And hasn't this particular set of symptoms, along with polio and many of the other infectious diseases grown much more serious in late years when it has appeared chiefly in adults rather than in children?

Then, take polio. How can anyone claim that infectious diseases are decreasing when "with bowed heads" as Dr. McLorinan says, we come to review "that most baffling and contradictory of all infectious diseases, polio." He is right; we have made little progress against polio. This used to be called "infantile paralysis." But today, the most serious cases of polio—and many of the fatal ones—occur among adults.

Decrease in Infections Due to More Vitamin C in the Diet

Dr. W. J. McCormick of Toronto takes almost exactly the opposite view in an article in the *Medical Record* for September, 1947. He asks, what is responsible for the really great decrease in infectious diseases? He gives us some arresting statistics. During the past 100 years, for instance, tuberculosis deaths have declined from 399 to 69 per hundred thousand in one city in England. The diphtheria death rate in Toronto was reduced from 132 to .3 per hundred thousand during the years of 1886 to 1945. Rheumatic fever death rates in New York City declined from 8.2 in 1900 to 1.3 in 1945.

Dr. McCormick asks, "where are the terrible diphtheria epidemics we used to dread?" Regarding typhoid fever, he reminds us that the acquisition of pure water and milk has of course had a favorable influence on these statistics, but fatalities from this disease were on the decline long, long before we began to chlorinate water and pasteurize milk. In regard to all the other infectious diseases, such as whooping cough, rheumatic fever, erysipelas and so forth—all these had decreased considerably in the early part of the century.

What, then, is the reason for the decline in contagious and infectious diseases—and how do you explain that many of them are now diseases of adults rather than children, as they used to be? Dr. McCormick says the reason is a change in nutrition. "The major change in nutrition in this period has been brought about by the tremendous increase in the production, distribution and consumption of citrus and other vitamin C containing fruits in North America and most of Europe, made possible by the gradual development of better transportation throughout the century—steamships, railways and motor highways." He tells us that the citrus fruit industry began in America in 1886 when the annual production was about 3 million bushels. In 1944, the total amounted to more than 278 million bushels. Production of tomato juice, also rich in vitamin C, rose from about 6 million pounds in 1932 to 924 million pounds in 1945. A hundred years ago, or even 50 years ago, fruits, especially tropical fruits, were a luxury, and no one in northern states had fresh fruit in the winter months. Today, mothers are well aware of the fact that their infants and young children must have vitamin C-rich foods.

Children Have the Benefit of This Reform

"This nutritional revolution has, perhaps, been applied more intensively in infancy and childhood than in the older age brackets," Dr. McCormick goes on. Fifty years ago, any infant who was not breast fed got cow's milk, condensed milk or some kind of prepared food in powder form. Fresh fruits were practically unheard of for infant feeding. Orange juice might possibly be given in very small quantity from the age of 10 months on. But often, mothers feared that any fruit juice would give the child "colic." Today, on the contrary, an infant one-month-old gets his orange juice daily, along with other fruits and vegetables, cereals enriched with wheat germ and so forth.

So today, babies, in general, get ample vitamin C to protect them against infectious diseases. But what of their older brothers and sisters? Dr. McCormick believes (and we agree with him) that "the infant in the nursery is given the full benefit of this nutritional reform, whereas, after this age, perverse dietary habits are gradually acquired through lack of parental guidance and inadequacy of public health education. The increased use of candy, carbonated beverages, tea, coffee, tobacco and alcohol by our juvenile and older age groups tends, generally, to displace the more wholesome nutritional habits of early childhood."

He goes on to talk about the use of vitamin C in treatment for various contagious and infectious diseases: tuberculosis, pneumonia, diphtheria, rheumatic fever, whooping cough and resistance to infection in general. It seems that the vitamin has been widely used in medicine to overcome infectious diseases.

It also seems that those who need especially to watch the vitamin C content of their diets are not the helpless babies who, today, are remarkably free from diseases caused by germs. However, older children and adults automatically assume that they are getting enough vitamin C in their diets (if they think of it at all) and as a result, are far more susceptible to the germ-caused disorders than the youngsters are. With proper

[949]

attention to sufficient vitamin C in the diet, perhaps we can finally do away with infectious diseases altogether.

We strongly advise against trying to get all your vitamin C requirements from citrus fruits. There is considerable evidence showing that too much citrus fruit (especially the juice) can have unfortunate effects on the teeth, gums and general health of those who are sensitive to it. We believe that many of these bad effects described may come from taking large quantities of citrus that has not been organically grown and may have been treated with dyes, as well as all the various insecticides, fungicides and so forth. Rose hip products and food supplements made from green peppers are excellent and reliable sources of vitamin C.

256. Many Disorders Associated with Salt Intake

Some people make more use of a salt shaker when they eat than they do of a knife and fork. The plate has hardly been set to rest on the table before they pass the salt shaker over everything on it. They put salt on watermelon and cantaloupe; ham and fish, often naturally too salty, get the full treatment anyway. Only the coffee escapes, and oftentimes the cook has taken care of that by adding salt to the grounds before brewing, to "enhance" the flavor. For such people, what lies under the salt is incidental. It could be a rubber sponge as well as a hamburger, or soap suds as well as mashed potatoes. If the consistency is similar, the taste will be the same—salty.

Of course, these people are missing a large part of the pleasure of eating—the subtle flavor of fresh foods, not masked by any condiments. If that were all they are missing, it would not be the concern of the nutritionist. Much more is involved, however. The addition of salt to foods is a health hazard so serious that death can result from its overuse.

"Salt" Never Given as Cause of Death

While it is true that no death certificate ever gave "salt" as cause of death, heart failure, hypertension, enlarged heart and kidney failure appear quite often, and any one of these can be the result of high salt intake. A quite convincing illustration of the dangers salt holds appeared in the *Annals of Internal Medicine* (November, 1953). In this article, 4 doctors reported on their findings in an experiment to determine the effect of various salt rations on a selected group of healthy rats. Seven groups were included in the test. The first group was fed a diet which contained about twice as much salt as the minimum considered absolutely necessary to sustain life. A second group ate a diet with the usual amount of salt used in all nutritional experiments. The amount was increased with each of the other five groups—20, 40, 50, 60 and 70 times the amount needed to sustain life.

After two months, 18 per cent of the rats in the 3 groups highest in salt intake had shown edema (unhealthy swelling) and an abrupt increase in weight. When these rats were sacrificed for further study, their kidneys were seen damaged in much the same fashion as in human cases of nephritis. The blood pressure of these rats had shown an increase and profound anemia was evident; blood protein was low.

The experiment continued. At the end of 9 months, hypertensive animals appeared in all of the 5 groups who had salt in their diets which exceeded the usual amount in laboratory diets. Most animals in the groups with the highest increases of salt had striking rises in blood pressure. It was obvious that the relationship between salt increase and blood pressure increase was proportionate. Chronic kidney failure was also common among the higher salt intake groups.

Of course, these experiments were carried on with rats, not people, and some will deny that the results apply to humans. But it must be admitted that salt does cause all tissue to hold water and increase body weight. Weight is a major factor in human heart disease because of the extra work it imposes on the heart. Excess sodium does create hardships for the kidneys. These facts hold good for men as well as rats, and we only show good sense when we heed the warnings presented by such experiments.

We All Need Some Salt

Without salt, the body's functioning would soon stop completely. We need a certain amount of it. But this amount is really quite small—two to three grams per day, according to R. Ackerly, M.D., in the *Proceedings of the Royal Society of Medicine*, 1910. We eat an average of 7 to 10 times that much and often more. Dr. L. Duncan Buckley, editor of the journal, *Cancer*, believes that one can do very well on 7 grams of added salt per week. We feel that these 7 grams come to one easily, without so much as touching the salt shaker. Just the sodium that is added to today's foods in processing would well fill the average family's needs. Add to this the salt used in the kitchen as the cook puts a meal together, and the 7 grams per week has been met and surpassed.

What do the experts predict for those who disregard the cautions against excessive amounts of salt in the diet? Cancer is one possibility, according to Dr. James Braithwaite of Leeds, England. He says that salt is not a food, but an inorganic material in dangerous oversupply, which harms tissue and is a powerful stimulant to cell metabolism. One of his patients showed an increase in the diameter of a tumor from 2⅜ inches to

3¼ inches on resumption of the daily use of salt. Frederick T. Marwood makes the interesting observation that, in Denmark, where consumption of salt fish is the highest in Europe, the cancer rate is highest in Europe as well.

In the June 5, 1959, issue of the *New England Journal of Medicine,* Lewis K. Dahl, M.D., gave some interesting information on salt and salt intake. He says that, while high blood pressure can be induced in animals by injecting certain chemicals, these chemicals will cause high blood pressure only if salt makes up two to four per cent of the daily diet. Dr. Dahl, along with Robert A. Love, M.D., also published a paper in the *Journal of the American Medical Association* (May 25, 1957), showing high blood pressure to be much more frequent among those humans who eat lots of salt as compared to those who are on low salt diets. They made careful observations on a total of 1,346 adults before writing this article. They divided the individuals (all employees of the laboratory) into 3 groups: those who denied ever adding salt to food at the table; those who added salt if, after tasting it, they found it "needed" salt; and those who automatically added salt to everything they ate without tasting it first. They called these groups "low," "average" and "high" in their consumption of salt—which seems to us a very fair way of naming them.

"Hypertension" was defined as blood pressure of at least 140/90. And of course, all figures over that level. The results of the observations (kept over a period of years) showed some very significant facts about salt eating and high blood pressure. The authors found: (1.) that individuals who are not overweight but are on a high-salt diet will have several times the incidence of hypertension, or high blood pressure, found in similar persons on a low-salt diet; (2.) among individuals who are on a high-salt diet, those who are overweight will have considerably more high blood pressure than those who are not overweight; (3.) those people who are both overweight and on a high-salt diet will have a much greater incidence of hypertension than will those not overweight and on a low-salt diet.

It is known, say the authors, that overweight individuals suffer from hypertension more commonly than do people of normal weight. Could it be, they ask, that in eating more food generally, more salt is taken? They feel this is one possible explanation.

In no case, was there any real craving for salt in patients whose intake was drastically reduced. For a week or so, they complained that food tasted flat, but after that, they became used to the new flavors and there were no more complaints. For some, the experience of giving up salt is similar to that of giving up smoking and drinking. For the first week or so the memory of old tastes persists, and after that, one simply forgets that they existed and has no desire for their return.

The high blood pressures indicated in the rats on salt diets, quoted above, have a counterpart in 21 patients reported on in *Ugeskrift For*

Laeger, a Copenhagen journal for March 30, 1950. These were treated with a low-salt diet for one to five months. In all cases, blood pressure was reduced 20 to 75 millimeters, usually within two to four weeks.

Dropsy, Pregnancy and Headaches

Dropsy, a disease which prompts the body to hoard water in abnormal amounts, is due to too much sodium in the body, according to Dr. Ferdinand R. Schemm. His salt-free diet in the treatment of this disease has won world-wide acceptance, and his tireless work in the field resulted in the establishment, in 1947, of the Western Foundation for Clinical Research.

Hospital Topics (1940) suggested that a lowering of salt intake can make pregnancy easier and less painful. Seventy patients put on a salt-free diet in the last weeks of pregnancy showed a definite decrease in the length of labor and in the severity of pains.

Dr. Max Goldzieher says migraine and other headaches may have their root in high salt intake. Dr. Goldzieher theorizes that there is a pressure on the nerves due to an increased flow of water to the tiny blood vessels of the head as a result of the water retention properties of the sodium.

Good Health magazine (no date) has also blamed salt, in part, for hives, epilepsy, nervous tension, rheumatic swelling and found that these conditions will respond to a restriction of salt intake.

One of the current arguments against salt intake is offered by Dr. Abraham E. Nizel in his book, *Nutrition and Clinical Dentistry.* He asserts that excess sodium chloride (salt) will enter into a struggle with calcium in the body and win. The result is less than an adequate amount of calcium for healthy teeth and bones. In this roundabout way, we have excessive use of salt to thank for dental caries.

Among other interesting effects of salt intake, we saw the strong guess by Dr. Eugene Foldes, printed in the *Medical Journal of Australia* (May 31, 1958), that baldness is one. Dr. Foldes did an experiment in which, in a closed environment, he actually counted the hairs falling from a subject eating salt without restriction. When the salt intake was reduced, the hairs falling out decreased in number. However, upon resumption of the unrestricted salt intake, the number of falling hairs increased in two days. Are you balding? Do you eat a lot of added salt?

Insomnia is also related to salt intake in the opinion of a French Army doctor Professor Coirault. In a speech before a conference on mental hygiene, he told of his theory, based on the fact that sodium and potassium are natural enemies in the body's chemistry. He said that a cell is in a state of repose when it rejects sodium and accepts potassium. It is in an active state when accepting sodium. This activity affects the nerves and causes insomnia. He described his success on treating sleeplessness by limiting or eliminating salt.

More evidence against the use of added salt is not hard to come by, but the above should convince anyone that salt is not conducive to good health. If your heart and kidneys are in good shape, stop using salt and help them stay that way. If you're already having such trouble, a salt reduction should improve your condition.

257. Diseases and the Medical Profession

The problem of doctor-induced diseases seems to grow with every so-called advance in medical technology. Treatments with modern drugs and X-ray apparatus create trouble faster than researchers can figure out how to combat it. Far from being a baseless charge brought forth by a group eager to embarrass physicians, the fact that such diseases exist is recognized by the doctors themselves, who have given these diseases a name—iatrogenic diseases.

Two Definitions by Medical Men

An exact definition for these diseases is a difficult thing to formulate. The *British Medical Journal* (August 30, 1958) carried an article which offered two definitions, neither of which was considered adequate. The first defines an iatrogenic disease as a "disorder unwittingly induced in the patient and based on a physician's examination, manner and discussion"; the second simply says "illness caused by a physician." The author says the definitions should be qualified, but any qualifications we make in the definition are not likely to mean very much to the patient or patient's family, when the actions of a physician have complicated an illness, rather than cured it.

The irony of this situation lies in the vast amount of publicity we hear which warns that a quick trip to the doctor is the only sure source of expert and unerring treatment. "Don't submit to anything but medically approved cancer treatment," they say, "follow your doctor's advice exclusively. Don't try to build yourself up with wheat germ, brewer's yeast or those other fad foods, consult your doctor for guidance that you can depend upon." So now, in the same newspapers and journals, we read that the medical profession quite candidly admits that it doesn't know what it's doing a lot of the time. Patients are treated, in many cases, with drugs whose results are uncertain or definitely dangerous. Routine procedures are followed in hospitals with calm assurance, and prove later to be the absolute cause of many deaths and serious diseases. These catastrophes caused by commonly employed medical practices should be noted by the public if only to serve as a guide for self-preservation in the event that a physician they consult should decide to use such questionable means of treatment on them.

Carelessness and Bungling Can't Be Excused

If all iatrogenic diseases were the result of honest mistakes, made by physicians familiar with every possible course of treatment and its result, one would find it easier to excuse them. Instead, we find that many serious diseases are the result of the physician's use of drugs with which he is not familiar. He knows nothing that is not printed in the sales brochures issued by the drug firm, and uses the preparation for the quick cure of a mild disease, without attempting to ascertain the patient's past experience with drugs and without any evidence of the drug's past performance. An unfortunate result in such a case can hardly be interpreted as an honest mistake. It is culpable carelessness.

What of the doctor who prescribes X-ray of the pelvic region for a pregnant woman, when absolute urgency is not the case? After all that has been written about the danger to the unborn child when X-ray is used on a pregnant woman, could such a prescription by a doctor be interpreted as anything but stupidity, carelessness or bungling?

The use of sulfa drugs is another area of seemingly irresponsible action on the part of our doctors. The supreme danger to the kidneys of these slow-to-dissolve drugs was the cause of a stoppage of urinary flow for 3 children *in a hospital,* seen by the author of an article in the September, 1957, issue of the *Practitioner.* A flushing of their kidneys through a uretic catheter was required before normal function could be restored. If this happened under hospital supervision, it can be reasonably supposed that the experience was repeated outside of hospitals hundreds of times throughout the country.

Hospital Procedures Proved Dangerous

The most famous, or infamous of the iatrogenic diseases is, of course, retrolental fibroplasia, a disease of premature infants which leads to complete blindness. The cause was found to be a hospital procedure considered quite normal up to the mid-1950's: The administration of large quantities of oxygen to premature infants. Oxygen was piped into the incubator units, whether needed or not, for a period of weeks, often causing severe damage to the retina, which resulted in blindness. The disease was known for approximately 5 years before the cause and hence, the preventive measure was discovered.

Kernicterus is another disease presented to premature babies by the medical profession. It is caused by overdosage of synthetic vitamin K, the coagulant vitamin, usually given to premature infants at birth, due to their greater danger of bleeding. It has since been discovered that an

[955]

ingredient of synthetic vitamin K is capable of destroying red blood cells when administered in large doses. The brain can become affected and the result is that the infants become spastic and mentally retarded. Natural vitamin K does not have this ingredient.

Vaccination Sometimes Fatal in Newborn Babies

We know that most newborn babies are vaccinated and such procedure is becoming common now. The *Practitioner* article (September, 1957) says that this is sometimes done to babies who have generalized eczema and notes that "the carrying out of vaccination in such a child causes harm and may even lead to the death of the child."

But among the greatest "helps" that can and have killed many persons are the antibiotics. They so alter intestinal flora as to interfere with, or abolish, synthesis of vitamins B and K. They can encourage a mucous membrane infection (thrush) which might become generalized and fatal, and are known to cause ulcerative colitis in some cases of prolonged use.

Penicillin—A Star Performer

Of course, penicillin is the star performer of the antibiotics. Its use has become so generalized that it is sometimes given no matter what the diagnosis "just to make sure there's no infection." Such indiscriminate use has resulted in a complete perversion of the intended use of penicillin. Its original purpose was to treat serious infections which were beyond the body's considerable powers of resistance. Penicillin was to be an emergency treatment. To think of using it as a preventive was certainly not in the discoverer's plans. Its effect on intestinal flora alone would dictate otherwise.

The question of tolerances soon arose. Not only would penicillin (and other antibiotics) not work on some patients after previous treatments with it, but penicillin would cause a violent reaction in the patient, with death as the final result in quite a number of cases. Even though all of this information appears quite commonly in the pages of medical journals all over the country, the chances that a doctor would hesitate to give you penicillin without going into your past experience with it, or search for an alternate treatment, if possible, are pretty slim. Many persons with a cold demand a penicillin shot and usually the doctor gives it to them, even though it is well known that penicillin has no effect whatsoever on colds. Who is responsible for any ill effects from such treatment? Can we say that the ill effects fit the definition "illness caused by a physician"? You bet we can.

At Last—Something to Neutralize Penicillin

On the subject of penicillin, there is an interesting development discussed in the *British Medical Journal* (August 2, 1958). It has been found that an enzyme formed by several species of bacteria, inactivates penicillin. This enzyme is called penicillinase and is now being used to destroy penicillin in the body, if such destruction should seem desirable, for example, when penicillin is causing a reaction in a sensitive patient. It was shown to be effective for this purpose in tests with 20 human subjects who were given 800,000 units of penicillin twice daily, and, after several days, a single injection of 800,000 units of penicillinase was given. The penicillin disappeared from the blood within one hour and remained undetectable for 4 to 7 days, even though the daily dosage of penicillin was continued as before.

At long last the wheel appears to have turned full-circle. A cure for penicillin, called the greatest cure of them all, has had to be found. And isn't it effective though! It seems to last and last. There is an aspect of the emergence of penicillinase that deserves exploration. Penicillinase is the enzyme to which the staphylococci germs owe their resistance to antibiotics. The staphylococcus infections run rampant when they occur, and no modern medication seems to be effective against them. The enzyme which makes this disease what it is, is the element needed to inactivate penicillin. If we're going to inject this enzyme into our bodies, an enzyme in which staphylococcus flourishes, how are we to get rid of it if staphylococcus infection should occur? Science will have to emerge with a drug more powerful than penicillin or penicillinase to get us out of that predicament. Crazy as it might sound to doctors, doesn't it seem simpler and safer to use penicillin on only the most serious cases, and eliminate its general use entirely where alternate treatment is possible?

The Court Recognizes an Iatrogenic Disease

Let this be one of the first reports on a brand new iatrogenic disease, which fits both definitions beautifully, and has been recognized as such by the Court of Appeals in New York. The story, which appears in the *AMA News* (October 20, 1958), tells us that the court ruled in favor of Mrs. Eleanor Ferrara to the tune of 15,000 dollars for mental anguish as the result of developing severe cancerophobia (fear of cancer.) The lady, suffering from bursitis in the right shoulder was treated for it with X-ray. The X-ray caused a skin reaction, and on a visit to a dermatologist, Mrs. Ferrara was advised to have her shoulder checked every 6 months because the X-ray burns might become cancerous.

The patient then sued the X-ray doctors for malpractice, alleging that too much X-ray was given, and evidence was introduced in court by a neuropsychiatrist showing that Mrs. Ferrara was suffering from a severe case of cancerophobia and that the symptoms of the scare might be permanent. This was indeed "an illness induced by a doctor." When bursitis turns into a cancer possibility due to the type of treatment used, it is not gross nor unfair to accuse the doctor in charge of dereliction of duty.

"Accepted" Cancer Treatments Backfire

An article in the *New York Times* (October 7, 1958) calls attention to accepted practices for treatment of cancer which actually speed the spread of cancerous tumors. The occasion for this revelation was the 44th Annual Clinical Congress of the American College of Surgeons. "In the treatment of patients with TSPA, nitrogen mustard, mechlorethamine, hydrochloride and nitromin, all synthetic compounds, and with Actinamycin D, an antibiotic, there was found, the report declared, an apparent stimulation of local cancer growth and spread." It is suggested that a test be performed before using a chemical agent to determine the sensitivity of a specific tumor to a specific agent. Such testing should not merely be suggested—it should be mandatory that the doctor do so. The horrible speed with which cancer spreads is efficient enough without any help from doctors upon whom we depend to slow down this march.

Corneal Ulcers through Carelessness

Still another disease due to medical treatment is corneal ulcers due to contaminated eye solutions administered by physicians. *Survey of Ophthalmology* (3: 203, June, 1958) makes this report and reminds doctors that solutions should be sterilized before use for each patient, and a sterile dropper used. That a medical journal finds it necessary to remind practicing doctors of these fundamental procedures is shocking.

Everybody makes mistakes, as the saying goes. Doctors make them, too. But mistakes and carelessness are not synonymous. The doctor who followed hospital procedure and gave an infant oxygen that caused retrolental fibroplasia can hardly be blamed for doing what was considered therapeutic. He was acting in the light of present knowledge and in good faith. But what excuse could there be for a penicillin reaction when no test was made for tolerance? What excuse for such an overdose of sulfa that kidney problems result, or what excuse for X-ray treatments for bursitis to the degree that serious burns that could lead to cancer result?

The list of diseases caused by physicians who cannot be excused, but must be labeled as careless, is still growing. The medical profession is losing respect and the confidence of patients because of this fact. If you are in doubt as to the procedure your doctor is using, say so to him. Let him know that you don't want to chance having the results of his treatment to be anything but beneficial.

258. Drugs Are Doing Us Little Good

The unrelieved use of drugs by doctors on their patients and by patients on their own, continues. They scarcely have time to try all of the various new preparations being put out almost daily by the big drug firms. But somehow these drugs do get tried and used by our physicians, and one of the major results turns out to be newer and more serious illnesses as the unforeseen effects of a great many of them.

In *Time* magazine (May 18, 1959), Dr. Maxwell Finland, Associate Professor of Medicine at Harvard Medical School, was quoted as saying that the antibiotic drugs have caused an actual increase in severe infections and deaths from hitherto harmless or uncommon germs. He suggested possible reasons for the awakening of these germs: possibly man's resistance to infection has been lowered because there are fewer infections around to give man a natural immunity or perhaps the sleeping germs in our organs may have been held in check all these years by substances secreted by killer germs. But with antibiotics destroying the killers, the natural barriers to the dormant germs have been broken.

Penicillin Again

Many of the results of antibiotics and other drugs are more immediately obvious. The *Medical Journal of Australia* (October 17, 1959) carries another of the growing list of reports on penicillin-induced fatalities. This time, a woman, 31 years of age, being treated for an inflammation of the ear lobe dropped dead following an injection of 900,000 units (not an unusual dose) into the arm. This reaction occurred in spite of fairly frequent previous injections of penicillin with no ill effects. No patient who is not tested for a reaction to penicillin before each treatment can feel sure that his reaction will be the expected one. Previous experience is not a sufficient indication of safety.

Penicillin is also showing up as a cause of mental illness, according to the *British Medical Journal* (May 21, 1960). Injections of procaine penicillin have been followed, on occasion, almost immediately by an hour or two of acute distress and several days of exhaustion. Hysterical behavior, fear of impending death and possibly hallucinations were noted. Three similar cases occurred from the use of oral tablets of probenecid penicillin. Both procaine and probenecid are considered "safe" drugs.

Antibiotic Therapy Induces Diarrhea

One of the common results of antibiotic therapy is diarrhea. This condition is due to the destruction of the friendly bacteria in the intestines along with the infective bacteria at which the antibiotic was aimed. This situation makes an unhealthy intestinal climate for the proper processing of food. *M. D.* (March, 1960) describes a new type of medication to combat this condition, which contains, as its base, a form of yogurt. Yogurt is valuable in maintaining the proper climate for the intestines. If one is taking a course of antibiotics, a daily dose would not be amiss. We mean pure yogurt, of course, not any drug preparation. Yogurt is cheap and easy to get. You can even make your own.

Tranquilizers are a challenge to antibiotics in the unwholesome side effects they cause. But each year Americans buy tranquilizers to the tune of 280,000,000 dollars as of January 30, 1960. In the *Tampa* (Florida) *Tribune* (January 29, 1960), Dr. W. C. Ballard of the Pinellas County Health Department, said of them: "The new stimulants and tranquilizers, swallowed as the mood dictates, create a type of addiction, less degrading, but comparable to that induced by alcohol and narcotics."

Even the Antidote Doesn't Work

The barbiturates, or sleeping pills, are close cousins to the tranquilizers and popular enough to sell 2,000 tons a year. In *Biochemical Pharmacology* (1959, p. 288), we learn that these drugs in sufficient quantity, are able to kill white blood cells. Cyanide is no more effective along these lines. The common antidote for barbiturate poisoning in humans does not have any effect in such a case.

Aspirin is one of our commonly used drugs, and in the *Archives of Physical Medicine and Rehabilitation* (June, 1960), we read the opinion that even when the most readily soluble aspirin preparations are used, there is an irritation of the stomach lining, accompanied by an intestinal loss of blood which shows up in the stool. Tests were made of the fecal waste of 140 patients who were receiving aspirin in dosages varying from 750 to 3,000 milligrams daily. The diet contained no meat and was as free from iron as possible. The patients were not even allowed to brush their teeth because of possibly bleeding gums. The stool specimens showed blood in 95 per cent of the patients while they were receiving aspirin. This irritation is experienced by millions of Americans yearly, and they don't even know it! Is there any wonder that the ulcer rate and intestinal cancer rate rises so steadily?

A Digitalis Story

Digitalis is the classic medication for a heart condition, although frequent reports of its serious bad effects come to us. One of the most recent appeared in the *Canadian Medical Association Journal* (July 1, 1959). It told of a 59-year-old woman who had been suffering from severe emotionalism and palpitations about 7 months before her admission. After a few months, the palpitations became more violent and her doctor prescribed digitalis. About a week later she began to vomit, but continued to take the digitalis for two months. Little or no solid food was retained by the patient during this period, but she drank great quantities of a beverage containing glucose. She lost more than 70 pounds in the 5 months before admission.

When she was admitted, she had excessive weakness and a mental disturbance. She was completely unaware of who she was or where she was; her pulse was rapid and bounding; her bladder was greatly swollen and she had no deep reflexes.

In view of this situation and others equally alarming, which frequently develop when common treatments for heart disease are used, we wonder why the medical men of the United States are so reluctant to give vitamin E a chance to show what it has done and can do. Certainly the element of risk is no factor, when such reports on the regularly accepted treatments are being seen. Vitamin E is a safe and effective treatment for heart disease as attested to by many international heart experts; ask your doctor to give it a chance.

Disenchanted Researchers

The disenchantment with cortisone and the other steroid drugs has long ago reached the researchers. It is the practicing physicians most of us consult who are either unaware of the dangers involved in their use or refuse to be influenced by the reports of the researchers. The entire situation was laid out neatly by Dr. Richard Freyberg, Professor of Medicine at Cornell University Medical School. In Denver, Colorado, for a series of clinics, he was quoted on his opinion of the steroids in the *Denver Post* (August 2, 1959).

Dr. Freyberg said that death can be one of the side effects of the use of these drugs. He told of a series of 168 patients treated with large amounts of steroids over a 5 year period. The disease was in no way stopped, but in many cases, pain was relieved and joint function maintained. The side effects shown in the same patients were so serious as to demand that doctors use them with the utmost caution and even avoid them whenever possible.

Between 7 and 8 per cent of the patients studied died, and there is strong suspicion, says Dr. Freyberg, that they died of the treatment, not the disease. Bone weaknesses which caused them to suffer frequent fractures were developed by 14 per cent, and 17 per cent came down with ulcers of the gastrointestinal tract. Other adverse effects included mental confusion and high susceptibility to infections.

Our files are bulging with material of this type. It happens every day, and, as can be imagined, only a small fraction of the cases are reported.

Cases Caused by X-Ray Treatments

One final note should not be omitted. It appeared in the *New England Journal of Medicine* (260/5: 197-202), and informed the reader that one-fifth of our cancer cases are caused by X-ray treatments for conditions that have nothing to do with malignancy. The article was based on the files and records of Massachusetts General Hospital. There was a latent period between irradiation and tissue breakdown. Cancer developed in 22 per cent of 165 cases studied.

The only recourse the patient has is to avoid drugs and other dangerous medical treatment whenever he can. He must ask his doctor why he is to receive this or that treatment. He must ask about possible side effects, and if there is a better-known safer treatment. Finally, he can always refuse a treatment he is convinced will do more harm than good. He can consult with one or several other doctors about a course of treatment to make certain of the first doctor's opinion. Such investigation might save his life!

259. Some Speculations on a Brand New Disease

Did you ever wonder how a new disease comes to be listed as such? After the process of recognition, it becomes necessary to describe the symptoms of the disease, all the results of laboratory tests and physical examinations of the patient. Then there ensues a search through the medical literature to see if any other physician has encountered and described these same symptoms in his practice. Experts in one field or another are consulted. They examine slides, study test results and analyses of tissues taken from the patient.

Finally, when it becomes apparent that this patient is not suffering from exactly the same set of conditions that characterizes one of the recognized and named diseases, it is decided that this is a new disease requiring new diagnosis and new treatment. Sometimes the disease is then named after the researcher who studies it first. Buerger's disease and Parkinson's disease are samples of this.

We have quite a file on new diseases. The reason we are interested in following all the various steps of the activity outlined above is that we have recently come upon an account of a brand new disease, hitherto undescribed, which seems to be related to something in the environment that the patient has inhaled. In fact, the researchers go so far as to speculate on whether the cause may be aerosols, insecticides or detergents.

The article, called "Pulmonary Alveolar Proteinosis," which appeared in the *New England Journal of Medicine* for June 5, 1958, describes this condition. It was written by 5 medical men from Washington, Boston and New Haven. The 20 pages of text and pictures leave no doubt in anyone's mind that this is really a new disease, unrelated to any other. The name given to the disease, which is also the name of the article, concerns

[962]

the protein material which gathers in the alveoli or air cells of the lungs. The patient complains of shortness of breath and persistent cough which produces mucus. Sometimes the mucus is blood-stained. Sometimes there is fever. Those patients who die apparently suffocate as a result of the blockage of the surface of the lungs. It is a chronic disease—nothing acute. In some patients, symptoms have persisted for from 5 to 35 months.

It would be easy, we suppose, for an unobservant or careless diagnostician to tell these folks they have grippe or flu, asthma or pneumonia. In fact, several of the patients discussed here were diagnosed as pneumonia patients until further tests revealed that they did not have true pneumonia symptoms.

The thoroughness of the tests given these patients is impressive. Truly, modern medicine has as a diagnostic aid an impressive array of tests which may indicate quite clearly to the expert diagnostician which body functions appear to be normal and which seem to be out of line. All the tests given are described in the *Journal* article. Twenty-seven patients are described. Throughout, there is no clue as to any possible cause of the disease.

What Causes This New Disease?

But, say the authors, "The possibility that a chemical inhalant is the inciting factor deserves consideration. . . . Perhaps some metal is involved. Moreover, innumerable new volatile solvents and plastics have been introduced in recent years. The use of aerosols and dispersing agents —in insecticides, for example—has enormously increased. Many detergents have also entered the market world. The role of recently developed antibiotics in altering tissue responses and in inducing allergic and other reactions, should also be considered. In other words, the new disease may be a penalty for the convenience of modern living."

Chemical magazines and the publications of the drug trade boast of the thousands—nay, hundreds of thousands—of new chemical compounds that have been developed and widely distributed over the face of the earth in the last 10 to 20 years. Undoubtedly this fact is a tribute to our technical excellence, but what may it be doing to our body cells? Where, in all the seemingly endless legions of new chemical substances can you start to look for the source of such a new disease? How large an army of investigators do you need to run down the possible harmfulness of hundreds of thousands of newly introduced chemicals to which we are exposed— to say nothing of astronomical numbers of combinations in which these substances might prove to be toxic?

One patient suffering from the new disease was a butcher and a sprayer of fruit. Another used a special cleaner in cleaning animal cages. Another worked in a toothpaste factory where he was exposed to silica flour. Another was exposed to considerable amounts of smoke from oil and kerosene in contact with hot metal. Another worked in a plastic factory. Possibly you might have at least some starting point—industrial hazards—in investigating these illnesses, but what about the 3-year-old baby who died of suffocation and whose lungs showed just the same characteristic conditions exhibited by the lungs of older people who died? Where do you start to look for the toxic substances which somehow entered this infant's lungs and caused death? Eight of the 27 known patients have died, incidentally.

Modern Technology Has Produced This Disease, It Seems

The authors of the article are convinced that something in the environment of all these patients was responsible for the diseases. If this premise is sound, then a chronic condition of the lungs would seem to indicate that whatever caused the disease was still around years later in the atmosphere. "Search for a causative agent by microbiologic, chemical and epidemiologic (having to do with epidemics) methods must be pursued with all vigor," say our authors, "since it is evident that the condition is not rare."

We have warned many times in our writings, top-flight experts in health have warned in Congressional investigations and medical men have sounded warning after warning throughout the pages of medical magazines: we are spreading abroad far too many new and possibly toxic chemical materials. We may already have reached the point where exposure to several or many of these is so nearly universal in this country, that we no longer have any individuals left as "controls"; that is, unexposed people whose physiology can be compared to that of the exposed people to see if abnormalities have been produced. When this point is finally reached, how will it be possible to track down the poisonous cause of *any* fatal poisoning?

We do not know how many years it will take to discover the cause of our new disease—Pulmonary Alveolar Proteinosis—or how many people will die from it first. Nor do we know what cautions to give our readers so that they may avoid "new diseases," except for the same warning we always give: avoid as much as you can any and all contacts with modern chemicals. Look with suspicion on the word "new" when it is used to advertise a product. "New" means—has to mean—untested, so far as possible toxicity goes. Eat food that has not been treated with insecticides, preservatives, artificial fat and colorings; breathe air as clean and pure as you can get and drink water uncontaminated by chemicals. If it is possible for you to live far out in the country and avoid all the many air pollutants that city dwellers have to put up with, then move to the country.

INDEX

A

Abdominal muscles
  exercise for strengthening, 11, 621-623
  massage of, and constipation, 623
  strain on, and hernia, 716
Acetylsalicylic acid. *See* Aspirin.
Acidosis
  in colds, 872
  in sinusitis, 872
Acrocyanosis, 168
Acroparasthesia, 168
ACTH
  arthritis and, 346
  effect on adrenal gland, 346
  side effects, 346
  ulcers and, 894
Adrenal gland
  alcoholism and, 324-325, 326
  civilization and, 412-413
  low blood sugar and, 762
Air
  polluted, and catalase, 455
  polluted, and lung cancer, 445-446, 478
  "stale," and colds, 594
Alcohol
  advisability of, in heart cases, 142-143, 214, 215
  choline appetite and, 488
  cirrhosis of the liver and, 250, 254
  effect on body, 142, 325
  experiment on rats and, 319-320
Alcoholic's Anonymous, 327
Alcoholism
  adrenocortical insufficiency and, 324-325, 326
  books on, 328
  change in thinking on, 323
  characteristics of alcoholics, 323-325
  diet for, 321-322
  high nutritional requirements and, 320-321, 748
  inheritance in, 320-321
  low blood sugar and, 325-326
  stress and, 327
  vitamin deficiency and, 320
Allergy
  difficulty in tracking down, 693
  epilepsy and, 691-692, 693
  food, and colds, 561
  food, and high blood pressure, 229-230
  food, and pruritus ani, 620
  food, and pulse, 148-149
  low blood sugar and, 694
  present in multiple sclerosis, 785-786
  smoking and, 944
  see also Asthma, Pulse test

Aluminum
  deposits, in artery walls, 211
  utensils, and pulse, 164
  source of, in foods, 212
Amino acids
  cataracts and, 39
  enlarged prostate and, 266-267
  foods high in, 268 (table)
  hearing and, 26-27
  muscular dystrophy and, 796
  see also Protein
Anemia
  bananas and, 930
  defined, 809
  folic acid and, 810-811
  types of, 809
  see also Aplastic anemia, Pernicious anemia
Aneurysm, 169
Anigoma, 169
Aniseikonia
  correction of, 119-120
  description of, 119
  discovery of, 119
  headaches and, 118
Antibiotics
  cancer and, 461
  catalase and, 454-455
  diarrhea and, 959-960
  dizziness and, 686
  given to CF victims, 632
  in fruits and vegetables, 462
  L. acidophilus and, 667-668
  lung cancer and, 478-479
  misuse of, 478, 604, 605
  results of widespread use of, 959
  staph resistant to, 875-876
  value of, 478
  yogurt when taking, 960
  see also Penicillin
Antihistamines
  colds and, 602
  death from, 602
  early tests of, 602
  impotence and, 603
  incidence of side reactions, 603
  side effects of, 603
Aplastic anemia
  causative agents, 741-742
  chloromycetin and, 742-743
  symptoms of, 741
Apoplexy. *See* Stroke.
Appendicitis
  cause of infection, 331
  deaths from, 329
  diagnostic difficulties, 330
  incidence of, 329
  refined foods and, 331-332
  stress and, 331
  symptoms of, 330

typical attack, 330

Appetite
  developing, 915
  faulty eating habits and, 909
  stress and, 909
  vitamin B and, 910

Apples
  for preventing tooth decay, 297-298
  heart disease and, 179-180
  pectin in, 179-180

Arrhythmia, 166

Arteries
  advantages of wide, 151-152
  coffee and, 145
  exercise and widening of, 151, 152
  health, and vitamin B, 239
  health, and thyroid gland, 240
  stress and, 154
  see also Blood vessels, Hardening of
    the arteries

Arteriosclerosis. See Hardening of the
  arteries.

Arthritis
  among farmers, 396
  bioflavonoids for, 358, 359, 396-397
  Brusch dietary regimen for, 351-356
  calcium-phosphorus ratio and, 349,
    350
  case histories, 367-370
  characteristics of arthritics, 340-342,
    366
  cold liver oil and, 351-352, 354
  conditions leading to, 349-350
  degenerative, 366
  diet and, 350-351, 352, 354
  drugs used for, 345-347, 390-391
  exercise and, 160-161
  gouty, and cherries, 348, 349
  heat and, 390, 391
  imbalanced feet and, 367-370
  low blood sugar and, 396
  mineral baths for, 391-392
  old-fashioned remedies for, 393-394
  posture and, 386
  rheumatoid, 366
  stress and, 340-342
  sulfur deficiency and, 391
  types of, 365
  vitamin A and, 335
  vitamin B and, 335-336
  vitamin C and, 336, 358, 359, 362-
    363
  vitamin D and, 336, 363
  see also Osteoarthritis, Rheumatism

Aschner, Dr. Bernard, 393-395

Aspirin
  asthma and, 405-406, 601
  bloody stools and, 960
  fatalities from, 601
  for children, 602
  effect in the body, 600-601
  poisoning, in children, 602
  side effects, 347, 601

thyroid gland and, 760
  vitamin K and, 601-602

Asthma
  aspirin and, 405-406, 601
  avoiding pollen, 399
  barometric pressure and, 404, 405
  cereal foods and, 407, 410
  common allergens, 398-399, 401
  cortisone and, 412
  defined, 398
  description of an attack, 407-408
  diet and, 403
  doctor's case of, 413-415
  drugs used for, 399, 409, 414
  exercise for, 411-412
  free of, during severe conditions, 410
  humidity and, 404-405
  ideal location for asthmatics, 406
  immunization, 399
  low blood sugar and, 401-402
  ordeal of Marcel Proust, 415-417
  patch tests, 408
  pattern of, 407
  physiology of, 408
  seeking ideal climate, 406-407
  serious consequences of, 398
  smoker's, 609-610
  stress and, 399-401, 406
  temperature and, 405
  testing for allergens, 408-409
  travel and, 406
  upside-down exercise for, 413
  see also Allergy

Atherosclerosis. See Hardening of the
  arteries.

Athlete's foot, 77, 282

Atropine
  side effects of, 63
  use of, 63

Aureomycin and the liver, 250-251

Auricular fibrillation, 166-167

Auricular flutter, 167

B

Bacillus Calmette Guering vaccine. See
  B. C. G.

Back
  construction of, 3
  exercise for strengthening muscles of,
    11-12
  rules for general hygiene of, 7-8

Backache
  bed and, 4
  causes of, 3
  foot disorders and, 370-372
  how it occurs, 3-4
  posture and, 3-4, 5, 6, 9

Bad breath
  causes of, 418-421
  experiment on garlic and, 419
  food and, 419-420
  in Roman times, 417

orally caused, 418
overcoming, 421
saliva and, 419-420
stress and, 420-421
systemically caused, 419
Baldness
inositol and, 110
long hair and, 110
lotions and, 111-112
male hormones and, 106, 111
pony-tail and, 111
salt and, 112-113, 953
scalp muscles and, 106, 109-110
sex differences in incidence of, 105
stress and, 110-111
traumatic, 111
vitamin A and, 106
Bananas
anemia and, 930
before and after operations, 931
colitis and, 930
constipation and, 929
diarrhea and, 654-655
for diabetics, 931
for typhoid fever patients, 931
gout and, 931
heart disease and, 931
kidney disease and, 931
nonallergenic properties of, 930
pellagra and, 930
ulcers and, 930
Barbiturates, 960
Barometric pressure and asthma, 404, 405
B. C. G.
advocates of, 888, 890
dietary deficiencies and infection from, 889
effectiveness of, 888, 890
fatalities from, 889
popularity of, overseas, 888
safety of, 888-889, 890
what it is, 888
see also Tuberculosis
Beard, Dr. Howard H., 457-459
Bed wetting
accompanying symptoms, 423, 424
anxiety and, 422-423
cause of, 423-424
characteristics of, 422
overtraining at toilet and, 422
treatment of, 424
Beriberi
compared to polio, 821
deafness in, 19-20
tinnitus in, 20
vitamin B deficiency and, 820
Biochemical individuality, 175-176, 320-321, 322-323
Bioflavonoids
arthritis and, 358, 359, 396-397
cancer and, 554

capillary fragility and, 358-359, 554, 555
colds and, 586-587
daily requirement of, 556
foods rich in, 557 (table)
gum disease and, 104
hemorrhage and, 554, 555
in natural vitamin C preparations, 104-105
labyrinthitis and, 686-687
ulcer and, 906
vitamin C and, 358, 555-556, 585-586
see also Rutin
Biotin in fat metabolism, 86
Blindness
cataracts and, 35
glaucoma and, 45
tobacco amblyopia and, 881, 940
Blood
chemicals and increase in diseases of, 741-743
chemistry, and mental illness, 753, 757
clotting of, and high-fat diet, 172
clotting of, and menthol, 605
clotting of, and vitamin E, 126, 127, 183, 184-185, 703, 918-919
clotting time, and starch, 222
clotting time in heart attack victims, 219
diseases, and insecticides, 741
flow, and smoking, 447, 881, 944
heat and, 193
normal level of sugar in, 787
pressure, and smoking, 944
ratio of weight to, and overweight, 803-804
stress and, 187
sugar, and adrenal gland, 762
sugar level, and multiple sclerosis, 787
transfusions, and undulant fever, 917-918
white cells, and barbiturates, 960
see also Anemia, Aplastic anemia, Hemoglobin, Leukemia, Lupus erythematosus, Pernicious anemia
Blood vessels
disorders, and dizziness, 684
disorders, and vitamin B_{12}, 550-552
disorders, in diabetics, 640
fragility of, and bioflavonoids, 554, 555
fragility of, and rutin, 130, 553-555
health, and vitamin C, 240
possible cause of disease of, 549
smoking and, 944
vitamin E and, 128, 183-186, 703
see also Arteries, Buerger's disease, Capillaries, Gangrene, Hardening of the arteries, Hemorrhage, Inter-

mittent claudication, Labyrinthitis, Phlebitis, Pulse, Stroke, Thrombosis, Varicose veins
Boines, Dr. George, 812-813, 814
Bones
  effect of osteoporosis on, 13
  fluoride deposition in, 776
  nature of, 14
  rebuilding in old age, 15
  spontaneous fractures of, 16
  vitamin C and formation of, 16, 17
  see also Osteoporosis
Bradycardia, 167
Breakfast, skipping, 132-133
Breast feeding
  acidified milk in place of, 653-654
  advice on, 651
  cancer and, 517-519
  reasons for not, 516-517, 651
  scurvy prevention and, 867
  substitutes for, 651-652
  sufficient vitamin E and, 635-636
Breathing
  colds and, 597, 598
  exercises, 411
  mouth, and malocclusion, 312, 315
  mouth, ill effects of, 315, 412
  physiology of, 411
  stress and, 598
Brewer's yeast
  constipation and, 626, 629, 630
  for vitamin B, 21
  vitamin D toxicity and, 364, 365
Brucellosis. See Undulant fever.
Bruising and vitamin C, 515
Bruxism
  causes of, 122
  defined, 121
  headaches and, 121-123
Buerger's disease
  course of, 425
  defined, 169
  gangrene and, 425, 704
  lung cancer and, 428
  rye bread and, 428
  smoking and, 425-426, 934, 944
  vitamin E and, 426-427, 428
Bunion, 77
Bush, Dr. Lucius, 565, 869-871
Buttermilk
  diarrhea and dysentery and, 652-653
  manufacture of, 652

C

Cabbage juice for ulcers, 894, 900-901
Caffeine
  arteries and, 145
  insomnia and, 734
  ulcers and, 892, 896
  see also Coffee
Calcium
  bone meal for, 17

cancer and, 462
can one get too much, 16-17
cataracts and, 39
deficiency, and constipation, 631
deposits, and vitamin C, 245-246
diabetes and, 639
excretion of, 14
factors in body's supply, 14
gum disease and, 96
hardening of the arteries and, 210
in the body, and salt, 589-590, 873, 953
metabolism, and exercise, 158
need for constant intake of, 15
nose cilia and, 565
osteoporosis and, 13-15
spontaneous fractures and lack of, 16
vitamin D and, 15
Calcium-phosphorus balance
  arthritis and, 349, 350
  infection and, 350
  menopause and, 350
  pyorrhea and, 101-102
  sugar and, 351
Calorie-counting, 798
Cancer
  air pollution and lung, 445-446, 478
  among gardeners, 493-494
  among Navajos, 487
  antibiotics and, 461
  antibiotics and lung, 478-479
  body electricity and, 495
  calcium and, 462
  case histories on Gerson's patients, 531-535
  catalase deficiency and, 453-454
  cervical, precautionary measures, 506
  character of discoverers of cancer "cures," 538-539
  chemicals in food and, 429-430, 440-442, 492
  choline and, 227-228, 487
  chymotrypsin and, 457, 458-459
  civilization and, 528-529
  coconut and, 462
  colds and susceptibility to lung, 561
  collagen degeneration in, 484, 513-514
  conditions considered precancerous, 508-509, 512
  diet and, 452-453, 484, 487-488, 489-490, 491, 528-530
  disturbance of inner respiratory system and, 491-492
  Drosnes-Lazenby treatment, 524-527
  epidemiology applied to, 443-444
  emotions and, 464-466
  factors in larnyx, 444
  factors in lung, 445-446
  factors in rectal, 444-445
  factors in skin, 444
  factors in stomach, 444

factors in uterine, 445, 505, 506
forecast of deaths from, 504 (illus.)
Frost's theory and treatment of, 536-537
garlic and, 507
geographical incidence of, 502-503
Gerson's treatment of, 530
Glyoxylide, 539-541
hair growth in victims, 468-469
heated fats and, 475-477
hormones and, 469
immature cell theory of, 450-452
increasing rate of, 429
Krebiozen, 519-523
lactation and breast, 517-519
lung, and Buerger's disease, 428
metastasis, and collagen, 514-515
"milk-factor" in, 460
need for impartial investigation of "cures," 535-536, 537, 541
new test for, 458
nutritional rules in light of, 485-486
of penis, and circumcision, 505-506
of prostate gland, 266
organic vs. chemical foods in, 485
overeating and, 483-484, 486, 487
oxidation-enzyme deficiency and, 490-491
personality of victims, 466
prevention of breast, 519
processed foods and, 482-483
radioactivity and, 430, 438-439, 961-962
riboflavin and, 482
rimless eyeglasses and skin, 480-481
role of the National Cancer Institute, 459
salt and, 488, 492
scientific outlook on, 527-528
smoking and lung, 445-446, 447-449, 478
statistics on breast and uterine, 518
steps necessary for preventing, 529-530
substances which cause, 432-435, 437-438, 440-441
sulfur and, 488
test for, involving electricity, 496
the liver and, 529, 530
thiamin and, 488-489
transplantation of, 515-516, 528
treatments which speed, 957-958
trophoblastic theory of, 458
virus, in milk and eggs, 461
virus, in polio vaccine, 470-471, 472
virus involved in, 460-461
vitamins and, 462-463, 487, 491
vitamin A and, 488
vitamin B and, 462
vitamin C deficiency in, 514
vitamin P and, 554
what befalls one who can "cure," 538
see also Carcinogens, Leukemia

Capillaries
fragility, and rutin, 553-555, 556
fragility, and stroke, 553, 554
fragility, and vitamin P, 554, 555
fragility, and vitamins C and P, 358-359
fragility, in arthritis, 358
fragility, results of, 357-358
importance of, 357, 813
structure, 358
weak, and ulcers, 905-906
see also Blood vessels, Hemorrhage, Labyrinthitis, Stroke
Carbohydrates
cancer and, 484
colds and, 560-561, 568
colitis and, 680-681
diet low in, for colitis, 670-673, 675-676
digestion, and thiamin, 724
fat deposits and, 174-175, 176
fermentation and dyspepsia, 730
heart disease and, 152, 153
low blood sugar and, 152
metabolism, and peptic ulcers, 670
tooth decay and, 306, 307
undigested, fermentation of, 673-674
undigested, in colitis, 674
see also Refined carbohydrates
Carcinogens
how we contact, 432-435
known, 432-435, 437-438, 440-441
need for information on, 436-437
suppression of information on, 436-439
see also Cancer
Carcinogens in food
difficulty in testing, 441-442
legislation on, 441-442
"safe" level of, 440, 442
suspected, 440-441
what must be done about, 442-443
Carob flour
diarrhea and, 649-650
history of cultivation, 650
uses of, 650
what it is, 650
Catalase
deficiency, and cancer, 453-454
destruction of, 454-455
function, in cell respiration, 453-454
hydrogen peroxide and, 454
Cataracts
age and, 36
amino acids and, 39
blindness from, 35
calcium and, 39
chlorophyll and, 40
dehydration of lens in, 39
description of, 34
detection of, 36-37
diet and, 39-41
dinitrophenol and, 35-36, 38

drugs and, 35-36
factors precipitating, 35-36
operation for, 35
origin of name, 37
riboflavin and, 38
smoke and, 36
sunlight and, 36
types of, 35
vitamin C and, 37-38
vitamin E and, 699
Celiac disease
  serious consequences of, 543
  symptoms of, 543
  treatment for, 543-544
  wheat gluten and, 544-545
Cellulose
  constipation and, 624-625
  effects of too much, 625
  foods high in, 625
Cereals
  asthma and, 407, 410
  colds and, 561, 567, 568, 569
CF. See Cystic fibrosis.
Chemicals
  increase in blood diseases and, 741-743
  myriads of new, 963
  tinnitus and, 32
Chemicals in food
  cancer and, 429-430, 440-442, 492
  catalase and, 454-455
  defense against, 431-432, 442-443
  ulcers and, 900
Cherries
  gouty arthritis and, 348, 349
  substances in, 348-349
Chilling and colds, 593-594
Chiropodists, 75
Chloramphenicol
  eyes and, 64
  use of, 64
Chloromycetin and aplastic anemia, 742-743
Chlorophyll
  cataracts and, 40
  compared to hemoglobin, 40
  cooking and, 490
  oxidation enzymes and, 490
Chloroquine
  arthritis and, 345
  side effects of, 345-346
Cholecystitis, 85
Cholelithiasis. See Gallstones.
Cholesterol
  deafness and, 20-21
  exercise and, 158, 172
  fats and, 134, 173, 207, 353-354
  function of, 133
  gallstones and, 85
  increase, and disease, 170-171
  inositol and, 86, 137
  lecithin and, 139, 140

level, and heart attacks, 178-179
  manufacture in the body, 207
  overweight and, 172
  pectin and, 179
  pyridoxine and, 202, 207
  smoking and, 144, 173
  stress and, 173
  unsaturated fatty acids and, 173, 207, 643-644
  vitamin C and, 134-136, 216
Choline
  alcohol and appetite for, 488
  cancer and, 227-228, 487
  deficiency, and muscular dystrophy in rabbits, 793-794
  fat deposits and, 136
  fat metabolism and, 86
  foods rich in, 228
  function, in the body, 343
  high blood pressure and, 227
  liver and, 252, 793
  removed from refined foods, 794
  sugar and appetite for, 488
Circulation. See Blood vessels.
Circumcision
  cancer of the penis and, 505-506
  cervical cancer and male, 506
Cirrhosis of the liver
  alcohol and, 250, 254
  incidence of, 254
  overeating and, 255-256
  protein and, 255
  synthetic B vitamins and, 254-255
Cleave, Dr. T. L., 922-926
Cleft palate
  cortisone during pregnancy and, 559
  defined, 558
  incidence of, 558
  prenatal diet and, 558-560
  vitamin A in prenatal diet and, 558
  vitamin B in prenatal diet and, 558-559
Climate
  glaucoma and, 54
  multiple sclerosis and, 785
  see also Weather
Coca Method. See Pulse test.
Cod liver oil and arthritis, 351-352, 354
Coffee
  effect on body, 145-146
  effect on nerves, 145-146
  glaucoma and, 48-49
  heart and, 145, 146
  iron absorption and, 145
  inositol and, 145
  thyroid gland and, 760
  see also Caffeine
Colds
  antihistamines and, 602
  bioflavonoids and, 586-587
  breathing exercises and, 597, 598
  Bush's treatment, 565
  cereals and, 561, 569

chilling and, 593-594
cold weather and, 574
cost of, 573
dancing and, 571-572
emotions and, 564-565, 568, 595-596
epidemics, and children, 573-574
exercise and, 568
fatigue and, 595
food allergies and, 561
garlic and, 587-588
heart failure and, 162-163, 562
high-carbohydrate diet and, 560-561,
    568, 613-614
history of Editor Rodale's, 563-564,
    565-566, 569, 570-572
home heating system and, 566
humidity and, 563, 592-593
miscellaneous suggestions on, 596
nasal temperature and, 566-567
overdressing and, 596, 599
prevention in the past, 592
prevention of, 163-164, 567-568
salt and, 589, 590, 873
smoking and, 609, 611
"stale" air and, 594
sugar and, 561
susceptibility to lung cancer and, 561
susceptibility to polio and, 574
system of baths for, 567
through contact, 562-563
tonsils and, 562
value of drugs for, 603
value of patented remedies, 599-600
vitamin A and, 576, 872
vitamin C and, 163-164, 563, 582-
    583, 586-587
"wet" walls and, 566
see also Flu

Colitis
bananas and, 930
fats for patients, 674
how a high-carbohydrate diet brings
    on, 672-673
laxatives and, 674, 675, 681
low-carbohydrate diet for, 675-676
milk and, 681-682
nervous tension and, 674
pyridoxine and, 301
Sandler's diet for, 670-671
undigested carbohydrates in, 674,
    680-681
value of Sandler's diet for, 671-672

Colitis, ulcerative
book on, 676
diarrhea in, 679
emotions and, 679-680
menu planning for sufferers, 678-679
mixed meals forbidden in, 677, 682
natural foods for, 677
runs in families, 680
symptoms of, 679

Collagen
degeneration, in cancer, 484, 513-514
degeneration, in rheumatism, 395
metastasis and, 514-515
vitamin C and, 395, 484, 514, 863
weakened, in nearsightedness, 57
smoking and, 944
Collagenosis, 920-921

Colon
fermentation of undigested carbohy-
    drates in, 673-674
normal contents of, 619

Color blindness
testing for, 881
tobacco amblyopia and, 881

Connective tissue. See Collagen.

Constipation
abdominal massage and, 623
bananas and, 930
calcium deficiency and, 631
causes of, 617-618
causes of atonic, 617
causes of spastic, 617
cellulose and, 624-625
diet for preventing, 718
diseases accompanied by, 619-620
exercise and, 621-623, 717
fats and, 626
fluids and, 625-626, 628-629
food supplements and, 626
heart disease and, 164-165
hemorrhoids and, 717
in an ancient Egyptian medical docu-
    ment, 616
in early times in England, 616-617
inositol and, 631
in the American colonies, 616
kinds of, 617
minerals and, 630
potassium deficiency and, 631
protein deficiency and, 631
pruritus ani and, 620
psychic causes, 619
refined foods and, 717
results of, 621
tips on avoiding, 717
varicose veins and, 923-924
vitamins and, 630
vitamin B and, 629, 630, 631, 718
who suffers from, 925-926

Copper
deposits, in artery walls, 211
liver disease and, 256
source of, in food, 212
Coronary infarction. See Heart attack.
Coronary thrombosis
accepted theories on, 213
alcohol and, 214, 215
defined, 213
incidence of, 213
refutation of accepted theories on,
    213-214

sex differences in incidence of, 216-217
smoking and, 214, 215-216, 217
survey of victims' habits, 214-215
theories of, 213-214
see also Heart disease

Cortisone
arthritis and, 346
asthma and, 412
during pregnancy, and cleft palate, 559
production, and lack of exercise, 160-161
pyridoxine and, 300-301
side effects of, 960-961
ulcer and, 894
walking and, 346-347

Cosmetics and skin disease, 276-277
Cretinism, 706
Crime and low blood sugar, 766-767
Crossed eyes
cause of, 42
importance of early correction of, 43
prenatal diet and, 42-43, 44-45
psychological causes of, 44
treatments for, 42, 43-44
vision with, 43

Cyanide
effect of, in the body, 710
goiter and, 708-710
in polluted water, 710
polio and, 709, 710

Cystic fibrosis
antibiotics in, 632
description of, 632
diagnosis of, 633
fat absorption in, 633
fatality record of, 632
fats in diets of victims, 637
incidence of, 633
pancreas and, 632-633
publicity on, 632
symptoms of, 633
vitamin deficiencies in, 635-636
vitamin E deficiency and, 633-634, 635

D

Dancing
colds and, 571-572
value of, to health, 572-573

Deafness
cholesterol and, 20-21
Eustachian tubes and, 29-30
extent of, in U. S., 21
in beriberi, 19-20
in pellagra, 19-20
nerve, and vitamin B, 19-21
vitamin A and, 21-24
vitamin C and, 25
see also Ear, Hearing

Dental caries. See Tooth decay.
Dental floss, 90

Dentistry
nutritional therapy and, 92-93
obligation of, 92

Dermatitis. See Skin disease.

Detergents
skin disease and, 279-280
tips on using, 280
see also Soap

Dextrocardia, 167

Diabetes
bananas in, 931
blood vessel disorders in, 640, 641-642
calcium and, 639
constipation in, 619
description of, 638
diet high in fruit for, 645-646
diet in, 638
exercise and, 640-641
fat metabolism and, 641, 642-643
fault in diet prescribed for, 644
gangrene and, 704
gangrene, and smoking, 937-938
incidence of, 638
thirst and, 639
unsaturated fatty acids and, 642-644
vitamin B and, 638-640
vitamin E and, 640
vitamin shortages in, 639
vitamin supplements in, 639
weather and, 646-648
see also Insulin

Diarrhea
antibiotics and, 959-960
bananas and, 654-655
buttermilk and, 652-653
carob flour and, 649-650
garlic and, 658, 659-660
in ulcerative colitis, 679
seriousness of, 543
vitamin deficiencies and, 656
see also Celiac disease, Dysentery, Steatorrhea

Diet
arthritis and, 350-351
asthma and, 403
breadless, and poison ivy, 569
Brusch, for arthritis, 351-356
cancer and, 452-453, 484, 487-488, 489-490, 491, 528-530
cataracts and, 39-41
difficulty in changing, 294
during pregnancy, and cleft palate, 558-560
during pregnancy, and crossed eyes, 42-43, 44-45
during pregnancy, and mental deficiency, 750, 751, 752
Evers', for multiple sclerosis, 788
fat in today's, 287-288
for alcoholism, 321-322
for eye health, 68-69

for low blood sugar, 328-329, 763-764, 768, 828-830
for muscular dystrophy patients, 795
for preventing colds, 567-568
for preventing constipation, 718
for reducing, 804-805
for starch dyspepsia, 730
for ulcer patients, 893, 894, 899, 901, 906
gallstones and, 85, 88
gray hair and, 107
hernia and, 721
high-carbohydrate, and colds, 560-561, 568
high in fruit, for diabetics, 645-646
high-protein, and nearsightedness, 58-59
high-protein, for TB patients, 886-887
in diabetes, 638-644
Jolliffe's, for mental patients, 748-749
lack of vitamin E in, 182
leucocytes and, 580-581
low-carbohydrate, and sinusitis, 612
low-carbohydrate, for colitis, 670-673, 675-676
low-carbohydrate, for TB patients, 613
low-protein, and low blood pressure, 224-225
low-sodium, and labyrinthitis, 686-687
of glaucoma patients, 50-51, 50 (table), 52-53
prescribed for Mongoloids, 781
pruritus ani and, 278
psoriasis and, 285, 286-287
pyridoxine in average, 201-202
raw food, for rheumatism, 337-339
rice-fruit, for high blood pressure, 229
Sandler's, for colitis, 670-672
Sandler's, for preventing heart disease, 177
Sandler's, for preventing polio, 828-830
scurvy and, 864, 865-866
shortcomings in supplementation, 822-823
starchless, and arthritis, 352, 354
Steyn's, for Parkinsonism, 807-808
stress and, 50
tooth decay and, 292-294, 302-303, 307, 308-309
value of bland, for ulcers, 896
vitamin C deficiency and, 864, 865-866
vitiligo and, 289-290
Waerland, 791-792
Waerland, for multiple sclerosis, 791
Digestion
aids to good, 725
carbohydrate, and thiamin, 724
enzymes in, 724

exercise and, 726
garlic and, 664-665, 728
mixed meals and, 677-678
Pavlov's experiments on, 677
posture and, 726
stomach acids in, 727-728
stress and, 725
vitamin B and, 724-725
Digestive tract
bacteria in, and bananas, 929
bacteria in, and pyridoxine, 301
damage, and polio susceptibility, 830
disorders, and garlic, 657-661, 728-729
disorders, and L. acidophilus, 666-667, 668
disorders, and vitamin deficiencies, 655
disorders, and wheat products, 731-732
garlic and, 657-658, 661, 728
protein and, 724
spread of bacteria from, 668
structure of, 723-724
value of L. acidophilus in, 666, 667
see also Colitis, Digestion, Dyspepsia, Elimination, Indigestion
Digitalis
careful supervision necessary, 242
effect of, on vision, 64
poisoning, 242
side effects of, 242, 960-961
use of, 64, 241-242
Dinitrophenol and cataracts, 35-36, 38
Disease
change in environment and, 945
decrease in infectious, and vitamin C, 948-950
difficulty in finding single cause of, 945-946
iatrogenic, see Iatrogenic disease
new infectious, 947-948
overlooked factors in, 946-947
process of determining a new, 962
Dizziness
causes of, 683-684, 685-686
Editor Rodale's experience with, 685-686
physiology of, 686
true indication of, 683
types of, 683
what to do about, 687-688
see also Labyrinthitis, Meniere's disease
Doctors and "faith healing," 413-414
Dropsy, 167, 953
Drosnes-Lazenby treatment,
campaign against, 525-527
discovery of mucorhicin, 524
tests of mucorhicin, 525, 526
Drugs
catalase and, 454

cataracts and, 35-36
dizziness and, 684
effects on eyes, 62-64
for arthritis, 345-347
for asthma, 399, 409, 414
for epileptics, 691
for heart disease, 241-244
headaches and, 115
misuse of, 62
pulse and, 147-148
reducing, dangerous, 798, 799
skin disease and, 277
tinnitus and, 32
"U" series, for Mongoloids, 780, 781
value of, for colds, 599-600, 603
see also ACTH, Antibiotics, Antihistamine, Aspirin, Cortisone, Digitalis, Menthol
Durovic, Dr. Steven, 519-520
Dysentery
buttermilk and, 653-654
garlic and, 658, 659, 662-663
Dyspepsia
causes of starch, 729-730
diet for starch, 730
garlic and, 660
symptoms of starch, 729

E

Ear
infection, and vitamin C, 25-26
inner, and dizziness, 683-684
sensitivity of, 31
vitamin C storage in, 25
see also Deafness, Dizziness, Eustachian tubes, Hearing, Labyrinthitis, Meniere's disease, Tinnitus
Edema, 167, 267
Effort syndrome, 167
Eggs
breakfast cereals vs., 345
cancer virus in, 461
lecithin in, 139
nutrients in, 344
rheumatic fever and, 343-344
Electricity
body as an aerial, 498-499
cancer and body, 495
exercise and, 496-497
high blood pressure and, 496
in cancer test, 496
in diagnosing disease, 499-500
in food, 497-498
in heart stimulation, 495-496
in the body, 494-495
in the soil, 500-501, 503
salt and body, 498
Elimination
exercises for strengthening muscles of, 621-623
role of muscles in, 621
see also Celiac disease, Constipation,

Diarrhea, Dysentery, Steatorrhea
Embolism, 169
Encephalitis
compared to polio, 820
history of incidence, 820
incidence, related to vitamin B deficiency, 821-822
Encephalopathy, 748
Endocarditis, 167
Enzymes
fluorine and, 774
gum disease and, 96-97
substrates and, 507-508
see also Oxidation enzymes
Epidemiology, 443
Epilepsy
allergies and, 691-692, 693
constipation in, 619
diagnosis of, 690
drugs used in, 691
heredity in, 694-695
incidence of, 689-690
low blood sugar and, 694
precipitating factors in seizures, 692
seizures, 690-691
superstition surrounding, 688-689
types of, 690-691
vitamin E and, 697-698
what it is not, 689
Eustachian tubes
deafness and, 29-30
function of, 28-29
see also Ear
Exercise
body electricity and, 496-497
breathing, 411
breathing, and colds, 597, 598
calcium metabolism and, 158
cholesterol and, 158
colds and, 568
constipation and, 621-623, 717
digestion and, 726
disease and lack of, 160-161
for abdominal muscles, 11, 621-623
for asthmatics, 411-412, 413
for back muscles, 11-12
for correcting posture, 5-6, 8-12
for correcting scoliosis, 12
for correcting sway-back, 11
for diabetics, 640-641
for eyes, 43-44
for obstructed nose, 410-411
glands and, 158
heart disease and, 155-160
hernia and, 721
muscle tone and, 157
overweight and, 799-800
oxygenation and, 157
phlebitis and, 921-922
sleep and, 157-158
varicose veins and, 921-922
vitamin absorption and, 158

widening of arteries and, 151, 152
see also Walking
Eye
  crossed, *see* Crossed eyes
  diagram of, 34
  diet for health of, 68-69
  effect of drugs on, 62-64
  exercise for, 43-44
  myelination of nerves, 42
  smoking and, 939
  virus disease of, 60-62
  vitamin deficiency symptoms in, 65-66, 68
  vitamins and, 37
  vitamin A deficiency and, 66, 68
  vitamin B deficiency and, 66-67
  vitamin C deficiency and, 67-68
  vitamin C in lens, 37
  see also Aniseikonia, Blindness, Cataract, Color blindness, Crossed eyes, Glaucoma, Nearsightedness, Shipyard eye, Tobacco amblyopia
Eyeglasses
  rimless, and skin cancer, 480-481
  rimless, reducing danger of, 480
Eyestrain
  headaches and, 116-117
  tension and, 41

F

Fallen arches, 71
Fat
  absorption in CF victims, 633
  animal, and multiple sclerosis, 785
  animal vs. vegetable, 134
  biotin and, 86
  blood clotting and, 172
  cholesterol level and, 134, 173, 207, 353-354
  choline and, 86, 136
  constipation and, 626
  deposits, and high-carbohydrate diet, 174-175, 176
  for colitis sufferers, 674
  gallstones and, 85-86
  gum disease and, 96
  heated, and cancer, 475-477
  heated, and ulcer, 896-897
  heated, use common, 474-475
  hydrogenated, 476
  importance of, 132, 474
  in diets of CF victims, 637
  inositol and, 86
  in today's American diet, 287-288
  metabolism, and pyridoxine, 202
  metabolism, in diabetics, 641, 642-643
  psoriasis and, 285, 287
  vitamins soluble in, 285
  vitamin B and, 285-286
  vitamin C and, 253

  see also Cholesterol, Lecithin, Unsaturated fatty acids
Fatigue and colds, 595
Feet
  badly treated, 70
  care of infants', 78
  dermatoses, and shoe linings, 283-284
  design of, 70
  rules for health of, 73-74
  see also Foot disorders, High-heeled shoes, Shoes
Flu
  Asiatic, or colds?, 701
  side effects of vaccine, 702
  value of vaccine for Asiatic, 701-702
  vitamin A and, 574-575
  vitamin C and, 702
Fluoridation
  advocates of, 777-778
  Mongolism and, 775, 776-777
  objections to, 308
  tooth decay and, 304
  variable factors in, 776
Fluorine
  deposited in bones, 776
  enzyme-inhibiting power of, 774
  passes through placenta, 774-775
Folic acid
  anemia and, 810-811
  mental deficiency in rats and, 750
Foot disorders
  among children, 75-76
  arthritis and, 367-370
  backache and, 370-372
  badly fitted shoes and, 71-73
  case histories, 367-374
  common, 77
  correction of, 368, 369, 370, 371-372
  high-heeled shoes and, 70-71
  incidence of, 75
  incorrect walking and, 71
  posture and, 71
  preventing, 80-81
  shoes and, 75-77, 79-80
  spinal deformities and, 372-374
  weight and, 374-375
Frost, Dr. I. N., 536-537
Fruit diet for diabetics, 645-646

G

Gall bladder
  disorders, 85
  disorders, and constipation, 619
  location and function, 84-85
  vitamin A and, 87
  vitamin K and, 87
Gallstones
  cholesterol and, 85
  diet and, 85, 88
  fat metabolism and, 85-86
  formation of, 85

vitamin C and, 87-88
Gamma globulin and hepatitis, 263
Gangrene
   Buerger's disease and, 425, 704
   diabetes and, 704
   diabetic, and smoking, 937-938
   vitamin E and, 704
Garlic
   bactericidal action of, 663
   cancer and, 507
   colds and, 587-588
   diarrhea and, 658, 659-660
   digestion and, 664-665, 728
   digestive disorders and, 657-661, 728-729
   digestive tract and, 657-658, 661, 728
   dosage, 588
   dysentery and, 658, 659, 662-663
   dyspepsia and, 660
   experiment on bad breath and, 419
   experiment on polio prevention and, 830-831
   grippe and, 588
   high blood pressure and, 130, 226-227, 664
   medicinal use of, 588, 657, 661-662, 663
   perles, 589
   running nose and, 588-589
   sore throat and, 588
   tablet from, 662
Gas on the stomach
   garlic and, 660, 728, 729
   L. acidophilus and, 667
Gerson, Dr. Max, 527-535
Glands
   disorders, and goiter, 712
   exercise and, 158
   see also Adrenal gland, Pancreas, Thyroid gland
Glaucoma
   as a deficiency disease, 54-55
   climate and, 54
   coffee and, 48-49
   description of, 45-47, 46 (illus.)
   detection of, 48
   diet of patients, 50-51, 50 (table), 52-53
   importance of early detection, 47-48
   incidence, 45
   rutin and, 555
   sleep therapy for, 53
   stress and, 48, 49-50
   summary of findings on, 55-56
   symptoms of, 47 (illus.)
   treatment of, 49
Glyoxylide, 539-541
Goiter
   cause of, 204
   clover that causes, 714
   conditions accompanying, 708

cyanide and, 708-710
geographical incidence of, 706-707
hardening of the arteries and, 204-205
iodine and, 706, 707-708
iodized salt and, 707-708
other gland disorders in, 712
polluted water and, 709
preventing, 711
salt and, 760
types of, 706
vitamin A deficiency and, 712-714
weather and, 714
see also Thyroid gland
"Gold therapy," 347
Gout
   bananas and, 931
   cherries and, 348, 349
Grand mal, 690-691
Gum disease
   calcium and, 96
   case histories, 90, 93-95
   causes of, 89
   enzymes and, 96-97
   fats and, 96
   nutritional deficiencies in, 96
   nutrition and, 97, 102-103
   protein and, 95-96
   smoking and, 939
   stress and, 94, 96
   Vitamin C-bioflavonoids for, 104
   see also Pyorrhea, Trench mouth
Gums
   bleeding, and vitamin C, 93-94
   habits which damage, 90-91, 94-95
   vitamin B and health of, 99-100

H

Hair
   dyes, and skin disease, 277
   effect of dyes on, 277
   gray, and copper, 107
   gray, and diet, 107
   growth in cancer patients, 468-469
   hormones and, 469
   loss of, see Baldness
   preparations, and health of, 107-108
   suggestions for care of, 108
   see also Baldness
Halitosis. See Bad breath.
Hardening of the arteries
   "abnormal" trace elements and, 210-211
   calcium and, 210
   chlorinated water and, 172
   civilization and, 203
   conflicting theories on, 208-209
   description of, 133
   diabetes and, 641-642
   essential food elements in preventing, 207
   fats and, 134, 171-172, 208, 239

overweight and, 803
posture and, 164
pyridoxine and, 136-137, 201
stress and, 154
suggestions for preventing, 204, 209-210
thyroid deficiency and, 204-205
vitamin C and, 135, 136
vitamin E and, 703
Harelip. *See* Cleft palate.
Headaches
aniseikonia and, 119
bruxism and, 121-123
causes of, 120
drugs and, 115
emotions and, 115-117
eyestrain and, 116-117
low blood sugar and, 117-118
milk and, 123-125
neck muscles and, 118
neck-stretching and, 118-119
refined carbohydrates and, 118
salt and, 953
sinusitis and, 871
statistics on, 114-115
suggestions on, 120-121
Hearing
age and, 23-24
amino acids and, 26-27
loss of, in U. S., 19
nutrition and, 24-25, 27
vitamin C and, 25
see also Deafness, Ear
Heart
amount of blood pumped by, 147
coffee and, 145, 146
electricity and, 495-496
enlargement of, 167-168
exercise and, 126
importance of, 125
murmur, 168
nasal obstruction and, 598-599
nutrition and, 125-126
palpitations, 168, 187
smoking and, 447, 933-934, 944
specific gravity of, 141
stress and, 187
thiamin deficiency and, 137-138
see also Blood vessels
Heart attack
activity and, 158-159
blood clotting time and, 219
cholesterol level and, 178-179
heat and, 194
hemoglobin level and, 219, 221
lactic acid and, 153
loss of fluids and, 221, 222
physiology of, 218
sun bathing and, 194-195
warning signal, 220
Heart disease
alcohol and, 142-143

apples in, 179-180
bananas in, 931
carbohydrates and, 152, 153
cause of neurotic, 188
cautions on use of vitamin E in, 241
colds and, 162-163, 562
constipation and, 164-165
Dr. Sandler's diet for preventing, 177
doctors and neurotic symptoms of, 189
drugs used in treating, 241-244
exercise and, 155-160
fats and, 133-134
food forbidden in, 126
general recommendations on, 165-166, 175
incidence of, 170
low blood sugar and, 152-153
oxygen lack and, 157
pains, and lactic acid, 153
pains, and low blood sugar, 176-177
pains, and oxygen lack, 153
pains, and threshold weight, 141
personality patterns of patients, 190-191
protein deficiency and, 177
side effects of drugs for, 242-243
simulated, 154-155
smoking and, 143-145, 172-173
soft water and, 195-196
stress and, 153-155, 188-192
symptoms of neurotic, 187-188
tallness and, 164
terms used in diagnosis of, 166-169
usual treatment of, 181
vitamin E and, 127-128, 180, 181-182
walking and, 149-151, 161-162
see also Coronary thrombosis, Heart attack, High blood pressure, Low blood pressure
Heat
arthritis and, 390
effect on blood, 193
effect on body, 193-194
heart attacks and, 194
Hemachromatosis, 818
Hemoglobin
compared to chlorophyll, 40
diet for lowering level of, 219-220, 221
function, 219
level, and loss of fluids, 221, 222
level, and starch, 222
level, in coronary patients, 219
Sahli test for, 219
Hemorrhage
blood vessel fragility and, 553
high blood pressure and, 553
in leukemia, 736, 737, 738
rutin and, 228-229, 553-555
vitamin P and, 554, 555

[977]

see also Stroke
Hemorrhoids
  avoiding, 718
  causes of, 716
  constipation and, 717
  defined, 716
  strain on abdominal muscles and, 716
Hepatitis
  deaths from, 259, 263
  defense against, 263-264
  gamma globulin and, 263
  incidence of, 259, 262-263
  polluted drinking water and, 261-262
  serum, 262
  spread of, 261-262, 263
  symptoms of, 259-260
  treatment of, 260-261
  types of, 259
Hernia
  causes of, 720
  common sites of, 719
  defined, 719
  diet and, 721
  exercise and, 721
  femoral, 720
  inguinal, 719-720
  serious consequence of, 720
  truss for, 720-721
  umbilical, 720
Hexamethonium, 243
High blood pressure
  choline and, 227
  consequences of, 128
  dizziness and, 684
  effectiveness of rauwolfia drugs in, 243
  electricity and, 496
  food allergies and, 229-230
  garlic and, 130, 226-227, 664
  hemorrhage and, 553
  overweight and, 131, 230, 802-803, 804, 952
  reduction, 129
  rice-fruit diet and, 229
  salt and, 129, 196-197, 229, 231-233, 234, 239, 952-953
  stress and, 154
  vitamin C and, 227
  vitamin E and, 228
High-heeled shoes
  foot disorders and, 70-71
  posture and, 5, 7
Hippocrates' tooth powder, 418
Histamine, 602-603
Hormones
  cancer and, 469
  deficiency, and enlarged prostate, 269
  hair growth and, 469
  male, and baldness, 106, 111
Hospitals
  cleanliness, and staph epidemics, 875
  overcrowding of nurseries and staph epidemics, 876
  recommendations for controlling staph epidemics in, 878-880
  staph epidemics in, 874-875, 877-878
Humidity
  asthma and, 404-405
  colds and, 563, 592-593
Hydralazine, 243
Hydrochloric acid
  Vitamin B_{12} absorption and, 811, 941
  vitiligo and, 289
Hydrogen peroxide
  catalase and, 454
  in cell respiration, 453-454
Hypertension. *See* High blood pressure.
Hypoglycemia. *See* Low blood sugar.
Hypokinetic disease, 161
Hypotension. *See* Low blood pressure.

I

Iatrogenic disease
  court recognition of, 957
  defined, 954
  examples of, 955-956, 958
  inexcusable, 955
  irony of, 954-955
Idiopathic nocturnal paresthesia, 383, 385
Indigestion
  avoiding, 725, 727
  functional, 723
  incidence of, 723
  niacin deficiency and, 724-725
  organic disorders causing, 723
  overeating and, 726-727
  symptoms of, 723
  see also Colitis, Dyspepsia
Infantile paralysis. *See* Polio.
Infection
  calcium-phosphorus ratio and, 350
  vitamin A and, 23, 577, 578
  vitamin C and, 582, 583, 584-585
  see also Disease, infectious
Influenza. *See* Flu.
Ingrown toenails, 77
Inositol
  baldness and, 110
  cholesterol and, 86, 137
  coffee and, 145
  constipation and, 631
Insecticides
  blood diseases and, 741
  dizziness and, 685-686
Insomnia
  caffeine and, 734
  Editor Rodale's experience with, 735
  hard mattress and, 735
  salt and, 953
  scientific relaxation to overcome, 733-734
  sleeping pills for, 732-733

stress and, 734
tips on overcoming, 735-736
Insulin
need, and diet high in fruit, 645
need, and exercise, 641
need, and unsaturated fatty acids, 643
need, and vitamin E, 704
need, and weather, 647-648
sugar not requiring, 644-645
vitamin C and, 639
zinc in, 273
see also Diabetes
Intermittent claudication
cause of, 546
effectiveness of vitamin E for, 547-548
symptoms, 546
test of vitamin E for, 546-547
vitamin B$_{12}$ and, 550, 552
Intestines. *See* Digestive tract.
Iodine
goiter and, 706, 707-708
in sea food, 708
polio prevention and, 833
shortage, and polio season, 833-834
sources of, 205-206
therapy, and polio, 832-833
thyroid gland and, 205, 705-706
use of, and vitamin A, 712
Ivy, Dr. Andrew C., 520-521, 522, 523

J

Juvenile delinquency and low blood sugar, 766

K

Keratomalacia, 66
Kernicterus, 955-956
Kidney
disease, and bananas, 931
smoking and, 937, 944
stones, and age, 244, 246
stones, and lack of exercise, 160
stones, and oxalic acid, 244
stones, and vitamin A, 244-245
stones, and vitamin C, 245, 246-247
Klein, Dr. Ernest, 218-222
Koch, Dr. William, 539-541
Korsakoff's psychosis, 856
Krebiozen
book on, 519
discovery of, 519-520
results of early tests of, 520
suppression of, 520-523

L

Labyrinthitis
bioflavonoids and, 686-687
low-sodium diet and, 686-687
symptoms of, 684

typical attack of, 686
see also Dizziness
Lactobacillus acidophilus
advantage of milk made with, 669
antibiotic action of, 667
antibiotics and, 667-668
common use of, in Europe, 666
digestive disorders and, 666-667, 668
manufacture of milk from, 668-669
post-operative gas pains and, 667
radiation injury and, 668
revival of interest in, 665
skin and, 667
ulcers and, 667
value of, in digestive tract, 666, 667
Larynx cancer, 444
Laxatives and colitis, 674, 675, 681
Lecithin
cholesterol and, 139, 140
destruction of, 139-140
in eggs, 139
manufacture of, 140
sources of, 140
Leprosy
disappearance of, 945
rampant in Middle Ages, 945
Leucocytes and diet, 580-581
Leukemia
breath and, 420
concurrent in mother and child, 737
factors pertaining to cause of, 736
hemorrhage in, 736, 737, 738
increased incidence of, 430-431, 736
radioactivity and, 431
scorbutic background in, 738-739
smoking during pregnancy and, 737, 738
see also Cancer
Lifting
proper, 8
rules for, 716, 721, 722 (illus.)
Lind, Dr. James, 858
Lip biting and malocclusion, 312, 315
Liver
aureomycin and, 250-251
cancer and, 529, 530
choline and, 252, 793
consequences of breakdown, 248
damage, and vitamin E assimilation, 793
function of, 248-249
lecithin manufacture in, 140
low blood sugar and, 767
nutrition and, 251-252
overweight and, 250
poisons, 256, 767
posture and, 257
protein and regeneration of, 256
recommendations for health of, 252, 258
regenerating power of, 249-250, 256
symptoms of breakdown, 248
vitamin C and, 252-253

zinc and, 250
see also Cirrhosis of the liver, Hepatitis, Pernicious anemia
Lordosis, 11
Low blood pressure
dizziness and, 684
in Addison's disease, 223
low-protein diet and, 224-225
postural, 223-224
significance of, 223, 224
thiamin deficiency and, 224
usually beneficial, 223
Low blood sugar
adrenal gland and, 762
alcoholism and, 325-326
allergy and, 694
arthritis and, 396
asthma and, 401-402
brain and, 767
cause of, 177, 402, 767, 898-899
conditions ascribed to, 762, 828
crime and, 766-767
diet for, 328-329, 763-764, 768, 828-830
epilepsy and, 694
headaches and, 117-118
heart disease and, 152-153
heart pains and, 176-177
high-carbohydrate diet and, 152
in juvenile delinquents, 766
in ulcer patients, 898
liver and, 767
mental symptoms and, 761, 764-765, 767-768
seriousness of, in children, 765
smoking and, 938, 944
symptoms of, 763, 787, 938
symptoms of, in children, 765-766
Lungs
colds and susceptibility to cancer of, 561
factors in cancer of, 445-446
polluted air and cancer of, 445-446, 478
smoking and cancer of, 445-446, 447-449, 478
Lupus erythematosus
defined, 740
detection of, 740-741
environmental agents and, 741
increased incidence, 740
vaccines and, 740
Lysozyme, 577

M

Malocclusion
causes of, 311-313, 315-316
defined, 309-310
dizziness and, 685
heredity or environment?, 313
incidence of, 310
preventing, 314

pyorrhea and, 98
refined foods and, 313-314
sugar and, 315-316
treatment of, 310
Masor, Dr. Nathan, 757
"McConkey Cocktail," 885
Meals, proper atmosphere for, 909
Meniere's disease
possible causes of, 685
sleep and, 685
symptoms of, 684-685
treatments for, 685
vitamin C and, 25
see also Dizziness
Menstruation
disorders, and polio, 825-826
disorders, and vitamin E, 826
Mental deficiency
diet during pregnancy and, 750, 751, 752
in rats, and folic acid, 750
in rats, and vitamin B_{12}, 750
nutrition and, 751-752
recognition of, 752
Mental illness
biochemical approach to, 757
blood chemistry and, 753, 757
case histories, 745-746
frustration of, 756
history of treatment, 756-757
incidence of, 744
Jolliffe's diet for patients, 748-749
nutrition and, 744-747
penicillin and, 959
pernicious anemia and, 753-754
symptoms, and low blood sugar, 761, 764-765, 767
symptoms, in pellagra, 747-748
thiamin deficiency and, 747-748
thyroid gland disorders and, 757-759
vitamin B_{12} and, 550-551, 552, 753-754, 755
vitamin E and, 696-697, 698-699
Menthol
blood clotting and, 605
effect on children, 606
inflammation from, 606-607
nasal congestion and, 607-608
use of, 605
Milk
advantages of *L. acidophilus,* 669
cancer virus in, 460, 461
colitis and, 681-682
cultured, differentiated, 665-666
manufacture of *L. acidophilus,* 668-669
"sick" headaches and, 123-125
substitutes for, 654
vitamin C in cow's and breast, 867
why you shouldn't drink, 682
see also Buttermilk
"Milk factor" in cancer, 460

Mineral baths
  for arthritis, 391-392
  in the past, 390
Minerals and constipation, 630
Miscarriage. *See* Spontaneous abortion.
Mixed meals
  faulty digestion of, 677-678
  forbidden in ulcerative colitis, 677, 682
Moccasins, 81
Mongolism
  abnormal chromosome in, 778
  appears early in pregnancy, 778
  characteristics of, 772
  contributing elements in, 772
  diet prescribed for, 781
  factors affecting treatment of, 779-780
  fluoridated water and, 775, 776-777
  goal of treatment, 779
  results of treatment with "U" drugs, 781
  "U" series of drugs for, 780
  vitamin E and, 772-773
  vitamin E deficiency during pregnancy and, 771, 773-774
Mononucleosis
  defined, 782
  incidence of, 782
  incubation period of, 783
  preventing, 783
  transmission of, 782-783
Mouth
  acids, and tooth decay, 302
  disorders, and vitamin B, 508-509, 512
  effect of pyridoxine in, 300
  vitamin deficiency symptoms in, 656
Mouth breathing. *See* Breathing, mouth.
Mucous membrane
  effect of smoking on, 610, 934, 944
  function of cilia, 577
  lysozyme secretions from, 577
  vitamin A and, 22, 577
Multiple sclerosis
  allergies present in, 785-786
  ammonia deposits in nerve cells and, 786
  animal fats and, 785
  blood sugar level and, 787
  case histories, 784, 790-791
  chemical fertilizers and, 787-788
  cold climate and, 785
  defined, 784-785
  development of, 784, 789
  Evers' diet and, 788, 790
  factors in cause of, 785
  nutritional deficiencies in, 786
  remission of, 785
  symptoms of, 789
  treatment of, 790
  vitamin B and, 786-787

Waerland diet for, 791-792
Muncie, Dr. Curtis H., 27-30
Muscles and vitamin E, 831-832
Muscular dystrophy
  amino acids and, 796
  diet for, 795
  factors in incidence of, 796
  in rabbits, and choline deficiency, 793-794
  in rabbits, and vitamin E deficiency, 792, 793
  symptoms of, 796
  wheat germ with vitamins B and C and, 794-795
Myocarditis, 168
Myopia. *See* Nearsightedness.
Myxedema, 706

N

Nail biting and malocclusion, 312
Navajos
  cancer among, 487
  diet of, 487
Nearsightedness
  description of, 56
  environmental factors in, 56-57
  higher-protein diet and, 58-59
  incidence of, 56
  serious consequences of, 58
  vitamin E and, 57-58
  weakened collagen in, 57
Nerves
  coffee and, 145
  diseases, and vitamin B, 821
  smoking and, 939
Neuritis
  drunkard's, 382
  sleep positions and, 379-382
Niacin
  deficiency, and encephalopathy, 748
  deficiency, and indigestion, 724-725
  multiple sclerosis and, 786-787
  trench mouth and, 99, 100
Nicotine
  intake, in smoking, 609, 932-933
  reproduction and, 936
  symptoms of poisoning, 933
  toxicity of, 609, 932, 944
  tolerance to, 933
  see also Smoking
Nicotinic acid. *See* Niacin.
Nose
  cilia, and calcium, 565
  cilia, function of, 565
  congestion, and menthol, 607-608
  functions of, 597-598
  obstructed, and heart trouble, 598-599
  obstructed, and sinusitis, 870, 871
  obstructed, exercise for, 410-411
  running, and garlic, 588-589
  temperature, and colds, 566-567

[981]

Numbness
 during sleep, 383
 spontaneous, during sleep, 383, 385
Nutritional therapy in dentistry, 92-93

O

Obesity. *See* Overweight.
Ochsner, Dr. Alton, 942-943
Operations
 bananas before and after, 931
 complications, and smoking, 611,
  935-936
 for cataract, 35
 for crossed eyes, 43
 for enlarged prostate, 266, 269
 gas pains after, and cultured milk,
  667
Organically grown foods
 cancer and, 485
 tooth decay and, 304-305
Osteoarthritis
 oxygenation and, 395-396
 vitamin B_{12} and, 335-336
 vitamin E and, 395
 see also Arthritis
Osteoporosis
 bones in, 13
 calcium and, 13-15
 childbirth and, 13
 physical activity and, 16
 prevention of, 18
 scurvy and, 17-18
 sex differences in incidence of, 13
 steatorrhea and, 14
 vitamin C and, 16, 18
 see also Bones
Overweight
 best plan for overcoming, 798-799
 blood-weight ratio and, 803-804
 danger of, 801
 danger of reducing drugs, 798, 799
 dieting, 131-133
 effectiveness of reducing drugs, 799
 effects on the body, 130-131
 emotions and, 800
 exercise and, 799-800
 hardening of the arteries and, 803
 high blood pressure and, 131, 230,
  802-803, 804, 952
 liver and, 250
 no easy way to overcome, 797-798
 objections to calorie-counting, 798
 personality and, 913, 914
 sex differences in, 800-801
 simplified diet for reducing, 804-805
 steam baths and, 800
 value of thyroid drugs for, 799
 why dieting overcomes, 798
 see also Specific gravity, Weight
Oxalic acid
 kidney stones and, 244
 sources of, 244

Oxidation enzymes
 chlorophyll and, 490
 deficiency, and cancer, 490-491
Oxygen
 importance of, 455-456
 in cell respiration, 453-454
Oxygenation
 disturbance of, and cancer, 490-491,
  492
 exercise and, 157
 heart pains and insufficient, 153
 osteoarthritis and, 395
 sugar and, 153
 vitamin E and, 127-128, 395-396,
  548, 698, 703-704
 see also Oxidation enzymes

P

PABA. *See* Para-amino-benzoic acid.
Painful shoulder
 causes of, 375-376
 one-sidedness and, 378
 personality of victims, 376-377
 prevention of, 378
 treatments, 378
Pamine, 894
Pancreas
 cystic fibrosis and, 632-633
 smoking and, 937-938
 zinc and, 273
Para-amino-benzoic acid and vitiligo,
 290-291
Paralysis agitans, 748
Parkinson's disease
 brain injection for, 806
 description of, 805
 pyridoxine and, 806-807
 Steyn's diet for, 807-808
Pasteur treatment
 effectiveness of, 855
 for rabies, 855
 hazards of, 855, 856-858
Pectin
 apples for, 180
 cholesterol level and, 179
 defined, 179
Pellagra
 bananas and, 930
 deafness in, 19-20
 mental symptoms in, 747-748
 tinnitus in, 20
Penicillin
 fatalities from, 959
 mental illness and, 959
 misuse of, 956
 neutralizer of, 956-957
 side effects of, 604
 see also Antibiotics
Penicillinase, 956-957
Periarteritis nodosa, 169
Periarthritis. *See* Painful shoulder.
Pericarditis, 168

[982]

Periodontal disease. *See* Gum disease.
Pernicious anemia
  immature red blood cells in, 450-451
  liver and, 809
  mental symptoms in, 753-754
  substances which cure, 451
  symptoms of, 809
  vitamin B₁₂ and, 810
Petit mal, 690
Phlebitis
  case histories, 919-920
  causes of, 919
  defined, 169
  exercise and, 921-922
  varicose veins and, 920, 921
  vitamin E and, 183-184, 919-920
Physostigmine
  eyes and, 63
  use of, 63
Placenta
  fluorides transferred through, 774-775
  function of, 770
  see also Pregnancy
Pneumonia and vitamin A, 575, 576
Poisons and vitamin C, 26
Poison ivy
  breadless diet and, 569
  diet and, 569
Polio
  appearance of, with steel-roller milling, 823
  astounding theories on, 815
  Boines' treatment of, 812-813
  civilization and, 815-817
  compared to beriberi, 821
  compared to encephalitis, 820
  cyanide and, 709, 710
  cyclical nature of, 836
  DDT and, 815
  early treatment of, 811
  experiment on garlic and prevention of, 830-831
  factors in incidence of, 838-839
  factors in 1955-1957 drop in, 843-844
  history of incidence, 820
  incidence of, 835
  incidence, related to vitamin B deficiency, 821-822
  increase in paralytic, 835, 844
  iodine therapy for, 832-833
  low blood sugar and, 827
  menstrual disorders and, 825-826
  new diagnosis criteria, 843
  new forms of diagnosis, 843-844
  polluted water and, 710
  prevention, and iodine, 833
  protein need in, 812-813
  results of Boines' treatment of, 814
  Sandler's diet for preventing, 828-830
  season, related to iodine shortage,

833-834
  Sister Kenny's treatment of, 812
  skin symptoms in, 818
  standard of living and, 815
  suggestions for protection from, 824
  susceptibility to, and colds, 574
  susceptibility to, and intestinal catarrh, 830
  value of quarantine in, 822
  vitamin A deficiency in, 817-818, 819
  vitamin C and, 813-814
  vitamin E therapy for, 825, 826
  see also Sabin vaccine, Salk vaccine
Poliomyelitis. *See* Polio.
Posture
  arthritis and, 386
  backache and, 3-4, 6, 9
  causes of poor, 5, 6-7
  correcting poor, 5-6, 8-12, 388, 389-390
  defects, 10-12
  digestion and, 726
  foot disorders and, 71
  good, 5, 7
  hardening of the arteries and, 164
  high-heeled shoes and, 5, 7
  how to check, 8
  liver disorders and, 257
  nutrition and, 9
  one-sidedness and, 389
  perfect, 386 (illus.)
  poor, 386 (illus.), 387-388
  results of poor, 7
  upright, and varicose veins, 922
  when doing housework, 388-389
Potassium iodate
  eyes and, 63
  use of, 63
Potatoes for ulcer, 894, 902-903
Prednisone and ulcer, 894
Pregnancy
  cortisone during, and cleft palate, 559
  diet during, and cleft palate, 558-560
  diet during, and crossed eyes, 42-43, 44-45
  diet during, and mental deficiency, 750, 751, 752
  easier, and low-salt diet, 953
  osteoporosis and, 13
  value of vitamin E in, 770-771
  see also Placenta, Spontaneous abortion
Price, Dr. Weston, 305-306, 313-314
Prostate gland
  cancer susceptibility of, 266
  enlarged, and amino acids, 266-267
  enlarged, and hormone deficiency, 269
  enlarged, and pumpkin seeds, 270-271, 272
  enlarged, and unsaturated fatty acids, 267

[983]

enlarged, operation for, 266, 269
enlarged, symptoms of, 265
enlarged, treatments for, 265-266
exercise and, 161
function of, 264-265
location of, 264
vitamin E and, 267
vitamin A and, 267
zinc in, 272, 273-274
Protein
  cirrhosis of the liver and, 255
  deficiency, and constipation, 631
  deficiency, and heart disease, 177
  deficiency, and low blood pressure, 224-225
  diet high in, for TB patients, 886-887
  digestive tract and, 724
  getting enough, 225
  gum disease and, 95-96
  nearsightedness and, 58-59
  need, and polio, 812-813
  regeneration of the liver and, 256
  utilization, and salt, 873
  see also Amino acids
Proust, Marcel
  asthmatic ordeal of, 415-416
  asthma treatments, 416
  death of, 417
  precautions to avoid chills, 416
Pruritus ani
  alkaline bowel movements and, 852-853
  Brooks' treatment for, 853-854
  causes of, 278
  constipation and, 620
  diet and, 278
  factors in, 278
  food allergies and, 620
  malt soup extract for, 853, 854
  treatment of, 278-279
  yogurt and whey for, 854
Psoriasis
  diet and, 285, 286-287
  fats and, 285, 287
  incidence of, 285
  research on, 286
  tips on avoiding, 288-289
Pulmonary alveolar proteinosis
  possible cause of, 963, 964
  symptoms of, 962-963
  victims of, 963-964
Pulse
  aluminum utensils and, 164
  defined, 147
  drugs and, 147-148
  emotions and, 147
  food allergies and, 148-149
  irregularities in, 168
  lowering, 147-150
  normal rate, 147
  rate, and longevity, 147
  smoking and, 147
  temperature and, 148

  vitamins and, 149
  walking and, 149-150
Pulse test, 148-149, 230, 403-404
Pumpkin seeds
  enlarged prostate and, 270-271, 272
  nutrients in, 271
Pyorrhea
  calcium-phosphorous balance and, 101-102
  causes of, 98
  description of, 97-98
  nutrition and, 101
  refined foods and, 102
  tooth loss in, 97, 104
  vitamin A and, 98-99
  vitamin C and, 100-101
  see also Gum disease
Pyridoxine
  cholesterol level and, 202
  cortisone and, 300-301
  effect of, in mouth, 300
  hardening of the arteries and, 136-137, 201
  in average diet, 201-202
  in fat metabolism, 202
  intestinal flora and, 301
  mucous colitis and, 301
  multiple sclerosis and, 787
  paralysis agitans and, 748
  Parkinson's disease and, 806-807
  shortage of, 137
  tooth decay and, 299-300, 301-302

Q

Quinidine, 242-243
Quinine
  effects on the eye, 64
  uses of, 63-64

R

Rabies
  defined, 854
  effectiveness of Pasteur vaccine, 855
  fatalities from Pasteur vaccine, 856-858
  hazards of Pasteur vaccine, 855
  Korsakoff's psychosis and, 856
  Pasteur vaccine for, 855
  rarity of, 855
  "scare," 857
  suggested treatment for dog bites, 857
  treatment of, 854-855
Radioactivity
  cancer and, 430, 438-439, 961-962
  injury, and L. acidophilus, 668
  leukemia and, 431
  what must be done about, 431
Raynaud's disease, 169
Rauwolfia drugs
  in blood pressure reduction, 243
  side effects of, 243

Rectum
  factors in cancer of, 444-445
  susceptible to skin disease, 278
Refined carbohydrates
  colds and, 613-614, 872-873
  diet low in, and sinusitis, 612
  diet low in, for TB patients, 613
  headaches and, 118
  sinusitis and, 872-873
  tooth decay and, 296-297
  vitamin B need and, 613
  see also Carbohydrates, Refined
    foods
Refined foods
  appendicitis and, 331-332
  cancer and, 482-483
  choline removed from, 794
  constipation and, 717
  malocclusion and, 313-314, 315
  pyorrhea and, 102
  sinusitis and, 872
  tooth decay and, 306
  ulcers and, 893
  varicose veins and, 925
  vitamin E removed from, 794
Retrolental fibroplasia, 955
Rheumatic fever
  eggs and, 343-344
  vitamin C and, 361, 362, 583
  vitamin E and, 336
Rheumatism
  collagen degeneration in, 395
  common symptoms of, 360
  incidence of, 333
  nature of, 333
  raw food diet for, 337-339
  stress and, 333-334
  treatments tried, 334-335
  types of, 334
  vitamin C and, 361, 395
  vitamin E and, 336-337
  see also Arthritis, Rheumatic fever
Riboflavin
  cataracts and, 38
  eyes and deficiency of, 67
Ringing in the ears. See Tinnitus.
Roberts, Dr. Sam E., 761
Roth, Dr. Harry, 91-95
Rowe, Dr. Albert H., 407-410
Rutin
  blood vessels and, 130
  capillary fragility and, 553-555, 556
  glaucoma and, 555
  hemorrhage and, 228-229, 553-555
  source of, 129-130, 556
  see also Bioflavonoids
Rye
  bread, and Buerger's disease, 428
  steatorrhea and, 15-16

S

Sabin vaccine

questions raised on, 839
results of field trials, 840
USPHS attitude towards, 840
Salk vaccine
  cancer virus in, 470-471, 472
  changes in manufacture of, 843
  claims for, 834-835, 836, 839, 848-
    849
  doubts concerning, 826-827
  effectiveness of, 472-473, 835, 845
  factors other than, in 1955-1957
    polio drop, 843-844
  mishandling of field-trial data, 842-
    843
  panel on, 841-847
  safety testing, 846-847
  USPHS role in promoting, 850-852
  value of field trials, 836-838
  variations in potency of, 471-472,
    843, 845-846, 848
  virus in, 840
Salt
  baldness and, 112-113, 953
  cancer and, 488, 492, 951-952
  colds and, 589, 590, 873
  diet low in, and labyrinthitis, 686-
    687
  dropsy and, 953
  easier pregnancy without, 953
  effect on body calcium, 589-590, 873,
    953
  effect on body electricity, 498
  experiment with rats and, 950-951
  getting along without, 233-236, 590
  goiter and, 760
  headaches and, 953
  high blood pressure and, 129, 196-
    197, 229, 231-233, 234, 952-953
  in common foods, 235 (table), 591
    (table)
  insomnia and, 953
  iodized, and goiter, 707-708
  need for, 590-591, 951
  protein utilization and, 873
  reduced intake, and health, 231, 233
  sinusitis and, 873
Sandler, Dr. Benjamin P., 670-673,
    827-830
Scoliosis, 12
Scotomata, 66
Scurvy
  breast feeding and prevention of, 867
  case histories, 865
  cause of, in infants, 867-868
  defined, 860-861
  diet and, 864, 865-866
  iatrogenic, 864
  incidence, in children, 861-862, 866-
    867
  incidence today, 861-862, 864
  in history, 858-859
  Lind's work on, 858
  osteoporosis and, 17-18

social, 863
subclinical, 861
symptoms of, 360, 859, 860, 864-865
symptoms of, in infants, 867
vitamin C and, 360, 860, 865, 868
Semen
prostate gland and, 264-265
zinc in, 273-274
Serum hepatitis, 262
Shipyard eye
appearance of, 60
cause of, 60-61
spread of, 61-62
symptoms of, 60
Shoes
advantages of non-deforming, 82-84
arch-support, 79
correct size, 72
evidence of badly fitted, 72
foot disorders and, 75-77
how often to change, 72
importance of correct size, 71-73
linings, and dermatitis, 283-284
men's, 80
new kind of, 73
non-deforming, 81-84
proper size for children's, 78-79
why we wear, 77, 81
women's, 79-80
see also High-heeled shoes
Shoulder
frozen, see Painful shoulder
painful, see Painful shoulder
susceptible to injury, 375
Sinuses
clearing of, 870
function of, 869
location of, 869
Sinusitis
acidosis in, 872
Bush's treatment for, 871
diet and, 871-872, 873-874
headaches and, 871
incidence of, 870-871
low-carbohydrate diet for, 612
obstructed nasal passages and, 870, 871
refined carbohydrates and, 872-873
salt and, 873
Sister Kenny, 812
Sitting
prolonged, and thrombosis, 156
proper, 4-5, 7
Skin
defenses of, 276
factors affecting acidity of, 281-282
factors in cancer of, 444
L. acidophilus and, 667
materials penetrating defenses of, 276
normal acidity of, 281
rimless eyeglasses and cancer of, 480-481
soap and acidity of, 281, 282

vitamins and, 287
Skin disease
alkaline condition and, 281-283
as indications of internal disorders, 818
cosmetics and, 276-277
detergents and, 279-280
drugs and, 277
food and, 279
hair dyes and, 277
incidence of, 276, 280, 281
in polio cases, 818
menthol and, 606-607
rectal area highly susceptible to, 278
soap and, 277, 281, 282
shoe linings and, 283-284
suggestions for protection from, 283
tracking down the cause of, 275-276
vitamin B$_{12}$ and, 552
see also Poison ivy, Pruritus ani, Psoriasis, Vitiligo
Sleep
exercise and, 157-158
glaucoma and, 53
Meniere's disease and, 685
numbness during, 383, 385
positions in, and bursitis, 382
positions in, and neuritis, 379-382
postures to avoid, 384 (illus.)
safe positions, 384 (illus.)
Sleeplessness. See Insomnia.
Smoking
allergy and, 944
arsenic residues in tobacco, 449-450
asthma from, 609-610
blackouts and, 880
blood flow and, 447, 881, 944
blood pressure and, 944
blood vessels and, 944
Buerger's disease and, 425-426, 934, 944
cholesterol and, 144, 173
cigarette consumption in U. S., 217
colds and, 609, 611
collagen and, 944
coronary thrombosis and, 214, 215-216, 217
diabetic gangrene and, 937-938
during pregnancy, and leukemia, 737, 738
effect on body, 143, 144, 215-216, 426
effect on children, 610, 937
effect on mucous membranes, 610, 934, 944
eyes and, 939
fetal heartbeat and, 737, 936-937
gum disorders and, 939
heart and, 447, 933-934, 944
heart disease and, 143-145, 172-173
hyperthyroidism and, 447, 760
intake of nicotine from, 609
intake of tobacco tars from, 608-609

irritation from, 609
kidney function and, 937, 944
list of disorders ascribed to, 944
low blood sugar and, 938, 944
lung cancer and, 445-446, 447-449, 478
malocclusion and, 316
minor disorders and, 609
nerves and, 938-939
nutrition to help stop, 943
pancreas and, 937-938
postnasal drip and, 934
post-operative complications and, 611, 935-936
pulse and, 147-148
sense of smell and, 939
sterility and, 935, 944
taste buds and, 944
temperature and, 881, 944
tips on giving up, 450
tuberculosis and, 934-935
ulcers and, 892, 896, 935, 942-943, 944
value of filters, 881-882
vitamin B and, 216
vitamin C and, 144, 216, 515, 944
vocal cord tumors and, 447
see also Nicotine, Tobacco amblyopia

Soap
getting clean without, 277
*p*H of some brands, 282
skin acidity and, 281, 282
skin disease and, 277, 281, 282
see also Detergents
Soft drink consumption in U. S., 762
Soft water
artificial, and nutrition, 199-200
artificial, and sodium, 196, 197-199, 200
corrosion of pipes and, 200
dangers of, 195-201
heart disease and, 195-196
Soil
electricity in, 500-501, 503
tooth decay and, 308
Sore throat and garlic, 588
Specific gravity
defined, 140-141
of the heart, 141
of the human body, 141
raising, 141-142
see also Weight
Spine
deformities, and foot imbalance, 372-374
one-sidedness in, 12
Spontaneous abortion
incidence, 769
question of abnormal birth, 769-770
vitamin E and, 770, 771
see also Pregnancy

Staph
balance of nature and, 879
carriers of, 877
deaths from, 878
epidemics, and hospital cleanliness, 875
epidemics, in hospitals, 874-875, 877-878
factors determining susceptibility to, 877
garlic and, 663
overcrowding of hospital nurseries and, 876
proposed solution to, 876
recommendations for controlling, 878-880
resistant to antibiotics, 875-876
symptoms of, 876-877
Staphylococcal infection. *See* Staph.
Steatorrhea
mineral loss in, 14
osteoporosis and, 14
rye and, 15-16
symptoms of, 542-543
wheat and, 15-16
Sterility
nicotine and, 936
smoking and, 935, 944
Steyn, Dr. Douw G., 806-808
Stockings, 79
Stomach cancer, 444
Strabismus. *See* Crossed eyes.
Stress
alcoholism and, 327
appendicitis and, 331
appetite and, 909
arthritis and, 340-342
asthma and, 399-401, 406
baldness and, 110-111
bed wetting and, 422-423
breathing and, 598
cancer and, 464-466
cholesterol level and, 173
colds and, 564-565, 568, 595-596
colitis and, 674, 679-680
constipation and, 619
dietary needs and, 51-52
digestion and, 725
dizziness and, 685
effect on body, 154, 186-187
eyestrain and, 41
glaucoma and, 48, 49-50
gum disease and, 94, 96
hardening of the arteries and, 154
headaches and, 115-117
heart disease and, 153-155, 188-192
high blood pressure and, 154
insomnia and, 734
overcoming, 41
overweight and, 800
painful shoulder and, 377
pulse and, 147

rheumatism and, 333-334
susceptibility to disease and, 466-467
ulcers and, 892-893
vitamins and, 155, 342
vitamin B in, 192-193
Stroke
aftereffects of, 237
capillary fragility and, 553, 554
causes of, 236
dizziness and, 684
little, as a danger signal, 237
little, symptoms of, 237-239
program of prevention, 239-240
see also Hemorrhage
Strontium 90 ingestion, 946
Sugar
calcium-phosphorus ratio and, 351
choline appetite and, 488
colds and, 561
consumption of, in U. S., 762-763
food vs. liver, in the body, 672-673
malocclusion and, 315-316
not requiring insulin, 644-645
oxygenation and, 153
overconsumption of, and low blood
sugar, 767-768
proposal to tax, 294-295
thirst and, 353
tooth decay and, 303
Sulfur
cancer and, 488
deficiency, and arthritis, 391
Sun
cataracts and, 36
heart disease and, 194-195
Sway-back, 11

T

Tabii, 82
Tachycardia, 168
Tartar
pyorrhea and, 98
vitamin C and, 245, 246
TB. See Tuberculosis.
Thiamin
cancer and, 488-489
carbohydrate digestion and, 724
deficiency, and low blood pressure,
224
deficiency, and mental symptoms,
747-748
deficiency, and refined carbohydrates,
137
deficiency, and the heart, 137-138
diet causing deficiency, 630
multiple sclerosis and, 786
smoking and, 216
symptoms of deficiency, 630
Thiouracil, 63
Thirst
diabetes and, 639
factors affecting, 627

sugar and, 353
Thong-type sandals, 81-82
Threshold age, 165
Threshold weight, 141
Thrombo-angiitis obliterans. See Buerger's disease.
Thrombosis
defined, 169
prolonged sitting and, 156
vitamin E and, 127, 184
Thyroid gland
artery health and, 240
aspirin and, 760
causes of disorders, 705-706, 760
deficiency, and hardening of the arteries, 204-205
disorders, and mental illness, 757-759
function of, 705
iodine and, 205, 705-706, 760
location of, 705
overweight and, 799
stimulants and, 447, 760
testing for malfunction of, 759
see also Goiter
Tinnitus
causes of, 31-33
central, 33
chemicals and, 32
drugs and, 32
entotic, 31-32
exotic, 31
in beriberi, 20
in pellagra, 20
reflex, 32-33
sounds of, 30-31, 33
types of, 31-33
vitamins and, 33
vitamin A and, 22, 23
see also Deafness, Hearing
Tobacco amblyopia
case histories, 880-881
factors determining severity of, 940
long known, 881
symptoms of, 880-881, 940
vitamin B_{12} and, 940-941
Tonsils and colds, 562
Tooth decay
AMA statement on, 306-308
ammoniated toothpastes and, 303-
304
apples for prevention of, 297-298
calcifying diet and, 302-303
carbohydrates and, 306, 307
diet and, 292-294, 307, 308-309
fluorides and, 304
"Health snacks" program of prevention, 295-296
Macmillan's prevention program,
296-297
mouth acids and, 302
organically grown foods and, 304-
305
pyridoxine and, 299-300, 301-302

refined foods and, 306
soil and, 308
sugar and, 303
toothbrushing and, 303
vitamins and, 307
see also Fluoridation
Toothpaste, ammoniated, 303-304
Tooth powder, 418
Trace elements
"abnormal," and hardening of the
arteries, 210-211
"abnormal," in the body, 202-203
Tranquilizers, 960
Trench mouth
description, 98
niacin and, 99, 100
see also Gum disease, Pyorrhea
Trichinosis
cooking pork to avoid, 883-884
incidence of, 883, 884
no attempt to detect trichina in pork,
882, 884
symptoms of, 883
transmission of, 883
Tuberculosis
high-protein diet for, 886-887
how infection operates, 889
low-carbohydrate diet for patients,
613, 614-615
premature births and, 886
regression of, 888
smoking and, 934-935
susceptibility to, and vitamins A and
C, 885-886
symptoms, and vitamin C, 583-584
vitamin A and, 575-576, 885, 886
vitamin C deficiency in, 885, 886
vitamin D and, 575-576
see also B. C. G.
Tujunga, 406
Turkel, Dr. Henry, 779-781

U

Ulcer
bananas and, 930
bioflavonoids and, 906
cabbage juice for, 894, 900-901
caffeine and, 892, 896
capillary weakness in, 905-906
case histories, 902, 905
constipation and, 619-620
development of, 891
diet for, 893, 894, 899, 901, 906
drugs and, 893, 894
food chemicals and, 900
heated fats and, 896-897
heredity in, 892
in children, 895, 899-900
incidence of, 892, 895
L. acidophilus and, 667
low blood sugar in, 898
nutrition and, 893

Pamine for, 894
peptic, and carbohydrate metabolism,
670
potatoes for, 894, 902-903
refined foods and, 893
sex differences in incidence, 895
sign of, 891
smoking and, 892, 896, 935, 942-943,
944
stress and, 892-893
theories on cause of, 892-893, 896-
897, 898, 900
types of, 892
value of bland diet for, 896
vitamin C and, 865, 902, 904-905
vitamin C deficiency in, 903-904
Ulcerative colitis. See Colitis, ulcerative.
Underweight
advice on, 912
conserving energy, 912
characteristics of "asthenic," 908
characteristics of "sthenic," 908
due to inability to absorb foods, 910-
911
due to lack of appetite, 909-910
food supplements for, 911-912
little information on, 908
personality, 913-914
types of, 908-909
undeveloped taste buds and, 913, 914
see also Weight
Undulant fever
cause of, 916
in history, 916
symptoms of, 916
transmission of, 916
transmission through blood transfusions, 917-918
vitamin C for, 916-917
United States Public Health Service
attitude on Sabin vaccine, 840
role in promoting Salk vaccine, 850-
852
Unsaturated fatty acids
cholesterol and, 173, 207, 643
defined, 138
diabetes and, 642-644
enlarged prostate and, 267
factors increasing need for, 171
function of, 138
hydrogenation of, 173-174
loss of, 208
saturation of, 138-139
sources of, 139
Uterine cancer
factors in, 445, 505, 506
statistics on, 518

V

Varicose veins
case histories, 921

constipation and, 923-924
defined, 169
development of, 920
exercise and, 921-922
favor left side of body, 923
incidence of, 922-923
individual differences in, 924
phlebitis and, 920, 921
refined foods and, 925
sex differences in incidence of, 924-925
upright posture and, 922
vitamin E and, 920, 921
Vertigo. *See* Dizziness.
Vincent's disease. *See* Trench mouth.
Vitamins
cancer and, 462-463
cause of inadequate intake, 511
constipation and, 630
deficiency, and alcoholism, 320
deficiency, and cancer, 491
deficiency, and diarrhea, 656
deficiency, and digestive disorders, 655
deficiency, and medications, 655-656
deficiency diseases, 55
deficiency, in cystic fibrosis, 635-636
deficiency, in diabetics, 639
deficiency symptoms, in eyes, 65-66, 68
deficiency symptoms, in the mouth, 656
fat-soluble, 285
loss, in cooking, 731
need, in alcoholism, 748
pulse and, 149
results of deficiency, 487
safety of large doses, 749
skin and, 287
stress and, 155, 342
supplements, for diabetics, 640
tinnitus and, 33
tooth decay and, 307
Vitamin A
absorption, and exercise, 158
antibody-forming ability and, 576
arthritis and, 335
baldness and, 106
bodily changes in deficiency, 818-819
cancer and, 488
cleft palate and, 558
colds and, 576, 872
deafness and, 21-24
deficiency, and age, 23-24
deficiency, and eyes, 66
deficiency, and goiter, 712-714
deficiency, in polio, 817-818, 819
deficiency, in TB, 885, 886
deficiency symptoms, 818
factors affecting body supply of, 99
flu and, 574-575
gall bladder and, 87
infection and, 23, 577, 578

kidney stones and, 244-245
level in blood, and susceptibility to TB, 885-886
mineral oil and, 24
mucous membrane and, 22, 577, 578
pneumonia and, 575, 576
poisoning, 579
prostate gland and, 267
pyorrhea and, 98-99
sources, 578, 819
supplements, 24, 578-579
tinnitus and, 22, 23
tuberculosis and, 575, 576
use of iodine and, 712
Vitamin B
appetite and, 909
arthritis and, 335-336
brewer's yeast for, 21
cancer and, 462
cleft palate and, 558-559
constipation and, 629, 630, 631, 718
deficiency, and beriberi, 820
deficiency, and eyes, 66-67
deficiency, related to polio incidence, 821-822
deficiency symptoms, 509
diabetes and, 638-640
difficulty in determining deficiency, 510-511
digestion and, 724-725
factors affecting body supply of, 99, 613, 821
fats and, 285-286
germ-resistant power and, 579-580
getting enough, 511-512, 581
gum health and, 99-100
isolation of, 820-821
mouth disorders and, 508-509, 512
muscular dystrophy and, 794-795
nerve deafness and, 19-21
nerve diseases and, 821
results of deficiency, 19
shortage, in our diets, 823
source of, 511-512, 513
storage, in the body, 822
stress and, 192-193
synthetic, and constipation, 631
zinc and, 274
see also Biotin, Choline, Folic acid, Inositol, Niacin, Para-amino-benzoic acid, Pyridoxine, Riboflavin, Thiamin, Vitamin B₁₂
Vitamin B₁. *See* Thiamin.
Vitamin B₂. *See* Riboflavin.
Vitamin B₆. *See* Pyridoxine.
Vitamin B₁₂
absorption, and hydrochloric acid, 811, 941
blood vessel disorders and, 550-552
diseases suggested for therapy with, 550
factors leading to deficiency in, 941

intermittent claudication and, 550, 552
intrinsic factor and, 810
mental deficiency in rats and, 750
mental confusion and, 550-551, 552
mental illness and, 753-754, 755
nervous deficiency symptoms, 754-755
osteoarthritis and, 335-336
paralysis and, 552
pernicious anemia and, 810
power of, 810
skin disorders and, 552
sources of, 811
therapeutic use of, 549
tobacco amblyopia and, 940-941
Vitamin C
arthritis and, 336, 358, 359, 362-363
bioflavonoids and, 104, 358, 555-556, 585-586
bleeding gums and, 92-93
blood vessel health and, 240
bone formation and, 16, 17
bruising and, 515
calcium deposits and, 245-246
capillary fragility and, 358-359
cataract and, 37-38
cholesterol and, 134-136, 216
colds and, 163-164, 563, 582-583, 586-587
cold weather and need for, 581-582
collagen and, 395, 484, 514, 863
content of cow's and breast milk, 867
cooking to preserve, 585
deafness and, 26
decrease in infectious disease and, 948-950
deficiency, and age, 69
deficiency, and diet, 864, 865-866
deficiency, and eyes, 67-68
deficiency, in background of leukemia, 738-739
deficiency, in TB, 885, 886
deficiency, in U. S., 18
deficiency symptoms, 516
destruction of, 246, 247, 253-254, 362
diphtheria susceptibility and, 583
factors affecting need for, 581-582, 866
fats and, 253
flu and, 702
for undulant fever, 916-917
function, in the body, 360
gum disease and, 104
hardening of the arteries and, 135, 136
hearing and, 25
high blood pressure and, 227
importance of, 25
infection and, 582, 583, 584-585
in lens of eye, 37
insulin and, 639

kidney stones and, 245, 246-247
level in blood, and susceptibility to, TB, 885-886
liver and, 252-253
massive doses of, 361-362
Meniere's disease and, 25
middle ear infection and, 25
minimum need of, 582, 864
osteoporosis and, 16, 18
poisons and, 26
polio and, 813-814
pyorrhea and, 100-101
rheumatic fever and, 361, 362, 583
rheumatism and, 361, 395
scurvy and, 360, 860, 865, 868
smoking and, 144, 216, 515, 944
sources of, 247, 359
stone formation and, 87-88, 245-246
storage, in body, 25
tartar on teeth and, 245, 246
tuberculosis symptoms and, 583-584
ulcers and, 865, 902-905
vitiligo and, 290
widespread deficiency, 362, 862-863
Vitamin D
antibody-forming ability and, 576
arthritis and, 336, 363
brewer's yeast and toxicity of, 364, 365
calcium and, 15
deficiency, and eyes, 68
massive doses of, 363-364
sources of, 15, 365
toxicity of, 364
tuberculosis and, 575-576
Vitamin E
anticlotting property of, 126, 127, 183, 184-185, 703, 918-919
benefits of, 428-429
blood vessels and, 128, 183-186, 703
breast feeding for sufficient, 637
Buerger's disease and, 426-427, 428
cataracts and, 699
cautions on use of, 241, 921
collateral circulation and, 919, 920
deficiency, and cystic fibrosis, 633-634
deficiency, and muscular dystrophy in rabbits, 792, 793
deficiency during pregnancy, and Mongoloid birth, 771, 773-774
deficiency, in infants, 636
deficiency symptoms, during pregnancy, 772
destruction of, 59
diabetes and, 640
doctors should use, 700
effects in the body, 772
epilepsy and, 697-698
FDA on, 59
foods containing, 60
gangrene and, 704
hardening of the arteries and, 703

heart disease and, 127-128, 180-182
high blood pressure and, 227
intermittent claudication and, 546-548
lack of, in average diet, 182
liver damage and assimilation of, 793
menstrual disorders and, 826
mental disorders and, 696-697, 698-699
miscarriage and, 770, 771
Mongolism and, 772-773
muscles and, 831-832
nearsightedness and, 57-58
necessity of, 59-60
need for supplements, 548
obliterative diseases and, 184
osteoarthritis and, 395
oxygenation and, 127-128, 395-396, 548, 698, 703-704
phlebitis and, 183-184, 919-920
psychosomatic diseases and, 699
removed from refined foods, 794
reproductive tract and, 267
rheumatic fever and, 336
rheumatism and, 336-337
scar tissue and, 128
sources, 705
strokes and, 240
substances accompanying, in food, 635
therapy, for polio patients, 825, 826
thrombosis and, 127, 184
value of, during pregnancy, 770-771
varicose veins and, 920, 921

Vitamin K
aspirin and, 601-602
blood clotting and, 601
gall bladder and, 87
synthetic, and kernicterus, 955-956

Vitamin P. *See* Bioflavonoids.

Vitiligo
description of, 289
diet and, 289-290
factors contributing to, 291
hydrochloric acid and, 289
para-amino-benzoic acid and, 290-291
vitamin C and, 290

W

Waerland diet, 791-792

Walking
barefoot on dewy grass, 501-502
correct, 71
heart disease and, 149-151, 161-162
incorrect, and foot disorders, 71
pulse and, 149-150

Water
after eating, 628
daily need for, 628
harm of ingesting too much, 627-628
in foods, 627
polluted, and goiter, 709, 710
polluted, and hepatitis, 261-262
polluted, and polio, 710
polluted, cyanide in, 710
see also Soft water

Weather
cold, and colds, 574
cold, and vitamin C need, 581-582
diabetes and, 646-648
health and, 646, 647
insulin need and, 647-648
see also Barometric pressure, Climate, Humidity

Weight
blood pressure and, 802 (table), 804
foot disorders and, 374-375
guideposts for correct, 801
"normal," 907
ratio of blood to, and overweight, 803-804
threshold, 141
see also Overweight, Specific gravity, Underweight

Wheat
digestive tract disorders and, 731-732
steatorrhea and, 15-16

Wheat germ
constipation and, 626
oil, and muscular dystrophy, 794-795

Williams, Dr. Roger, 319-323

X

Xerophthalmia, 66

X-ray
prenatal, and leukemia, 737
treatment, and cancer, 961-962
see also Radioactivity

Y

Yogurt
constipation and, 626
when taking antibiotics, 960

Z

Zinc
daily need for, 274
foods containing, 274-275
function, in the body, 272, 273
in insulin, 273
in prostate gland, 272, 273-274
in semen, 273-274
liver and, 250
pancreas and, 273
symptoms of deficiency, 272-273
vitamin B and, 274